Intracranial Aneurysms

Vol. II

Intracranial Aneurysms

Volume II

John L. Fox, M.D.
Professor of Neurosurgery
West Virginia University
School of Medicine
Morgantown, West Virginia

With 354 Illustrations, 111 in Full Color

Springer-Verlag New York Berlin Heidelberg Tokyo

John L. Fox, M.D.
Professor of Neurosurgery
West Virginia University
Medical Center
Morgantown, West Virginia 26506

Library of Congress Cataloging in Publication Data
Fox, John L., 1934–
Intracranial aneurysms.
Includes bibliographies and index.
1. Intracranial aneurysms. 2. Intracranial aneurysms—Surgery.
I. Title. [DNLM: 1. Cerebral aneurysm. WL 355
I609]
RC693.F69 1983 616.8′1 83–834

Softcover reprint of the hardcover 1st edition 1983

9 8 7 6 5 4 3 2 1

ISBN-13: 978-1-4612-5583-3 e-ISBN-13: 978-1-4612-5581-9
DOI: 10.1007/ 978-1-4612-5581-9

Dedicated to our patients
who sought to be made well again
and to our families and colleagues
who gave their time and encouragement

Contents of Volume II

24 Anesthesiology. *II* Induced Hypotension 662

Author: Richard L. Keenan, M.D.

25 Craniotomy for Aneurysm. *I* Control of Intracranial Pressure and Circulation 669

26 Craniotomy for Aneurysm. *II* Instrumentation 678

27 Craniotomy for Aneurysm. *III* Aneurysm Clips 708

28 Craniotomy for Aneurysm. *IV* Protective Coatings 735

29 Craniotomy for Aneurysm. *V* Cranial Approaches 750

30 Craniotomy for Aneurysm. *VI* Tissue Section and Resection 800

31 Craniotomy for Aneurysm. *VII* Special Methods of Treating the Aneurysm 812

32 Craniotomy for Aneurysm. *VIII* Operative Complications and Postoperative Care 846

33 Carotid Artery Ligation in the Neck 860

Contents of Volume I

Contents of Volume III—Appendices

Foreword

Professor Fox has undertaken the monumental task of compiling the available data on intracranial arterial aneurysms. The magnitude and extent of the undertaking attest to the tremendous amount of information which has accumulated in the past few decades and to the accelerated pace at which the field has expanded, particularly since the end of World War II.

Our heritage can be traced to many sources, among whom should be mentioned such notables as Willis, Quincke, Blackall, Moniz, Dott, Dandy, Hounsfield, and others. The modern era includes a number of investigators and clinicians, some of whom have contributed to this magnificent tome. The bibliography of over 4000 references represents the increasing interest in this subject on the part of many investigators. However, the neurosurgical community should be given particular credit for developing and expanding surgical techniques which now place the operative results within a very respectable range, in contrast to the high mortality and morbidity experienced by patients several decades ago.

In his Preface, Dr. Fox has quoted Cannon and Rosenblueth in questioning where to stop the record. One can only document progress to date—and certainly the advances in this field are noteworthy—and then make some cautious predictions for the future. They have correctly made note that the overall morbidity and mortality of these aneurysm patients remains unacceptably high, largely as a result of the secondary complications of the subarachnoid hemorrhage itself. More attention should be directed in the future to the recognition of those patients with unruptured aneurysms and those with minimal bleeds. Hopefully information will be forthcoming as to which individuals are at risk because of some unusual congenital, metabolic, or acquired defect. Much more work needs to be done!

A.L. Sahs, M.D.
Professor Emeritus
Department of Neurology
College of Medicine
University of Iowa
Iowa City, Iowa

Preface

The first book written on the subject of intracranial aneurysms was authored by Walter Dandy in 1944 (2). Dandy at that time published the first series of cases treated for this problem. An important contribution to Dandy's text was the section on cerebrovascular embryology and anatomy by Dorcas Padget (7). In 1952 Wallace Hamby's treatise portrayed his experiences and the significant advances already taking place (6). A more recent book (excluding symposia [3,8] and publication reproductions [10,11]) was that written by J. Lawrence Pool and D. Gordon Potts (9). This noteworthy collaboration between a neurosurgeon and a radiologist was published in 1965.

Our book on intracranial aneurysms surveys the state of the art through modern times and adds several new dimensions. These include a statistical analysis of related variables, an update on the phenomenon of vasospasm, a discussion of etiology and pathogenesis, a presentation of variations in vascular anatomy, a description of advances in neuroradiologic diagnosis and therapy, a portrayal of the role of neuroanesthesia and advanced life-support systems, considerations of prognosis and timing, and an account of the evolution of medical and surgical therapies. Of particular interest for neurosurgeons and anatomists is the emphasis on microvascular techniques and anatomy. Several chapters are devoted to surgical techniques well illustrated with color photographs of live anatomy taken through the operating microscope and providing a valuable surgical atlas.

In this second volume (Chapters 21–39) we cover the prognosis and timing of therapy, medical treatment, anesthetic techniques, and surgical therapy of intracranial aneurysms. The last six chapters provide a color atlas of microsurgical photography.

In their 1937 preface Cannon and Rosenblueth reminded us (1),

> "The preparation of a summary of progress when progress is rapidly continuing involves hazards. In the quick movement of events the maintenance of a proper perspective is an almost impossible achievement. Discrimination between what is important and what is unimportant, which always requires perspicacious judgement, becomes especially difficult, and if attempted, is liable to wide error. Also there appears acutely the problem of deciding where to stop the record; even while we are writing and seeing the book through the press, new and, it may be, highly significant discoveries are being reported."

This is even more true in our modern era with the explosion of knowledge and technical advances. Yet we believe this book still serves as a reliable base upon which further discoveries and change can occur.

The bibliography at the end of the chapters and appendices represents an accumulation and review of over 4000 references. In addition, the appendices (especially Appendix 2) contain a fairly complete collection of aneurysm case report material from the world literature; these patient profiles, analyzed in Chapters 3 and 4, are available for further reference, analysis, and criticism by anyone in the future.

The overall morbidity and mortality of these aneurysm patients remains unacceptably high. In large part this is due to the secondary complications of the subarachnoid hemorrhage. It is this circumstance that prompted the dedication of this book to our patients. This brings to mind words of one of my teachers, James W. Watts, who said of those under his care (4), "—I am filled with admiration at the way they face disability and death. I often wonder at the source of their courage.—I hope that when my time comes that I will behave as well as many of my patients."

This book had its inception during the 1973–74 academic year when, after nine years of active neurosurgical practice in Washington, D.C., I became a student again to study microsurgical techniques under M. Gazi Yaşargil in Zurich, Switzerland. G. Robert Nugent subsequently appointed me to the Cerebrovascular Section of the Department of Neurosurgery at the West Virginia University Medical Center where work on this book progressed toward completion. The surgical technique as illustrated here is based in part upon my early residency training and observations of Walter Dandy's disciples, including George Hayes at the Walter Reed Army Medical Center and Hugo Rizzoli at the George Washington University Medical Center. Hence, the reader will recognize modifications of the original "Dandy flap" in the approach to the circle of Willis. My early association with Ludwig Kempe reinforced this approach. In addition, the application of more recent microsurgical techniques required unlearning old habits and relearning new ones (Chapter 20), a much easier process if the student is still in his formative years. In Professor Yaşargil's laboratory is a visitor's signature record (spring, 1974) into which was copied a quotation from George Garrett's book entitled *Death of the Fox* (5),

> "You who would know something of the truth of kings, who stir dust and peruse the leaves of faded documents, seeking to retail the chronicle of dead kings and queens—yes, especially you who meddle with the dead, must first strip and simplify yourselves, becoming as the basest subjects who are content to love, honor, and obey their rulers.
>
> "You who would begin to conceive of kings, living or dead, must change yourselves to do so. *Must unlearn all to learn again.** And then perhaps you may come to some dim understanding—like that of an infant in a cradle of the tall alien world of faces which lean hugely close, then vanish without rhyme or reason—not of kings or the mysteries of kingship, but of the dream of kings."

In this era of specialization it is impossible for any person to maintain up-to-date knowledge in all aspects relating to intracranial aneurysms. A special tribute to the contributors is appropriate (in order of chapter presentation):

Robert J. Hacker and **John M. Krall** Statistical Data (3 and 4)
Richard P. White Vasospasm (9)
William E. Stehbens Pathology (11), Etiology and Pathogenesis (12)
T.A. Lie Anatomical Variations (15)
John R. Hesselink Radiology (17 and 18)
Richard L. Keenan Anesthesiology (23 and 24)

Finally, I owe a special debt of gratitude to Ludwig G. Kempe for his advice and encouragement.

Bibliography

1. Cannon WB, Rosenblueth A: Autonomic Neuroeffector Systems. New York: Macmillan, 1937
2. Dandy WE: Intracranial Arterial Aneurysms. New York/London: Hafner; and Ithaca, New York: Comstock, 1944, reprinted 1969
3. Fields WS, Sahs AL (eds): Intracranial Aneurysms and Subarachnoid Hemorrhage. Springfield, Illinois: Charles C Thomas, 1965
4. Fox JL: Professor James W. Watts—teacher, scientist, physician. GW Medicine (Washington, DC), Summer 1969, pp 18–20
5. Garrett G: Death of the Fox. New York: Doubleday, 1971, p 41
6. Hamby WB: Intracranial Aneurysms. Springfield, Illinois: Charles C Thomas, 1952
7. Padget DH: The circle of Willis. Its embryology and anatomy. In Dandy WE: Intracranial Arterial Aneurysms. New York/London: Hafner; and Ithaca, New York: Comstock, 1944, reprinted 1969, pp 67–90
8. Pia HW, Langmaid C, Zierski J (eds): Cerebral Aneurysms. Advances in Diagnosis and Therapy. Berlin/Heidelberg/New York: Springer-Verlag, 1979
9. Pool JL, Potts DG: Aneurysms and Arteriovenous Anomalies of the Brain. Diagnosis and Treatment. New York/Evanston/London: Harper & Row, 1965
10. Sahs AL, Perret GE, Locksley HB, Nishioka H (eds): Intracranial Aneurysms and Subarachnoid Hemorrhage. A Cooperative Study. Philadelphia/Toronto: JB Lippincott, 1969
11. Suzuki J (ed): Cerebral Aneurysms. Tokyo: Neuron, 1979

John L. Fox

* My italics

Contributors

John L. Fox, M.D., Department of Neurosurgery, West Virginia University Medical Center, Morgantown, West Virginia 26506, U.S.A. (Principal author and editor of book)

Robert J. Hacker, M.D., Suite 202, Merrill Lynch Plaza, 10330 Regency Parkway Drive, Omaha, Nebraska 68144, U.S.A. (Co-author of Chapters 3 and 4)

John R. Hesselink, M.D., Department of Radiology (Neuroradiology), Massachusetts General Hospital and Harvard Medical School, Boston, Massachusetts 02114, U.S.A. (Author of Chapters 17 and 18)

Richard L. Keenan, M.D., Department of Anesthesiology, Medical College of Virginia, Richmond, Virginia 23298, U.S.A. (Author of Chapters 23 and 24)

John M. Krall, Ph.D., Department of Community Medicine, West Virginia University Medical Center, Morgantown, West Virginia 26506, U.S.A. (Co-author of Chapters 3 and 4)

T.A. Lie, M.D., Department of Neurosurgery, St. Elizabeth Hospital, Tilburg, The Netherlands (Author of Chapter 15)

William E. Stehbens, M.D., D.Phil., Department of Pathology, Wellington Clinical School of Medicine and Wellington Cancer and Medical Research Institute, Wellington, New Zealand (Author of Chapters 11 and 12)

Richard P. White, Ph.D., Department of Pharmacology, University of Tennessee Center for Health Sciences, Memphis, Tennessee 38163, U.S.A. (Author of Chapter 9)

The work on this book was completed while Dr. J.L. Fox was Professor of Neurosurgery at the Downstate Medical Center and Kings County Hospital in Brooklyn, New York, during the academic year 1982–83. The senior author is grateful for their support during this period.

Artists

Barbara L. Gould, Department of Photography and Illustration, West Virginia University Medical Center, Morgantown, West Virginia 26506, U.S.A.

Jno Randall, Department of Neurological Surgery, George Washington University Medical Center, Washington, District of Columbia 20037, U.S.A.

Computer Technicians (West Virginia University)

Paul Hshieh and Yu-Lein F. Kung, graduate students

Administrative and Technical Personnel (West Virginia University)

Ruby A. Bryan, Chauna S. Bucklew, Helen L. Crane, Betty L. Davis, Lila B. Flint, Linda D. Hemingway, Joyce E. Herschberger, Joette G. Mateer, Robin E. Metheny, and N. Darlene Rukse

Table I
Symbols and Abbreviations

A

A *angiogram* for head injury (under symptoms column); *aborted* (under comment column in appendices)
A-1 or A_1 horizontal segment of anterior cerebral artery
A_1AA or A1AA aneurysm of A-1 or horizontal segment of anterior cerebral artery
A-2 or A_2 initial part of ascending segment of anterior cerebral artery
Abs or ABS absent internal carotid artery
AC caesarian section, done before aneurysm surgery (under comment column)
aca anterior cerebral artery distribution of AVM
acha anterior choroidal artery distribution of AVM
AChA anterior choroidal artery
AChAA or ACHAA anterior choroidal artery aneurysm (not at internal carotid artery)
achaICAA or ACHA-ICAA internal carotid artery aneurysm at anterior choroidal artery take-off
ACeA anterior cerebral artery (including A-1 or horizontal part as well as parts distal to anterior communicating artery)
ACeAA or ACEAA anterior cerebral artery aneurysm located distal to the anterior communicating artery
ACoA anterior communicating artery
ACoAA or ACOAA anterior communicating artery aneurysm
AComA anterior communicating artery
AD adults
ADH antidiuretic hormone
Aei or AEI anastomosis, extra-intracranial
Age or AGE agenesis of corpus callosum
aica anterior inferior cerebellar artery distribution of AVM
AICA anterior inferior cerebellar artery
AICAA anterior inferior cerebellar artery aneurysm
aicaBAA or AICA-BAA basilar artery aneurysm at anterior inferior cerebellar artery take-off
AMCA amino methylcyclohexane carboxylic acid (tranexamic acid) or accessary middle cerebral artery
amcaICAA or AMCA-ICAA internal carotid artery aneurysm at accessary middle cerebral artery take-off
anACeAA or AN-ACEAA aneurysm of an anomalous anterior cerebral artery
Ant or ANT A-1 artery clipping or ligation
Aor or AOR aortic stenosis (coarctation)
AP anterior-posterior
Aqu or AQU aqueduct stenosis
Art or ART arteritis
as aspergillus fungus
astro astrocytoma
AT abscess tap
AV vaginal delivery, done before aneurysm surgery
A-V block atrial-ventricular block in heart
AVM arteriovenous malformation
azACeAA or AZ-ACEAA aneurysm of an azygous anterior cerebral artery

B

B bruit
BA basilar artery
BAA basilar artery aneurysm
Bal or BAL balloon occlusion
Bas or BAS basilar artery ligation
bBAA or B-BAA basilar artery aneurysm at terminal bifurcation of basilar artery
BC before Christ
bg basal ganglia
bICAA or B-ICAA internal carotid artery aneurysm at terminal bifurcation of the internal carotid artery
bif bifurcation
bm brucella melitensis
BP blood pressure (in appendices and tables: 0 means not hypertensive, + means hypertensive, − means no information)

Bra or BRA brain abscess
BTH bitemporal hemianopia

C

c cerebral
C *centigrade* (Celsius) measurement of temperature or *caesarian section* (under comment column)
ca *candida albicans* fungus or *carcinoma* or *circa* (approximately)
Case-no or CASE-NO case number
Case # case number
CAT computed axial tomogram (or computerized axial tomography)
Cav or CAV cavernous sinus thrombophlebitis
cav-s cavernous sinus
cb corynebacterium
CBF cerebral blood flow
cblm cerebellum
CBV cerebral blood volume
C-C carotid-cavernous
CCA common carotid artery
Cer or CER cervical carotid artery ligation
ch cardiobacterium hominis or choriocarcinoma
CH children
Chi or CHI child (age less than 20 years)
CI craniotomy injury
Clp or CLP clipping or ligation of aneurysm
cm centimeter
CMA callosal-marginal artery
C_{max} maximal contraction
$CMRO_2$ cerebral metabolic rate (oxygen utilization)
CN cranial nerve (e.g., CN-7 means 7th cranial nerve)
CO_2 carbon dioxide
Cot or COT cotton wrapping
CPK creatine phosphokinase
CPP cerebral perfusion pressure
Cra or CRA craniotomy done but no details regarding aneurysm
craniopharyng craniopharyngioma
CRA central retinal artery
CRV central retinal vein
cs cavernous sinus
csICAA aneurysm on segment of internal carotid artery within the cavernous sinus
CSF cerebrospinal fluid
CSF-P cerebrospinal fluid pressure
CT *computed tomogram* (or computerized tomography) or *cranial tongs*
CVP central venous pressure
CVR cerebrovascular resistance
CWA circle of Willis aneurysm

D

D died
DC direct current (galvanic current)
Dec or DEC decompression (cranial) only
DIC disseminated intravascular coagulapathy
DID delayed ischemic deficit
Dis or DIS distally located aneurysm
Dup or DUP duplication number (assigned to every case reported to have more than one aneurysm in Appendix 02)
Dx diagnosis

E

E epileptic seizure
EACA epsilon aminocaproic acid or Amicar®
ECA external carotid artery
Echo—EG echoencephalogram
EDS Ehler-Danlos Syndrome
EEG electroencephalogram
EKG electrocardiogram
EM electron microscopy
Emb or EMB embryo
en enterococcus
End or END endocarditis
ependym ependymoma
et al. and others
Exc or EXC excision of aneurysm
Exp or EXP exploration only

F

f frontal
F female; carotid-cavernous fistula; fair clinical status
FDP fibrin degradation products
FMD fibromuscular dysplasia
fp or f-p frontoparietal
FPA frontopolar artery
front frontal

G

g giant
G good clinical status
Gel or GEL gelfoam wrapping
GI giant

Gia or GIA giant
glioblast glioblastoma
gm grams
GOT glutamate-oxalacetic transaminase
Gr or GR *grade* (clinical status of patient or *Greek*

H

h hour
H hypoxia/ischemia
Heu or HEU at heubner's artery
Hg mercury
HI head injury
Hrt heart
Hx history
hypopit signs of hypopituitism
Hz Hertz or cycles per second

I

I incidental
ICA internal carotid artery
ICAA internal carotid artery aneurysm
ic/csICAA or IC/CS-ICAA aneurysm on infraclinoid segment of internal carotid artery, presumably within cavernous sinus
ICH intracerebral hematoma
Ico or ICO internal cotton packing
ICP intracranial pressure
IHF interhemispheric fissure
Imu or IMU internal muscle packing
INF infundibulum of pituitary stalk
infra vide see below
Iox or IOX internal oxycellulose packing
ISADH inappropriate secretion of antidiuretic hormone
Isi or ISI internal silk suture placement
Isy or ISY internal synthetic packing
IVH intraventricular hematoma
Iwi or IWI internal wire insertion

K

Kgm or kgm kilogram

L

L *left* side; *living* infant; *labor* (childbirth)
Lar or LAR large
lat lateral
LMWD low molecular weight dextran
LP lumbar puncture
lv lateral ventricle
LW lessor wing of sphenoid

M

M male
M-1 or M_1 first segment of middle cerebral artery
M-2 or M_2 primary divisions of middle cerebral artery after M-1 bifurcation
MAP mean arterial pressure
Marfans Marfan's syndrome
mca middle cerebral artery distribution of AVM
MCA middle cerebral artery
MCAA middle cerebral artery aneurysm
Med or MED medulloblastoma
medullo medulloblastoma
Men or MEN meningitis
mening meningioma
mEq or meq milliequivalents
mes mesencephalon
met metastatic
mg milligrams
mi micrococcus
MI mastoidectomy injury
micro microtechnique; operating microscope used
min minute
ml milliliter
mm millimeter
mOm milliosmoles
Moy or MOY moyamoya collaterals
MU multiple
Mus or MUS muscle wrapping
my myxoma
Myc or myc mycotic aneurysm

N

N *nosebleed* = epistaxis (under symptoms column) or *nothing done* (under comment column)
Neg or NEG no aneurysm operation
neurin neurinoma
NPH normal pressure hydrocephalus
ns neisseria meningiditis
NS non-specific signs

O

o occipital
O otic (ear) bleed
O_2 oxygen
OA ophthalmic artery
OAA ophthalmic artery aneurysm (not at internal carotid artery)
oaICAA or OA-ICAA internal carotid artery aneurysm at ophthalmic artery take-off
Obs or OBS observation (number)
olf olfactory
oligo oligodendroglioma
Onc or onc oncotic aneurysm
OR operating room
Orb or ORB orbital infection
OS orbital surgery
Ost or OST osteomyelitis
OWR Osler-Weber-Rendu disease
Oxy or OXY oxycellulose wrapping

P

p parietal
P poor clinical status; pressure
P-1 or P_1 horizontal segment of posterior cerebral artery (mesencephalic artery)
P-2 or P_2 first portion of posterior cerebral artery after junction with posterior communicating artery
PA posterior-anterior
P_1AA or P1AA aneurysm of P-1 or horizontal segment of the posterior cerebral artery
PAC premature atrial contractions of heart
$PaCO_2$ arterial carbon dioxide pressure
PaO_2 arterial oxygen pressure
PC caesarian section, done after aneurysm surgery
pca posterior cerebral artery distribution of AVM
pcaICAA PCA-ICAA internal carotid artery aneurysm at posterior communicating artery take-off
pcaPCeAA or PCA-PCEAA posterior cerebral artery aneurysm at junction of posterior communication artery
PCeA posterior cerebral artery
PCeAA or PCEAA posterior cerebral artery aneurysm distal to the posterior communicating artery
PChA posterior choroidal artery
PChAA or PCHAA posterior choroidal artery aneurysm
PCK polycystic kidneys
pCO_2 carbon dioxide pressure
PCoA posterior communicating artery
PCoAA or PCOAA posterior communicating artery aneurysm (not at internal carotid artery)
PComA posterior communicating artery
PEG pneumoencephalogram
Pel or PEL pellet to aneurysm neck
perfAA or PERF-AA aneurysm of perforating arteries of circle of Willis
PG prostaglandin
Phy or PHY phycotic aneurysm
PI projectile injury
PICA posterior inferior cerebellar artery
PICAA posterior inferior cerebellar artery aneurysm (not on vertebral artery)
picaVAA or PICA-VAA vertebral artery aneurysm at posterior inferior cerebellar artery take-off
Pil or PIL pilojection (hairs shot into aneurysm)
Pit or PIT pituitary adenoma
pm penicillium fungus
pn pneumococcus
po or p-o parieto-occipital
post-op postoperative
pp petrous pyramid
ppICAA or PP-ICAA aneurysm on segment of internal carotid artery within petrous pyramid
PR pregnancy related
Pre or PRE pregnant patient
pre-op preoperative
PrHA primitive hypoglossal artery
PrHAA or PR-HAA primitive hypoglossal artery aneurysm
Pro or PRO proximal clipping or ligation of parent artery
PrOA primitive otic artery
PrOAA primitive otic artery aneurysm
PrTA primitive trigeminal artery
PrTAA or PR-TAA primitive trigeminal artery aneurysm
PV vaginal delivery, done after aneurysm surgery
PVC premature ventricular contractions of heart
PXE pseudoxanthoma elasticum

Q

q every
quadrig quadrigeminal

R

R right side; reference
RBC red blood cells
rCBF regional cerebral blood flow
R-date or R-DATE reference date (year of publication)
Re Reynolds number
Ref or REF reference (number)
Ref # reference number
Report # report number
RIND reversible ischemic neurologic deficit
RN scan radionuclide scan (or radioactive brain scan)

S

S subarachnoid hemorrhage
sa staphylococcus
SAH subarachnoid hemorrhage
SAP systemic arterial pressure
SAS subarachnoid space
sca superior cerebellar distribution of AVM
SCA superior cerebellar artery
SCAA superior cerebellar artery aneurysm (not on basilar artery)
scaBAA or SCA-BAA basilar artery aneurysm at superior cerebellar artery take-off
Scl or SCL stereotaxic clipping of aneurysm
SDH subdural hematoma
se streptococcus
Sep or SEP septicemia
SGOT serum glutamate-oxalacetic transaminase
Sin or SIN sinusitis
Sir or SIR stereotaxic iron injection
Ski or SKI skin abscess
Sma or SMA small or standard (i.e., not giant) size aneurysm
SNP sodium nitroprusside
sph sphenoid
S/S signs and symptoms
ST subdural taps
STA superficial temporal artery
supra vide see above
Surg or SURG surgical procedure
SW stab wound
Swi or SWI stereotaxic wire injection
Sx or SX signs and symptoms
Syn or SYN synthetic wrapping

T

t temporal
T tumor signs
tb tubercle bacilli
Tc-99m radioactive technetium isotope
temp temporal
Ten or TEN tentorial section
Thr or THR thrombectomy
thrChAA or THR-CHAA aneurysm of choroidal arteries in roof of 3rd ventricle
TIA transient ischemic attack
to or t-o tempero-occipital
tp or t-p temperoparietal
Tra or TRA *trapping* procedure; *traumatic* aneurysm
trBAA or TR-BAA basilar artery aneurysm involving trunk of basilar artery but more specific origin not given
Tri or TRI trigeminal rhizotomy
TS transnasal, transphenoidal, or transethmoidal surgery
tuber tuberculum
TV television
Tx treatment; thromboxane

U

UC caesarian section, time unknown in relation to aneurysm surgery
Unk unknown origin
uo unknown origin (site not specified)
uoBAA or UO-BAA basilar artery aneurysm of unknown origin (site not specified)
uoICAA or UO-ICAA internal carotid artery aneurysm of unknown origin (site not specified)
uoVAA or UO-VAA vertebral artery aneurysm of unknown origin (site not specified)
Ure or URE urethane foam embolization
Utr uterus
UV vaginal delivery, time unknown in relation to aneurysm surgery

V

v ventricle
V vaginal delivery
3v third ventricle
VA vertebral artery
VAA vertebral artery aneurysm

vaBAA or VA-BAA basilar artery aneurysm at union of vertebral arteries (or vertebral artery aneurysm at union of vertebral arteries)
V-B vertebro-basilar
Ver or VER vertebral artery ligation
vg vein of Galen
vICAA or V-ICAA ventral or paraclinoid position of internal carotid artery aneurysm
VT ventricular tap

W

WBC white blood cells
WVUMC West Virginia University Medical Center

X

X midline; magnification

Table II
Instrument and Drug Companies

Abbott Laboratories, North Chicago, Illinois
Aesculap Instruments, New York, New York, and Tuttlingen, West Germany
American Sterilizer Company, Erie, Pennsylvania
Ayerst Laboratories, New York, New York
Boehringer Ingelheim Ltd., Ridgefield, Connecticut
Bristol Laboratories, Syracuse, New York
Burroughs Wellcome Co., Research Triangle Park, North Carolina
Carl Zeiss, Inc., New York, New York, and Oberkochen, West Germany
C.G.R. Medical Corporation, Pittsburgh, Pennsylvania
Ciba Pharmaceutical Co., Summit, New Jersey
Circon Corporation, Goleta, California
Codman and Shurtleff Company, Randolph, Massachusetts
Davis and Geck Co., Danbury, Connecticut
DePuy Company, Warsaw, Indiana
Designs for Vision, Inc., New York, New York
Downs Surgical, Inc., Niagara Falls, New York
Edward Weck & Company, Inc., Long Island City, New York
Eli Lilly and Company, Indianapolis, Indiana
Ethicon, Inc., Somerville, New Jersey
Hall International, Inc., Santa Barbara, California
Hoechst—Roussel Pharmaceuticals, Inc., Somerville, New Jersey
Kees Surgical Speciality Co., Wilder, Kentucky
Kerr Sybron Corporation, Romulus, Michigan
Lederle Laboratories, Wayne, New Jersey
Mathys & Sohn, Zurich, Switzerland
Merck Sharpe & Dohme, Inc., West Point, Pennsylvania
Parke—Davis Company, Morris Plains, New Jersey
Pfizer Laboratories, New York, New York
Phelan Manufacturing Corp., Minneapolis, Minnesota
Richmond Dental Cotton Co., Charlotte, North Carolina
Roche Laboratories, Nutley, New Jersey
Ruggles Corporation, Boston, Massachusetts
Searle Laboratories, Chicago, Illinois
Smith Kline & French Laboratories, Philadelphia, Pennsylvania
Sparta Instrument Corp., Fairfield, New Jersey
Spinger & Tritt, Jestetten, West Germany
Squibb & Sons, Inc., Princeton, New Jersey
Storz Instrument Company, St. Louis, Missouri
Stryker Corporation, Kalamazoo, Michigan
Upjohn Company, Kalamazoo, Michigan
Urban Engineering Co., Inc., Burbank, California
V. Mueller Company, Chicago, Illinois
Winthrop Laboratories, New York, New York
Wyeth Laboratories, Philadelphia, Pennsylvania
Zimmer Company, Warsaw, Indiana

21
Prognosis and Timing

Regardless of the treatment a physician selects for his patient, he cannot be privy to every possible untoward occurrence that may evolve. We try to minimize morbidity and mortality risk by gaining knowledge and experience. But, like in Heisenberg's Uncertainty Principle of physics (128), knowledge of all possible events and consequences of treatment (or no treatment) is impossible, for both therapies and natural histories of disease and host are in a continual state of evolution and change. The treating physician is confronted daily with Murphy's Law: the principle that whatever can possibly go wrong will (26). The following apparently is the origin of Murphy's Law as told to Arthur Bloch by George E. Nichols:

> The event occurred in 1949 at Edwards Air Force Base, Muroc, California, during Air Force Project MX981. This was Col. J.P. Stapp's experimental crash research testing on the track at North Base. . . . The Law's namesake was Capt. Ed Murphy, a development engineer from Wright Field Aircraft Lab. Frustration with a strap transducer which was malfunctioning due to an error in wiring the strain gauge bridges caused him to remark—"If there is any way to do it wrong, he will"—referring to the technician who had wired the bridges at the Lab. . . . Col. Stappp indicated . . . that our fine safety record during several years of simulated crash force testing was the result of a firm belief in Murphy's Law, *and our consistent effort to deny the inevitable.* (26)

The prognosis of a patient harboring an intracranial aneurysm—whether ruptured, tumorous, or incidental—has been and continues to be the subject of much discussion and argument. Such discussions are not merely academic, for proper conclusions will help guide the physician toward a more proper therapy. Unfortunately, the studies and bases upon which these discussions are held often are both unreliable and invalid, since the statistics vary greatly from author to author and adequate scientific controls are missing. It does seem fairly well accepted that if a patient has had a SAH of unknown cause and complete and adequate cerebral angiography is normal, the chances of a poor prognosis and rebleed are minimal and certainly better than if an aneurysm was found (5,77,164,173,247).

Nonoperative Prognosis

Through the years there have been many studies and opinions, often biased, regarding the prognosis, particularly the rebleed and death from rebleed incidence (3, 6, 7, 9, 18, 25, 31, 45, 46, 65, 67, 70, 71, 84, 93, 124, 129, 146, 155, 161, 189, 192, 208, 217, 224–227, 232, 245, 270–273, 282a, 301, 316, 317, 330, 335, 337, 339, 352–354). Since most patients with an intracranial aneurysm are discovered after the first bleed, any therapy directed at the aneurysm is strictly prophylactic: to prevent a rebleed. In 1971 Drake (65) concluded that if a person under the age of 60 years unknowingly harbors an intracranial aneurysm greater than 6 mm in diameter, this aneurysm is very likely to kill him. His rule of five was as follows: "If 5 patients with primary subarachnoid haemorrhage from rupture of an aneurysm are left untreated, at the end of a year only one will be alive and well, another will be disabled and 3 will be dead" (65). Drake (67) later went on to opine, "Even after a year, fatal rebleeding occurs at the rate of about 3% per year. One can imagine the alterations in the life-style of an informed patient who has been asked to live with this ever-hovering threat to his being."

There is much confusion when the reader tries to assimilate previous data: early and late rebleed rates, early and late death rates from any cause, early and late death rates from rebleed, death rate from first bleed versus death from early rebleed, etc. Consequently, the resulting numbers vary widely, as Tönnis and Walter (335) found in their review of publications between 1930 and 1960: mortality rates after the first SAH ranged from 10 to 75%. I will now summarize *in chronological order* the conclusions of some authors. Most percentages are rounded off to the nearest 5%. In none of these cases was surgery instituted.

Chronological Reports

In 1950 Hyland (146) studied 191 cases of SAH, most with proven aneurysms. Fifty percent were dead within 6 months of the first SAH. Of 67 patients followed for an average of 6.1 years, 20% died of recurrent bleed (or about 3% per year). In 1955 Hazouri (124) retrospectively analyzed 63 hospitalized cases: 45% died of the first bleed and 55% of the survivors died of a rebleed while still in the hospital. Only 10% survived to leave the hospital. In 1959 Alexander et al. (7) reported that 50% of 115 cases studied had had a rebleed. Three-fourths of these rebleeds occurred within 42 days, with the average period being 15 days post-SAH. In the same year Logue (192) stated that 90% of his 62 rebleed ACoAA cases rebled in the first 8 weeks; 10% rebled during the ninth to twelfth week. The majority (60%) rebled during the first 2 weeks, with half in the first week.

In 1962 Tappura (330) studied 115 cases surviving the first bleed. Fifty-five percent had rebled with a 75% mortality. Forty percent of the rebleeds occurred in the first 4 weeks; 30% occurred after 18 months (the longest being 9 years). Tappura found no correlation between rebleed and age or blood pressure, but positive correlation with increase in size of aneurysm. In 1964 Boldrey (31) mentioned 12 patients of whom 50% died of rebleed between 5 months and 9 years of the first SAH.

In 1966 Locksley (189,189a) summarized the results of a cooperative study performed with his co-workers in which 2951 cases of aneurysm with SAH and 314 cases of aneurysm without SAH were analyzed from 24 medical centers. They define three populations of patients with ruptured aneurysm: (a) those dying from their first bleed, (b) those at high risk of death from rebleed during first 6 weeks (an average of 6.6% per day died during this period), and (c) those at low risk from rebleed after the first 6-week period. They found 10–15% of these patients fell in the first population group, i.e., 10–15% died from their first bleed (189,189a). Basically these are patients in whom the cerebral injury and secondary complications of the bleed were so devastating as to make survival unlikely. However, the actual mortality for the initial bleed is probably about 40% when one considers patients who die prior to becoming a hospital statistic (245). Of these early deaths from the first bleeding, Locksley (189,189a) found 20% died within the first 48 h, 40% within the first week, and nearly 70% within the first 3 weeks.

Locksley (189,189a) reported on the aneurysm rebleed rate of the anterior circle of Willis in the 1966 Cooperative Study (Fig. 21.1): first week, 10% of all surviving patients; second week, 12%; third week, 7%; fourth week, 8%; fifth through twelfth weeks, 1.8% of surviving patients per week. The rebleed rate for the first 2 weeks was about 25%. Within the first year 35% of all nonoperated aneurysm cases rebled, with a death rate of 40% of those who rebled (these figures are rounded off to the nearest 5%). Ten percent of second bleeding episodes occurred more than 1 year after the first SAH. They also studied 34 cases of asymptomatic unruptured aneurysms: 25% subsequently had a fatal rebleed.

In the same 1966 Cooperative Study Nishioka (232,232a) found that ACeAA cases had the worst prognosis in terms of morbidity/mortality from both the initial and subsequent bleeds. There was no significant difference in the rebleed incidence between anterior circulation aneurysms and vertebro-basilar (V-B) aneurysms except that the former tended to rebleed earlier (within the first few weeks of the first SAH) and the latter tended to rebleed later (months or years later). Nishioka and co-workers found little evidence to suggest that other nonruptured aneurysms in the multiple-aneurysm patient would rupture later—at least during the 7 years of the study. (This seems to counter the statement by the previous author that 25% of asymptomatic unruptured aneurysms subsequently had a fatal rebleed.)

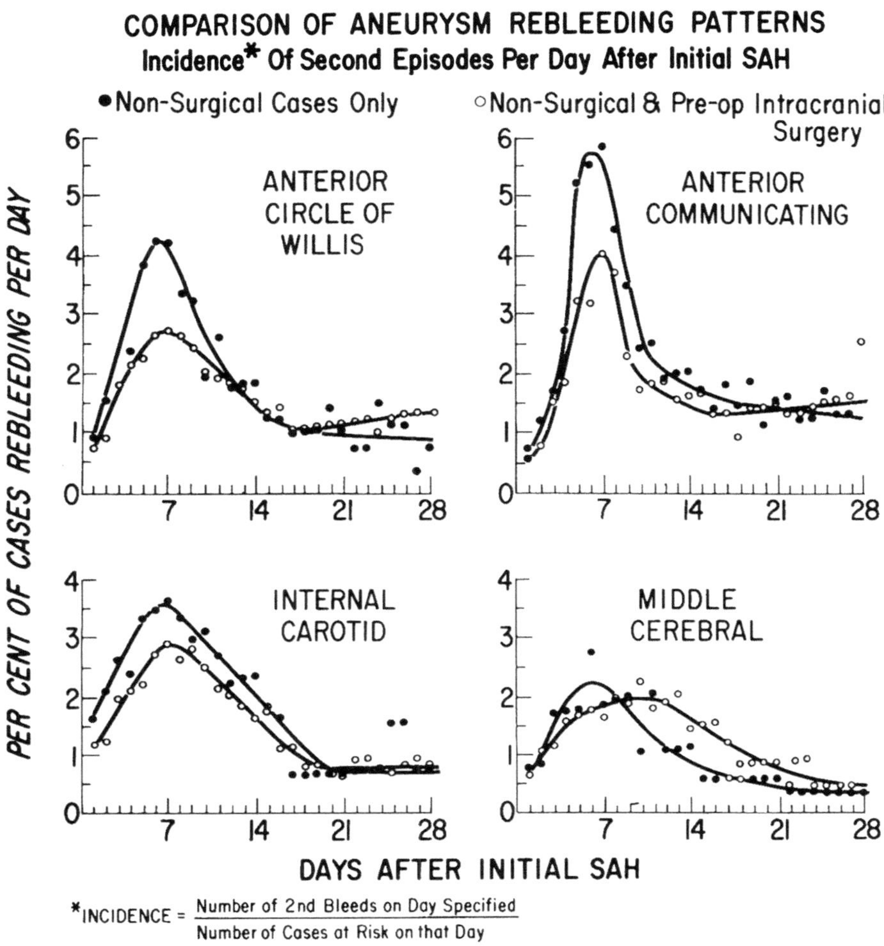

Fig. 21.1. (From ref. 189)

Another very significant study, the Helsinki Study, was conducted by Pakarinen (245) and published in 1967. He found that nearly 45% of 389 ruptured intracranial aneurysm cases died from the initial bleed. This study included patients who died before admission to a hospital as well as those admitted; his figure probably more closely approaches the true death rate. Most (30% of all ruptured aneurysm cases) died within the first 24 h. Of those surviving the initial bleed, 75% rebled later (55% within the first 8 weeks). Since these cases apparently were not considered for surgical therapy, there is some case selection preventing comparison with results of surgery. A second bleed was lethal in 65% of second-bleed cases. A third bleed was lethal in 85% of third-bleed cases (245).

In the first year of Pakarinen's study (245) 35% of nonoperated cases died of a rebleed (25% of nonoperated cases died of a rebleed the first month). There was an additional 25% who died during the second through fifth years post-SAH. He concluded that about half of the survivors of the first bleed would die of a rebleed during the next 5 years. The risk of death decreased by 5% per week in the first 5 weeks. Ten percent more died during the period of the sixth week to the end of the first year. Thereafter, about 5% more died per year through the end of the fifth year. Added to these grim statistics are the *serious disabilities* encountered by the survivors; the original article should be read for details (245).

In 1967 Ahmed and Sedzimir (6) reported that 30% of their grades 1–2 (at time of admission) aneurysm cases subsequently died, and 65% of their grades 3–5 aneurysm cases died. This confirms the poorer prognosis for the poorer-grade patient. In the same year Trumpy (339) described 73 cases. Mortality on rebleed was 60%. This death rate on rebleed, like Pakarinen's (245), is considerably higher than that of 40% gleaned from the 1966 Cooperative Study (129). In 1971 Fujinaga et al. (93) examined 120 nonoperated cases and reconfirmed that the maximum incidence of rebleed was at the end of the first week post-SAH. In the same year Troupp (337) reviewed 20 bBAA cases; 40% died of rebleed 4 to 52 months after surviving the initial hemorrhage. In 1973 af Björkesten (3) reviewed 207 cases; he concluded that the risk of death from rebleed drops from 35% in the first week to 10% in the sixth week to nearly 0% by the end of the first year. In 1975 Mingrino et al. (217) reviewed 100 cases that survived 3 weeks; 6% died of late rebleed months to years later (13% if deaths of unknown etiology are included). In the same year Cioffi et al. (45,46) reported on 30 grade 1 unoperated cases; 55% had recurrent SAH and 40% of the total died of SAH. Most of these deaths were in the first 6 months.

In 1973 and again in 1977 Winn, Richardson, and Jane (155,352,353) assessed the rebleed and death-from-rebleed rate in 213 patients who had survived 6 months. These were pcaICAA and ACoAA patients not treated by surgery. They made five observations:

1. Rebleeding occurred at an average of 3.5% per year for the first 10 years.
2. The mortality rate for the second bleed was 67%.
3. There was a positive correlation between rebleed tendency and both female sex and high blood pressure only in the pcaICAA cases.
4. The younger patient took longer to rebleed than did the older patient.
5. There was no correlation between an increase in aneurysm size and rebleed tendancy.

They *summarized* by estimating the rebleed rate at 3% per year and the death-from-rebleed rate at 2% per year in these cases. In a separate study the same authors found that after 6 months from the initial SAH there was little continued improvement in morbidity of the survivors (354). Late morbidity correlated positively with initial grading, hypertension, presence of hematoma, and vasospasm.

In 1974–1975 Nibbelink et al. (225,226) reported a 20% rebleed rate during the first 14 days. Their highest rebleed period was from the fifth through the ninth days (227). They opined that this increase in rebleed incidence (especially among the poorer-risk patients in their cases) was associated with increased fibrinolytic activity in the sicker patient. Unlike most previous authors, Suzuki and co-workers (316,317) claimed that most rebleeds occurred before the fourth day and after the fourteenth day in the initially unconscious patient. They felt that in these cases neurologic deterioration between the fourth and fifteenth days is usually due to ischemia from vasospasm. On the other hand, if the patient was conscious, rebleeds occurred at random frequency during the first 2 weeks. In 1976 Drake (71) stated that 18% of his cases rebled while awaiting surgery. Sengupta et al. (301) had a 26% early-rebleed rate; Fodstad and Thulin (84), a 39% early-rebleed rate; and Maurice-Williams (208), a 56% early-rebleed rate. Interestingly, Matson (207) never saw early rebleed in 16 cases of children with intracranial aneurysm.

In 1977 Nibbelink and colleagues (227) reviewed 187 patients treated by bedrest only in a cooperative study. Over a 6.5-year period about 35% died from proven rebleed; an additional 15% died from either unproven rebleeds or from other causes. There was not much of a statistically significant difference in rebleed rate among the various grades. The increased death rate in the worse grades was related to other factors (e.g., blood pressure, medical condition, brain damage, etc.). The rebleed rate was highest for MCAA, intermediate for ACoAA and ACeAA, and lowest for ICAA cases. In 1977 Henderson and co-workers (129) analyzed the same 187 cases as in the above cooperative study. Thirty percent rebled in the first month and 45% rebled during the first 5 years (i.e., 15% rebled after the first month). Thus their rebleed rate approximates the 3% per year found by Winn et al. (353). The rebleed morbidity/mortality was worse if the patient was a male, if the interval between bleeds was short, and if vascular hypertension existed. In 1978 Kaste and Troupp (161) reported that 17%, of the ruptured aneurysm cases who en-

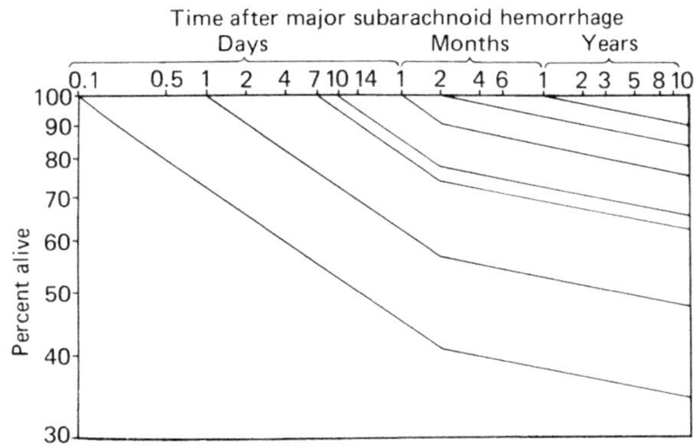

Fig. 21.2. Survival rates of patients admitted to the study at particular times after their initial major SAH. (From ref. 9, copyright 1928–42–43–59–22, American Medical Association)

tered their study an average of 7 weeks post-SAH died of rebleed over the subsequent 5-year period. Again, the long-term rebleed rate of at least 3% per year seems likely here.

Survival Probabilities and Risk Factors

The survival probabilities of aneurysm patients after their most recent SAH were analyzed by Alvord et al. (9). Figure 21.2 and Table 21.1 summarize their study. One might determine, for example, that about 37 out of 100 aneurysm patients will survive 2 years after their most recent SAH. However, if the patient has already survived 1 month, then about 82 out of 100 such patients will survive 2 years. Thirty percent of surviving patients die in each ten-fold cycle of time during the first 2 months. Ten percent of patients alive at 2 months are dead in 2 years. Their long-term death rate after 6 months is 1% per year (one-half that of Winn et al. (353).

From Table 21.1 one can make a more exact estimate based on the patient's *clinical grade.* For example, a grade 1 or 2 patient (i.e., alert, oriented, and otherwise healthy) who has survived 10 days has a 90–95% probability of surviving 2 years. A grade 3 patient who has survived 10 days has only a 75% probability of surviving 2 years. Thus it is obvious that the clinical grade has a profound effect on the mortality rate of nonoperative therapy just as it does on the mortality rate of operative therapy. Alvord and Thorn (10) summarize this in Figure 21.3. Of even greater import may be not only the grade on admission but also the *dynamic trend.* A patient going from a grade 3 to a grade 2 has a better prognosis than one going from a grade 2 to a grade 3 (85).

In the meantime, Richardson and colleagues (270–273) worked out a formula for predicting the chance of rebleed. They gave weightings to prognostic factors, which in their formula for ACoAA patients were sex (slightly worse for males), alertness (worse if less alert), direction aneurysm points (worse the more upward it points), shape of aneurysm (worse the rounder the aneurysm is; better if elongated), days since first bleed (worse in first 40 days), age (slightly worse if older), and blood pressure (worse if diastolic blood pressure is elevated). They found the risk factors for pcaICAA rebleed were different: sex (much worse if female), hematoma (worse if present), vasospasm (worse if present), and size of aneurysm (worse if aneurysm greater than 9 mm in diameter).

More recently (1981) Torner et al. (335a)

Table 21.1. Percentage of Probability for Survival for 2 Years after Subarachnoid Hemorrhage (SAH) from Aneurysm

Clinical Grade	*Days after SAH* 0–1	1–3	3–7	7–21	21–60	60+	All Intervals
I	65	80	90	95	95	95	90
II	55	70	75	90	95	95	75
III	45	55	65	75	85	95	65
IV	30	4	45	50	60	70	45
V	5	5	5	5	5	5	5
All grades	45	55	65	75	85	95	65

Note: For 2-month survival probabilities, add 5%.
Nishioka's grading system is used (see number 16 of Appendix 1). The grade is applied at the time the probability is calculated (not necessarily at the time of the SAH). (From ref. 9)

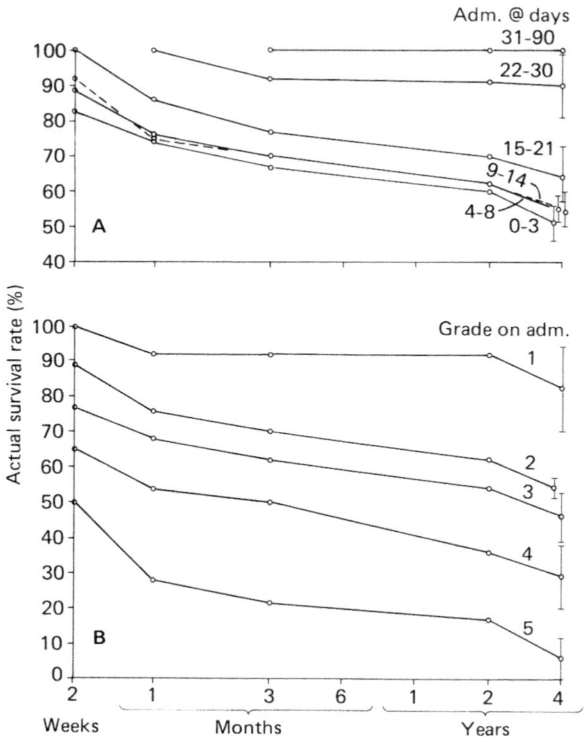

Fig. 21.3. Actual survival rates (% ± standard error indicated at 4 years) for the most common types of patients admitted. **A** The results in all 601 patients admitted in grade 2 status at various times after their SAH. **B** The results of 370 patients admitted 4 to 8 days after their SAH in various grades. (From ref. 10)

summarized the findings of another cooperative study. Whereas overall mortality was related to a worse admission neurologic grade, an elevated diastolic BP, a delay in treatment, a greater degree of vasospasm, and a poorer general medical condition, occurrence of *rebleed* was principally related to a worse admission neurologic grade, an elevated systolic BP, a delay in treatment, and a female sex. See Chapter 11 for additional details.

Summary

The information so far presented in this chapter is an attempt to set the stage for comparative studies regarding prognosis for neurosurgical intervention. Unfortunately, many of the prognostic figures by different authors are quite variable and occasionally contradictory. Part of this is due to the lumping together of all aneurysm subtypes, of cases admitted at variable times post-SAH, and of many other clinical factors. Richardson et al. (270–273) attempted to separate out some of these specific factors. Some of the large cooperative studies also looked at the effect of these factors on prognosis (129, 189,227,232). Others tended to average out variables and come up with an average statistic (9,245).

One does get the sense, however, that an untreated intracranial aneurysm is a "time bomb" whose lethality is nearly 40% when it first bleeds and possibly 60% if and when it rebleeds. Approximately 40% of untreated survivors of the initial bleed will rebleed during the first year. At bedrest but untreated medically or surgically, about 25% of survivors of the initial bleed will rebleed in the first 2 weeks. This same initial 2 week period has the greatest rebleed rate, with the rate markedly decreasing over the next 6 weeks. Beyond this 6-week period the rebleed rate is probably about 3% per year. Survivors of the first bleed have a higher death rate if their clinical grade on admission is worse, *a fact of paramount importance when comparing operative statistics with nonoperative statistics.* Finally, there may be a tendency for recurrent bleed to be less in recent years. Better medical therapy may be causally related in part; but perhaps the fact that aspirin, a known platelet antiadhesive drug, is no longer given for headache after SAH is responsible!

Reported Operative Results

This section will summarize the results of surgery by craniotomy (mainly clipping, ligature, parent artery ligation, or trapping) for treatment of the aneurysm. See Chapter 33 for results of carotid artery ligation. The results of unusual techniques (stereotaxic methods, etc.) were insufficiently documented or too low in numbers to make any reasonable comparisons at this time.

In early years, beginning with Walter Dandy's series in 1944 (53), many surgeons tended to tackle most anterior circulation aneurysms without regard to the clinical condition (grade) of the patient. Anesthetic and life support techniques were in their infancy. It took years for any one surgeon to gain experience in these cases. Radiologic methods of localization were in evolution. Microtechnique was unknown to the neurosurgeon. Hence, it is little wonder that mortality and morbidity rates were high—even up until the late 1960s. In 1941 Dandy (54) himself was pessimistic and lamented:

> It is highly improbable that more than an occasional aneurysm of this [middle cerebral] vessel can ever be cured without a permanent hemiplegia, and treatment of this character would not be considered. . . . Some aneurysms of the anterior cerebral artery . . . are amenable to treatment, although none have as yet been cured. . . . There are little prospects of cure [of vertebrobasilar aneurysms] by surgical means. . . .

Dandy (54) was more optimistic about internal carotid artery aneurysms, the subject of that same paper.

In 1964 Logue (190) echoed frustrations at attempts to make meaningful correlations from surgical statistics. He noted that previous statistics often had shown a poor prognosis, but lack of adequate information (especially the timing of surgery) and the degree of neurologic damage, or grade, just prior to surgery made it difficult to decipher and correlate such statistics. A number of authorities have pointed out that while *operative* mortality and morbidity statistics may have some value, a patient is just as dead if he died while awaiting surgery rather than as a complication of surgery. That is, the *management* mortality and morbidity is needed to make reasonable comparisons among series of cases with no treatment, with various medical treatments, and with various surgical treatments (104,189,219,226,266,276, 298,304,344,346). Morley (219) reminded us that

> not all centers keep a tally of their "total management" results; unless this information is available, figures of results following any particular form of treatment must be regarded with skepticism.

Statistics between any two surgeons are meaningless unless both preoperative and postoperative mortality and morbidity are included. A preoperative death may have been prevented by earlier surgery; a postoperative death may have been avoided by delaying or omitting surgery. In some series, operative results appear better due to case selection—without similar case selection for another operative series or for a control nonoperative series. Locksley (189,189a) cautioned that

> removal from the bed rest category of a more favorable spectrum of patients for surgery tends to make these prognostic data for bed rest more pessimistic than would be obtained in a completely unselected natural history population.

After early experience with high operative mortalities and making nursing home rounds on postoperative survivors, many physicians relegated the poor-risk patient to a nonoperative series, a factor that later skewed the results in favor of surgery and against medical treatment or against no specific treatment. Poppen (264) eloquently stated the physicians' dilemma:

> If in the execution of the excision or trapping, however, a patient is hopelessly and permanently crippled or his usefulness has been permanently damaged, one might wish that he had taken a completely conservative course rather than carry out a surgical procedure.

Clearly, the results of both medical and surgical treatment correlate closely with the patient's grade upon admission or upon institution of treatment. Surgical obliteration does have the advantage [not in every case however (73a,161)] of permanently removing or defusing the "time bomb." Contrariwise, the patient destined to die from a future rebleed may have lived an extra few years instead of being a possible statistical death from a surgical mishap.

Reported Surgical Mortalities

At this juncture it is worthwhile to review some of the reported mortalities from intracranial surgery. Adequate morbidity statistics are impossible to compare in most instances. Nevertheless, in the 1966 Cooperative Study where 979 cases of intracranial operation were analyzed, the overall surgical mortality of single aneurysm cases was 30%, and an *additional* 25% were functionally disabled (303). This left only about 45% of operated cases which really may have benefited from surgery (and this neglects those surviving and dead cases who never would have rebled without surgery anyway). Regardless of whether or not one accepts this multicentric study as valid for those years (1958–1965), it does emphasize the nearly 1:1 ratio of disabilities to deaths. Hopefully, with more modern therapies and adjuncts, the drop in mortality is being matched by a similar drop in morbidity. More recent (1975) statistics support this contention where, for example, a mortality statistic of 4% was nearly equaled by a poor result statistic of 5% (355).

In their 1966 review Tönnis and Walter (335) found reported operative mortalities to range from 5 to 45%. Table 21.2 gives some of the reported operative mortalities gleaned from various series from 1944 to 1979. One notices a definite trend: half of the patients died from surgery in the early 1950s; this gradually dropped, especially in the 1970s, to mortality rates of about 5–10%. The earlier surgeons worked under difficult circumstances without the advantage of cumulative experience and more modern techniques. Yet there was one surgeon, Gösta Norlén, who repeatedly reported mortality rates of less than 10% (see Table 21.2). He had gained considerable experience, certainly an important factor. But of equal importance was the factor of case selection: Norlén and Barnum (236) pointed out that

> our series . . . is weighted as to time in that not more than 6 patients were operated on during the first 3 weeks after hemorrhage, because of problems of transportation and bed capacity.

In 1968 Norlén (233) was still of the opinion that it may be best for the patient if intracranial surgery was delayed 3 weeks after the SAH.

By the mid-1960s many neurosurgeons were convinced that their operative mortality was lower than the nonoperative mortality, and the surgical treatment of aneurysms continued for better or for worse. Then, in 1966, the results of the multicenter Cooperative Study (303a) came out: a 30% mortality rate with only a 45% useful, functional patient survival.

Discussion

The results of the 1966 Cooperative Study only served to confirm Hamby's (115) earlier opinion that the neurosurgeon attacking an intracranial aneurysm on many occasions "was much in the position of the hunter arousing a tiger when stalking a deer." Whereas we all look to hunt down our own tiger, Drake (69) warned that

> the challange of this small deadly sac, churning with bright blood, has undoubtedly brought out a degree of rashness in many of us in our determination to obliterate it and to protect the patient. . . . Our failures must be examined carefully in order to understand the reasons and institute measures for their prevention.

Gradually, surgical results did improve (Table 21.2). There were many reasons. Much credit was given to the use of the operating microscope (see "micro" under Comment column in Table 21.2). Recently, a study group concluded:

> In the opinion of this study group, it is advisable that patients with ruptured intracranial aneurysms be considered for aneurysmal ligation intracranially by microtechnique. Slosberg's [304] study of 99 aneurysm patients given long term hypotensive treatment (without surgery), among whom 18 aneurysm-related deaths occurred, does not provide definitive evidence that medical therapy is superior to the surgical therapy recommended here. Both medical therapy and carotid artery ligation in the neck provide alternative therapies when expert microsurgical treatment is either unavailable or infeasible or when a specific contraindication to surgical therapy exists. Present day transportation facilities permit safe transfer of a stable, good risk aneurysm patient by air or ambulance to an appropriate neurosurgical center.
>
> Many of the contraindications for surgery are relative. The consensus of the study group and of most neurosurgeons who see cases of aneurysm in large numbers is that patients in Grades III, IV, and V should not be operated upon intracranially for the purpose of ligating an aneurysm. . . . Some types of aneurysms, due to their size, location, configuration, or clot content, are generally considered inoperable in terms of ligation or excision. With the advent of microtechnique and the application of newer anesthetic methods in aneurysm surgery, however, many of these cases formerly considered inoperable are now regarded as operable in the hands of the highly skilled neurosurgeon. Some lesions are amenable to specific techniques that thrombose or otherwise reinforce the wall of the aneurysm either internally or externally.
>
> The patient's age is not in itself a contraindication to this surgery. Botterell placed the patient older than 50 years (as are most patients with aneurysm) in a less favorable grade, and in some instances this may delay operation. When a patient's age exceeds 65 years, the value of surgery is judged according to individual risks: physiological age, other medical problems, and the probabilities of rebleeding. Surgery might have to be deferred in any patient with a medical problem not under good control. . . . Pregnancy in itself is

Table 21.2. Operative Mortality for Intracranial Aneurysm Surgery

Year	Authors and References	Total Cases	Mortality (%)[a]	Comment
1944	Dandy (53)	32	60	
1952	Bassett et al. (22)	25	40	
1952	Hamby (115)	15	60	
1953	Norlén and Barnum (236)	24	8	
1955	Graf (105)	55	45	
1955	Magladery (198)	37	65	
1955	Rowe et al. (281)	34	20	
1956	Hamby (120)	39	20	
1956	Logue (191)	37	15	
1957	Calvert (40)	31	20	
1957	Frugoni and Ruberti (92)	22	25	
1958	Botterell et al. (35)	73	25	
1958	Höök and Norlén (134)	55	10	MCAA only
1959	Krayenbühl and Weber (174)	45	50	ACoAA only
1960	Frugoni and Morello (91)	26	20	ACoAA only
1960	Poppen and Fager (265)	95	20	
1960	Uihlein and Lippert (341)	88	15	
1961	Laitinen and Troupp (184)	226	9	
1962	Davis (57)	75	20	
1962	Hunt et al. (143)	55	15	
1962	Karlsberg and Adams (160)	54	40	
1962	Lang and Poppen (185)	31	40	ACoAA only
1963	Lougheed et al. (194)	133	25	
1963	Norlén (235)	65	5	ACoAA only
1964	Austin (17)	20	35	
1964	Höök and Norlén (132)	67	7	ACoAA only
1964	Höök and Norlén (133)	50	15	ICAA only
1962	McKissock et al. (212)	52	25	MCAA only
1965	Lougheed et al. (197)	310	25	
1965	Maspes and Marini (204)	81	20	
1966	Hunt et al. (144)	93	15	
1966	Sachs (282)	52	40	MCAA only
1966	Skultety and Nishioka (303a)	979	30	
1968	Bartal et al. (21)	25	50	bBAA only
1968	Drake (66)	226	25	
1968	French et al. (89)	260	15	
1968	Hunt and Hess (141)	156	15	
1968	Jamieson (153)	28	40	V-B aneurysms
1968	Marshall et al. (200)	401	20	
1968	Maspes and Marini (205)	159	20	
1968	Morello (218)	231	15	
1968	Norlén (233)	95	5	ACoAA only
1969	Lapras et al. (185a)	31	30	ACoAA only
1970	Bohm and Hugosson (30)	185	8	
1970	Gass (97)	100	30	
1970	Hamby (117)	173	15	

Continued

not considered a contraindication to operation; however, because temporary hypotensive anesthesia may be required, close fetal monitoring is essential. An incidental carotid artery stenosis or occlusion is not a contraindication to aneurysm surgery; however, each case must be assessed individually regarding risks during anesthesia. Glaucoma is not a contraindication, but, subsequent to hypotensive anesthesia in the presence of uncontrolled glaucoma, visual loss is possible.

In preparation for surgery, the risks and alternative methods of therapy should be detailed to the patient or the nearest of kin. For the usual ruptured aneurysm on a vessel of the anterior circulation, the operating surgeon should be able to state that there are approximately a 5% chance

Table 21.2. Operative Mortality for Intracranial Aneurysm Surgery (*Continued*)

Year	*Authors and References*	*Total Cases*	*Mortality (%)*[a]	*Comment*
1970	Laine et al. (183)	100	25	MCAA only
1970	Paul and Arnold (250)	186	40	
1971	Galbraith and White (95)	212	15	
1971	Sano (291)	200	5	micro[b]
1972	Arseni et al. (13)	328	30	
1972	Cotsou et al. (52)	72	30	
1972	Krayenbühl et al. (178)	250	5	micro
1973	Cophignon et al. (48)	48	8	micro
1973	Cophignon et al. (49)	50	8	micro
1973	Corkill and Hodgson (51)	20	10	micro
1973	Dinning (62)	198	7	
1973	Hollin and Decker (130)	42	5	micro
1973	Hugosson (138)	43	9	
1973	Lougheed and Marshall (195)	497	20	
1973	Pertuiset et al. (252)	41	4	micro
1973	Saito et al. (284)	150	7	micro
1974	Chou and Ortiz-Suarez (44)	20	30	V-B aneurysms
1974	Duffy (76)	30	10	
1974	French and Ortiz-Suarez (90)	97	15	
1974	Graf and Nibbelink (107)	228	35	
1974	Jones (156)	41	15	
1975	Infuso et al. (147)	678	15	
1975	Martinez Coll and Del Corral (202)	65	5	
1975	Thomas and Paterson (333)	30	25	ACeAA only
1975	Yaşargil and Fox (355)	505	4	micro
1976	Adams et al. (2)	100	15	micro
1976	Deruty et al. (60)	60	15	micro
1976	Drake (64)	319	8	V-B aneurysms
1976	Kaufman and Tabaddor (162)	123	20	
1976	Kikuchi (167)	93	15	micro
1976	Loach and De Azevedo Filho (188)	133	10	micro
1976	Miller et al. (215)	249	10	
1976	Suzuki (314)	1000	6	
1977	Fukumitsu et al. (94)	27	7	
1977	Hollin and Decker (131)	70	4	ICAA only, micro
1977	Ito et al. (150)	113	6	
1977	Post et al. (266)	86	8	micro
1977	Saito et al. (287)	400	6	micro
1977	Sundt (308)	323	5	micro
1977	Zlotnik et al. (361)	137	6	micro
1978	Bohm and Hugosson (29)	366	8	
1978	Suzuki (312)	1000	6	
1979	Nornes and Wikeby (239a)	468	5	micro

[a] The mortality rate is given to the nearest 5% if it was reported over 10%.
[b] "micro" means that the operating microscope was used.

of death and a 5% chance of serious neurological deficit after the operation. The percentages might drop in future years.

Both reports in the recent literature and the increasing use of the microscope by neurosurgeons confirm the opinion and experience of study group members that the application of the operating microscope and microtechnique has markedly reduced the mortality and morbidity associated with intracranial aneurysm surgery. Parallel improvements in equipment have contributed additionally to these results. The cardinal factors, however, are the training, experience, and expertise of the operating surgeon who utilizes these new techniques and the capabilities of his operative team.

Equally important are the morbidity statistics. Members of this study group believe that considerably less mortality and morbidity are experienced by all operated aneurysm patients when the operating microscope and microtechnique are used by neurosurgeons experienced in their application. This opinion is supported by many publications.

In summary, early angiography is advisable for all patients with SAH to permit appropriate medical therapy to be instituted while the patient awaits surgery if a ruptured aneurysm is found. The new medical regimens seem to be reducing the number of early episodes of rebleeding so that some surgeons now believe it to be safer, even in the Grade I and II patients, to wait 1 or 2 weeks before operating on the aneurysm. Others believe that early, even immediate, surgery should be done on Grade I to Grade II patients. Thus, even among highly experienced neurosurgeons the question of timing is still controversial. Such surgery should be performed with the aid of a well trained operating team, including nurses and an anesthesiologist. Patients in Grade III or Grade IV categories (i.e., confused, lethargic, or obtunded) ought to have operation delayed until they have improved to a Grade I or II (Hunt's or Botterell's) or Grade I-a (Hunt's) status. Hamby further suggests that the CSF pressure should be less than 200 mm H_2O. However, hydrocephalus or hematoma may cause a CSF pressure greater than this—a condition that may even aid surgical exposure once the CSF is drained or the clot is removed at operation. The study group is unaware of any convincing evidence at present showing that either stereotactic procedures on the aneurysm, ligation of the carotid artery in the neck or of the A-1 anterior cerebral artery intracranially, or therapeutic catheterization procedures have allowed ruptured intracranial aneurysms to be treated earlier with greater safety. However, some of these treatments are still under investigation. (87)

However, several surgeons have reported equally low statistics without the use of the operating microscope (30,62,76,202,215,314). What other factors are playing a role here? We must conclude that advances in diagnostic accuracy (radiology), life support and monitoring systems (anesthesiology and intensive care units), and preoperative care play a significant role. Several authors have concluded that personal experience with a significant number of cases, subspecialization among neurosurgeons, and referral patterns to medical centers seeing many of these cases are important (20,86,87, 117,147,162,214,307,336). Even as far back as 1952 Oscar Sugar (307) noted:

> One of the most important things is that one's results improve with experience. . . . It is clear to me that the more aneurysms one treats, the better one gets at it. Perhaps it is because one learns on which to operate and which to leave alone.

A key to obtaining good results must certainly be not only case selection factors but also timing factors, which often are reported insufficiently to allow adequate and meaningful comparison of different series. A patient surviving the period of planning and transportation to a tertiary referral center must, of necessity, be in better condition for surgery (and for medical therapy).

Factors Affecting Surgical Risk

Timing of Intracranial Surgery

If one discusses the optimum time to clip or ligate an intracranial aneurysm (ignoring the grade 5 patient whose survival from the first bleed is unlikely), the general consensus of neurosurgical opinion has been to delay surgery until the patient is in good medical and neurologic condition. This generally means waiting until the second week post-SAH. af Björkesten (3) analyzed 886 operated cases and 207 nonoperated cases (Fig. 21.4). He concluded that in

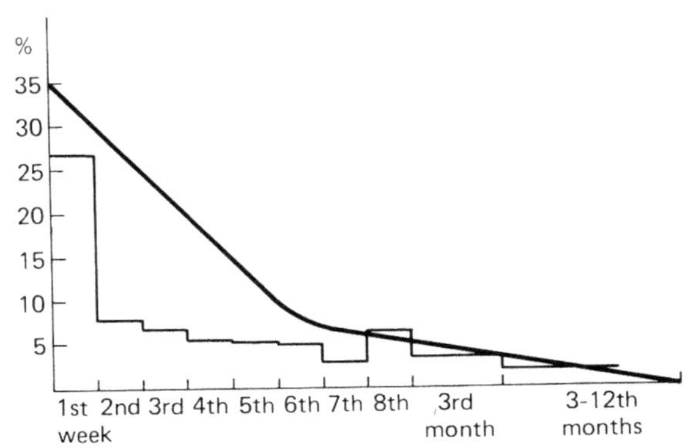

Fig. 21.4. The risk of death from rebleeding (*smooth thick curve*) and operative mortality (*irregular step-shaped line*). The smooth curve represents an unselected series of 207 aneurysm patients taken from the Helsinki Study (245) who were not operated on and were followed for several years. The operative mortality occurred in 886 aneurysm operations between 1954 and 1968. (From ref. 3)

the first week the operative and nonoperative rebleed mortality rates were nearly the same. After the fifth week both the nonoperative rebleed mortality and the operative mortality were low and again nearly equal. He therefore concluded that one is most justified in operating during the second through fifth weeks, and that the best management results would occur by operating during the second week. This does ignore the patient's grade and recent advances in surgical therapy, for some surgeons believe that very early operation is indicated in the grade 1 or 2 patient.

The list of references favoring delayed surgery (7–14 days after the SAH are commonly reported waiting periods) in most patients is quite voluminous (3, 30, 55, 59, 63, 65, 67, 69, 70,76, 78, 82, 102, 105, 110, 112, 120, 132, 133, 136, 139, 147, 150, 160, 177, 184, 186, 188, 193–196, 207, 223, 230, 237, 240, 253, 266, 268, 278, 281, 283, 284, 299, 302, 308, 310, 327, 340, 348). These advocates point out that, in their opinion, the mortality risk of early brain surgery in the face of cerebral edema, cerebrovascular dysautoregulation, and possible vasospasm and ischemia equals or exceeds the chance of death from failure to operate early. This is especially true as medical therapy (see Chapter 22) to inhibit early rebleed becomes more effective. Norlén (233,234) took the position that the surgery should be delayed 3 weeks. Other surgeons have specified that if the patient is alert and in good condition (grade 1 or 2), early operation (as soon as possible or at least within the first 3 days) is advisable to prevent rebleed; otherwise, surgery is delayed until he is in a grade 1 or 2 condition (33, 36, 44, 50, 51, 87, 99, 111, 112, 137, 140–142, 145, 154, 172, 178, 251, 255, 258–261, 263, 290a, 325, 349, 355–357). Unfortunately, some authors would include grades 3 and even 4 as "favorable" conditions for surgery; most indicate grade 1 or 2 as "favorable." Another body of opinion leaned toward early surgery (as soon as possible or within the first 3 days) in most cases, except those that were moribund (35, 94, 96, 112, 113, 168, 182, 244, 248).

Galera et al. (96) in 1967, Tindall and Odom (334) in 1972, and Guidetti (112) in 1973 suggested that early surgery within the first 3 days may be relatively safe, for vasospasm does not begin until after that period. However, Tindall and Odom (334) felt that the patient should be alert and in good condition if such early surgery were to be undertaken. Otherwise they recommended waiting until after the tenth day post-SAH. Subsequently, beginning in 1976, a number of reports further suggested that surgery could be carried out during the first 3 days or after the eighth day. Between these time boundaries is a period of vasospasm and ischemia during which surgery is too hazardous (135, 242, 287, 289, 292–295, 311, 312, 314, 315, 318, 321, 323). Contrariwise, some recommended surgery during these "forbidden" third to ninth days (47,62), indicating that the issue of proper timing of surgery remains far from settled. The value of early operation, late operation, or no operation will depend on comparative *management* mortality and morbidity statistics rather than just operative statistics. Unfortunately, tertiary referral centers select out many poor-grade and rebleed patients, so that management mortality may also be skewed in favor of surgery. The statistician in such cases will not have access to patients not transferred for medical or other reasons.

There are two interesting but diverging views regarding the timing of aneurysm surgery in *children*. Matson (207) stated that he never saw an early rebleed in his 16 childhood cases and recommended delaying surgery. Shulman and Tabaddor (302) delayed surgery 14 days in children. Contrariwise, Orozco et al. (244) carry out early surgery because (a) it is difficult to control blood pressure and intracranial pressure changes due to crying, etc., and (b) the results of early surgery on the childhood brain are better than on the adult brain.

Some surgeons have used additional information to determine optimum timing of surgery. Hamby (114,116–119,121), Klafta and Hamby (172), Klafta (170,171), and Ballantine and Klein (19) were in favor of delaying surgery if the *CSF pressure* was measured in excess of 200 mm H_2O by standard lumbar puncture. In 1969 Klafta and Hamby (172) concluded that in 112 operated aneurysm cases CSF pressure was not a significant indicator of surgical risk if the patient was grade 1 or 2. If the CSF pressure in the grade 3 patient exceeded 200 mm H_2O, then surgery should be delayed because then the risk was excessive. Thus they operated on grade 1 or 2 cases as soon as possible regardless of the CSF pressure. Many of these cases very likely had hydrocephalus as a contributing factor to the high CSF pressure. In these cases

CSF drainage at surgery would be an advantage.

Nornes and Magnaes (238,239) recorded extradural pressures in patients with ruptured aneurysms (see Chapter 8). They found that if extradural pressure peaks (returning toward the baseline) occur, this heralds a rebleed within 24 h; they would do emergency surgery in this circumstance. If they have a threatening clot or hydrocephalus, early operation may be done, although they will often use ventricular drainage in the latter circumstance. Nornes (238) agreed with Hamby that the results of surgery are better if the intracranial pressure is below 200 mm H_2O, although he will operate with less than 400 mm ICP provided the patient is in good condition.

Other authors described the use of circulation time, angiographic evidence of spasm, or cerebral blood flow studies to determine timing of surgery. Bohm and Hugosson (30) delayed surgery until slowed *arm-to-brain circulation time* (using radioactive isotope) returned to normal. Drake (65,67) recommended repeating the angiogram and delaying attack on the aneurysm if significant *angiographic vasospasm* is seen. *Dynamic radionuclide (RN) scans* were investigated by Goodman and Hayes (103) and Kelly et al. (165,166). The early scanning phase often showed reduced cerebral perfusion associated with a high incidence of infarcts (166). There was no correlation between perfusion deficits and angiographic evidence of spasm (165), but there was close correlation with the operative result: a poorer result if perfusion was slow, a better result if perfusion had returned to normal. In addition there was a higher incidence of rebleed once the perfusion, as seen on the dynamic RN scan, had returned to normal.

Cerebral blood flow (CBF) using radioactive isotopes was employed by Heilbrun and Olesen (125), Bohm and Hugosson (29), and Ishii (148). These authors recommended delay of surgery until a normal CBF returned. Ishii (148) avoided operation until the CBF exceeded 30 ml per 100 g per min, *and* normal cerebrovascular reactivity to CO_2 challenge and normal autoregulation returned. It would appear that a body of evidence is accumulating that shows that poor *cerebrovascular reactivity* (to CO_2 and blood pressure changes), whether vasospasm is present or not, prevents the brain from tolerating surgical intervention and anesthesia without adverse reaction.

Another useful test is *computed tomography* (CT). Obvious edema and tight ventricles (Fig. 21.5) would lead the surgeon to delay surgery,

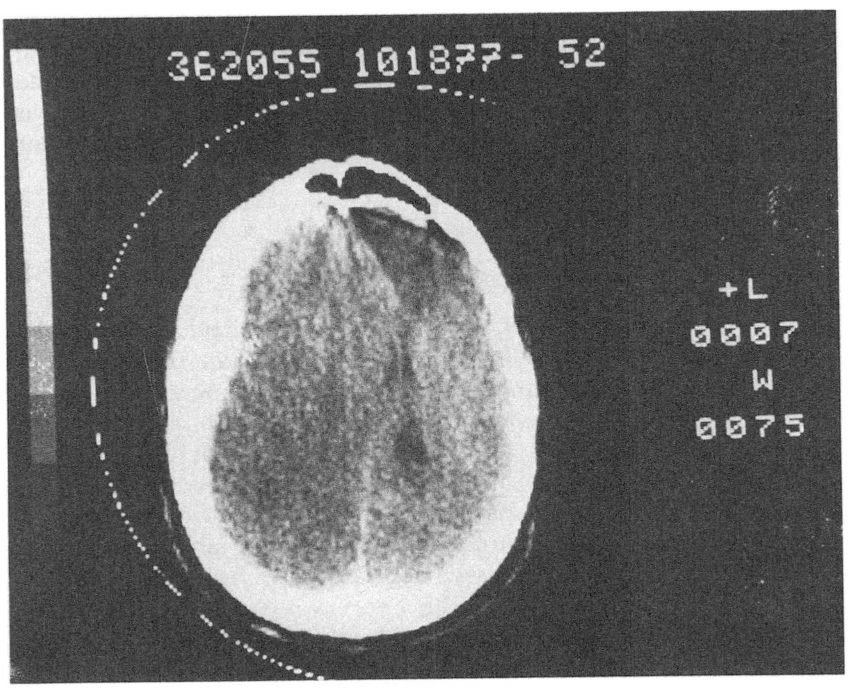

Fig. 21.5. Computed tomogram of the brain following rupture of the left ICAA. There is obvious left subdural hematoma, severe edema, and shifted (to the right), tight ventricles. This 29-year-old man died 24 h after his bleed. Only the hematoma was removed.

whereas hydrocephalus may provide good brain relaxation as the CSF is drained. If severe hemorrhage is seen on CT scan and is a predictor of future vasospasm, surgery might also be delayed in this circumstance.

Grade of the Patient

The grading of the aneurysm patient has become important mainly for purpose of comparisons among patients and among various treatment and prognostic series. There are many types of grading classifications (see Appendix 1 and Chapter 5). [This book uses the 1973 modified Botterell classification (number 25 in Appendix 1) unless otherwise stated.] There is rather universal agreement that the results of intracranial surgery (like the results of nonoperative treatment) are better when the patient is in a good grade (1, 6, 8, 29, 30, 32–34, 38, 40, 42–44, 47, 60, 66, 70, 87, 90, 95, 97, 101, 107, 111, 132, 133, 136, 140–142, 147, 154, 159, 160, 163, 167, 178, 183–185, 185a, 188, 194, 195, 199, 200, 202, 210, 211, 228, 235, 250, 256, 278, 290a, 293, 299, 300, 306, 308–310, 312, 314, 325, 335, 340, 348, 355, 358).

In 1967 Gillingham (101), like most surgeons, came to the conclusion that

> the most important single factor that came out of our earlier experience in determining the success or failure of operative treatment in intracranial aneurysm was the conscious level of the patient before operation.

This factor, the patient's grade, is of necessity very closely related to timing, for many patients tend to improve their grade status with time (235). This, of course, excludes events such as later deterioration from rebleed, vasospasm, hematoma, edema, hydrocephalus, etc. Yet it is the expected improvement in the patient's grade which stays the hand of many surgeons who look for a better operative result. However, the question of better total management result remains unsettled in the minds of many.

Other Medical Factors

A number of clinicians found that *vascular hypertension* makes the operative risk greater (60, 170, 171, 188, 205, 210, 211, 261, 278). There was an occasional dissenter (164). A problem is differentiating chronic hypertension from the commonly present acute hypertension related to stress, elevated catecholamines, and the Cushing reflex. Most authors have not clarified this; indeed, this may be difficult to differentiate immediately post-SAH.

Certainly a patient with cardiac hypertrophy, chronic renal disease, and long-standing hypertension is not an ideal surgical candidate. Furthermore, the patient with the acute elevation in blood pressure often associated with vasospasm, EKG changes, pulmonary edema, or increased ICP is already in an unfavorable grade. Unfortunately, it is this patient who not only is at greater risk for surgery but also is at greater risk for rebleed as the blood pressure rises.

Another factor which increased operative risk in most series was increased *age* (6, 11, 29, 35, 107, 147, 162, 163, 183, 196, 205, 210, 211, 227, 261, 303, 312, 314, 335, 348, 358). Most authors found that the mortality rate increased if the patient was older than 50 years. An exception was Hugosson (138) who found no significant increase in mortality in 43 patients (out of 300 total) aged 60–70 years. Amacher and colleagues (11) found only an increase in mortality from 11% in 494 grade 1 and 2 patients under 60 years of age to 15% in 93 grade 1 and 2 patients over 60 years of age. The generally accepted increase in mortality in the older age group relates to many obvious factors including cardiovascular status and other age-related risk factors. Of interest is the finding by Nibbelink et al. (227) that there is a higher incidence of vasospasm in the older age group.

Vasospasm

One of the most serious secondary complications of ruptured intracranial aneurysm is vasospasm. This phenomenon is more thoroughly discussed in Chapters 9 and 10. It is of import here, for when the spasm reaches a certain point, ischemia, infarction, and edema (Fig. 21.6) may result in serious neurologic impairment, making both surgical and nonsurgical prognosis worse. Vasospasm has generally been assumed to be a narrowing of the lumen of the conducting cerebral arteries due to smooth muscle constriction. It is usually diagnosed by cerebral angiography or direct observation at surgery. It may be suspected by the clinical course and by measured reduction in regional cerebral blood flow and impaired cerebral circulation time. It may be mimicked or aggravated by edema of the vessel wall and by marked increases in intracranial pressure. Its onset is rarely seen prior to the third day post-SAH (Fig. 21.7), commonly becomes symptomatic on the fifth to the eighth day, commonly becomes maximum within 48 h, and usually recedes by the eleventh to fourteenth day (30, 61, 70, 81, 88, 96, 108, 157, 169, 179, 181, 201, 262, 267, 284, 285, 287, 289, 292–294, 311, 313, 316, 342, 347, 350).

There has been considerable variation in opinion among authors in terms of which specific ruptured aneurysm most commonly causes vasospasm (30,35,61,108,203,229,285,227). Although there may be a tendancy for ACoAA to have a higher incidence, this does not appear to be statistically significant.

Whereas one may believe that vasospasm, due to its effect on cerebral blood flow, would reduce the tendency to rebleed, such is not the case. du Boulay and Gado (75) and Henderson et al. (129) noted no such correlation. In fact Nibbelink et al. (224,226) found an increased incidence of aneurysm rebleed in the presence of vasospasm (21%) as opposed to no vasospasm (11%).

There is almost universal agreement that vasospasm is bad and, when present, worsens the prognosis for a good surgical result (14, 23, 37, 65, 69, 73, 105, 110, 123, 139, 141–143, 182, 188, 191, 193, 195, 231, 234, 237, 243, 261, 268, 292, 295, 334, 345). Pool (257) in 1958, French et al. (89) in 1968, and Suzuki (311) in 1976 recommended that in some cases early or immediate surgery may even reduce the risk of vasospasm by irrigation or toilet of the subarachnoid space (clot and breakdown product removal) and by removal of the aneurysm wall from stretching under the pressure of the bloodstream. Others such as Yasargil et al. (355,356), Suzuki et al. (319,320,322), Graf and Nibbelink (107), Braakman (36), Prakash et al. (267), Richardson (275), and Millikan (216) found no correlation between the *radiologic* evidence of vasospasm and surgical mortality. Many of these authors considered the state of alertness and clinical grade a better indicator of prognosis. Very likely there is no contradiction. It may not be the vasospasm per se that predicts the prognosis but rather its severity (see Fig. 10.1): diffuse, severe vasospasm invariably will be seen only in the confused or unconscious patient of grade 3 level or worse. Ransohoff et al. (268) concluded that "secondary cerebral vasospasm remains the major obstacle to early recovery and definitive surgery for ruptured intracranial aneurysms."

Surgery carried out just prior to the onset of signs of vasospasm may aggravate the condition, with surgery being blamed for a clinical picture already in the making. Such a clinical picture, however, may be worsened by hematoma, hydrocephalus, cerebral thrombosis, and edema, all of which in themselves can create ischemic lesions and mimic signs of vasospasm.

A number of autopsy studies and clinicopathologic correlations have strongly suggested that vasospasm is at least one of the significant factors creating ischemic lesions, infarcts, and abnormal vessel wall permeability (15, 16, 35, 41, 79, 122, 187, 209, 277, 296, 297, 305). Schneck (296) suggested that a greater role was played by surgical retraction, compression by subarachnoid or intracerebral hematoma, shock, and other events which comprised cerebral blood flow already made tenuous by vasospasm. The presence of reduced cerebral perfusion, blood-brain barrier abnormalities, and infarcts in the presence of vasospasm has been further documented by RN (12,103,165, 166,351) and CT scans (286) in these patients.

Surgery Versus Conservative Treatment

Surgeons have frequently assumed, often on the basis of scant scientific evidence, that the aneurysm patient is better off having surgical treatment. Unfortunately this assumption, whether valid or not, has been supported by statistics which do not compare management mortalities between equally comparable operated and nonoperated series. For example, some authors present nonoperative mortalities in the neighborhood of 50% and then use such as the yardstick against which to compare their lower operative mortalities (13,174–176,199). Many of these nonoperated cases were already excluded from possible surgery by their poor

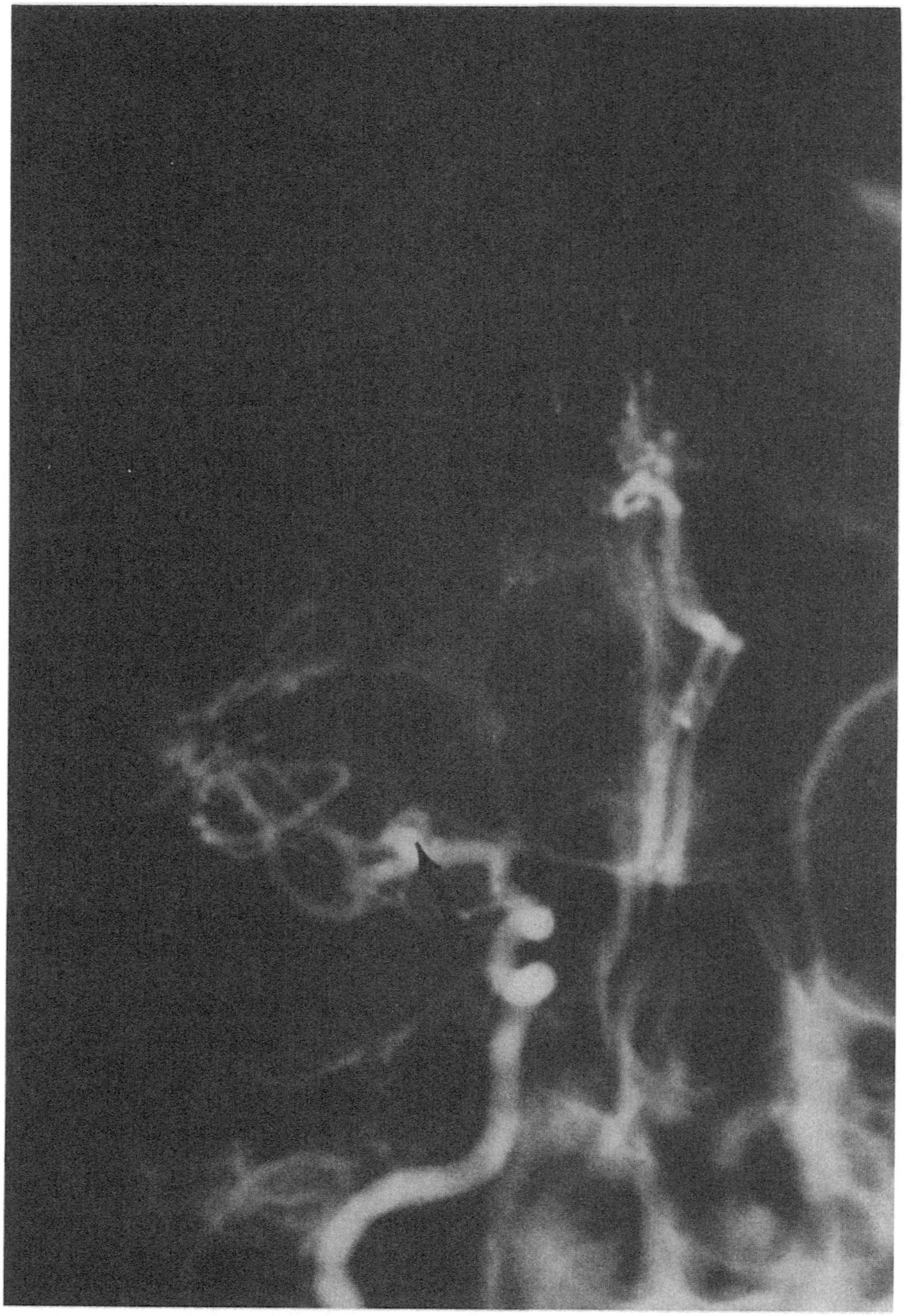

Fig. 21.6. A AP view (transorbital) of the right carotid angiogram in a 51-year-old lady (*arrow:* MCAA).

grade status, and none benefited from modern conservative therapy. In the randomized prospective study by McKissock et al. (212) in 1962, they found that the 23% operative mortality in 52 MCAA cases treated by direct attack on the aneurysm was less than the nonoperative mortality. The same authors did not find this to be true of ACoAA cases (211).

There have been a number of authors presenting data suggesting that the surgical risk is no better than the nonsurgical risk. In 1955 Magladery (198) compared 189 nonsurgical cases with 37 surgical cases. The surgical mortality was 65%; the nonsurgical mortality of those 52 cases surviving 24 h after their SAH was 20%. The latter dropped to 12% if they

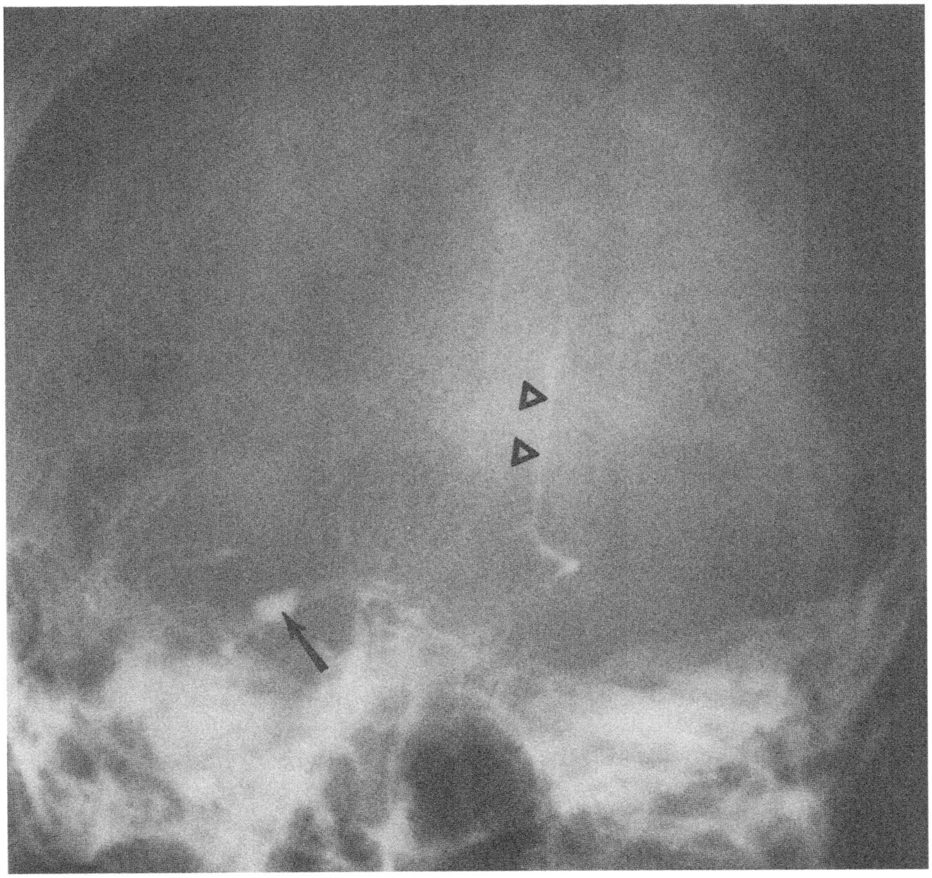

Fig. 21.6. B Repeat angiogram of the same patient 11 days after her SAH. This AP view (Towne) demonstrates the aneurysm (*arrow*) and severe, delayed vasospasm with edema and shift of the anterior cerebral artery (*two triangles*) under the falx.

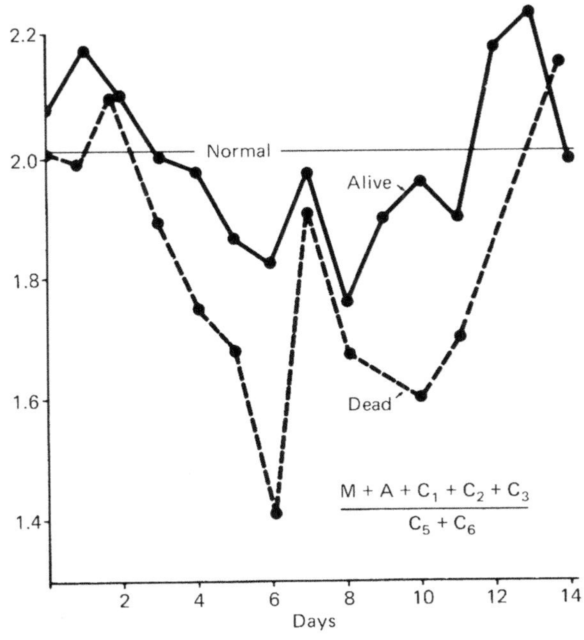

Fig. 21.7. Curve for reduction in ratio of the caliber of vessels in the subarachnoid space to those outside versus time. Based on 429 angiograms done posthemorrhage and preoperatively; there is more constriction in 120 angiograms on patients who died (*broken line*) than in 309 survivors (*continuous line*). (From ref. 347)

had already survived 1 week. In 1956 Roberts (276) found a 14% nonsurgical mortality among 113 cases surviving 24 h after their SAH. He believed this could not be bettered by surgery. In 1958 Benson (24) compared 22 operated and 18 nonoperated cases. He concluded the prognosis was equal if one excluded nonoperated cases dying prior to the safe time for surgery. In 1962 Davis (57) reviewed a series of 75 surgical cases operated an average of 30 days post-SAH. He concluded the mortality rate of 20% did not justify surgery.

In 1960 McKissock and co-workers (210) again did a retrospective study comparing 119 nonoperated cases and 385 operated cases (craniotomy or carotid ligation). The mortality rates were equal (28%) in both series. They kept certain factors such as age, blood pressure, and clinical grade similar in the two series. However, when they separated out the various cases based on aneurysm site, they found that MCAA patients benefited from direct attack but ACoAA patients did not benefit from surgery in terms of the first 6-month survival post-SAH (211,212,274,343).

In 1968 af Björkesten and Troupp (4) analyzed 123 cases divided into surgical (direct operation) and nonsurgical categories 2–6 weeks after the SAH. Except for ICAA cases in good condition, there was no difference in mortality rates. Troupp and af Björkesten (338) and Kaste and Troupp (161) then followed 178 grade 1 ruptured aneurysm cases from 1964 to 1969. Patients were admitted to the randomized study an average of 7 weeks after the SAH. They were matched according to age, sex, blood pressure, grade, and site of aneurysm. Among the nonoperated cases 17% died of rebleed during the time of the study. Among the operated cases there was one operative death, but 7% died of later rebleed (due to unsatisfactory surgery, presumably). But deaths from all causes (especially cardiovascular disease) resulted in little difference in the ultimate mortality between the two groups during the period of observation: 20% if operated, 24% if not operated. They concluded that

> despite the significant difference in numbers of deaths from rebleeding, we were unable to reduce the total mortality significantly by operation: in the surgical group more people died from cardiovascular disease, which evened out the small difference achieved by surgery. (161)

Keller (164) came to a similar conclusion after analyzing 5-year survivorship of operated and unoperated cases. This study reviewed matched cases treated in United States Veterans Administration Hospitals from 1958 through 1962. The survey likewise found no significant difference in ultimate survivorship between operated and nonoperated cases.

In 1977 Alvord and Thorn (10) subjected previously reported operative series to comparative analysis (see Fig. 21.3). They summarize as follows:

> Mortality rates by themselves are misleading, since they are affected by the clinical condition (grade) of the patient and the time after hemorrhage that he has already survived when he appears for treatment. In fact, when these two major determinants of the patient's prognosis were considered together, no great difference in the number of survivors (the inverse of mortality) could be detected in previously reported series of cases regardless of the method of treatment, site or number of aneurysms, or any other factor which could then be analyzed.

Heiskanen and Martilla (127) and Paterson and Bond (249) came to similar conclusions when cases with multiple aneurysms were studied.

Incidental Intracranial Aneurysms

Nishioka (232) in the 1966 Cooperative Study concluded that there was little to suggest that a patient with multiple aneurysms would suffer a future bleed from the untreated aneurysm(s). This was based on a 7-year period of study. Bailey and Loeser (18) opined that surgery for incidental intracranial aneurysms was not justified. More recently, Heiskanen (126a) followed 61 patients with multiple aneurysms where only the ruptured one was clipped; the death-from-rebleed rate over an average of 16 years was 11.5%. Romy et al. (280) investigated the cerebral vessels in 11,696 autopsies and found 145 incidental aneurysms (1.22%). Fifty percent of these aneurysms had evidence of previous bleed: 70% if ACoAA and 30% if pcaICAA. The incidence was much higher if the patient was older or hypertensive. They advised surgical therapy for incidental aneurysms.

In various reported series of patients having their incidental aneurysm (one of multiple aneurysms after a previous SAH or one discovered without prior suspicion) attacked intracranially, the morbidity and mortality rates have been extremely low or absent: no mortality in 26 cases (64), in 10 cases (151), in 24 cases (220–222), and in 49 cases (290). Accordingly, the following was the opinion of a recent study group:

> In experienced hands, the unruptured aneurysm in a patient with multiple aneurysms or an aneurysm incidentally found during angiography for other reasons can be ligated safely. The patient

should be told (with individual exceptions based on the physician's judgment) that the natural mortality statistics are unknown for persons with incidentally found aneurysms; that the aneurysm represents a perpetual threat to his life; that such a threat is greatest under conditions of emotional or physical stress, including sexual intercourse; and that in experienced hands the surgical mortality rate is less than 5% and probably less than 1% for a Grade 0 patient. Bailey and Loeser [18], on the basis of statistical estimates of the incidence of future rupture of aneurysms found incidentally, believe that these should not be treated surgically. However, the skill of the surgical team and results of the surgery performed in the past should be considered in reaching a decision. The giant aneurysm, the basilar artery aneurysm, and certain unusual aneurysms are special phenomena requiring individual judgment. The mortality and morbidity rates for both surgical and nonsurgical therapy are inevitably higher in these instances. (87)

Summary

Recent advances in both medical and surgical treatment of intracranial aneurysms have allowed better protection of the patient from an early rebleed while the patient's brain and cerebrovascular system normalize to a state better tolerating permanent surgical obliteration of the aneurysm. The high surgical mortality rates of earlier years are not acceptable now. Likewise, the continuous threat of an aneurysm capable of causing cerebral destruction is not acceptable. Modern neurosurgical treatment of the aneurysm is the preferred therapy at present. Details of the timing of surgery and various technical aspects remain under discussion in the literature.

Bibliography

1. Abe H, Tsuru M, Tashiro K, et al.: Ruptured aneurysms with intracerebral hematoma. Neurol Surg (Tokyo) 5:527–535, 1977
2. Adams CBT, Loach AB, O'Laoire SA: Intracranial aneurysms: analysis of results of microneurosurgery. Brit Med J 2:607–609, 1976
3. af Björkesten G: The timing of aneurysm operations. J Neurosurg Sci 17:11–13, 1973
4. af Björkesten G, Troupp H: A controlled trial of delayed surgery for intracranial arterial aneurysms. First results. Progr Brain Res 30:353–356, 1968
5. af Björkesten G, Troupp H: Prognosis of subarachnoid hemorrhage. A comparison between patients with verified aneurysms and patients with normal angiograms. J Neurosurg 14:434–441, 1957
6. Ahmed RH, Sedzimir CB: Ruptured anterior communicating aneurysms. A comparison of medical and specific surgical treatment. J Neurosurg 26:213–217, 1967
7. Alexander E Jr, Davis CH Jr, Kester NC: Intracranial aneurysms. Methods of treatment; value of hypothermia in the surgical approach. Arch Neurol Psychiat 81:684–692, 1959
8. Allégre G, Vigouroux R: Le traitement chirurgical des anévrysmes supra-clinoïdiens. Neurochirurgia (Stuttgart) 1:215–242, 1959
9. Alvord EC Jr, Loeser JD, Bailey WL, et al.: Subarachnoid hemorrhage due to ruptured aneurysms. A simple method of estimating prognosis. Arch Neurol 27:273–284, 1972
10. Alvord EC Jr, Thorn RB: Natural history of subarachnoid hemorrhage: Early prognosis. Clin Neurosurg 24:167–175, 1977
11. Amacher AL, Ferguson GG, Drake CG, et al.: How old people tolerate intracranial surgery for aneurysm. Neurosurgery 1:242–244, 1977
12. Arseni C, Constantinovici A, Mihăilă G: Evaluation of ischemia disturbances due to spasms caused by rupture of cerebral vascular malformations. In Fusek I, Kunc Z (eds.): Proceedings of the Fourth European Congress of Neurosurgery. Present Limits of Neurosurgery. 1972, pp. 255–259
13. Arseni C, Constantinovici A, Mihăilă G, et al.: Cerebral vascular diseases. Cerebral aneurysms. Our experience with 482 cases. Neurol Psihiatr Neurochir 17:395–418, 1972
14. Arseni C, Nash F: Cerebral ischemia in the course of ruptured aneurysms. Europ Neurol 1:308–323, 1968
15. Arutyunova AS: Morphological studies of the brain in aneurysms of the anterior communicating artery. Vop Neirokhir 32:4–10, Jan.–Feb. 1968
16. Arutyunova AS, Konovalov AN: Some data of morphological investigation in aneurysms of the arteries of the base of the brain. Vop Neirokhir 29:15–19, March–April 1965
17. Austin DC: A review of intracranial aneurysms. Henry Ford Hosp Med Bull 12:251–271, 1964
18. Bailey WL, Loeser JD: Intracranial aneurysms. JAMA 216:1993–1996, 1971
19. Ballantine HT Jr, Klein DM: Management of spontaneous intracranial subarachnoid hemorrhage. Circulation 17:1123–1136, 1958
20. Ballenger OM, Salcman M, Ducker TB, et al.:

Prognosis of surgically treated intracranial arterial aneurysm patients. JAMA 237:1845–1847, 1977
21. Bartal A, Schiffer J, Weinstein M: A successful case of basilar bifurcation aneurysm surgery. Acta Neurochir 19:163–170, 1968
22. Bassett RC, List CF, Lemmen LJ: Surgical treatment of intracranial aneurysm. Surg Gynec Obstet 95:701–708, 1952
23. Beck OJ, Weiser HX: Die Bedeutung des Vasospasmus für die Prognose nach Aneurysmablutung. Zbl Neurochir 35:21–34, 1974
24. Benson DF: Conservative vs. surgical treatment of cerebral aneurysms. Neurology 8:852–856, 1958
25. Bevan B, Caird FI, Hughes IE: Subarachnoid haemorrhage in the army. Lancet 1:133–135, 1960
26. Bloch A: Murphy's Law. Los Angeles, Price/Stern/Sloan, 1977, pp. 4–5
27. Bloor BM, Majzoub HS, Nugent GR, et al.: Cerebrovascular hemodynamics in intracranial hemorrhage. Excerpta Med No 293:46, 1973
28. Bohm E, Aronson G, Hugosson R, et al.: Cerebral circulatory conditions in patients with ruptured aneurysms measured by an intravenous radioactive indicator technique. Acta Neurol Scand 44:33–42, 1968
29. Bohm E, Hugosson R: Experiences of surgical treatment of 400 consecutive ruptured cerebral arterial aneurysms. Acta Neurochir 40:33–43, 1978
30. Bohm E, Hugosson R: Results of surgical treatment of 200 consecutive cerebral arterial aneurysms. Acta Neurol Scand 46:43–52, 1970
31. Boldrey E: Long-term follow-up of aneurysms of the internal carotid-middle cerebral system. Western J Surg 72:126–129, 1964
32. Bonnal J, Stevenaert A: Indications actuelles de l'abord direct des anévrysmes artériels du polygone de Willis. Acta Neurol Belg 70:240–268, 1970
33. Bonnal J, Stevenaert A: Operability limits of anterior arterial aneurysms of the Willis circle. In Fusek I, Kunc Z (eds.): Proceedings of the Fourth European Congress of Neurosurgery. Present Limits of Neurosurgery, Vol 1. Prague, Avicenum, Czechoslovak Medical Press, 1972, p. 267
34. Bonnal J, Stevenaert A, Brotchi J, et al.: Bilan de neuf ans d'expérience de la chirurgie des anévrysmes artériels intracrâniens. Acta Neurol Belg 74:337–355, 1974
35. Botterell EH, Lougheed WM, Morley TP, et al.: Hypothermia in the surgical treatment of ruptured intracranial aneurysms. J Neurosurg 15:4–18, 1958
36. Braakman R: Present-day treatment of subarachnoid hemorrhage in the Netherlands. Results of an inquiry. Psychiat Neurol Neurochir 75:429–436, 454, 1972
37. Bromowicz J, Danilewicz B, Jedlińska M: Angiospasms in subarachnoid haemorrhages from ruptured intracranial aneurysms. Neurol Neurochir Pol 8:249–255, 1974
38. Brown AS, Horton JM: Elective hypotension with intracardiac pacemaking in the operative management of ruptured intracranial aneurysms. Acta Anaesth Scand Suppl 23:665–670, 1966
39. Bull JWD: Massive aneurysms at the base of the brain. Brain 92:535–570, 1969
40. Calvert CA: Experiences in the treatment of ruptured intracranial aneurysms. J Neurol Neurosurg Psychiat 20:159–164, 1957
41. Cambria S, Daum S: Le ramollissement cérébral au cours de l'évolution des anévrismes intra-craniens rompus. Sem Hôp Paris 42:220–227, 1966
42. Castaigne P, Buge A, Lhermitte F, et al.: Résultats et indications du traitement chirurgical des anévrysmes artériels intracraniens rompus d'aprés 90 cas personnels. Presse Med 74:2397–2400, 1966
43. Charlez V, Dawson BH: Study of anterior communicating aneurysm. J Neurol Neurosurg Psychiat 38:406, 1975
44. Chou SN, Ortiz-Suarez HJ: Surgical treatment of arterial aneurysms of the vertebrobasilar circulation. J Neurosurg 41:671–680, 1974
45. Cioffi FA, Tomasello F: Long-term prognosis in a group of patients with ruptured unoperated intracranial arterial aneurysms. J Neurosurg Sci 19:69, 1975
46. Cioffi FA, Tomasello F, Albanese V: Prognosi a distanza di un gruppo di pazienti con aneurismi intracranici rotti non trattati chirurgicamente. Acta Neurol (Napoli) 30:638–643, 1975
47. Clark K: Complications of aneurysm surgery. Clin Neurosurg 23:342–356, 1976
48. Cophignon J, Rey A, Thurel C, et al.: Microchirurgie des anévrysmes artériels de la partie antérieure du polygone de Willis. Étude d'une série consécutive de 48 cas. Neuro-chirurgie Paris 19:519–530, 1973
49. Cophignon J, Rey A, Thurel C, et al.: Microchirurgie des anévrysmes intracrâniens. Etude d'une série consécutive de 50 cas. Nouv Presse Méd 2:2935–2938, 1973
50. Corkill G: Earlier operation and antifibrinolytic therapy in the management of aneurysmal subarachnoid haemorrhage. Review of recent experience in Tasmania. Med J Australia 1:468–470, 1974
51. Corkill G, Hodgson MJH: Hypotension with sodium nitroprusside in the surgery of cerebral aneurysms. Anaesthesia 28:191–194, 1973

52. Cotsou S, Schliack H: Über die Therapie der intrakraniellen sackförmigen Aneurysmen. Ein Bericht über 200 Fälle. Fortschr Neurol Psychiatr 40:113–135, 1972
53. Dandy WE: Intracranial Arterial Aneurysms. New York, Hafner; Ithica, New York, Comstock Publishing, 1944 (reprinted 1969)
54. Dandy WE: The surgical treatment of intracranial aneurysms of the internal carotid artery. Ann Surg 114:336–340, 1941
55. David M, Pertuiset B, Guyot JF: La cure radicale des anévrysmes de la communicante antérieure sans résection cérébrale ni hypothermie chez le malade conscient. Considérations sur la mortalité et les troubles du comportement postopératoires. Press Med 76:1467–1470, 1968
56. David M, Sachs M: Les anéurysmes de la bifurcation de la carotide interne. Neurochirugia (Stuttgart) 10:96–105, 1967
57. Davis RA: The results of delayed intracranial surgery in a series of 75 selected cerebral aneurysms. Quart Bull Northwest Univ Med Sch 36:237–244, 1962
58. Deborsu FL: Quand faut-il opérer un anévrysme supra-clinoidien rompu? Neuro-chirurgie (Paris) 4:95–106, 1958
59. Dereymaeker A: La chirurgie des angiomes et anévrysmes intracrâniens. Bruxelles-Méd 40:175–183, 1960
60. Deruty R, Dechaume J-P, Lecuire J, et al.: Traitement microchirurgical d'une série d'anévrysmes artériels intra-crâniens sus-tentoriels. Neuro-chirurgie (Paris) 22:227–238, 1976
61. Dickmann GH, Zamboni O, Driollet Laspiur R, et al.: Aneurysms and vasospasm: Clinico-radiological correlation. In Fusek I, Kunc Z (eds.): Proceedings of the Fourth European Congress of Neurosurgery. Present Limits of Neurosurgery. Prague, Avicenum, Czechoslovak Medical Press, 1972, pp. 229–232
62. Dinning TAR: Timing of surgery for leaking cerebral aneurysms: Clinical, radiological and radio-isotopic considerations. Proc Australian Assoc Neurol 9:219–226, 1973
63. Dott NM: Intracranial aneurysmal formations. Clin Neurosurg 16:1–15, 1969
64. Drake CG: Cerebral aneurysm surgery—an update. In Scheinberg P (ed.): Cerebrovascular Diseases. Tenth Princeton Conference. New York, Raven Press, 1976, pp. 289–310
65. Drake CG: Discussion. In Toole JF, Moossy J, Janeway R (eds.): Cerebral Vascular Diseases. New York, Grune & Stratton, 1971, pp. 241–244, 249
66. Drake CG: Discussion of : Risk related to time of surgery in intracranial aneurysms. J Neurosurg 28:19–20, 1968
67. Drake CG: Intracranial aneurysms. In Tower DB (ed.): The Nervous System. The Clinical Neurosciences, Vol 2. New York, Raven Press, 1975, pp. 287–295
68. Drake CG: Management of aneurysms of posterior circulation. In Youmans JR (ed.): Neurological Surgery, Vol 2. Philadelphia, Saunders, 1973, pp. 787–806
69. Drake CG: On the surgical treatment of ruptured intracranial aneurysms. Clin Neurosurg 13:122–155, 1965
70. Drake CG: Ruptured intracranial aneurysms. Proc Roy Soc Med 64:477–481, 1971
71. Drake CG: In Summary of the Tenth Princeton conference on cerebral vascular diseases, January 7–9, 1976. Stroke 7:235–238, 1976
72. Drake CG: Surgical treatment of vertebrobasilar aneurysms. In Koos WT, Böck FW, Spetzler RF (eds.): Clinical Microneurosurgery. Stuttgart, Georg Thieme Verlag, 1976, pp. 213–219
73. Drake CG: The surgical treatment of vertebral-basilar aneurysms. Clin Neurosurg 16:114–169, 1969
73a. Drake CG, Allcock JM: Postoperative angiography and the "slipped" clip. J Neurosurg 39:683–689, 1973
74. du Boulay G: Distribution of spasm in the intracranial arteries after subarachnoid haemorrhage. Acta Radiol [Diagn] 1:257–266, 1963
75. du Boulay G, Gado M: The protective value of spasm after subarachnoid haemorrhage. Brain 97:153–156, 1974
76. Duffy G: The surgical treatment of anterior communicating artery aneurysms. Austral NZ J Surg 44:257–260, 1974
77. Dunsmore RH, Polcyn JL: Subarachnoid hemorrhage: prognostic factors. J Neurosurg 13:165–169, 1956
78. Ectors L: La neurochirurgie fait le bilan des anévrysmes supratentoriels rompus. Déductions thérapeutiques. Acta Neurol Belg 67:431–451, 1967
79. Falconer MA: Surgical pathology of spontaneous intracranial haemorrhage due to aneurymsm and arteriovenous malformations. Proc Roy Soc Med 47:693–700, 1954
80. Fisher CM, Roberson GH, Ojemann RG: Cerebral vasospasm after ruptured aneurysm. Stroke 8:11, 1977
81. Fisher CM, Roberson GH, Ojemann RG: Cerebral vasospasm with ruptured saccular aneurysm—the clinical manifestations. Neurosurgery 1:245–248, 1977
82. Fleischer AS, Tindall GT: Preoperative management of ruptured cerebral aneurysms. Contemp Neurosurg 1:1–6, 1978
83. Fletcher TM, Taveras JM, Pool JL: Cerebral vasospasm in angiography for intracranial

aneurysms. Incidence and significance in one hundred consecutive angiograms. Arch Neurol 1:38–47, 1959
84. Fodstad H, Thulin C-A: Use of tranexamic acid (AMCA) in the preoperative management of patients with ruptured intracranial aneurysms. Excerp Med ICS No 418:98, 1977
85. Fox JL: From files on personal experience, 1979
86. Fox JL: Neurosurgical training. J Neurosurg 40:137–139, 792–795, 1974
87. Fox JL, Albin MS, Bader DCH, et al.: Microsurgical treatment of neurovascular disease. Neurosurgery 3:285–337, 1978
88. Fox JL, Ko JP: Cerebral vasospasm: a clinical observation Surg Neurol 10:269–275, 1978
89. French LA, Chou SN, Long DM: The direct approach to intracranial aneurysms. Clin Neurosurg 15:117–132, 1968
90. French LA, Ortiz-Suarez HJ: Anterior communicating artery aneurysms: technique of operation and results. Clin Neurosurg 21:115–119, 1974
91. Frugoni P, Morello G: Considérations sur le traitement des anévrysmse de l'artère communicante antérieure. Neuro-chirurgie (Paris) 6:25–29, 1960
92. Frugoni P, Ruberti R: Considérations sur le traitement chirurgical des anévrismas sacculaires intracraniens de la carotide interne et de ses branches. Neuro-chirurgie (Paris) 3:241–252, 1957
93. Fujinaga R, Mizukami M, Araki G, et al.: Prognosis of ruptured intracranial aneurysm treated by the conservative method. Brain Nerve (Tokyo) 23:1265–1270, 1971
94. Fukumitsu T, Miwa Y, Tokuriki Y, et al.: Emergency operation for the ruptured intracranial aneurysms—within 5 days after subarachnoid hemorrhage. Neurol Med Chir (Tokyo) 17 (Part 2):227–232, 1977
95. Galbraith JG, White RL: Surgical treatment of intracranial aneurysms. Am Surg 37:600–604, 1971
96. Galera R, Greitz T, Bergvall U: Angioespasmo cerebral consecutivo a la ruptura de aneurismas arteriales intracraneales. Consideraciones hemodinámicas y terapéuticas. Acta Neurol Lat Am 13:283–294, 1967
97. Gass H: The risks in intracranial obliteration of berry aneurysms. Mich Med 69:479–484, 1970
98. Gelmers HJ, Beks JWF, Journée HL: Regional cerebral blood flow in patients with subarachnoid haemorrhage. Acta Neurochir 47:245–251, 1979
99. Giannotta SL, Kindt GW: Total morbidity and mortality rates of patients with surgically treated intracranial aneurysms. Neurosurgery 4:125–128, 1979
100. Gillingham FJ: The management of ruptured intracranial aneurysm. Ann Roy Coll Surg 23:89–117, 1958
101. Gillingham FJ: The management of ruptured intracranial aneurysms. Scot Med J 12:377–383, 1967
102. Gillingham FJ: Twenty-five years' experience with middle cerebral aneurysms. J Neurol Neurosurg Psychiat 38:405, 1975
103. Goodman SJ, Hayes M: Value of cerebral isotope flow studies in timing of surgery for ruptured aneurysms when there is vasospasm and neurologic deficit. J Nucl Med 15:1113–1116, 1974
104. Graf CJ: Prognosis for patients with nonsurgically-treated aneurysms. Analysis of the cooperative study of intracranial aneurysms and subarachnoid hemorrhage. J Neurosurg 35: 438–443, 1971
105. Graf CJ: Results of direct attack on nonfistulous intracranial aneurysm with remarks on statistics. J Neurosurg 12:146–153, 1955
106. Graf CJ: Surgical treatment of angiographically localized intracranial aneurysms. A follow-up report. Neurology 6:686–692, 1956
107. Graf CJ, Nibbelink DW: Cooperative study of intracranial aneurysms and subarachnoid hemorrhage. Report on a randomized treatment study. III. Intracranial surgery. Stroke 5:557–601, 1974
108. Griffith HB, Cummins BH, Thomson JLG: Cerebral arterial spasm and hydrocephalus in leaking arterial aneurysms. Neuroradiology 4:212–214, 1972
109. Grubb RL, Raichle ME, Eichling JO, et al.: Effects of subarachnoid hemorrhage on cerebral blood volume, blood flow, and oxygen utilization in humans. J Neurosurg 46:446–453, 1977
110. Guidetti B: Considerazioni sul trattamento chirurgico degli aneurismi sacculari intracranici. Revista di Neurol (Napoli) 27:609–638, 1957
111. Guidetti B: Microsurgical treatment of intracranial saccular aneurysms. Acta Neurochir 43:153–162, 1978
112. Guidetti B: Results of 98 intracranial aneurysm operations performed with the aid of an operating microscope. Acta Neurochir 29:65–71, 1973
113. Guidetti B: Surgical treatment of aneurysms of the anterior communicating artery. Progr Brain Res 30:303–307, 1968
114. Hamby WB: Intracranial surgery for aneurysms. Progr Neurol Surg 3:1–65, 1969
115. Hamby WB: Intracranial Aneurysms. Spring-

field, Ill., Charles C Thomas, 1952
116. Hamby WB: Intracranial surgical procedures in subarachnoid hemorrhage and intracranial aneurysms. In Fields WS (ed.): Pathogenesis and Treatment of Cerebrovascular Disease. Springfield, Ill., Charles C Thomas, 1961, pp. 496–507
117. Hamby WB: Remarks concerning intracranial aneurysm surgery. Clin Neurosurg 17:1–17, 1970
118. Hamby WB: Subarachnoid hemorrhage from congenital aneurysm of the circle of Willis. Postgrad Med 34:317–322, 1963
119. Hamby WB: The surgical management of intracranial aneurysms. Acta Neurol Latinoamer 4:341–346, 1956
120. Hamby WB: The surgical treatment of intracranial aneurysms. Results in angiographically located aneurysms. Arch Neurol Psychiat 75:345–349, 1956
121. Hamby WB: The surgical treatment of intracranial vascular lesions. Bull NY Acad Med 45:339–350, 1969
122. Hanau J, Foncin J-F, Le Beau J: Sir le rôle de l'ischémie cérébrale dans l'évolution fatale des ruptures anévrismales supra-tentorieles. Neuro-chirurgie (Paris) 15:353–368, 1969
123. Hawkes CD, Ogle WS: Vasospasm with subarachnoid hemorrhage from intracranial aneurysm. Arch Surg 90:404–409, 1965
124. Hazouri LA: A review of 75 intracranial aneurysms. J Med Assoc Georgia 44:15–19, 1955
125. Heilbrun MP, Olesen J: Regional cerebral blood flow studies in subarachnoid hemorrhage. Europ Neurol 8:1–7, 1972
126. Heilbrun MP, Olesen J, Lassen NA: Regional cerebral blood flow studies in subarachnoid hemorrhage. J Neurosurg 37:36–44, 1972
126a. Heiskanen O: Risk of bleeding from unruptured aneurysms in cases with multiple intracranial aneurysms. J Neurosurg 55:524–526, 1981
127. Heiskanen O, Martilla I: Risk of rupture of a second aneurysm in patients with multiple aneurysms. J Neurosurg 32:295–299, 1970
128. Heitler W: The departure from classical thought in modern physics. In Schilpp PA (ed.): Albert Einstein: Philosopher-Scientist. Evanston, Ill., Library of Living Philosophers, 1949, pp. 179–198
129. Henderson WG, Torner JC, Nibbelink DW: Intracranial aneurysms and subarachnoid hemorrhage—Report on a randomized treatment study. IV-B. Regulated bed rest—statistical evaluation. Stroke 8:579–589, 1977
130. Hollin SA, Decker RE: Microsurgical treatment of cerebral aneurysms. Mt Sinai J Med NY 40:91–103, 1973
131. Hollin SA, Decker RE: Microsurgical treatment of internal carotid artery aneurysms. J Neurosurg 47:142–149, 1977
132. Höök O, Norlén G: Aneurysms of the anterior communicating artery. Acta Neurol Scand 40:219–240, 1964
133. Höök O, Norlén G: Aneurysms of the internal carotid artery. Acta Neurol Scand 40:200–218, 1964
134. Höök O, Norlén G: Aneurysms of the middle cerebral artery. A report of 80 cases. Acta Chir Scand Suppl 235:1–39, 1958
135. Hori S, Suzuki J: Early and late results of intracranial direct surgery of anterior communicating artery aneurysms. J Neurosurg 50:433–440, 1979
136. Horwitz NH, Rizzoli HV: Aneurysms and arteriovenous fistulas. In Postoperative Complications in Neurosurgical Practice. Recognition, Prevention, and Management. Baltimore, Williams & Wilkins, 1967, pp. 83–129
137. Hudson CH, Raaf J: Timing of angiography and operation in patients with ruptured intracranial aneurysms. J Neurosurg 29:37–41, 1968
138. Hugosson R: Intracranial arterial aneurysms. Considerations on the upper age limit for surgical treatment. Acta Neurochir 28:157–164, 1973
139. Hugosson R, Högström S: Factors disposing to morbidity in surgery of intracranial aneurysms with special regard to deep controlled hypotension. J Neurosurg 38:561–567, 1973
140. Hunt WE: Grading of risk in intracranial aneurysms. Excerp Med ICS No 320:169–175, 1974
141. Hunt WE, Hess RM: Surgical risk as related to time of intervention in the repair of intracranial aneurysms. J Neurosurg 28:14–20, 1968
142. Hunt WE, Kosnik EJ: Timing and perioperative care in intracranial aneurysm surgery. Clin Neurosurg 21:79–89, 1974
143. Hunt WE, Meagher JN, Barnes JE: The management of intracranial aneurysms. J Neurosurg 19:34–40, 1962
144. Hunt WE, Meagher JN, Hess RM: Intracranial aneurysm. A nine-year study. Ohio Med J 62:1168–1171, 1966
145. Hunt WE, Miller CA: The results of early operation for aneurysm. Clin Neurosurg 24:208–215, 1977
146. Hyland HH: Prognosis in spontaneous subarachnoid hemorrhage. Arch Neurol Psychiat 63:61–78, 1950
147. Infuso L, Bettinelli A, De Benedittis G: Evaluation of indications for direct surgical management in SAH due to ruptured intracranial aneurysms. Immediate and long-term results

in a cooperative study of 678 cases. J Neurosurg Sci 19:47–53, 1975
148. Ishii R: Regional cerebral blood flow in patients with ruptured intracranial aneurysms. J Neurosurg 50:587–594, 1979
149. Ishii R, Kobayashi K, Aoki H, et al.: Changes in cerebral blood flow following rupture of intracranial aneurysms. Part 1. Mean hemispheric values. Neurol Med Chir (Tokyo) 18 (No 3, Part 2):183–190, 1978
150. Ito K, Yoshihama Y, Terakado Y, et al.: Intentional delayed surgery for ruptured intracranial aneurysms. Excerp Med ICS No 418:93, 1977
151. Jain KK: Surgery of intact intracranial aneurysms. J Neurosurg 40:495–498, 1974
152. James IM: Changes in cerebral blood flow and in systemic arterial pressure following spontaneous subarachnoid haemorrhage. Clin Sci 35:11–22, 1968
153. Jamieson, KG: Aneurysms of the vertebrobasilar system. Further experience with nine cases. J Neurosurg 28:544–555, 1968
154. Jamieson KG: Direct operation for intracranial aneurysm: some technical problems and attempts at their solution. Neurol Med Chir (Tokyo) 11:1–10, 1971
155. Jane JA, Winn HR, Richardson AE: The natural history of intracranial aneurysms: rebleeding rates during the acute and long term period and implication for surgical management. Clin Neurosurg 24:176–184, 1977
156. Jones RAC: Problems in the management of multiple intracranial aneurysms. J Neurol Neurosurg Psychiat 37:1281, 1974
157. Kågström E, Greitz T, Hanson J, et al.: Changes in cerebral blood flow after subarachnoid haemorrhage. Excerp Med Int Congr Series 110:629–633, 1966
158. Kak VK, Taylor AR: Cerebral blood-flow in subarachnoid hemorrhage. Lancet 2:875–877, 1967
159. Karasawa J, Kikuchi H, Furuse S, et al.: Surgery of multiple intracranial aneurysms. Neurol Surg (Tokyo) 2:763–769, 1974
160. Karlsberg P, Adams JE: Value of hypothermia and arterial occlusion in the treatment of intracranial aneurysms. J Neurosurg 19:665–674, 1962
161. Kaste M, Troupp H: Subarachnoid haemorrhage: long-term follow-up results of late surgical versus conservative treatment. Brit Med J 1:1310–1311, 1978
162. Kaufman DM, Tabaddor K: Intracranial surgery for cerebral artery aneurysms. Five years' experience. JAMA 236:1707–1710, 1976
163. Kayama T, Yoshimoto T, Uchida K, et al.: Intracranial saccular aneurysms. Surgical results of 1,000 consecutive cases. Tohoku J Exp Med 126:117–124, 1978
164. Keller AZ: Hypertension, age and residence in the survival with subarachnoid hemorrhage. Am J Epidem 91:139–147, 1970
165. Kelly PJ, Gorten RJ, Grossman RG, et al.: Cerebral perfusion, vascular spasm, and outcome in patients with ruptured intracranial aneurysms. J Neurosurg 47:44–49, 1977
166. Kelly PJ, Gorten RJ, Rose JE, et al.: Radionuclide cerebral angiography and the timing of aneurysm surgery. Neurosurgery 5:202–207, 1979
167. Kikuchi H: Operative indication and surgical technique of the cerebral aneurysm. Neurol Med Chir (Tokyo) 16 (No 6, Part 2):479–486, 1976
168. Kikuchi H, Furuse S, Karasawa J: Microsurgery of cerebral aneurysm in acute phase (within 1 week after subarachnoid hemorrhage). In Koos TH, Böck FW, Spetzler RF (eds.): Clinical Microneurosurgery. Stuttgart, Georg Thieme Verlag, 1976, pp. 202–203
169. Kim H, Mizukami M, Kawase T, et al.: Time course of vasospasm—its clinical significance. Neurol Med Chir 19:95–102, 1979
170. Klafta LA Jr: Intracranial aneurysms; factors effecting survival—Part I. Med Trial Tech Q: pp 286–293, 1971
171. Klafta LA Jr: Intracranial aneurysms; factors effecting survival—Part II. Med Trial Tech Q: pp 392–399, 1971
172. Klafta LA Jr, Hamby WB: Significance of cerebrospinal fluid pressure in determining time for repair of intracranial aneurysms. J Neurosurg 31:217–219, 1969
173. Klinlger M: Zur Prognose des blutenden Aneurysma der Gehirnbasis bei konservativer Therapie. Schwiez med Wschr 87:1389–1392, 1957
174. Krayenbühl H, Weber G: Résultats comparatifs des différentes méthodes. In Krayenbühl H, et al. (eds.): L'Anévrysme de l'Artère Communicante Antérieure. Paris, Masson et Cie, 1959, pp. 110–112
175. Krayenbühl H, Weber G, Yaşargil MG: Pronostic de l'anévrysme rompu sans traitement chirurgical. In Krayenbühl H, et al. (eds.): L'Anévrysme de l'Artère Communicante Antérieure. Paris, Masson et Cie, 1959, pp. 91–95
176. Krayenbühl H, Weber G, Yaşargil MG: Traitement chirurgical et pronostic. In Krayenbühl H, et al. (eds.): L'Anévrysme de l'Artère Communicante Antérieure. Paris, Masson et Cie, 1959, pp. 96–107
177. Krayenbühl H, Yaşargil MG: Diagnosis and therapy of intracranial aneurysms. In Cooper

P, Nyhus LM (eds.): Surgery Annual. New York, Appleton-Century-Crofts, 1970, pp. 327–343
178. Krayenbühl H, Yaşargil MG, Flamm ES, et al.: Microsurgical treatment of intracranial saccular aneurysms. J Neurosurg 37:678–686, 1972
179. Kutsuna M, Someda K, Morita K, et al.: Ischemic cerebral symptoms after subarachnoid hemorrhage due to aneurysm rupture. No Shinkei Geka 6:543–548, 1978
180. Kutsuzawa T, Takahashi S, Saito C, et al.: Studies of cerebral hemodynamics in subarachnoid hemorrhage. Tohoku J Exp Med 94:407–415, 1968
181. Kwak R, Niizuma H, Ohi T, et al.: Angiographic study of cerebral vasospasm following rupture of intracranial aneurysms. Part I. Time of the appearance. Surg Neurol 11:257–262, 1979
182. Laine E: Arterial vertebro-basilar aneurysms. Progr Brain Res 30:323–346, 1968
183. Laine E, Andreussi L, Delandsheer J-M, et al.: Anévrysmes de l'artère cérébrale moyenne. Étude anatomique, clinique et thérapeutique. A propos d'une série de 116 cas dont 100 ont été opérés. Neuro-chirurgie (Paris) 16:181–201, 1970
184. Laitinen L, Troupp H: Reliability of partial ligation in the treatment of intracranial arterial aneurysm. Acta Neurol Scand 37:62–66, 1961
185. Lang EF, Poppen JL: Aneurysms of the anterior communicating artery: Results of surgical treatment. Surg Clin N Am 42:793–805, 1962
185a. Lapras C, Goutelle A, Dechaume J-P, et al.: Pronostic des anévrysmes de la communicante antérieure traités par abord direct. Neuro-chirurgie (Paris) 15:369–378, 1969
186. Le Beau J: Anévrismes de l'artère communicante antérieure. Ruptures et indications neurochirurgicales. Neurochirurgia (Stuttgart) 5:38–57, 1962
187. Le Beau J, Wolinetz E, Barré Y: Observation anatomo-clinique d'un cas de ramollissement cérébral signe trompeur d'une rupture anévrismale. Rev Neurol 110:415–418, 1964
188. Loach AB, De Azevedo Filho HRC: Some observations on the microneurosurgical treatment of intracranial aneurysms. Acta Neurochir 35:97–103, 1976
189. Locksley HB: Natural history of subarachnoid hemorrhage, intracranial aneurysms and arteriovenous malformations. Based on 6,368 cases in the cooperative study. In Sahs AL, Perret GE, Locksley HB, Nishioka H (eds.): Intracranial Aneurysms and Subarachnoid Hemorrhage. A Cooperative Study. Philadelphia, Lippincott, 1969, pp. 37–108
189a. Locksley HB: Report on the cooperative study of intracranial aneurysms and subarachnoid hemorrhage. Section V. Natural history of subarachnoid hemorrhage, intracranial aneurysms and arteriovenous malformations. Based on 6,368 cases in the cooperative study. J Neurosurg 25: 219–239, 321–368, 1966
190. Logue V: Posterior fossa aneurysms. Clin Neurosurg 11:183–207, 1964
191. Logue V: Surgery in spontaneous subarachnoid haemorrhage. Operative treatment of aneurysms on the anterior cerebral and anterior communicating artery. Brit Med J 1:473–479, 1956
192. Logue V: Traitement chirurgical des anévrysmes des artères communicante et cérébrale antérieures pendant la phase aiguë. In Krayenbühl H, et al. (eds.): L'Anévrysme de l'Artère Communicante Antérieure. Paris, Masson et Cie, 1959, pp. 113–130
193. Lougheed WM: Selection, timing, and technique of aneurysm surgery of the anterior circle of Willis. Clin Neurosurg 16:95–113, 1969
194. Lougheed WM, Botterell EH, Morley TP: Results of the direct attack in the surgical management of internal carotid and middle cerebral aneurysms. Clin Neurosurg 9:193–200, 1963
195. Lougheed WM, Marshall BM: Management of aneurysms of the anterior circulation by intracranial procedures. In Youmans JR (ed.): Neurological Surgery, Vol 2. Philadelphia, Saunders, 1973, pp. 731–767
196. Lougheed WM, Morley TP, Tasker RR: The results of surgical treatment of ruptured berry aneurysms. Excerp Med ICS NO 110:681–684, 1966
197. Lougheed WM, Morley TP, Tasker RR, et al.: The results of surgical treatment of ruptured berry aneurysms. In Fields WS, Sahs Al (eds.): Intracranial Aneurysms and Subarachnoid Hemorrhage. Springfield, Ill., Charles C Thomas, 1965, pp. 295–307
198. Magladery JW: On subarachnoid bleeding—an appraisal of treatment. J Neurosurg 12:437–449, 1955
199. Marini G, Maspes PE: Survey of the long-term fate of 192 consecutive cases of primary subarachnoid haemorrhage. Comparison between operated and non-operated patients. Acta Neurochir 18:208–215, 1968
200. Marshall BM, Lougheed WM, Gordon RA: Evaluation of the effect of anaesthetic techniques on survival after intracranial surgery for ruptured aneurysms. Canad Anaesth Soc J 15:227–231, 1968

201. Marshall WH Jr: Delayed arterial spasm following subarachnoid hemorrhage. Radiology 106:325–327, 1973
202. Martinez Coll A, Del Corral JF: Experiences in intracranial surgery for aneurysms. Surg Neurol 3:191–193, 1975
203. Maspes PE, Marini G: Intracranial arterial spasm related to supraclinoid ruptured aneurysms. Acta Neurochir 10:630–638, 1962
204. Maspes PE, Marini G: Surgery of cerebral arterial aneurysms. Results of direct intracranial approach in 103 surgical cases. Panminerva Med 7:215–221, 1965
205. Maspes PE, Marini G: Surgical experience and results on 159 consecutive cases of intracranial direct attack to saccular aneurysms of the internal carotid and its branches. Progr Brain Res 30:317–321, 1968
206. Mathew NT, Meyer JS, Hartmann A: Diagnosis and treatment of factors complicating subarachnoid hemorrhage. Neuroradiology 6:237–245, 1974
207. Matson DD: Neurosurgery of Infancy and Childhood, 2nd ed. Springfield, Ill., Charles C Thomas, 1969, pp. 741–748
208. Maurice-Williams R: Prolonged antifibrinolysis—an effective non-surgical treatment for ruptured intracranial aneurysms? J Neurol Neurosurg Psychiat 41:188, 1978
209. McCormick WF: Intracranial arterial aneurysm: a pathologist's view. Stroke 8:15–19, 1973
210. McKissock W, Paine KWE, Walsh LS: An analysis of the results of treatment of ruptured intracranial aneurysms. Report of 772 consecutive cases. J Neurosurg 17:762–776, 1960
211. McKissock W, Richardson A, Walsh L: Anterior communicating aneurysms. A trial of conservative and surgical treatment. Lancet 1:873–876, 1965
212. McKissock W, Richardson A, Walsh L: Middle-cerebral aneurysms. Further results in the controlled trial of conservative and surgical treatment of ruptured intracranial aneurysms. Lancet 2:417–421, 1962
213. McKissock W, Richardson A, Walsh LS, et al.: Multiple intracranial aneurysms. Lancet 1:623–626, 1964
214. McMurtry JG III, Housepian EM, Bowman FO Jr, et al.: surgical treatment of basilar artery aneurysms. Elective circulatory arrest with thoracotomy in 12 cases. J Neurosurg 40:486–498, 1974
215. Miller RH, MacCarty CS, Kerr FWL, et al.: Letter to the editor on the analysis of subarachnoid hemorrhage data. Arch Neurol 33:309, 1976
216. Millikan CH: Cerebral vasospasm and ruptured intracranial aneurysm. Arch Neurol 32:433–449, 1975
217. Mingrino S, Salar G, Scanarini M: Long-term results of non-operative management of ruptured intracranial aneurysms. J Neurosurg Sci 19:54–58, 1975
218. Morello G: Remarks on the direct attack on intracranial aneurysms. Progr Brain Res 30:347–349, 1968
219. Morley TP: Current Controversies in Neurosurgery. Philadelphia, Saunders, 1976, pp. 257–258
220. Mount LA, Brisman R: Treatment of multiple and asymptomatic aneurysms. In Schmidek HH, Sweet WH (eds.): Current Techniques in Operative Neurosurgery. New York, Grune & Stratton, 1977, pp. 19–23
221. Mount LA, Brisman R: Treatment of multiple aneurysms—symptomatic and asymptomatic. Clin Neurosurg 21:166–170, 1974
222. Mount LA, Brisman R: Treatment of multiple intracranial aneurysms. J Neurosurg 35:728–730, 1971
223. Mullan S, Hanlon K, Brown F: Management of 136 consecutive supratentorial berry aneurysms. J Neurosurg 49:794–804, 1978
224. Nibbelink DW: Cooperative aneurysm study: antihypertensive and antifibrinolytic therapy following subarachnoid hemorrhage from ruptured intracranial aneurysm. In Whisnant JP, Sandok BA (eds.): Cerebral Vascular Disease. New York, Grune & Stratton, 1975, pp. 155–165
225. Nibbelink DW, Knowler LA: Cooperative study of intracranial aneurysms and subarachnoid hemorrhage. Report on a randomized treatment study. II. Objectives and design of randomized aneurysm study. Stroke 5:552–556, 1974
226. Nibbelink DW, Torner JC, Henderson WG: Intracranial aneurysms and subarachnoid hemorrhage. A cooperative study. Antifibrinolytic therapy in recent onset subarachnoid hemorrhage. Stroke 6:622–629, 1975
227. Nibbelink DW, Torner JC, Henderson WG: Intracranial aneurysms and subarachnoid hemorrhage—Report on a randomized treatment study. IV-A. Regulated bed rest. Stroke 8:202–218, 1977
228. Niemeyer P: Resultados da microcirurgia em 54 aneurismas intracranianos. Arq Neuro-psiquiat 32:175–186, 1974
229. Niizuma H, Kwak R, Otabe K, et al.: Angiographic study of cerebral vasospasm following rupture of intracranial aneurysms. Part II. Relation between the site of aneurysm and the occurrence of the vasospasm. Surg Neurol 11:263–267, 1979

230. Nikiforov BM Several findings on the surgical treatment of sacculated aneurysms of the anterior section of the circle of Willis. Vop Neirokhir 31:9–13, May–June 1967
231. Nilsson BW: Cerebral blood flow in patients with subarachnoid haemorrhage studied with an intravenous isotope technique. Its clinical significance in the timing of surgery of cerebral arterial aneurysm. Acta Neurochir 37:33–48, 1977
232. Nishioka H: Evaluation of the conservative management of ruptured intracranial aneurysms. In Sahs AL, Perret GE, Locksley HB, Nishioka H (eds.): Intracranial Aneurysms and Subarachnoid Hemorrhage. A Cooperative Study. Philadelphia, Lippincott, 1969, pp. 125–142
232a. Nishioka H: Report on the cooperative study of intracranial aneurysms and subarachnoid hemorrhage. Section VII, Part I. Evaluation of the conservative management of ruptured intracranial aneurysms. J Neurosurg 25:574–592, 1966
233. Norlén G: Aneurysm of the anterior communicating artery. Prog Brain Res 30:295–302, 1968
234. Norlén G: Klinik und chirurgische Behandlung der sackförmigen Hirnaneurysmen. Dtsch Z Nervenheilk 170:446–459, 1953
235. Norlén G: Some aspects of the surgical treatment of intracranial aneurysms. Clin Neurosurg 9:214–222, 1963
236. Norlén G, Barnum AS: Surgical treatment of aneurysms of the anterior communicating artery. J Neurosurg 10:634–650, 1953
237. Norlén G, Olivecrona H: The treatment of aneurysms of the circle of Willis. J Neurosurg 10:404–415, 1953
238. Nornes H: Monitoring of patients with intracranial aneurysms. Clin Neurosurg 22:321–331, 1975
239. Nornes H, Magnaes B: Intracranial pressure in patients with ruptured saccular aneurysm. J Neurosurg 36:537–547, 1972
239a. Nornes H, Wikeby P: Results of microsurgical management of intracranial aneurysms. J Neurosurg 51:608–614, 1979
240. Odom GL: Neurological surgery—current needs. In Fields WS, Moossy J (eds.): Stroke. Diagnosis and Management. Current Procedures and Equipment. St Louis, Warren H Green, 1973, pp. 249–254
241. Onuma T, Suzuki J: Surgical treatment of giant intracranial aneurysms. J Neurosurg 51:33–36, 1979
242. Onuma T, Yoshimoto T, Hori S, et al.: Early operation for ruptured intracranial aneurysms, within 48 hours after the last subarachnoid hemorrhage. Excerp Med ICS No 418:93, 1977
243. Orosz É, Pasztor E, Juhász J: Angiospasm as a limiting factor in the surgery of intracranial aneurysms. In Fusek I, Kunc Z (eds.): Proceedings of the Fourth European Congress of Neurosurgery. Present Limits of Neurosurgery. Prague, Avicenum, Czechoslovak Medical Press, 1972, pp. 237–239
244. Orozco M, Trigueros F, Quintana F, et al.: Intracranial aneurysms in early childhood. Surg Neurol 9:247–252, 1978
245. Pakarinen S: Incidence, aetiology, and prognosis of primary subarachnoid haemorrhage. A study based on 589 cases diagnosed in a defined urban population during a defined period. Acta Neurol Scand 43 (Suppl 29):1–128, 1967
246. Parkes JD, James IM: Electroencephalographic and cerebral blood flow changes following spontaneous subarachnoid haemorrhage. Brain 94:69–76, 1971
247. Parkinson D: The problem of spontaneous subarachnoid hemorrhage with proven aneurysms. J Neurosurg 12:565–569, 1955
248. Paterson A: Direct surgery in the treatment of posterior communicating aneurysms. Lancet 2:808–811, 1968
249. Paterson A, Bond MR: Treatment of multiple intracranial arterial aneurysms. Lancet 1:1302–1304, 1973
250. Paul RL, Arnold JG Jr: Operative factors influencing mortality in intracranial aneurysm surgery: analysis of 186 consecutive cases. J Neurosurg 32:289–294, 1970
251. Pertuiset B, Cabezas C: Contre-indications et indications de l'abord direct des anévrismes sacculaires rompus du carrefour artériel communicante antérieure-cérébrale antérieure. Ann Chir (Paris) 15:1165–1172, 1961
252. Pertuiset B, van Effenterre R, Caruel N, et al.: Les résultats de l'abord direct des anévrysmes intra-crâniens sus-tentoriels en fonction de l'hypotension contrôlée, de la coagulation bipolaire et de la magnification optique. Rev Neurol 129:57–59, 1973
253. Pertuiset B, van Effenterre R, Robert G: Chronologie des actes diagnostiques et thérapeutiques dans les trois semaines suivant la rupture d'un anévrisme sacculaire intra-cranien (d'apres 316 cas). Rev Neurol (Paris) 134: 22–34, 1978
254. Pitts LH, Macpherson P, Wyper DG, et al.: Cerebral blood flow, angiographic cerebral vasospasm, and subarachnoid hemorrhage. Acta Neurol Scand 56 (Suppl 64):334–335, 1977
255. Pool JL: Aneurysms of the anterior communicating artery. Bifrontal craniotomy and rou-

tine use of temporary clips. J Neurosurg 18:98–111, 1961
256. Pool JL: Bifrontal craniotomy for anterior communicating artery aneurysms. J Neurosurg 36:212–220, 1972
257. Pool JL: Cerebral vasospasm. New Engl J Med 259:1259–1264, 1958
258. Pool JL: Direct attack on intracranial aneurysms. In Fields WS, Sahs AL (eds.): Intracranial Aneurysms and Subarachnoid Hemorrhage. Springfield, Ill., Charles C Thomas, 1965
259. Pool JL: Early treatment of ruptured intracranial aneurysms of the circle of Willis with special clip techniques. Bull NY Acad Med 35:357–369, 1959
260. Pool JL: Timing and techniques in the intracranial surgery of ruptured aneurysms of the anterior communicating artery. J Neurosurg 19:378–388, 1962
261. Pool JL, Potts DG: Aneurysms and Arteriovenous Anomalies of the Brain. Diagnosis and Treatment. New York, Harper & Row, 1965
262. Pool JL, Ransohoff J, Yahr MD, et al.: Early surgical treatment of aneurysms of the circle of Willis. Neurology 9:478–486, 1959
263. Poppen JL: Operative treatment for aneurysms of the anterior communicating artery. Clin Neuorsurg 11:8–13, 1964
264. Poppen JL: Specific treatment of intracranial aneurysms. Experience with 143 surgically treated patients. J Neurosurg 8:75–102, 1951
265. Poppen JL, Fager CA: Intracranial aneurysms. Results of surgical treatment. J Neurosurg 17:283–296, 1960
266. Post KD, Flamm ES, Goodgold A, et al.: Ruptured intracranial aneurysms. Case morbidity and mortality. J Neurosurg 46:290–295, 1977
267. Prakash B, Kristiansen K, Amundsen P: Subarachnoid hemorrhage and vasospasm. In Fusek I, Kunc Z (eds.): Proceedings of the Fourth European Congress of Neurosurgery. Present Limits of Neurosurgery. Prague, Avicenum, Czechoslovak Medical Press, 1972, pp. 233–235
268. Ransohoff J, Goodgold A, Benjamin MV: Preoperative management of patients with ruptured intracranial aneurysms. J Neurosurg 36:525–530, 1972
269. Ransohoff J, Guy HH, Mazzia VDB, et al.: Deliberate hypotension in surgery of cerebral aneurysm and correlative animal studies. NYS J Med 69:913–918, 1969
270. Richardson AE: The natural history of patients with intracranial aneurysm after rupture. Prog Brain Res 30:269–273, 1968
271. Richardson AE, Jane JA, Payne RM: Assessment of the natural history of anterior communicating aneurysms. J Neurosurg 21:266–274, 1964
272. Richardson AE, Jane JA, Payne PM: The prediction of morbidity and mortality in anterior communicating aneurysms treated by proximal anterior cerebral ligation. J Neurosurg 25:280–283, 1966
273. Richardson AE, Jane JA, Yashon D: Prognostic factors in the untreated course of posterior communicating aneurysms. Arch Neurol 14:172–176, 1966
274. Richardson AE, McKissock W, Walsh L: Anterior communicating aneurysms. In Fields WS, Sahs AL (eds.): Intracranial Aneurysms and Subarachnoid Hemorrhage. Springfield, Ill., Charles C Thomas, 1965, pp. 467–485
275. Richardson JTE: Arterial spasm and recovery from subarachnoid haemorrhage. J Neurol Neurosurg Psychiat 39:1134–1136, 1976
276. Roberts JG: Surgery of intracranial aneurysms. Brit Med J 1:1107, 1956
277. Robertson EG: Cerebral lesions due to intracranial aneurysms. Brain 72:150–185, 1949
278. Robinson RG: Ruptured aneurysms of the middle cerebral artery. J Neurosurg 35:25–33, 1971
279. Rohe S, Austin G, Laffin D, et al.: Effects of subarachnoid hemorrhage on cerebral blood flow measured by an intravenous isotope technique. In Koos WT, Böck FW, Spetzler RF (eds.): Clinical Microneurosurgery. Stuttgart, Georg Thieme Verlag, 1976, pp. 191–202
280. Romy M, Werner A, Wildi E: De la fréquence des anévrysmes artériels intra-crâniens et de leur rupture, d'après une série d'autopsies de routine. Neuro-chirurgie (Paris) 19:611–626, 1973
280a. Rousseaux P, Scherpereel B, Bernard MH, et al.: Fever and cerebral vasospasm in ruptured intracranial aneurysms. Surg Neurol 14:459–465, 1980
281. Rowe SN, Grunnagle JF, Susen AF, et al.: Results of direct attack on intracranial aneurysm. J Neurosurg 12:475–486, 1955
282. Sachs M: Les anévrismes de l'artère sylvienne. A propos de 75 observations. Ann Chir 20:998–1019, 1966
282a. Sahs AL, Nibbelink DW, Torner JC (eds.): Aneurysmal Subarachnoid Hemorrhage. Report of the Cooperative Study. Baltimore, Urban & Schwarzenberg, 1981
283. Saito I, Basugi N, Sano K: Surgical treatment of intracranial aneurysms in the acute stage. Neurol Med Chir (Tokyo) 12:344, 1972
284. Saito I, Basugi N, Sano K: Surgical treatment of intracranial aneurysms in the acute stage, with special reference to pre- and postoperative vasospasm. Excerp Med No 293:160, 1973

285. Saito I, Sano K: Vasospasm following rupture of cerebral aneurysms. Neurol Med Chir (Tokyo) 19:103–107, 1979
286. Saito I, Shigeno T, Aritake K, et al.: Vasospasm assessed by angiography and computerized tomography. J Neurosurg 51:466–475, 1979
287. Saito I, Ueda Y, Sano K: Significance of vasospasm in the treatment of ruptured intracranial aneurysms. J Neurosurg 47:412–429, 1977
288. Sakurai Y, Ito Z, Uemura K: Pathophysiological aspects of acute stage patients with ruptured intracranial aneurysms. Part II. Relationships between neurological prognosis and sequential changes of cerebral blood flow dynamics. Brain Nerve (Tokyo) 27:1213–1221, 1975
289. Sakurai Y, Yoshimoto T, Hori S, et al.: Causes of death in intracranial aneurysm cases with direct surgery. Neurol Med Chir (Tokyo) 17 (Part 2):153–161, 1977
290. Samson DS, Hodosh RM, Clark WK: Surgical management of unruptured asymptomatic aneurysms. J Neurosurg 46:731–734, 1977
290a. Samson DS, Hodosh RM, Reid WR, et al.: Risk of intracranial aneurysm surgery in the good grade patient: early versus late operation. Neurosurgery 5:422–426, 1979
291. Sano K: Surgery of intracranial aneurysm. Brain Nerve (Tokyo) 23:1252–1264, 1971
292. Sano K, Saito I: Follow-up results of microsurgery of intracranial aneurysms. Brain Nerve (Tokyo) 29:977–985, 1977
293. Sano K, Saito I: Indication and timing of surgery for ruptured intracranial aneurysms with vasospasm. Neurosurgery 1:65, 1977
294. Sano K, Saito I: Microsurgery of ruptured intracranial aneurysms. Relation to cerebral vasospasm. Seara Méd Neurocir 7:175–184, 1978
295. Sano K, Saito I: Timing and indication of surgery for ruptured intracranial aneurysms with regard to cerebral vasospasm. Acta Neurochir 41:49–60, 1978
296. Schneck SA: On the relationship between ruptured intracranial aneurysm and cerebral infarction. Neurology 14:691–702, 1964
297. Schneck SA, Kricheff II: Intracranial aneurysm rupture, vasospasm, and infarction. Arch Neurol 11:668–680, 1964
298. Sencer W, Andiman R: A clinical study of intracranial aneurysms. Mt Sinai J Med (NY) 40:72–81, 1973
299. Sengupta RP: Anatomical variations in the origin of the posterior cerebral artery demonstrated by carotid angiography, and their significance in the direct surgical treatment of posterior communicating aneurysms. Neurochirurgia (Stuttgart) 18:33–42, 1975
300. Sengupta RP, Chiu JSP, Brierley H: Quality of survival following direct surgery for anterior communicating artery aneurysms. J Neurosurg 43:58–64, 1975
301. Sengupta RP, So SC, Villarejo-Ortega FJ: Use of epsilon aminocaproic acid (EACA) in the preoperative management of ruptured intracranial aneurysms. J Neurosurg 44:479–484, 1976
302. Shulman K, Tabaddor K: Intracranial vascular disease in childhood. In O'Brien MS (ed.): Pediatric Neurological Surgery. New York, Raven Press, 1978, pp. 45–49
303. Skultety FM, Nishioka H: The results of intracranial surgery in the treatment of aneurysms. In Sahs AL, Perret GE, Locksley HB, Nishioka H (eds.): Intracranial Aneurysms and Subarachnoid Hemorrhage. A Cooperative Study. Philadelphia, Lippincott, 1969, pp. 173–194
303a. Skultety FM, Nishioka H: Report on the cooperative study of intracranial aneurysms and subarachnoid hemorrhage. Section VIII, Part 2. The results of intracranial surgery in the treatment of aneurysms. J Neurosurg 25:683–704, 1966
304. Slosberg PS: Nonoperative management of ruptured intracranial aneurysms. Clin Neurosurg 21:90–99, 1974
305. Smith B: Cerebral pathology in subarachnoid haemorrhage. J Neurol Neurosurg Psychiat 26:535–539, 1963
306. Stevens WW: Intracranial aneurysms: An experience in treatment. Va Med 104:314–315, 1977
307. Sugar O: Discussion. Arch Neurol Psychiat 68:843–844, 1952
308. Sundt TM Jr: Cerebral vasospasm following subarachnoid hemorrhage: evolution, management, and relationship to timing of surgery. Clin Neurosurg 24:228–239, 1977
309. Sundt TM Jr, Murphey F: Clip-grafts for aneurysm and small vessel surgery. Part 3. Clinical experience in intracranial internal carotid artery aneurysm. J Neurosurg 31:59–71, 1969
310. Sundt TM Jr, Whisnant JP: Subarachnoid hemorrhage from intracranial aneurysms. Surgical management and natural history of disease. New Engl J Med 299:116–122, 1978
311. Suzuki J: Direct surgery of intracranial aneurysms: experience with over 1000 cases. Proc Inst Neurol Madras 6:15–23, 1976
312. Suzuki J: Intracranial saccular aneurysms. Surgical results of 1,000 consecutive cases. Seara Méd Neurocir 7:185–195, 1978
313. Suzuki J: Mechanism of occurrence of cerebral vasospasm. Nippon Ronen Igakkai Zasshi 14:382–385, 1977
314. Suzuki J: Operative indication and surgical

technique of the cerebral aneurysm. 3. Neurol Med Chir (Tokyo) 16 (No 6, Part 2):487–495, 1976
315. Suzuki J: Surgery of ruptured intracranial aneurysm. Timing and grading. Neurol Surg (Tokyo) 6:459–470, 1978
316. Suzuki J, Hori S: Prediction of reattacks following rupture of intracranial aneurysms. Neurologia Medico-Chirurgica 15 (Part I):35–39, 1975
317. Suzuki J, Hori S, Mori T: "Reattack" following the rupture of intracranial aneurysms. Clin Neurol (Tokyo) 14:823–828, 1974
318. Suzuki J, Onuma T, Yoshimoto T: Results of early operation on cerebral aneurysms. Surg Neurol 11:407–412, 1979
319. Suzuki J, Takaku A, Kodama N: Prognostic correlation with the cerebral vasospasm and the direct operation for the intracranial aneurysm. Jpn J Surg 1:210–215, 1971
320. Suzuki J, Takaku A, Yoshimoto T: Early operation of ruptured intracranial aneurysms. Brain Nerve (Tokyo) 23:1281–1286, 1971
321. Suzuki J, Yoshimoto T: Early operation for the ruptured intracranial aneurysms—especially the cases operated within 48 hours after the last subarachnoid hemorrhage. Neurol Surg (Tokyo) 4:135–141, 1976
322. Suzuki J, Yoshimoto T: Early operation for the ruptured intracranial aneurysm. Jpn J Surg 3:149–156, 1973
323. Suzuki J, Ohara H: Clinicopathological study of cerebral aneurysms. Origin rupture, repair, and growth. J Neurosurg 48:505–514, 1978
324. Symon L: Disordered cerebro-vascular physiology in aneurysmal subarachnoid haemorrhage. Acta Neurochir 41:7–22, 1978
325. Symon L: Subarachnoid haemorrhage from intracranial aneurysm and angioma. In Russell RWR (ed.): Cerebral Arterial Disease. Edinburgh, Churchill Livingstone, 1976, pp. 231–261
326. Symon L: Vascular spasm. Excerp Med 293:55, 1973
327. Symon L: Vasospasm in aneurysm. In Toole JF, Moossy J, Janeway R (eds.): Cerebral Vascular Disease. New York, Grune & Stratton, 1971, pp. 232–240
328. Symon L, Ackerman R, Bull JWD, et al.: The use of the xenon clearance method in subarachnoid haemorrhage. Post-operative studies with clinical and angiographic correlation. Europ Neurol 8:8–15, 1972
329. Symon L, Rees J: Clinical assessment of regional cerebral perfusion and correlation of xenon clearance with anatomico-pathological data in subarachnoid haemorrhage. In Fusek I, Kunc Z (eds.): Proceeding of the Fourth European Congress of Neurosurgery. Present Limits of Neurosurgery. Prague, Avicenum, Czechoslovak Medical Press, 1972, pp. 225–228
330. Tappura M: Prognosis of subarachnoid haemorrhage. A study of 120 patients with unoperated intracranial arterial aneurysms and 267 patients without vascular lesions demonstrable in bilateral carotid angiograms. Acta Med Scand Suppl 392:1–75, 1962
331. Taylor AR, Kak VK: Cerebral blood flow in subarachnoid hemorrhage. In Meyer JS, Lechner H, Eichhorn O (eds.): Research on the Cerebral Circulation. Third International Salzburg Conference. Springfield, Ill., Charles C Thomas, 1969, pp. 364–374
332. Taylor AR, Kak VK: Cerebral circulation times in subarachnoid haemorrhage. Prog Brain Res 30:289–294, 1968
333. Thomas DGT, Paterson A: Results of surgical treatment of pericallosal aneurysms. J Neurol Neurosurg Psychiat 38:826, 1975
334. Tindall GT, Odom GL: Saccular aneurysms of the brain. Surgical treatment. In Vinken PJ, Bruyn GW (eds.): Handbook of Clinical Neurology. Vol 12, Vascular Diseases of the Nervous System, Part II. Amsterdam, North Holland; New York, American Elsevier, 1972, pp. 205–226
335. Tönnis W, Walter W: Die Behandlung der sackförmigen intrakraniellen Aneurysmen. In Olivecrona H, Tönnis W (eds.): Klinik and Behandlung der raumbeengenden intrakraniellen Prozesse. Handbuch der Neurochirurgie, Vol 4, Part 2. Berlin, Springer-Verlag, 1966, pp. 212–363
335a. Torner JC, Kassell NF, Wallace RB, et al.: Preoperative prognostic factors for rebleeding and survival in aneurysm patients receiving antifibrinolytic therapy: report of the cooperative aneurysm study. Neurosurgery 9:506–513, 1981
336. Troupp H: The management of intracranial arterial aneurysms in the acute stage. In Krayenbühl H (ed.): Advances and Technical Standards in Neurosurgery, Vol 3. New York, Springer-Verlag, 1976, pp. 35–46
337. Troupp H: The natural history of aneurysms of the basilar bifurcation. Acta Neurol Scand 47:350–356, 1971
338. Troupp H, af Björkesten G: Results of a controlled trial of late surgical versus conservative treatment of intracranial arterial aneurysms. J Neurosurg 35:20–24, 1971
339. Trumpy JH: Subarachnoid haemorrhage. Time sequence of recurrences and their prognosis. Acta Neurol Scand 43:48–60, 1967
340. Tytus JS, Haven H: Present day concepts in the management of intracranial aneurysms. Rev Surg 20:230–240, 1963

341. Uihlein A, Lippert RG: Surgical treatment of verified intracranial aneurysms. Arch Surg 81:1005–1012, 1960
342. Van der Werf AJM: The clinical significance of arterial spasm in subarachnoid hemorrhage. In Fusek I, Kunc Z (eds.): Proceedings of the Fourth European Congress of Neurosurgery. Present Limits of Neurosurgery. Prague, Avicenum, Czechoslovak Medical Press, 1972, pp. 251–254
343. Walsh L: Experience in the conservative and surgical treatment of ruptured intracranial aneurysms. Res Publ Assoc Res Nerv Ment Dis 41:169–178, 1966
344. Walsh LS: Trials of treatment of intracranial aneurysms. Psychiatr Neurol Neurochir 75:437–440, 1972
345. Walter W, Schütte W: Über die Gefässpasmen bei frisch rupturierten sackförmigen Aneurysmen der Hirnarterien. Acta Neurochir 11: 631–652, 1964
346. Walton JN: The prognosis and management of subarachnoid haemorrhage. Canad Med Assoc J 72:165–175, 1955
347. Weir B, Grace M, Hansen J, et al.: Time course of vasospasm in man. J Neurosurg 48:173–178, 1978
348. Weir B, Rothberg C, Grace M, et al.: Relative prognostic significance of vasospasm following subarachnoid hemorrhage. Canad J Neurol Sci 2:109–114, 1975
349. Wilkins RH: The role of intracranial arterial spasm in the timing of operations for aneurysm. Clin Neurosurg 24:185–207, 1977
350. Wilkins RH, Alexander JA, Odom GL: Intracranial arterial spasm: a clinical analysis. J Neurosurg 29:121–134, 1968
351. Wilkins RH, Wilkinson RH, Odom GL: Abnormal brain scans in patients with cerebral arterial spasm. J Neurosurg 36:133–140, 1972
352. Winn HR, Richardson AE, Jane JA: Late morbidity and mortality in cerebral aneurysms: a ten-year follow-up of 364 conservatively treated patients with a single cerebral aneurysm. Trans Am Neurol Assoc 98:148–150, 1973
353. Winn HR, Richardson AE, Jane JA: The long-term prognosis in untreated cerebral aneurysms: I. The incidence of late hemorrhage in cerebral aneurysm: a 10-year evaluation of 364 patients. Ann Neurol 1:358–370, 1977
354. Winn HR, Richardson AE, O'Brien W, et al.: The long-term prognosis in untreated cerebral aneurysms: II. Late morbidity and mortality. Ann Neurol 4:418–426, 1978
355. Yaşargil MG, Fox JL: The microsurgical approach to intracranial aneurysms. Surg Neurol 3:7–14, 1975
356. Yaşargil MG, Fox JL, Ray MW: The operative approach to aneurysms of the anterior communicating artery. In Krayenbühl H (ed.): Advances and Technical Standards in Neurosurgery, Vol 2. New York, Springer-Verlag, 1975, pp. 113–170
357. Yaşargil MG, Smith RD: Surgery on the carotid system in the treatment of hemorrhagic stroke. In Thompson RH, Green JR (eds.): Advances in Neurology. Vol 16, Stroke. New York, Raven Press, 1977, pp. 181–209
358. Yoshimoto T, Uchida K, Kaneko U, et al.: An analysis of follow-up results of 1000 intracranial saccular aneurysms with definitive surgical treatment. J Neurosurg 50:152–157, 1979
359. Zingesser LH, Schechter MM, Dexter J, et al.: On the significance of spasm associated with rupture of a cerebral aneurysm. The relationship between spasm as noted angiographically and regional blood flow determinations. Arch Neurol 18:520–528, 1968
360. Zingesser LH, Schechter MM, Dexter J, et al.: Regional cerebral blood flow in patients with subarachnoid hemorrhage. Acta Radiol 9:573–588, 1969
361. Zlotnik EI, Oleshkevich FV, Stolkarts JZ: Microsurgical technique in the treatment of intracranial aneurysms. J Neurosurg 46:591–595, 1977

22

Preoperative and Medical Therapy

In their Preface, Pool and Potts (133) warned:

> It is now recognized . . . that an aneurysm, whether large or small, is like a time bomb which may explode at any time unless suitably treated.

If a patient with a ruptured aneurysm is to undergo surgical treatment, there will usually be a period of time during which various medical therapies will be in progress to prevent a rebleed and to optimize the patient's condition for the stress of anesthesia and surgery. Should surgical treatment be contraindicated for the patient, then the medical regime will be prolonged. In either case, there may be urgent medical or surgical measures needed to combat secondary complications (see Chapter 8) such as hydrocephalus, hematoma, edema, vasospasm, ischemia and infarction, fluid and electrolyte disorders, seizures, gastrointestinal hemorrhage, pulmonary edema, cardiovascular irregularities, and preexisting medical diseases such as diabetes and hypertension. These will not be detailed in this chapter.

The medical treatment of ruptured intracranial aneurysms began many years ago. The lack of medical knowledge concerning pathophysiology forced physicians to apply historical remedies, however inappropriate. It is only in the recent past that administration of aspirin for headache after subarachnoid hemorrhage was determined to be not only inappropriate but even dangerous due to its tendency to impair platelet aggregation within the rent in the aneurysm. In 1842 A.T. Thomson (184) had a patient with multiple aneurysms on both internal carotid arteries. The applied treatment (?!) for this unfortunate patient included cupping the nape of the neck and temples; wrapping in blankets; a foot warmer; a blister to the nape of the neck; enemas; medication consisting of calomel, croton oil, and oil of caraway after the enema; calomel q 4 h by mouth; sesquicarbonate of ammonia q 4 h by mouth; ice to the shaven scalp; tartar-emetic ointment to the scalp; and iodide of potassium by mouth! In spite of such efforts the patient died. In 1875 W.E. Humble (73) continued the usual treatment of potassium iodide daily (starting at 9 grains and increasing to 36 grains daily); he was delighted when this therapy resulted in the much-hoped-for consolidation of the suspected "aneurism" as the patient heard several "cracks" in her head followed by disappearance of the bruit. Medical thinking on the subject forged ahead when, as early as 1888, W.R. Gowers (60) quite succinctly presaged much of today's opinion:

> If an intracranial aneurism is suspected, it is important to avoid as far as possible all influences which tend to increase the arterial pressure. . . . The bowels should be kept loose, and the patient should sleep with head and shoulders well raised. . . . More reasonable measures are those designed to favor coagulation in the sac.

A wealth of material has been written relating to the medical treatment of intracranial aneurysms (1–204). Of particular importance is the role of the nursing staff (19,20,40,94, 95,132). The care of the aneurysm patient requires the nurse to have considerable neurosurgical knowledge and experience in specialized care and monitoring. Table 22.1 summarizes some of the measures to be considered in the medical and preoperative management of these patients.

Routine Care

Bedrest

An essential element of therapy is rest, quietude, and absence of exertion. The patient is often agitated and easily stressed by noise and discomfort. Any agitation raises blood pressure, thus increasing the transmural pressure across the wall of the aneurysm. A clot is organizing within the rent in the aneurysm (Fig. 22.1), and this must be protected. Hence, most physicians recommend a quiet, semidarkened private room with reasonable sensory deprivation (36,44,61–64,87,139,143,144,152,186,196). In the absence of surgery this period of bedrest is recommended to be 4–8 weeks (average of 6 weeks) to allow time for the clot in the rent in the aneurysm to firmly organize. During this time the increased fibrinolytic activity in the blood and CSF returns to normal (see pages 645–647 in this chapter).

The patient should be turned frequently if he is unconscious, and should receive passive motion to the limbs and pulmonary percussion therapy as needed. Elastic stockings or leg wrappings are advisable to forestall thrombophlebitis if the patient is not active. The head should be elevated moderately to improve cranial venous drainage, reduce brain swelling,

Table 22.1. Measures to be Considered in Preoperative Management of the Patient with Ruptured Intracranial Aneurysm

Bedrest
Quiet, darkened private room
Nursing care on one-to-one basis
Moderate elevation of the head
Sedatives or tranquilizers
Analgesics
Gentle laxatives, stool softeners
Antihypertensive agents
Controlled partial ligation of cervical carotid artery
Glucocorticosteroids
Antifibrinolytic agents
Anticonvulsants
Repeated lumbar punctures

(From Fox et al., ref. 40.

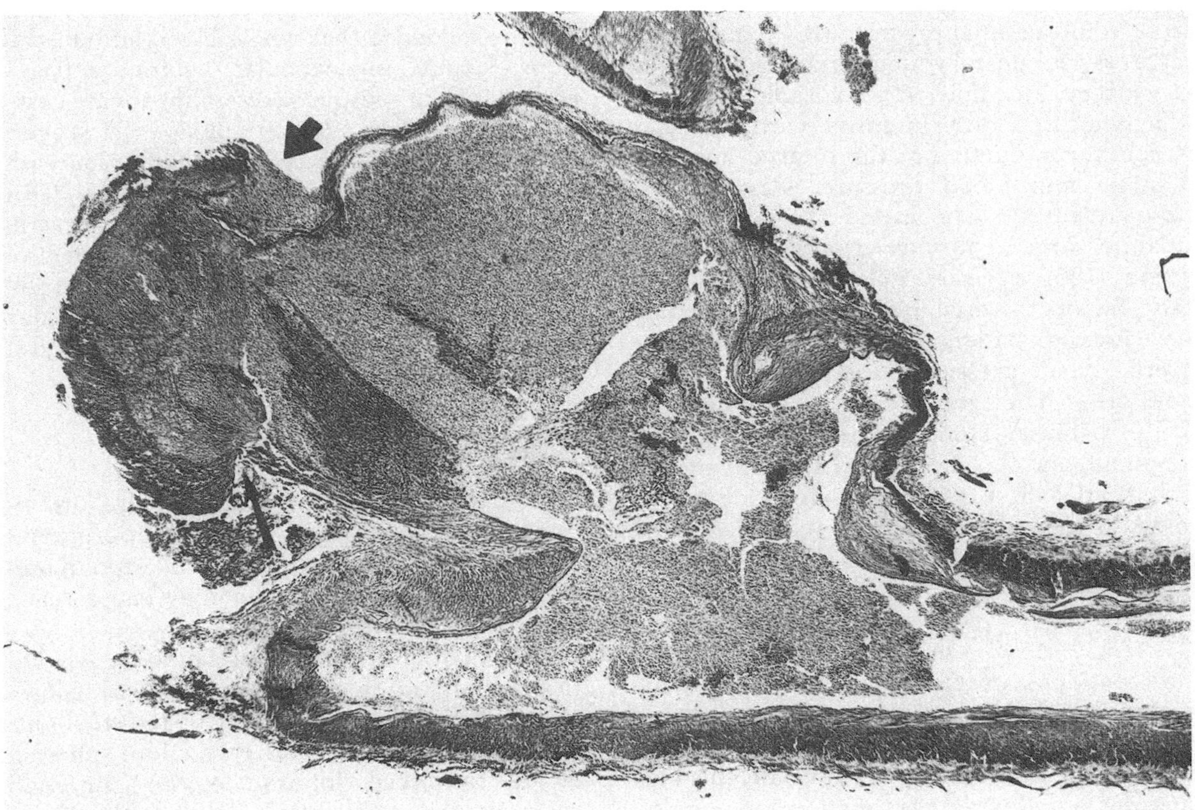

Fig. 22.1. A plug of thrombus (between *arrows*) is extruding from a rupture in an aneurysm. Laminated mural thrombus is also present in the lower part of the sac. (From ref. 22a)

reduce intracranial blood pressure, and limit abdominal pressure on the respiratory diaphragm. Occasionally the horizontal "coma position" (three-quarter prone position) may be necessary in the unconscious patient if respiratory secretions are a problem.

Financial and insurance constraints or unavailability of nursing personnel may interdict the presence of a private duty nurse. However, from a medical standpoint it is optimum if private duty, or one-to-one, nursing is present to monitor and to tend to the many needs of this ill patient. Long waits for medication, personal assistance, etc. only serve to further aggravate the distraught patient and raise his blood pressure.

Monitoring

In the past most neurosurgeons have relied on routine monitoring of neurologic and vital signs by nursing staff in a private or quiet, semiprivate hospital room. Most likely this is still standard practice. The physical and psychological stress of intracranial pressure (ICP), intra-arterial pressure, central venous pressure or pulmonary artery, etc., lines in a favorable grade patient lying in a busy intensive care unit may be counterproductive to the desired lowering of stress and blood pressure. Nevertheless, there are authors who are now recommending such measures to various extents (53,115,125). Nornes (125) suggested following blood hemostatic factors, arterial blood gases and pH in the comatose patient, EEG, EKG, direct-line arterial blood pressures, and continuous ICP monitoring. The extent of monitoring depends on the patient's clinical state, the physician's judgment, and the expertise of the nursing and technician staff. A quiet intensive care unit devoted to these specific problems is ideal but often unavailable when needed.

Diet and Fluids

If the patient is awake and alert, a low-residue diet with vitamins and minerals has been recommended by some (61,63,186). The purpose is to reduce intestinal bulk. However, this may cause some undesired constipation and unpalatable food for some patients. The confused or unconscious patient is best fed by intravenous lines, for vomiting and aspiration pneumonitis is an ever-present hazard.

The preoperative and postoperative intravenous fluid intake orders are similar. Standard orders have been, for example, about 80 ml/h (or 2000 ml/day) of 5% dextrose in half-normal saline. This represents mild fluid restriction, appropriate for those patients who are often susceptible to various degrees of inappropriate secretion of ADH (see pages 123–125). Mild to moderate fluid restriction to avoid aggravation of brain edema has been advised by some (121,156). Nibbelink (121) noted a correlation between fluid restriction and a lower mortality rate. Recently, there has been interest in expanding blood volume with crystalloid and/or colloid solutions and even blood transfusions to improve cerebral arterial perfusion in the face of the expected vasospasm (53,92,93). Maroon and Nelson (92,93) pointed out that SAH patients placed at bedrest develop a reduced red blood cell mass and blood volume, a factor aggravating the effects of vasospasm. Whether to give a high-fluid intake to combat vasospasm or a low-fluid intake to limit cerebral edema remains somewhat controversial. There is some evidence that whole-blood administration expands intravascular volume and increases cardiac output without improving cerebral blood flow (CBF) (202a). However, reducing blood viscosity by hemodilution with plasma expanders appears to increase CBF while at the same time tending to raise intracranial pressure. We have adopted the policy of giving 5% Plasmanate (Cutter Laboratories, Inc.), 250 ml daily, starting on the third day after SAH in all cases of ruptured aneurysm until the risk of vasospasm has passed.

Bowel and Bladder Care

Unconscious patients usually require an indwelling urinary catheter to allow appropriate drainage and adequate intake and output monitoring. A distended bladder may cause reflex elevation in blood pressure.

Constipation and diarrhea should be avoided to prevent straining and irritation with consequent effects on blood pressure. Mild stool softeners such as Colace (dioctyl sodium sulfosuccinate by Mead Johnson & Co.) or mild laxatives such as Ducolax (bisacodyl by Boehringer Ingelheim Ltd.) are usually effective. In 1941 Richardson and Hyland (144) warned against overstraining on the bedpan. For the conscious patient, a bedside commode is preferable to a bedpan. Benton et al. (14) noted that more effort and energy was expended using the bedpan than the commode. In 1952 Hamby (63) regarded the bedpan as "an especially lethal weapon in patients having spontaneous subarachnoid hemorrhage."

Respiratory Care

Other than pulmonary physical therapy, interdiction of smoking, and respiratory status evaluation in the patient with chronic lung problems, the alert patient should require little additional support. Patients with pulmonary disease will need their surgery delayed until their condition is assessed and under good medical control.

The obtunded or deeply comatose patient, especially if the brainstem respiratory centers are compromised, may require repeated blood gas evaluation and machine-assisted ventilation via endotracheal tube or tracheostomy. In this situation one must weigh the risk of inducing coughing and aneurysm rupture against the risk of cerebral hypoxia and hypercarbia aggravating brain edema and ischemia (35,40,45, 52,115,180). The review by Frost (47) on respiratory problems in the head-injured patient is highly recommended and equally applicable to the patient with a ruptured intracranial aneurysm.

Intracranial Pressure Control

Lumbar Puncture

A common method of lowering intracranial pressure (and thus improving arterial perfusion) is with lumbar spinal fluid drainage by one or more spinal taps or by an indwelling lumbar catheter. In 1933 Andrews (5) treated all cases of SAH by lumbar puncture (LP) to keep intracranial pressure well below arterial blood pressure. There have been several advocates of repeated LP to reduce ICP, relieve headache and agitation, remove blood from CSF, and reduce the chance of hydrocephalus (5,7,22,25,70,71,77,89,90,103,104,147,197,200). Most of these authors recommended serial LP as a major part of the treatment. This was common practice by many in earlier years; the CSF pressure was usually reduced to one-half its original level by releasing sufficient CSF. In 1932 Howell (71) stated:

> The treatment of these cases at present consists in keeping the patient during the recent condition at rest with morphia, and reducing the intracranial pressure by lumbar puncture and by intravenous glucose. Enemas of magnesium sulfate may also prove useful.

In 1933 Dott (25) agreed, saying:

> Conservative treatment by rest and morphia in the earlier days following a single subarachnoid haemorrhage may be supplemented by lumbar puncture.

Many other neurosurgeons have hesitated carrying out repeated LP for fear of reducing ICP sufficiently to cause the aneurysm to rupture again. However, Merritt (103), Walton (197), and Heidrich (70) found no evidence of increase in rebleed tendency from the use of repeated LP. In 1938 Merritt (103) concluded (perhaps erroneously) that

> The danger of lumbar puncture in these cases has been overemphasized. There is no adequate physiological basis for hypothesis that removal of fluid by lumbar puncture tends to increase the hemorrhage. . . .

He got some support from Lindsay (89) who calculated that a drop in CSF pressure of 100 mm H_2O over a 1-min period is the same as raising the blood pressure by 7.3 mm Hg over the same time period. He felt, therefore, that the danger of rupture following LP was much less than the danger of rupture from coughing, straining, and blood pressure elevation—especially when one considers that the normal pulse pressure itself exceeds 7.3 mm Hg in a much shorter period of time.

If many physicians recommended routine serial LP, an equal number opposed the practice, fearful of precipitating a rebleed (9,42,56, 152,179). Meredith (102) studied animals and patients in terms of ridding the CSF of blood by serial intermittent lumbar drainage. He found that in actual practice only a small fraction of the total blood could be removed. Sprong (175) noted that in 15 cases of traumatic SAH, daily CSF removal of 15–37 ml resulted in no detectable difference in the rate of disappearance of blood from the CSF compared with control subjects not so treated. At present, most neurosurgeons do not agree with routine daily LP due to the risk of excess lowering of ICP around the aneurysm and due to the questionable evidence for adequate removal of blood products from the CSF. However, there is considerable agreement that in the SAH patient agitated with meningismus and severe headache, removal of CSF by spinal puncture is frequently helpful as symptomatic treatment resulting in more comfort and less risk of vascular hypertension (36,41,44,45,61,63,64,101,139, 144,179,186,197).

Ventricular Drainage

Ventricular drainage may be lifesaving in situations of acute hydrocephalus after SAH (see pages 185–195). Bellotti et al. (12) and Suzuki et al. (178) have described its routine use in cases of severe hemorrhage or where the patient is very ill from the SAH and blood breakdown products in the CSF.

Positioning and Respiratory Care

Elevation of the head and respiratory care have already been described (see previous page). Carbon dioxide retention, hypoxia, and excess respiratory effort with its attendant energy requirements serve to dramatically raise ICP. Hence, controlled passive hyperventilation via endotracheal tube or tracheostomy may be useful in the seriously ill case of respiratory distress.

Controlled Vascular Hypotension

The use of antihypertensive agents to reduce intracranial blood pressure and hence brain capillary hydrostatic pressure will be discussed later in this chapter (see pages 642–645).

Glucocorticosteroids

The use of steroids such as methylprednisolone or dexamethasone has been popular (11,35, 36,43,45,46,52,53,64,75,134,141,146,156,172, 186,196). Whereas there is ample documentation that steroids reduce cerebral edema in patients with brain neoplasms, there is little convincing evidence that these drugs do so for patients with SAH or head injury. For this reason there is no universal agreement that steroids and their attendant risks should be used routinely (we do not use them routinely before surgery).

Steroids may play an important role, however, in minimizing the aseptic meningitis and arachnoid adhesions, thus reducing the chances of future hydrocephalus. Contrariwise, these drugs may mask fever from pneumonitis or pulmonary embolism, induce gastritis or peptic ulcers, suppress normal adrenal gland function, and inhibit scar formation around the wall of the aneurysm. It may be worthwhile to administer antacids and/or Tagamet (cimetadine by Smith Kline & French Laboratories), the latter being a histamine H-2 receptor antagonist suppressing gastric acid secretions.

Osmotic Agents

Hypertonic mannitol is rarely indicated as preoperative therapy in most cases of SAH. Nevertheless, the evolution of severe cerebral edema unresponsive to other measures may require agents which increase the osmotic gradient from brain to blood (35,40,64,71,115,134,141, 186).

In earlier years glucose, magnesium sulfate, or albumin solutions were used (71). Glycerol has not become popular yet. Low molecular weight dextran has been advocated by some (141). Intravenous 15% mannitol drip (0.5–4 mg/kg body weight) remains the mainstay of osmotic therapy (39,40). The smaller doses are generally used. It may require titration against a continuous ICP monitor. These agents operate by osmotically pulling water out of the brain across the blood-brain barrier as well as by reducing total body water through diuresis. They have the advantage of transiently reducing blood viscosity and red blood cell aggregation, and the disadvantage of causing dehydration and possible rebound in ICP.

Loop Diuretics

Presently, Lasix (furosemide by Hoechst-Roussel Pharmaceuticals Inc.) is a commonly used diuretic, reducing total body water via kidney loop diuresis. It also appears to have some direct effect on reduction of CSF formation, probably at the choroid plexus level. This drug has been used in cases of SAH to help reduce blood pressure as well as ICP. As with the osmotic diuretics, these drugs may disturb fluid and electrolyte balance and confuse the clinical picture where hypophyseal functions are already compromised (especially antidiuretic hormone disturbances).

Summary

There are numerous methods of reducing ICP in these cases; Table 22.2 summarizes these methods. Operative treatments such as subtemporal decompression are uncommonly used now. Frequently, hematomas must be removed or CSF diversion (internal shunt or external drainage for hydrocephalus) carried out. Rarely, the aneurysm itself is so large as to act as a tumor requiring excision to reduce ICP.

Other Medications and Adjuncts

Sedatives and Analgesics

Mild to moderate sedation of the conscious or agitated patient is universally recommended. Phenobarbital has been very popular due to its additional anticonvulsant effect and low incidence of side effects. Tranquilizers may be added or substituted as needed. Valium (diazepam by Roche Laboratories) also has some

Table 22.2. Control of Intracranial Pressure: Practical and Theoretical

I. Maintenance of functioning body-organ systems (respiratory, cardiac, vascular, renal, hepatic, endocrinologic, and balance of nutrition and electrolytes)

II. Removal of reaction force to distending action force of intracranial contents
- A. Remove envelope—mechanical operative decompression
- B. Reduce vascular hydrostatic pressure
  1. Elevation of head
  2. Induction of controlled vascular hypotension—antihypertensive agents
  3. Reduction of body temperature—hypothermia
  4. Reduction of CO_2 pressure
     - a. Controlled passive hyperventilation
     - b. Tracheostomy

III. Removal of distending action force
- A. Reduce size of space-taking lesion
  1. Mechanical operative decompression
  2. Hemostasis
- B. Reduce vascular volume (same methods as II,B)
- C. Reduce size of brain parenchyma
  1. Reduce total body water
     - a. Restriction of intake of fluid
     - b. Stimulation of diuresis (osmotics, mercurials, chlorothiazides, xanthines, furosemide, carbonic-anhydrase inhibitors, cation-exchange resins)
  2. Reduce vascular hydrostatic pressure (same methods as II,B)
  3. Increase vascular osmotic pressure—infusion of osmotic agents (urea, mannitol, salts, sugars, albumin, glycerol, dextran)
  4. Reduce osmotic pressure of brain water and impermeability of cell membrane (surface tension)
     - a. Limitation of iatrogenic physical and physiological brain trauma
     - b. Administration of cortisone drugs
     - c. Reduction of CO_2 pressure (same methods as II,B)
  5. Reduce metabolism of brain cells
     - a. Prevent hyperthermia
     - b. Induce hypothermia
  6. Avoid anaerobic metabolism of brain cells—adequate perfusion, oxygenation, and nutrition of brain
  7. Counteract toxins of brain cells (anticholinergics—atrophine; antiserotonin agents—methysergide, antihistamines, antiadrenergic agents, antienzymes, cortisone)
  8. Encourage removal of exudates
     - a. Elevation of head
     - b. Use of proteolytic enzymes
     - c. CSF drainage
- D. Reduce size of compartment of cerebrospinal fluid
  1. Direct—drainage of cerebrospinal fluid (ventricular, cisternal, spinal)
  2. Indirect (consider cerebrospinal fluid as "extracellular fluid")
     - a. Same methods as III,C
     - b. Inhibition of carbonic anhydrase (Diamox, Cardrase)
     - c. Loop diuretic (Lasix)

Modified from Fox JL, ref. 39.

additional anticonvulsant effects. Thorazine (chlorpromazine by Smith Kline & French Laboratories) has some additional vascular hypotensive effects. Serpasil (reserpine by Ciba Pharmaceutical Co.) is a tranquilizer, has some vascular hypotensive effects, and interferes with serotonin and catecholamine synthesis (therefore it has also been used by some physicians to prevent vasospasm). However, reserpine has side effects which has limited its popularity for cases of SAH.

Most analgesics used in patients with ruptured aneurysm also have some hypnotic or sedative effects. Narcotics such as Demerol (meperidine by Winthrop Laboratories) are quite useful in this regard. Respiratory depression and hypotension may occur with the larger dosages or in combination with other drugs, especially in elderly patients. Codeine is useful but may have a greater tendency to cause constipation. Aspirin, once in common use for headache from SAH (63,144,152,170), is now usually considered to be contraindicated. Aspirin increases the fibrinolytic activity of blood, increases bleeding time, and impairs platelet aggregation (111,199). (Many other drugs will also have these effects to some extent.) Since the aim of therapy is to protect the patient from rebleeding, aspirin should be avoided if possible.

Anticonvulsants

Prophylactic administration of anticonvulsants such as phenobarbital and Dilantin (phenytoin by Parke-Davis Co.) is recommended by some physicians (40,41,136,139,180,186). However, such prophylaxis does not appear to be universally adopted.

Vasodilators

Other than improving cerebral perfusion by expanding blood volume and/or raising the blood pressure, there has been no universally accepted therapy for vasospasm. Past and recent trends are reviewed in Chapters 9 and 10. Needless to say, low blood volumes and vascular hypotension should be reversed if vasospasm threatens the patient. The dilemma revolves around elevation of the blood pressure in the unprotected aneurysm as well as in the perfusing arteries. Vasodilators tested in the past have had inadequate effect on cerebral vessels in normal dosages and have had serious side effects such as systemic vascular hypotension.

Antihypertensive Agents and Techniques

Some studies have shown that reduction in the patient's blood pressure reduces the risk of rebleed, but the statistical evidence is not dramatic in the 1966 Cooperative Study (145, 145a), Meyer and Bauer's investigation in 1962 (105), and Nibbelink's report in 1974 (121). Nevertheless, a large number of physicians recommend antihypertensive agents (Table 22.3) for medical or preoperative treatment to prevent rebleed (1,2,4,8,11,34–36,40,41,52,53, 64,75,76,79,83,91,96,105,112,113,115,136,139, 146,154,156,159–170,172,180,186,196).

The arterial pulse pressure is the blood pressure added to the diastolic tone by the contraction of the heart; systolic pressure is the result. With each systolic pressure wave through the intracranial artery and its aneurysm, the aneurysm is seen during surgical exposure to expand

Table 22.3. Antihypertensive Medications

Generic Name	*Trade Name*	*Company*
Methyldopa	Aldomet	Merck Sharpe & Dohme, Inc.
Hydralazine	Apresoline	Ciba Pharmaceutical Co.
Reserpine	Serpasil	Ciba Pharmaceutical Co.
Chlorothiazide	Diuril	Merck Sharpe & Dohme, Inc.
Propranolol	Inderol	Ayerst Laboratories
Chlorpromazine	Thorazine	Smith Kline & French Laboratories
Trimethaphan	Arfonad	Roche Laboratories
Nitroprosside	Nipride	Roche Laboratories
Clonidine	Catapres	Boehringer Ingelheim Ltd.
Prazosin	Minipress	Pfizer Laboratories

as the blood swirls through it. When the cranium is closed, each pulsation in the aneurysm is buttressed by a similar increase in pressure outside the aneurysm. However, because the aneurysm is on the more proximal conducting arteries, the pressure inside it will slightly precede the general increase in intracranial pressure. The latter is effected by the systolic thrust into the more distal and smaller perfusing arteries of greater resistance. This will allow for an early, transient pressure gradient across the wall of the aneurysm (89,127). Atkinson (8) believed the commonly found atherosclerosis in these arteries stiffens them, causing the systolic pulse to be inadequately dampened by the wall of the artery. The studies of Moritake et al. (107–110) on elastic tubes and on aneurysms at autopsy support this. The thin-walled and often brittle aneurysm then takes the brunt of the pulsatile force, which Atkinson believed can be lessened by antihypertensive agents.

During exposure of an ACoAA, Martinez Coll et al. (96) measured the intra-aneurysmal blood pressure. They discovered that the pressure fell from 78/58 to 52/42 mm Hg, with significant reduction of the pulse wave during induced hypotension. Inside a MCAA they found the blood pressure dropped from 90/60 to 78/50 mm Hg, again with prominent reduction of the pulse wave during induced hypotension. This effect on the pulse wave suggests that a reduction in blood pressure while awaiting surgery would reduce the risk of rebleed. Ferguson (28) measured the blood pressure inside four aneurysms at surgery and found the mean intra-aneurysmal pressure to equal the systemic blood pressure, suggesting that these sacs are subjected to the full force of the systemic blood pressure. Wright (203) measured the pressures inside three MCAAs and found the pressure inside his patients' aneurysms to be less than that in the systemic arteries. Bakay and Sweet (10) studied the pressures inside arteries of brain tumor patients; the pressures inside the M-1, M-2, A-1, and A-2 arteries were only minimally less than the internal carotid artery pressures.

Black and German (17) concluded that the strain on the wall of an intracranial aneurysm is equal to the sum of various stresses including hydrostatic pressure, pulsatile nature of blood flow, turbulence, and jet action. According to the law of Laplace, the tangential tension (T) in the wall of a sphere (aneurysm) is equal to RP/2, where R is the radius of the sphere and P is the transmural pressure; hence the blood pressure inside the aneurysm will have a direct effect on the tension of the wall (27,80,176,201). Notice also that the larger the aneurysm radius (R), the greater the tension (T) in the wall risking rupture. It is for this reason that aneurysms less than 6 mm in diameter uncommonly rupture (26,176). At surgery, the remarkably forceful pulsation of the giant aneurysm compared to the smaller aneurysm can be explained by a modification of the law of Laplace by Early and Fink (27): the force (F) expanding the aneurysmal sac is equal to $\pi R^2 P$. This force is proportional to the internal blood pressure (minus any external buttressing pressure) and to the second power of the radius. One can see that a considerably greater drop in blood pressure may be needed to reduce the force distending the sac of larger aneurysms compared to that needed for smaller aneurysms. Such a reduction in blood pressure may be particularly important if the observations of Scott (153) and Ferguson (29) are correct: the walls of aneurysms are more rigid (or less distensible) than the walls of the parent arteries (Fig. 22.2). This places a much greater tension on the aneurysm wall compared to the arterial wall with each systolic thrust. Hence, as Slosberg (166) put it, "The blood pressure has been considered to be a major factor (although not the only one) in the rupture of an intracranial aneurysm."

There has been considerable discussion among various authors regarding the role of flow, turbulence, and vibration in the etiology, expansion, and rupture of intracranial aneurysms (17,29,30,48,49,51,72,74,80,84,100,126, 128,137,158,176,177). Each systolic spurt of blood into the orifice of the aneurysm has an impulse component (proportional to the square of the velocity) pushing the aneurysm away from the artery and an opposite reaction tending to tear the artery away from the aneurysm (17). Any sudden increase in this systolic pulse (pulse pressure) from adverse psychological or physical factors (185) or during rapid eye movement (REM) sleep cycles (142) may stress and weaken the aneurysm wall to rupture at its weakest point. Besides the ever-changing and pulsatile blood pressures inside the aneurysm, there appears to be flow-related turbulence (Fig. 22.3) which may or may not be sufficient

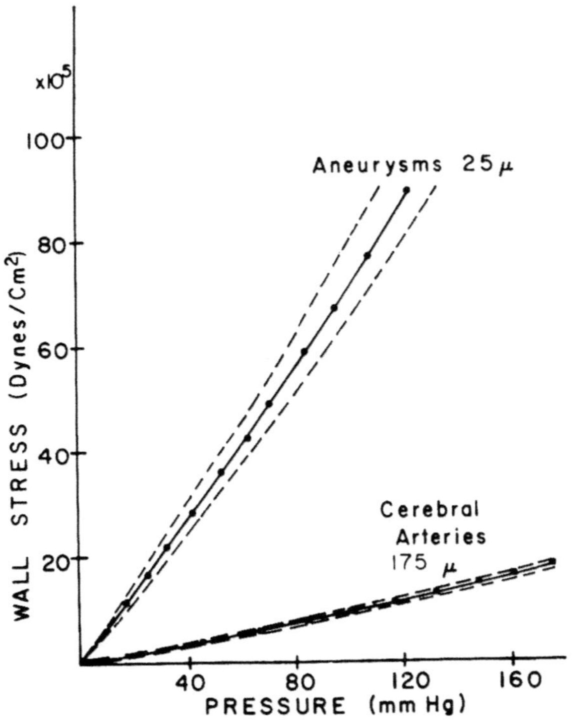

Fig. 22.2. Relationship between the stress on the walls of cerebral aneurysms and arteries and the internal hydrostatic pressure induced in autopsy specimens. (From ref. 29)

to set off sonic waves (vibrations)—possibly even to the point of destructive resonance in the wall of the aneurysm. A greater systolic thrust increases the pulsatile flow rate; this increases turbulence in the aneurysm. Lowering the blood pressure would dampen this postulated threat to the wall of the aneurysm.

Whereas there is no question that there is a high incidence of vascular hypertension after rupture of an intracranial aneurysm, much of it may be acute and secondary to stress, elevated catecholamines (13,118,130), and the Cushing reflex induced by elevated ICP (23). The incidence and role of chronic hypertension is controversial. Peet et al. (131) believed there is a high incidence of preexisting hypertension in patients with aneurysm. Black and Hicks (16) found a 47% incidence and Stehbens (175a) a 54% incidence of evidence for chronic hypertension in autopsy cases. The evidence consisted of left ventricular hypertrophy of the heart, contracted granular kidneys, and/or documented history of a preexisting blood pressure exceeding 150/100 mm Hg. Keller (85), McCormick and Schmalstieg (99), and Wolfe (202), on the other hand, could find no significant differences between cases with aneurysms and a matched control series. Andrews and Spiegel (6) came to similar conclusions, except females 18–54 years of age had a higher incidence of hypertension if they also had aneurysms. Under the age of 55 years, both male and female (especially female) hypertensive patients were twice as likely to have *multiple* aneurysms.

If it is agreed that, in the absence of threatening vasospasm or other causes of reduced cerebral perfusion, a patient with a previously ruptured aneurysm is less likely to rebleed with a lower blood pressure, which methods of control are best? In 1932 Freeman (42) suggested venesection, now an outmoded therapy. Elevation of the head and tranquility are advisable. In addition, antihypertensive drugs are often necessary. Table 22.3 lists some of the more commonly used drugs in patients with ruptured aneurysms. There are others which are either newer or more hazardous; their use in SAH remains to be established. Trimethaphan and sodium nitroprusside require close observation and intra-arterial lines to monitor blood pressure. They are given by titrated intravenous drip, and they are not used routinely unless the patient has uncontrolled hypertension. Methyldopa, with or without chlorthiazide, has been commonly prescribed. However, Mullan et al. (112,115) have felt methyldopa caused occasional problems with cerebral perfusion [possibly related to combination therapy with ε-aminocaproic acid (EACA)].

Adams and co-workers (2) and Snyckers (172) have used propranolol, a beta-adrenergic blocking agent. We have found this to be an extremely effective drug, but worry about its possible adverse effects on cerebral vasospasm, for beta-adrenergic–*stimulating* drugs have been used to treat vasospasm. Spence et al. (174a) studied the effects of various antihypertensive agents in monkeys. They reported that propranolol and clonidine not only reduce blood pressure but also reduce blood flow, whereas methyldopa and hydralazine reduce blood pressure but increase blood flow through their cardiac and vascular effects. Therefore, if one wishes to increase blood flow to maintain good cerebral perfusion or if one wishes to reduce blood flow to reduce turbulence in the aneu-

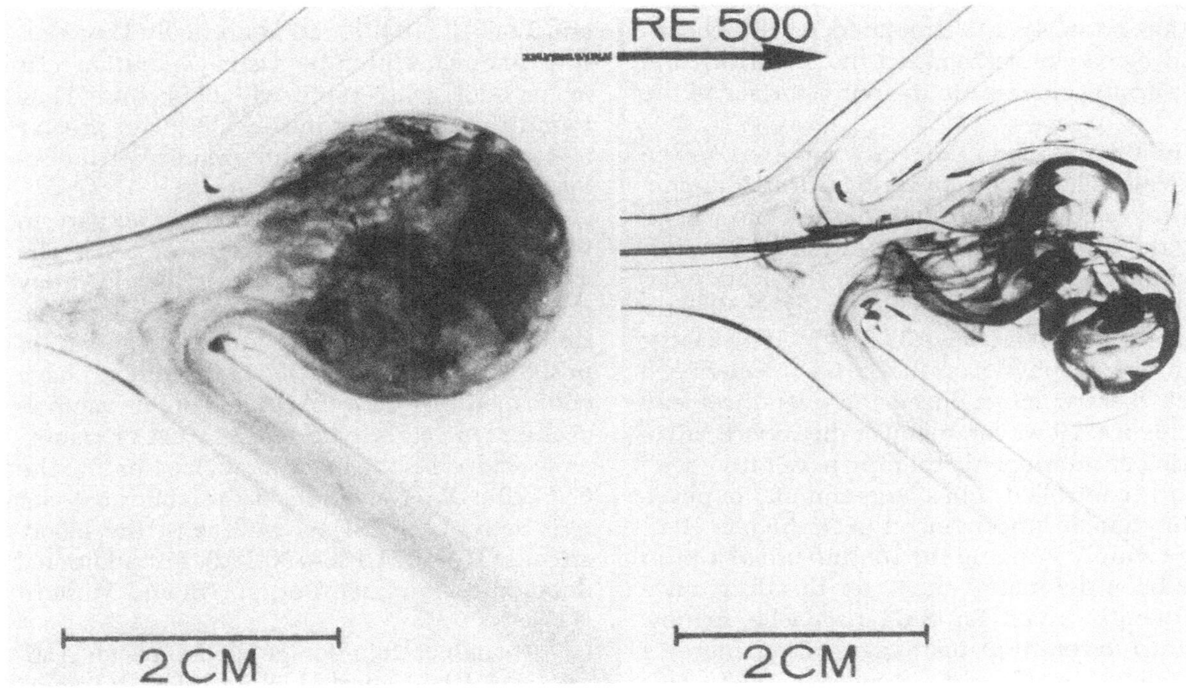

A B

Fig. 22.3. **A** Turbulence in the sac of a large, spherical, glass model aneurysm. The Reynolds number (Re 500) corresponds to the flow rate when the photograph was taken. The direction of flow is shown by the *arrow*. Evans blue dye has been injected to demonstrate flow patterns. **B** Turbulence in both loculi of the large, bilocular, glass model aneurysm. Flow in the stem and both branches is streamlined. (From ref. 30)

rysm, then a more definitive antihypertensive drug may have to be ordered. Regarding the preoperative treatment of the patient's blood pressure, a study group concluded:

> A blood pressure (BP) of 200 mm Hg systolic should be reduced to 130 to 150 mm Hg if the patient has no adverse reaction. Most neurosurgeons agree that control of an elevated BP is mandatory, although precipitous drops in BP should be avoided for the protection of the brain if the arteries are atherosclerotic or spastic. The initial BP elevation due to the hemorrhage itself often recedes after rest and sedation. Lowering systolic BP to 90 to 100 mm Hg in a normotensive patient with a BP of 120 mm Hg may be difficult, but some physicians and surgeons believe that the attempt should be made. (40)

Long-term antihypertensive therapy instead of surgery has been advocated by Slosberg. The reader is referred to his many writings on the subject for details of his management (159–170).

Partial Carotid Artery Ligation

This technique of lowering the blood pressure on the side of blood flow to the aneurysm was first described by Dandy in 1944 (24). He had four cases of ICAA. The internal carotid artery was only partially ligated; the aneurysms later were clipped. In 1963 Jain (81) did experimental work on dogs which showed that partial ligation of the internal carotid artery was helpful in reducing the distal pulsatile force of the blood. More recently Mullan (113,115) advocated partial common carotid artery occlusion by a screw clamp to reduce local blood pressure in ICAA or MCAA cases while the patient awaits definitive repair.

Antifibrinolytic Drugs

In 1886 Bramwell (18) was undertaking the autopsy of a case with a ruptured internal carotid artery aneurysm. He made an important observation, noting that "a laminated, partly decolorized blood-clot surrounded the aneurism, and was firmly adherent to the outer surface of the sac."

In 1965 Mullan et al. (116) reported on the possible value of administering a drug (ε-aminocaproic acid) to retard lysis of the clot protecting the ruptured aneurysm. Although a few reports have suggested that such medication has not reduced rebleed incidence (their dosages may have been too low) (57,58,138,195), a large number of physicians have been convinced such therapy has reduced the overall rebleed incidence. However, many of the reports advocating antifibrinolytic therapy have often been poorly controlled, and a large number of physicians remain unconvinced of its benefit. Perhaps simply stopping the routine use of aspirin has been the main benefit, for this drug, once frequently given for SAH headache, is now known to retard platelet aggregation, increase bleeding time, and accelerate clot lysis (111,117,199). Certainly we can say that use of anticoagulants (sometimes necessary where the risk of death from pulmonary embolism exceeds the risk of a rebleed) would undoubtedly be fatal if rebleed occurs, even though Finney and Gholston (33) reported just such a patient who survived!

Hematomas in the subarachnoid spaces tend to organize more slowly than they do in muscle or in the peritoneal cavity (148). As early as 1942 Globus and Schwab (59) mentioned that CSF has anticoagulant properties which are, in part, responsible for failure of blood to clot early. Since then a number of investigations have shown that fibrinolytic activity can be detected in blood and CSF following injury and/or SAH (15,31,69,78,88,106,117,135,171,181, 183,187–192). Normally pia, dura, arachnoid, endothelium, and choroid plexus contain the plasminogen activator which, when released, catalyzes the conversion of the blood plasminogen to plasmin. CSF also contains plasminogen activator but has no plasminogen until blood is released into the CSF from hemorrhage. Plasmin assists in clot dissolution or lysis.

Normally blood and CSF contain little or no clot lysis (fibrinolysis) activity unless plasmin is present. Plasmin, a proteolytic enzyme, attacks fibrin (formed from fibrinogen to join platelets and red blood cells in forming the clot network). Plasmin can also attack other clotting factors, which in part may explain why Uttley and Buckell (194) found abnormally long clotting times with thromboplastin generation tests in patients with ruptured aneurysms. They found the incidence statistically even greater in cases of rebleeding, and greater yet the severer the bleed.

Adults have greater fibrinolytic activity in blood and CSF than children after SAH. The rise in activity begins on about the third day post-SAH and lasts for 2–3 weeks. (Note the similarity of this time sequence to that of post-SAH vasospasm.) Several authors have confirmed that both EACA and amino methylcyclohexane carboxylic acid (AMCA or tranexamic acid) cross the blood-brain barrier into the CSF after SAH and retard the abnormal clot lysis activity in CSF as well as in the bloodstream (31,88,171,188–190,192). For additional detailed reviews, see Bergin (15) and Mustard (117).

Although certain dosage guidelines for Amicar (EACA by Lederle Laboratories) or tranexamic acid (AMCA; not available for patients in the United States as of 1979) are available, many authors recommended testing the patient's streptokinase blood clot lysis time to determine proper dosage. The normal range is about 3 h. The Therapeutic range is over 16 h, and some recommended sufficient drug to keep the streptokinase clot lysis time at 48–72 h (50,112,113,119,122,123). [See Nibbelink (119) for details of the techniques.] Watanabe et al. (198) have used streptokinase euglobulin lysis time, keeping it at 130–150 s.

There are now a number of reports testifying to the efficiency of both EACA (1,2,11,32, 34–36,41,50,55,75,82,86,91,112–116,119–123, 124,136,139,146,154–157,171,180,186,196) and AMCA (3,21,37,38,54,79,97,98,149–151,188–190,192,198) as worthwhile agents reducing by one-half the 25% incidence of rebleed during the first 2 weeks after rupture of an intracranial aneurysm. There are also a number of neurosurgical centers not using this therapy, but their negative opinions have not yet been published, except for a few (57,58,138,195). In other words, a large body of opinion feels that there may be other factors responsible for the apparent reduction in incidence of early rebleed and many studies with EACA and AMCA have had inadequate controls. Hence, the final judgment is not yet in on the practical clinical value of these antifibrinolytic agents in terms of prophylaxis against rebleed.

Someda and co-workers (173) examined cerebral arteries of patients dying after rupture of an aneurysm. With the scanning electron microscope they noted a high incidence of endothelial injury, denudation of elastica, and mural thrombus formation (mistaken for "vasospasm" on angiography). They warned about the indiscriminate use of antifibrinolytic drugs in these situations (as a cause of cerebral thrombosis). Sonntag and Stein (174) presented three EACA-treated patients with arteriopathic complications (cerebral arteritis and thrombosis). Bergin (15) reviewed some of the reported complications of EACA therapy (including deep-vein thrombosis and disseminated thrombosis). In terms of percentages, however, the actual high-risk complication rate must be extremely low in the usual dosage setting. Giammusso and Vassallo (52) recommended not using antifibrinolytic therapy in very old patients. Mullan (112) wondered if the combination of EACA with methyldopa increased the adverse effects. Although not necessarily a complication, antifibrinolytic therapy seems to firm up the clot around the perianeurysmal dissection area at surgery. Patterson and Harpel (129) found that EACA and AMCA increase the strength of the hematoma inside experimental rat aortic pouches. Maurice-Williams (98) has seen fibrous tissue encasing aneurysms at surgery; he attributed this protective tissue to the preoperative use of AMCA.

EACA can be given intravenously or by mouth. Although there are many suggested regimes by various authors, a reasonable one is to give 6 g q 3 h for the first day post-SAH (i.e., 48 g total) and then 3 g q 3 h thereafter (i.e., 24 g daily until surgery or for 6 weeks). The regime will vary for an individual depending on the blood streptokinase clot lysis time. This clot lysis time should be at least between 16 and 24 h, but Mullan (112) recommended keeping it at 48 h. If no surgery is to be carried out, Mullan (112) used high total daily dosages of 48 g for 2 weeks post-SAH, then 36 g daily for 2 weeks, and finally 24 g daily for 2 weeks. Some physicians recommend continuous drip, hourly infusions, or q 2 h infusions rather than the q 3 h infusions mentioned above.

As with EACA, there is variance of dosage of AMCA among authors. A reasonable dosage intravenously is 1 g q 4 h for the first week post-SAH and 1 g q 6 h for the remaining time (until surgery or until the end of 6 weeks). A few physicians have added proteinase inhibitors to the AMCA regime (149–151,157), but such has not become common practice.

Summary

As the surgical treatment to prevent intracranial aneurysm rebleed advanced, so indeed has the medical treatment. The two must go hand-in-hand as best judged by the attending physician in order not only to remove this terrible threat to brain and life but also to do it with preservation of function and a useful quality to the patient's future.

Bibliography

1. Acosta-Rua GJ, et al.: Cerebral aneurysm. J Florida Med Assoc 63:847–849, 1976
2. Adams CBT, Chir M, Fearnside MR, et al.: An investigation with serial angiography into the evolution of cerebral arterial spasm following aneurysm. J Neurosurg 49:805–815, 1978
3. Aiba T, Kumagai N, Nakamura O, et al.: Antifibrinolytic therapy of patients with ruptured intracranial aneurysms for preoperative management. Excerp Med ICS No 418:98–99, 1977
4. Allcock JM, Drake CG: Ruptured intracranial aneurysms—The role of arterial spasm. J Neurosurg 22:21–29, 1965
5. Andrews MC: Blood pressure and subarachnoid haemorrhage. Lancet 2:1087–1089, 1933
6. Andrews RJ, Spiegel PK: Intracranial aneurysms. Age, sex, blood pressure, and multiplicity in an unselected series of patients. J Neurosurg 51:27–32, 1979
7. Ask-Upmark E, Ingvar D: A follow-up examination of 138 cases of subarachnoid hemorrhage. Acta Med Scand 138:15–31, 1950
8. Atkinson WJ: New approach to management of intracranial aneurysms. Lancet 1:5–9, 1975
9. Ayer WD: So-called spontaneous subarachnoid hemorrhage. A resumé with its medicolegal consideration. Am J Surg 26:143–151, 1934
10. Bakay L, Sweet WH: Cervical and intracranial intra-arterial pressures with and without vascular occlusion. Surg Gynec Obstet 95:67–75, 1952
11. Ballenger OM, Salcman M, Ducker TB, et al.: Prognosis of surgically treated intracranial ar-

terial aneurysm patients. JAMA 237:1845–1847, 1977
12. Bellotti C, Formaggio G, Arrigone M: Observations on the use of early external ventriculostomy in recent subarachnoid haemorrhage. Acta Neurochir 36:153–154, 1977
13. Benedict CR, Loach AB: Clinical significance of plasma adrenaline and noradrenaline concentrations in patients with subarachnoid haemorrhage. J Neurol Neurosurg Psychiat 41:113–117, 1978
14. Benton JG, Brown H, Rusk HA: Energy expended by patients on the bedpan and bedside commode. JAMA 144:1443–1447, 1950
15. Bergin JJ: The complications of therapy with epsilon-aminocaproic acid. Med Clin N Am 50:1669–1678, 1966
16. Black BK, Hicks SP: The relation of hypertension to arterial aneurysms of the brain. US Armed Forces Med J 3:1813–1818, 1952
17. Black SPW, German WJ: The treatment of internal carotid artery aneurysms by proximal arterial ligation. A follow-up study. J Neurosurg 10:590–601, 1953
18. Bramwell B: Clinical and pathological memoranda. IV.—Case of aneurism of the right internal carotid artery. Edinburgh Med J 32:97–108, 1886
19. Breunig KA: After the blowup—How to care for the patient with a ruptured cerebral aneurysm. Nursing 6:37–46, 1976
20. Carini E, Owens G: Neurological and Neurosurgical Nursing, 6th ed. St. Louis, Mosby, 1974, pp. 249–250
21. Chandra B: Treatment of subarachnoid hemorrhage from ruptured intracranial aneurysm with tranexamic acid: a double-blind clinical trial. Ann Neurol 3:502–504, 1978
22. Collier J: Observations on cerebral haemorrhage due to causes other than arteriosclerosis. Brit Med J 2:519–521, 1931
22a. Crompton MR: Recurrent haemorrhage from cerebral aneurysms and its prevention by surgery. J Neurol Neurosurg Psychiat 29:164–170, 1966
23. Cushing H: Some experimental and clinical observations concerning states of increased intracranial tension. Amer J Med Sci 124:375–400, 1902
24. Dandy WE: Intracranial Arterial Aneurysms. New York, Hafner; Ithica, New York, Comstock Publishing, 1944 (reprinted 1969)
25. Dott NM: Intracranial aneurysms: Cerebral arterio-radiography: surgical treatment. Edinburgh Med J 40 (section on Trans Med-Chir Soc Edinburgh):219–234, 1933
26. Drake CG: Cerebral aneurysm surgery—an update. In Scheinberg P (ed.): Cerebrovascular Diseases. Tenth Princeton Conference. New York, Raven Press, 1976, pp. 289–310
27. Early CB, Fink LH: Some fundamental applications of the law of Laplace in neurosurgery. Surg Neurol 6:185–189, 1976
28. Ferguson GG: Direct measurement of mean and pulsatile blood pressure of operation in human intracranial saccular aneurysms. J Neurosurg 36:560–563, 1972
29. Ferguson G: Physical factors in the initiation, growth, and rupture of human intracranial saccular aneurysms. J Neurosurg 37:666–677, 1972
30. Ferguson GG: Turbulence in human intracranial saccular aneurysms. J Neurosurg 33:485–497, 1970
31. Filizzolo F, D'Angelo V, Collice M, et al.: Fibrinolytic activity in blood and cerebrospinal fluid in subarachnoid hemorrhage from ruptured intracranial saccular aneurysm before and during EACA treatment. Eur Neurol 17:43–47, 1978
32. Filizzolo F, d'Angelo VA, Donati MB, et al.: Monitoring of antifibrinolytic therapy in subarachnoid haemorrhage from ruptured intracranial saccular aneurysms. Acta Neurochir 36:154–155, 1977
33. Finney LA, Gholston D: Cerebral aneurysm rupture during anticoagulant therapy with survival. JAMA 200:1127–1128, 1967
34. Flamm ES: Parasurgical treatment of aneurysms. Clin Neurosurg 24:240–247, 1977
35. Fleischer AS, Tindall GT: Preoperative management of ruptured cerebral aneurysms. Contemp Neurosurg 1:1–6, 1978
36. Fleischer AS, Tindall GT: Preoperative treatment of ruptured cerebral aneurysms. J Med Assoc Georgia 66:151–154, 1977
37. Fodstad H, Liliequist B, Schannong M, et al.: Tranexamic acid in the preoperative management of ruptured intracranial aneurysms. Surg Neurol 10:9–15, 1978
38. Fodstad H, Thulin C-A: Use of tranexamic acid (AMCA) in the preoperative management of patients with ruptured intracranial aneurysms. Excerp Med ICS No 418:98, 1977
39. Fox JL: Development of recent thoughts on intracranial pressure and the blood-brain barrier. J Neurosurg 21:909–967, 1964
40. Fox JL, Albin MS, Bader DCH, et al.: Microsurgical treatment of neurovascular disease. Neurosurgery 3:285–337, 1978
41. Fox JL, Nugent GR: Recent advances in intracranial aneurysm surgery. West Virginia Med J 72:104–105, 1976
42. Freeman W: Intracranial aneurisms. Med Ann DC 1:206–212, 1932
43. French LA: The use of steroids in the treat-

ment of cerebral edema. Bull NY Acad Med 42:301–311, 1966
44. French LA, Blake PS: Subarachnoid hemorrhages and intracranial aneurysms. J Lancet 70:459–466, 1950
45. French LA, Chou SN, Long DM: The direct approach to intracranial aneurysms. Clin Neurosurg 15:117–132, 1968
46. French LA, Ortiz-Saurez HJ: Anterior communicating artery aneurysms: technique of operation and results. Clin Neurosurg 21:115–119, 1974
47. Frost EAM: Respiratory problems associated with head trauma. Neurosurgery 1:300–306, 1977
48. German WJ, Black SPW: Experimental production of carotid aneurysms. New Engl J Med 250:104–106, 1954
49. German WJ, Black SPW: Intra-aneurysmal hemodynamics—jet action. Circ Res 3:463–468, 1955
50. Geronemus R, Herz DA, Shulman K: Streptokinase clot lysis time in patients with ruptured intracranial aneurysms. J Neurosurg 40:499–503, 1974
51. Geyer K-H: Strömungsverhaltnisse im grossen Karotisaneurysma. Fortschr Roentgenstr 103:440–443, 1965
52. Giammusso V, Vassallo A: Medical treatment of subarachnoid hemorrhage due to cerebral aneurysm in old patients. J Neurosurg Sci 19:70–71, 1975
53. Giannotta SL, Kindt GW: Total morbidity and mortality rates of patients with surgically treated intracranial aneurysms. Neurosurgery 4:125–128, 1979
54. Gibbs JR, Corkill AGL: Use of an anti-fibrinolytic agent (tranexamic acid) in the management of ruptured intracranial aneurysms. Postgrad Med J 47:199–200, 1971
55. Gibbs JR, O'Gorman P: Fibrinolysis in subarachnoid haemorrhage. Postgrad Med J 43:779–784, 1967
56. Gilchrist AR: Discussion of Dott NM: Intracranial aneurysms: Cerebral arterio-radiography: surgical treatment. Edinburgh Med J 40 (section on Trans Med-Chir Soc Edinburgh):235–236, 1933
57. Girvin JP: The failure of antifibrinolytic agents to improve the operative treatment of ruptured intracranial aneurysms. In Morley TP (ed.): Current Controversies in Neurosurgery. Philadelphia, Saunders, 1976, pp. 279–281
58. Girvin JP: The use of antifibrinolytic agents in the preoperative treatment of ruptured intracranial aneurysms. Trans Am Neurol Assoc 98:150–152, 1973
59. Globus JH, Schwab JM: Intracranial aneurysms. Their origin and clinical behavior in a series of verified cases. J Mt Sinai Hosp 8:547–578, 1942
60. Gowers WR: A Manual of Diseases of the Nervous System, Vol. 2. London, Churchhill, 1888, pp. 494–504
61. Graf CJ: Surgical treatment of angiographically localized intracranial aneurysms. A follow-up report. Neurology 6:686–692, 1956
62. Grinker RR, Bucy PC, Sahs AL: Neurology, 5th ed. Springfield, Ill., Charles C Thomas, 1960, pp. 773–784
63. Hamby WB: Intracranial Aneurysms. Springfield, Ill., Charles C Thomas, 1952
64. Hamby WB: Intracranial surgery for aneurysms. Progr Neurol Surg 3:1–65, 1969
65. Hamby WB: Remarks concerning intracranial aneurysm surgery. Clin Neurosurg 17:1–17, 1970
66. Hamby WB: Subarachnoid hemorrhage from congenital aneurysm of the circle of Willis. Postgrad Med 34:317–322, 1963
67. Hamby WB: The surgical treatment of intracranial vascular lesions. Bull NY Acad Med 45:339–350, 1969
68. Hamby WB: Treatment of ruptured intracranial aneurysms. Surg Clin N Am 34:1063–1075, 1954
69. Hassler O, Fodstad H: Fibrinolytic activity in the walls of cerebral saccular aneurysms. Acta Neurochir 37:49–55, 1977
70. Heidrich R: Subarachnoid haemorrhage. In Vinken PJ, Bruyn GW (eds.): Handbook of Clinical Neurology. Vol 12, Vascular Diseases of the Nervous System, Part II. Amsterdam, North Holland Publ; New York, American Elsevier Publ, 1972, pp. 68–204
71. Howell CMH: Some notes on cerebral aneurysms. Barth Hosp J 39:130–133, 1932
72. Hugh AE, Fox JA: Circulatory cavitation. "Bubbles in the blood." Lancet 2:717–718, 1963
73. Humble WE: Intra-cranial aneurism. Lancet 2:489–490, 874, 1875
74. Hung EJ, Botwin MR: Mechanics of rupture of cerebral saccular aneurysms. J Biomech 8:385–392, 1975
75. Hunt WE, Kosnik EJ: Timing and perioperative care in intracranial aneurysm surgery. Clin Neurosurg 21:79–89, 1974
76. Hunter AR: Neurosurgical Anaesthesia, 2nd ed. Philadelphia, Lippincott, 1975, pp. 161–192
77. Hyland HH: Spontaneous subarachnoid haemorrhage (with report of twelve cases). Canad Med Assoc J 29:145–149, 1933
78. Imanaga H, Osugi T, Kagawa M, et al.: Fibrinolytic activity of cerebrospinal fluid in sub-

arachnoid hemorrhage. Neurol Surg (Tokyo) 5:51–58, 1977

79. Ito K, Yoshihama Y, Terakado Y, et al.: Intentional delayed surgery for ruptured intracranial aneurysms. Excerp Med ICS No 418:93, 1977
80. Jain KK: Mechanism of rupture of intracranial saccular aneurysms. Surgery 54:347–350, 1963
81. Jain KK: Partial carotid occlusion as treatment for intracranial internal carotid aneurysms. Canad Med Assoc J 88:247–251, 1963
82. Jain KK: Surgery of anterior communicating aneurysms: experience with various techniques and evolution of a modified approach. Surg Neurol 2:31–33, 1974
83. Jamieson KG: Treatment of cerebral aneurysms. Med J Australia 1:198–200, 1976
84. Jerrard W, Burton AC: Demonstration of hemodynamic principles in particular of turbulent and stream-line flow. J Appl Physiol 4:620–622, 1952
85. Keller AZ: Hypertension, age and residence in the survival with subarachnoid hemorrhage. Am J Epidem 91:139–147, 1970
86. Khilko VA, Shklyarova ED: A method of artificial thrombosis of arterial aneurysms using epsilon-aminocaproic acid and other coagulants in addition to regionally retarded circulation (preliminary report). Vop Neirokhir 33:6–11, July–August 1969
87. Kirgis HD, Echols DH: Management of intracranial arterial aneurysms. Surg Clin N Am 33:1003–1021, 1953
88. Levy BJ, Silver D: Treatment of subarachnoid hemorrhage: the ability of epsilon aminocaproic acid to cross the blood brain barrier and reduce the spinal fluid fibrinolytic activity. Surg Forum 19:413–414, 1968
89. Lindsay JSB: Some observations on spontaneous subarachnoid haemorrhage. N Zealand Med J 49:722–731, 1950
90. Logue V: Posterior fossa aneurysms. Clin Neurosurg 11:183–207, 1964
91. Lougheed WM, Marshall BM: The diploscope in intracranial aneurysm surgery: results in 40 patients. Canad J Surg 12:75–82, 1969
92. Maroon JC: Comment. Neurosurgery 4:128, 1979
93. Maroon JC, Nelson PB: Hypovolemia in patients with subarachnoid hemorrhage: therapeutic implications. Neurosurgery 4:223–226, 1979
94. Martin MA: Case of a patient with a cerebral aneurysm. Am J Nursing 65:90–95, April 1965
95. Martin MA: Nursing management of a patient with cerebral aneurysm. J Nurs Educ 6:27–39, 1967
96. Martinez Coll A, Del Corral JF, Yazawa S, et al.: Intra-aneurysmal pressure differences in human saccular aneurysms. Surg Neurol 6:93–96, 1976
97. Maurice-Williams R: Prolonged antifibrinolysis: an effective non-surgical treatment for ruptured intracranial aneurysms? Br Med J 1:945–947, 1978
98. Maurice-Williams R: Prolonged antifibrinolysis—an effective non-surgical treatment for ruptured intracranial aneurysms? J Neurol Neurosurg Psychiat 41:188, 1978
99. McCormick WF, Schmalstieg EJ: The relationship of arterial hypertension to intracranial aneurysms. Arch Neurol 34:285–287, 1977
100. McDonald DA: Murmurs in relation to turbulence and eddy formation in the circulation. Circulation 16:278–281, 1957
101. Meadows SP: Intracranial aneurysms. In Feiling A (ed.): Modern Trends in Neurology. London, Butterworth, 1951, pp. 391–465
102. Meredith JM: The inefficiency of lumbar puncture for the removal of red blood cells from the cerebrospinal fluid. Surgery 9:524–533, 1941
103. Merritt HH: The diagnosis and treatment of vascular lesions in brain. Med Clin N Am 22:577–589, 1938
104. Merwarth HR, Freiman IS: Hydrocephalus following subarachnoid hemorrhage. Report of a case with pathologic study. Brooklyn Hosp J 1:149–157, 1939
105. Meyer JS, Bauer RB: Medical treatment of spontaneous intracranial hemorrhage by the use of hypotensive drugs. Neurology 12:36–47, 1962
106. Moltke P: Plasminogen activator in animal meninges. Proc Soc Exp Biol Med 98:377–379, 1958
107. Moritake K: Biomechanical studies on the pathogenesis of cerebral aneurysms and the mechanism of their growth and rupture. Part I. Structure and mechanical behaviors of cerebral arteries. Arch Jpn Chir 44:87–107, 1975
108. Moritake K: Biomechanical studies on the pathogenesis of cerebral aneurysms and the mechanism of their growth and rupture. Part II. Hemodynamics at cerebral arterial bifurcations and in cerebral aneurysms. Arch Jpn Chir 44:108–123, 1975
109. Moritake K, Handa H, Okumura A, et al.: Stiffness of cerebral arteries—its role in the pathogenesis of cerebral aneurysms. Neurol Med Chir (Tokyo) 12 (Part 1):47–53, 1974
110. Moritake K, Hazama F, Handa H, et al.: Variation of the circle of Willis related to the pathogenesis of cerebral aneurysm. Neurol Med Chir (Tokyo) 16 (Part 2): 427–435, 1976
111. Moroz LA: Increased blood fibrinolytic activity after aspirin ingestion. New Engl J Med 296:525–529, 1977

112. Mullan S: Conservative management of the recently ruptured aneurysm. Surg Neurol 3:27–32, 1975
113. Mullan S: The initial medical management of ruptured intracranial aneurysms. In Morley TP (ed.): Current Controversies in Neurosurgery. Philadelphia, Saunders, 1976, pp. 259–269
114. Mullan S, Dawley J: Antifibrinolytic therapy for intracranial aneurysms. J Neurosurg 28:21–23, 1968
115. Mullan S, Hanlon K, Brown F: Management of 136 consecutive supratentorial berry aneurysms. J Neurosurg 49:794–804, 1978
116. Mullan S, Raimondi AJ, Dobben G, et al.: Electrically induced thrombosis in intracranial aneurysms. J Neurosurg 22:539–547, 1965
117. Mustard JF: Platelets and thrombosis in acute myocardial infarction. Hospital Practice 115–128, January 1972
118. Neil-Dwyer G, Cruickshank J, Stott A, et al.: The urinary catecholamine and plasma cortisol levels in patients with subarachnoid haemorrhage. J Neurol Sci 22:375–382, 1974
119. Nibbelink DW: Antifibrinolytic activity during administration of epsilon-aminocaproic acid. Stroke 2:555–558, 1971
120. Nibbelink DW: Cooperative aneurysm study: antihypertensive and antifibrinolytic therapy following subarachnoid hemorrhage from ruptured intracranial aneurysm. In Whisnant JP, Sandok BA (eds.): Cerebral Vascular Disease. New York, Grune & Stratton, 1975, pp. 155–165
121. Nibbelink DW: The role of fluid restriction in treatment of acute subarachnoid hemorrhage following ruptured intracranial aneurysm. Neurology 24:372–373, 1974
122. Nibbelink DW, Knowler LA: Cooperative study of intracranial aneurysms and subarachnoid hemorrhage. Report on a randomized treatment study. II. Objectives and design of randomized aneurysm study. Stroke 5:552–556, 1974
123. Nibbelink DW, Torner JC, Henderson WG: Intracranial aneurysms and subarachnoid hemorrhage. A cooperative study. Antifibrinolytic therapy in recent onset subarachnoid hemorrhage. Stroke 6:622–629, 1975
124. Norlén G, Thulin C-A: The use of antifibrinolytic substances in ruptured intracranial aneurysms. Neurochirurgia (Stuttgart) 12:100–102, 1969
125. Nornes H: Monitoring of patients with intracranial aneurysms. Clin Neurosurg 22:321–331, 1975
126. Nornes H, Grip A, Wikeby P: Intraoperative evaluation of cerebral hemodynamics using directional Doppler technique. Part 2. Saccular aneurysms. J Neurosurg 50:570–577, 1979
127. Nornes H, Magnaes B: Intracranial pressure in patients with ruptured saccular aneurysm. J Neurosurg 36:537–547, 1972
128. Olinger CP, Wasserman JF: Electronic stethoscope for detection of cerebral aneurysm, vasospasm and arterial disease. Surg Neurol 8:298–312, 1977
129. Patterson RH Jr, Harpel P: The effect of epsilon aminocaproic acid and tranexamic acid on thrombus size and strength in a simulated arterial aneurysm. J Neurosurg 34:365–371, 1971
130. Peerless SJ, Kassell NF: ICP, aneurysms and subarachnoid hemorrhage. J Canad Sci Neurol 3:263, 1976
131. Peet MM, Isberg EM, Bassett RC: Hypertension complicated spontaneous subarachnoid hemorrhage. Am J Surg 78:912–917, 1949
132. Pia HW, Pertuiset B, Brihaye J: Neurosurgical training in Europe. Acta Neurochir 40:335–344, 1978
133. Pool JL, Potts DG: Aneurysms and Arteriovenous Anomalies of the Brain. Diagnosis and Treatment. New York, Harper & Row, 1965
134. Poppen JL: Operative treatment for aneurysms of the anterior communicating artery. Clin Neurosurg 11:8–13, 1964
135. Porter JM, Acinapura AJ, Kapp JP, et al.: Fibrinolysis in the central nervous system. Neurology 19:47–52, 1969
136. Post KD, Flamm ES, Goodgold A, et al.: Ruptured intracranial aneurysms. Case morbidity and mortality. J Neurosurg 46:290–295, 1977
137. Potter JM, McDonald DA: Cerebral haemodynamics. Lancet 2:919–920, 1954
138. Profeta G, Castellano F, Guarnieri L, et al.: Antifibrinolytic therapy in the treatment of subarachnoid haemorrhage caused by arterial aneurysms. J Neurosurg Sci 19:77–78, 1975
139. Ransohoff J, Goodgold AL: Nonoperative management of aneurysms. In Youmans JR (ed.): Neurological Surgery, Vol 2. Philadelphia, Saunders, 1973, pp. 724–730
140. Ransohoff J, Goodgold AL, Benjamin MV: Preoperative management of patients with ruptured intracranial aneurysms. J Neurosurg 36:525–530, 1972
141. Ransohoff J, Guy HH, Mazzia VDB, et al.: Deliberate hypotension in surgery of cerebral aneurysm and correlative animal studies. NYS J Med 69:913–918, 1969
142. Richardson DW, Honour HJ, Fenton GW, et al.: Variation in arterial pressure throughout the day and night. Clin Sci 26:445–460, 1964
143. Richardson JC: Discussion of Hamby WB: Spontaneous subarachnoid hemorrhage of aneurysmal origin. JAMA 136:527–528, 1948
144. Richardson JC, Hyland HH: Intracranial aneu-

rysms. A clinical and pathological study of subarachnoid and intracerebral hemorrhage caused by berry aneurysms. Medicine 20:1–83, 1941
145. Sahs AL: Hypotension and hypothermia in the treatment of intracranial aneurysms. In Sahs AL, Perret GE, Locksley HB, Nishioka H (eds.): Intracranial Aneurysms and Subarachnoid Hemorrhage. A Cooperative Study. Philadelphia, Lippincott, 1969, pp. 143–149
145a. Sahs AL: Report on the cooperative study of intracranial aneurysms and subarachnoid hemorrhage. Section VII. Hypotension and hypothermia in the treatment of intracranial aneurysms. J Neurosurg 25:593–600, 1966
146. Salazar JL: Treatment of ruptured and unruptured internal carotid artery aneurysms. Surg Neurol 11:451–455, 1979
147. Sands IJ: Diagnosis and management of subarachnoid hemorrhage. Arch Neurol Psychiat 46:973–1005, 1941
148. Schemm GW: Blood clot absorption and organization in the cerebrospinal fluid. Surg Forum 17:423–425, 1966
149. Schisano G: Antifibrinolytics in the treatment of subarachnoid hemorrhage due to rupture of arterial aneurysm. J Neurosurg Sci 18:39–46, 1974
150. Schisano G: Antifibrinolytics in the treatment of subarachnoid hemorrhages due to ruptured aneurysms. J Neurosurg Sci 19:79–80, 1975
151. Schisano G: The use of antifibrinolytic drugs in aneurysmal subarachnoid hemorrhage. Surg Neurol 10:217–222, 1978
152. Schwartz HG: Subarachnoid hemorrhage and intracranial aneurysm. Postgrad Med 4:307–314, 1948
153. Scott RM, Ballantine HT Jr: Spontaneous thrombosis in a giant middle cerebral artery aneurysm. Case report. J Neurosurg 37:361–363, 1972
154. Selverstone B: Coating of intracranial aneurysms with nontoxic adherent plastics. In Schmidek HH, Sweet WH (eds.): Current Techniques in Operative Neurosurgery. New York, Grune & Stratton, 1977, pp. 31–40
155. Sengupta RP, So SC, Villarejo-Ortega FJ: Use of epsilon aminocaproic acid (EACA) in the preoperative management of ruptured intracranial aneurysms. J Neurosurg 44:479–484, 1976
156. Shields CB: Current trends in management of cerebral aneurysms. J Ky Med Assoc 75:529–535, 1977
157. Sicuteri F: Treatment of subarachnoid and other intracranial hemorrhages with proteinase inhibitors. Ann NY Acad Sci 146:682–700, 1968
158. Simkins TE, Stehbens WE: Vibrational behavior of arterial aneurysms. Letters in Applied and Engineering Sciences 1:85–100, 1973
159. Slosberg PS: Hypotensive therapy in acute intracranial bleeding. J Mt Sinai Hosp 23:825–831, 1956
160. Slosberg PS: Hypotensive therapy of acute intracranial hemorrhage: further studies. J Mt Sinai Hosp 26:553–561, 1959
161. Slosberg PS: Medical management of intracranial aneurysm. Heart Bull 11:73–77, 1962
162. Slosberg PS: Medical treatment of intracranial aneurysm. An analysis of 15 cases. Neurology 10:1085–1089, 1960
163. Slosberg PS: Nonoperative management of ruptured intracranial aneurysms. Clin Neurosurg 21:90–99, 1974
164. Slosberg PS: On some aspects of vascular anomalies of the circle of Willis. Confin Neurol 19:273–301, 1959
165. Slosberg PS: Subarachnoid hemorrhage with vertebro-basilar aneurysm. Report of eight cases with medical management; no deaths. Acta Neurol Scand 42:515–536, 1966
166. Slosberg PS: The current status of medical treatment of intracranial aneurysms. Prog Neurol Surg 3:230–248, 1969
167. Slosberg PS: Treatment and prevention of stroke. I. Subarachnoid hemorrhage due to ruptured intracranial aneurysm. NYS J Med 73:279–288, 1973
168. Slosberg PS: Treatment of intracranial aneurysm in the older patient. Geriatrics 18:557–564, 1963
169. Slosberg PS: Treatment of ruptured intracranial aneurysms by induced hypotension. Mt Sinai J Med (NY) 40:82–90, 1973
170. Slosberg PS: Treatment of ruptured aneurysms with induced hypotension. In Fields WS, Sahs AL (eds.): Intracranial Aneurysms and Subarachnoid Hemorrhage. Springfield, Illinois, Charles C Thomas, 1965, pp. 221–233
171. Smith RR, Upchurch JJ: Monitoring antifibrinolytic therapy in subarachnoid hemorrhage. J Neurosurg 38:339–344, 1973
172. Snyckers FD: The treatment of cerebral aneurysms. A report on 51 cases. S Afr Med J 50:835–839, 1976
173. Someda K, Morita K, Yamanouchi Y, et al.: Mural thrombus as a cause of prolonged so-called vasospasm following aneurysmal rupture. Excerp Med ICS No 418:98, 1977
174. Sonntag VKH, Stein BM: Arteriopathic complications during treatment of subarachnoid hemorrhage with epsilon aminocaproic acid. J Neurosurg 40:480–485, 1974
174a. Spence JD, Pesout J, Melmon KL: Effects of antihypertensive drugs on blood velocity in Rhesus monkeys. Stroke 8:589–594, 1977
175. Sprong W: The disappearance of blood from

the cerebrospinal fluid in traumatic subarachnoid haemorrhage. The ineffectiveness of repeated lumbar punctures. Surg Gynec Obstet 58:705–710, 1934

175a. Stehbens WE: Hypertension and cerebral aneurysms. Med J Aust 49:8–10, 1962

176. Stehbens WE: Pathology of the Cerebral Blood Vessels. St. Louis, Mosby, 1972

177. Stehbens WE: Turbulence of blood flow. Quart J Exp Physiol 44:110–117, 1959

178. Suzuki J, Yoshimoto T, Hori S: Continuous ventricular drainage to lessen surgical risk in ruptured intracranial aneurysm. Surg Neurol 2:87–90, 1974

179. Symonds CP: Spontaneous subarachnoid haemorrhage. Quart J Med 18:93–122, 1924–1925

180. Sypert GW: Intracranial aneurysms: natural history and surgical management. Compr Ther 4:64–73, 1978

181. Takashima S, Koga M, Tanaka K: Fibrinolytic activity of human brain and cerebral spinal fluid. Brit J Exp Path 50:533–539, 1969

182. Tamaki N, Kusunoki T, Ohi S, et al.: Clinical study on rebleeding of cerebral aneurysms—with special reference to the warning signs of rebleeding and antifibrinolytic treatment during waiting time for surgery. Neurol Surg (Tokyo) 3:647–654, 1975

183. Tang B-H, McKenna PG, Rovit RL: Primary fibrinolytic syndrome associated with subarachnoid hemorrhage. A case report. Angiology 24:627–634, 1973

184. Thomson AT: A case of aneurisms within the skull, terminating in apoplexy and paralysis, with clinical remarks. Lond Edinburgh Monthly J Med Sci 2:557–563, 1842

185. Tomonaga M, Fukushina T, Tanaka A, et al.: Clinical and pathological study of rebleeding of intracranial aneurysm. Based on 7 cases expired by rebleeding during hospital stay. Neurol Med Chir (Tokyo) 18:49–55, 1978

186. Toole JF, Patel AN: Cerebrovascular Disorders, 2nd ed. New York, McGraw-Hill, 1974, pp. 280–313

187. Tovi D: Fibrinolytic activity of human brain. A histochemical study. Acta Neurol Scand 49:152–162, 1973

188. Tovi D: Preoperative management of patients with aneurysmal subarachnoid hemorrhage. J Neurosurg Sci 19:59–64, 1975

189. Tovi D: The use of antifibrinolytic drugs to prevent early recurrent aneurysmal subarachnoid haemorrhage. Acta Neurol Scand 49:163–175, 1973

190. Tovi D, Nilsson IM, Thulin C-A: Fibrinolysis and subarachnoid haemorrhage. Inhibitory effect of tranexamic acid. A clinical study. Acta Neurol Scand 48:393–402, 1972

191. Tovi D, Nilsson IM, Thulin C-A: Fibrinolytic activity of the cerebrospinal fluid after subarachnoid haemorrhage. Acta Neurol Scand 49:1–9, 1973

192. Tovi D, Thulin C-A: Ability of tranexamic acid to cross the blood-brain barrier and its use in patients with ruptured intracranial aneurysms. Acta Neurol Scand 48:257, 1972

193. Troupp H: The management of intracranial arterial aneurysms in the acute stage. In Krayenbühl H (ed.): Advances and Technical Standards in Neurosurgery, Vol 3. New York, Springer-Verlag, 1976, pp. 35–46

194. Uttley AHC, Buckell M: Biochemical changes after spontaneous subarachnoid haemorrhage. Part III. Coagulation and lysis with special reference to recurrent haemorrhage. J Neurol Neurosurg Psychiat 31:621–627, 1968

195. Van Rossum J, Wintzen AR, Endtz LJ, et al.: Effect of tranexamic acid on rebleeding alter subarachnoid hemorrhage: a double-blind controlled clinical trial. Ann Neurol 2:242–245, 1977

196. Wallace CT: Anesthesia for intracranial aneurysms. South Med J 68:725–729, 1975

197. Walton, JN: Subarachnoid Haemorrhage. Edinburgh, E & S Livingstone, 1956

198. Watanabe H, Ito M, Chigasaki H, et al.: Antifibrinolytic therapy in ruptured intracranial aneurysm through repeated monitoring of fibrinolytic activity of blood. Neurol Med Chir (Tokyo) 16 (Part 1):91–96, 1976

199. Weiss HJ: Antiplatelet drugs—A new pharmacologic approach to the prevention of thrombosis. Am Heart J 92:86–102, 1976

200. Wilson SAK, Bruce NA: Neurology, 2nd ed, Vol 3. Baltimore, Williams & Wilkins, 1955, pp. 1485–1496, 1522–1523

201. Wolf AV: Demonstration concerning pressure-tension relations in various organs. Science 115:243–244, 1952

202. Wolfe HRI: Spontaneous subarachnoid haemorrhage. A surgical challenge. Brit J Surg 40:319–325, 1953

202a. Wood JH, Snyder LL, Simeone FA: Failure of intravascular volume expansion without hemodilution to elevate cortical blood flow in region of experimental focal ischemia. J Neurosurg 56:80–91, 1982

203. Wright RL: Intraaneurysmal pressure reduction with carotid occlusion. Observations in three cases of middle cerebral aneurysms. J Neurosurg 29:139–142, 1968

204. Zucker MB: Platelet agglutination and vasoconstriction as factors in spontaneous hemostasis in normal, thrombocytopenic, heparinized and hypoprothrombinemic rats. Am J Physiol 148:275–289, 1947

23

Anesthesiology

I. Management

Richard L. Keenan

Evaluation and Preparation

The preanesthetic evaluation of patients scheduled for surgical repair of intracranial aneurysm begins with the neurologic status. The patient's level of consciousness is important in determining the need for premedicant drugs and in planning the emergence phase of anesthesia after operation. Presence of mass lesions (such as hematoma), hydrocephalus, or brain swelling should be noted since these will make more difficult the production of a "slack" brain during surgery.

In anticipation of the use of induced hypotension, the patient's cardiovascular system is evaluated with a careful history looking especially for evidence of ischemic heart disease (previous infarction, angina), a 12-lead electrocardiogram, and a chest x-ray (to determine any presence of cardiac enlargement). A previous history of hypertension and its medical treatment should be noted. Antihypertensive drugs, if employed, are continued up to the day of operation (57). It is useful to review the range of blood pressures recorded on the hospital chart. Hypertension, while not contraindicating the use of induced hypotension, may modify the lowest acceptable level of blood pressure during operation (27,54).

Renal function, and in particular the presence of impaired function, is best determined from blood urea nitrogen and creatinine levels. If renal function is unimpaired, deep hypotension can be undertaken without fear of kidney damage (47).

Respiratory function is evaluated as for any major operation. If the patient has been awake and alert for several days, no special problems need be anticipated. However, if a previous intracerebral bleed has made the patient stuporous, clearance of tracheobronchial secretions may not have been optimal; atelectasis and pulmonary infection may be present. While this does not contraindicate necessary surgery, it will increase the risk. Moreover, knowing about it in advance gives the anesthesiologist the opportunity to improve matters by aggressive suctioning and hyperinflation of the lungs after anesthetic induction and tracheal intubation.

Adequate hydration and a normal circulating blood volume are also less likely in a stuporous, bedridden patient than in one who is awake and ambulatory. Fluid deficits make the conduct of induced hypotension more difficult and are best corrected (or avoided) with adequate preoperative intravenous therapy.

Preanesthetic medication of patients scheduled for intracranial aneurysm repair is variable. Those with normal neurologic function and without an elevated intracranial pressure may safely be given any traditional premedicant drug. However, in the presence of any cerebral dysfunction, all depressant drugs are best avoided (40). A prudent approach would be to prescribe an antianxiety drug such as a benzodiazepine or barbiturate in those patients who are alert and anxious, and to use nothing in stuporous patients. Anticholinergic drugs such as atropine or glycopyrrolate may be safely used in any patient if desired; a drying agent prior to general anesthesia is no longer considered mandatory (53).

In the immediate preoperative period, just before anesthetic induction, venous cannulation is performed. Since it is possible that a large volume of blood might have to be given rapidly, at least one and preferably two large-bore (14- or 16-guage) cannulae will be required. Blood-warming coils and pumping devices should be tested and ready. A minimum of two units of whole blood or packed red cells should be immediately available.

Monitoring

Cardiovascular Monitoring

With the widespread use of induced hypotension during cerebral aneurysm surgery, direct arterial pressure monitoring has become universally accepted (1,4,17,34,39,41,60,62,71). The continuous display of an accurate pressure determination (especially in very low ranges) represents an important advance over the indirect, or cuff, method in that adjusting the drip rate of a rapidly acting and evanescent drug such as sodium nitroprusside is greatly facilitated by direct arterial pressure monitoring. Indeed, an automated servo device which uses continuous arterial pressure information to control the drip rate of a hypotensive agent may soon be available (5).

The radial artery is the preferred site of cannulation for pressure monitoring. When a small cannula (20 gauge or less) is used and adequate collateral flow via the ulnar artery is demonstrated, radial artery cannulation is remarkably safe (7,9). The dorsalis pedis artery may be safely used as an alternative (4); brachial artery cannulation has a slightly higher incidence of postcannulation thrombosis (6) and should be used only as a last resort.

The position of the transducer in an arterial pressure recording system is normally not as critical as in venous pressure determination. However, with deep hypotension (pressures of 30–40 torr) the "zero" level does become important. Aitken and Drake (4) have recommended that the arterial transducer be placed at the level of the cerebral cortex in order to obtain the perfusion pressure of the brain. Moreover, in discussing arterial blood pressure, especially regarding the end-point of a hypotensive technique, it is important to specify whether "systolic" or "mean" pressure is meant. Mean arterial pressure (MAP), which is readily obtained from electronic recording systems currently used for direct arterial pressure monitoring, is preferable since it more accurately represents tissue perfusion pressure than does systolic pressure.

Because control of arterial pressure (especially avoidance of hypertension) is an important aspect of anesthetic induction and tracheal intubation in patients with cerebral aneurysms, arterial cannulation should be performed and monitoring begun prior to induction.

Central venous pressure monitoring is useful in determining the existence of any preoperative fluid deficit and in following the patient's volume status during any period of blood loss and its replacement. A central venous catheter may be inserted after induction by any convenient route other than via the jugular system. The catheter tip should lie within the thorax, and the "zero" point of the recording device should be placed at the level of the right atrium (e.g., the anterior axillary line). Recent evidence suggests that significant inaccuracy is inherent in water manometers (16,43); an electronic transducer system is more accurate and, with the display of the waveform, provides the additional information of the venous pressure waves and the effect of ventilation.

Pulmonary artery catheterization is not normally required for cerebral aneurysm surgery. However, it should be considered in any patient with cardiac disease in which left ventricular function is (or may be) impaired, since in these cases central venous pressure monitoring may not be a reliable guide to cardiac filling pressure (43).

Electrocardiographic monitoring is now routine during any general anesthetic, craniotomy being no exception. In cerebral aneurysm surgery, where induced hypotension is planned, careful lead placement can yield useful information in addition to that of rate and rhythm. A precordial lead (V5) or a 3-lead monitoring system with the positive lead over the precordium can be useful in diagnosing ischemia during surgery (44), provided the electronic display system does not distort the S-T segment. This can be of considerable value in the assessment of coronary perfusion during induced hypotension in a patient with known coronary artery disease.

Electrocardiographic abnormalities suggestive of myocardial ischemia (S-T segment and T-wave changes) have been reported after subarachnoid hemorrhage (46,48,72), and they may be related to sympathetic overactivity. Plasma catecholamine levels have been found to be elevated (10). Similar EKG changes have been reported with severely elevated intracranial pressure from other causes (29). It is therefore possible, though not yet proven, that these ST-T changes represent myocardial ischemia in susceptible patients caused by the arterial hypertension frequently seen with severe intracranial insults.

Respiratory Monitoring

Arterial blood gas analysis is the definitive measure of adequate ventilatory function during craniotomy, and its ready availability is as much an indication for arterial cannulation as is pressure monitoring. End-tidal CO_2 monitoring is not mandatory, but it can afford the anesthetist a convenience early in the course of the anesthetic by guiding him in the initial setting and adjustment of the mechanical ventilator.

When a volume-limited ventilator is used, the airway pressure (as read from the breathing system pressure gauge) provides useful information regarding compliance and airway resistance. Accumulation of secretions or a kinking endotracheal tube will be manifested by a rising airway pressure. System leaks and partial disconnects will result in a fall in pressure. In addition, monitoring of breath sounds with an esophageal stethoscope is widely practiced.

Neurologic Monitoring

Currently, intraoperative monitoring of neurologic function during aneurysm surgery is of uncertain value. Intracranial pressure (ICP) monitoring is normally not necessary since ICP is usually not elevated, and the cranium is eventually opened in any event. The electroencephalogram (EEG) is known to reflect the effects of anesthesia (11,20,26) as well as those due to cerebral ischemia during cardiac surgery (69), and the EEG has been used successfully as a monitor of cerebral perfusion during carotid endarterectomy (64). However, in a recent series, scalp encephalography during intracranial aneurysm surgery with deep hypotension (MAP 55 torr) failed to predict three of four severe postoperative neurologic deficits (42). A more fruitful approach for the future might be that of Eisenberg and his colleagues (25) in which cortical electrodes were used to measure responses evoked by direct cortical stimulation during induced hypotension. The cortical evoked responses were seen to diminish as mean arterial pressure fell; the level of hypotension at which cortical responses disappeared varied from patient to patient.

Miscellaneous Monitoring

Body temperature should be monitored during aneurysm surgery, as with all major procedures—and especially if hypothermia is intended. Urine volume should also be recorded; all patients should have an indwelling catheter placed prior to operation and connected to a calibrated collection system. Induced hypotension, anesthetics, hyperosmotic agents, and changes in fluid volume will all affect urine volume. Additionally, measurement of urinary electrolytes and osmolality can be made easily.

Serum electrolyte levels and osmolality should be determined, especially when diuretic therapy with hyperosmolar agents is used or when surgery is prolonged. Blood glucose levels are useful in diabetic patients and are superior to urinary glucose values.

Anesthetic Agents and Techniques

Two basic principles must be considered in all decisions regarding anesthetic drugs or methods: (a) As with any craniotomy, the intracranial pressure and brain size must be kept minimal and (b) the aneurysm must not be induced to rupture. Obviously, a smooth anesthetic, without coughing or straining and without dramatic increases in blood pressure in response to stress, subserves both principles. In addition, anesthetic agents which decrease cerebral blood flow and metabolic rate may be used to minimize brain size while anesthetics which are cerebral vasodilators are avoided; the blood pressure within the aneurysm can be kept artificially low with hypotensive drugs.

Induction and Tracheal Intubation

For the anesthesiologist, this is the most critical and stressful period of the entire operation. He must therefore be thoroughly organized and prepared before he begins, must not allow himself to be rushed, and must have the undivided attention of at least one assistant during the induction period.

Unconsciousness is best produced with a barbiturate such as thiopental since, in addition to their hypnotic properties, barbiturates produce a 50% fall in cerebral metabolic rate and cerebral blood flow in doses sufficient to cause sleep (56). Furthermore, rapid intravenous barbiturate infusion is associated with a fall in ICP in those patients with space-occupying lesions (63). Large bolus doses are often also associated with a fall in arterial pressure, which in the context of cerebral aneurysm surgery is beneficial. Diazepam has a similar effect on cerebral blood flow (18), as does Althesin (70), and these may be used as an alternative to barbiturate induction. Ketamine, however, is a potent cerebral vasodilator and has no place in neuroanesthesia (30).

Prior to tracheal intubation it is important that steps be taken to block any cardiovascular hyperdynamic response to that powerful stimulus. Intravenous narcotics or narcotic-tranquilizer combinations (neuroleptoanalgesia) are useful in this regard and are associated with modest decreases in intracranial pressure (28). Lidocaine, given as an intravenous bolus in a dose of 1.5 mg/kg, may also be added. Bedford and his colleagues (8) have shown that this modality completely blocks the increase in ICP often seen with laryngoscopy and intubation and blunts the rise in arterial pressure as well.

Muscular relaxation at the time of intubation must be profound in order to prevent coughing or straining. Succinylcholine is felt by some to be contraindicated in neuroanesthesia since elevated ICP has been reported in association with its use (32,68). This association, however, may be spurious, and in fact several groups have routinely used succinylcholine to facilitate intubation prior to aneurysm surgery (4,22, 34,58,62,65). Curare, and more recently pancuronium, are also used (17,22,31,60) and have the advantage that, being longer lasting, they prevent coughing during head positioning and shaving.

Maintenance

The general rule of neuroanesthesia, that cerebral vasodilators are to be avoided and cerebral vasoconstrictors used where possible, must be modified in aneurysm surgery in order to facilitate induced hypotension. Moreover, intracranial pressure and compliance are often normal. Nevertheless, attempts should be made where possible to minimize cerebral vasodilation in order to present the surgeon with a "slack" brain.

The volatile agents—halothane, enflurane, and isoflurane—all increase cerebral blood flow (21,49,76). However, in low concentrations and in the presence of hypocarbia they can be employed without increasing intracranial pressure (2,3). Halothane in particular has been used for aneurysm surgery either with other hypotensive techniques (4,22,34,41,65,71) or as a sole hypotensive agent (22,39). Nitrous oxide has a modest but clinically insignificant effect on intracranial pressure (36) and may be considered safe for use during craniotomy.

Respiratory Management

With the patient paralyzed and anesthetized, it is a simple matter to achieve hyperventilation by mechanical means for prolonged periods. For most anesthetists this represents the safest course of respiratory management. The near-universal employment of hyperventilation to Pa_{CO_2} levels of 25–30 torr during craniotomy is based on the well-documented fact that hypocarbia is associated with reduced cerebral blood flow in normal human subjects (45,76) and with a lowered intracranial pressure in some pathologic conditions (59). Its value during craniotomy is more difficult to prove scientifically (61), but its association with a relaxed brain has been a distinct clinical impression for years (35).

So widespread is the use of hyperventilation during intracranial aneurysm surgery that a notable exception is worth special mention. Aitken, Drake, and their colleagues at the University of Western Ontario have performed aneurysm surgery on a large number of patients breathing spontaneously under general anesthesia (4,23,62). By combining local analgesia with very light halothane anesthesia (0.3–0.7% inspired concentration), arterial CO_2 tensions near normal (40–50 torr) were maintained with unassisted spontaneous ventilation—even with profound hypotension induced with sodium nitroprusside. As a guide to the adequacy of brainstem perfusion during hypotension or after interrupting a major artery, spontaneous ventilation was felt to be of particular value in cases of basilar artery aneurysms (62). Spinal fluid drainage and mannitol were routinely used as adjuncts to control brain size. However, caution should be employed by any clinician wishing to apply this technique; great skill, close communication, and an understanding of each other's problems are required of both anesthesiologist and surgeon.

Cardiovascular Management

Induced hypotension has been heralded as a major advance in the surgical treatment of intracranial aneurysms (23,74) and is now used universally. While the use of halothane (22,39), trimethaphan (4,41,71), hexamethonium (34), and (more recently) nitroglycerin (15) have been described, the distinct preference during the past decade has been sodium nitroprusside (1,4,17,60,65).

By lowering the arterial pressure, the tendency of the aneurysm to rupture is lessened, particularly during dissection of the sac (23). In addition, the entire vasculature becomes softer and more mobile, making dissection around the aneurysm easier (23,39). Furthermore, should the aneurysm rupture during dissection, induced hypotension will diminish the volume of blood lost. Typically, moderate hypotension is produced (MAP 70–90 torr) as the dura is opened and the aneurysm approached; then, as the aneurysm is dissected, deep hypotension (MAP 50 torr) is achieved. Finally, as the aneurysm is clipped, hypotension to MAP levels below 50 torr for short periods are recommended by some groups (39,60,62,65). Should the aneurysm rupture, the infusion of hypotensive drug is not interrupted, but blood is replaced as rapidly as possible. Once the aneurysm has been successfully obliterated, the blood pressure is allowed to return to normal.

Unfortunately, precise data as to how low the pressure may be safely allowed to go, and for how long, are not available and undoubtedly vary from patient to patient. Although evidence from animal studies (51) suggests that a MAP of 50 torr is well-tolerated by the brain regardless of the method of hypotension, Nornes et al. (54) have found, using trimethaphan during cerebral aneurysm surgery, that cerebral blood flow began to decrease when mean arterial pressures were lowered to an average of 62 torr in Botterell grades 1 and 2 patients. However, the range of MAP at which flow began to fall was 35–85 torr. Furthermore, in grade 3 patients who had higher initial blood pressures, cerebral flow began to fall at even higher pressures (average 76 torr). Despite these findings, however, values of MAP below those levels are usually well-tolerated during aneurysm surgery (60,62,66). For a more detailed discussion of induced hypotension, see Chapter 24.

It is generally recommended that blood volume be replaced as it is lost. Normally, blood replacement is required only if the aneurysm ruptures. Intravenous fluid therapy should be held to maintenance levels (1.5 ml/kg/h) unless a preexistent deficit exists and should consist of isotonic salt solutions (normal saline, lactated Ringer's solution). Hypotonic or salt-free solutions are avoided because they may result in hyponatremia and cerebral edema (75).

Ancillary Therapy

In positioning the patient for operation, elevation of the head 10–20° promotes cerebral venous drainage and may also facilitate induced hypotension. If the head is turned, care must be taken that jugular venous blood flow is not restricted; a support under one shoulder is often useful. Support stockings or leg wraps will reduce the incidence of postoperative deep-vein thrombosis.

If desired, spinal drainage may be instituted by placing a subarachnoid needle (18-gauge) in one or two lumbar interspaces. The needle may then be connected to sterile plastic tubing with stopcocks at the other end to control the drainage of fluid (34). Fluid is removed, if necessary, only after the cranial bone flap has been lifted.

Hyperosmolar diuretic therapy, particularly with 20% mannitol (1.5 g/kg) given rapidly intravenously, has been used to decrease the brain bulk during intracranial aneurysm surgery (60,62,71). The nonosmotic "loop" diuretic, furosemide, has been recommended to reduce intracranial pressure during craniotomy (19), but its value in aneurysm surgery has not been determined.

Barbiturate therapy has been shown in animals to protect the brain in regional ischemic insults (38,50,67). With this in mind, Hoff and his colleagues (37) administered large doses of pentobarbital (15 mg/kg/24 h) to seven patients undergoing aneurysm surgery when occlusion of a major cerebral artery was required. Four of the seven patients recovered with no neurologic deficit, suggesting that barbiturate therapy might have afforded some protection. It should be noted, however, that as with many studies of barbiturate protection of the brain to date (52), this series lacked controls. While no definite clinical conclusions can be made at present, the fact remains that acute regional cerebral ischemia is the one form of ischemia in which barbiturate protection has been demonstrated in animals (50). Thus, in a desperate situation which requires occlusion of a major cerebral artery, intravenous barbiturate administration is not unreasonable.

Hypothermia by surface cooling has been used in the operative management of intracranial aneurysms (12) and was quite popular in the 1950s. Deep hypothermia with cardiopulmonary bypass (24,55) and selective brain cooling (31,73) have also been tried. However, these cumbersome and time-consuming techniques have not improved outcome (24,33) and, accordingly, have been abandoned by most centers. Normal or near-normal body temperature can be maintained with the use of circulating water blankets, humidification of anesthetic gases (14), and the administration of blood warmed to body temperature (13).

Emergency and Early Postoperative Care

Once the dura is closed, the decision as to whether or not to waken the patient must be made. Patients of preoperative grade 1 or 2 usually present little problem, especially if the aneurysm has not ruptured intraoperatively and anesthesia has gone well. In these cases full return of consciousness may be expected shortly after discontinuation of the anesthetic. The ventilation should be decreased in order to allow a gradual return of Pa_{CO_2} to normal during closure. In order to ensure a smooth emergence, suctioning of the tracheobronchial tree should be performed while the patient has some degree of neuromuscular blockade; the anesthetic may be discontinued as the head wrap is applied. It may be helpful to administer a bolus of intravenous lidocaine (1.5 mg/kg) just prior to extubation of coughing is considered hazardous.

If, because of preoperative neurologic depression, difficulty with the operative procedure, or anesthetic problems, the patient is expected to have significant postoperative CNS depression, it is then advisable to continue endotracheal cannulation and mechanical ventilation, perhaps even muscular paralysis, into the postoperative period. Problems of respiratory depression, retention of tracheobronchial secretions, and aspiration are thus avoided.

Bibliography

1. Adams CBT, Loach AB, O'Laoire SA: Intracranial aneurysms: analysis of results of microneurosurgery. Brit Med J 2:607–609, 1976
2. Adams RW, Cucchiara RF, Gronert GA, et al.: Isoflurane and cerebrospinal fluid pressure in neurosurgical patients. Anesthesiology 54:97–99, 1981
3. Adams RW, Gronert GA, Sundt TM Jr, et al.: Halothane, hypocapnia, and cerebrospinal fluid pressure in neurosurgery. Anesthesiology 37:510–517, 1972
4. Aitken RR, Drake CG: A technique of anesthesia with induced hypotension for surgical correction of intracranial aneurysms. Clin Neurosurg 21:107–114, 1974
5. Auer L: Microprocessor control of drug infusion for automatic blood pressure control. Medical Biolog Engineering Computing (in press, 1981)
6. Barnes RW, Foster EJ, Jansen GA, et al.: Safety of brachial artery catheters as monitors in the intensive care unit—prospective evaluation with the Doppler ultrasonic velocity detector. Anesthesiology 44:260–264, 1976
7. Bedford RF: Radial artery function following percutaneous cannulation with 18-gauge and 20-gauge catheters. Anesthesiology 47:37–39, 1977
8. Bedford RF, Winn HR, Park TS, et al.: Lidocaine prevents increased ICP after endotracheal intubation. In Shulman K, Marmaran A, Miller JD, et al. (eds.): Intracranial Pressure IV. New York, Springer-Verlag, 1980, pp. 595–598
9. Bedford RF, Wollman H: Complications of radial artery cannulation. Anesthesiology 38:228–236, 1973
10. Benedict GR, Loach AB: Clinical significance of plasma adrenaline and noradrenaline in patients with subarachnoid hemorrhage. J Neurol Neurosurg Psychiat 41:113–117, 1978

11. Bickford RG: Use of frequency discrimination in the automatic electroencephalographic control of anesthesia (servo-anesthesia). Electroencephalogr Clin Neurophysiol 3:83–86, 1951
12. Botterell EH, Lougheed WM, Morley TP, et al.: Hypothermia in the surgical treatment of ruptured intracranial aneurysms. J Neurosurg 15:4–18, 1958
13. Boyan CP, Howland WS: Cardiac arrest and temperature of bank blood. JAMA 183:58–60, 1963
14. Chalon J, Patel C, Ali M, et al.: Humidity in the anesthetized patient. Anesthesiology 50:195–198, 1979
15. Chestnut JS, Albin MS, Gonzalez-Abola E, et al.: Clinical evaluation of intravenous nitroglycerin for neurosurgery. J Neurosurg 48:704–711, 1978
16. Civetta JM: Invasive catheterization. In Shoemaker WC, Thompson WL (eds.): Critical Care: State of the Art, Part I (B). Fullerton, California, Society of Critical Care Medicine, 1980, pp. 6–8
17. Corkill G, Hodgson MJH: Hypotension with sodium nitroprusside in the surgery of cerebral aneurysms. Anaesthesia 28:191–194, 1973
18. Cotev S, Shalit MN: Effects of diazepam on cerebral blood flow and oxygen uptake after head injury. Anesthesiology 43:117–122, 1975
19. Cottrell JE, Robustelli A, Post K, et al.: Furosemide and mannitol induced changes in ICP and serum osmolality and electrolytes. Anesthesiology 47:28–30, 1977
20. Courtin RF, Bickford RG, Faulconer A Jr: The classification and significance of electro-encephalographic patterns produced by nitrous oxide-ether anesthesia during surgical operations. Proc Staff Mtg Mayo Clin 25:197–206, 1950
21. Cucchiara RF, Theye RA, Michenfelder JD: The effects of isoflurane on canine cerebral metabolism and blood flow. Anesthesiology 40:571–574, 1974
22. Doll WA, Jenkins LC: A review of anesthetic techniques for the surgical treatment of intracranial aneurysms. Can Anaesth Soc J 18:310–318, 1971
23. Drake CG: Ruptured intracranial aneurysms. Proc Roy Soc Med 64:477–481, 1971
24. Drake CG, Barr HWK, Coles JC, et al.: The use of extracorporeal circulation and profound hypothermia in treatment of ruptured intracranial aneurysm. J Neurosurg 21:575–581, 1964
25. Eisenberg HM, Turner JW, Teasdale G, et al.: Monitoring of cortical excitability during induced hypotension in aneurysm operations. J Neurosurg 50:595-602, 1979
26. Faulconer A, Pender JW, Bickford RG: The influence of partial pressure of nitrous oxide on the depth of anesthesia and the electroencephalogram in man. Anesthesiology 10:601–609, 1949
27. Finnerty FA Jr, Witkin L, Fazekas JF: Cerebral hemodynamics during cerebral ischemia induced by acute hypotension. J Clin Invest 33:1227–1232, 1954
28. Fitch W, Barker J, Jennett WB, et al.: The influence of neuroleptanalgesic drugs on cerebrospinal fluid pressure. Brit J Anaesth 41:800–806, 1969
29. Galloon S, Rees GAD, Briscoe CE, et al.: Prospective study of electrocardiographic changes associated with subarachnoid hemorrhage. Brit J Anaesth 44:511–516, 1972
30. Gardner AE, Olson BE, Lichtiger M: Cerebrospinal fluid pressure during dissociative anesthesia with ketamine. Anesthesiology 35:226–228, 1971
31. Gissen AJ, Matteo RS, Housepian EM, et al.: Elective circulatory arrest during neurosurgery for basilar artery aneurysms. JAMA 207:1315–1318, 1969
32. Gordon E (ed.): A Basis and Practice of Neuroanesthesia. Amsterdam, Excerpta Medica, 1975, p. 178
33. Hamby WB: Intracranial surgery for aneurysm. Effect of hypothermia upon survival. J Neurosurg 20:44–45, 1963
34. Hart W, Willatts S: An anesthetic technique for intracranial aneurysms. Anaesthesia 30:233–234, 1975
35. Hayes GJ, Slocum HC: The achievement of optional brain relaxation by hyperventilation techniques of anesthesia. J Neurosurg 19:65–69, 1962
36. Henriksen HT, Jörgensen PB: The effect of nitrous oxide on intracranial pressure in patient with intracranial disorders. Brit J Anaesth 45:486–492, 1973
37. Hoff JT, Pitts LH, Spetzler R, et al.: Barbiturates for protection from cerebral ischemia in aneurysm surgery. Acta Neurol Scand 56 (Suppl 64):158–159, 1977
38. Hoff JT, Smith AL, Hankins HL, et al.: Barbiturate protection from cerebral infarction in primates. Stroke 6:28–33, 1975
39. Hugosson R, Högström S: Factors disposing to morbidity in surgery of intracranial aneurysms with special regard to deep controlled hypotension. J Neurosurg 38:561–567, 1973
40. Hunter AR: Neurosurgical Anaesthesia, 2nd ed. Philadelphia, Lippincott, 1975, p. 171
41. Ishimori S, Oshida K, Sankawa H: Hypervolemic hypotension in surgical treatment of intracranial aneurysm. Surg Neurol 11:119–122, 1979
42. Jones TH, Chiappa KH, Young RR, et al.: EEG monitoring for induced hypotension for surgery of intracranial aneurysms. Stroke 10:292–294, 1979
43. Kaplan JA: Hemodynamic monitoring. In Kaplan JA (ed.): Cardiac Anesthesia. New York, Grune & Stratton, 1979, pp. 71–153
44. Kaplan JA, King SB III: The precordial electro-

cardiographic lead (V5) in patients who have coronary artery disease. Anesthesiology 45:570–574, 1976
45. Kety SS, Schmidt CF: The effects of altered tensions of carbon dioxide and oxygen on cerebral blood flow and cerebral oxygen consumption of normal young men. J Clin Invest 27:487–492, 1948
46. Kreus KE, Kemilä SF, Takala JK: Electrocardiographic changes in cerebrovascular accidents. Acta Med Scand 185:327–334, 1969
47. Lindop MJ: Complications and morbidity of controlled hypotension. Brit J Anaesth 47:799–803, 1975
48. McIntyre WR, Dobson D, Weir BKA, et al.: Monitoring under anesthesia with reference to subarachnoid hemorrhage and the T-wave as an electrocardiographic manifestation. Can Anaesth Soc J 18:293–297, 1971
49. Michenfelder JD, Cucchiara RF: Canine cerebral oxygen consumption during enflurane anesthesia and its modification during induced seizures. Anesthesiology 40:575–580, 1974
50. Michenfelder JD, Milde JH, Sundt TM Jr: Cerebral protection by barbiturate anesthesia. Use after middle cerebral artery occlusion in Java monkeys. Arch Neurol 33:345–350, 1976
51. Michenfelder JD, Theye RA: Canine systemic and cerebral effects of hypotension induced by hemorrhage, trimethaphan, halothane, or nitroprusside. Anesthesiology 46:188–195, 1977
52. Miller JD: Barbiturates and raised intracranial pressure. Ann Neurol 6:189–193, 1979
53. Mirakhur RK, Dundee JW, Connolly JDR: Studies of drugs given before anesthesia. XVII: Anticholinergic premedicants. Brit J Anaesth 51:339–345, 1979
54. Nornes H, Knutzen HB, Wikeby P: Cerebral arterial blood flow and aneurysm surgery. Part 2. Induced hypotension and autoregulatory capacity. J Neurosurg 47:819–827, 1977
55. Patterson RH Jr, Ray BS: Profound hypothermia for intracranial surgery. Laboratory and clinical experiences with extracorporeal circulation by peripheral cannulation. Ann Surg 156:377–393, 1962
56. Pierce EC, Lambertsen CJ, Deutsch S, et al.: Cerebral circulation and metabolism during thiopental anesthesia and hyperventilation in man. J Clin Invest 41:1664–1671, 1962
57. Prys-Roberts C, Meloche R, Foex P: Studies of anesthesia in relation to hypertension. I. Cardiovascular responses of treated and untreated patients. Brit J Anaesth 43:122–136, 1971
58. Rollason WN, Latham JW: Anaesthesia for intracranial aneurysms. Anaesthesia 18:498–502, 1963
59. Rowed DW, Leech PJ, Reilly PL, et al.: Hypocapnia and intracranial volume-pressure relationship. A clinical and experimental study. Arch Neurol 32:369–373, 1975
60. Rudehill A, Gordon E, Lagerkranser M: Sodium nitroprusside as a hypotensive agent in intracranial aneurysm surgery. Acta Anaesth Scand 23:404–410, 1979
61. Schettini A, Cook AW, Owre ES: Hyperventilation in craniotomy for brain tumor. Anesthesiology 28:363–371, 1967
62. Sellery GR, Aitken RR, Drake CG: Anesthesia for intracranial aneurysms with hypotension and spontaneous respiration. Can Anaesth Soc J 20:468–478, 1973
63. Shapiro HM, Wyte SR, Harris AB: Acute intraoperative intracranial hypertension in neurosurgical patients. Anesthesiology 37:399–405, 1972
64. Sharbrough FW, Menick JM, Sundt TM Jr: Correlation of continuous electroencephalograms with cerebral blood flow measurements during carotid endarterectomy. Stroke 4:674–683, 1973
65. Siegel P, Moraca PP, Green JR: Sodium nitroprusside in the surgical treatment of cerebral aneurysms and arteriovenous malformations. Brit J Anaesth 43:790–795, 1971
66. Siqueira EB, Behnia R: Prolonged, profound hypotension produced safely with sodium nitroprusside. Surg Neurol 6:169–172, 1976
67. Smith AL, Hoff JT, Nielsen SL, et al.: Barbiturate protection in acute focal cerebral ischemia. Stroke 5:1–7, 1974
68. Sondergard W: Intracranial pressure during general anaesthesia. Dan Med Bull 8:18–25, 1961
69. Stockard JJ, Bickford RG, Myers RR, et al.: Hypotension-induced changes in cerebral function during cardiac surgery. Stroke 5:730–746, 1974
70. Turner JM, Coroneos NJ, Gibson RM, et al.: The effect of althesin on intracranial pressure in man. Brit J Anaesth 45:168–172, 1973.
71. Wallace CT: Anesthesia for intracranial aneurysms. South Med J 68:725–729, 1975
72. Wilkins RH, Alexander JA, Odom GL: Intracranial arterial spasm. A clinical analysis. J Neurosurg 29:121–134, 1968
73. Williams BN, Turner EA: Report on 10 operations under local cerebral hypothermia. J Neurol Neurosurg Psychiat 33:647–655, 1970
74. Wilson CB, Spetzler RF: Factors responsible for improved results in the surgical management of intracranial aneurysms and vascular malformations. Am J Surg 134:33–38, 1977
75. Wise BI: Fluids and Electrolytes in Neurological Surgery. Springfield, Ill., Charles C Thomas, 1965
76. Wollman H, Alexander SC, Cohen PJ, et al.: Cerebral circulation of man during halothane anesthesia. Effects of hypocarbia and of d-tubocurarine. Anesthesiology 25:180–184, 1964

24
Anesthesiology

II. Induced Hypotension

Richard L. Keenan

Induced hypotension is now an integral part of the anesthetic management for intracranial aneurysm surgery (24,88), ranking with microsurgery as an important advance in the surgical treatment of aneurysms (88). The development of rapidly acting vasodilator drugs has done much to make induced hypotension effective and reasonably safe. Before these drugs are discussed, earlier techniques will be briefly reviewed since they have contributed to an understanding of the hazards and limits of hypotension.

Early Techniques and Drugs

Hemorrhage with vasoconstriction was noted and used to advantage by Cushing (20) as early as 1917 to produce a dry surgical field. Using arteriotomy as previously described in animals (45), Gardner (31) in 1946 found that arterial pressure could be lowered to 80 torr with the withdrawal of 1600 ml of blood, which was later reinfused. Like Cushing, Gardner recognized that "vasoconstriction (as in shock) rather than hypotension gave the dry field" (31). Despite this, arteriotomy was used in neurosurgery during the 1950s since it produced excellent operating conditions and its effect was certain: the pressure always fell (7,10,38). Since this was nothing more than hemorrhagic shock, arteriotomy was discarded as safer methods of lowering the blood pressure were developed.

Total sympathetic blockade with high spinal anesthesia as a means of deliberate hypotension was first reported by Griffiths and Gillies (33) in 1948. In their patients blood pressure was unrecordable at times, pulse rate was 40–50 beats/min, and the surgical field was dry. Studies later done by Sancetta et al. (68) revealed that the hypotension due to high spinal anesthesia was a result not only of decreased peripheral resistance but also of a fall in cardiac index, presumably due to venous pooling. Arteriovenous oxygen differences were increased, suggesting some degree of hypoperfusion. Payne (62) found that the situation was aggravated by blood loss and emphasized adequate volume replacement during induced hypotension. Extradural block has also been used for controlled hypotension, and it is especially effective in lowering blood pressure when combined with general anesthesia (9,34). Although spinal and extradural blockade continue to be used for induced hypotension in some forms of surgery (71), they have not found a place in craniotomy.

With the advent of halothane in 1956, induced hypotension with a general anesthetic became possible. The degree of hypotension produced by halothane is directly proportional to its inspired concentration (39). Originally, ganglionic blockade (66) and peripheral vasodilatation (11) were believed to be the mechanisms of hypotension. Indeed, patients under deep halothane anesthesia appear to be pink, warm, and well-perfused despite systolic pressures of 80 torr. However, evidence that halothane reduces myocardial contractile force (58) and cardiac output (8,73) began to accumulate, and it is now recognized that halothane hypotension is mainly a result of myocardial depression (65). This realization, combined with a growing concern with hepatotoxicity (2) and the availability of specific vasodilator agents, has resulted in the curtailment of the use of halothane as a sole hypotensive agent, although it continues to be used as an anesthetic and an adjunct to hypotension produced by other means.

Pharmacologic ganglionic blockade to induce hypotension was introduced by Enderby (25) in 1950 using pentamethonium. Hexamethonium, because of its more certain action, replaced it shortly thereafter (74). Hemodynamically, the ganglionic blocking drugs have proved to be similar to high spinal anesthesia: in addition to a fall in peripheral resistance, a fall in cardiac output is seen as well (3,90) due to venous pooling. This effect can actually be enhanced in order to increase the hypotensive effect of the drug during surgery by using a head-up position and continuous positive airway pressure (26) to retard venous return.

Pentolinium, another ganglioplegic drug, is much more potent and less prone to tachyphylaxis than hexamethonium (46). Both drugs, however, are relatively prolonged in their action (20–45 min) and have now been superseded by the shorter-acting and more controllable ganglionic blocking drug, trimethaphan (Arfonad) (60), which is discussed in detail below.

Pacemaker-induced hypotension has been suggested by Dimant and his colleagues (23). A transvenous cardiac pacemaker is used to produce tachycardia of approximately 175 beats/min, which in turn leads to hypotension due to a fall in cardiac output. Its use has not been widely accepted, presumably on the basis that it represents a form of cardiogenic shock.

Drugs in Use

Trimethaphan Camsylate

Trimethaphan camsylate (Arfonad) is a ganglionic blocking drug which also has a direct vasodilating action and releases histamine, effects which contribute to hypotension (63,85). Its half-life is 1–2 min due to rapid inactivation by plasma cholinesterase. It is best administered by continuous intravenous infusion. A 0.2% solution (2 mg/ml) is prepared by dissolving 500 mg in 250 ml of 5% dextrose in water. Infusion rates of 0.5–5 mg/min are normally required to obtain adequate levels of hypotension. Obviously, the dosage must be titrated against a continuously monitored direct mean arterial pressure. On discontinuation, blood pressure returns to normal within a few minutes—although with large doses delays up to 30 min may be experienced. Clinicians should be warned that continued ganglioplegia during this time will also cause widely dilated pupils. As with other ganglionic blocking drugs, tachyphylaxis frequently develops with trimethaphan, a fact which limits its usefulness (46). Use of adjuvant drugs (halothane, propranolol) or techniques (position, positive airway pressure) improve its efficacy (26).

Hemodynamically, trimethaphan resembles the other ganglioplegic drugs in that cardiac output tends to fall with hypotension (22,40,79). Although myocardial depression has been suspected, venous pooling is more likely a cause since cardiac output falls more in the head-up position than when patients are kept horizontal (70).

Cerebral blood flow during trimethaphan hypotension falls modestly (3), and autoregulation appears to be well-maintained (61). Unlike sodium nitroprusside, trimethaphan hypotension does not usually produce a rise in intracranial pressure in patients with intracranial masses (83). For this reason trimethaphan may be the hypotensive drug of choice if intracranial compliance is poor.

That trimethaphan might have a direct cerebral toxic effect was suggested by Magness, Yashon, and their colleagues (51,89) and by Michenfelder and Theye (54). Both groups, working with dogs, found increased cerebral lactic acid levels during trimethaphan hypotension not seen at comparable levels of halothane or nitroprusside hypotension. The clinical significance of these findings is unclear, but they could simply be the result of cerebral ischemia.

Nitroglycerin

Nitroglycerin, or glyceryl trinitrate (GTN), has traditionally been used to relieve angina pectoris. The mechanism by which angina is relieved is known to be a reduction in blood pressure (53). GTN can also be given as an intravenous infusion and has been employed as a hypotensive agent during coronary artery surgery (42), hip arthroplasty (27), and neurosurgery (12). GTN is now available for use in intravenous form. A good hypotensive response is usually seen at an infusion rate of 2 μ/kg/min. Onset of action is rapid (within a minute), and its half-life in plasma is about 2 min; it is rapidly metabolized in the liver. Although methemoglobinemia is a possible toxicity, it has not been observed in total doses of up to 200 mg (18).

Hemodynamically, GTN resembles trimethaphan rather than sodium nitroprusside. With hypotension, cardiac output falls as a result of vasodilatation of capacitance vessels, although peripheral resistance falls as well (53). There is no myocardial depression (57). Pulse rate does not increase significantly (12).

The effect of GTN on cerebral blood flow is not yet known, but one would expect little change similar to trimethaphan since arterial dilatation is not a major component of its action. Studies of its effect on intracranial pressure are conflicting. Chestnut et al. (12) reported good results in using GTN to control blood pressure during craniotomy in 64 patients, many of whom had tumors. Conversely, Cottrell and Turndorf (19) and more recently Traystman and Rogers (82) have observed increases in intracranial pressure during GTN-induced hypotension, possibly as a result of venous pooling in the cranium.

Perhaps the most serious drawback of GTN as a hypotensive agent in aneurysm surgery is the uncertainty of its action. Fahmy (27) found that hypotensive levels were not as profound with GTN as with sodium nitroprusside, although they were sufficient for hip arthroplasty. In the series of Chestnut and his colleagues (12) GTN failed to produce low enough pressures to clip a cerebral aneurysm on three occasions. At present, the proper role of GTN in neurosurgery is unclear, but its usefulness in the production of profound hypotension seems doubtful.

Sodium Nitroprusside

Sodium nitroprusside (SNP) is currently the most popular hypotensive agent not only in neurosurgery (1,14,35,67,72,75,76,88) but also in orthopedic surgery to minimize blood loss (6,48,80), and it is commonly used in cardiology and cardiac surgery to reduce left ventricular afterload (13,81) in patients with impaired myocardial oxygen supply.

The chemical formula of sodium nitroprusside is $Na_2Fe(CN)_5NO \cdot 2H_2O$. Obviously, cyanide is contained in the molecule; and, especially in the presence of sulfhydryl groups, cyanide ions can be released. Fortunately, cyanide released in the body is converted by rhodonase enzymes to relatively nontoxic thiocyanate in the presence of thiosulfate. But, because conversion to thiocyanate is rate-limited by thiosulfate availability (and thiocyanate itself is toxic in high concentrations), cyanide toxicity with SNP is a possibility and at least one death has been reported (21). Although various antidotes have been suggested for use with SNP (15, 36,55), limitation of the rate of administration of SNP to a known safe level renders antidote therapy unnecessary. This is readily achievable in the clinical setting when SNP hypotension is supplemented with halothane (4), enflurane (5), or propranolol (6). SNP doses of less than 1 mg/kg/h are now advocated for safe administration (17,84). Early toxicity is manifested by tachyphylaxis and the development of metabolic acidosis. Whenever increasing doses of SNP are required to maintain hypotension, arterial blood gas analysis to determine the metabolic acid-base status helps to confirm or rule out cyanide toxicity. For a thorough discussion of SNP toxicity see the excellent review by Tinker and Michenfelder (81).

Because SNP is unstable in solution, it is supplied in powder form in vials of 50 mg which, when mixed with 500 ml of dextrose in water, provides a 0.01% mixture or 100 μg/ml. The mixture should be protected from light and discarded after 4 h. SNP is given by continuous infusion; because both onset (within 60 s) and length of action (90 s or less) are surprisingly swift, extreme care must be taken with the initial administration. Dramatic swings in pressure from too low one minute to too high the next, both of which can be disastrous during cerebral aneurysm surgery, are to be avoided. A calibrated drip regulator or infusion pump is mandatory. In addition, washing in of the drug via a freely running intravenous line must be assured and unchanging. A port of injection in the intravenous line as close to the vein as possible is preferred in order to shorten the "lag time" in adjustment of infusion rates.

Hemodynamically, SNP differs from all other commonly used hypotensive agents in that cardiac output during hypotension falls only slightly in awake subjects (69) and actually increases in patients under general anesthesia (77,87). This is probably due to the mechanism of action of SNP, which is believed to be direct depression of the contractile mechanism of vascular smooth muscle (59). No evidence of myocardial depression has been found (69), and resistance vessels (arterioles) are affected more than capacitance vessels (30). Heart rate typically increases about 20% with SNP hypotension (87), and tachycardia can occasionally be troublesome. However, it is readily corrected with small doses of intravenous propranolol (6).

One would expect a reduction in coronary artery blood flow during hypotension with SNP, but the fall in perfusion pressure is more than offset by a reduced workload and lowered oxygen need—at least down to some as-yet-unspecified mean arterial pressure. On this basis SNP has been widely and successfully used to treat left ventricular failure due to ischemic heart disease (13,30) and is being increasingly used for induced hypotension in elderly patients undergoing hip arthroplasty (48,80) with little or no cardiac morbidity (49). Similarly, hepatic and renal complications, although implicated in an earlier series (50), have not been a problem with SNP or indeed with any hypotensive technique in recent years (49).

Cerebral effects of SNP include a rise in intracranial pressure (16,52,83) which, in the presence of intracranial mass lesions, can be of sufficient magnitude to interfere with surgery (83). Turner et al. (83) have shown that the rise in intracranial pressure seen in their patients was maximal when hypotension was moderate (MAP at 80–90% of control), but fell back to control levels when more profound hypotension was reached (MAP less than 70% of control). The likeliest explanation for this phenomenon is that SNP, by abolishing cerebral arteriolar tone, allows an initial sharp increase in cerebral blood flow and cerebral blood volume. Then, as blood pressure falls, cerebral blood flow falls back toward normal—and even below normal if blood pressure falls low enough. Ivankovich et al. (37) have shown in goats that SNP abolishes pressure autoregulation of cerebral blood flow, and Weiss et al. (86) recently demonstrated in cats that this loss of autoregulation with SNP can outlast the hypotensive effect of the drug when its infusion is stopped. Thus both hypoperfusion and hyperperfusion of the brain is theoretically possible when SNP is used. How often this occurs in practice is unclear. However, in one study of cerebral blood flow during cerebral aneurysm surgery with SNP hypotension (32), normal cerebral blood flow was found to be preserved despite significantly decreased cerebrovascular resistance; cerebral oxygen uptake was also normal.

It is known that a cerebral blood flow of 20 ml/100 g/min is sufficient to maintain cerebral function (78). According to Lassen and Christensen (47) such a flow is maintained with a mean arterial pressure of 40 torr (corresponding to a cerebral perfusion pressure of 30 torr, if intracranial pressure is normal) in lightly anesthetized healthy subjects. However, higher pressures are required to maintain the same flow in patients with hypertension. Furthermore, increased sympathetic tone, as in hypovolemia, increases the pressure at which adequate cerebral blood flow is maintained by causing vasoconstriction of the larger cerebral arteries (29). Despite these considerations, mean arterial pressures of 40 torr or less seem to be well-tolerated during cerebral aneurysm surgery, especially when SNP is used. This can be partly explained by the fact that with the cranium open the intracranial pressure is zero, making mean arterial pressure the same as cerebral perfusion pressure. Furthermore, nitroprusside itself is associated with a low critical perfusion pressure. Not only does it not cause sympathetic cerebral vasoconstriction, but it will also actually block constriction from any cause such as hypovolemia or conceivably even essential hypertension. In any event, reports of severe neurologic deficits due solely to induced hypotension are rare (49).

Tachyphylaxis in the absence of cyanide toxicity is occasionally observed with SNP (28), necessitating an increase in dosage to maintain an acceptable level of hypotension. In addition, an overshoot of blood pressure to hypertensive levels when SNP is discontinued has also been noted (43). These effects are likely caused by increased plasma renin activity (28,41,43,64) resulting from lowered kidney perfusion (41) during hypotension. Pretreatment of patients with propranolol has been shown to block renin release during SNP hypotension (44), and recently Bedford et al. (6) found that small intravenous doses of propranolol (0.01–0.02 mg/

kg) given at the time of surgery dramatically reduced the amount of SNP required to maintain hypotension. Moreover, blood cyanide levels were lowered as well.

Bedford has also shown in dogs that halothane (4) and enflurane (5) anesthesia sharply reduces the amount of SNP required to produce a given level of hypotension when compared to awake animals or those anesthetized with nitrous oxide and morphine. Cardiac output was well-maintained. The mechanism by which the volatile anesthetics potentiate SNP is unclear, but renin activity caused by SNP hypotension may be blocked (56). Whatever the mechanism, the addition of an inhalent such as halothane, enflurane, or isoflurane is an important clinical consideration when SNP is used to induce hypotension since it allows dosages of SNP well below those at which cyanide toxicity is observed. It is not surprising that in several of the reported series of intracranial aneurysm surgery in which SNP was used to induce hypotension, halothane was used as a part of the anesthetic technique (2,35,67,75).

In summary, sodium nitroprusside has become the current hypotensive agent of choice because its effect is rapid, certain, and readily reversible. Its use is associated with a well-maintained cardiac output, and although effects on cerebral blood flow are variable, cerebral perfusion appears to be maintained down to profound levels of hypotension. While cyanide toxicity is possible, it can be avoided by limiting the dose of sodium nitroprusside required with the concomitant use of propranolol or a potent inhalation anesthetic.

Bibliography

1. Adams CBT, Loach AB, O'Laoire SA: Intracranial aneurysms. Analysis of results of microneurosurgery. Brit Med J 2:607–609, 1976
2. Aitken RR, Drake CG: A technique of anesthesia with induced hypotension for surgical correction of intracranial aneurysms. Clin Neurosurg 21:107–114, 1974
3. Aviado DM: Hemodynamic effects of ganglion blocking drugs. Circ Res VIII:304–314, 1960
4. Bedford RF: Increasing halothane concentrations reduce nitroprusside dose requirement. Anesth Analg 57:457–462, 1978
5. Bedford RF: Sodium nitroprusside: Hemodynamic dose-response during enflurane and morphine anesthesia. Anesth Analg 58:174–178, 1979
6. Bedford RF, Berry FA Jr, Longnecker DE: Impact of propranolol on hemodynamic response and blood cyanide levels during nitroprusside infusion. A prospective study in anesthetized man. Anesth Analg 58:466–469, 1979
7. Bilsland WL: Controlled hypotension by arteriotomy in intracranial surgery. Anaesthesia 6:20–25, 1951
8. Black GW, McArdle L: The effects of halothane on the peripheral circulation in man. Brit J Anaesth 34:2–10, 1962
9. Bromage PR: Vascular hypotension in 107 cases of epidural analgesia. Anaesthesia 6:26–29, 1951
10. Brown AS: Pre-operative exsanguination in intracranial surgery. Anaesthesia 9:17–20, 1954
11. Burn JH, Epstein HG: Hypotension due to halothane. Brit J Anaesth 31:199–204, 1959
12. Chestnut JS, Albin MS, Gonzalez-Abola E, et al.: Clinical evaluation of intravenous nitroglycerin for neurosurgery. J Neurosurg 48:704–711, 1978
13. Cohn JN: Progress in vasodilator therapy for heart failure. New Engl J Med 302:1414–1416, 1980
14. Corkill G, Hodgson MJH: Hypotension with sodium nitroprusside in the surgery of cerebral aneurysms. Anaesthesia 28:191–194, 1973
15. Cottrell JE, Casthely P, Brodie JD, et al.: Prevention of nitroprusside-induced cyanide toxicity with hydroxocobalamine. New Engl J Med 298:809–811, 1978
16. Cottrell JE, Patel K, Turndorf H, et al.: Intracranial pressure changes induced by sodium nitroprusside in patients with intracranial mass lesions. J Neurosurg 48:329–331, 1978
17. Cottrell JE, Turndorf H: Anesthesia and Neurosurgery. St. Louis, Mosby, 1980, p. 390
18. Ibid, p. 393
19. Ibid, p. 394
20. Cushing H: Tumors of the Nervus Acusticus. Philadelphia, Saunders, 1917
21. Davies DW, Kadar D, Steward DJ, et al.: A sudden death associated with the use of sodium nitroprusside for induction of hypotension during anesthesia. Can Anaesth Soc J 22:547–552, 1975
22. Didier EP, Clagett OT, Theye RA: Cardiac performance during controlled hypotension. Anesth Analg (Cleve) 44:379–386, 1965
23. Dimant S, Piper CA, Murphy TO: Pacemaker-controlled hypotension in surgery. Surgery 62:663–669, 1967
24. Drake CG: Ruptured intracranial aneurysms. Proc Roy Soc Med 64:477–481, 1971
25. Enderby GEH: Controlled circulation with hypotensive drugs and posture to reduce bleeding in surgery. Preliminary results with pentamethonium iodide. Lancet 1:1145–1147, 1950
26. Enderby GEH: Pharmacological blockade. Postgrad Med J 50:572–575, 1974
27. Fahmy NR: Nitroglycerin as a hypotensive drug

during general anesthesia. Anesthesiology 49:17–20, 1978
28. Fahmy NR, Sunder N, Moss J, et al.: Tachyphylaxis to nitroprusside: Role of the renin-angiotensin system and catecholamines in its development. Anesthesiology 51:S72, 1979
29. Fitch W: Sodium nitroprusside and the cerebral circulation. Brit J Anaesth 49:399–400, 1977
30. Franciosa JA, Guiha NH, Limas CJ, et al.: Improved left ventricular function during nitroprusside infusion in acute myocardial infarction. Lancet 1:650–654, 1972
31. Gardner WJ: The control of bleeding during operation by induced hypotension. JAMA 132:572–574, 1946
32. Griffiths DPG, Cummins BH, Greenbaum R, et al.: Cerebral blood flow and metabolism during hypotension induced with sodium nitroprusside. Brit J Anaesth 46:671–679, 1974
33. Griffiths HWC, Gillies J: Thoracolumbar splanchnicectomy and sympathectomy; anaesthetic procedure. Anaesthesia 3:134–146, 1948
34. Henley J, Kritchman M: Total sympathetic blockade as an adjunct to anesthesia. NY J Med 62:348–355, 1962
35. Hoff JT, Pitts LH, Spetzler R, et al.: Barbiturates for protection from cerebral ischemia in aneurysm surgery. Acta Neurol Scand 56(Suppl 64):158–159, 1977
36. Ivankovich AD, Braverman B, Kanuru RP, et al.: Cyanide antidotes and methods of their administration in dogs. A comparative study. Anesthesiology 52:210–216, 1980
37. Ivankovich AD, Miletich DJ, Albrecht RF, et al.: Sodium nitroprusside and cerebral blood flow in the anesthetized and unanesthetized goat. Anesthesiology 44:21–26, 1976
38. Jackson I: Arteriotomy in neurosurgery. Anaesthesia 9:13–16, 1954
39. Johnstone M: The human cardiovascular response to fluothane anaesthesia. Brit J Anaesth 28:392–410, 1956
40. Jordan WS, Graves CL, Boyd WA, et al.: Cardiovascular effects of three techniques for inducing hypotension during anesthesia. Anesth Analg (Cleve) 50:1059–1068, 1971
41. Kaneko Y, Takeda T, Ikeda T, et al.: Effect of ganglion-blocking agents on renin release in hypertensive patients. Circ Res 7:97–103, 1970
42. Kaplan JA, Dunbar RW, Jones EL: Nitroglycerin infusion during coronary artery surgery. Anesthesiology 45:14–21, 1976
43. Khambatta HJ, Stone JG, Khan E: Hypertension following sodium nitroprusside. Physiologist 21:64, 1978
44. Khambatta HJ, Stone JG, Khan E: Propranolol abates nitroprusside-induced renin release. Anesthesiology 51:S74, 1979
45. Kohlstaedt KG, Page IH: Hemorrhagic hypotension and its treatment by intra-arterial and intravenous infusion of blood. Arch Surg 47:178–191, 1943
46. Larson AG: Deliberate hypotension. Anesthesiology 25:682–706, 1964
47. Lassen NA, Christensen MS: Physiology of cerebral blood flow. Brit J Anaesth 48:719–734, 1976
48. Lawson NW, Thompson DS, Nelson CL, et al.: Sodium nitroprusside-induced hypotension for supine total hip replacement. Anesth Analg 55:654–662, 1976
49. Lindop MJ: Complications and morbidity of controlled hypotension. Brit J Anaesth 47:799–803, 1975
50. Little DM Jr: Induced hypotension during surgery and anesthesia. Anesthesiology 16:320–332, 1955
51. Magness A, Yashon D, Locke G, et al.: Cerebral function during trimethaphan-induced hypotension. Neurology 23:506–509, 1973
52. Marsh ML, Shapiro HM, Smith RW, et al.: Changes in neurologic status and intracranial pressure associated with sodium nitroprusside administration. Anesthesiology 51:336–338, 1979
53. Mason DT, Zelis R, Amsterdam EA: Actions of the nitrates on the peripheral circulation and myocardial oxygen consumption: significance in the relief of angina pectoris. Chest 59:296–305, 1971
54. Michenfelder JD, Theye RA: Canine systemic and cerebral effects of hypotension induced by hemorrhage, trimethaphan, halothane, or nitroprusside. Anesthesiology 46:188–195, 1977
55. Michenfelder JD, Tinker JH: Cyanide toxicity and thiosulfate protection during chronic administration of sodium nitroprusside in the dog. Anesthesiology 47:441–448, 1977
56. Miller ED, Ackerley JA, Vaughan ED Jr, et al.: The renin-angiotensin system during controlled hypotension with sodium nitroprusside. Anesthesiology 47:257–262, 1977
57. Miller RR, Vismara LA, Zelis R, et al.: Clinical use of sodium nitroprusside in chronic ischemic heart disease. Circulation 51:328–336, 1975
58. Morrow DH, Morrow AG: The effects of halothane on myocardial contractile force and vascular resistance. Direct observations made in patients during cardiopulmonary bypass. Anesthesiology 22:537–541, 1961
59. Needleman P, Jakschik B, Johnson EM: Sulfhydryl requirement for relaxation of vascular smooth muscle. J Pharmacol Exp Ther 187:324–331, 1973
60. Nicholson MJ, Sarnoff SJ, Crehan JP: The intravenous use of a thiophanium derivative (Arfonad-RO2-2222) for the production of flexible and rapidly reversible hypotension during surgery. Anesthesiology 14:215–225, 1953

61. Nornes H, Knutzen HB, Wikeby P: Cerebral arterial blood flow and aneurysm surgery. Part 2. Induced hypotension and autoregulatory capacity. J Neurosurg 47:819–827, 1977
62. Payne JP: Controlled hypotension in theory and practice. Brit J Anaesth 25:134–154, 1953
63. Payne JP: Histamine release during controlled hypotension with arfonad. Proc World Congr Anesthesiologists (Scheveningen, The Netherlands, September 5–10, 1955), Minneapolis, Burgess Publ, 1956, p. 80
64. Pettinger WA, Keeton K: Altered renin release and propranolol potentiation of vasodilatory drug hypotension. J Clin Invest 55:236–243, 1975
65. Prys-Roberts C, Gersh BJ, Baker AB, et al.: The effects of halothane on the interactions between myocardial contractility, aortic impedence, and left ventricular performance. I. Theoretical considerations and results. Brit J Anaesth 44:634–649, 1972
66. Raventos J: The action of fluothane—a new volatile anaesthetic. Brit J Pharmacol 11:394–410, 1956
67. Rudehill A, Gordon E, Lagerkranser M: Sodium nitroprusside as a hypotensive agent in intracranial aneurysm surgery. Acta Anaesth Scand 23:404–410, 1979
68. Sancetta SM, Lynn RB, Simeone FA, et al.: Studies of hemodynamic changes in humans following induction of low and high spinal anesthesia. I. General considerations of the problem. The changes in cardiac output. Brachial arterial pressure, peripheral and pulmonary oxygen contents and peripheral blood flows induced by spinal anesthesia in humans not undergoing surgery. Circulation VI:559–571, 1952
69. Schlant RC, Tsagaris TS, Robertson RJ Jr: Studies on the acute cardiovascular effects of intravenous sodium nitroprusside. Amer J Cardiol 9:51–59, 1962
70. Scott DB, Stephen GW, Marshall RL, et al.: Circulatory effects of controlled arterial hypotension with trimetaphan during nitrous oxide/halothane anaesthesia. Brit J Anaesth 44:523–527, 1972
71. Sculco TP, Ranawat C: The use of spinal anesthesia for total hip replacement arthroplasty. J Bone Joint Surg 57:173–177, 1975
72. Sellery GR, Aitken RR, Drake CG: Anesthesia for intracranial aneurysms with hypotension and spontaneous respiration. Can Anaesth Soc J 20:468–478, 1973
73. Severinghaus JW, Cullen SC: Depression of myocardium and body oxygen consumption and fluothane. Anesthesiology 19:165–177, 1958
74. Shackleton RPW: The reduction of surgical haemorrhage. Some observations on controlled hypotension with methonium compounds. Brit Med J 1:1054–1056, 1951
75. Siegel P, Moraca PP, Green JR: Sodium nitroprusside in the surgical treatment of cerebral aneurysms and arteriovenous malformations. Brit J Anaesth 43:790–795, 1971
76. Siqueira EB, Behnia R: Prolonged, profound hypotension produced safely with sodium nitroprusside. Surg Neurol 6:169–172, 1976
77. Styles M, Coleman AJ, Leary WP, et al.: Some hemodynamic effects of sodium nitroprusside. Anesthesiology 38:173–176, 1973
78. Sundt TM Jr, Sharbrough FW, Anderson RE, et al.: Cerebral blood flow measurements and electroencephalograms during carotid endarterectomy. J Neurosurg 41:310–320, 1974
79. Theye RA, Tuohy FG: Effect of trimetaphan on haemodynamics and oxygen consumption during halothane anaesthesia in man. Brit J Anaesth 37:144–152, 1965
80. Thompson GE, Miller RD, Stevens WC, et al.: Hypotensive anesthesia for total hip arthroplasty: a study of blood loss and organ function (brain, heart, liver, and kidney). Anesthesiology 48:91–96, 1978
81. Tinker JH, Michenfelder JD: Sodium nitroprusside. Pharmacology, toxicology and therapeutics. Anesthesiology 45:340–354, 1976
82. Traystman RJ, Rogers MC: The effect of nitroglycerin on cerebral blood flow and cerebrospinal fluid pressure in normoxic and hypoxemic dogs. Crit Care Med 9:245, 1981
83. Turner JM, Powell D, Gibson RM, et al.: Intracranial pressure changes in neurosurgical patients during hypotension induced with sodium nitroprusside or trimetaphan. Brit J Anaesth 49:419–424, 1977
84. Vesey C, Cole P: Dose limits to acute nitroprusside therapy challenged. Anesthesiology 49:55–56, 1978
85. Wang HH, Liu LMP, Katz RL: A comparison of the cardiovascular effects of sodium nitroprusside and trimethaphan. Anesthesiology 46:40–48, 1977
86. Weiss MH, Spence J, Apuzzo MLJ, et al.: Influence of nitroprusside on cerebral pressure autoregulation. Neurosurgery 4:56–59, 1979
87. Wildsmith JAW, Marshall RL, Jenkinson FL, et al.: Hemodynamic effects of sodium nitroprusside during nitrous oxide/halothane anesthesia. Brit J Anaesth 45:71–74, 1973
88. Wilson CB, Spetzler RF: Factors responsible for improved results in the surgical management of intracranial aneurysms and vascular malformations. Am J Surg 134:33–38, 1977
89. Yashon D, Stone W, Magness A, et al.: Evidence of preservation of aerobic cerebral metabolism during halothane-induced hypotension. J Neurosurg 39:712–717, 1973
90. Zimmerman BG, Brody MJ, Beck L: Mechanism of the cardiac output reduction by hexamethonium. Amer J Physiol 199:319–324, 1960

25

Craniotomy for Aneurysm

I. Control of Intracranial Pressure and Circulation

Chapters 23 and 24 detail the role of the anesthesiologist in providing circulatory management and control of intracranial pressure (ICP). Table 25.1 summarizes techniques of reducing ICP during aneurysm surgery. This chapter will discuss only CSF drainage as one method of ICP control.

Cerebrospinal Fluid Drainage

The most common method of CSF removal during aneurysm surgery has been lumbar puncture (LP) with drainage by needle or indwelling catheter. A number of authors have described its use (1,6,7,9,10,13,14,17,20,22,24, 31,32,35,36,38,41,43,44,50,52,54–56,66,69,71, 76,80,81,95,106–108,115,116,119,126,127,133, 134,136,140,141,141a,143,144).

Aitken and Drake (7) warned that too rapid removal of CSF may cause an undesirable blood pressure elevation, especially if the patient is in a lateral position. Tindall and Odom (133) cautioned against excessive drainage, which may result in brain shifting and premature aneurysm rupture. For the same reason Sundt and Murphy (127) suggested that the LP needle or catheter not be opened until the dura is opened.

As noted by a study group in 1978 (31), spinal fluid most commonly is removed by aspiration from the basilar cisterns and/or lumbar CSF space. Many surgeons routinely insert a lumbar spinal needle for CSF drainage to be started as the dura is opened. Some surgeons believe that excess CSF drainage by lumbar puncture may have several results: (a) it may cause excessive brain shrinkage and increase the risk of tearing a bridging vein or the olfactory nerve; (b) it may cause cerebral and vascular tissues to dehydrate too rapidly; and (c) it may prevent diffusion of blood, thereby promoting clotting in basal cisterns and later hydrocephalus. We prefer to use LP drainage only initially and when the brain is tight owing to hydrocephalus. The CSF bathing the aneurysm and keeping its walls from becoming dry and brittle is better than extensive use of saline irrigations. In the presence of hydrocephalus, commonly due to adhesions in the region of Liliequist's membrane, the surgeon can open this membrane between the optic nerve and carotid artery or between the oculomotor nerve and carotid artery. Otherwise the membrane is left intact (unless a basilar artery bifurcation aneurysm is attacked by the frontolateral approach), because it acts as a protective barrier to the passage of blood into the posterior cisterns. Occasionally, in pronounced hydrocephalus, the lamina terminalis can be punctured. A ventricular tap is rarely necessary; however, in the past it has been used on occasion by a number of surgeons (1,4,17,18,39,52,54,60,76,91,100,104,117,118, 120,120a,142,143).

Comment

We have utilized most of the methods described in Table 25.1. Patients who are grade 3 or worse have surgery delayed until they are grade 1 or 2. The patient's head is elevated 10–15° (a higher elevation conflicts with the operating microscope focal distance). Mannitol 15% (about 300 ml for an adult patient) is started during induction; this not only helps with brain shrinkage but also retards red blood

Table 25.1. Methods to Control ICP During Aneurysm Surgery

1.	Operate on grade 1 or grade 2 patient
2.	Minimize trauma to brain
	Use less retraction
	Gentle microtechnique
3.	Prevent vasospasm
	Atraumatic vessel manipulation
	Topical papaverine or phentolamine
	Minimize blood in cisterns
	Avoid cold irrigating solutions
4.	Avoid increasing venous pressure
	Elevate head
	Avoid compromising jugular veins
	Minimize sectioning of bridging veins
	Ventilatory control
5.	Use osmotic agents
	Mannitol 15% most commonly used; also urea or glycerol
	Also decreases blood viscosity
6.	Use hypothermia
	Less commonly used now
7.	Use glucocorticosteroids
	Probably helpful (not proved)
	Omit if peptic ulcer is present
	Dexamethasone or methylprednisolone most commonly used
8.	Use controlled ventilation
	Maintain arterial P_{CO_2} at 25–35 mm Hg
9.	Use chemical diuretics (e.g., furosemide)
10.	Avoid overhydration and recognize inappropriate secretion of ADH
11.	Develop CSF drainage
	Spinal tap
	Cisternal tap
	Aspiration from cisterns
	Puncture of Liliequist's membrane
	Puncture of lamina terminalis
	Ventricular tap
12.	Induce vascular hypotension
13.	Evacuate clot

From Fox JL, Albin MS, Bader DCH, et al., ref. 31.

cell aggregation. Hypothermia is not used. Steroids are begun during surgery to help reduce arachnoid inflammation and adhesions. Unlike their beneficial effect on brain neoplasm edema, steroids have only questionable effect on the edema of SAH and vasospasm. Controlled passive hyperventilation is routine; arterial blood gases are monitored and the P_{CO_2} kept at 25–30 mm Hg. Furosemide is used occasionally. An indwelling urinary catheter is kept in place. Fluid intake is kept normal; that is, under- or overhydration is not routinely practiced, although the patient may receive additional crystalloid fluids to compensate for urinary losses and colloid solutions or blood to maintain mild volume expansion (therapy for vasospasm). The use of CSF drainage has already been detailed. Induced vascular hypotension is commonly used. Technique and discussions are given elsewhere (see below and previous two chapters). An indwelling arterial line for monitoring blood pressure is standard. A central venous pressure line is not placed routinely.

Controlling Circulation

Induced Hypotension

Methods used by the anesthesiologist to control the circulation, including induced hypotension, are described in the previous two chapters. The use of controlled hypotension may be hazardous in older patients, in patients placed in the sitting position, and in the presence of marked preoperative hypertension, pregnancy, glaucoma, severe atherosclerosis (renal, coronary, cerebral), increased ICP from any cause, vasospasm, carotid or vertebral artery stenosis or occlusion, excess brain retraction pressure, giant aneurysms compressing the brainstem, and temporary arterial occlusion or trapping procedures.

Active measures (beyond sufficient anesthesia) to reduce BP during aneurysm surgery often are not started until after the dura is opened and the approach to the aneurysm begun, for in many patients the craniotomy procedure causes a response that interferes with lowering the BP. Similarly, rapid administration of osmotic agents at the same time hypotensive agents are given may cause an expansion of blood volume that offers resistance to the reduction in BP. The method, duration, amount, and timing of induced hypotension are determined by consultation between the surgeon and anesthesiologist.

Proximal Cervical Carotid/Vertebral Control

The purpose of reducing systemic BP is to: (a) reduce the pulsatile flow and force of blood within the aneurysm, thereby preventing premature rupture; and (b) retard hemorrhage already occurring through a rent in the aneurysm wall. An extension of this principle is temporary ligature of the cervical carotid and/or vertebral arteries to retard cranial flow while preserving systemic flow.

Hamby (53) sometimes used a Poppen–Blaylock clamp to close the cervical carotid artery 24 h prior to craniotomy. After the aneurysm was ligated, he then released the clamp. Several authors described exposure of the CCA or ICA (unilaterally or bilaterally) in the neck at surgery. They placed temporary ligatures around these vessels and used them either in case the aneurysm ruptured or temporarily while dissecting the aneurysm (29,47,48,52,55,89,91, 97,104,108,111,112). Others exposed both carotid arteries and both vertebral arteries in the neck (mainly for BAA cases) (8,11,12,17,21, 25,32,62,75,77,88) or reached into the chest (from above or via a median sternotomy) and applied temporary ligatures about the innominate, left subclavian, and left common carotid arteries with the patient under hypothermia (2,3,46,63).

Temporary Cardiac Arrest

During the 1960s cardiac arrest with moderate (28–32°) to profound (10–15°) hypothermia was utilized by teams of neurosurgeons, cardiac surgeons, and anesthesiologists for treatment of difficult aneurysm cases (15,16,27,40,42,58, 65,73,78,79,83–87,92–94,98,114,122,124,135, 137–139). These included open- and closed-chest techniques with cardiopulmonary bypass. Such methods were largely abandoned, for the benefits of cerebral protection from ischemia, a slack brain, and absence of blood flow were negated by the untoward complications—especially blood coagulation defects and bleeding during the rewarming phase. Recently there has been renewed interest in these techniques (84,120a).

Temporary Ligature/Clips

In 1953 Campbell and Burklund (14) described the use of temporary occlusion of the M-1 artery during middle cerebral aneurysmorrhaphy. They placed a 00 silk suture around the middle cerebral artery and then passed both ends through an eyelet at the tip of a silver probe. An assistant tightened the sutures around the MCA and against the probe tip while the aneurysm was obliterated. Laine (70) placed silk ligatures around the anterior communicating artery on either side of an ACoAA. He temporarily arrested blood flow into the aneurysm by a single tie of the sutures. The aneurysm was then ligated and the temporary sutures released. Hamby (49,51) reported his method (a snare) of using silk suture through a polyethylene tube to temporarily stop blood flow (Fig. 25.1). White et al. (141a) used a similar method. Subsequently Drake (23) described a similar technique using 3-0 prolene suture passed through a polyethylene tube. He extended the application of this method by leaving the tube *in situ* with the free end placed under the scalp; in this way the artery could be permanently closed later, thereby effecting a Hunterian ligature proximal to the aneurysm. This is performed while the patient is awake and under arteriographic monitoring.

In 1952 Hamby (48) published an account of his use of a ⅞-inch serafine clamp specially altered for use as a temporary intracranial vascular clamp; it was applied by a long-handled tonsil forceps. Gibbs (38) used a large special clamp held by an assistant. Jamieson (60–62) applied a lady's hair-curling clip for temporary intracranial vessel occlusion. Martinez Coll and Del Corral (80) invented a special clip with a spring cable. This clip was tightened on the artery by a screw mechanism turned via the spring cable. It was not until the early 1950s when, with the development of the Schwartz clip, temporary clipping of intracranial arteries during aneurysm surgery became commonplace (30,82). A number of authors subsequently reported on the use of temporary clips (5,32–34,45,57,59–62,64,72,74–77,80,81,89–91, 96,99–105,109,110,113,123,129–132,140,145, 146).

One of the proponents of the temporary spring clip was Pool (99–104), who used the Mayfield spring clip, a modification of the Schwartz clip (30). He warned that induced vascular hypotension should not be used if temporary clips are to be applied (99). By 1972 Pool (100) had stopped routine use of temporary clips. Connolly (19) had already warned of creating ischemic deficits with the use of temporary clips. The 1966 Cooperative Study (121, 121a) found no improvement in surgical mortality in cases where such clips were used. Temporary clips may cause vessel irritation, vasospasm, endothelial damage, focal dissecting aneurysms, and thrombus formation (28,37, 67,68).

The design of temporary clips is improving, and neurosurgeons now find their application beneficial in selected cases (90,129,145). Aihara

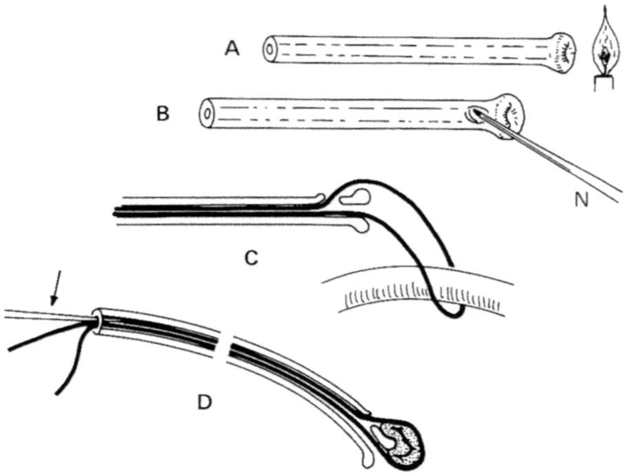

Fig. 25.1. Hamby snare employed for temporary occlusion of cerebral arteries. **A** Flaring of the tip of polyethylene tube by flame. **B** Side opening made with hot needle. **C** Ligature surrounding artery with the suture drawn through the aperatures in the plastic tube. **D** Details of arterial constriction against tip of tube, the ligature being secured by a toothpick (*arrow*) in free end of tube. From Hamby WB, ref. 51.

(5) found that one could safely occlude paren vessels up to 60 min during normotensive, normothermic conditions. Suzuki et al. (132) determined that the time limit was 20–60 min depending on the temperature (extended with hypothermia) and the collateral circulation. Intravenous mannitol may be helpful by reducing the tendency of blood cells to adhere. Intermittent release of temporary clips helps prolong the total occlusion time. If one uses prolonged occlusion of major vessels, the use of induced hypothermia may be considered. We have used induced *hyper*tension (and no hypothermia) without ill effects in some patients undergoing prolonged temporary trapping or occlusion. We prefer the Heifetz aneurysm clip for temporary occlusion of intracranial arteries at or near the circle of Willis, for this clip places less force on the arterial wall than do many other aneurysm clips (125). The use of temporary clips undoubtedly has greater risk in the presence of vasospasm or excess brain retraction pressure.

Bibliography

1. Adams CBT, Chir M, Fearnside MR, et al.: An investigation with serial angiography into the evolution of cerebral arterial spasm following aneurysm. J Neurosurg 49:805–815, 1978
2. Adams JE: Clinical experiences with hypothermia. In Fields WS, Sahs AL (eds.): Intracranial Aneurysms and Subarachnoid Hemorrhage. Springfield, Ill., Thomas, 1965, pp. 275–294
3. Adams JE, Wylie EJ: Value of hypothermia and arterial occlusion in the treatment of intracranial aneurysms. Surg Gynecol Obstet 108:631–635, 1959
4. Ahmed RH, Sedzimir CB: Ruptured anterior communicating aneurysms. A comparison of medical and specific surgical treatment. J Neurosurg 26:213–217, 1967
5. Aihara H: The direct surgical treatment of ruptured intracranial aneurysms—utilizing temporary occlusion of the cerebral artery under normothermic, normotensive anesthesia. Excerpta Medica ICS No. 418:198, 1977
6. Aitken RR: Hypotension in the operative treatment of intracranial aneurysm. In Arias A (ed.): Recent Progress in Anaesthesiology and Resuscitation. Amsterdam, Excerpta Medica, 1975, pp. 779–783
7. Aitken RR, Drake CG: A technique of anesthesia with induced hypotension for surgical correction of intracranial aneurysms. Clin Neurosurg 21:107–114, 1974
8. Alexander E Jr, Davis CH Jr, Kester NC: Intracranial aneurysms. Methods of treatment; value of hypothermia in the surgical approach. Arch Neurol Psychiatry 81:684–692, 1959
9. Ballenger OM, Salcman M, Ducker TB, et al.: Prognosis of surgically treated intracranial arterial aneurysm patients. JAMA 237:1845–1847, 1977
10. Bassett RC, List CF, Lemmen LJ: Surgical treatment of intracranial aneurysm. Surg Gynecol Obstet 95:701–708, 1952
11. Botterell EH, Lougheed WM, Morley TP, et al.: Hypothermia in the surgical treatment of ruptured intracranial aneurysms. J Neurosurg 15:4–18, 1958
12. Botterell EH, Lougheed WM, Scott JW, et al.: Hypothermia, and interruption of carotid, or carotid and vertebral circulation, in the surgical management of intracranial aneurysms. J Neurosurg 13:1–42, 1956
13. Cademartori MS, Ferreira NP, Wainer F, et al.: Tratamento dos aneurismas do sistema de artéria cerebral anterior. Neuropsiquiatr (Sao Paulo) 32:24–30, 1074
14. Campbell E, Burklund CW: Aneurysms of the middle cerebral artery. Ann Surg 137:18–28, 1953
15. Campkin TV: Moderate hypothermia and circulatory arrest for neurosurgical operations. Br J Anaesth 37:528–532, 1965

16. Campkin TV, Dallas SH: Elective circulatory arrest in neurosurgical operations. Br J Anaesth 40:527–531, 1968
17. Chou SN, Ortiz-Suarez HJ: Surgical treatment of arterial aneurysms of the vertebrobasilar circulation. J Neurosurg 41:671–680, 1974
18. Choudhury AR: Proximal occlusion of the dominant anterior cerebral artery for anterior communicating aneurysm. J Neurosurg 45: 484–490, 1976
19. Connolly C: Aneurysms of the middle cerebral artery. J Neurol Neurosurg Psychiatry 22:77–78, 1959
20. De Grood MPAM: Neurosurgical technique in saccular aneurysms. Psychiatr Neurol Neurochir 75:425–428, 1972
21. Drake CG: Bleeding aneurysms of the basilar artery. Direct surgical management in four cases. J Neurosurg 18:230–238, 1961
22. Drake CG: Cerebral aneurysm surgery—an update. In Scheinberg P (ed.): Cerebrovascular Diseases. Tenth Princeton Conference. New York, Raven Press, 1976, pp. 289–310
23. Drake CG: Giant intracranial aneurysms: experience in 174 patients. Clin Neurosurg 26:12–95, 1979
24. Drake CG: On the surgical treatment of ruptured intracranial aneurysms. Clin Neurosurg 13:122–155, 1965
25. Drake CG: Surgical treatment of rupture of aneurysms of the basilar artery. Experience with 14 cases. J Neurosurg 23:457–473, 1965
26. Drake CG: The surgical treatment of aneurysms of the basilar artery. J Neurosurg 29:436–446, 1968
27. Drake CG, Barr HWK, Coles JC, et al.: The use of extracorporeal circulation and profound hypothermia in treatment of ruptured intracranial aneurysm. J Neurosurg 21:575–581, 1964
28. Dujovny M, Osgood CP, Barrionuevo PJ, et al.: SEM evaluation of endothelial damage following temporary middle cerebral artery occlusion in dogs. J Neurosurg 48:42–48, 1978
29. Elvidge AR, Feindel WH: Surgical treatment of aneurysm of the anterior cerebral and the anterior communicating arteries diagnosed by angiography and electroencephalography. J Neurosurg 7:13–32, 1950
30. Fox JL: Vascular clips for the microsurgical treatment of stroke. Stroke 7:489–500, 1976
31. Fox JL, Albin MS, Bader DCH, et al.: Microsurgical treatment of neurovascular disease. Neurosurgery 3:285–337, 1978
32. French LA, Chou SN, Long DM: The direct approach to intracranial aneurysms. Clin Neurosurg 15:117–132, 1968
33. French LA, Chou SN, Story JL, et al.: Aneurysm of the anterior communicating artery. J Neurosurg 24:1058–1062, 1966
34. French LA, Zarling ME, Schultz EA: Management of aneurysms of the anterior communicating artery. J Neurosurg 19:870–876, 1962
35. Gallagher JP: Obliteration of intracranial aneurysms by pilojection. JAMA 183:231–236, 1963
36. Gass HH, McGuire JF, Simmons DR: Intracranial eradication of middle cerebral aneurysms. J Neurosurg 15:223–233, 1958
37. Gertz SD, Kurgan H, Wajnberg RS, et al.: Endothelial cell damage and thrombus formation following temporary arterial occlusion. J Neurosurg 50:578–586, 1979
38. Gibbs JR: On the advantages of opening certain intracranial aneurysms. J Neurol Neurosurg Psychiatry 20:165–171, 1957
39. Gillingham FJ: The management of ruptured intracranial aneurysm. Ann R Coll Surg 23:89–117, 1958
40. Gissen AJ, Matteo RS, Housepian EM, et al.: Elective circulatory arrest during neurosurgery for basilar artery aneurysms. JAMA 207:1315–1318, 1969
41. Glasauer FE: Cerebral aneurysms. Surgical treatment. NY State J Med 74:1781–1786, 1974
42. Gonski A, Johnston JB: Profound hypothermia as an adjunct in the surgical management of intracranial aneurysms. Report of eight cases. Pacific Med Surg 74:259–263, 1966
43. Guidetti B: Microsurgical treatment of intracranial saccular aneurysms. Acta Neurochir (Wien) 43:153–162, 1978
44. Guidetti B: Results of 98 intracranial aneurysm operations performed with the aid of an operating microscope. Acta Neurochir (Wien) 29:65–71, 1973
45. Guidetti B: Surgical treatment of aneurysms of the anterior communicating artery. Prog Brain Res 30:303–307, 1968
46. Gye R, Segelov J, Nicks R, et al.: Control of the cerebral circulation in the surgical treatment of ruptured intracranial aneurysms. Med J Aust 1:263–268, 1969
47. Hamby WB: A method for control of carotid cerebral circulation during operation. J Neurosurg 2:241–244, 1945
48. Hamby WB: Intracranial Aneurysms. Springfield, Illinois, Thomas, 1952
49. Hamby WB: Intracranial surgery for aneurysms. Prog Neurol Surg 3:1–65, 1969
50. Hamby WB: Intracranial surgical procedures in subarachnoid hemorrhage and intracranial aneurysms. In Fields WS (ed.): Pathogenesis and Treatment of Cerebrovascular Disease. Springfield, Ill., Thomas, 1961, pp. 496–507
51. Hamby WB: Remarks concerning intracranial

aneurysm surgery. Clin Neurosurg 17:1–17, 1970
52. Hamby WB: The modern treatment of intracranial aneurysms. NY State J Med 52:2497–2502, 1952
53. Hamby WB: The surgical management of intracranial aneurysms. Acta Neurol Latinoam 4:341–346, 1956
54. Harris P: Aneurysms of the anterior communicating artery. Cincinnati J Med 42:1–7, 1961
55. Harris P, Udvarhelyi GB: Aneurysms arising at the internal carotid-posterior communicating artery junction. J Neurosurg 14:180–191, 1957
56. Hart W, Willatts S: An anaesthetic technique for intracranial aneurysms. Anaesthesia 30: 233–234, 1975
57. Hoff JT, Pitts LH, Spetzler R, et al.: Barbiturates for protection from cerebral ischemia in aneurysm surgery. Acta Neurol Scand [Suppl 64] 56:158–159, 1977
58. Housepian EM, Bowman FO Jr, Gissen AJ: Elective circulatory arrest in intracranial surgery. Successful treatment of an aneurysm of the basilar artery with a method of open-chest circulatory arrest. J Neurosurg 26:594–597, 1967
59. Jain KK: Surgery of anterior communicating aneurysms: experience with various techniques and evolution of a modified approach. Surg Neurol 2:31–33, 1974
60. Jamieson, KG: Aneurysms of the vertebrobasilar system. Further experience with nine cases. J Neurosurg 28:544–555, 1968
61. Jamieson KG: Aneurysms of the vertebrobasilar system. Surgical intervention in 19 cases. J Neurosurg 21:781–797, 1964
62. Jamieson KG: Direct operation for intracranial aneurysm: some technical problems and attempts at their solution. Neurol Med Chir (Tokyo) 11:1–10, 1971
63. Karlsberg P, Adams JE: Value of hypothermia and arterial occlusion in the treatment of intracranial aneurysms. J Neurosurg 19:665–674, 1962
64. Kempe LG: Operative Neurosurgery, Vol 1: Cranial, Cerebral, and Intracranial Vascular Disease. Berlin, Springer-Verlag, 1968, pp. 1–75, 203–214
65. Khambatta HJ, Matteo RS, McMurtry JG III, et al.: Anesthesia for basilar arterial aneurysm with elective circulatory arrest and moderate hypothermia. Anesthesiology 41:512–516, 1974
66. Krayenbühl HA, Yaşargil MG, Flamm ES, et al.: Microsurgical treatment of intracranial saccular aneurysms. J Neurosurg 37:678–686, 1972
67. Kristiansen K: Methods of circulatory arrest. Prog Brain Res 30:377–382, 1968
68. Kunc Z: Aneurysms of carotid and posterior communicating artery. Prog Brain Res 30: 309–315, 1968
69. Laine E: Arterial vertebro-basilar aneurysms. Prog Brain Res 30:323–346, 1968
70. Laine E: Traitement chirurgical des anévrysmes de l'artère communicante antérieure. In Krayenbühl H, et al.: L'Anévrysme de l'Artère Communicante Antérieure. Paris, Masson et Cie, 1959, pp. 131–182
71. Laine E, Allègre GE, Goutelle A, et al.: Les anévrysmes vertébro-basilaires: choix de la voie d'abord. Problème de adjuvants per-opératoires. Neurochirurgie 18:317–332, 1972
72. Le Beau J: Anévrismes de l'artère communicante antérieure. Ruptures et indications neurochirurgicales. Neurochirurgia (Stuttg) 5:38–57, 1962
73. Leblanc G, Bertho E: Résection d'un anévrisme cérébral à l'aide de l'hypothermie profonde, l'arrêt circulatoire total et l'exsanguination. Laval Med 33:414–418, 1962
74. Lougheed WM: Selection, timing, and technique of aneurysm surgery of the anterior circle of Willis. Clin Neurosurg 16:95–113, 1969
75. Lougheed WM, Botterell EH, Morley TP: Results of the direct attack in the surgical management of internal carotid and middle cerebral aneurysms. Clin Neurosurg 9:193–200, 1963
76. Lougheed WM, Marshall BM: Management of aneurysms of the anterior circulation by intracranial procedures. In Youmans JR (ed.): Neurological Surgery, Vol 2. Philadelphia, Saunders, 1973, pp. 731–767
77. Lougheed WM, Marshall BM: The place of hypothermia in the treatment of intracranial aneurysms. Prog Neurol Surg 3:115–148, 1969
78. MacCarty CS: The application of profound hypothermia to the treatment of cerebrovascular disorders. Res Publ Assoc Res Nerv Ment Dis 41:126–144, 1966
79. MacCarty CS, Michenfelder JD, Uihlein A: Treatment of intracranial vascular disorders with the aid of profound hypothermia and total circulatory arrest: three years' experience. J Neurosurg 21:372–377, 1964
80. Martinez Coll A, Del Corral JF: Experiences in intracranial surgery for aneurysms. Surg Neurol 3:191–193, 1975
81. Maspes PE, Marini G: Aneurysms of the anterior communicating artery. Result of direct surgical treatment. Acta Neurochir (Wien) 11:479–494, 1963
82. Mayfield FH, Kees G Jr: A brief history of the development of the Mayfield clip. J Neurosurg 35:97–100, 1971
83. McMurtry JG III: Basilar artery aneurysms [letter]. J Neurosurg 45:361, 1976
84. McMurtry JG III, Housepian EM, Bowman FO

Jr, et al.: Surgical treatment of basilar artery aneurysms. Elective circulatory arrest with thoracotomy in 12 cases. J Neurosurg 40:486–498, 1974
85. Michenfelder JD, Kirklin JW, Uihlein A, et al.: Clinical experience with a closed-chest method of producing profound hypothermia and total circulatory arrest in neurosurgery. Am Surg 159:125–131, 1964
86. Michenfelder JD, Terry HR Jr, Daw EF, et al.: Profound hypothermia in neurosurgery: open-chest versus closed-chest techniques. Anesthesiology 24:177–184, 1963
87. Michenfelder JD, Uihlein A, MacCarty CS, et al.: Profound hypothermia and total circulatory arrest in neurosurgery: methods, results and physiologic effects. Acta Neurochir [Suppl] (Wien) 13:159–174, 1964
88. Moyes PD: Basilar aneurysm associated with agenesis of the left internal carotid artery. Case report. J Neurosurg 30:608–611, 1969
89. Moyes PD: Management and surgical treatment of ruptured intracranial aneurysms. Can Med Assoc J 94:13–18, 1966
90. Nornes H, Wikeby P: Results of microsurgical management of intracranial aneurysms. J Neurosurg 51:608–614, 1979
91. Northfield DWC: The Surgery of the Central Nervous System. Oxford, Blackwell, 1973, pp. 346–401
92. Obrador S, Rábago G, Córdoba A, et al.: Multiple cerebral arterial aneurysms operated under cardiac arrest. Bull Inst Res Univ Madrid 18:57–70, 1965
93. Patterson RH Jr, Ray BS: Profound hypothermia for intracranial surgery: laboratory and clinical experiences with extracorporeal circulation by peripheral cannulation. Ann Surg 156:377–393, 1962
94. Patterson RH Jr, Ray BS: Profound hypothermia for intracranial surgery using a disposable bubble oxygenator. J Neurosurg 23:184–190, 1965
95. Peerless SJ: The surgical approach to middle cerebral and posterior communicating aneurysms. Clin Neurosurg 21:151–165, 1974
96. Pertuiset B, van Effenterre R, Goutorbe J, et al.: Management of aneurysmal rupture during surgery, using bipolar coagulation, deep hypotension, and the operating microscope. Acta Neurochir (Wien) 30:195–205, 1974
97. Pertuiset B, Vouyouklakis D, Guyot JF, et al.: Les résultats du traitement chirurgical des anévrysmes artériels sus-tentoriels rompus. D'après 81 cas personnels. Neurochirurgie 12: 421–436, 1966
98. Pia HW: Neue Wege in der Behandlung cerebralen Aneurysmen. Dtsch Z Nervenheilk 184:459–472, 1963
99. Pool JL: Aneurysms of the anterior communicating artery. Bifrontal craniotomy and routine use of temporary clips. J Neurosurg 18: 98–111, 1961
100. Pool JL: Bifrontal craniotomy for anterior communicating artery aneurysms. J Neurosurg 36:212–220, 1972
101. Pool JL: Early treatment of ruptured intracranial aneurysms of the circle of Willis with special clip techniques. Bull NY Acad Med 35: 357–369, 1959
102. Pool JL: Timing and techniques in the intracranial surgery of ruptured aneurysms of the anterior communicating artery. J Neurosurg 19:378–388, 1962
103. Pool JL, Housepian EM: Temporary clip occlusion of major cerebral arteries during intracranial aneurysm surgery: clinical and postmortem data. Surg Forum 10:791–794, 1960
104. Pool JL, Potts DG: Aneurysms and Arteriovenous Anomalies of the Brain. Diagnosis and Treatment. New York, Harper & Row, 1965
105. Poppen JL: Discussion. Clin Neurosurg 11: 183–219, 1964
106. Poppen JL: Operative treatment for aneurysms of the anterior communicating artery. Clin Neurosurg 11:8–13, 1964
107. Poppen JL, Fager CA: Anterior communicating aneurysms: improved surgical mortality and morbidity. Lahey Clin Found Bull 19:1–7, 1970
108. Rand RW: *Microneurosurgery.* St. Louis, Mosby, 1969, pp. 198–209
109. Ransohoff J: Treatment of subarachnoid hemorrhage. Current status. NY State J Med 63:2494–2501, 1963
110. Robinson RG: Ruptured aneurysms of the middle cerebral artery. J Neurosurg 35:25–33, 1971
111. Rousseaux R, Lepoire J: Anévrismes vestigiaux du segment supraclinoidien de la carotide. Neurochirurgie 2:254–270, 1956
112. Rowe SN, Grunnagle JF, Susen AF, et al.: Results of direct attack on intracranial aneurysm. J Neurosurg 12:475–486, 1955
113. Sato O: Microsurgical techniques of clipping of IC-PC aneurysms with a broad neck. Excerpta Medica ICS No. 418:105, 1977
114. Selker RG, Wolfson SK Jr, Maroon JC, et al.: Preferential cerebral hypothermia with elective cardiac arrest: resection of "giant" aneurysm. Surg Neurol 6:173–179, 1976
115. Sellery GR, Aitken RR, Drake CG: Anaesthesia for intracranial aneurysms with hypotension and spontaneous respiration. Can Anaesth Soc J 20:468–478, 1973
116. Selverstone B: Coating of intracranial aneurysms with nontoxic adherent plastics. In Schmidek HH, Sweet WH (eds.): Current Techniques in Operative Neurosurgery. New York, Grune & Stratton, 1977, pp. 31–40

117. Shephard RH: Operation for aneurysms of the middle cerebral artery. In Logue V (ed.): Operative Surgery, Vol 14: Neurosurgery, 2nd ed. Philadelphia, Lippincott, 1971, pp. 172–177
118. Shephard RH: Ruptured cerebral aneurysms. Proc R Soc Med 64:481–483, 1971
119. Shields CB: Current trends in management of cerebral aneurysms. J Ky Med Assoc 75: 529–535, 1977
120. Shiobara R, Toya S, Iisaka Y, et al.: [An evaluation of the continuous ventricular drainage for ruptured cerebral aneurysms.] Neurol Med Chir (Tokyo) 17 (Part 2):145–152, 1977
120a. Silverberg GD, Reitz BA, Ream AK: Hypothermia and cardiac arrest in the treatment of giant aneurysms of the cerebral circulation and hemangioblastoma of the medulla. J Neurosurg 55:337–346, 1981
121. Skultety FM, Nishioka H: The results of intracranial surgery in the treatment of aneurysms. In Sahs AL, Perret GE, Locksley HB, et al. (eds.): Intracranial Aneurysms and Subarachnoid Hemorrhage. A Cooperative Study. Philadelphia, Lippincott, 1969, pp. 173–194
121a. Skultety FM, Nishioka H: Report on the cooperative study of intracranial aneurysms and subarachnoid hemorrhage. Section VIII, Part 2. The results of intracranial surgery in the treatment of aneurysms. J Neurosurg 25:683–704, 1966
122. Small JM, Stephenson SCF: Circulatory arrest in neurosurgery. Lancet 1:569–570, 1966
123. Speakman TJ, Barlass JL: The bifrontal approach to aneurysms of the anterior communicating artery. Can J Surg 6:237–243, 1963
124. St Ville JM, Tobias E: Intracranial surgery. Profound hypothermia and cardiac arrest. Arch Surg 92:573–575, 1966
125. Sugita K, Hirota T, Iguchi I, et al.: Comparative study of the pressure of various clips. J Neurosurg 44:723–727, 1976
126. Sundt TM Jr: Clip-grafts for aneurysm and small vessel surgery. Part 4. Relative application to various aneurysms and repair of anterior communicating aneurysms using a right-angle clip holder. Technical note. J Neurosurg 37:753–758, 1972
127. Sundt TM Jr, Murphy F: Clip-grafts for aneurysm and small vessel surgery. Part 3. Clinical experience in intracranial internal carotid artery aneurysm. J Neurosurg 31:59–71, 1969
128. Sundt TM Jr, Nofzinger JD: Clip-grafts for aneurysm and small vessel surgery. Part 1. Repair of segmental defects with clip-grafts; laboratory studies and clinical correlations. Part 2. Clinical application of clip-grafts to aneurysms; technical considerations. J Neurosurg 27:477–489, 1967
129. Suzuki J: Direct surgery of intracranial aneurysms: experience with over 1000 cases. Proc Inst Neurol Madras 6:15–23, 1976
130. Suzuki J: Operative indication and surgical technique of the cerebral aneurysm. 3. Neurol Med Chir (Tokyo) 16 (6 Part 2):487–495, 1976
131. Suzuki J, Kowada M, Asahi H, et al.: [Surgical treatment of aneurysms of the anterior communicating artery.] Brain Nerve (Tokyo) 16:391–397, 1964
132. Suzuki J, Kwak R, Okudairo Y: The safe time limit of temporary clamping of cerebral arteries in the direct surgical treatment of intracranial aneurysm under moderate hypothermia. Tohoku J Exp Med 127:1–7, 1979
133. Tindall GT, Odom GL: Saccular aneurysms of the brain. Surgical treatment. In Vinken PJ, Bruyn GW (eds.): Handbook of Clinical Neurology, Vol 12: Vascular Diseases of the Nervous System, Part II. Amsterdam, North Holland, 1972, pp. 205–226
134. Tytus JS, Haven H: Present day concepts in the management of intracranial aneurysms. Rev Surg 20:230–240, 1963
135. Uihlein A: Profound hypothermia and circulatory arrest in operations for intracranial aneurysms. Ann Chir Thorac Cardiovasc 1:811–812, 1962
136. Uihlein A, Hughes RA: The surgical treatment of intracranial vestigial aneurysms. Surg Clin North Am 35:1071–1083, 1955
137. Uihlein A, MacCarty CS, Michenfelder JD, et al.: Deep hypothermia and surgical treatment of intracranial aneurysms. A five-year survey. JAMA 195:639–641, 1966
138. Uihlein A, MacCarty CS, Svien HJ, et al.: Intracranial aneurysms. Operations with hypothermia of less than 15 C and perfusion with the open and closed thorax. JAMA 183:599–601, 1963
139. Uihlein A, Michenfelder JD: Profound hypothermia in neurologic surgery. Prog Neurol Surg 3:249–273, 1969
140. Uihlein A, Thomas RL, Cleary J: Aneurysms of the anterior communicating artery complex. Proc Mayo Clin 42:73–87, 1967
141. Wallace CT: Anesthesia for intracranial aneurysms. South Med J 68:725–729, 1975
141a. White R, Yashon D, Olbin M: [The treatment of cerebral aneurysms employing temporary parent vessel isolation.] Vopr Neirokhir, pp. 3–7, Jan–Feb 1975
142. Wilson CB, Christensen FK, Subrahmanian MV: Intracranial aneurysms at the pericallosol artery bifurcation. Am Surg 31:386–393, 1965
143. Wilson CB, U HS: Surgical treatment for aneurysms of the upper basilar artery. J Neurosurg 44:537–543, 1976
144. Yaşargil MG: Microsurgery Applied to Neuro-

surgery. Stuttgart, Georg Thieme Verlag, 1969, pp. 119–143
145. Yaşargil MG, Fox JL: The microsurgical approach to intracranial aneurysms. Surg Neurol 3:7–14, 1975
146. Yaşargil MG, Smith RD: Surgery on the carotid system in the treatment of hemorrhagic stroke. Adv Neurol 16:181–209, 1977
147. Yoshimoto T, Suzuki J: Intracranial definitive aneurysm surgery under normothermia and normotension—utilizing temporary occlusion of major cerebral arteries and preoperative mannitol administration. Neurol Surg (Tokyo) 4:775–783, 1976

26
Craniotomy for Aneurysm

II. Instrumentation

This chapter describes some of the instrumentation commonly used for intracranial aneurysm surgery. In parts it gives the bias of the author (JLF). Commercial sources are given in the appendix of another monograph (50) as well as in a table in the front matter of this book.

External Instrumentation

Operating Room Table

For aneurysms about the circle of Willis we place the patient on the American Sterilizer OR table so that the patient's head is at the foot end of the table (Fig. 26.1). This has several advantages: (a) the table pedals are not in the way of the sitting surgeon's feet (the anesthesiologist or circulating nurse manipulates these as needed); (b) there is more room for the base of the microscope (which we position to the left of the surgeon); (c) the normal opening in the OR table lies under the lumbar region of the patient's back, facilitating lumbar CSF drainage without turning the patient. The only disadvantage of this alignment is that the main weight of the patient is off the center of gravity for the OR table. An assistant must lift up on the table under the patient's shoulders when the patient's head is raised (table flexed) to its final position (about 10–15° elevation of the patient's head). This lightens the unbalanced load on the table while the table is flexed. One must be careful to avoid sliding the buttocks into the opening, which would risk sciatic nerve pressure in short patients.

For vertebral artery aneurysms the patient may be either in the standard sitting position on the OR table, with the surgeon using the head rest as an arm rest (Fig. 26.2) or in the three-quarter prone position (see Fig. 29.60) with the patient's head at the head end of the table. In either case the surgeon may be sitting.

Head Holder

In the present era of microsurgical technique and self-retaining retractors, it is essential that the head be immobilized by three-point skull fixation. We use the Mayfield–Kees skull clamp (Kees Surgical Specialty Company). This clamp (Fig. 26.3) is inserted into the normal foot end of the American Sterilizer table for patients with circle of Willis aneurysms. The horizontal part of the head holder should be nearly parallel with the floor. We prefer to have the two-point side of the clamp on the side of the surgery, as the opposite one-point side may project out too far. All joints are tightened securely, and the head is immobilized throughout the operation.

A study group stated (51):

> Under the surgical microscope, the slightest movement of the patient's head is magnified considerably. Microsurgery demands a precisely maintained position of the firmly fixed cranium throughout the entire operation, whether one operates with the patient in the sitting, supine, or prone position. This is best achieved by a pinion head holder, in which the essential element is a clamp made to accommodate three relatively sharp pins. The pins penetrate the scalp and are then firmly fixed to the outer table of the skull. When placing the pins, the surgeon should take care to avoid a spinal fluid shunt, surface vessels, thin bone (such as over the frontal and mastoid sinuses), and the thick temporal muscle where

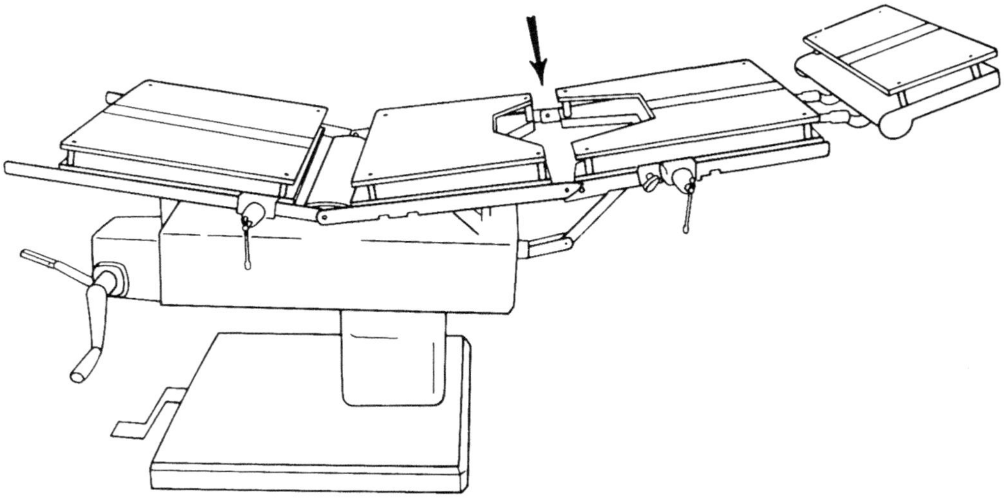

Fig. 26.1. **A** Sketch of American Sterilizer operating room (OR) table. The usual head end is to the observer's left. The head rest has been removed from this end and placed at the normal foot end on the observer's right. The patient's head initially rests on the head rest on the observer's right with that end elevated 10–15° and with the lumbar region of the patient's back resting over the opening (*arrow*) in the table.

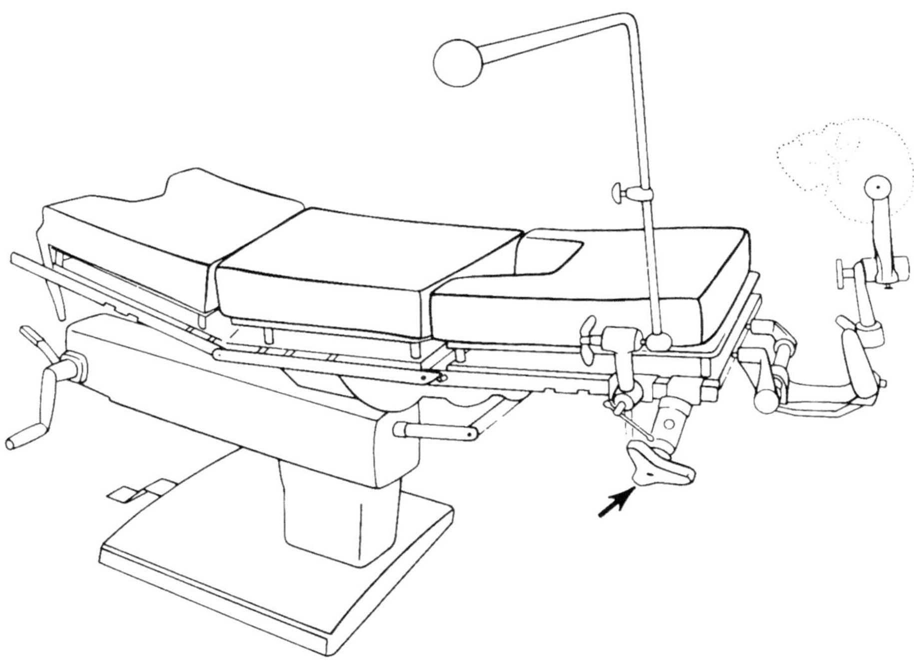

B Same after specially made mattress is in place with opening for lumbar CSF drainage. A model skull (see Fig. 26.3) is held by the skull clamp (replacing the head rest). An "ether screen" (bar with knob projecting toward observer) projects away from the left side of the patient to later hold the drapes and suction tubes. The Leyla self-retaining retractor bar (see Fig. 26.15) attaches (*arrow*) to the OR table just cephalad to the "ether screen" attachment. The microscope stands just cephalad to the "ether screen," and the anesthesiologist is positioned caudal to the "ether screen." (*Continued*).

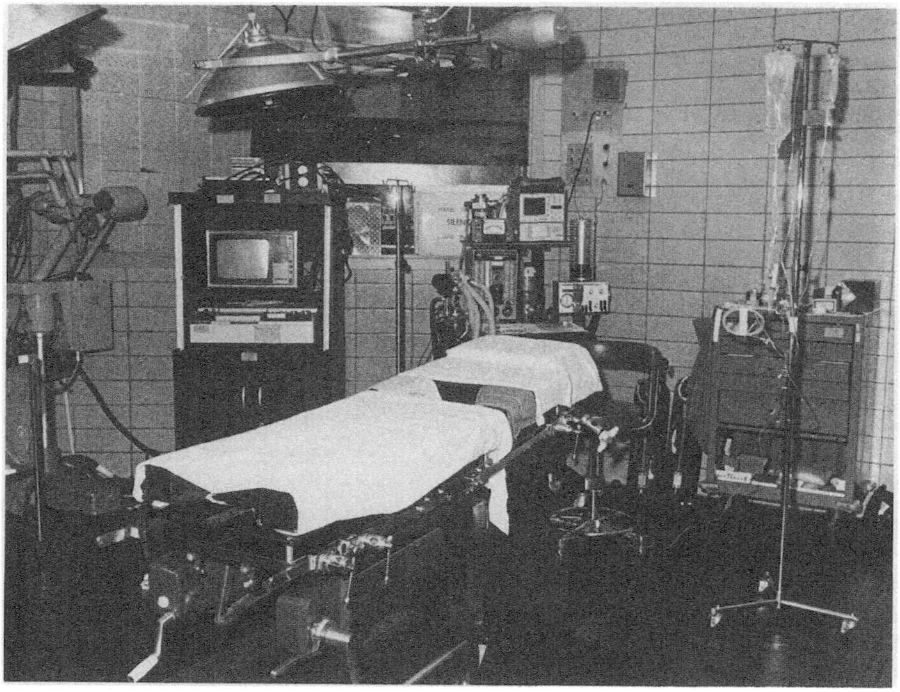

Fig. 26.1 **C** OR table in position for induction of anesthesia. Rather than move the anesthesiologist's equipment, the OR table later is turned counterclockwise 90° so that the anesthesiologist is on the left side of the patient.

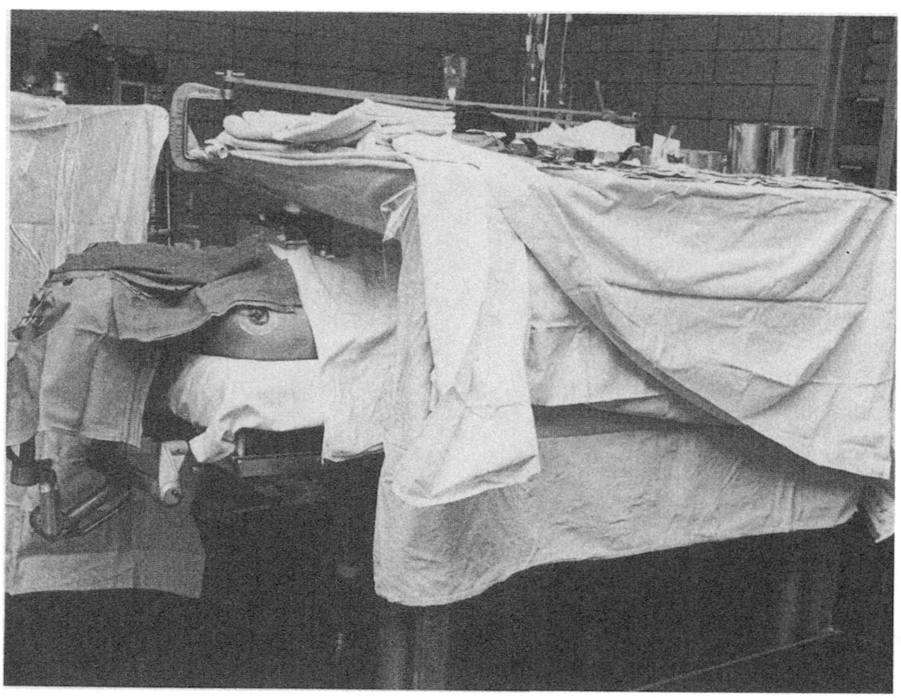

D Preliminary draping of patient. Instruments are placed on the overhead instrument table (Phelan Manufacturing Corp., Minneapolis). Note the sterilized "C-clamps" at each end with rubber tubing stretched between. These are covered after final draping and prevent instruments from falling off into the anesthesiologist's nonsterile field.

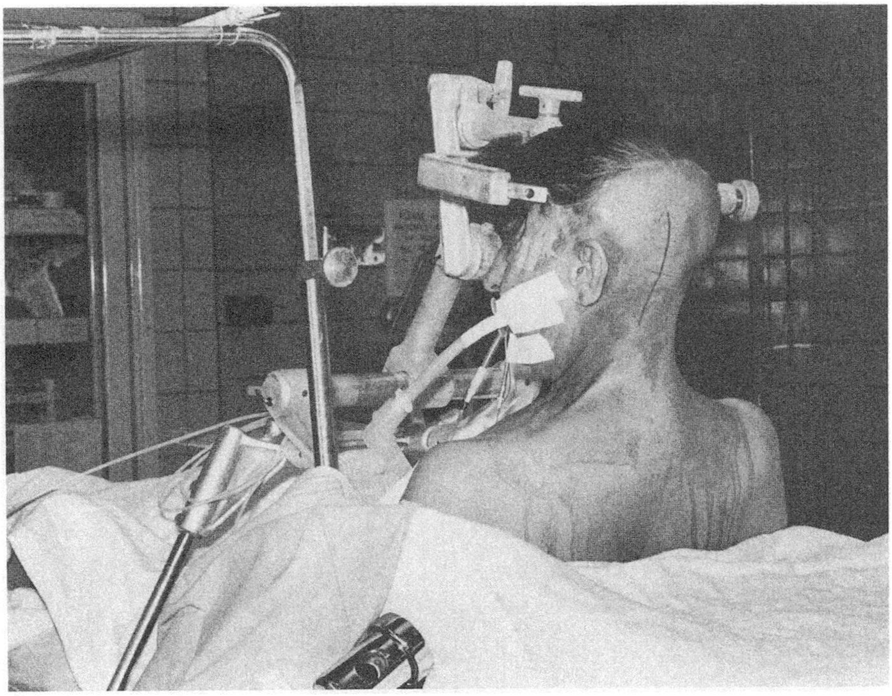

Fig. 26.2. Patient with left VAA in sitting position. Head rest with white sheets turned down is to be used as surgeon's arm rest. Incision is marked halfway between midline and left mastoid area. Head is turned leftward. Mayfield–Kees head support and Yaşargil–Aesculap (Leyla) retractor-bar connector are in place.

the position of the pin tends to remain unstable, however tightly the clamp is applied. A pin on the forehead should, of course, be well away from the eye, and when the clamp is positioned too close to the incision a pin-casing can be a hindrance. Special smaller pins available for infants can also be used for patients who have thin skulls. Particular attention should be given to patients who have had a long history of hydrocephalus. Having secured the clamp, the surgeon holds the head in the desired position while the final attachment to the operating table is made. Manipulation of the head holder accurately and with safety may be difficult at first, but with experience any obstacles encountered can usually be surmounted. This method of skull fixation avoids the pressure injuries that may occur to the scalp or face when the head has been resting on rubber pads for long periods.

The time of insertion of the points into the scalp and skull is a critical period. The head must be perfectly positioned according to the approach used by the surgeon. Any deficiency will cause defective alignment of the target (aneurysm), cranial opening, microscope, and surgeon's eyes. The alignment must be such that there will be a clear view of the aneurysm at the focal point of the microscope with the surgeon in a comfortable position. Upon insertion of the points, the patient's blood pressure will rise unless he is properly anesthetized and his blood pressure is under control. Control is necessary to avoid the risk of premature rupture of the aneurysm at this time. The surgeon must notify the anesthesiologist before he inserts the points. Colley and Dunn (26) recommended local anesthesia in the scalp at the point-insertion sites.

Surgeon's Chair

Surgeons' chairs are available from various companies, e.g., Storz Instrument Company, Stryker Corporation, and V. Mueller Co. Yaşargil et al. (181) reported on their special chair. We prefer the pneumatic lift chair (style P390244) available from the C.G.R. Medical Corporation of Pittsburgh (Fig. 26.4). A hard cushion may be placed on the seat to give the surgeon a bit more height. The stool height is adjustable by pressing on the foot bar.

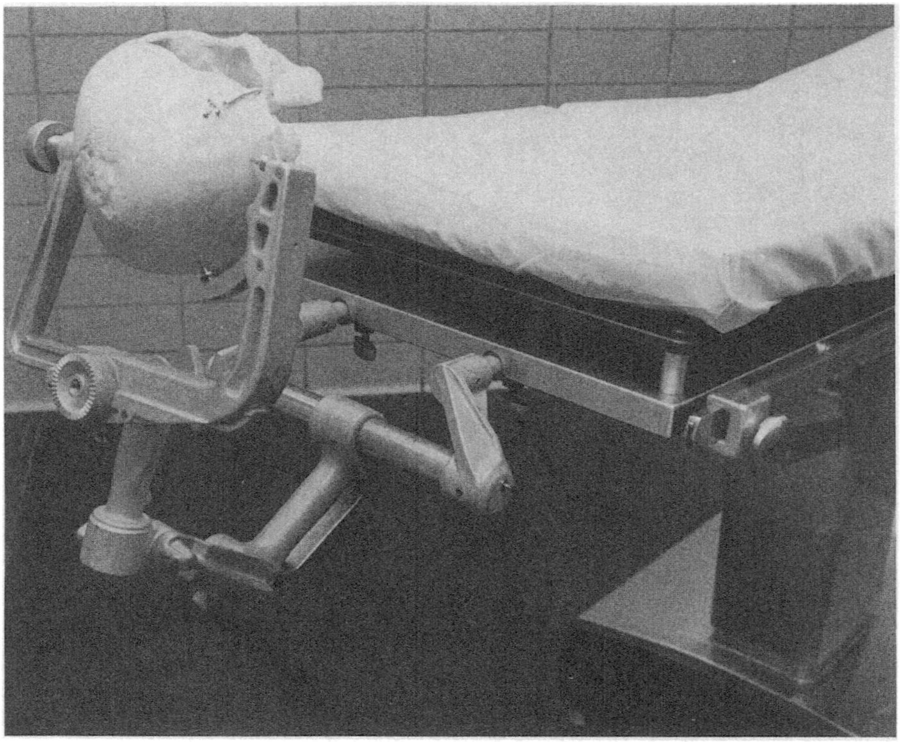

Fig. 26.3. A Mayfield–Kees headholder with demonstration skull (bone flap removed) in position for right frontolateral craniotomy.

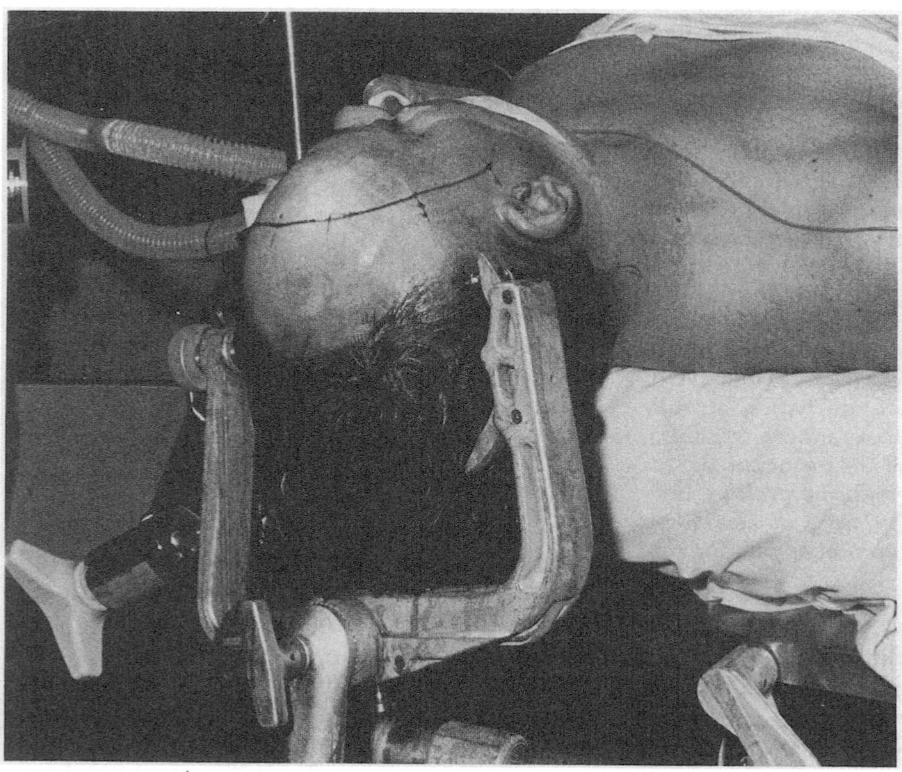

B Patient in position with head turned in 40° to left, tilted 15° to left, and dropped back 15°.

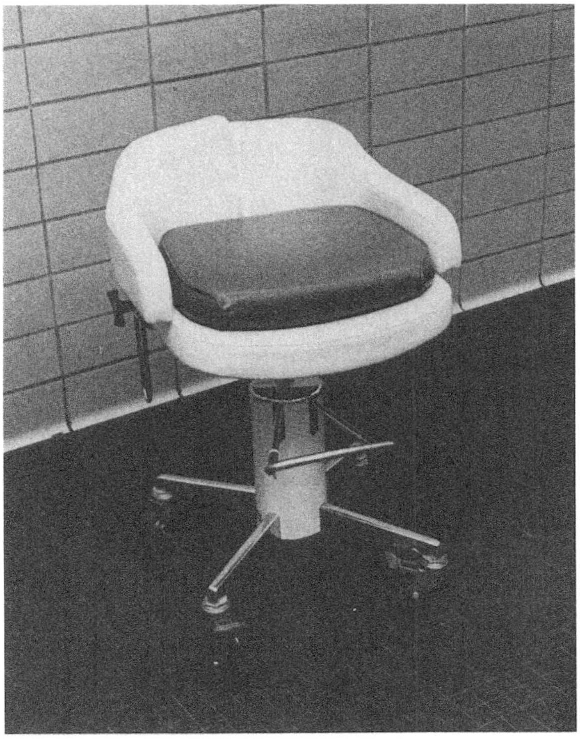

Fig. 26.4. Pneumatic lift chair (C.G.R. Medical Corporation, Pittsburgh). The dark cushion is added for extra height.

Loupes and Headlight

Some surgeons prefer surgical loupes (Fig. 26.5), also called "operating telescopes," to the operating microscope. Designs for Vision, Inc. makes loupes with up to 8× magnification. This amount of magnification is nearly equivalent

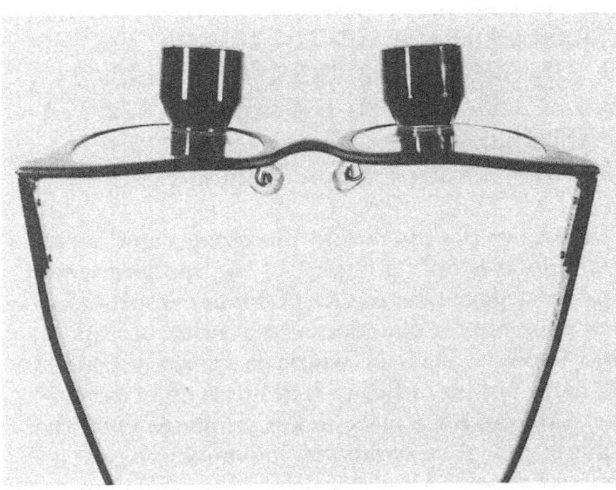

Fig. 26.5. Example of surgical loupes (Designs for Vision, Inc.).

to the true magnification given by our own Zeiss operating microscope with a 275 mm objective lens, 12.5× eyepieces, and the dial set at its third magnification setting. The loupes are used in conjunction with a fiberoptic headlight.

Loupes have a few disadvantages: When the surgeon turns his head the visual field and focus on target are temporarily lost, whereas with the microscope they remain unchanged. Slight movements of the surgeon's head are distracting. Moreover, there are no observer's tubes and no satisfactory method of televising the operation; photographic techniques are inferior. A new pair of loupes must be purchased when the refraction of the surgeon's eyes changes, and loupes of high magnification can be heavy and uncomfortable for the surgeon. Loupes do have the advantage of lower cost and convenience, however, and floor space is not taken up by a floor-mount microscope.

Bischoff (16) used loupes in 1863 at 3× to 12× magnification for dissecting cranial nerves in the laboratory. Donaghy (37) and Yaşargil (171) produced good historical reviews on the subject. A number of surgeons have now used loupes during craniotomy for intracranial aneurysms (9,11,40–43,70,70a,84,102,113,120,160).

Operating Microscope

> The remarkable new surgical world revealed under the operating microscope and the beautiful instruments available to work in it have undoubtedly played a major role in placing the safety and scope of aneurysm surgery where they are today (39).

> However, it should never be forgotten that there is much more to microtechnique in neurosurgery than the possession of a highly perfected optical instrument. This alone is of little value without special methods of bipolar coagulation, carefully adapted instruments, and, above all, atraumatic operation techniques (171).

In 1865 Bischoff (16) published his work on dissections of the cranial nerves. He began with loupes and later graduated to the dissecting microscope with up to 50× power. The evolution of the use of the operating microscope in surgery is detailed in other publications (37,51, 92,101,108,124,125,171). Its application to intracranial aneurysms first began with anatomists and pathologists who studied details of cerebral vascular anomalies and their environ-

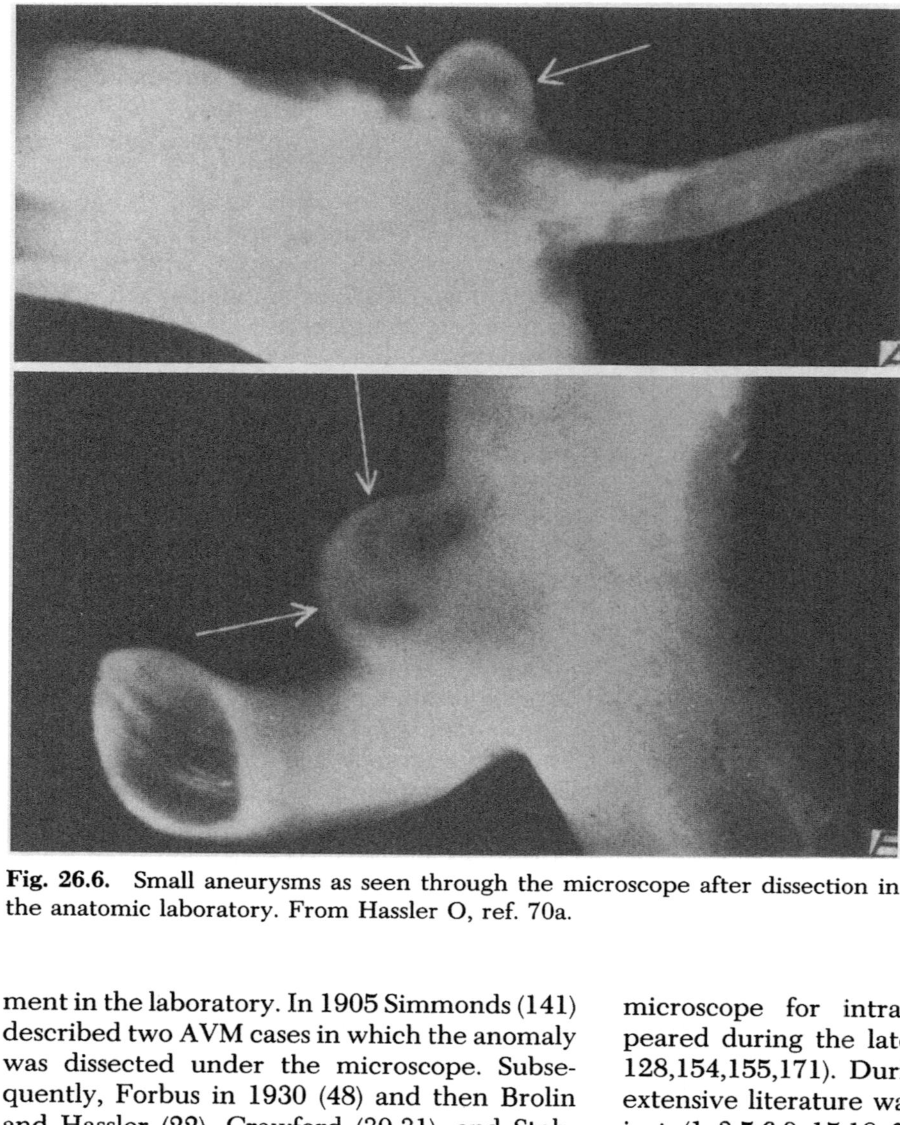

Fig. 26.6. Small aneurysms as seen through the microscope after dissection in the anatomic laboratory. From Hassler O, ref. 70a.

ment in the laboratory. In 1905 Simmonds (141) described two AVM cases in which the anomaly was dissected under the microscope. Subsequently, Forbus in 1930 (48) and then Brolin and Hassler (22), Crawford (30,31), and Stehbens (144) wrote about aneurysms dissected under the microscope in anatomic laboratories (Fig. 26.6).

By the early 1960s Lougheed (51) was already using the operating microscope in the treatment of some aneurysms. In 1964 Adams and Witt (4) reported on the use of the otological operating microscope for intracranial aneurysms. In 1965 Tovi was photographed clipping an aneurysm; he was looking through a microscope at the time (104). In 1965 Pool (121,122) published the first scientific description of the clinical application of the microscope for intracranial aneurysms. In 1967 Rand and Jannetta (127) were the first to report on use of the microscope in cases with basilar artery aneurysms. A few additional reports on use of the operating microscope for intracranial aneurysms appeared during the late 1960s (96,98,124,126–128,154,155,171). During the next decade an extensive literature was published on the subject (1–3,5,6,9–15,18–21,23–25,27–29,33,34,36, 39,44,47,51–53,56,65,66,71–74,78–80,82,85–87,89,90,95,97,103,105–107,109–120,123,125, 129,131–138,142,143,145,146,148,148a,149, 152,153,156–159,161–164,166–170,172,174–180,182,183).

In 1978 a study group concluded (51):

> The use of the operating microscope and microtechnique is only one part of the modern trend in the surgical treatment of certain cerebrovascular problems. Coincidentally a team of experts has evolved, each of whom is specially trained to carry out his or her task in this type of surgery. . . . Although we place major emphasis upon the microsurgical techniques, advances have occurred as well in anesthesiology, nursing care, radiological diagnostic methods, pharmacology, and available monitoring systems. Certainly the judi-

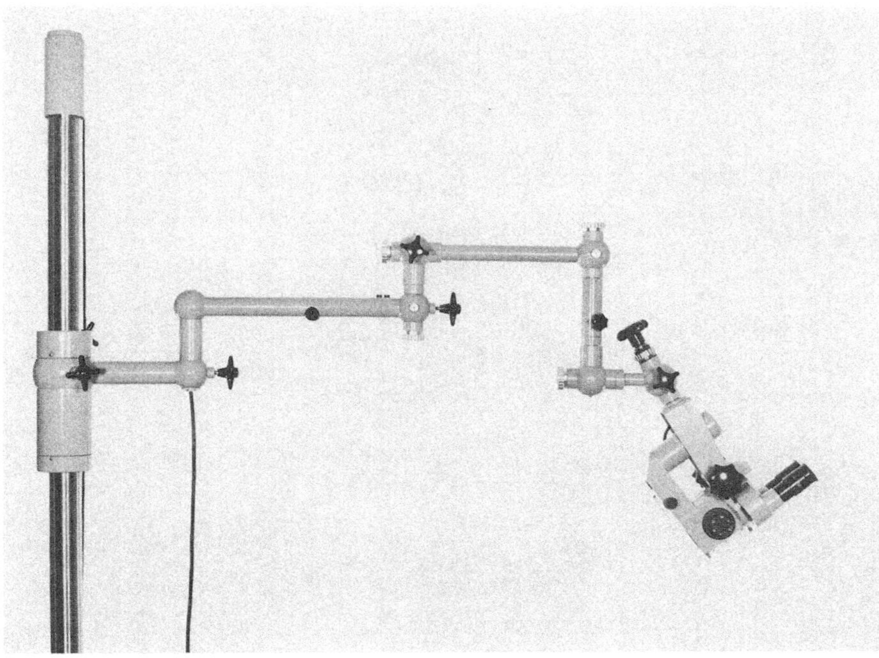

A

Fig. 26.7. Standard OPMI-1 model of the Zeiss operating microscope. Courtesy of Carl Zeiss, Inc.

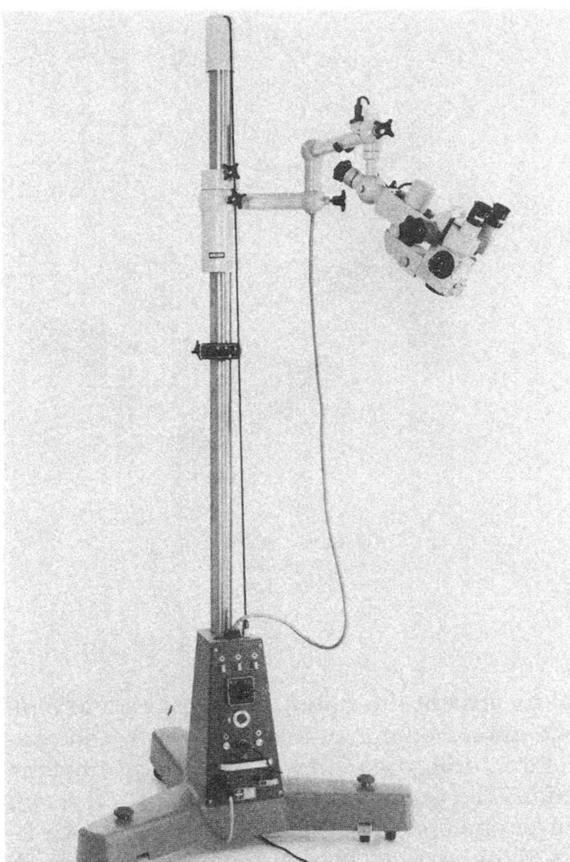

B

cious use of vascular hypotension and of techniques to control intracranial pressure has helped greatly to reduce patient morbidity. Some operations would be extremely difficult if not impossible to perform without today's sophisticated personnel. . . . Both reports in the recent literature and the increasing use of the microscope by neurosurgeons confirm the opinion and experience of study group members that the application of the operating microscope and microtechnique has markedly reduced the mortality and morbidity associated with intracranial aneurysm surgery. Parallel improvements in equipment have contributed additionally to these results. The cardinal factors, however, are the training, experience, and expertise of the operating surgeon who utilizes these new techniques and the capabilities of his operative team.

Some of the technical aspects of optics, supports, accessories, use, care, and sterilization of the microscope and its accessories are given elsewhere (38,49,51,91,93,100,101,124,125, 171,181). The Zeiss operating microscope (Carl Zeiss, Inc.) is the unit most commonly used at this time (Figs. 26.7–26.9).

We have been using the counterbalanced Zeiss–Contraves unit (Figs. 26.8 and 26.9) with electronic switches which release magnetic locks, immobilizing the microscope in any desired position (181). Our preference is the OPMI No. 1 Zeiss magnification system rather than the zoom lens system attached to the Con-

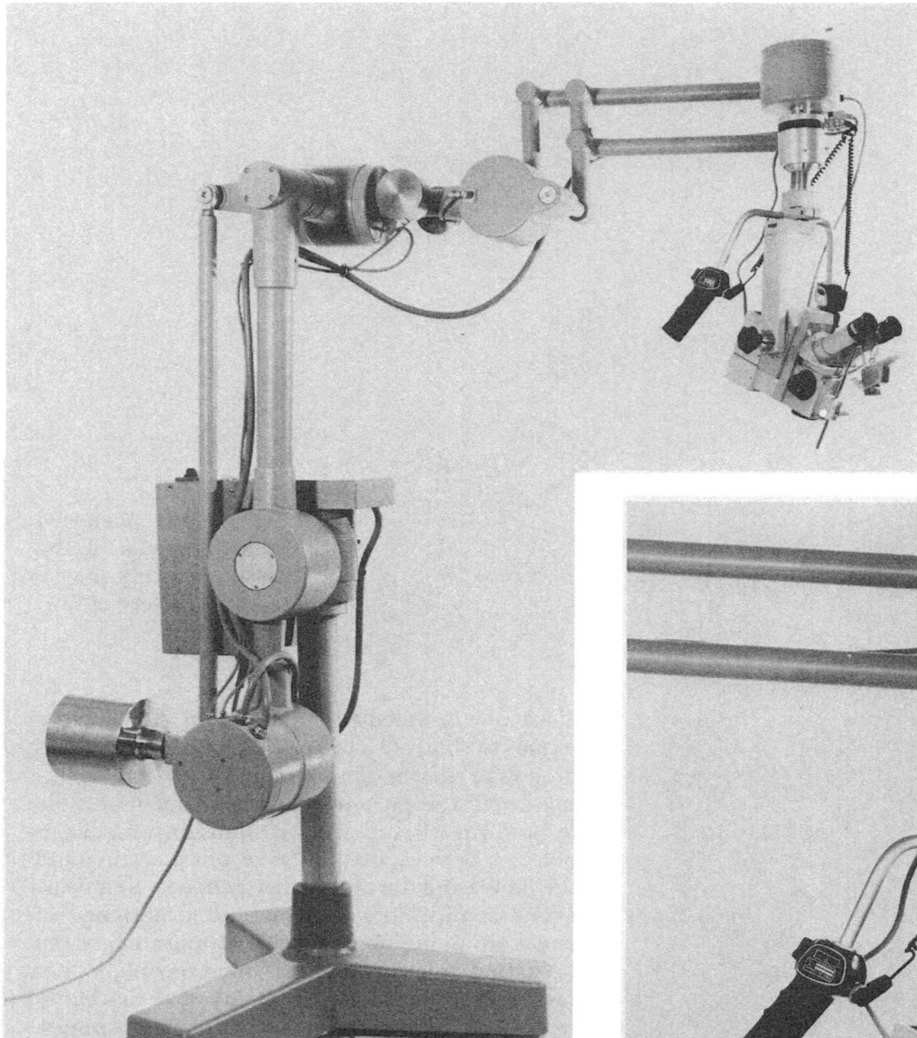

A

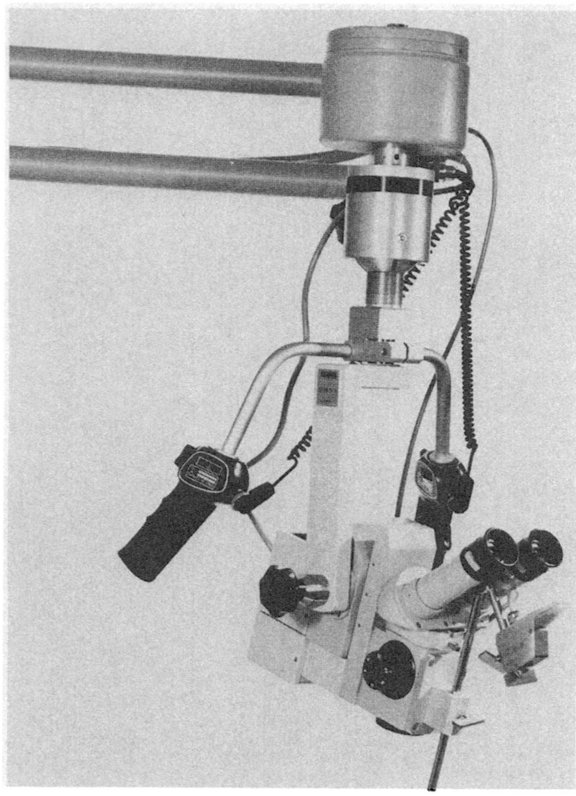

B

Fig. 26.8. Counterbalanced Zeiss–Contraves operating microscope. Courtesy of Carl Zeiss, Inc.

traves stand. We also prefer the floor mount to the ceiling mount. In our OR the television camera is attached to the left side of the beam splitter, and the binocular observation tube is attached to the right side. For still camera photography we temporarily replace the observer tube with the still camera and its adapter. Prior to more stringent U.S. government restrictions, we (JLF) cold-gas-sterilized our entire microscope (except the stand), still camera and film, television camera, and cables, lenses, and connectors using two ampoules of pure ethylene oxide. The gas was allowed to dissipate through three enclosing (air tight) plastic bags for 12–18 h overnight. If the same microscope is needed twice the same day, it is then draped in the usual manner for the second operation. In over 10 years of satisfactory experience with

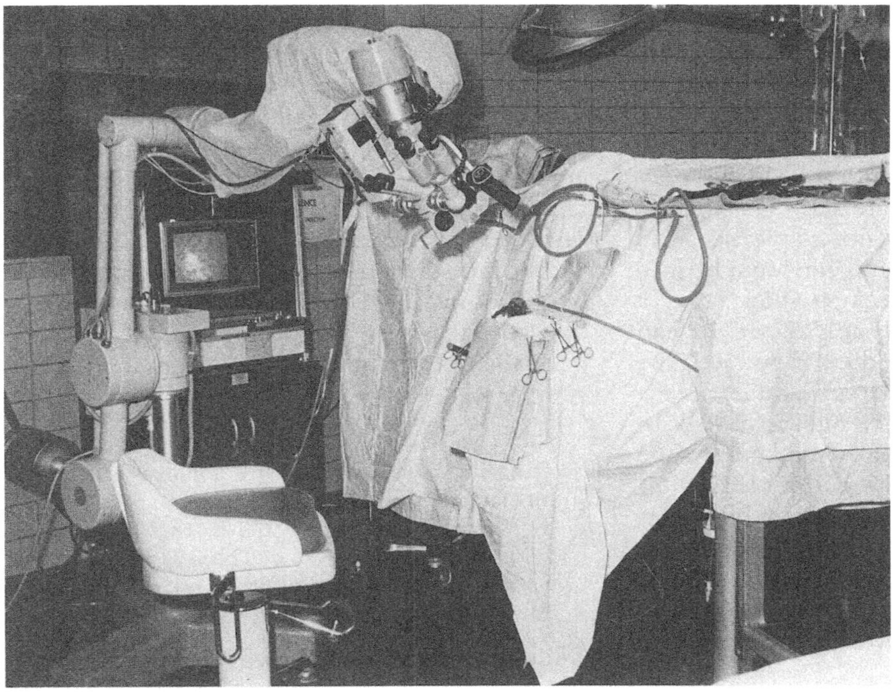

Fig. 26.9. A Zeiss–Contraves operating microscope in position at surgery. It has been cold-gas-sterilized overnight with ethylene exide. Draping is completed. The bone flap has been turned. Note the rubber tubing that holds the drapes firmly down and caudally. Above are two suction tubes in readiness. In the background is a television monitor.

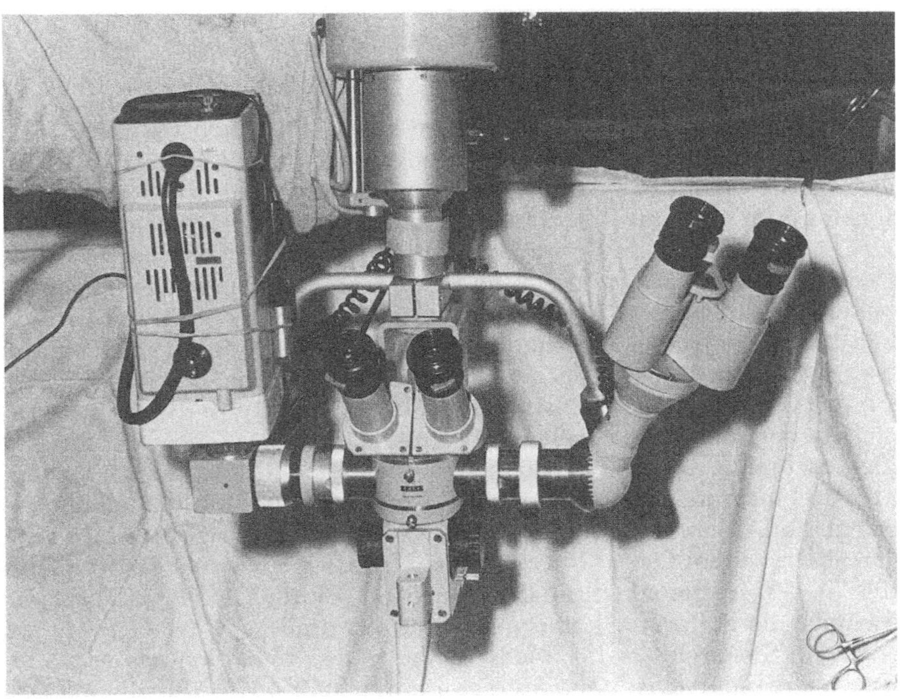

B Close-up view of microscope and attachments. *Left:* television camera and microphone. *Center:* Binocular system and beam-splitter. *Right:* assistant's observation tube. The latter is removed temporarily when still camera photographs are made.

this type of sterilization of many microscopes used by several surgical services prior to 1980, we have had no sterilization-related injury to any parts of the microscope or attendant personnel. Other details of our technique are given below under the sections on television and photographic methods and materials.

Although agreement is not universal as to when the microscope should be brought into the operative field, experience shows that a more gentle, accurate, and rapid dissection can be carried out if, once the dura is opened, the entire approach to the aneurysm and its dissection are carried out under the microscope. With the patient supine, the angled binocular tube is used most often. With the patient sitting for posterior fossa surgery, the straight binocular tube is used. With experience, the surgeon often finds that he routinely uses the same higher magnification (e.g., 6× or 8× true magnification) for the approach to the aneurysm as he does for its dissection.

Several *disadvantages* of the operating microscope have been mentioned (51,173): special training is required for using the microscope, microtools, and microsuture; it necessitates operating in a deep, narrow gap; it requires longer adaptation time; it does not permit good tissue palpation (instruments are used, not fingers) and requires visual manipulation; work is indirect; work is tiring to the eyes; stiff neck, shoulders, and back generally result; distractions are poorly tolerated; equipment and training are expensive; it takes up space in the operating room; and the operating time for most surgeons is longer.

Advantages for the neurosurgeon far outweigh any drawbacks, however (51,173): Fewer parallax problems occur because the objective lens brings the target closer to the surgeon's vision; binocular vision is improved; illumination is increased; the focus is sharper; and magnification permits a smaller craniotomy, less brain retraction, a smaller cortical incision, and better delineation of normal and abnormal anatomy. Structures that are better identified by the microscope are (51,173): the arachnoid space, compartments, and bands; the perforating arteries; vascular variations in the circle of Willis; aneurysmal anatomy; microaneurysms; the impending rupture of an aneurysm; small bleeding points for bipolar coagulation; and the nerves. The advantages to the patient are a smaller wound, better repair of nerves and vessels, the fact that some inoperable lesions become operable, optimal hemostasis, fewer surgical lesions, and fewer postoperative complications (51,173). Educational advantages include use of the observer tube, television with tape recording, and cinematography or still photography. In addition, the television system allows the scrub nurse and anesthesiologist to know the state of the surgery from moment to moment.

As the microsurgical era in intracranial aneurysm treatment began, Drake in 1965 stated (41):

> The ability to see the minute details of the structures about an aneurysm has been, in my opinion, the source of much trouble in this as in other fields of neurosurgery . . . There is a new world waiting for us. The dissecting microscope with its superb illumination is ideal. . . .

Gillingham cautioned, however (60):

> This is a moment to reflect on the use of magnification. It may make us ten times more gentle but it leads to obsessive over dissection in an endeavor to find the neck of a sac which is nonexistent or excessive manipulation in the region of the neck. . . .

Television

As mentioned above, television has important educational advantages (live visualization of microanatomy and taping procedures for future teaching) as well as practical advantages (51,77). Operating room physicians and nurses alter their anesthetic techniques and ongoing activities as well as more efficiently prepare for anticipated operative events based on information received from the television monitor. Figure 26.10 illustrates the clarity of these modern television systems.

Color television systems (Fig. 26.9B) for the microscope are in a state of rapid evolution in terms of image clarity and brightness, weight, durability, and freedom from need for frequent repairs. Hence it is pointless to recommend specific systems at this time.

Many of the newer television cameras can operate at a lower light level. Yet it is still advantageous to obtain good lighting to allow a smaller diaphragm opening and consequently a greater depth of field and a sharper focus.

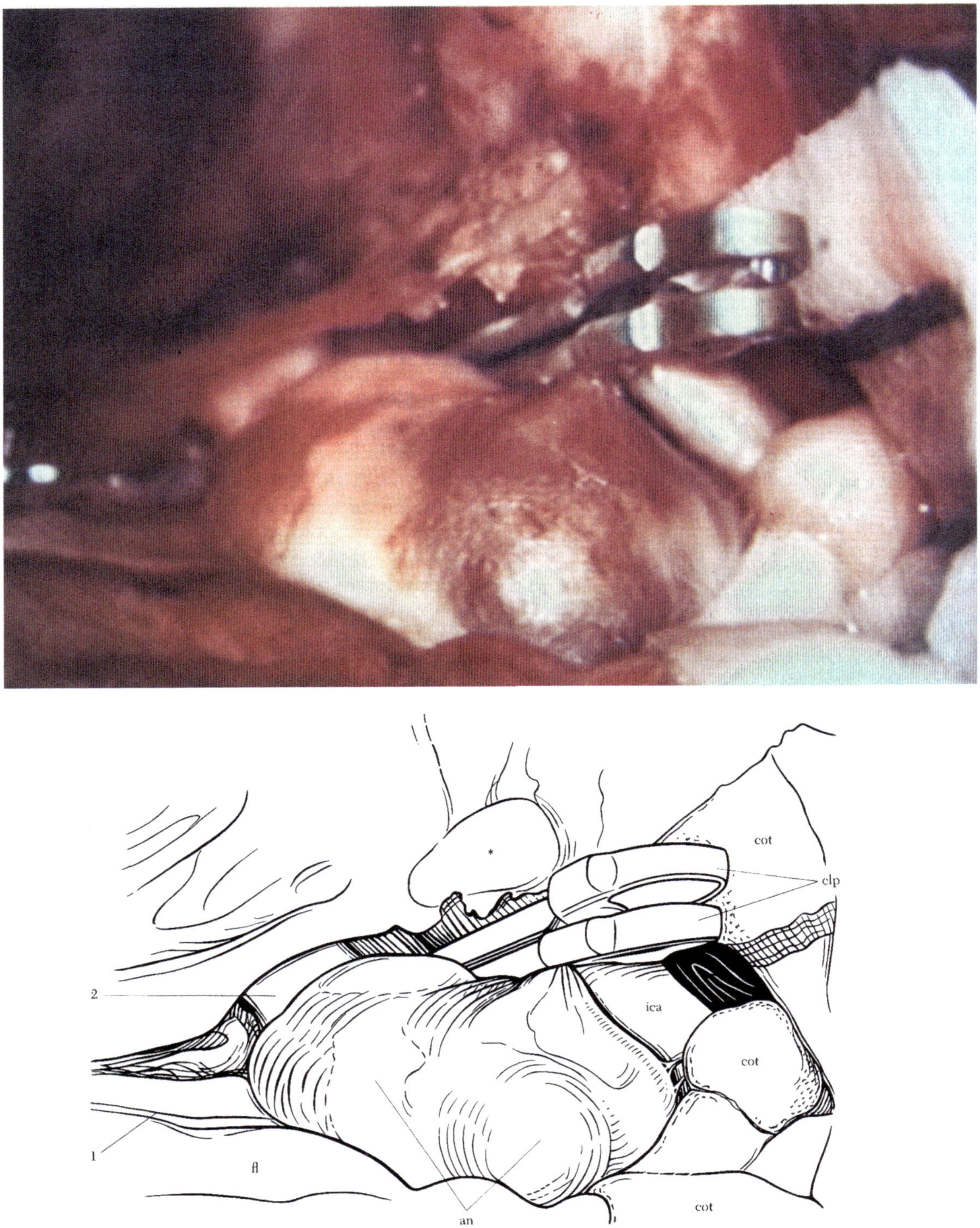

Fig. 26.10. Television screen showing right frontolateral view of giant internal carotid artery aneurysm (*an*) at take-off of ophthalmic artery. *fl*, frontal lobe. *1*, olfactory tract. *2*, optic nerve. *, anterior clinoid process (dura removed). *cot*, cottonoids. *clp*, clips (Yaşargil type). *ica*, internal carotid artery. On close scrutiny can one detect horizontal television lines. (See Fig. 34.1 for orientation of patient's head.)

Table 26.1. Methods of Improving Lighting for the Surgeon and/or Cameras[a]

1. Increase voltage in transformer (shortens bulb life).
2. Use an efficient lighting system (currently in state of improvement).
3. Keep bulbs and optical system clean.
4. Discard bulbs with blue or dark spots in light image.
5. Use add-on light sources.
6. Use short focal length objective lens.
7. Avoid zoom lens system, which absorbs more light.
8. Turn off bright lights in operating room (better contrast; surgeon's pupils are dilated, requiring less light).
9. Make use of internal reflections in surgical wound; avoid reflections back into the microscope.
10. Remove black paint border around glass light deflector behind objective lens (present in some microscopes).
11. Use 30–70 beam splitter (70% to side arms, only 30% to surgeon) instead of 50–50 beam splitter.
12. Use greater magnification in eyepieces, thereby requiring less magnification (hence less light loss) inside microscope unit.
13. Open diaphragm to camera (with loss of sharpness and depth of focus).
14. Properly adjust TV camera power supply and TV monitor.
15. Select efficient TV camera or film that can operate with less light.

[a] Certain methods listed have particular value in some circumstances, whereas in others they may prove unnecessary or impractical. Items 1–10 also increase brightness for the surgeon. Item 11 decreases image brightness to the surgeon. From Fox JL, Albin MS, Bader DCH, et al., ref. 51.

Table 26.1 summarizes some methods to improve lighting for the surgeon and for the television or photographic cameras.

Cinemaphotography

With the advent of television cameras for the operating microscope and their taping facilities, movie films of microneurosurgical operations are less common now. Television tape is cheaper, easier to copy and edit, and more convenient to use in the operating room; it also can be edited and converted to movie film for presentation to large audiences. Such a process is expensive, but so is multiple movie film editing.

Still Cameras

The still color photographs of aneurysm anatomy shown elsewhere in this book (Chapters 34–39) and in a previous article (49) were reproduced from 35-mm color slides. The following two paragraphs are taken in part from a previous article by Fox (49).

For photography, we used a Zeiss OPMI-1 operating microscope equipped with a 275 mm objective lense, a 160-mm focal-length binocular tube, 12.5× eyepieces, a 30/70 beam splitter (70% of the light is deflected and divided equally between the film on the right and the television camera on the left; 30% goes to the surgeon's eyes), a Zeiss camera adapter and 2× magnification attachment, a Nikon camera back, and ASA 160 (tungsten) Ektachrome 35-mm film. A 30- or 50-watt incandescent light bulb was used without auxiliary lighting but with the transformer constantly on "overload" (about 9 volts) throughout the operation. (If the heat is allowed to escape directly into the room, the light bulb usually lasts throughout several operations.) Prior to 1980 no drapes were used, but the microscope, camera, film, and television system were cold-gas-sterilized for 12–18 h with pure ethylene oxide gas. (New federal regulations have now restricted this method of sterilization.) Any black-paint border around the glass prism deflecting the light through the objective lens was removed. Overhead lights in the operating room were turned off to provide better contrast and to facilitate dilation of the surgeon's pupils.

Photographs were made during the expiratory phase of the automatic respirator with 1-sec exposures and with the *f*-stop on the Zeiss photoadapter set at 44. The brief systolic pulsations of intracranial arteries are not sufficient to blur the image. Self-retaining retractors and white cottonoids were positioned to provide light reflections within the wound while avoiding reflections toward the microscope. Unless otherwise indicated, the photographs presented were made with the Zeiss magnification dial set at No. 16 (or at its third magnification setting), providing a true 6× magnification for the surgeon. Although the photographs do not provide stereoscopic vision and sufficient depth of field, which may be 6 cm from the skull surface, it is hoped that the reader's knowledge of anatomy will compensate for this.

We have tried some of the special adaptors which allow connection with both a television camera and a still camera. Photographs of poorer quality resulted; until a better system is available, we have continued to sacrifice the inconvenience of temporarily changing the right-sided observer tube with the still camera adapter when we wish to photograph. Also, when the still camera is placed on the left side, we found the image on the slide to be reversed. The techniques we use to provide good lighting (without add-on sources) have allowed us to use the small *f*-stop opening of 44, which explains the sharpness, brightness, and depth of field seen in many of the photographs. To use a brighter lighting system and shorten the time may be self-defeating, for shorter time exposures (unless one can reduce the time to 1/1000 s at a 44 *f*-stop or less without overheating the operative field) often catch the arterial pulsations during systole, blurring the image. The 1-s exposures average out this arterial movement of short duration. A wider diaphragm opening (*f*-stop number is smaller) allows in more light but causes loss of depth of field, a flatness to the picture, and a greater fuzziness at the edge of the image. If certain nonincandescent light sources are used, one may have to use daylight (instead of tungsten) color film for better color reproduction.

Intraoperative Instrumentation

Fishhooks

The use of improvised tissue retraction hooks, or "fishhooks," connected to rubber bands has been used by many surgeons to retract scalp, muscle, and dura. More recently a fishhook retractor device using springs (Aesculap Instrument Co.) instead of rubber bands has been suggested (181). We prefer the "disposable" Weck Durahooks (Edward Weck & Co.), although, we remove their rubber bands and substitute our own thicker rubber bands for repeated use.

The hooks are used to retract the frontotemporal scalp flap turned over the patient's forehead as follows (Fig. 26.11): The sterile drapes between the overhead table (neurosurgical instrument table; Phelan Manufacturing Corp., Minneapolis) and the patient's head are held firmly downward and caudally by standard rubber suction tubing of appropriate length. The ends of this tubing are secured to each side of the OR table. This tube (a) firmly holds the drapes in place and (b) allows a convenient site of attachment for the rubber bands that retract both the scalp hooks and then the bone flap. In this way the drapes of the perioperative field are smooth, firm, and clear of unnecessary clamps and other retractors.

Suction and Suction–Irrigation Devices

Suction tubes usually are sized (diameter) by the "French" (Fr) designation: a 3-Fr size has an outer diameter of 1 mm; a 9-Fr size is 3 mm; etc. Standard sizes for aneurysm surgery are 3-Fr, 7-Fr, 9-Fr, and 11-Fr, although there are many other variations. There are a multitude of types of suction tube with variations in length, angulation, tip configuration, and vacuum pressure (10,17,51,68,69,128a,178, 181).

A suction system with a mechanism to control the negative pressure at very low levels is essential. The suction should be finely adjusted to eliminate the hazard of small anatomical structures being entrapped and damaged. Many neurosurgical suction tubes are constructed to allow regulation of suction strength by adjusting the degree to which the thumb occludes the air hole. These holes can be enlarged (17,69), and/or venting needles can be placed in rubber suction tubes. The trap bottles can have pressure-regulating gauges. When dissecting delicate structures, it may be advisable to use special smooth-tipped suction tubes and negative pressures of about 2 meters of water (approximately 0.2 atm) (181). In place of wall suction, some surgeons prefer an electric suction pump, easily regulated by adjusting the dials on the pump.

Irrigating fluid in conjunction with the suction apparatus is essential during the surgical procedure. In addition to keeping tissues from drying and the aneurysm wall from becoming brittle, it discourages the formation of small blood clots and their adherence to the dissected surfaces; it also increases the effectiveness of bipolar coagulation and reduces tissue adhesiveness. Constant bathing with CSF has the same effect. Some surgeons prefer a combination suction–irrigation unit.

We usually use an angulated Frazier suction tube of varying lengths. The 11-Fr and 9-Fr sizes are used for cranial work and the 7-Fr for aneurysm dissection. We use the 7-Fr size rather than smaller suction tubes because of

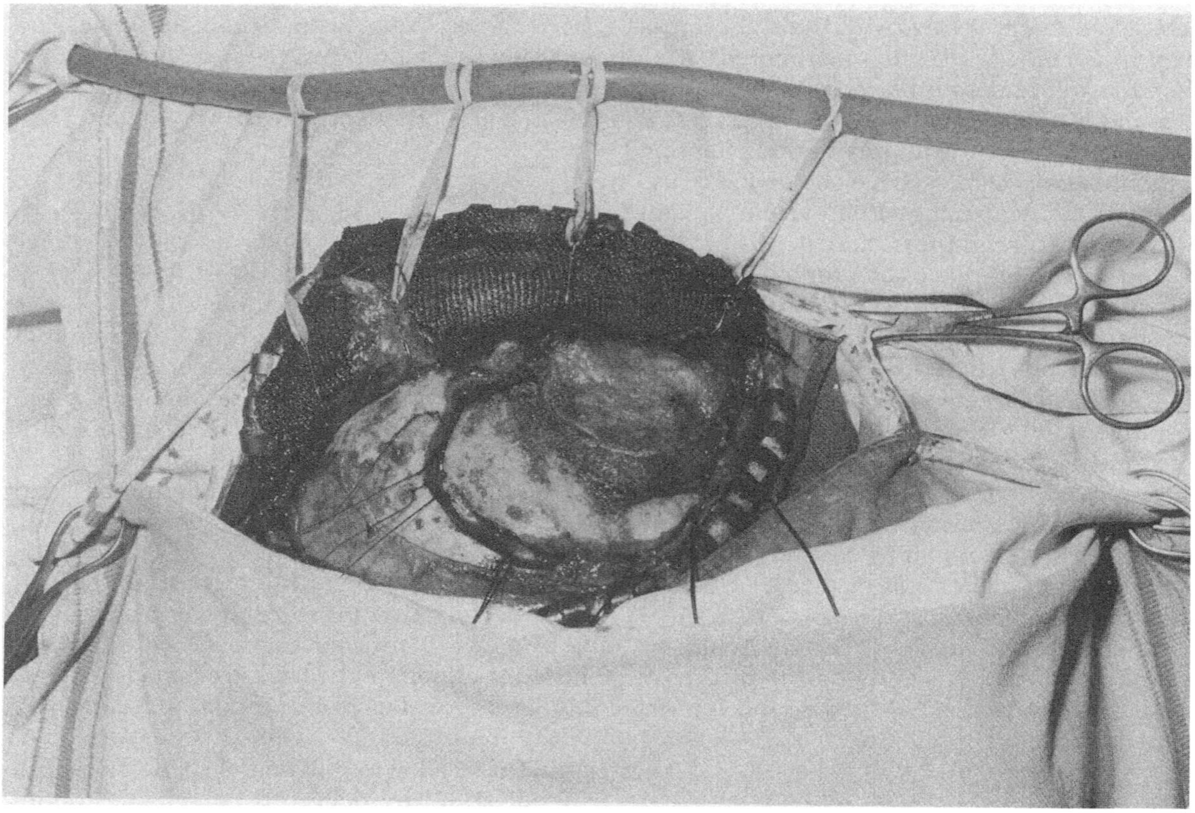

Fig. 26.11. Close-up view of rubber tube holding drapes firmly (see Fig. 26.9A). Here the same tubing is used to attach the rubber bands holding the fishhooks. These fishhooks retract the oxycellulose-covered scalp flap forward. The right frontolateral bone flap is attached to the temporalis muscle (at *center* of figure). Dural tack-up sutures and bone flap sutures are in place in the cranium before the dura is opened.

its use as a dissector and retractor as well as a suction device. Moreover, the larger diameter provides less air and liquid velocity for the same vacuum pressure. The metal suction tube also can be used for resting microscissors or other instruments to reduce tremor when making a delicate dissection. The suction tube is held in the surgeon's left hand, often with his hand or fifth finger resting on the Leyla retractor bar or the skull. The suction is often used against small dental cotton balls (Richmond Dental Cotton Co., Charlotte, North Carolina) or small cottonoids for suction protection and retraction. Rubber tubing is preferred to plastic tubing, the latter being too stiff for comfortable use. We routinely put 1000 units of heparin in each liter of irrigating solution to limit clotting, which could cause obstruction within the tubing; this practice may retard undesirable clotting in the basilar cisterns as well. The only time we use a suction–irrigation apparatus (House–Radpour unit) is during bone (sphenoid wing or anterior clinoid process) drilling.

Bone Removal Instruments

In 1930 Rogers (130) gave an excellent historical account of craniotomy methods. He noted that the Horsley trephine had its origins in the time of Hippocrates (ca. 400 years B.C.). The technique of bone flap removal made a significant advance with Gigli's application of the wire saw (the Gigli saw, Fig. 26.12) in 1894 (57,58). This saw is still routinely used by many surgeons—especially in elderly patients where the dura may be stuck to the inner table of the skull. The present-day use of power (pneumatic or electric) drills and craniotomy for lifting skull flaps is well known and requires no further discussion here. However, one must use

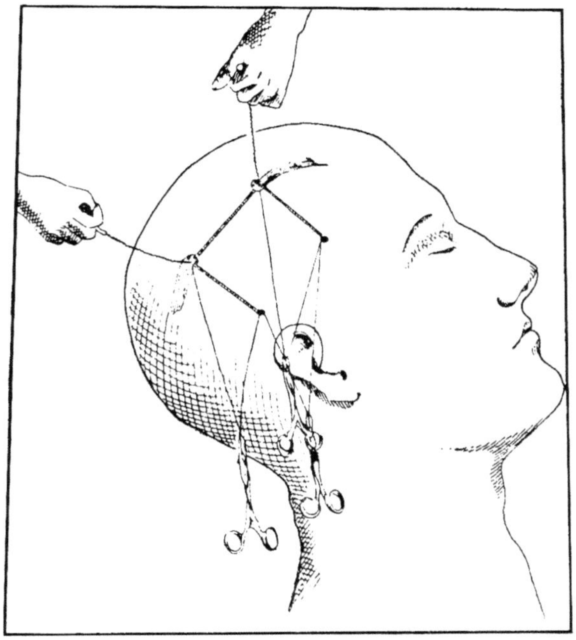

Fig. 26.12. Original Gigli wire saw. From Gigli L, ref. 58.

caution in the commonly performed breaking or cracking of the base of a frontotemporal flap under the temporalis muscle. The vibration at that moment may be transmitted to the aneurysm, causing its premature rupture.

Rongeurs for biting away the base of the bone flap are standard in any craniotomy set. We commonly use the Leksell, Echlin, and Lempert rongeurs for frontotemporal craniotomy, where bone is rongeured away at the base. The flat-jawed Lempert rongeur is especially helpful for removing that portion of the sphenoid wing sticking out as a ridge toward the sylvian fissure.

The neurosurgeon needs a small, high-speed electric or pneumatic drill for removing the sphenoid ridge, the clinoid process, and other protrusions of the cranial base; however, only after he has become acquainted with and skilled in its application in the laboratory should he use a high-speed drill in a neurosurgical operation (51). A drill that can reverse its direction is preferred by some to one that cuts in only one direction. A constant suction–irrigation system with physiological saline can be used to cool the drill; otherwise, heat is transmitted to nearby neural structures. One obtains a more accurate and controlled use of the drill when it is operated at high speeds; only very slight pressure should be used to remove the bone. Dangerous skidding may occur at slow speeds or with dull drill bits because of the greater pressure needed to cut bone. When using lightweight drills or burrs, steel burrs are used when the drilling is remote from the dura. Diamond burrs are safer close to the dura or vital structures, for they tend less to tear soft tissue. We use oxycellulose rather than cotton sponges to cover the nearby galea, muscle, and bone flap, as no harm occurs if these get caught in the drill. Cotton, on the other hand, may cause serious damage if caught in the drill.

There are several types of small, high-speed drills. We prefer the Codman 100,000 rpm air drill (Codman & Shurtleff Co.), although there are many good models and improvements are being made continually.

Removal of skull bone requires a satisfactory method to stop bone bleeding. The time-honored application of bone wax (Horsley's "antiseptic wax" or its modification) remains the most common method (75,76,94). In 1890 Keen reported (83):

> Not uncommonly after trephining, the cut edge of the bone bleeds very freely. To arrest this, Mr. Horsley informs me that he uses a paste or putty made as follows: Melt repeatedly one part of yellow wax and four of vasoline. Next, add carbolic acid one part to twenty of the wax and vasoline, and mix intimately. Then add sufficient white wax to make a mass that will be hard when cold, but that can be quickly softened by the fingers. With this (kept disinfected, of course) he "putties up" the vessels in the edge of the bone.

Horsley subsequently modified his bone wax so it was composed of the now well-known beeswax, almond oil, and salicylic acid, as he noted in 1892 (75):

> The antiseptic wax which Mr. Rushton Parker refers to . . . has the following composition: beeswax, 7 parts; almond oil, 1 part; salicylic acid, 1 per cent. It is the outcome of experiments made in 1885, when, remembering the practice of Magendie and others at the commencement of the century in stopping the sinuses with wax, I tried the effect of "smudging" modelling wax worked soft in the fingers on the free bleeding cut surface of the cranial bones in dogs. As such a proceeding instantly arrested the bleeding, I tried to make an antiseptic compound for operations on man, and the formula was published. It was not, however, satisfactory in my opinion, and I asked Mr. P. W. Squire kindly to make experiments so as

> to arrive nearly at the tenacity of modeling wax. This, I think, he has perfectly succeeded in with the above formula. I have very often used it, and without the least inconvenience. I need hardly say that it is always sterilized by boiling before use, and kept in covered stoppered bottles.

Since then bone wax has been modified somewhat by a few producers. For example, Ethicon, Inc. (Somerville, New Jersey) (46) has used refined beeswax and isopropyl palmitate.

When using bonewax under the microscope, we have found the following to be helpful: The scrub nurse applies a small bit of bonewax to one side of a small cottonoid and hands it by bayonet forceps to the center of the surgeon's operative field. The surgeon then can use his bipolar forceps (without current applied) or his finger to push the cottonoid against the wax, which is pressed into the bleeding bone. Usually we use this technique on the sphenoid wing after drilling it under magnification.

Electrocautery

Electrocautery for coagulation of vessels and vascular tissues has been an integral part of neurosurgery ever since the advent of the "Bovie" electrosurgical unit, reported by Cushing and Bovie in 1928 (32). Light (94) gave a good historical overview of the subject in 1945. In 1967 Malis (99) reviewed the developments and evolution of bipolar electrocoagulation since the time of Greenwood in 1940 (63).

"Monopolar" electrocoagulation has been and continues to be commonly used to coagulate or cut tissues. (Of course, it is really bipolar: One pole is the "ground plate" and the other is the hand-held electrode.) Bipolar electrocoagulation of the type where both poles are in the forceps was developed by Greenwood (61–64) to cauterize small blood vessels on the spinal cord, where minimal heat and electrical spread was essential. Accordingly, the bipolar forceps basically consists of a modification of ordinary bayonet or jewelers' forceps in which each blade of the forceps is one of the electrodes or poles; the blades are isolated from each other by insulation, which separates them at their base.

For microvascular and intracranial aneurysm surgery, bipolar electrocautery units have become essential. There have been many modifications in both the forceps and the power supply (35,45,55,61–64,67,81,88,99,139,150,151,178,181). Malis (99) improved the power supply to provide a damped wave spark unit which was electrically better isolated. This unit, (Codman and Shurtleff Co.) has been one of the more popular and reliable units for neurosurgery (and is preferred by us). The unit was designed specifically to provide the best coagulation at the lowest voltage with the least muscle stimulation; at the same time, it restricts the current to the shortest path between the tips of the two blades of the forceps, with no current of consequence flowing from tip to ground or tip to patient. The greater safety of bipolar coagulation compared to monopolar coagulation around brainstem structures was demonstrated by Gestring et al. (55).

Some tried to provide a single unit for both monopolar and bipolar electrocoagulation (55, 67). Sugita et al. (150,151) used a thermister at the tip of their forceps to automatically cut off the electric current when a preset temperature was reached. Others developed a suction (139) or irrigation (45,88) system attached to one blade of their forceps. DeLong and Fox (35) described an automatic cycling on–off bipolar electrocautery power supply.

We used to prefer the Yaşargil bipolar forceps (178,181) (Mathys & Sohn, Zurich, Switzerland), but we now use the stainless steel Fox bipolar bayonet forceps (V. Mueller Co., Chicago) (Fig. 26.13). These forceps come in 16, 18, and 20 cm lengths and with 0.5 and 1.0 mm tip diameters. Other popular bipolar forceps for aneurysm surgery include the Rhoton round-handled forceps and the Malis forceps with the blades slightly angled downward rather than parallel to the handle. Titanium or stainless steel are commonly used metals, the former being lighter. We prefer the heavier weight of the stainless steel forceps for better balance, comfort, and proprioceptive feedback. It is important not to sterilize titanium and stainless steel instruments in the same package, for the different metals in close proximity may create an electrical potential conducive to rusting and corrosive activity.

DeLong and Fox (35) recommended the following care of these forceps to limit the sticking of tissues to their tips:

1. Do not short-circuit the electric current by touching the forceps tips together.

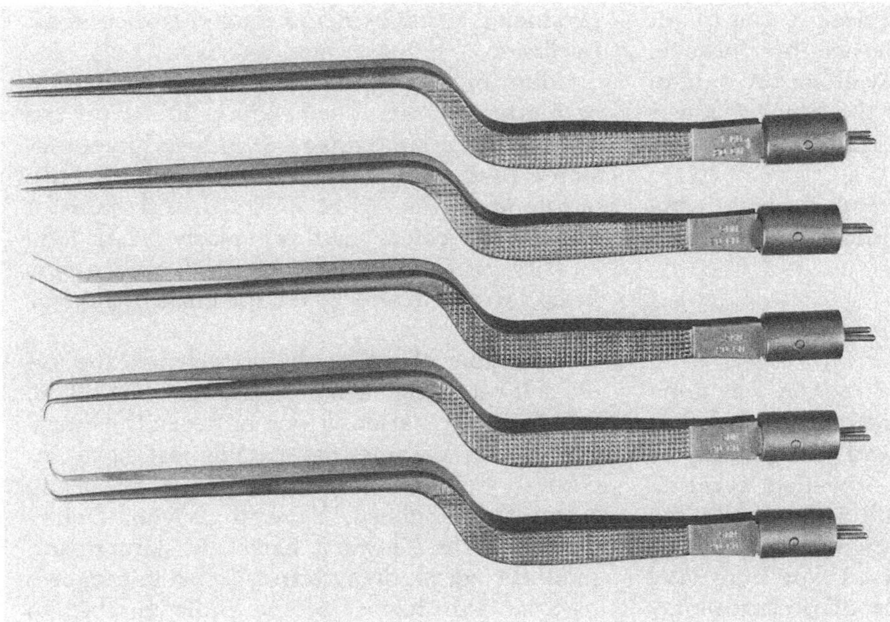

Fig. 26.13. Fox bipolar electrocautery forceps in three lengths: 16, 18, and 20 cm. Each of the straight forceps comes in 0.5 and 1.0 mm diameter tips; curved and angled tips also are available. Courtesy of V. Mueller Company, Chicago.

2. Clean the tips frequently only with a damp cloth (not with the scalpel!).
3. Polish the tips periodically (or obtain new forceps) when the tips become pitted and rough.
4. "Knead" the tissue between the forceps tips by gently squeezing and releasing the forceps blades.
5. Lift the forceps from tissue contact frequently.
6. Keep the tissue moist with CSF or saline.
7. Avoid high current settings.
8. Apply the current in short bursts to allow heat dissipation.

We use the bipolar forceps as the principal dissecting and tissue-separating instrument intracranially. For this reason the blades of the forceps must have proper spreading tension, yet not be so tense as to make tip approximation uncomfortable. They must not rotate inappropriately in the surgeon's hand. In terms of time, its actual application for electrocauterization is quite short compared to its use as a tissue dissector, perforator, spreader, separater, and grasper. It is used to place and remove cottonoids, cotton balls, gelfoam, oxycellulose, and rubber or plastic sheets. For us, the suction tube (in the surgeon's left hand) and the bipolar electrocautery forceps (in the right hand) have become the main microsurgical instruments (in terms of frequency and duration of use) during intracranial aneurysm surgery.

For most of our extracranial cauterization we use either the monopolar or bipolar unit with the Malis power supply dial set at 30 or 35. On cerebral cortex we use the Malis bipolar power supply dial at the 25–30 settings; on the brainstem we use the 15–25 settings. Finer-tipped forceps increase the current density at the tips. If higher settings are required, the spark gap in the unit probably needs resetting. With faulty spark gap distances or other electrical problems, one can use higher power settings to obtain more current, but the quality (wave forms) of the electrical output will be poor, resulting in poor coagulation and a tendency for vessels to explode or be incised. Prolonged or intensive use, even in one patient, may result in a need for an electrical overhaul. Therefore two or more such bipolar power supplies should be available. We use a 15-foot cord between the power supply and the forceps. Longer cords may cause defective electrical output at the forceps. We set the power supply at the foot of the OR table. In this position it does not add to the instrument clutter near the surgeon, and its electromagnetic noise emission is a sufficient distance from the television system so as to not create any significant audiovisual interference. For the same reason, the wall socket plug-in sites for the television and the bipolar power supply units should be at a considerable distance from each other.

The use of the bipolar forceps for narrowing the neck of an aneurysm is described in Chapter 31.

Retractors

In past years most brain retraction was done by assistant surgeons. Such retraction was often inconsistent, inaccurate, and dangerous, as brain retraction pressure exceeded cerebral perfusion pressure. In 1958 Gillingham (59) warned that bleeding from an aneurysm at surgery (causing reversal of blood flow from vital brain tissues and a drop in blood pressure) may result in ischemia of nearby brain tissue. He warned that this would be aggravated by excess or prolonged brain retraction. Additionally, he cautioned that inaccurate or excessive retraction may place traction on vital perforators, producing vasospasm and inadequate cerebral perfusion.

Albin et al. (7,8,51) have shown that brain retraction pressures exceeding 20 torr cause underlying brain damage. If induced hypotension is used, even less brain retraction pressure is tolerated. Fig. 26.14 illustrates CT scans of patients operated years previously. Their low-density zones may have resulted from excess brain retraction and/or compromise of a major artery.

A number of authors have described the use of self-retaining brain retractors (51,69,70, 100,112,181). Various types, either in the literature or in commercial catalogues, have included the de Martel, Dott (Edinburgh), Hamby, Greenberg, Yaşargil (Leyla), Dohn–Carton, Malis, Cloward, Enker, Miskimon, and Jannetta retractor systems. Self-retaining retractors also have become indispensable to aneurysm surgery because they allow the surgeon to work in a relatively confined space unhindered by the presence of an assistant's hands, which are less dependable for maintaining constant retraction of the brain. Self-retain-

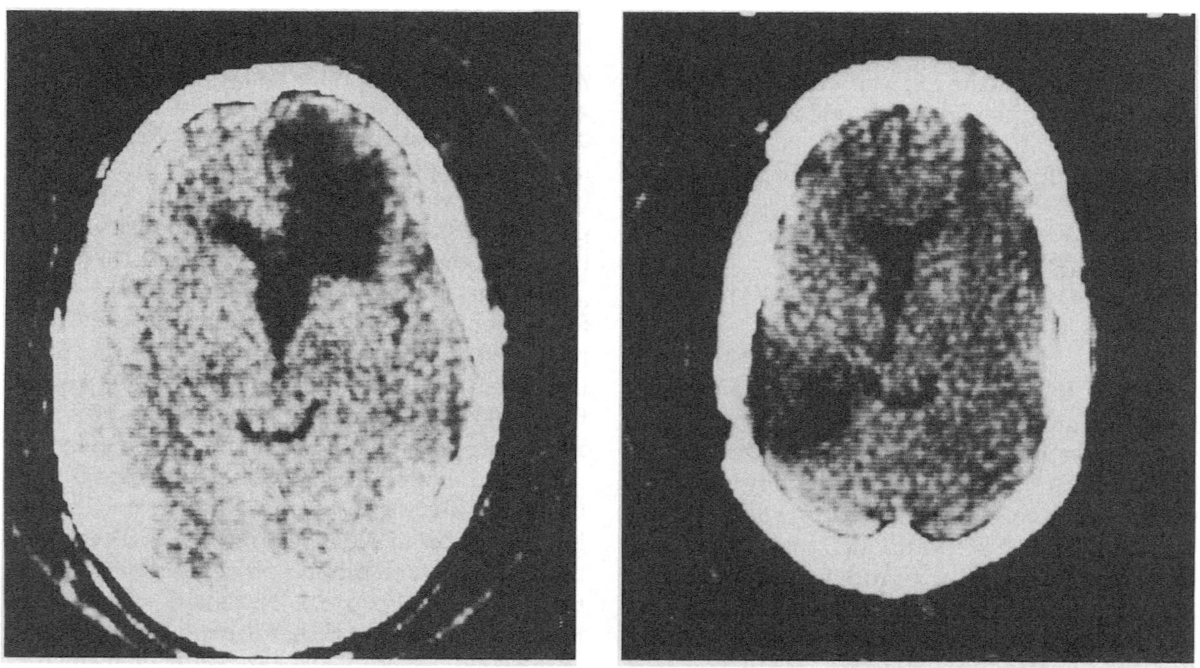

A **B**

Fig. 26.14. **A** CT scan taken 3 years after clipping of an ACoAA. The right frontal lobe had been retracted. **B** CT scan taken 5 years after clipping of bBAA. The left temporal lobe had been retracted.

ing brain retractors are of two basic types (51). One is comprised of a series of straight shafts attached by small clamps to give the correct arm length and configuration required for holding the brain spatula in place. The other consists of a series of ball-and-socket units that resemble a chain of pearls with an internal cable which, when tightened, remains in the desired position.

Of greatest importance in aneurysm surgery is the minimal brain retraction necessary (Table 26.2), ascribable not only to use of the surgical microscope and microtechnique but also to improvements in exposure techniques that allow a lower, basal, and tangential approach to the circle of Willis, aided in part by removal of a portion of the sphenoid wing and the use of special self-retaining brain retractors. However, these aids would be totally useless without a relaxed brain effected by proper timing of surgery and by superior anesthetic and life support methods.

The selection of a self-retaining retractor system is up to the individual surgeon's preference and habit. Many prefer systems that attach only to the skull. They are concerned that table-mounted retractors may move relative to the brain even if the skull is immobilized by three-point fixation (100). We have found that the Aesculap–Yaşargil (Leyla) retractor system (Fig. 26.15) is ideal for most cases of intracranial aneurysm surgery. We attach the bar to the left side of the OR table just cranial to the "ether screen" attachment (which holds drapes that separate the microscope from the anesthesiologist). Two or three flexible (unless tightened) retractor arms are attached to the connector on the bar. All joints must be firmly tightened to avoid drift.

Firstly, set the retractor blade (in the flexible arm) near the planned retraction site. Then tighten the flexible bar by turning the screw which pulls the internal wire taut. Lastly, "toe-in" the retractor blade to its desired position and retraction pressure and then tighten its wing-nut. Drift is minimal or absent if done properly. With the patient in the sitting position, have the flexible arm (from the bar on the left) for the right side rest on the patient's head to minimize downward drift. Always have the point of connection between the retractor blade and flexible bar *away* from the cranial opening. This requires attaching the flexible arm near the end of the retractor blade and bending the blade at its proper point for descent into the cranial cavity. This maneuver gives better intracranial exposure without the ends of the flexible retractor arms being in the way.

Table 26.2. Minimal Brain Retraction

Permitted by
1. Use of microscope, microtechnique
2. Low basal, tangential approach
3. Self-retaining brain retractor
4. CSF drainage
5. Neuroanesthetic techniques
Avoids
1. Removal of significant brain for exposure of lesion
2. Cutting of olfactory nerve
3. Dividing of some bridging veins
4. Secondary brain contusion or edema, vascular spasm
5. Vascular compression by retractor or stretched arachnoidal bands
6. Traction on aneurysm
7. Unnecessary exposure of A-1 and M-1 arterial segments

From Fox JL, Albin MS, Bader DCH, et al., ref. 51.

Although these retractors usually are applied against brain tissue or its coverings, on occasion a narrow retractor can be used to gently retract aneurysms or arteries such as the ICA or M-1 artery during frontotemporal approaches to the bBAA (49,148,148a). Such retraction requires displacement and protection of these arteries without occluding them.

Other Microsurgical Instruments

There now are a large number of microsurgical instruments in the field of neurosurgery. We cannot review all of them in this rapidly changing field.

Figures 26.16 and 26.17 illustrate some of the instruments we most commonly use for microdissection of intracranial aneurysms. The jewelers' forceps is used to pick up the arachnoid over the sylvian fissure to initiate opening of this fissure. The Aesculap bayonet scissors (curved and straight) come in three lengths (16 cm for surface work, 18 cm for work about the anterior circle of Willis, and 20 cm for deeper work, e.g., about the posterior circle of Willis). There is also a 22-cm scissor. The bipolar forceps have been described in the earlier section

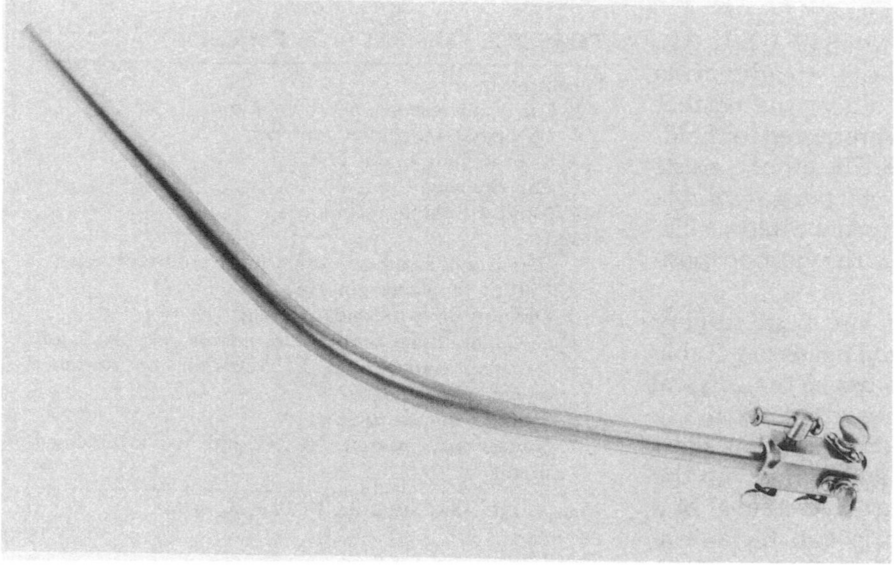

A

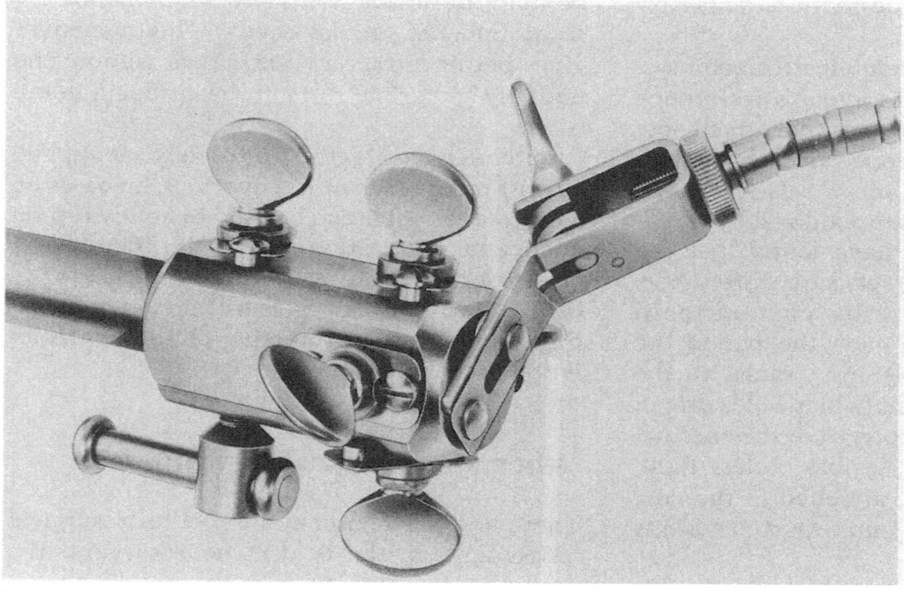

B

Fig. 26.15. A–C Leyla (Yaşargil) retractor system. Courtesy of Aesculap-Werke AG, Tuttlingen, West Germany. **B** Close-up view of attachment head between the bar (*left*) and retractor arm connector (*right*). **C** Close-up view of connector between bar and OR table. **D** Retractor bar and attachment head in preliminary position. Above is the draped scalp with an outline of a right frontolateral craniotomy incision.

on electrocautery. The Rhoton instruments shown in Fig. 26.17 are the four types most commonly used by us. The "long flat instrument" (a "micro-Penfield No. 4") is used to retract nerves, arteries, and the aneurysm. The "short flat instrument" is ideal for separating adhesions between the aneurysm and adjacent tissues because the edges of its angled, flat end are somewhat sharp. The 40° hook is safer to use than the right-angled hook, for it will not catch and tear tissues upon its removal from the field.

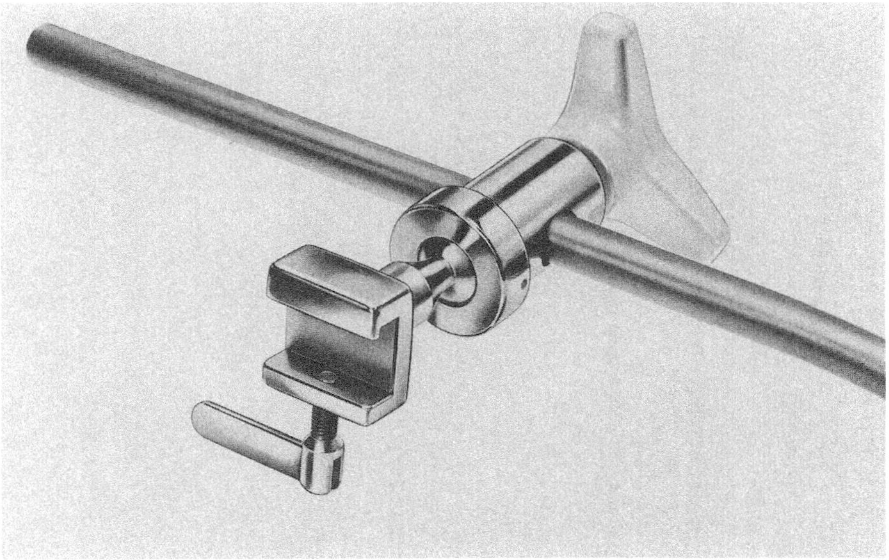

C

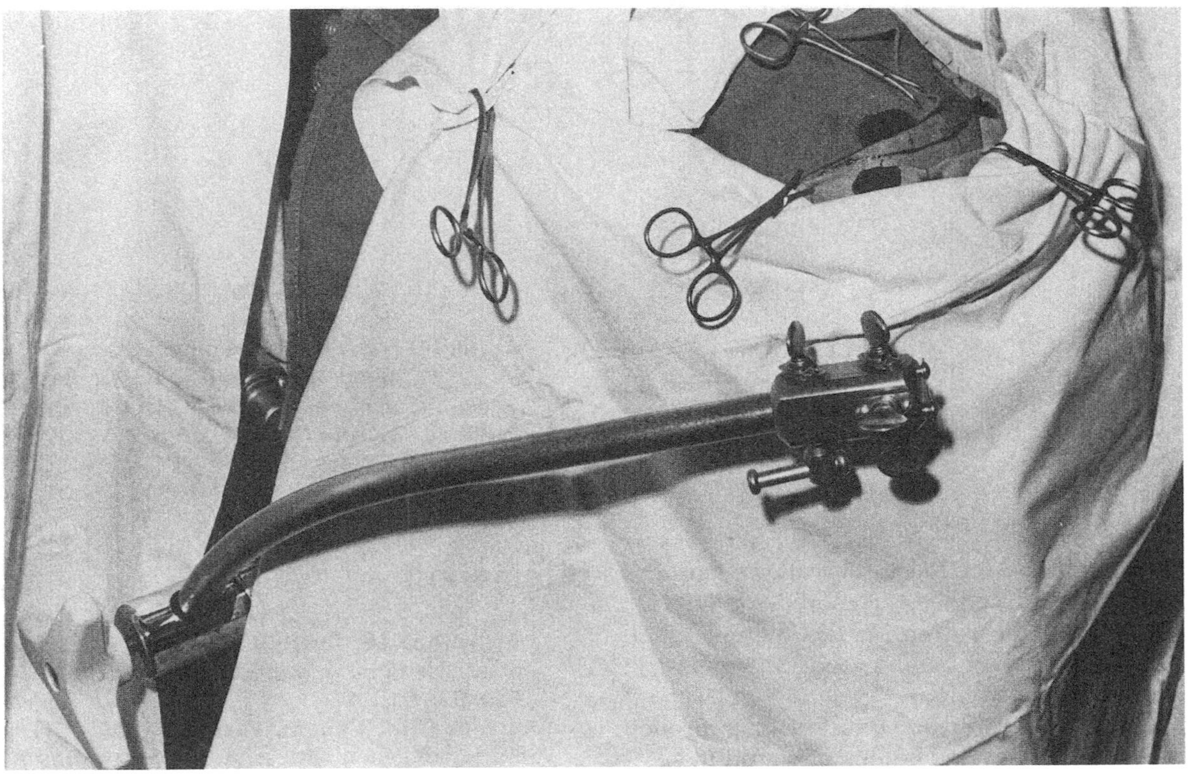

D

Instruments and suture for reanastomosing or repairing blood vessels and nerves should be available along with the expertise to do so. These are detailed in many articles on microvascular anastomosis.

These microsurgical instruments require some training and experience in their use and manipulation through a small opening and inside a deep narrow cavity. The surgeon can rest his hand on the skull or on the Leyla bar which holds the self-retaining retractors. Often the surgeon rests only his fifth finger as a point

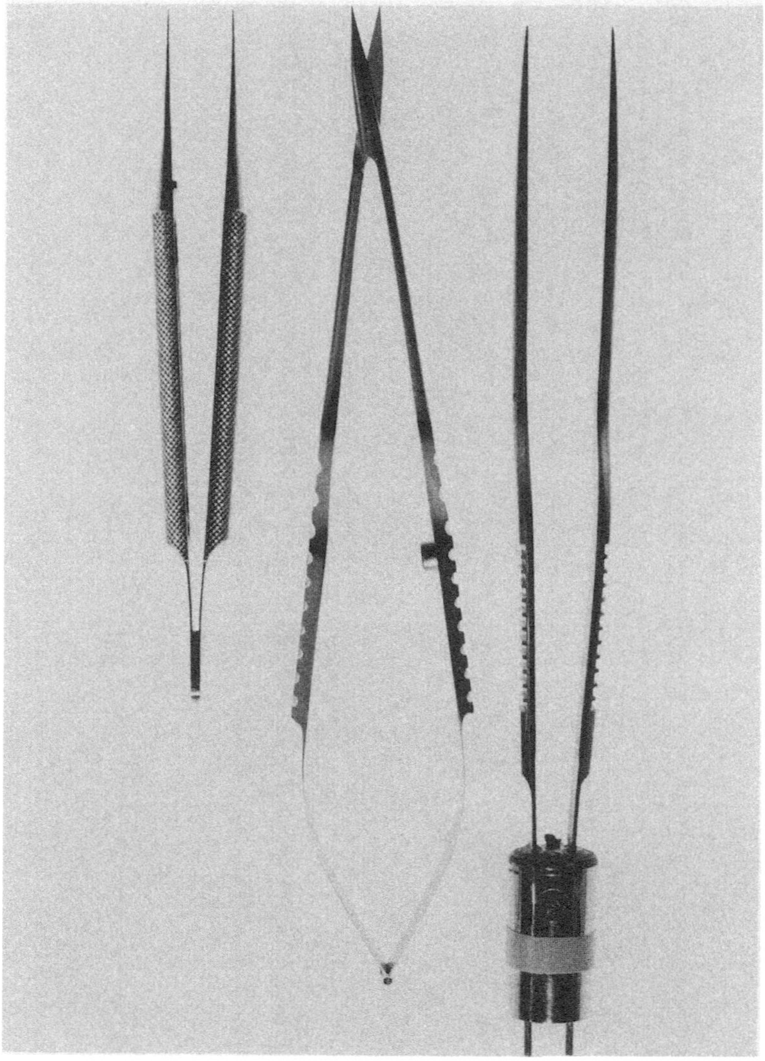

Fig. 26.16. *Left:* Jewelers' forceps (Edward Weck & Co.). *Center:* Bayonet shaped microscissors (Aesculap Instruments). *Right:* Bayonet shaped bipolar electrocautery forceps (Mathys & Sohn).

of proprioceptive feedback. This allows sensory orientation and reduces tremor. One instrument can also be rested on the suction tube of the surgeon's left hand to reduce tremor in critical moments.

On occasion a mirror at the tip of a probe can be useful for seeing behind and around vessels or aneurysms. Wilson and Spetzler (165) used a dental mirror, Sugita et al. (147) a 5-mm mirror, and Yaşargil and colleagues (181) a mirror which can change positions by squeezing the grip handle.

Clips

See Chapter 27.

Bibliography

1. Acosta-Rua GJ, Lyerly JG Sr, Sullivan EJ Jr, et al.: Cerebral aneurysm. J Fla Med Assoc 63:847–849, 1976
2. Adams CBT, Chir M, Fearnside MR, et al.: An investigation with serial angiography into the evolution of cerebral arterial spasm following aneurysm. J Neurosurg 49:805–815, 1978
3. Adams CBT, Loach AB, O'Laoire SA: Intracranial aneurysms: analysis of results of microneurosurgery. Br Med J 2:607–609, 1976
4. Adams JE, Witt J: The use of otologic microscope in the surgery of aneurysms. Presented at the Neurosurgical Society of America meeting on January 25, 1964

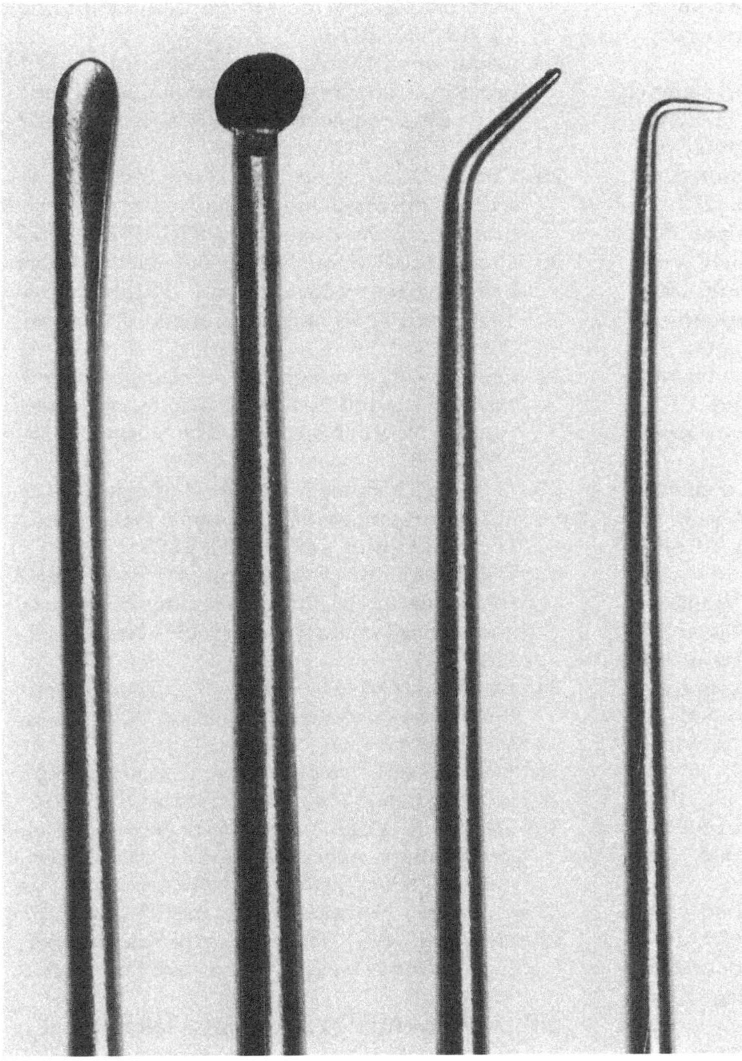

Fig. 26.17. Enlarged view of microsurgical dissecting instruments (Rhoton type; V. Mueller Co.). *Left end:* No. 7, or "long flat instrument." *Left center:* No. 2, or "short flat instrument." *Right center:* No. 11, or "40° hook." *Right end:* No. 10, or "right angle hook."

5. Aiba T: [Operative indication and surgical technique of the cerebral aneurysm. 1.] Neurol Med Chir (Tokyo) 16 (6 Part 2):467–478, 1976
6. Aiba T: [Operative procedures of aneurysm of the middle cerebral artery.] Neurol Surg (Tokyo) 3:205–217, 1975
7. Albin MS, Bunegin L, Bennett MH, et al.: Clinical and experimental brain retraction pressure monitoring. Acta Neurol Scand [Suppl 64] 56:522–523, 1977
8. Albin MS, Bunegin L, Dujovny M, et al.: Brain retraction pressure during intracranial procedures. Surg Forum 26:499–500, 1975
9. Almeida GM, Bianco E, Shibata MK: Anterior communicating artery aneurysms. J Neurosurg 33:53–57, 1976
10. Bader DCH: Micro-surgical treatment of intracranial aneurysms. J Neurosurg Nurs 7:25–27, 1975
11. Ballenger OM, Salcman M, Ducker TB, et al.: Prognosis of surgically treated intracranial arterial aneurysm patients. JAMA 237:1845–1847, 1977
12. Benedetti A, Curri D: Direct attack on carotid ophthalmic and large internal carotid aneurysms. Surg Neurol 8:49–54, 1977
13. Berger E, Duval C, Kyriazidou M: Intracranial aneurysm surgery using the surgical microscope and hypotensive technique. In Koos TH, Böck FW, Spetzler RF (eds.): Clinical Microneurosurgery. Stuttgart, Georg Thieme Verlag, 1976, pp. 204–209
14. Berger E, Duval C, Kyriazidou M: Per-operative angiography in aneurysm and angioma surgery, using the microscope and deep hypo-

tension, acute fibrinolysis as a possible complication. In Handa H (ed.): Microneurosurgery. Tokyo, Igaku Shoin, 1975, p. 27
15. Berger E, Kyriazidou M: Intraoperative angiography in cerebral aneurysm and angioma surgery. In Koos TH, Böck FW, Spetzler RF (eds.): Clinical Microneurosurgery. Stuttgart, Georg Thieme Verlag, 1976, pp. 209–213
16. Bischoff EPE: Mikroskopische Analyse der Anastomosen der Kopfnerven. Munich, Verlag der JJ Lentner'schen Buchhandlung, 1865 (see Microscopic Analysis of the Anastomosis Between the Cranial Nerves, translated by Sachs E Jr, Valtin EW. Hanover, New Hampshire, University Press of New England, 1977)
17. Bondurant CP: Alteration of suction tip pressure. J Neurosurg 46:559, 1977
18. Bonnal J, Stevenaert A: Indications actuelles de l'abord direct des anévrysmes artériels du polygone de Willis. Acta Neurol Belg 70:240–268, 1970
19. Bonnal J, Stevenaert A: Operability limits of anterior arterial aneurysms of the Willis circle. In Fusek I, Kunc Z (eds.): Proceedings of the Fourth European Congress of Neurosurgery. Present Limits of Neurosurgery, Vol 1. Prague, Avicenum, Czechoslovak Medical Press, 1972, p. 267
20. Bonnal J, Stevenaert A, Brotchi J, et al.: Bilan de neuf ans d'expérience de la chirurgie des anévrysmes artériels intracrâniens. Acta Neurol Belg 74:337–355, 1974
21. Brenner H, Böck FW: Prognosis of aneurysms after microsurgery. In Koos TH, Böck FW, Spetzler RF (eds.): Clinical Microneurosurgery. Stuttgart, Georg Thieme Verlag, 1976, pp. 183–191
22. Brolin SE, Hassler O: Minute aneurysms, detected by microdissection of basal cerebral arteries. Acta Pathol Microbiol Scand 44:59–63, 1958
23. Bromowicz J, Danilewicz B: [Case of double aneurysm located at the bifurcation of the basilar artery.] Neurol Neurochir Pol 11:389–393, 1977
24. Chou SN, Ausman JI, Erickson DL, et al.: Microneurosurgery at the University of Minnesota Hospital. Minn Med 57:580–586, 1974
25. Ciric I: Application of microneurosurgery in the treatment of cerebral aneurysm. Proc Inst Med Chicago 29:319, 1973
26. Colley PS, Dunn RC Jr: Prevention of blood pressure response to skull-pin head holder by local anesthesia. Anesth Analg (Cleve) 58:241–243, 1979
27. Cophignon J, Rey A, Thurel C, et al.: Microchirurgie des anévrysmes artériels de la partie antérieure du polygone de Willis. Étude d'une série consécutive de 48 cas. Neurochirurgie 19:519–530, 1973
28. Cophignon J, Rey A, Thurel C, et al.: Microchirurgie des anévrysmes intracrâniens. Étude d'une série consécutive de 50 cas. Nouv Presse Med 2:2935–2938, 1973
29. Corkill G, Hodgson MJH: Hypotension with sodium nitroprusside in the surgery of cerebral aneurysms. Anaesthesia 28:191–194, 1973
30. Crawford T: Some aspects of subarachnoid haemorrhage: a symposium. II. Intracranial aneurysms—pathological aspects. Br J Radiol 32:84, 1959
31. Crawford T: Some observations on pathogenesis and natural history of intracranial aneurysms. J Neurol Neurosurg Psychiatry 22:259–266, 1959
32. Cushing H, Bovie WT: Electro-surgery as an aid to the removal of intracranial tumors. Surg Gynecol Obstet 47:751–784, 1928
33. Danilewicz B: [Evaluation of microsurgical technique in operative treatment of cerebral aneurysms.] Neurol Neurochir Pol 12:197–201, 1978
34. De Klerk DJJ, De Villiers JC: Microsurgery for aneurysms on the circle of Willis. S Afr Med J 48:825–830, 1974
35. DeLong WB, Fox JL: Automatic cycling bipolar coagulator. Surg Neurol 8:15–16, 1977
36. Deruty R, Dechaume J-P, Lecuire J, et al.: Traitement microchirurgical d'une série d'anévrysmes artériels intra-crâniens sustentoriels. Neurochirurgie 22:227–238, 1976
37. Donaghy RMP: The history of microsurgery in neurosurgery. Clin Neurosurg 26:619–625, 1979
38. Donaghy RMP, Yaşargil MG: Micro-vascular Surgery. Stuttgart, Georg Thieme, 1967
39. Drake CG: Cerebral aneurysm surgery—an update. In Scheinberg P (ed.): Cerebrovascular Diseases. Tenth Princeton Conference. New York, Raven Press, 1976, pp. 289–310
40. Drake CG: Further experience with surgical treatment of aneurysms of the basilar artery. J Neurosurg 29:372–392, 1968
41. Drake CG: On the surgical treatment of ruptured intracranial aneurysms. Clin Neurosurg 13:122–155, 1965
42. Drake CG: Surgical treatment of ruptured intracranial aneurysms. In Cooper P (ed.): The Craft of Surgery, Vol III, 2nd ed. Boston, Little, Brown, 1971, pp. 1765–1784
43. Drake CG: The surgical treatment of vertebral-basilar aneurysms. Clin Neurosurg 16: 114–169, 1969
44. Drake CG: The treatment of aneurysms of the posterior circulation. Clin Neurosurg 26:96–144, 1979

45. Dujovny M, Vas R, Osgood CP, et al.: Automatically irrigated bipolar forceps. Technical note. J Neurosurg 43:502–503, 1975
46. Ethicon Inc: Personal communication, March 13, 1978
47. Faleiro LCM, Rodrigues PA, Rodrigues JA, et al.: Tratamento microcirúrgico de aneurismas da artéria communicante anterior. Arq Neuropsiquiatr 31:264–270, 1973
48. Forbus WD: On the origin of miliary aneurysms of superficial cerebral arteries. Bull Johns Hopkins Hosp 47:239–284, 1930
49. Fox JL: Microsurgical exposure of intracranial aneurysms. J Microsurg 1:2–31, 1979
50. Fox JL: Microvascular Anastomosis Techniques: The Carotid Artery of the Rat. Fairfield, New Jersey, Sparta Instrument Corp, 1976
51. Fox JL, Albin MS, Bader DCH, et al.: Microsurgical treatment of neurovascular disease. Neurosurgery 3:285–337, 1978
52. Fox JL, Nugent GR: Recent advances in intracranial aneurysm surgery. W Va Med J 72: 104–105, 1976
53. Freidberg SR, Walsh JW: Use of microscopic techniques in neurosurgery. Surg Clin North Am 56:781–795, 1976
54. Gestring G, Koos W: A mobile microsurgical unit. Excerpta Medica ICS No. 418:105, 1977
55. Gestring GF, Koos WT, Boeck FW: Bipolar coagulation with modified conventional electrocoagulators. Technical note. J Neurosurg 37:501–504, 1972
56. Giannotta SL, Kindt GW: Total morbidity and mortality rates of patients with surgically treated intracranial aneurysms. Neurosurgery 4:125–128, 1979
57. Gigli L: Über ein neues Instrument zum Durchtrennen der Knochen, die Drahtsäge. Zentralbl Chir 21:409–411, 1894
58. Gigli L: Zur Technik der temporären Schädelresektion mit meiner Drahtsäge. Zentralbl Chir 25:425–428, 1898
59. Gillingham FJ: The management of ruptured intracranial aneurysm. Ann R Coll Surg 23:89–117, 1958
60. Gillingham FJ: Twenty-five years' experience with middle cerebral aneurysms. Rev Inst Nacl Neurol (Mex) 10:16–21, 1976
61. Greenwood J Jr: Electrocoagulation in neurosurgery. Surg Neurol 2:4, 1974
62. Greenwood J Jr: Two point coagulation. A follow-up report on a new technique and instrument for electrocoagulation in neurosurgery. Arch Phys Ther 23:552–554, 1942
63. Greenwood J Jr: Two point coagulation. A new principle and instrument for applying coagulation current in neurosurgery. Am J Surg 50:267–270, 1940
64. Greenwood J Jr: Two-point or interpolar coagulation. Review after a twelve-year period with notes on addition of sucker tip. J Neurosurg 12:196–197, 1955
65. Guidetti B: Microsurgical treatment of intracranial saccular aneurysms. Acta Neurochir (Wien) 43:153–162, 1978
66. Guidetti B: Results of 98 intracranial aneurysm operations performed with the aid of an operating microscope. Acta Neurochir (Wien) 29:65–71, 1973
67. Gurdjian ES, Thomas LM, Gurdjian ES: A single unit for bipolar, monopolar coagulation, and cutting. J Neurosurg 29:567–568, 1968
68. Hamby WB: Intracranial Aneurysms. Springfield, Ill., Thomas, 1952
69. Hamby WB: Intracranial surgery for aneurysms. Prog Neurol Surg 3:1–65, 1969
70. Hamby WB: Remarks concerning intracranial aneurysm surgery. Clin Neurosurg 17:1–17, 1970
70a. Hassler O: On the etiology of intracranial aneurysms. In Fields WS, Sahs AL (eds.): Intracranial Aneurysms and Subarachnoid Hemorrhage. Springfield, Ill., Thomas, 1965, pp. 25–39
71. Helme WB: Infrequent aneurysm surgery. Neurosurgery 3:210–212, 1978
72. Hollin SA, Decker RE: Effectiveness of microsurgery for intracranial aneurysms. Postoperative angiographic study of 50 cases. J Neurosurg 39:690–693, 1973
73. Hollin SA, Decker RE: Microsurgical treatment of cerebral aneurysms. Mt Sinai J Med NY 40:91–103, 1973
74. Hollin SA, Decker RE: Microsurgical treatment of internal carotid artery aneurysms. J Neurosurg 47:142–149, 1977
75. Horsley V: Antiseptic wax [letter]. Br Med J 1:1165, 1892
76. Horsley V: On the technique of operations on the central nervous system. Br Med J 2: 411–423, 1906
77. Housepian EM, Unger WH, Scharff TB, et al.: Experience with videotape monitoring of microscopic neurosurgical procedures. J Neurosurg 42:204–208, 1975
78. Inaba Y, Fukushima Y, Tachibana N, et al.: Microneurosurgery in cerebral aneurysms. Neurol Med Chir 12:204–205, 1972
79. Ito Z: Microsurgical interhemispheric approach for ruptured aneurysm of anterior communicating artery in acute stage. Excerpta Medica ICS No. 418:73, 1977
80. Iwabuchi T, Suzuki S, Sobata E: Intracranial direct operation for carotid-opthalmic aneu-

rysm by unroofing of the optic canal. Acta Neurochir 43:163–169, 1978
81. Jacques S, Bullara LA, Pudenz RH: Microvascular bipolar coagulator. Technical note. J Neurosurg 44:523–524, 1976
82. Jain KK: Surgery of anterior communicating aneurysms: experience with various techniques and evolution of a modified approach. Surg Neurol 2:31–33, 1974
83. Keen WW: Intracranial lesions. Med News (NY) 57:439–449, 1890
84. Kempe LG: Operative Neurosurgery, Vol 1: Cranial, Cerebral, and Intracranial Vascular Disease. Berlin, Springer-Verlag, 1968, pp. 1–75, 203–214
85. Kikuchi H: [Operative indication and surgical technique of the cerebral aneurysm.] Neurol Med Chir (Tokyo) 16 (6 Part 2):479–486, 1976
86. Kikuchi H, Furuse S, Karasawa J: Microsurgery of cerebral aneurysm in acute phase (within 1 week after subarachnoid hemorrhage). In Koos TH, Böck FW, Spetzler RF (eds.): Clinical Microneurosurgery. Stuttgart, Georg Thieme Verlag, 1976, pp. 202–203
87. Kikuchi H, Furuse S, Karasawa J: Surgical experience with basilar aneurysms. In Koos TH, Böck FW, Spetzler RF (eds.): Clinical Microneurosurgery. Stuttgart, Georg Thieme Verlag, 1976, p. 220
88. King TT, Worpole R: Self-irrigating bipolar diathermy forceps. J Neurosurg 37:246–247, 1972
89. Krayenbühl H, Yaşargil MG: Diagnosis and therapy of intracranial aneurysms. In Cooper P, Nyhus LM (eds.): Surgery Annual. New York, Appleton-Century-Crofts, 1970, pp. 327–343
90. Krayenbühl HA, Yaşargil MG, Flamm ES, et al.: Microsurgical treatment of intracranial saccular aneurysms. J Neurosurg 37:678–686, 1972
91. Krieger AJ: The Use of the Operating Microscope. New York, Carl Zeiss, 1978
92. Kurze T: Microtechniques in neurological surgery. Clin Neurosurg 11:128–137, 1964
93. Kurze T, Apuzzo MCJ, Weiss MH, et al.: Experiences with sterilization of the operating microscope. J Neurosurg 47: 861–863, 1977
94. Light RU: Hemostasis in neurosurgery. J Neurosurg 2:414–434, 1945
95. Loach AB, De Azevedo Filho HRC: Some observations on the microneurosurgical treatment of intracranial aneurysms. Acta Neurochir (Wien) 35:97–103, 1976
96. Lougheed WM: Selection, timing, and technique of aneurysm surgery of the anterior circle of Willis. Clin Neurosurg 16:95–113, 1969
97. Lougheed WM, Marshall BM: Management of aneurysms of the anterior circulation by intracranial procedures. In Youmans JR (ed.): Neurological Surgery, Vol 2. Philadelphia, Saunders, 1973, pp. 731–767
98. Lougheed WM, Marshall BM: The diploscope in intracranial aneurysm surgery: results in 40 patients. Can J Surg 12:75–82, 1969
99. Malis LI: Bipolar coagulation in microsurgery. In Donaghy RMP, Yaşargil MG (eds.): Micro-Vascular Surgery. Stuttgart, Georg Thieme Verlag, 1967, pp. 126–130
100. Malis LI: Instrumentation and techniques in microsurgery. Clin Neurosurg 26:626–636, 1979
101. Malis LI: In press
102. Martinez Coll A, Del Corral JF: Experiences in intracranial surgery for aneurysms. Surg Neurol 3:191–193, 1975
103. McMurtry JG III, Housepian EM, Bowman FO Jr, et al.: Surgical treatment of basilar artery aneurysms. Elective circulatory arrest with thoracotomy in 12 cases. J Neurosurg 40:486–498, 1974
104. Nilsson L, Nordfeldt S: Operation pågår med nedkyld patient. Vecko J 48:30–32, Dec 3, 1965
105. Nornes H, Wikeby P: Results of microsurgical management of intracranial aneurysms. J Neurosurg 51:608–614, 1979
106. Nukui H, Miyagi O, Nojiri K, et al.: [Psychiatric symptoms in cases with ruptured anterior communicating aneurysms before and after surgery.] Neurol Med Chir (Tokyo) 17 (part 2):335–341, 1977
107. Nukui H, Tanaka S, Miyagi O, et al.: Psychiatric symptoms of ruptured anterior communicating aneurysms before and after operation. Excerpta Medica ICS No. 418:206, 1977
108. Nylen CO: The microscope in aural surgery. Its first use and later development. Acta Otolaryngol [Suppl] (Stockh) 116:226–240, 1954
109. Paillas JE, Bonnal J: Anévrysmes artériels. In Patel J, Leger L (eds.): Nouveau Traité de Technique Chirurgicale, Vol 6. Paris, Masson & Cie, 1975, pp 237–277
110. Papo I, Caruselli G, Salvolini U: Aneurysm of the superior cerebellar artery. Surg Neurol 7:15–17, 1977
111. Pecker J, Guy G, Fardoun R: La place des anti-agrégants et des macromolécules dans le traitement des anévrismes arteriels cérébraux. Anesth Analg (Paris) 3:653–658, 1976
112. Peerless SJ: The surgical approach to middle cerebral and posterior communicating aneurysms. Clin Neurosurg 21:151–165, 1974
113. Penzholz H, Piscol K: Experiences with the operating microscope in the treatment of intracranial aneurysms and angiomas. In Koos

TH, Böck FW, Spetzler RF (eds.): Clinical Microneurosurgery. Stuttgart, Georg Thieme Verlag, 1976, pp. 179–183
114. Pertuiset B, Houtteville J-P, van Effenterre R, et al.: Chirurgie des anévrysmes artériels sus-tentoriels. Réduction par coagulation bipolaire sous hypotension profonde et exclusion par clip autobloquant: (52 cas opérés sous microscope). Nouv Presse Med 3:1649–1652, 1974
115. Pertuiset B, van Effenterre R, Caruel N, et al.: Les résultats de l'abord direct des anévrysmes intra-crâniens sus-tentoriels en fonction de l'hypotension contrôlée, de la coagulation bipolaire et de la magnification optique. Rev Neurol (Paris) 129:57–59, 1973
116. Pertuiset B, van Effenterre R, Goutorbe J, et al.: Management of aneurysmal rupture during surgery, using bipolar coagulation, deep hypotension, and the operating microscope. Acta Neurochir (Wien) 30:195–205, 1974
117. Peterschmitt O, Racenberg E, Fechner R: Anästhesieverfahren bei Operationen von Gehirngesfässaneurysmen. Prakt Anaesth 12: 393–400, 1977
118. Pia HW: Microsurgical treatment of cerebral aneurysms. Neurosurg Rev 1:15–24, 1978
119. Pia HW: The microsurgical treatment of intracerebral aneurysms. In Koos TH, Böck FW, Spetzler RF (eds.): Clinical Neurosurgery. Stuttgart, Georg Thieme Verlag, 1976, pp. 177–179
120. Pool JL: Bifrontal craniotomy for anterior communicating artery aneurysms. J Neurosurg 36:212–220, 1972
121. Pool JL: New dimension in aneurysm surgery. Columbia Univ Phys Surg Q 10:18–20, 1965
122. Pool JL, Colton RP: The dissecting microscope for intracranial vascular surgery. J Neurosurg 25:315–318, 1966
123. Post KD, Flamm ES, Goodgold A, et al.: Ruptured intracranial aneurysms. Case morbidity and mortality. J Neurosurg 46: 290–295, 1977
124. Rand RW: Microneurosurgery. St. Louis, Mosby, 1969, pp. 198–209
125. Rand RW: Microneurosurgery, 2nd ed. St. Louis, Mosby, 1978, pp. 43–44, 311–324
126. Rand RW, Jannetta PJ: Microneurosurgery: application of the binocular surgical microscope in brain tumors, intracranial aneurysms, spinal cord disease, and nerve reconstruction. Clin Neurosurg 15:319–342, 1968
127. Rand RW, Jannetta PJ: Micro-neurosurgery for aneurysms of the vertebral-basilar artery system. J Neurosurg 27:330–335, 1967
128. Rand RW, Jannetta PJ: Microneurosurgery for aneurysms of the vertebral-basilar artery system. In Donaghy RMP, Yaşargil MG (eds.): Micro-Vascular Surgery. Stuttgart, Georg Thieme Verlag, 1967, p. 148
128a. Rhoton AL, Merz W: Suction tubes for conventional and microscopic neurosurgery. Surg Neurol 15:120–124, 1981
129. Richardson JTE: Arterial spasm and recovery from subarachnoid haemorrhage. J Neurol Neurosurg Psychiatry 39:1134–1136, 1976
130. Rogers L: The history of craniotomy: an account of the methods which have been practiced and the instruments used for opening the human skull during life. Ann Med Hist 2:495–514, 1930
131. Saito I, Basugi N, Sano K: Surgical treatment of intracranial aneurysms in the acute stage, with special reference to pre- and postoperative vasospasm. Excerpta Med No. 293:160, 1973
132. Saito I, Tamura A, Sano K: [Follow-up results of cases with anterior communicating aneurysm operated on in the acute stage—with special reference to time-course of morbidity after operations.] Neurol Med Chir (Tokyo) 17 (part 2):233–341, 1977
133. Sakaki T, Kikuchi H, Furuse S, et al.: [Carotid-ophthalmic aneurysm. A study of 5 cases.] Neurol Surg (Tokyo) 2:553–558, 1974
134. Samson DS, Hodosh RM, Reid WR, et al.: Risk of intracranial aneurysm surgery in the good grade patient: early versus late operation. Neurosurgery 5:422–426, 1979
135. Sano K: [Surgery of intracranial aneurysm.] Brain Nerve (Tokyo) 23:1252–1264, 1971
136. Sano K, Saito I: Follow-up results of microsurgery of intracranial aneurysms. Brain Nerve (Tokyo) 29:977–985, 1977
137. Sano K, Saito I: Indication and timing of surgery for ruptured intracranial aneurysms with vasospasm. Neurosurgery 1:65, 1977
138. Scalais M, Collignon R, Vandresse JH, et al.: Anévrysmes triples bilatéraux, opérés en deux temps. Deux observations. Acta Neurol Belg 77:144–150, 1977
139. Scarff TB: A new bipolar suction-cautery forceps for microneurosurgical use. Surg Neurol 2:213, 1974
140. Shields CB: Current trends in management of cerebral aneurysms. J Ky Med Assoc 75: 529–535, 1977
141. Simmonds M: Über das Angioma racemosum und serpentinum des Gehirns. Virchows Arch [Pathol Anat] 180:280–288, 1905
142. Snyckers FD: The treatment of cerebral aneurysms. A report on 51 cases. S Afr Med J 50:835–839, 1976
143. Someda K, Yasui N, Moriwaki Y, et al.: Extravasation of contrast material into subdural space from internal carotid aneurysm during

angiography. Case report. J Neurosurg 42: 473–477, 1975
144. Stehbens WE: Aneurysms and anatomical variation of cerebral arteries. Arch Pathol 75:45–64, 1963
145. Stroobandt G, Cornelis G, Thauvoy C: Les anévrismes intracrâniens multiples. I. Evolution et orientation actuelle du traitement chirurgical. Acta Neurol Belg 73:298–310, 1973
146. Stroobandt G, Cornelis G, Thauvoy C: Les anévrismes intracrâniens multiples. II. Problèmes posés par les lésions de petite taille. Acta Neurol Belg 73:311–319, 1973
147. Sugita K, Hirota T, Tsugane R: Application of nasopharyngeal mirror for aneurysm operation. Technical note. J Neurosurg 43:244–246, 1975
148. Sugita K, Kobayashi S, Shintani A, et al.: Microneurosurgery for aneurysms of the basilar artery. J Neurosurg 51:615–620, 1979
148a. Sugita K, Kobayashi S, Takemae T, et al.: Direct retraction method in aneurysm surgery. J Neurosurg 53:417–419, 1980
149. Sugita K, Shintani A, Mutsuga N, et al.: [Microsurgery for vertebrobasilar aneurysms.] Neurol Med Chir (Tokyo) 17 (part 2):351–360, 1977
150. Sugita K, Tsugane R: Bipolar coagulator with automatic thermocontrol. Technical note. J Neurosurg 41:777–779, 1974
151. Sugita K, Tsugane R, Kageyama N: Bipolar coagulator with automatic thermocontrol and some improvements of microsurgical instruments. In Handa H (ed.): Microneurosurgery. Baltimore, University Park Press, 1975, p. 17
152. Sundt TM Jr: Clip-grafts for aneurysm and small vessel surgery. Part 4. Relative application to various aneurysms and repair of anterior communicating aneurysms using a right-angle clip holder. Technical note. J Neurosurg 37:753–758, 1972
153. Sundt TM Jr: Intracranial aneurysms and subarachnoid hemorrhage: a subject review for the clinician. Mayo Clin Proc 45:455–466, 1970
154. Sundt TM Jr, Murphey F: Clip-grafts for aneurysm and small vessel surgery. Part 3. Clinical experience in intracranial internal carotid artery aneurysm. J Neurosurg 31: 59–71, 1969
155. Sundt TM Jr, Nofzinger JD: Clip-grafts for aneurysm and small vessel surgery. Part 1. Repair of segmental defects with clip-grafts; laboratory studies and clinical correlations. Part 2. Clinical application of clip-grafts to aneurysms; technical considerations. J Neurosurg 27:477–489, 1967
156. Sundt TM Jr, Pluth JR, Gronert GA: Excision of a giant basilar aneurysm under profound hypothermia. Report of a case. Mayo Clin Proc 47:631–634, 1972
157. Sundt TM Jr, Whisnant JP: Subarachnoid hemorrhage from intracranial aneurysms. Surgical management and natural history of disease. N Engl J Med 299:116–122, 1978
158. Symon L: Subarachnoid haemorrhage from intracranial aneurysm and angioma. In Russell RWR: Cerebral Arterial Disease. Edinburgh, Churchill Livingstone, 1976, pp. 231–261
159. Sypert GW: Intracranial aneurysms: natural history and surgical management. Compr Ther 4:64–73, 1978
160. Taylor JC, Choudhury AR, Shephard RH: Surgery of aneurysms of the middle cerebral artery: a comparison of results of "wrapping" and "clipping" procedures. J Neurol Neurosurg Psychiatry 40:200, 1977
161. Thurel C, Rey A, Thiébaut JB, et al.: Anévrysmes carotido-ophtalmiques. Neurochirurgie 20:25–39, 1974
162. VanderArk GD, Kempe LG, Smith DR: Anterior communicating aneurysms: the gyrus rectus approach. Clin Neurosurg 21:120–133, 1974
163. Viale GL, Pau A: Carotid-choroidal aneurysms: remarks on surgical treatment and outcome. Surg Neurol 11:141–145, 1979
164. Wilson CB, Spetzler RF: Factors responsible for improved results in the surgical management of intracranial aneurysms and vascular malformations. Am J Surg 134:33–38, 1977
165. Wilson CB, Spetzler RF: Operative approaches to aneurysms. Clin Neurosurg 26: 232–247, 1979
166. Wilson CB, U HS: Surgical treatment for aneurysms of the upper basilar artery. J Neurosurg 44:537–543, 1976
167. Wilson DH: Limited exposure in cerebral surgery. Technical note. J Neurosurg 34:102–106, 1971
168. Yada K, Owada T: [Aneurysms of the internal carotid artery.] Neurol Surg (Tokyo) 3:459–465, 1975
169. Yaşargil MG: Die Behandlung der intrakraniellen sackförmigen aneurysm. Ophthalmologica 167:189–192, 1973
170. Yaşargil MG: Intracranial microsurgery. Clin Neurosurg 17:250–255, 1970
171. Yaşargil MG: Microsurgery Applied to Neurosurgery. Stuttgart, Georg Thieme Verlag, 1969, pp. 119–143
172. Yaşargil MG: Microsurgical approach to the cerebrovascular diseases. In Fusek I, Kunc Z (eds.): Proceedings of the Fourth European Congress of Neurosurgery. Present Limits of Neurosurgery. Prague, Avicenum, Czechoslovak Medical Press, 1972, pp. 357–361
173. Yaşargil MG: Presented at the University of

Florida Symposium on Microneurosurgery. Tarpon Springs, Florida, May 9–11, 1974

174. Yaşargil MG, Antic J, Laciga R, et al.: Microsurgical pterional approach to aneurysms of the basilar bifurcation. Surg Neurol 6:83–91, 1976
175. Yaşargil MG, Boehm WB, Ho REM: Microsurgical treatment of cerebral aneurysms at the bifurcation of the internal carotid artery. Acta Neurochir (Wien) 41:61–72, 1978
176. Yaşargil MG, Carter LP: Saccular aneurysms of the distal anterior cerebral artery. J Neurosurg 39:218–223, 1974
177. Yaşargil MG, Fox JL: The microsurgical approach to intracranial aneurysms. Surg Neurol 3:7–14, 1975
178. Yaşargil MG, Fox JL, Ray MW: The operative approach to aneurysms of the anterior communicating artery. In Krayenbühl H (ed.): Advances and Technical Standards in Neurosurgery, Vol 2. New York, Springer-Verlag, 1975, pp. 113–170
179. Yaşargil MG, Gasser JC, Hodosh RM, et al.: Carotid-ophthalmic aneurysms: direct microsurgical approach. Surg Neurol 8:155–165, 1977
180. Yaşargil MG, Smith RD: Surgery on the carotid system in the treatment of hemorrhagic stroke. Adv Neurol 16:181–209, 1977
181. Yaşargil MG, Vise WM, Bader DCH: Technical adjuncts in neurosurgery. Surg Neurol 8:331–336, 1977
182. Yaşargil MG, Yonas H, Gasser JC: Anterior choroidal artery aneurysms: their anatomy and surgical significance. Surg Neurol 9:129–138, 1978
183. Zlotnik EI, Oleshkevich FV, Stolkarts JZ: Microsurgical technique in the treatment of intracranial aneurysms. J Neurosurg 46:591–595, 1977

27

Craniotomy for Aneurysm

III. Aneurysm Clips

The ancient and modern history as well as the evolution of vascular clamps or clips used by vascular surgeons and neurosurgeons are detailed by Jacobson and McAllister (76), McFadden (102), Mayfield and Kees (96), and Fox (51). These reports are highly recommended to the reader.

The first modern vascular clip used in neurosurgery was the Cushing silver clip (Fig. 27.1) described in 1911 (20). Although Cushing used it for hemostasis and not for aneurysms, this clip has been applied to the necks of aneurysms by others. In 1927 McKenzie (104) reported some modifications (Fig. 27.2), including the use of flat instead of round wire, and the clip became more popular. Most clips are obtained from suppliers, although some surgeons have purchased the roll of wire and clip-making outfit and made their own. McKenzie clips are now sterling silver or tantalum (51).

In 1938 Dandy (21–23) introduced the technique of directly occluding the neck of an aneurysm with a metal (silver) clip. The first patient so cured had the clip applied to the neck of a pcaICAA (see Fig. 29.1). As only the phrase "silver clip" was used, we do not know whether Dandy used a Cushing or a McKenzie clip. The enormous importance of Dandy's surgical feat was recognized the same year (1938) by Matas (94), who told us that on

> . . . March 23, 1937, the clip was . . . used intracranially to obliterate the pedicle of the aneurysm from the internal carotid with which it was connected. . . . [T]he silver clip was substituted for the ligature and from the purely technical viewpoint alone, Dandy's procedure is a unique and important performance because it greatly simplifies the operation itself in one of its most essential features.

Figures 27.1–27.33 demonstrate various aneurysm clips of the three categories (malleable, screw, spring), and Table 27.1 provides a guide to their references in the literature. Their component materials and commercial sources have been reported previously (51).

Types of Clips

Malleable Clips

The Cushing (20) clip (Fig. 27.1) and the McKenzie (104) clip (Fig. 27.2) are described above. Duane (43) modified the McKenzie V-shaped clip into a U-shaped one so that it surrounded the vessel more effectively during closure; unlike the V-shaped clip, this new design closed first at the tips of the blades (Fig. 27.2). Drew (42) used both V- and U-shaped clips and developed a special clip applier. Sugar (51) used McKenzie clips that were 7 mm long. These malleable clips originally were made from silver, but some manufacturers have used tantalum.

Tovi (171) also developed a U-shaped silver clip with a special applicator (Fig. 27.3). Samuels et al. (135,136) used a modified U-shaped design (Fig. 27.4) which, like the Tovi clip, permitted the tips of the blades of the clip to come together so as to trap the vessel during clip closure; this tantalum clip has become known as the Samuels–Weck Hemoclip (Edward Weck & Co., Inc.). Codman and Shurtleff, Inc., altered the design (Vesclip) in such a way that the clip

Much of the material for this chapter is taken from a previous article by JLF (51) with the permission of the American Heart Association, Inc.

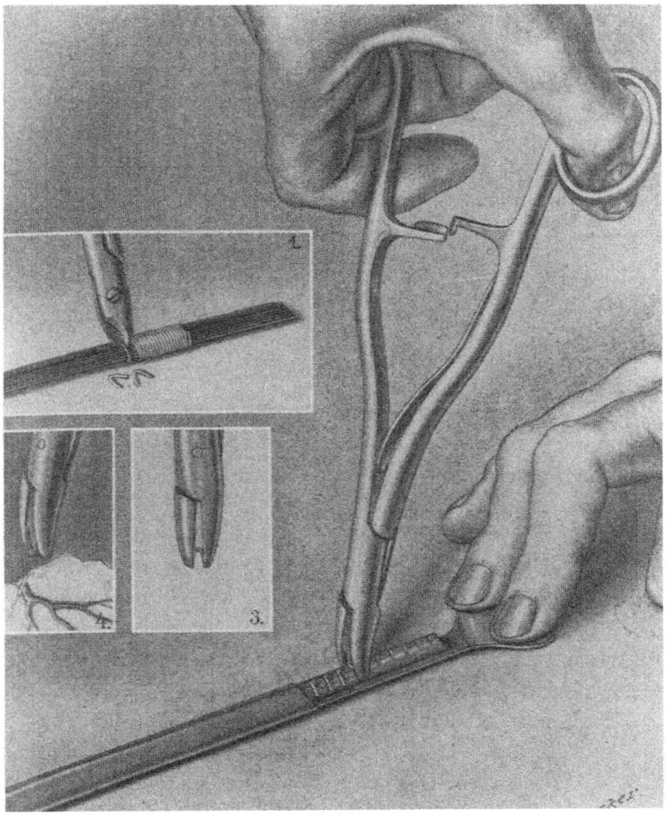

Fig. 27.1. Original Cushing silver clip. From Cushing H, ref. 20.

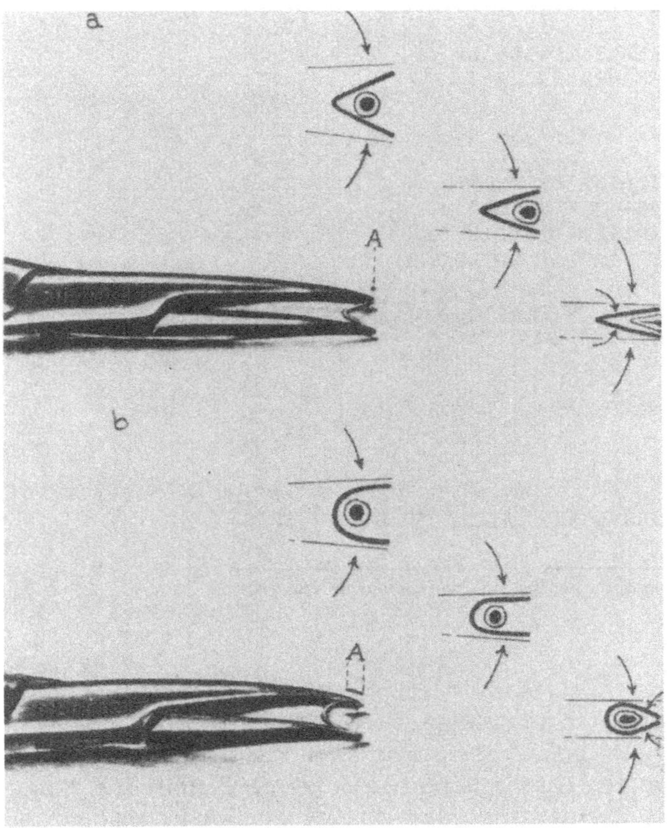

Fig. 27.2. McKenzie clip: the original (*top*) and as modified by Duane (*bottom*). From Duane W Jr, ref. 43.

Table 27.1. Intracranial Aneurysm Clips

Type	*References*	*Figure*
Cushing clip	4,20,25,42,51,52,54,56,64,149,174,176	27.1
McKenzie clip	6,32,33,35,42,51,52,63,104,109,146	27.2
Sugar–McKenzie clip	51,52	—
Duane–McKenzie clip	42,43,51,63	27.2
Tovi clip	51,52,171	27.3
Samuels–Weck Hemoclip	2,9,51,52,117,124,135–137,156,157,181,184	27.4
Ethicon Ligaclip	51,52	27.4
Early tantalum clips	48,51,52,178	27.5
Gold dental plate clip	51,52,79	27.6
Olivecrona clip	1,4,13,14,25,32,35,51,52,56,57,60,61, 63,73,75,79,105,106,109,111,119,120, 125–127,134,137,146,148,150,152,154, 156,167,170,172,173,176,179	27.7 27.8
Nyström clip	116	—
Housepian clip	51,52,105	27.9
Pool–Pfeiffer locking clip	51,52,126	27.10
Iwabuchi memory clip	74	—
Crutchfield screw clip	19,51,52,63	27.11
Nyström screw clip	115	—
Schwartz spring clip	51,52,65,88,96,102	27.12
Mayfield–Kees spring clip	3,4,14,24,32–35,37,38,51–53,61,63–65, 78,80,84–86,88,93,96,102,105,110,117, 121,125,131,133,137,142,146,151,152, 155,168,169,180	27.13 27.14
Corrugated Mayfield–Kees clip	51,52	27.15
Chaffee–Mayfield spring clip	15,51,52	—
Shahbabian–Mayfield clip	145	27.16
McFadden Silastic-coated clip	51,52,101	—
McFadden–Kees spring clip	7,24,51,52,101,112,113,133	27.17
Drake–Kees spring clip	24,31,34,36,39,40,50–52,132,133	27.18
Graf spring clip	51,52,58	27.19
Yaşargil–Aesculap clip	2,6–8,12,24,29,51,52,62,77,110,117,118, 121–125,132,133,138,142,156,177,182–185	27.20 27.21
New McFadden–Kees clip	51,52,98	27.22
Sugita spring clip	39,51,133,156,158	27.23
New Yaşargil–Aesculap clip	186	27.24
Lougheed–Kerr spring clip	51,52,63,87,89–92,121,133,153,154,156	27.25
Scoville–Lewis spring clip	2,6,7,16,24,29,34,38,39,44,51,52,61–63, 66,73,79,83–85,93,102,105,110,113,117,121, 124,125,128,133,137,141,156,158,165,177,181,183	27.26
Nyström spring clip	116	27.27
Heifetz–Weck spring clip	2,7,9,11,24,29,39,47,51,52,55,59,67–69, 72,77,84,95,97,105,107,117,124,125,130, 132,133,137,138,142,144,147,156–158,166,177	27.28
Sparta spring clip	51,52	27.29
Codman Vari-Angle clip	51,52	27.30
V. Mueller Pivot clip	51,52	27.30
Suzuki spring clip	82,163,164	—
Smith encircling spring clip	51,52,102	27.31
Sundt–Kees encircling clip	6,7,29,51,52,72,93,103,108,114,121,132,137,159–162	27.32 27.33

In part from Fox JL, ref. 51. See ref. 51 for commercial sources of these clips and their component materials.

stayed more firmly in the clip applier during transfer and then encircled the vessel (51). This identical tantalum clip (name changed to Ligaclip) has been available from Ethicon, Inc. (Fig. 27.4).

Several authors (48,129,135,178) reported that tantalum was preferable for malleable vascular clip construction (Fig. 27.5) owing to the tissue reaction to silver (100,103), and today many of today's malleable clips are made from

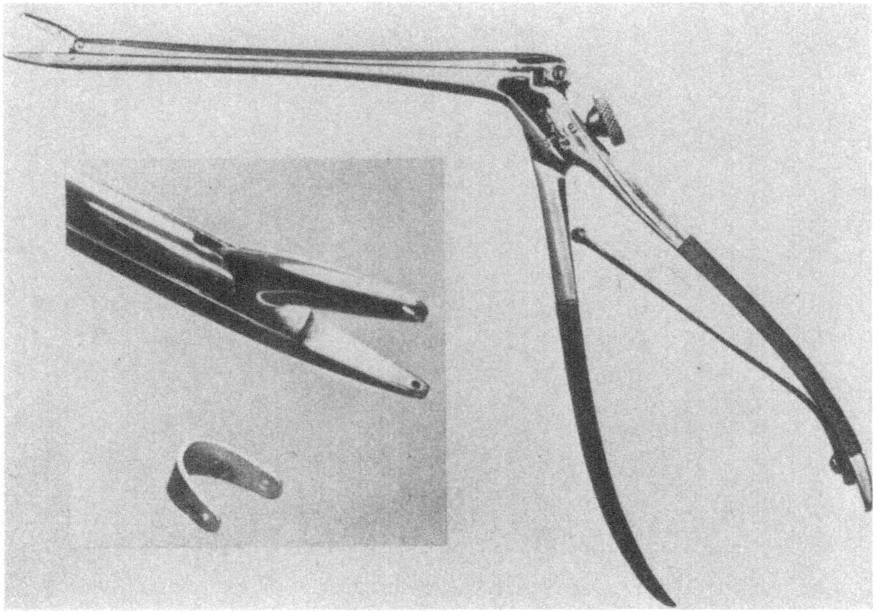

Fig. 27.3. Tovi clip. From Tovi D, ref. 171.

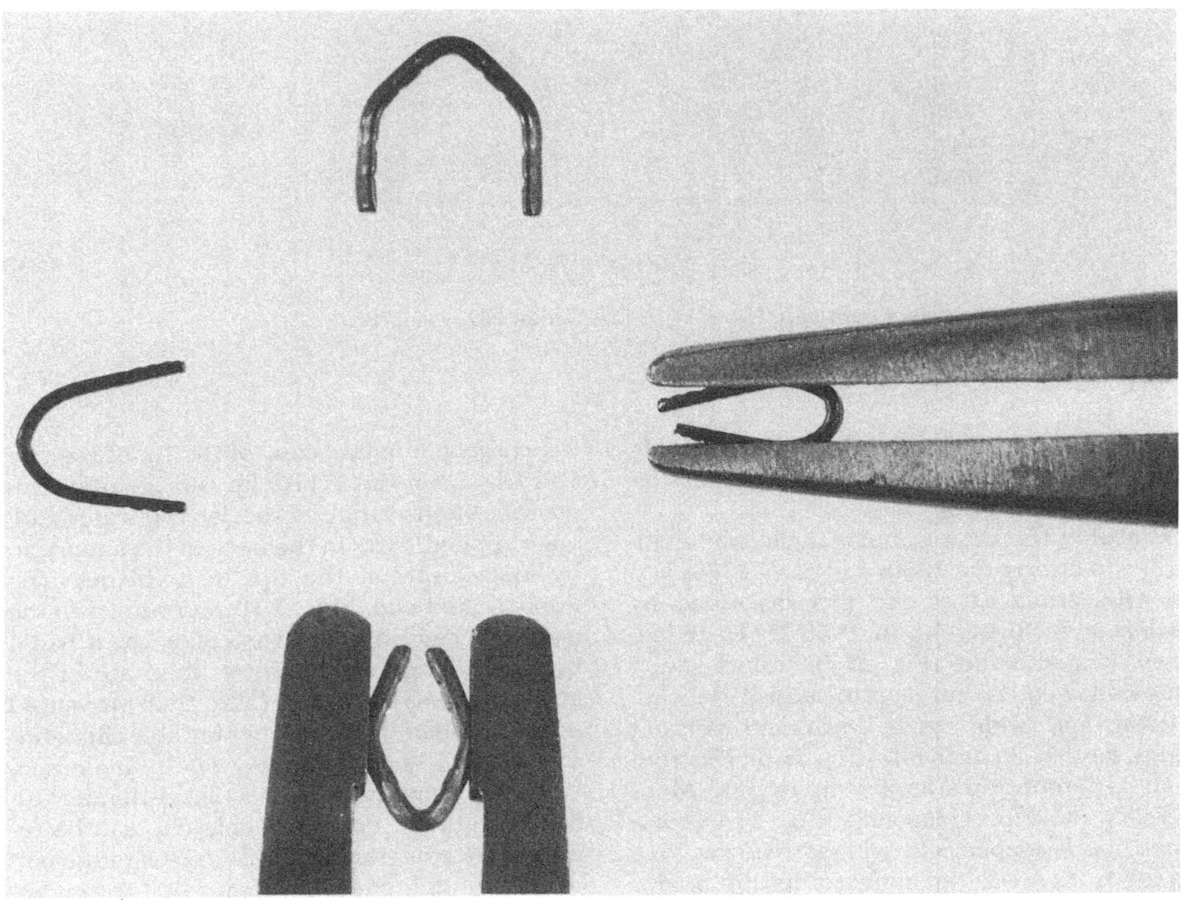

Fig. 27.4. Samuels–Weck Hemoclip appears at top and bottom; the Ethicon Ligaclip is on the right and left. From Fox JL, ref. 51.

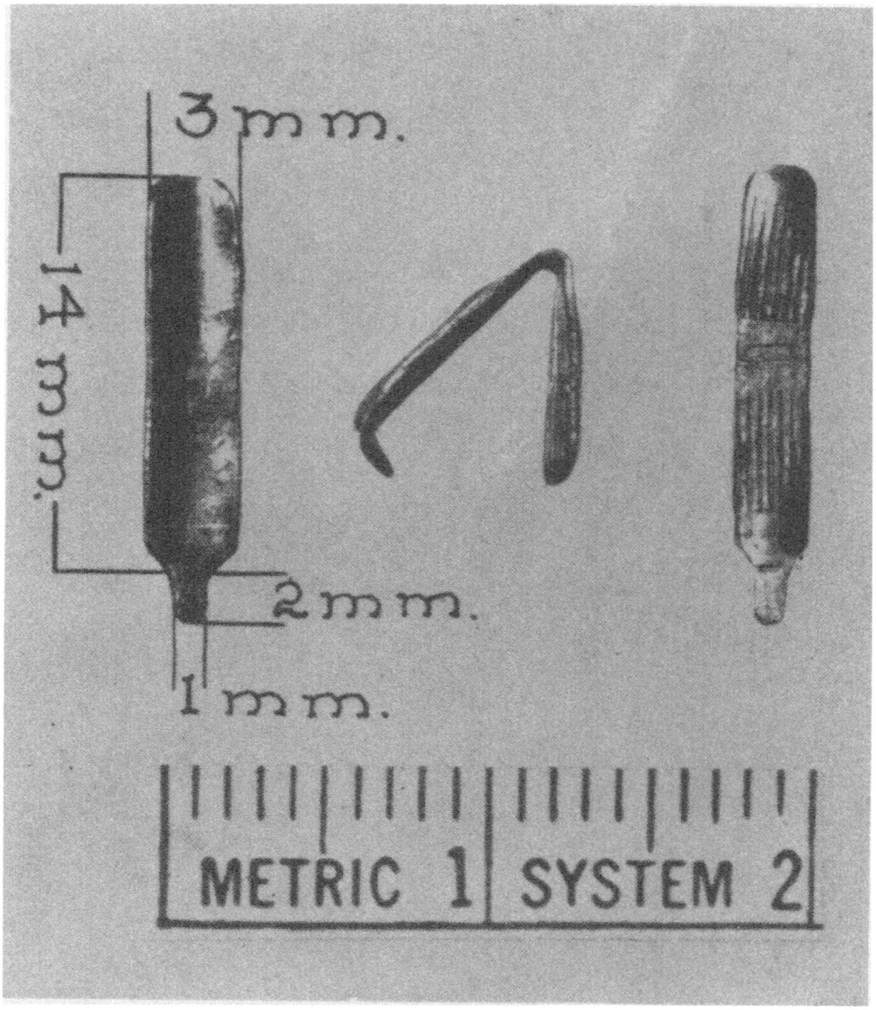

Fig. 27.5. Wise–Green tantalum clip. From Wise BL, Green ED, ref. 178.

tantalum. Some surgeons fashion malleable clips from gold plates obtained from dental supply houses (Fig. 27.6).

Probably the most popular malleable aneurysm clip during the 1950s and early 1960s was the Olivecrona silver clip first described by Norlén and Olivecrona in 1953 (111). It featured winged blades (Fig. 27.7), an innovation which allowed the surgeon to reopen the clip. Narrow and wide types, with and without wings, have been available (Fig. 27.8). Nyström et al. (116) reported a similar clip in 1962. More recently the Housepian clip (Fig. 27.9) combined the U-shaped and winged features (51). An innovation was the ability of its clip holder to grasp the clip more caudally, thereby giving the surgeon a better view of the tip of the clip and the aneurysm. This clip can be angled in any direction within its special applicator and, once applied, locks in the neck of the aneurysm by first closing at the tips of its blades. The Pool–Pfeiffer clip (Fig. 27.10) was similar to the narrow, wingless Olivecrona clip, but it had a unique locking mechanism as the neck of the aneurysm was encircled (126) that prevented arterial pulsations from opening the clip later.

Iwabuchi et al. (74) developed an unusual "memory" clip made from a nickel-titanium alloy (55 nitinol). This malleable clip can be removed by applying heat (79–107°C) to the clip which results in the clip opening up to its preapplied shape.

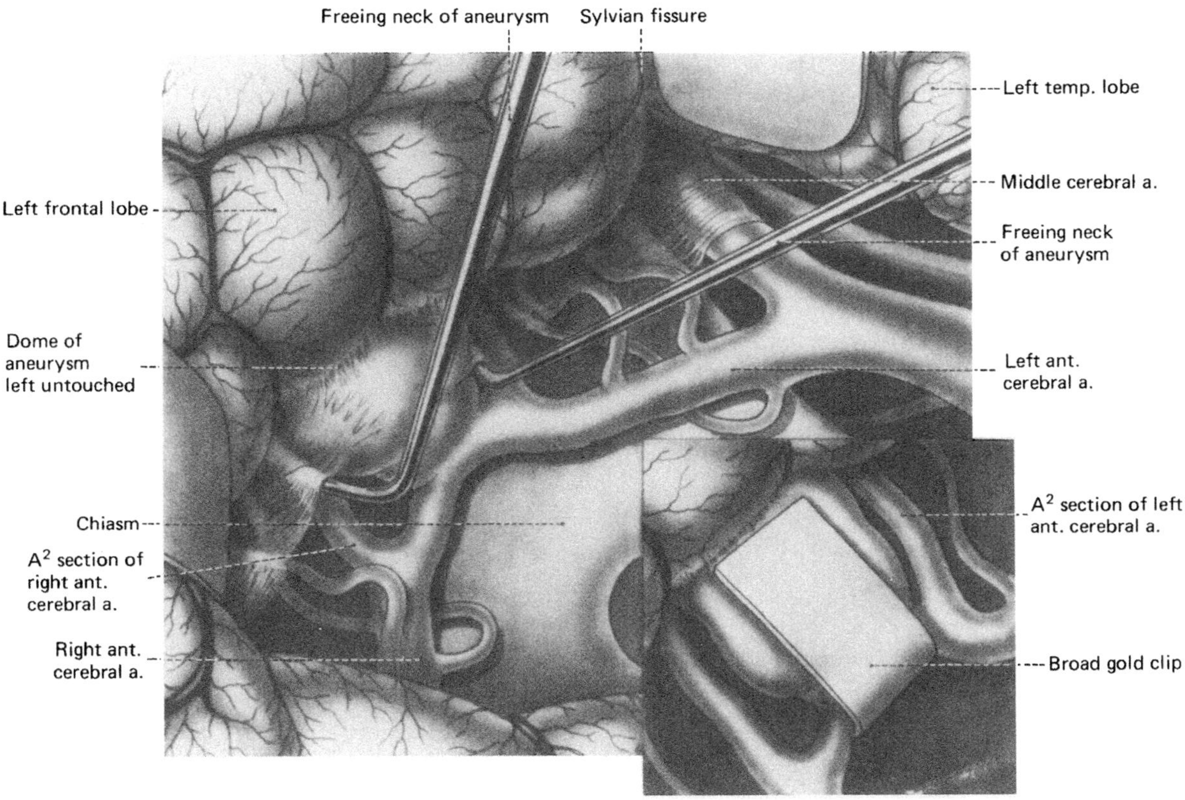

Fig. 27.6. Gold clip made from dental gold plate. From Kempe LG, ref. 79.

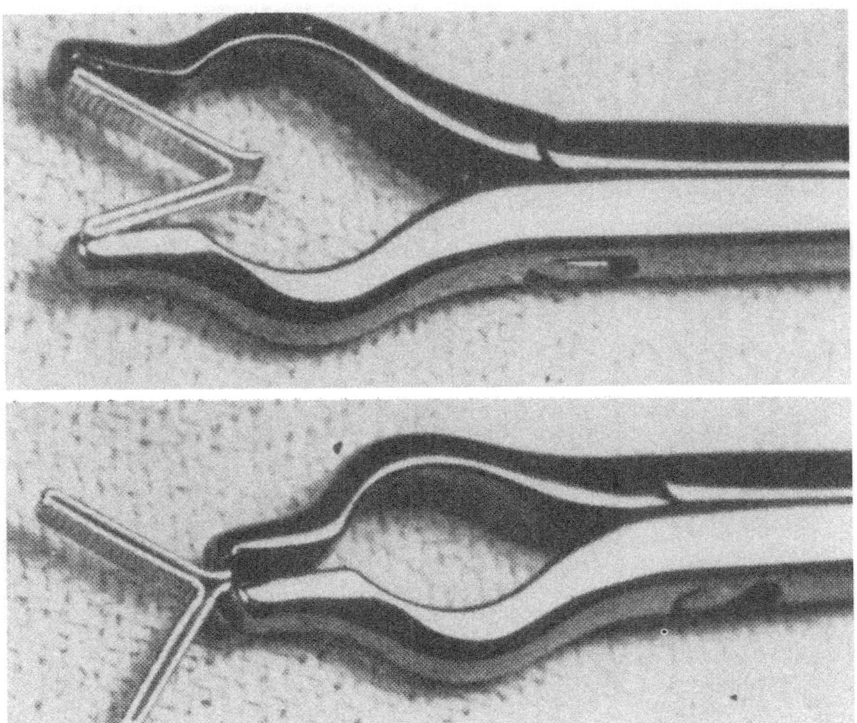

Fig. 27.7. Original Olivecrona clip with wings. From Norlén G, Olivecrona H, ref. 111.

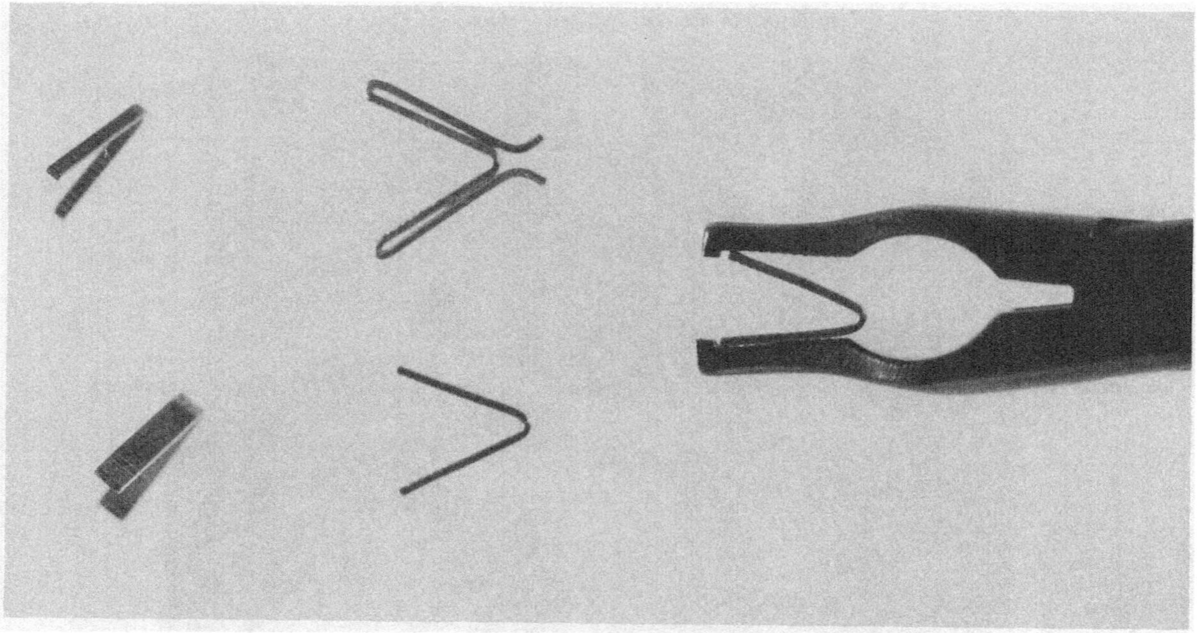

Fig. 27.8. Four types of Olivecrona clip: narrow (with and without wings) and wide (with and without wings). A narrow wingless clip is held in the Hayes–Olivecrona clip applier. From Fox JL, ref. 51.

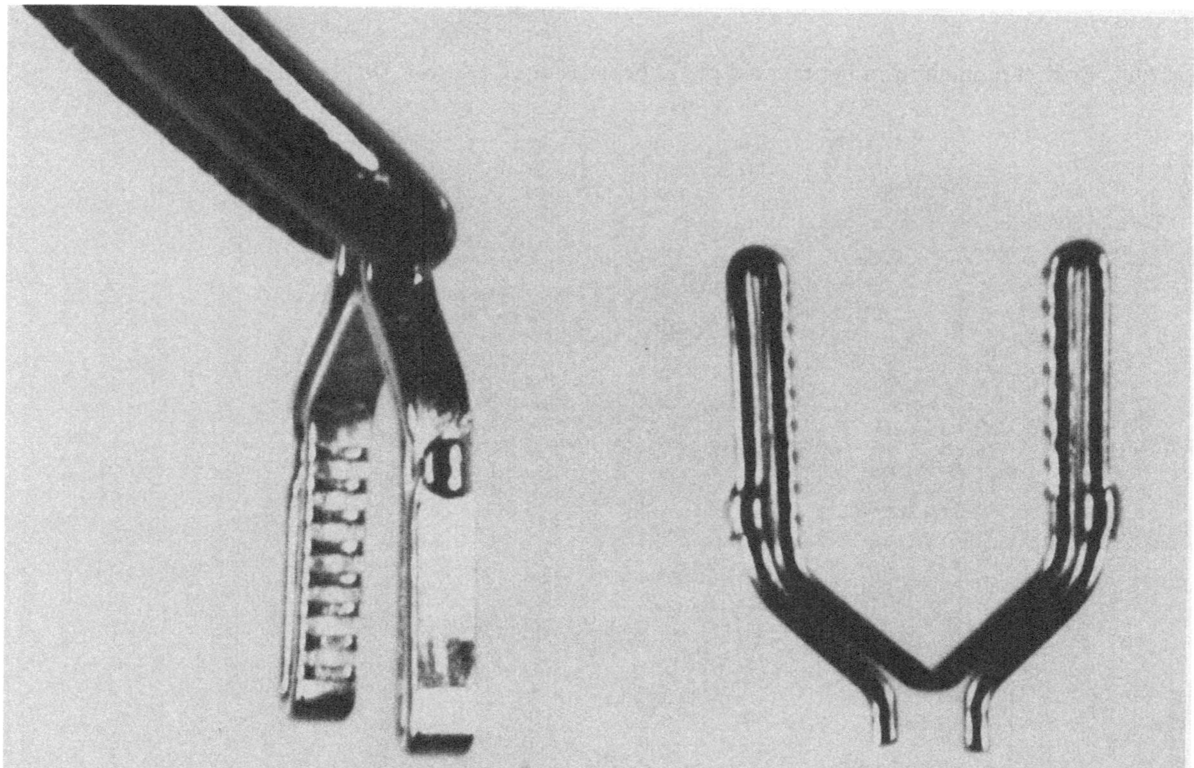

Fig. 27.9. Housepian clip. From Fox JL, ref. 51.

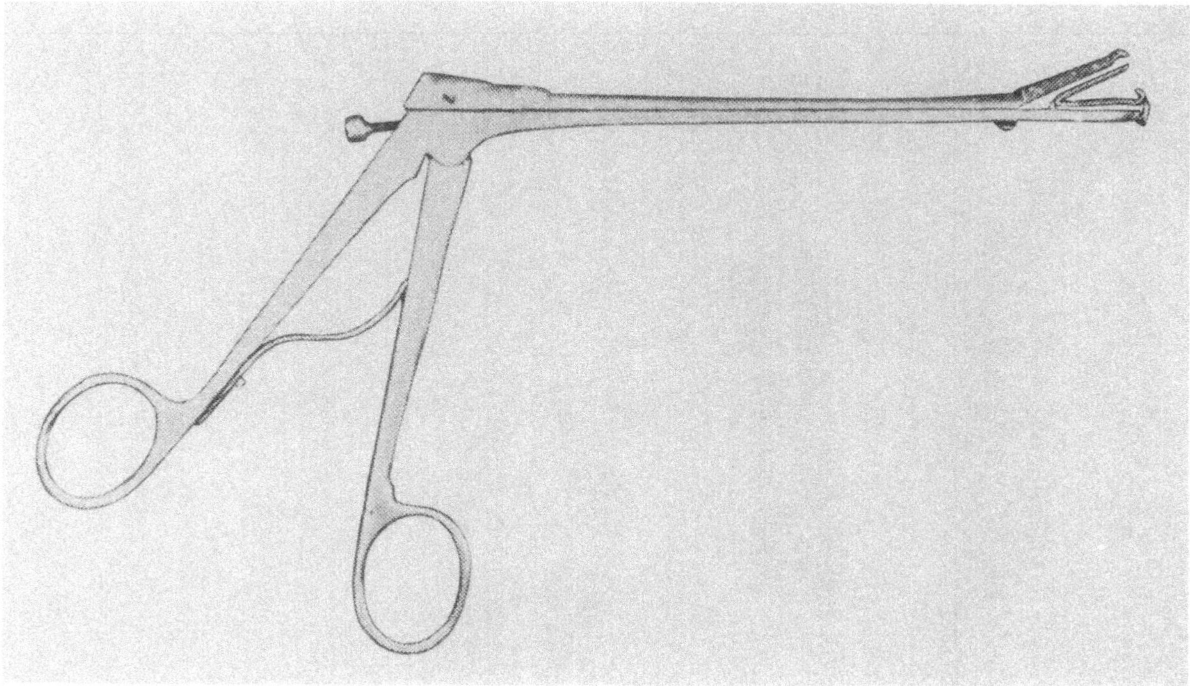

Fig. 27.10. Pool–Pfeiffer locking clip. From Pool JL, Potts DG, ref. 126.

Screw Clips

Unlike the malleable clips described above (Figs. 27.1–27.10), Crutchfield (19) developed a clip (or clamp) which screwed down to occlude a vessel or aneurysm (Fig. 27.11). Various other types of screw clip have been designed, e.g., Nyström clip (115), Berci–Nyhus clip (10), and Martinez Coll–Del Corral clip (93), but none have become popular.

Spring Clips

Spring clips are the most commonly used clips for aneurysm occlusion and temporary occlusion of vessels in microvascular surgery. During the early 1950s Schwartz developed a cross-action, or crossed-legged, clip (Fig. 27.12) intended to be used for temporary vascular occlusion (96). This clip has three basic parts: a shank (which is held by the clip applier), the crossing

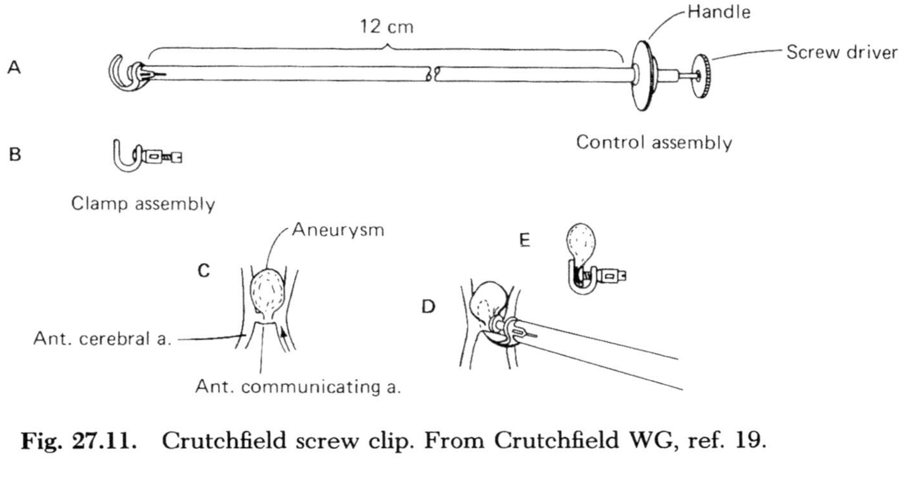

Fig. 27.11. Crutchfield screw clip. From Crutchfield WG, ref. 19.

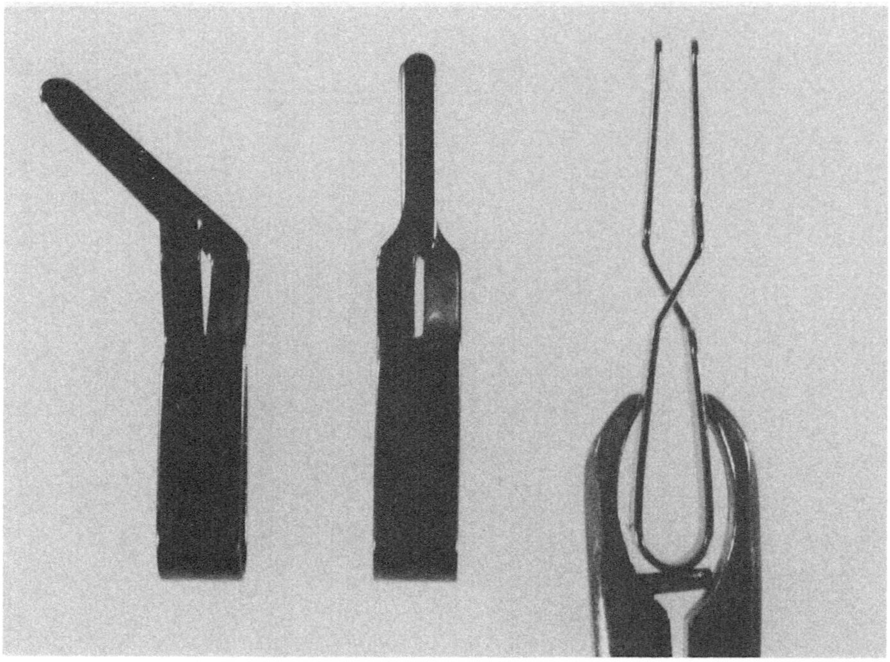

Fig. 27.12. Schwartz spring clip. The opened clip is held by a modified Mayfield clip holder. From Fox JL, ref. 51.

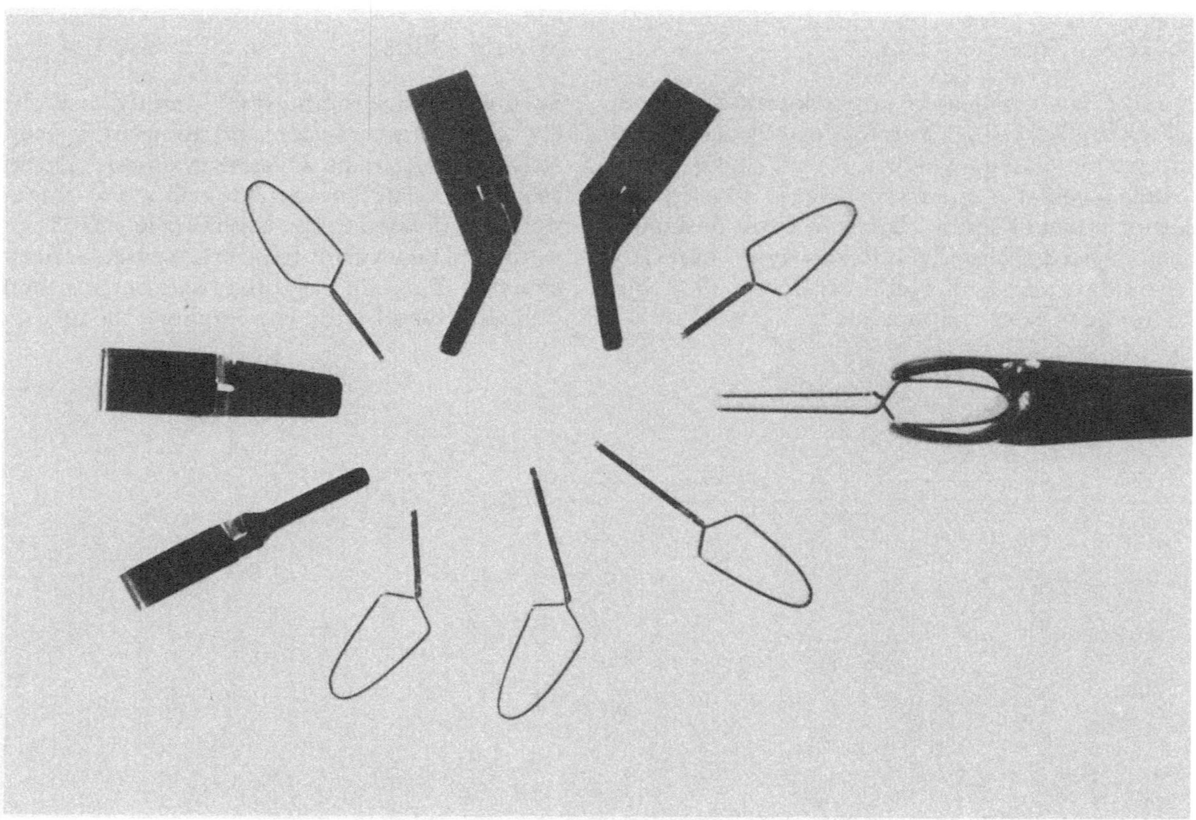

Fig. 27.13. Mayfield–Kees spring clips. From Fox JL, ref. 51.

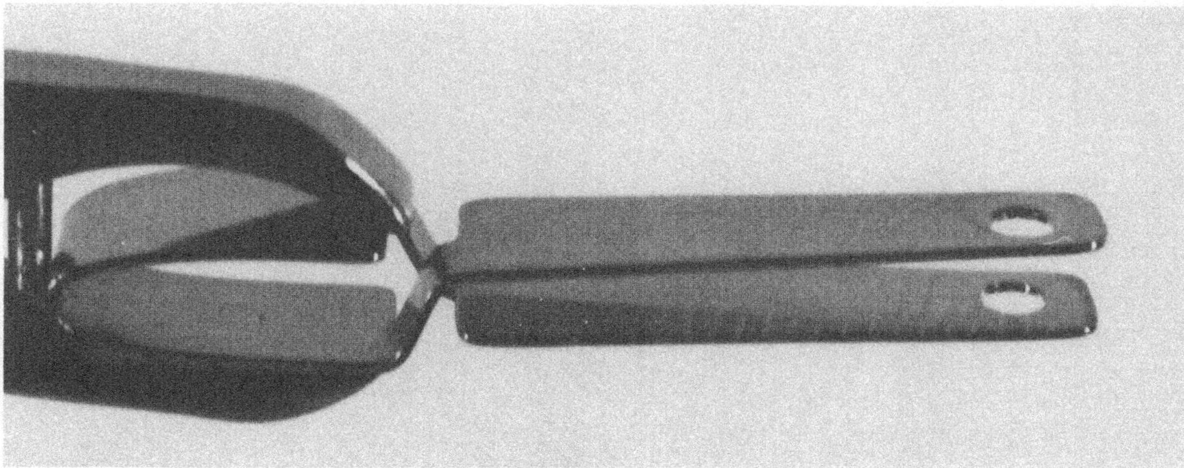

Fig. 27.14. Mayfield–Kees spring clip with a suture hole at the tip of the blade. From Fox JL, ref. 51.

zone of the blades, and the opposing zone of the blades. Subsequently Mayfield and Kees designed a similar clip for permanent occlusion of an aneurysm. It had the advantage of a comparatively smaller shank that can be held by the clip applier during transfer and application (96). During the 1950s and 1960s the Mayfield clip (Fig. 27.13) (Kees Surgical Specialty Company) seemed to have been the most popular spring clip for dealing with an intracranial aneurysm or for temporary occlusion of arteries (51). The original version tended to have a scissoring action, risking severance of the vessel (3); this was modified so that the blades do not touch along the crossing zone. Many sizes and configurations have evolved (Fig. 27.13). A clip with a hole at the end of the blades was made for certain large aneurysms with broad necks (Fig. 27.14), thereby allowing the surgeon to tie the blades of the clip firmly together to prevent the clip from opening. Because there have been a few reports of spring clips slipping off the aneurysmal neck (41), the Mayfield–Kees clip also comes with corrugated inner blade surfaces, and the blades tend to be somewhat narrower (Fig. 27.15). Chaffee (15) modified the

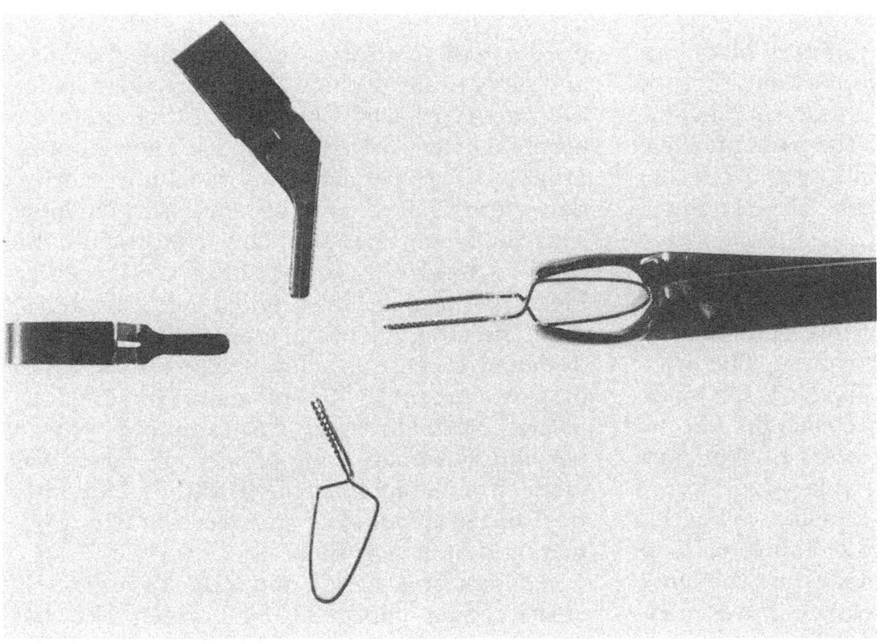

Fig. 27.15. Corrugated Mayfield–Kees spring clip in various configurations. From Fox JL, ref. 51.

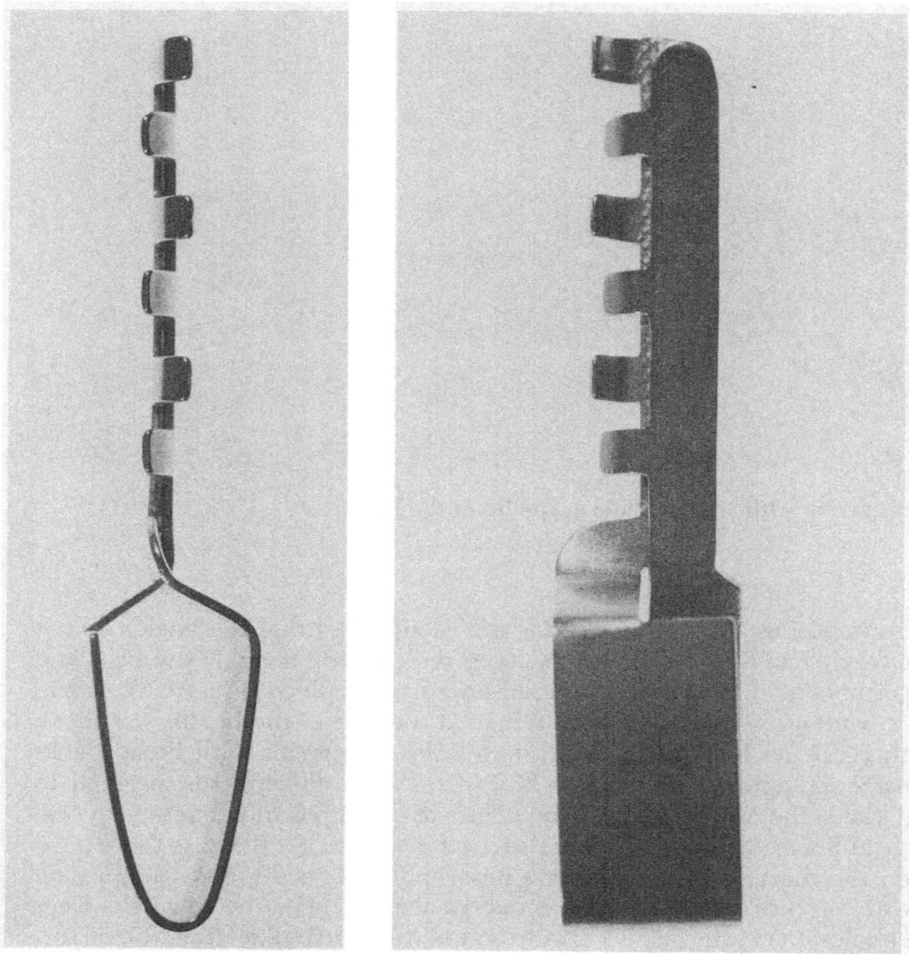

A B

Fig. 27.16. Shahbabian–Mayfield spring clip.

Mayfield clip to permit the tapering blade tips to bypass each other after application, thereby entrapping the neck of the aneurysm. Shahbabian and Mayfield (145) used the basic Mayfield design but added teeth which would prevent slippage from the broad necks of large aneurysms (Fig. 27.16).

McFadden (101) tried to prevent tissue reaction to the clip by coating the modified Mayfield clip with silicone-rubber, but this made the clip blades too slippery for practical use. The original McFadden–Kees spring clip (101) is a modification of the Mayfield cross-action clip in which the blades are narrower, thicker, and stronger (Fig. 27.17). The Drake–Kees spring clip (34,40) is similar to the straight McFadden modification except that an opening, or loop, has been created between blades and the cross-action zone (Fig. 27.18). Drake's clip was made by Kees one night in time for Drake to re-expose a basilar artery aneurysm the next day and successfully occlude the otherwise inoperable aneurysm while preserving the posterior cerebral artery (51). This clip has allowed preservation of parent arteries, branching arteries, perforators, nerves, and other clips in the loop. This loop concept, also now adapted to the Heifetz–Weck clip, is not unlike Graf's earlier idea as he evolved his original clip (Fig. 27.19) (58). The Graf clip (not a cross-action type) was designed in part to allow passage of a vessel in close proximity to an aneurysm (51). Although originally made as a temporary clip of beryllium–copper composition, it later was made from stainless steel (Hastings Laboratories) and distributed as an aneurysm clip (Codman and Shurtleff, Inc.).

Another cross-action clip is the Yaşargil–Aesculap spring clip (183,184), which also has strong, narrow, corrugated blades but, in addi-

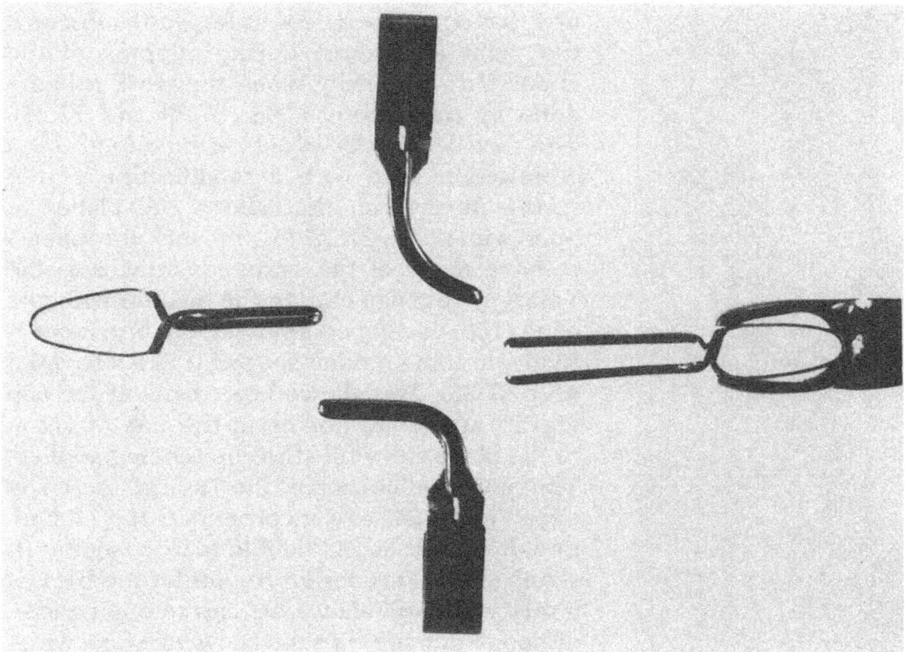

Fig. 27.17. Original McFadden–Kees spring clip in various configurations. From Fox JL, ref. 51.

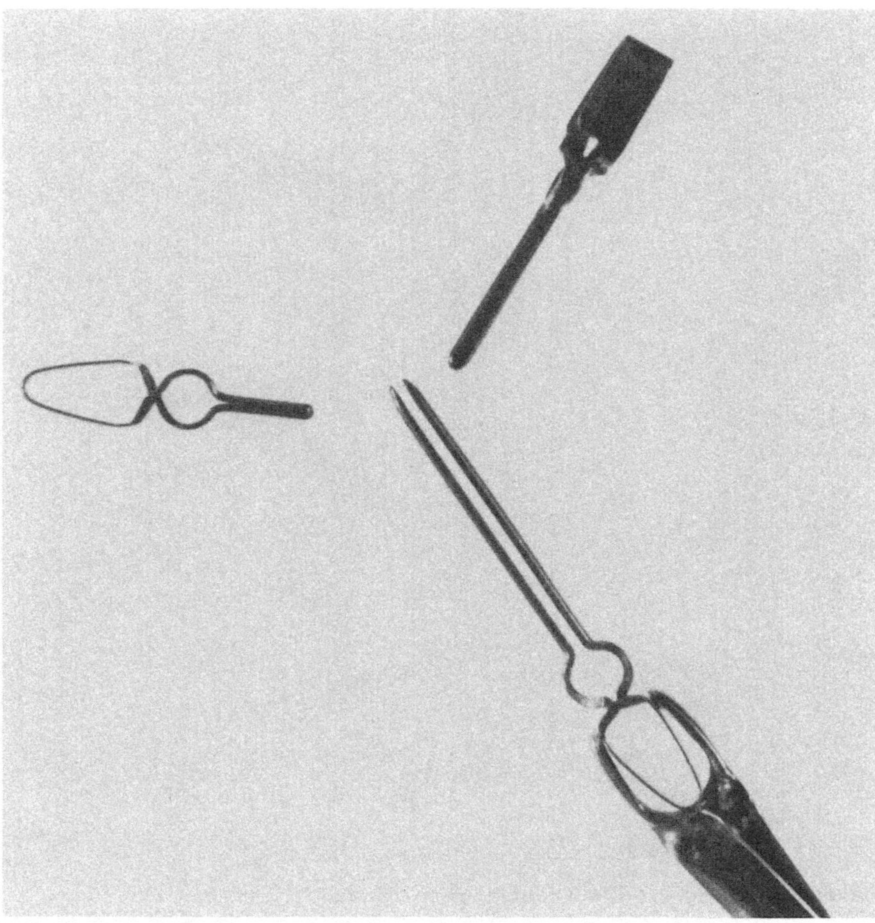

Fig. 27.18. Drake–Kees spring clip. From Fox JL, ref. 51.

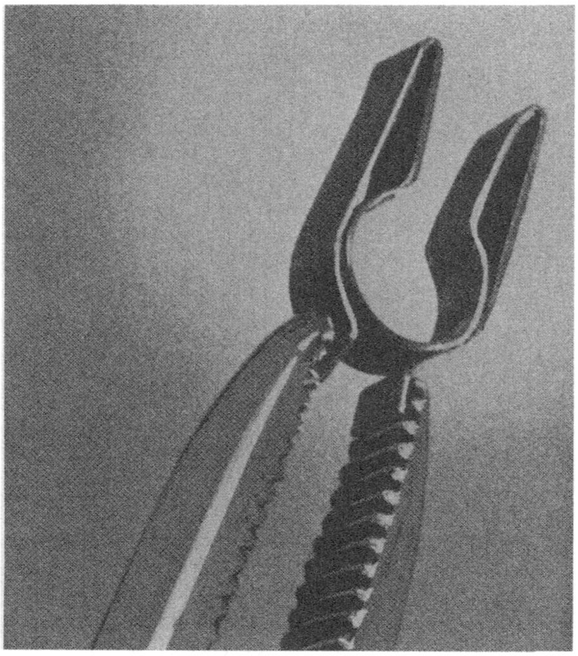

Fig. 27.19. Graf spring clip. From Graf CJ, ref. 58.

tion, has a narrow base that less easily obscures the point of interest during clipping of the aneurysm—especially when the work is being done by microscopy (Figs. 27.20 and 27.21). The new McFadden–Kees spring clip also is a cross-action type with a modification of the spring mechanism that allows the blades to open wider (Fig. 27.22) (51,98); this clip appears to have many of the same advantages as the Yaşargil–Aesculap clip. In the meantime Sugita et al. (156) developed a similar clip but, innovatively, in some models shaped it like a bayonet (Fig. 27.23). This allowed the shank of the clip and its applier to not be in the line of vision to the blade tips while the clip is being applied. The new modification of the Yaşargil–Aesculap clip (Fig. 27.24) also incorporated the McFadden–Kees and Sugita double helix design in its shank (186). This design resembles the back of a safety pin and allows the clip to open wider, although in some clips the allowance for a wider opening causes a loss of some closing force in its application to the neck of the aneurysm.

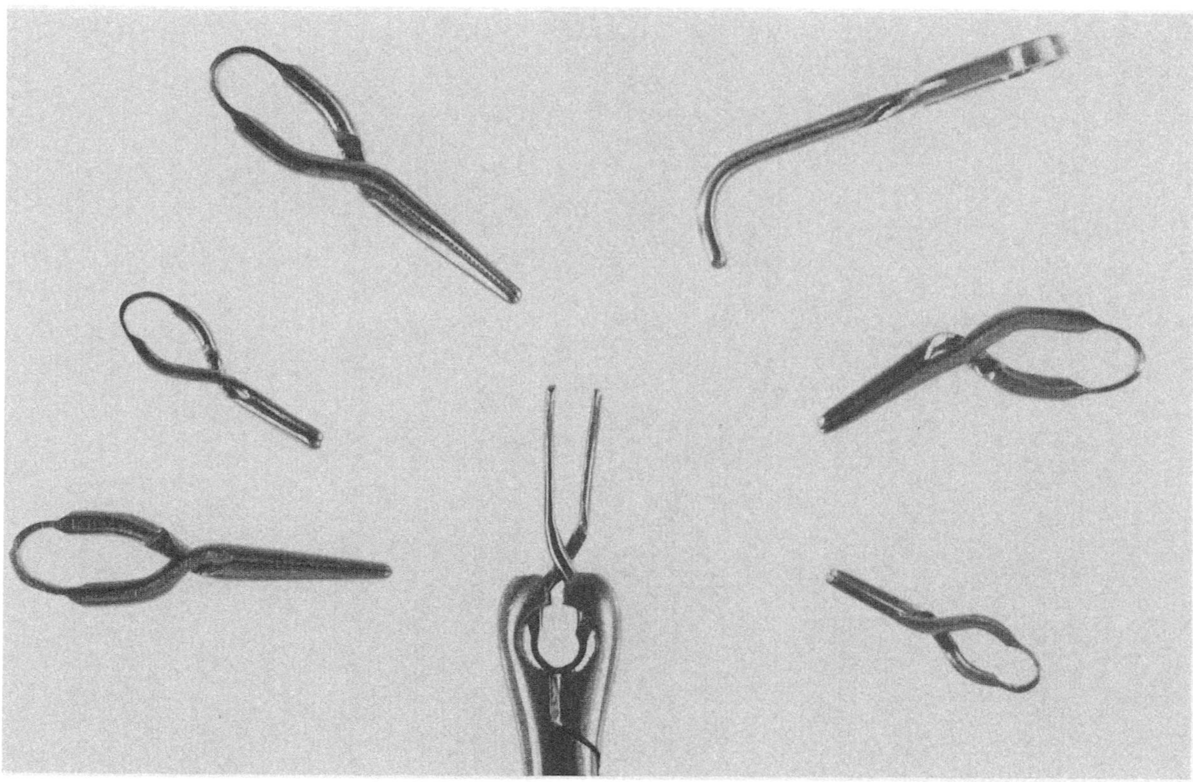

Fig. 27.20. Original Yaşargil–Aesculap spring clip in various configurations. From Fox JL, ref. 51.

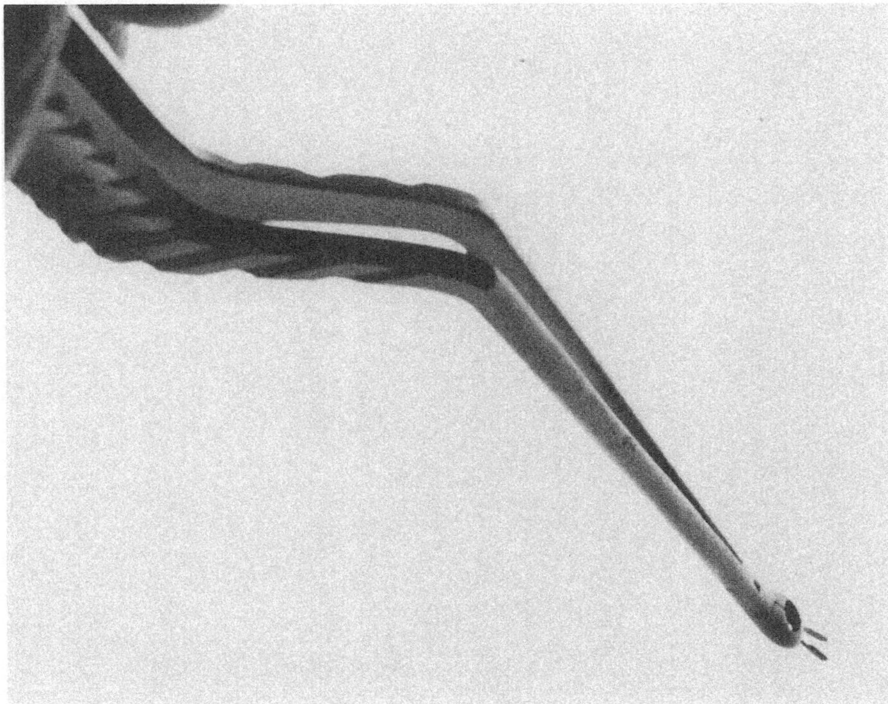

Fig. 27.21. Yaşargil–Aesculap clip applier, emphasizing the bayonet shape preferred by some for vascular surgery under the microscope. From Fox JL, ref. 51.

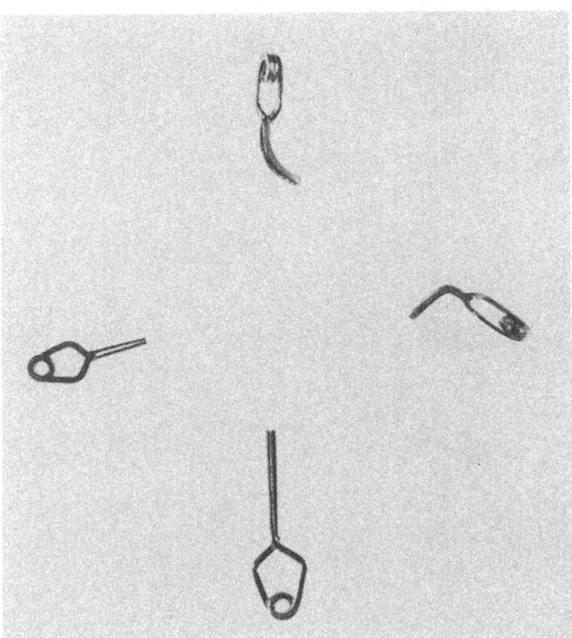

Fig. 27.22. Vari-Angle McFadden clip (Codman & Shurtleff, Inc.) in various configurations. From Fox JL, ref. 51.

The Lougheed–Kerr spring clip (89) was unique in that it gained its spring action from an attached ring (Fig. 27.25), which can be moved to change the force of the spring. Furthermore, the clip can be swiveled in any direction in the clip holder, an advantage also found in the Scoville–Lewis, Sparta, and Codman Vari-Angle or V. Mueller Pivot clips (see below). The Scoville–Lewis spring clip (141) has a coiled spring whose axis is set parallel to the line of clip action (Fig. 27.26), a unique torsion bar mechanism that also acts as a small base, or shank, making visualization easier.

In 1962 Nyström et al. (116) reported their spring clip with corrugated blades, the first aneurysm clip to use an internal spring to hold the clip closed (Fig. 27.27). In 1969 Heifetz (69) described a similar clip (Fig. 27.28), which has been quite popular among neurosurgeons. This spring is inside a fairly small shank. The opposing surfaces of the Heifetz–Weck clip blades were slightly rounded (to prevent cutting the tissue) and serrated (to avoid slipping of the blades). The Sparta clip (51) (Fig. 27.29) and the Codman Vari-Angle or V. Mueller Pivot

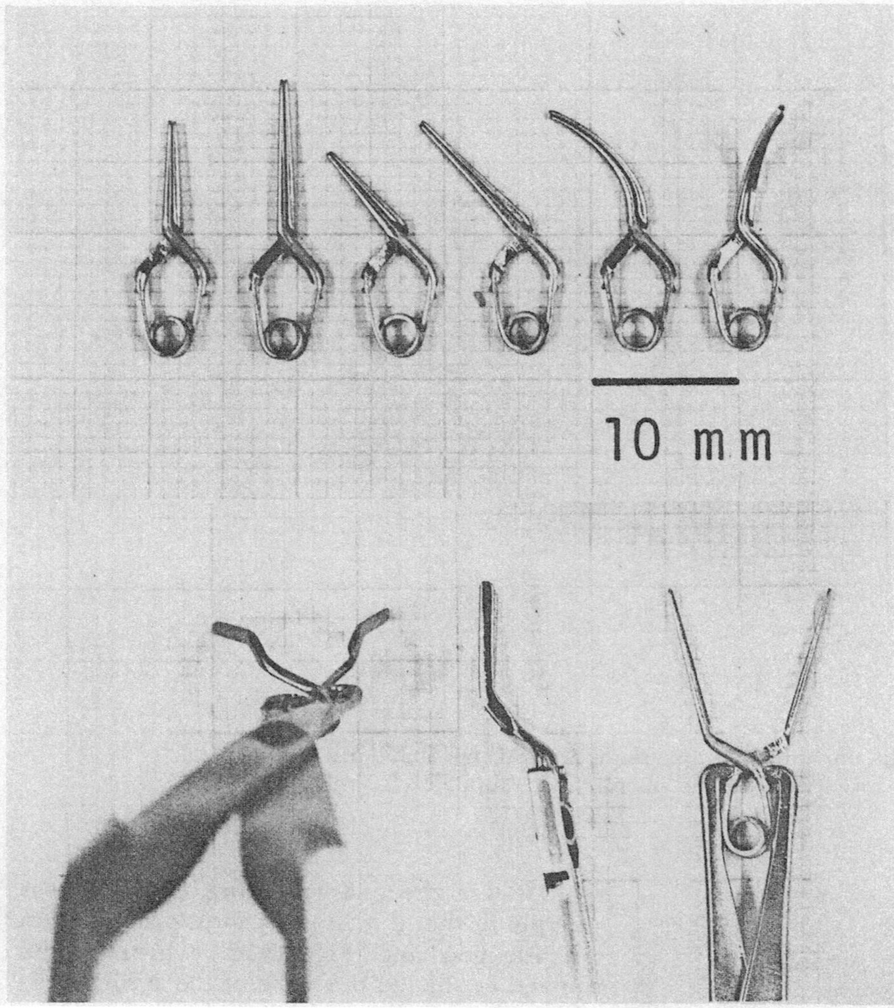

Fig. 27.23. Sugita clip in various configurations. Note the bayonet shape of some. From Sugita K, Hirota T, Iguchi I, et al., ref. 156.

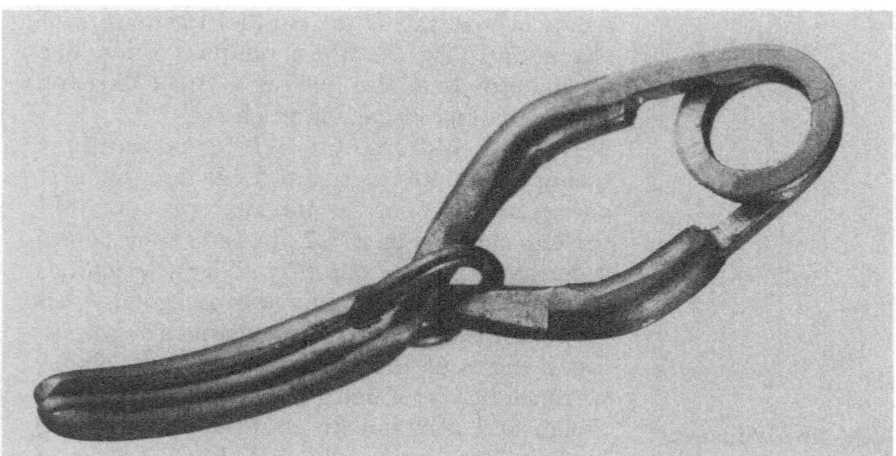

Fig. 27.24. Modified Yaşargil–Aesculap spring clip.

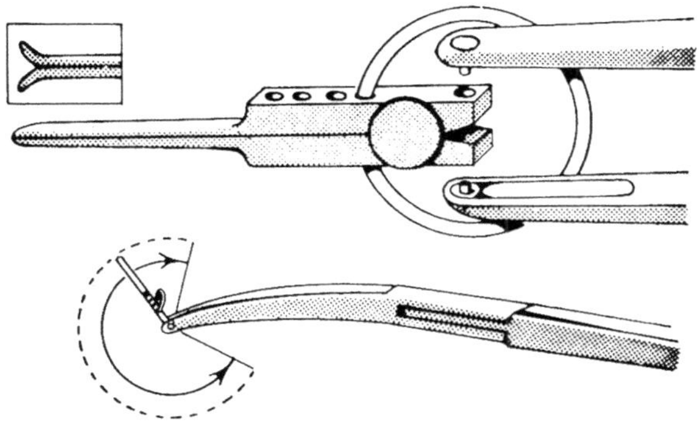

Fig. 27.25. Lougheed–Kerr spring clip. From Lougheed WM, Khodadad G, ref. 89.

spring clips (Fig. 27.30) have similar internal spring mechanisms. Such mechanisms have somewhat weaker blade closure forces than many of the cross-action (cross-legged) clips (24,26,30,156).

In 1969 Khodadad (82) reported his microvascular spring clip, which has a silicone-rubber band just in front of the pivot point (or fulcrum) of the blades. This band held the blades together. Later Suzuki et al. (163,164) described a similar clip (Suzuki clip) for use on intracranial aneurysms.

The next major innovation, developed by George W. Smith, was based on the concept of obliterating an aneurysm on the arterial wall opposite to the surgeon by the use of a vessel-encircling clip (Fig. 27.31) (51,102). The next logical step was the encircling clip-graft described by Sundt et al. (162), the principle of which is illustrated in Fig. 27.32; examples are shown in Fig. 27.33. The Heifetz–Weck clip models used a similar design (Fig. 27.28).

Other Clip Data

Performance Characteristics

Lougheed and Marshall (90) stated that intracranial aneurysm clips ideally should have the following characteristics:

1. Be available in various sizes
2. Have edges and ends polished and of sufficient thickness to prevent cutting or tearing
3. Have sufficient blade strength to prevent torsion or bending with pulsation of the aneurysm
4. Possess a narrow body and blade to allow minimal aneurysm neck dissection
5. Have opposing surfaces of blades slightly serrated for good holding power
6. Contain clip blades that close by their own tension
7. Be available in various angles, shapes, and types
8. Possess the capability of having various mounting angles in the clip holder
9. Be able to be released from the clip holder in a smooth and efficient fashion

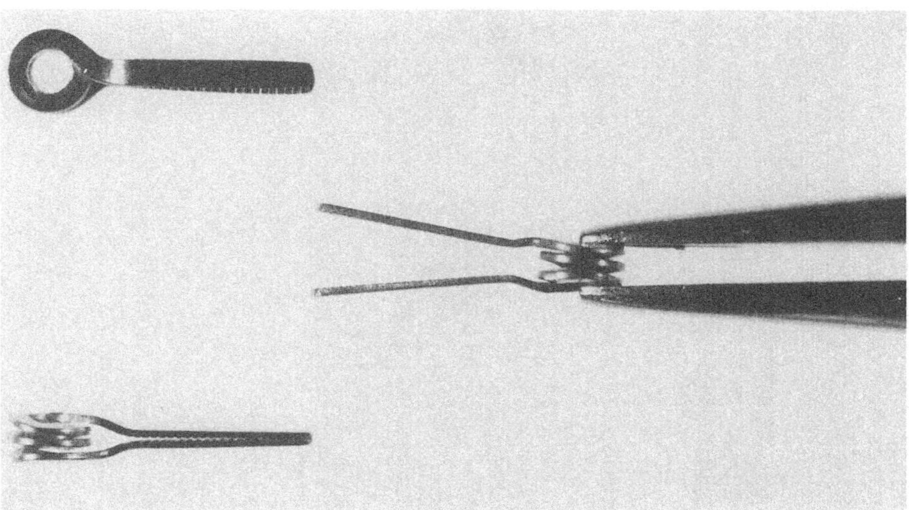

Fig. 27.26. Scoville–Lewis spring clip. From Fox J, ref. 51.

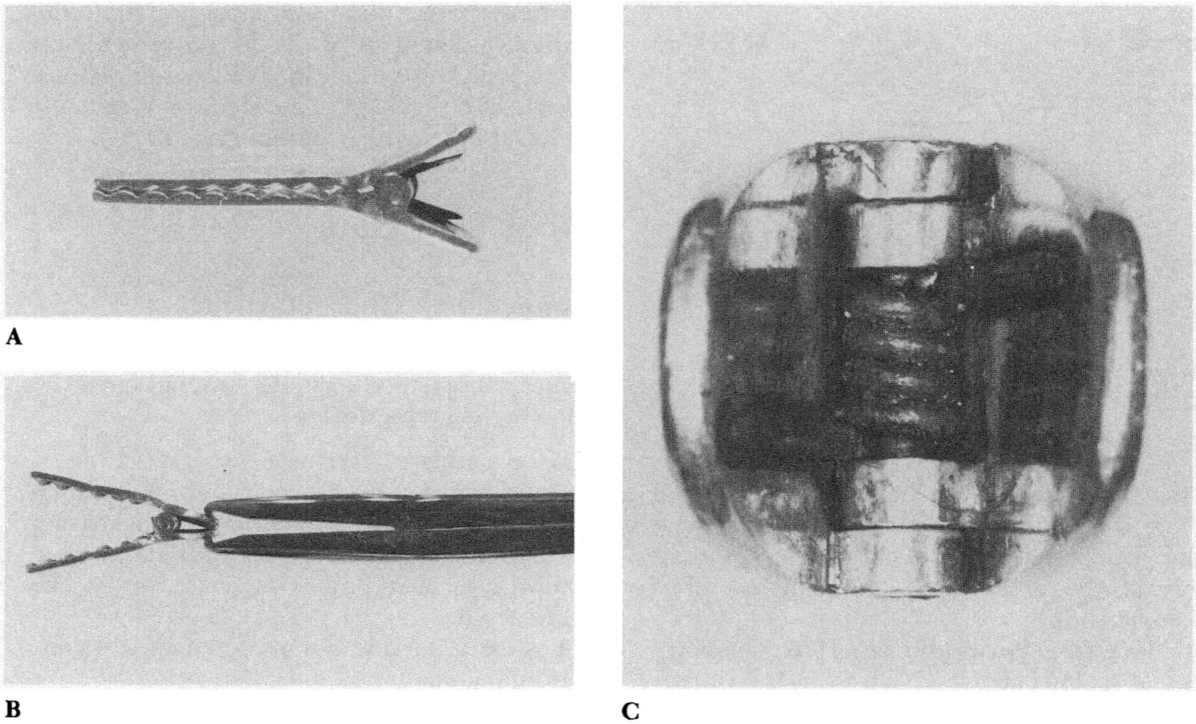

Fig. 27.27. This Nyström clip was reported in 1962 (116). Courtesy of S.H.M. Nyström.

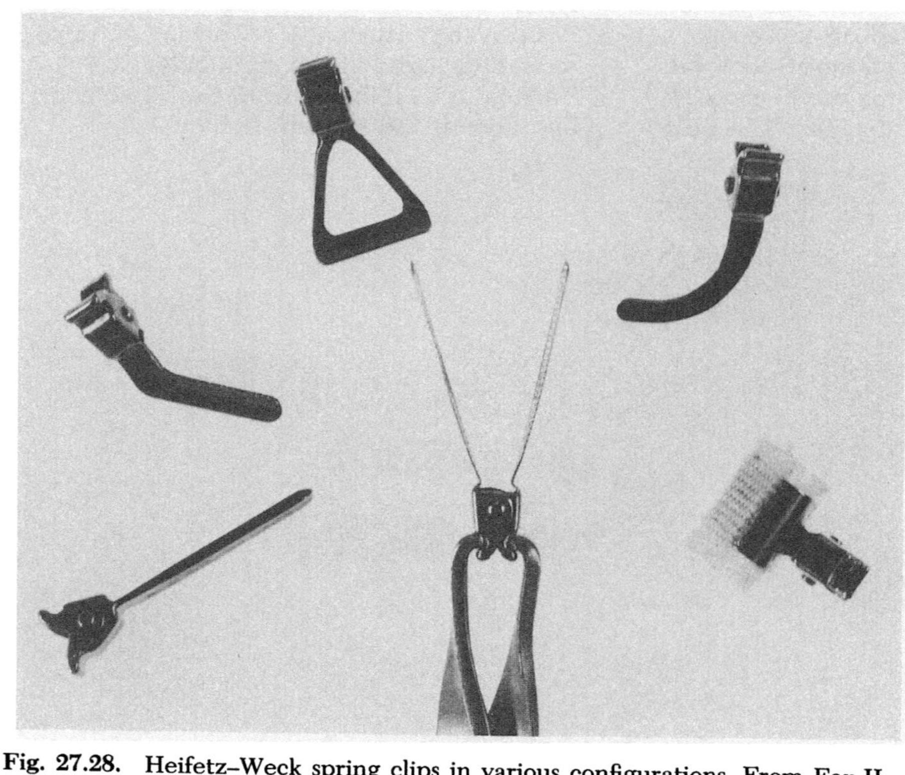

Fig. 27.28. Heifetz-Weck spring clips in various configurations. From Fox JL, ref. 51.

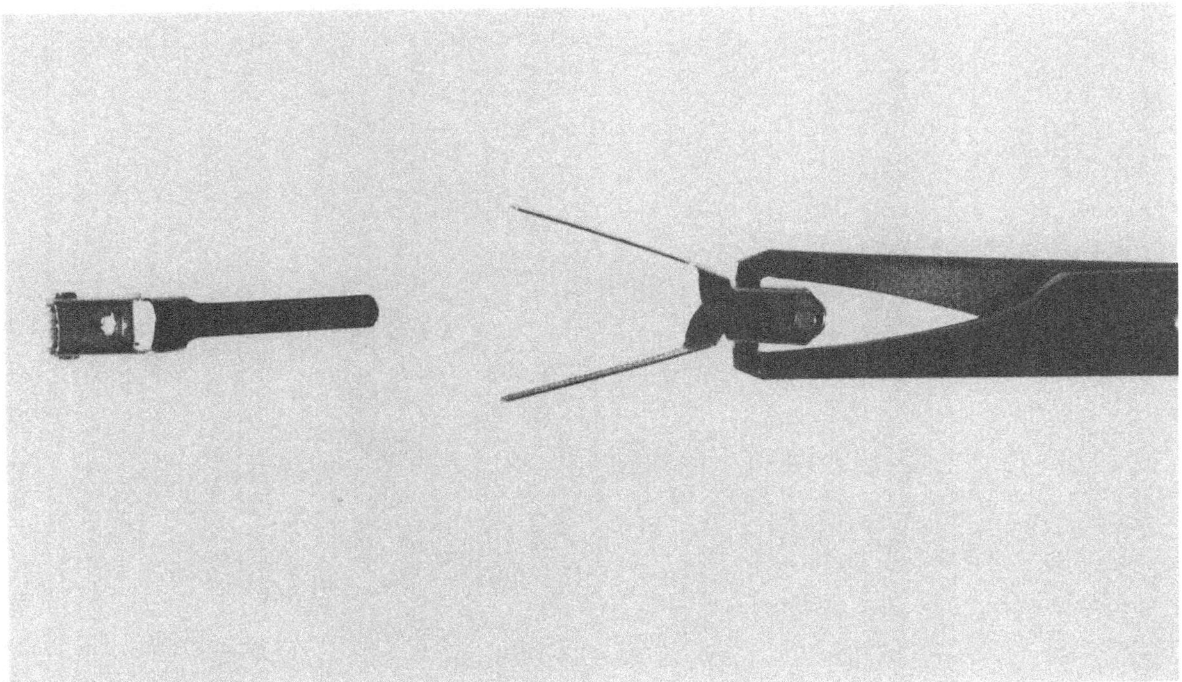

Fig. 27.29. Sparta spring clip. From Fox JL, ref. 51.

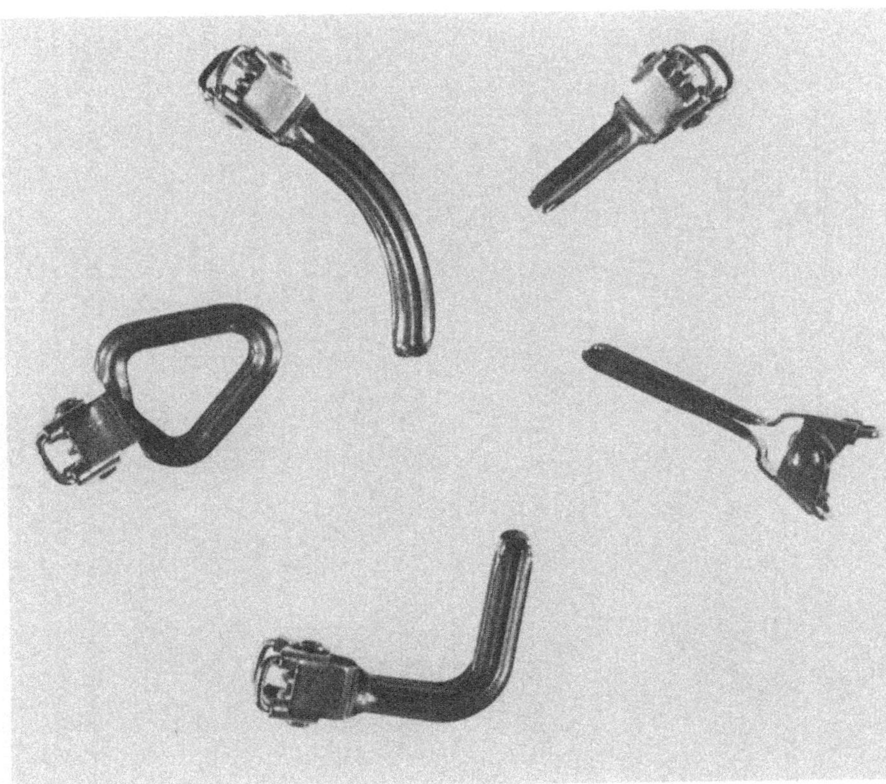

Fig. 27.30. These clips were originally called Sundt–Kees spring clips (51), but they have been sold as the Codman Vari-Angle clip and later as the V. Mueller Pivot clip. From Fox JL, ref. 51.

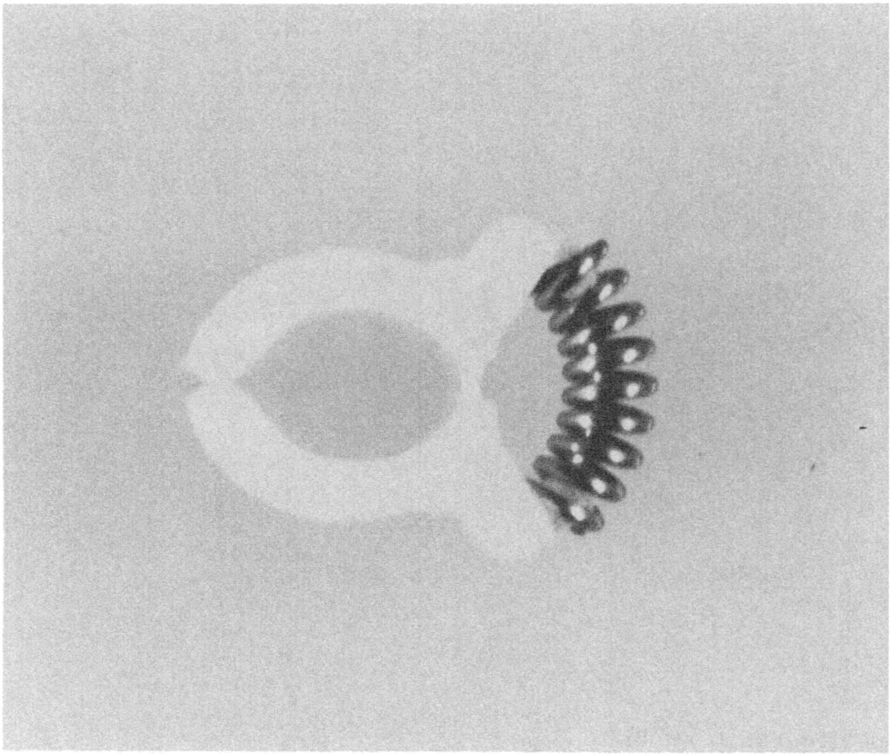

Fig. 27.31. The Smith encircling spring clip is molded from polyethylene plastic. From Fox JL, ref. 51.

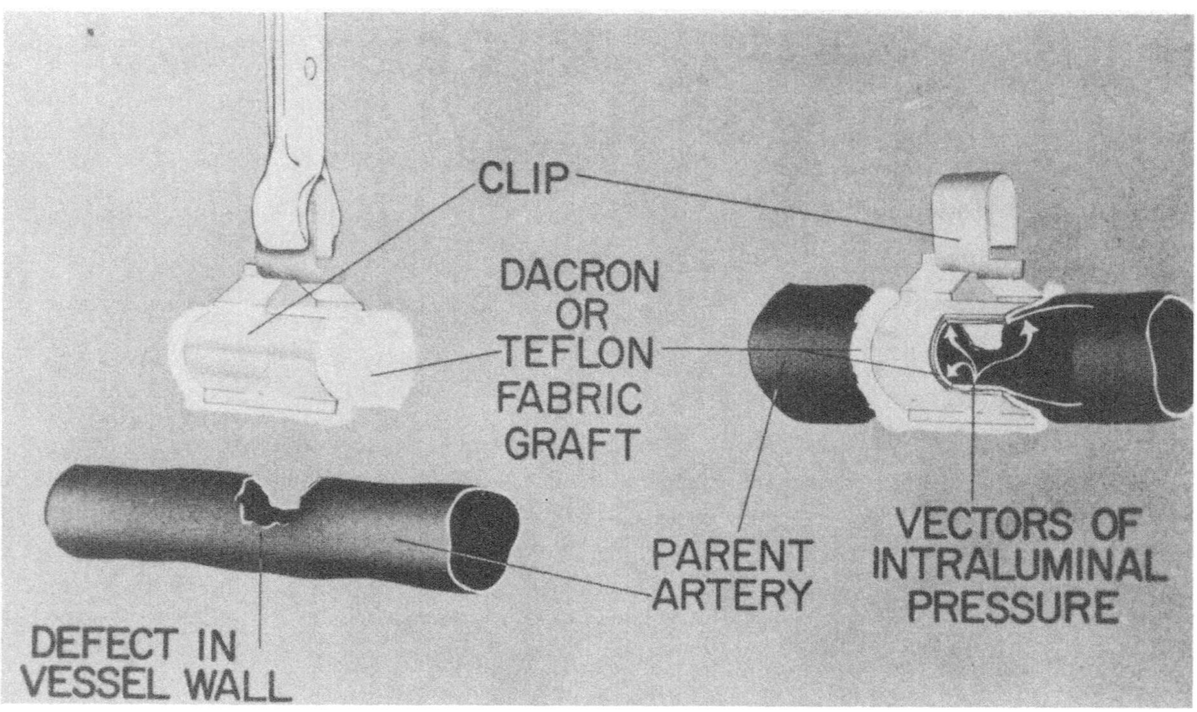

Fig. 27.32. Principle behind the use of the Sundt–Kees clip-grafts (encircling clips). From Sundt TM Jr, Nofzinger JD, ref. 162.

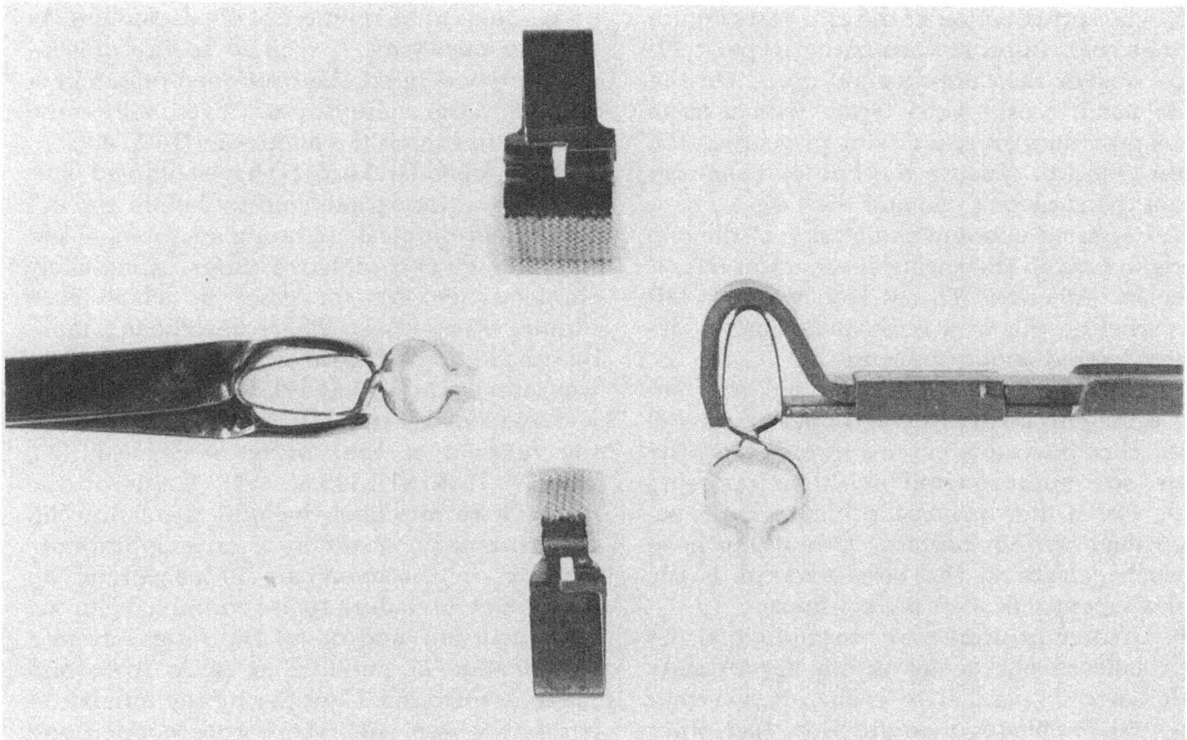

Fig. 27.33. Sundt–Kees encircling clip, or clip-graf. From Fox JL, ref. 51.

Other characteristics could be added, e.g., those relating to metallurgy; the materials composing the clip ideally should be nonreactive with each other and with the intracranial tissues. A clip with parts made from different metals may corrode owing to electrochemical reactions (83a). The reader is referred to studies on principles of tissue reaction and metallurgy (27,100,103); see also a previous article for a listing of materials found in various clips (51). Finally, von Holst and colleagues (175) found that titanium clips caused little artifact interference on CT scans and suggested that his material might be considered.

Clip Strength

The closing pressure of aneurysm spring clip blades, an essential feature that prevents blood from entering the aneurysm, is dependent on many variables. Some of these, difficult to measure, include the following (24,26,27,30,46,49, 133,156):

1. As the clip blade lengthens, there may be less pressure exerted at its tip. On the other hand, as the aneurysm neck is located closer to the spring clip fulcrum, greater pressure is exerted to occlude the aneurysm.

2. A wide clip blade may exert less pressure (force per unit area) than a narrow blade, as the force generated by the spring action may be distributed over a wide area. Most clip strength measurements are in terms of force (e.g., dynes or grams), as it is difficult to calculate pressures due to geometric problems: The clip blades are curved, round, irregular, or serrated, and the aneurysm wall contact varies considerably in configuration and texture.

3. Clips composed of highly elastic materials have less plasticity or "give" and hence more strength. However, the manufacture of clips with certain metals of high elasticity may be difficult, with compensating weakness occurring as the metals are heated and/or bent into position.

4. Thin blades have less elasticity than thick ones and hence are weaker for the reasons given above. However, excessively thick blades are difficult to negotiate between the aneurysm neck and nearby vital structures.

5. The spring action of the clip plays an important role. Internal wire spring types tend to be weaker than cross-legged types. On the other hand, cross-legged types, with a large shank providing greater closing pressure in the blades, tend to obscure the line of vision between the surgeon's eye and the target.

6. Repeated opening and closing of the clip tends to fatigue the spring mechanism (i.e., it loses its resilience). This is true whether OR personnel do this or a large, pulsating, inadequately closed aneurysm causes it.

7. Clip pressures vary with the state in which the clip blades are held open or closed. Some clips have low closure forces when the blades are approximated but their opposing blade forces increase as the blades are separated (high spring constant). Other clips have no such change in the force exerted as the blades separate (low spring constant).

8. Greater pressures are exerted when the clip blades about an aneurysm approximate each other in parallel to each other—rather than with the blades diverging from each other distal to the shank. (Perhaps the closing blade tips should slightly approach each other, occluding the opposite side of the aneurysm before its proximal side.)

Certainly most neurosurgeons dealing with intracranial aneurysms are well acquainted with the individual clip characteristics from a practical viewpoint. Long and extensive experience with thousands of patients in the history of aneurysm surgery has proved the practical value and safety of the vast majority of properly applied aneurysm clips. Whether detailed mechanical and mathematical analysis of clinically proved aneurysm clips will alter patient care for the better remains to be seen.

Early, Fink, and their colleagues (46,49) have analyzed the target (aneurysm) factors that affect clip closure. They have shown that, in keeping with the law of La Place, the larger the neck of an aneurysm, the more closing pressure any given clip requires to maintain closure. A large aneurysm has not only a greater pulsatile counterforce within it but also thicker walls which resist approximation. Large aneurysms require large clips, but clips with longer and broader blades have less blade pressure (force per square millimeter). For this reason and because of irregularities in the thickness of the aneurysm wall, it is not uncommon for two or more clips in parallel or in overlapping series (in tandem) to be used to totally occlude necks of large aneurysms. If such an aneurysm is incompletely clipped, the continued pulsation of blood into the aneurysm may eventually cause the clip to slip off the aneurysm (139,140).

Allcock and Drake (5,41) have obtained postoperative arteriograms (mostly before the era of the neurosurgical operating microscope) and found a high percentage of either inadequately clipped aneurysms or cases in which clips slipped after surgery. There have been a number of additional reports where an applied clip was later found to have dislodged, sometimes with evidence of stress fractures of a blade near the fulcrum of the spring mechanism (24, 47,68,70,71,80,81,130,143,144). Some of the factors here very likely include: (a) a faulty clip mechanism; (b) selection of an inappropriate clip for a given aneurysm; (c) inaccurate clip placement; (d) failure to use additional clips on one aneurysm; and/or (e) clip fatigue from a combination of pulsatile or static stress and metallic corrosion. Considering the number of patients whose aneurysms were clipped and cured without evidence of clip failure, these few case reports of clip failure are relatively inconsequential statistically. However, they do indicate the need for further improvement.

Some surgeons have added muscle or cotton fibers to create adhesions around the clip for future security. Others have applied tissue adhesives (14,18,97,184). It is doubtful that muscle has much beneficial effect (28), and tissue adhesives have adverse effects in some cases (17,45).

Summary

The development and application of clips to occlude aneurysms has been a major advance in the evolution of the surgical treatment of intracranial aneurysms during the twentieth century. Most of these clips are illustrated and described here. Innovations and refinements continue.

Bibliography

1. Adams JE, Wylie EJ: Value of hypothermia and arterial occlusion in the treatment of intracranial aneurysms. Surg Gynecol Obstet 108:631–635, 1959
2. Aiba T: [Operative indication and surgical

technique of the cerebral aneurysm. 1.] Neurol Med Chir (Tokyo) 16 (6 Part 2):467–478, 1976
3. Alexander E Jr, Adams JE, Davis CH Jr: Complications in the use of temporary intracranial arterial clip. J Neurosurg 20:810–811, 1963
4. Alexander E Jr, Davis CH Jr, Kester NC: Intracranial aneurysms. Methods of treatment; value of hypothermia in the surgical approach. Arch Neurol Psychiatry 81:684–692, 1959
5. Allcock JM, Drake CG: Postoperative angiography in cases of ruptured intracranial aneurysm. J Neurosurg 20:752–759, 1963
6. Almeida GM, Pindaro J, Plese P, et al.: Intracranial arterial aneurysms in infancy and childhood. Childs Brain 3:193–199, 1977
7. Almeida GM, Shibata MK, Bianco E: Carotid-ophthalmic aneurysms. Surg Neurol 5:41–45, 1976
8. Bader DCH: Micro-surgical treatment of intracranial aneurysms. J Neurosurg Nurs 7:25–27, 1975
9. Benedetti A, Curri D: Direct attack on carotid ophthalmic and large internal carotid aneurysms. Surg Neurol 8:49–54, 1977
10. Berci G, Nyhus LM: A new vessel clamp for micro-surgery. Med Pharmacol Exp (Basel) 16:45–48, 1967
11. Bongartz EB, Nau HE, Grote W: Successful operative treatment of an aneurysm on a left persistent hypoglossal artery. Neurochirurgia (Stuttg) 20:169–173, 1977
12. Bonnal J, Stevenaert A, Brotchi J, et al.: Bilan de neuf ans d'expérience de la chirurgie des anévrysmes artériels intracrâniens. Acta Neurol Belg 74:337–355, 1974
13. Botterell EH, Lougheed WM, Scott JW, et al.: Hypothermia, and interruption of carotid, or carotid and vertebral circulation, in the surgical management of intracranial aneurysms. J Neurosurg 13:1–42, 1956
14. Carton CA, Kennady JC, Heifetz MD, et al.: The use of a plastic adhesive (methyl-2-cyanoacrylate monomer) in the management of intracranial aneurysms and leaking cerebral vessels: a report of 15 cases. In Fields WS, Sahs AL: Intracranial Aneurysms and Subarachnoid Hemorrhage. Springfield, Ill., Thomas, 1965, pp. 372–440
15. Chaffee BA: Modified aneurysm clip. J Neurosurg 26:449, 1967
16. Choki J, Yamaguchi T, Ueda K, et al.: Vertebral artery aneurysm presenting as a lateral medullary syndrome. Report of a case. Neurol Surg (Tokyo) 5:785–789, 1977
17. Chou SN: Use of cyanoacrylates [letter]. J Neurosurg 46:226, 1977
18. Clarke P: Breaking of an aneurysm clip [letter]. J Neurosurg 48:318, 1978
19. Crutchfield WG: Instruments for use in the treatment of certain intracranial vascular lesions. J Neurosurg 16:471–475, 1959
20. Cushing H: The control of bleeding in operations for brain tumors. With the description of silver "clips" for the occlusion of vessels inaccessible to the ligature. Ann Surg 54:1–19, 1911
21. Dandy WE: Intracranial aneurysm of internal carotid artery, cured by operation. Ann Surg 107:654–659, 1938
22. Dandy WE: Intracranial Arterial Aneurysms. New York, Hafner, 1944, reprinted 1969
23. Dandy WE: The surgical treatment of intracranial aneurysms of the internal carotid artery. Ann Surg 114:336–340, 1941
24. Daniels AU, Gardiner RJ, Klingler DR: Final Report. Aneurysm Clip Data Collection and In Vitro Testing. Washington, DC, US Government Printing Office, 1978
25. Davis L, Davis RA: Intracranial aneurysms. In Principles of Neurological Surgery. Philadelphia, Saunders, 1963, pp. 184–192.
26. DeLong WB: A simple method of measuring aneurysm clip tension. Technical note. J Neurosurg 47:788–789, 1977
27. DeLong WB, Ray RL: Metallurgical analysis of aneurysm and microvascular clips. J Neurosurg 48:614–621, 1978
28. Dencker H, Flyger G: The histological reaction of hammered muscle applied to the brain. In experimental investigation in rabbits (with special reference to the "wrapping" of arterial cerebral aneurysms). Acta Chir Scand 118: 178–183, 1960
29. Deruty R, Dechaume J-P, Lecuire J, et al.: Traitement microchirurgical d'une série d'anévrysmes artériels intra-crâniens sus-tentoriels. Neurochirurgie 22:227–238, 1976
30. Dolan EJ, Tator CH: A new method for testing the force of clips for aneurysms or experimental spinal cord compression. J Neurosurg 51:229–233, 1979
31. Drake CG: Advances in the neurosurgical treatment of aneurysms, arteriovenous malformations, and hematomas of the vertebral circulation. Adv Neurol 16:211–225, 1977
32. Drake CG: Bleeding aneurysms of the basilar artery. Direct surgical management in four cases. J Neurosurg 18:230–238, 1961
33. Drake CG: Further experience with surgical treatment of aneurysms of the basilar artery. J Neurosurg 29:372–392, 1968
34. Drake CG: Management of aneurysms of posterior circulation. In Youmans Jr (ed.): Neurological Surgery, Vol 2. Philadelphia, Saunders, 1973, pp. 787–806
35. Drake CG: Surgical treatment of rupture of aneurysms of the basilar artery. Experience

with 14 cases. J Neurosurg 23:457–473, 1965
36. Drake CG: Surgical treatment of vertebrobasilar aneurysms. In Koos WT, Böck FW, Spetzler RF (eds.): Clinical Microneurosurgery. Stuttgart, Georg Thieme Verlag, 1976, pp. 213–219
37. Drake CG: The surgical treatment of aneurysms of the basilar artery. J Neurosurg 29:436–446, 1968
38. Drake CG: The surgical treatment of vertebral-basilar aneurysms. Clin Neurosurg 16:114–169, 1969
39. Drake CG: The treatment of aneurysms of the posterior circulation. Clin Neurosurg 26:96–144, 1979
40. Drake CG: Vertebral basilar aneurysms. A progress report. In Scientific Program Manuscript of the American Association of Neurological Surgeons, paper 61, 1971, pp. 1–8
41. Drake CG, Allcock JM: Postoperative angiography and the "slipped" clip. J Neurosurg 39:683–689, 1973
42. Drew JA: An applicating forceps in which clips cannot stick or jam. J Neurosurg 10:439–440, 1953
43. Duane W Jr: A modification of the McKenzie silver clip. J Neurosurg 7:92–93, 1950
44. Duffy G: The surgical treatment of anterior communicating artery aneurysms. Aust NZ J Surg 44:257–260, 1974
45. Dujovny M, Kossovsky N, Kossowsky R, et al.: Heifetz clip failure. A metallurgical study. J Neurosurg 50:368–373, 1979
46. Early CB, Fink LH: Some fundamental applications of the law of La Place in neurosurgery. Surg Neurol 6:185–189, 1976
47. Edner GF, Ericson K, Forster DMC, et al.: The broken clip. Acta Neurochir (Wien) 40:145–149, 1978
48. Elvidge AR, Feindel WH: Surgical treatment of aneurysm of the anterior cerebral and the anterior communicating arteries diagnosed by angiography and electroencephalography. J Neurosurg 7:13–32, 1950
49. Fink LH, Flandry RE: Pratt RA, et al.: A comparative study of performance characteristics of cerebral aneurysm clips. Surg Neurol 11:179–186, 1979
50. Fox JL: Microsurgical exposure of intracranial aneurysms. J Microsurg 1:2–31, 1979
51. Fox JL: Vascular clips for the microsurgical treatment of stroke. Stroke 7:489–500, 1976
52. Fox JL, Albin MS, Bader DCH, et al.: Microsurgical treatment of neurovascular disease. Neurosurgery 3:285–337, 1978
53. Fox JL, Luessenhop AJ: Hydrocephalus secondary to hemorrhage from a basilar artery aneurysm. With a note on embolization technique. Acta Neurochir (Wien) 17:228–235, 1967
54. Froman C: A congenital aneurysm of the circle of Willis associated with polycystic kidney. S Afr J Surg 7:72–73, 1969
55. Fuchs EC, Grumme T: Über die klinische Bedeutung von Manschettenclips in der Neurochirurgie. Neurochirurgia (Stuttg) 19:129–132, 1976
56. Gillingham FJ: The management of ruptured intracranial aneurysm. Ann R Coll Surg 23:89–117, 1958
57. Gillingham FJ: The management of ruptured intracranial aneurysms. Scott Med J 12:377–383, 1967
58. Graf CJ: A clip for temporary occlusion of cerebral arteries. Am J Surg 100:587–588, 1960
59. Grode ML, Saunders M, Carton CA: Subarachnoid hemorrhage secondary to ruptured aneurysms in infants. Report of two cases. J Neurosurg 49:898–902, 1978
60. Guidetti B: Il trattamento chirurgico degli aneurismi della comunicante anteriore. Minerva Neurochir 2:4–14, 1958
61. Guidetti B, La Torre E: Carotid-ophthalmic aneurysms. A series of 16 cases treated by direct approach. Acta Neurochir (Wien) 22:289–304, 1970
62. Guidetti B, La Torre E: Management of carotid-ophthalmic aneurysms. J Neurosurg 42:438–442, 1975
63. Hamby WB: Intracranial surgery for aneurysms. Prog Neurol Surg 3:1–65, 1969
64. Hamby WB: Intracranial surgical procedures in subarachnoid hemorrhage and intracranial aneurysms. In Fields WS (ed.): Pathogenesis and Treatment of Cerebrovascular Disease. Springfield, Ill., Thomas, 1961, pp. 496–507
65. Hamby WB: Multiple intracranial aneurysms. Aspects of treatment. J Neurosurg 16:558–563, 1959
66. Hammer WJ, Luessenhop AJ, Weintroub AM: Observations on the electrocardiographic changes associated with subarachnoid hemorrhage with special reference to their genesis. Am J Med 59:427–433, 1975
67. Handa J, Aoyama I, Handa H: Extravasation from an intracranial aneurysm during angiography. Case report. Arch Jpn Chir 43:302–306, 1974
68. Hayakawa I, Sasaki A, Fujiwara K, et al.: Ein ungewöhnliches Aneurysmarezidiv nach Verclippung—ein struktureller Fehler des Clips? Acta Neurochir (Wien) 35:271–277, 1976
69. Heifetz MD: A new intracranial aneurysm clip. J Neurosurg 30:753, 1969
70. Heiskanen O: Cerebral circulatory arrest caused by acute increase of intracranial pres-

sure. A clinical and roentgenological study of 25 cases. Acta Neurol Scand [Suppl 7] 40:1–57, 1964
71. Heiskanen O, Marttila I: Risk of rupture of a second aneurysm in patients with multiple aneurysms. J Neurosurg 32:295–299, 1970
72. Hollin SA, Decker RE: Microsurgical treatment of internal carotid artery aneurysms. J Neurosurg 47:142–149, 1977
73. Howe JF, Harris AB, Sypert GW: Giant aneurysm of the middle cerebral artery. Surg Neurol 6:231–233, 1976
74. Iwabuchi T, Suzuki S, Ebina K, et al.: Memory clip for intracranial aneurysm surgery. Technical note. J Neurosurg 42:733–735, 1975
75. Jackson JR, Tindall GT, Nashold BS Jr: Rupture of an intracranial aneurysm during carotid arteriography. A case report. J Neurosurg 17:333–336, 1960
76. Jacobson JH II, McAllister FF: A method for the controlled occlusion of larger blood vessels. Ann Surg 145:334–343, 1957
77. Jefferson A: The significance for diagnosis and for surgical technique of multiple aneurysms of the same internal carotid artery. Acta Neurochir (Wien) 41:23–37, 1978
78. Kak VK, Gleadhill CA, Bailey IC: The familial incidence of intracranial aneurysms. J Neurol Neurosurg Psychiatry 33:29–33, 1970
79. Kempe LG: Operative Neurosurgery, Vol 1: Cranial, Cerebral, and Intracranial Vascular Disease. Berlin, Springer-Verlag, 1968, pp. 1–75, 203–214
80. Kessler LA, Wholey MH: Internal carotid occlusion for treatment of intracranial aneurysms. A new percutaneous technique. Radiology 95:581–583, 1970
81. Khambatta HJ, Matteo RS, McMurtry JG III, et al.: Anesthesia for basilar arterial aneurysm with elective circulatory arrest and moderate hypothermia. Anesthesiology 41:512–516, 1974
82. Khodadad G: Microvascular surgery. In Rand RW (ed.): Microneurosurgery. St Louis, Mosby, 1969, pp. 170–182
83. Klemme WM: Hemorrhage from a previously undemonstrated intracranial aneurysm as a late complication of carotid artery ligation. Case report. J Neurosurg 46:654–658, 1977
83a. Kossowsky R, Dujovny M, Kossovsky N: Metallurgical evaluation of the compatibility of surgical clips with their appliers. Acta Neurochir (Wien) 59:95–109, 1981
84. Laine E, Allègre GE, Goutelle A, et al.: Les anévrysmes vertébro-basilaires: choix de la voie d'abord. Problème de adjuvants per-opératoires. Neuro chirurgie 18:317–332, 1972
85. Lanigan JP, Carey PC, Pate AR: Subarachnoid haemorrhage and the surgical treatment of intra-cranial aneurysms. A ten years' survey. J Irish Med Assoc 66:55–64, 1973
86. Le Beau J: Indications opératories et traitement chirurgical des anévrismes artériels intra-craniens sus-tentoriels. Ann Chir 15:1153–1163, 1961
87. Lougheed WM: Selection, timing, and technique of aneurysm surgery of the anterior circle of Willis. Clin Neurosurg 16:95–113, 1969
88. Lougheed WM, Botterell EH, Morley TP: Results of the direct attack in the surgical management of internal carotid and middle cerebral aneurysms. Clin Neurosurg 9:193–200, 1963
89. Lougheed WM, Khodadad G: A new clip for surgery of intracranial and small blood vessels. J Neurosurg 22:397–398, 1965
90. Lougheed WM, Marshall BM: Management of aneurysms of the anterior circulation by intracranial procedures. In Youmans JR (ed.): Neurological Surgery, Vol 2. Philadelphia, Saunders, 1973, pp. 731–767
91. Lougheed WM, Morley TP, Tasker RR: The results of surgical treatment of ruptured berry aneurysms. Excerpta Medica ICS No. 110:681–684, 1966
92. Lougheed W, Morley T, Tasker R, et al.: The results of surgical treatment of ruptured berry aneurysms. In Fields WS, Sahs AL (eds.): Intracranial Aneurysms and Subarachnoid Hemorrhage. Springfield, Illinois, Thomas, 1965, pp. 295–307
93. Martinez Coll A, Del Corral JF: Experiences in intracranial surgery for aneurysms. Surg Neurol 3:191–193, 1975
94. Matas R: Aneurysms of the circle of Willis. A discussion of Dr. Dandy's intracranial occlusion of the internal carotid for aneurysms of the circle of Willis, with supplementary remarks. Ann Surg 107:660–680, 1938
95. Maxwell RE, Chou SN: Aneurysmal tumors of the basifrontal region. J Neurosurg 46:438–445, 1977
96. Mayfield FH, Kees G Jr: A brief history of the development of the Mayfield clip J Neurosurg 35:97–100, 1971
97. Mazur JB, Salazar JL: Late thrombosis of middle cerebral artery following clipping and coating of aneurysms. Surg Neurol 10:131–133, 1978
98. McFadden JT: Aneurysm clips. J Neurosurg 46:129, 1977
99. McFadden JT: Chocked-clip aneurysmorrhaphy. Surg Gynecol Obstet 132:898, 1971
100. McFadden JT: Metallurgical principles in neurosurgery. J Neurosurg 31:373–385, 1969
101. McFadden JT: Modifications of cross-action in-

tracranial clips. Technical note. J Neurosurg 32:116–118, 1970
102. McFadden JT: The origin and evolutionary principles of spring forceps. Surg Gynecol Obstet 130:356–368, 1970
103. McFadden JT: Tissue reactions to standard neurosurgical metallic implants. J Neurosurg 36:598–603, 1972
104. McKenzie KG: Some minor modifications of Harvey Cushing's silver clip outfit. Surg Gynecol Obstet 45:549–550, 1927
105. McMurtry JG III, Housepian EM, Bowman FO Jr, et al.: Surgical treatment of basilar artery aneurysms. Elective circulatory arrest with thoracotomy in 12 cases. J Neurosurg 40:486–498, 1974
106. Merrem G, Goldhahn W-E: Neurochirurgische Operation. Leipzig, Johann Ambrosius Barth, 1966, pp. 84–87
107. Mizukami M, Kin H, Araki G, et al.: Is angiographic spasm real spasm. Acta Neurochir (Wien) 34:247–259, 1976
108. Morrison G, Hegarty WM, Brausch CC, et al.: Direct surgical obliteration of a persistent trigeminal artery aneurysm. Case report. J Neurosurg 39:249–251, 1974
109. Moyes PD: Basilar aneurysm associated with agenesis of the left internal carotid artery. Case report. J Neurosurg 30:608–611, 1969
110. Niemeyer P: Resultados da microcirurgia em 54 aneurismas intracranianos. Arq Neuropsiquiatr 32:175–186, 1974
111. Norlén G, Olivecrona H: The treatment of aneurysms of the circle of Willis. J Neurosurg 10:404–415, 1953
112. Nornes H: Cerebral arterial flow dynamics during aneurysm haemorrhage. Acta Neurochir (Wien) 41:39–48, 1978
113. Nornes H, Wikeby P: Cerebral arterial blood flow and aneurysm surgery. Part 1. Local arterial flow dynamics. J Neurosurg 47:810–818, 1977
114. Nutik S: Carotid paraclinoid aneurysms with intradural origin and intracavernous location. J Neurosurg 48:526–533, 1978
115. Nyström SHM: Some aspects of the treatment of intracranial aneurysms. Int Surg 45:19–23, 1966
116. Nyström S, Snellman A, Mäkelä T: Sur le traitement des anévrysmes de la "communicante anterieure." A propos d'une série de cent quarante-sept cas opérés. Neurochirurgie 8:414–422, 1962
117. Paillas JE, Bonnal J: Anévrysmes artériels. In Patel J, Leger L (eds.): *Nouveau Traité de Technique Chirurgicale,* Vol 6. Paris, Masson & Cie, 1975, pp. 237–277
118. Papo I, Caruselli G, Salvolini U: Aneurysm of the superior cerebellar artery. Surg Neurol 7:15–17, 1977
119. Paterson A: Direct surgery in the treatment of posterior communicating aneurysms. Lancet 2:808–811, 1968
120. Paterson A: Direct surgery of posterior communicating aneurysms. In Logue V (ed.): Operative Surgery, Vol 14: Neurosurgery, 2nd ed. Philadelphia, Lippincott, 1971, pp. 167–171
121. Peerless SJ: The surgical approach to middle cerebral and posterior communicating aneurysms. Clin Neurosurg 21:151–165, 1974
122. Pertuiset B, Houtteville J-P, van Effenterre R, et al.: Chirurgie des anévrysmes artériels sus-tentoriels. Réduction par coagulation bipolaire sous hypotension profonde et exclusion par clip autobloquant: (52 cas opérés sous microscope). Nouv Presse Med 3:1649–1652, 1974
123. Pertuiset B, van Effenterre R, Goutorbe J, et al.: Management of aneurysmal rupture during surgery, using bipolar coagulation, deep hypotension, and the operating microscope. Acta Neurochir (Wien) 30:195–205, 1974
124. Pia HW: Microsurgical treatment of cerebral aneurysms. Neurosurg Rev 1:15–24, 1978
125. Pia HW: The microsurgical treatment of intracerebral aneurysms. In Koos TH, Böck FW, Spetzler RF (eds.): Clinical Neurosurgery. Stuttgart, Georg Thieme Verlag, 1976, pp. 177–179
126. Pool JL, Potts DG: Aneurysms and Arteriovenous Anomalies of the Brain. Diagnosis and Treatment. New York, Harper & Row, 1965
127. Poppen JL: An Atlas of Neurosurgical Techniques. Philadelphia, Saunders, 1960, pp. 156–181
128. Portnoy HD, Avellanosa A: Carotid aneurysm and contralateral carotid stenosis with successful surgical treatment of both lesions. Case report. J Neurosurg 32:476–482, 1970
129. Pudenz RH: The use of tantalum clips for hemostasis in neurosurgery. Surgery 12:791–797, 1942
130. Quest DO, Countee RW: Fractured aneurysm clip. Case report. J Neurosurg 47:466–468, 1977
131. Raimondi AJ, Yashon D, Reyes C, et al.: Intracranial false aneurysms. Neurochirurgia (Stuttg) 11:219–233, 1968
132. Rhoton AL, Jackson FE, Gleave J, et al.: Congenital and traumatic intracranial aneurysms. Clin Symp 29:1–40, 1977
133. Rosenbaum TJ, Sundt TM Jr: Interrelationship of aneurysm clips and vascular tissue. J Neurosurg 48:929–934, 1978
134. Rowe SN, Grunnagle JF, Susen AF, et al.: Re-

sults of direct attack on intracranial aneurysm. J Neurosurg 12:475–486, 1955
135. Samuels, PB, Concotti JJ: The use of hemostatic clips in vascular surgery. J Cardiovasc Surg 9:150–153, 1968
136. Samuels PB, Roedling H, Katz R, et al.: A new hemostatic clip. 2-year review of 1007 cases. Ann Surg 163:427–431, 1966
137. Sano K: [Surgery of intracranial aneurysm.] Brain Nerve (Tokyo) 23:1252–1264, 1971
138. Sato O, Kamitani H: Giant aneurysm of the middle cerebral artery: angiographic analysis of blood flow. Surg Neurol 4:27–31, 1975
139. Sato S, Onuma T, Suzuki J: [A consideration of incomplete surgical treatment of intracranial aneurysm.] Brain Nerve (Tokyo) 23:157–162, 1971
140. Sato S, Suzuki J: Prognosis in cases of intracranial aneurysm after incomplete direct operations. Acta Neurochir (Wien) 24:245–252, 1971
141. Scoville WB: Miniature torsion bar spring aneurysm clip. J Neurosurg 25:97, 1966
142. Selverstone B: Coating of intracranial aneurysms with nontoxic adherent plastics. In Schmidek HH, Sweet WH (eds.): Current Techniques in Operative Neurosurgery. New York, Grune & Stratton, 1977, pp. 31–40
143. Sencer W: A study of subarachnoid hemorrhage and intracranial aneurysm. J Mt Sinai Hosp NY 30:302–323, 1963
144. Servo A, Puranen M: Delayed breaking of a Heifetz aneurysm clip. Case report. J Neurosurg 47:463–465, 1977
145. Shahbabian S, Mayfield FH: Modification of intracranial aneurysm clip J Neurosurg 49:935–936, 1978
146. Sharkey PC, Apostolcu A: Intracranial aneurysms: a partial community study. South Med J 59:185–191, 1966
147. Shields CB: Current trends in management of cerebral aneurysms. J Ky Med Assoc 75:529–535, 1977
148. Simmons DR, Portnoy HD, Gurdjian ES: Packing with muscle of internal carotid artery for aneurysm with immediate occlusion and subsequent establishment of flow. J Neurosurg 20:1000–1004, 1963
149. Sjöqvist O: Thread ligature of intracranial saccular aneurysms. In Proceedings of the 5th Congress of Neurology, Vol 3. Lisbon, 1953, pp. 108–115
150. Smith KR Jr, Bardenheier JA III: Aneurysm of the pericallosal artery caused by closed cranial trauma. Case report. J Neurosurg 29:551–554, 1968
151. Speakman TJ, Barlass JL: The bifrontal approach to aneurysms of the anterior communicating artery. Can J Surg 6:237–243, 1963
152. Steven JL: Postoperative angiography in treatment of intracranial aneurysms. Acta Radiol [Diagn] (Stockh) 5:536–548, 1966
153. Stroobandt G, Cornelis G: Intrasellar carotid-ophthalmic aneurysm. Angiotomographic demonstration and surgical cure. Neurochirurgia (Stuttg) 14:220–224, 1971
154. Stroobandt G, Cornelis G, Vermonden J: Le traitement chirurgical des anévrysmes sylviens. Acta Neurol Belg 69:661–680, 1969
155. Sugar O, Tsuchiya G: Plastic coating of intracranial aneurysms with "EDH-adhesive." J Neurosurg 21:114–117, 1964
156. Sugita K, Hirota T, Iguchi I, et al.: Comparative study of the pressure of various clips. J Neurosurg 44:723–727, 1976
157. Sugita K, Hirota T, Tsugane R: Application of nasopharyngeal mirror for aneurysm operation. Technical note. J Neurosurg 43:244–246, 1975
158. Sugita K, Kobayashi S, Shintani A, et al.: Microneurosurgery for aneurysms of the basilar artery. J Neurosurg 51:615–620, 1979
159. Sundt TM Jr: Clip-grafts for aneurysm and small vessel surgery. Part 4. Relative application to various aneurysms and repair of anterior communicating aneurysms using a right-angle clip holder. Technical note. J Neurosurg 37:753–758, 1972
160. Sundt TM Jr: Intracranial aneurysms and subarachnoid hemorrhage: a subject review for the clinician. Mayo Clin Proc 45:455–466, 1970
161. Sundt TM Jr, Murphey F: Clip-grafts for aneurysm and small vessel surgery. Part 3. Clinical experience in intracranial internal carotid artery aneurysm. J Neurosurg 31:59–71, 1969
162. Sundt TM Jr, Nofzinger JD: Clip-grafts for aneurysm and small vessel surgery. Part 1. Repair of segmental defects with clip-grafts; laboratory studies and clinical correlations. Part 2. Clinical application of clip-grafts to aneurysms; technical considerations. J Neurosurg 27:477–489, 1967
163. Suzuki J, Kodama N, Homma M: New clip and flexible clip forceps for neurosurgery. Excerpta Medica ICS No. 418:146, 1977
164. Suzuki J, Kodama N, Homma M: New clip and flexible clip forceps for neurosurgery. In Suzuki J (ed.): *Cerebral Aneurysms.* Tokyo, Neuron, 1979, pp. 386–388
165. Symon L: Disordered cerebro-vascular physiology in aneurysmal subarachnoid haemorrhage. Acta Neurochir (Wien) 41:7–22, 1978
166. Takahara Y, Ikeda K, Kageyama N, et al.: [HeiFetz's clip in surgery of cerebral aneurysm.] Shujutsa 25:1131–1135, 1971
167. Thierry A, Ballivet J, Binnert D, et al.: Les

anévrysmes sacciformes de l'artère cérébelleuse moyenne (artère cérébelleuse antérieure et inférieure). Présentation d'un cas opéré avec succès et revue de la littérature. Neurochirurgie 17:137–142, 1971
168. Thierry A, Ballivet J, Dumas R, et al.: Les cas familiaux d'anévrysmes intra-craniens. Revue de la littérature et présentation d'une observation. Neurochirurgie 18:267–276, 1972
169. Thierry A, Ballivet D, Dumas R, et al.: Une complication peu connue de la chirurgie intracrânienne des anévrysmes: hydrocéphalie aiguë traitée par dérivation ventriculo-jugulaire. J Med Lyon 53:1381–1385, 1972
170. Todd EM, Sheldon CH, Crue BL Jr, et al.: Plastic jackets for certain intracranial aneurysms. JAMA 179:935–939, 1962
171. Tovi D: New instrument to obliterate intracranial saccular aneurysm. J Neurosurg 12:525–527, 1955
172. Tytus JS, Haven H: Present day concepts in the management of intracranial aneurysms. Rev Surg 20:230–240, 1963
173. Uihlein A, Theye RA, Dawson B, et al.: The use of profound hypothermia, extracorporeal circulation and total circulatory arrest for an intracranial aneurysm. Preliminary report with reports of cases. Proc Mayo Clin 35:567–576, 1960
174. Vanderfield G: Periodic headache associated with cerebral aneurysm, with report of a case successfully treated by surgery. Med J Aust 2:289–290, 1957
175. Von Holst H, Bergström M, Möller A, et al.: Titanium clips in neurosurgery for elimination of artefacts in computer tomography (CT). A technical note. Acta Neurochir (Wien) 38:101–109, 1977
176. Williamson WP, Brackett CE Jr: Management of intracranial aneurysms of the anterior communicating artery. Am Surg 22:100–107, 1956
177. Wilson CB, U HS: Surgical treatment for aneurysms of the upper basilar artery. J Neurosurg 44:537–543, 1976
178. Wise BL, Green ED: A new type of tantalum clip for occluding cerebral blood vessels. J Neurosurg 11:633–634, 1954
179. Wissinger JP, Danoff D, Wisiol ES, et al.: Repair of an aneurysm of the basilar artery by a transclival approach. Case report. J Neurosurg 26: 417–419, 1967
180. Wright WH, Todd EM, Duemler LP, et al.: Simultaneous direct operations for bilateral internal carotid artery aneurysms. Surg Neurol 2:355–358, 1974
181. Yaşargil MG: Microsurgery Applied to Neurosurgery. Stuttgart, Georg Thieme Verlag, 1969, pp. 119–143
182. Yaşargil MG, Antic J, Laciga R, et al.: Microsurgical pterional approach to aneurysms of the basilar bifurcation. Surg Neurol 6:83–91, 1976
183. Yaşargil MG, Fox JL: The microsurgical approach to intracranial aneurysms. Surg Neurol 3:7–14, 1975
184. Yaşargil MG, Fox JL, Ray MW: The operative approach to aneurysms of the anterior communicating artery. In Krayenbühl H (ed.): *Advances and Technical Standards in Neurosurgery,* Vol 2. New York, Springer-Verlag, 1975, pp. 113–170
185. Yaşargil MG, Smith RD: Surgery on the carotid system in the treatment of hemorrhagic stroke. Adv Neurol 16:181–209, 1977
186. Yaşargil MG, Vise WM, Bader DCH: Technical adjuncts in neurosurgery. Surg Neurol 8:331–336, 1977

28

Craniotomy for Aneurysm

IV. Protective Coatings

It has been common practice to apply some form of protective coating to the aneurysm to prevent future bleeding and expansion. Although this is less commonly done now (clipping being preferred), there are aneurysms with a broad base where clipping may not be possible. Such cases may be treated by wrapping or coating the aneurysm. However, it is essential that: (a) the aneurysm is entirely covered by the material used; and (b) the material safely prevents future bleeding and expansion of the aneurysm.

There are some problems involved. Often it is difficult or impossible to expose and cover the entire aneurysm, and in the attempt to do so the aneurysm may rupture. The material may be poorly reactive and offer inadequate protection (e.g., muscle, gelatin sponge, or oxycellulose) or it may be histotoxic and markedly reactive (some tissue adhesives).

Autogenous Tissue

Muscle

Cushing is often credited with introducing the use of muscle to control bleeding during brain surgery, but in 1911 Cushing himself quoted Lund as having seen Horsley demonstrate the hemostatic action of muscle fragments in the laboratory (19). In 1914 Horsley (82) recommended the application of cut muscle pressed against a bleeding vessel for hemostasis, but he doubted it would maintain protection against a blood pressure in excess of 60–80 mm Hg.

In 1933 Dott (25) noted, "We were accustomed to deal successfully with quite formidable intracranial hemorrhages during operations by applying to the bleeding point a fragment of fresh muscle which formed a secure scaffolding for the clot, and became organized into fibrous tissue with it. Why not expose a bleeding aneurysm and deal with it after this fashion?"—as he had done successfully in 1931 (25). It was a case of a bICAA (at the M-1 artery), the first reported case in history directly operated successfully after an SAH from an aneurysm diagnosed prior to surgery. Upon exposure of the aneurysm, the aneurysm ruptured, whereupon it was tamponaded with muscle and then wrapped in muscle. The patient did well.

During the 1930s the technique of wrapping an aneurysm developed (25,47,88,170,172,179) more often than not perforce, for the pressure of a piece of muscle was often necessary to stem the tide of blood from an inadvertently ruptured aneurysm. In other cases it seemed the only way to deal with a giant aneurysm. Subsequently a number of authors described the use of cut autogenous muscle, hammered (or not) into smashed pieces, to coat or wrap an intracranial aneurysm (1,2,5,8,15,20,24,28,30–32,38–44,46,48,54–58,60–63,71,73,77–79,81, 83, 95–99, 104, 113, 115–117, 119–122, 126, 127, 129, 130, 133–135, 138, 139, 143, 155–158, 171,176).

For individual case reports of aneurysms treated by muscle coating, see the *Surg* column (symbol *MUS*) in Appendix 2.

It now appears that muscle coating of aneurysms is ineffective treatment, as a number of cases of rebleed have been reported (2,15, 31,143); several authors, after gaining experience with the technique, concluded that the aneurysm was poorly protected (21,37,99, 105,121,122). Moreover, histologic studies of

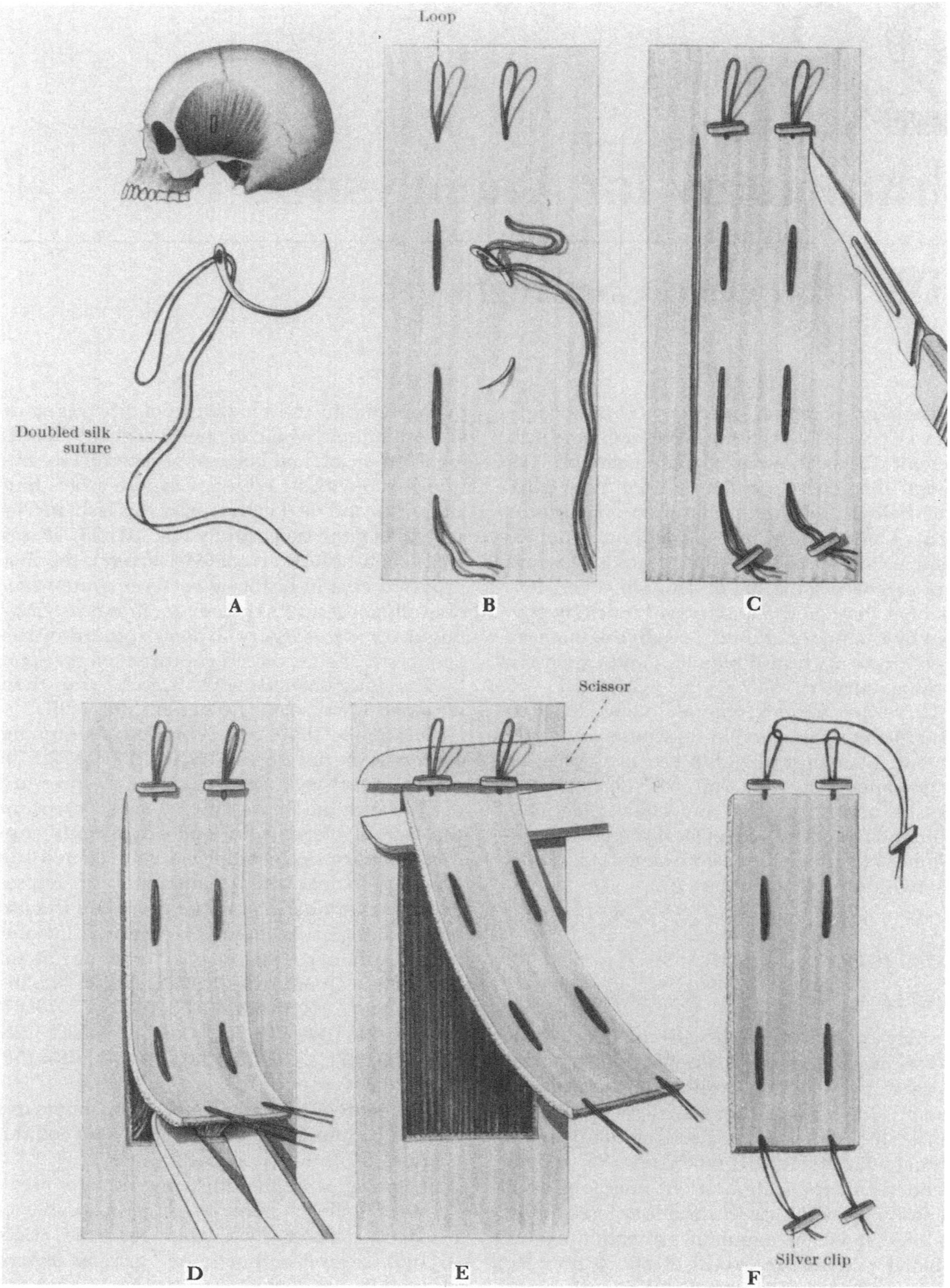

Fig. 28.1. Wrapping a ruptured ICAA in a temporalis fascial sling. **A–F** Taking fascial sling from temporalis fascia.

tissue reaction to autogenous muscle have revealed poor adhesion formation and an absence of satisfactory fibrous envelopment (21,143). Regarding the use of hammered muscle to surround the sac of an intracranial aneurysm, Logue (105) concluded that it was "a procedure which surely must have more effect on the surgeon's peace of mind, than on the aneurysm."

Other Tissues

Occasionally fibrous tissues, e.g., dura or temporalis fascia (Fig. 28.1), have been used to wrap an aneurysm (91).

Gelatin Sponge

Gelatin sponge (Gelfoam) has been a standard material used for hemostasis in neurosurgery, a subject well reviewed by Light (103). Several surgeons have used Gelfoam to cover aneurysms (44,61,73,101,102,121,134,158), although the material evokes minimal tissue reaction or adhesions (85) and hence is not recommended as a protective wrap. However, it may be used in conjunction with other materials, perhaps to separate nerves from the materials used to coat the aneurysm.

For individual case reports of aneurysms treated by gelfoam wrapping see the *Surg* column (symbol *GEL*) in Appendix 2.

Cotton

Cotton fibers are known to evoke a fibrous, granulomatous reaction which provides a fairly prominent coat around the aneurysm within about 2–3 weeks (18,143,178). This reaction is rarely harmful so long as it does not involve adjacent nerves or brain. Jaeger (87) in 1950 was one of the first to report this technique. Shortly thereafter others—Falconer (39), Gillingham (49), Graf (53), Hamby (62), Jefferson (89), and Northfield (123)—described the application of wisps of cotton fibers or pieces of fine mesh cotton gauze (muslin) to the walls of aneu-

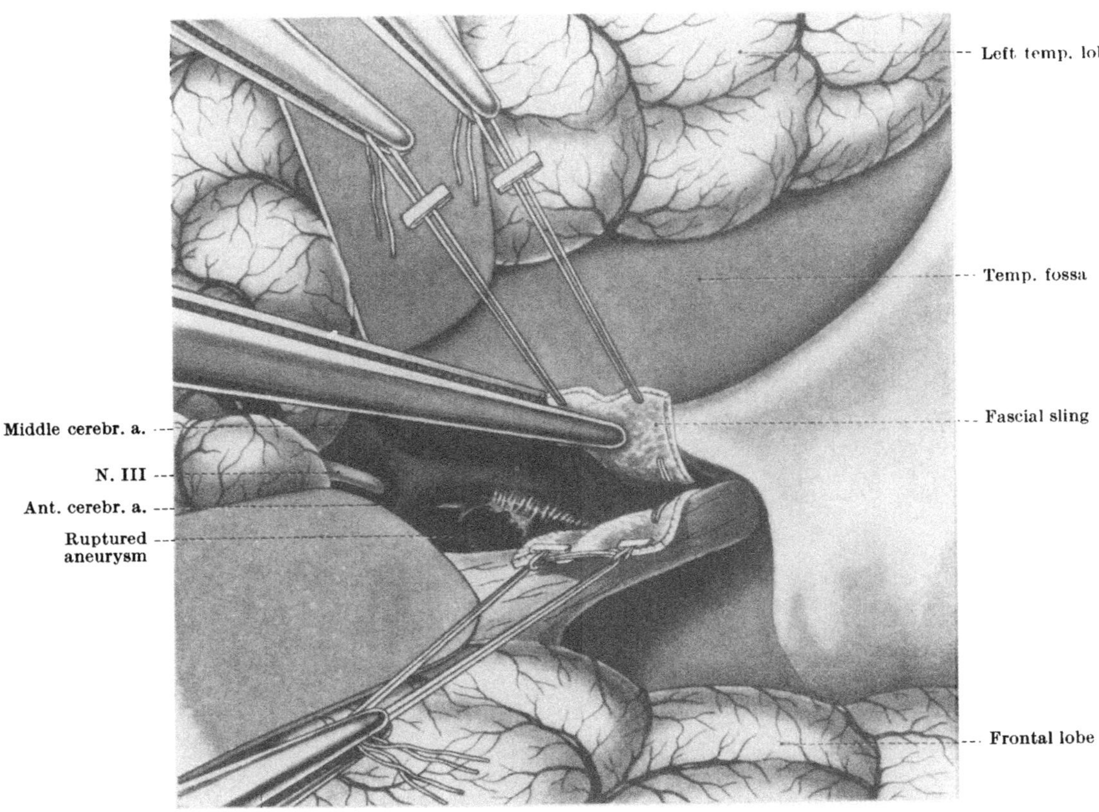

G–J Placing sling around ICA and its aneurysm and maintaining with Olivecrona clips. From Kempe LG, ref. 91 (*continued*).

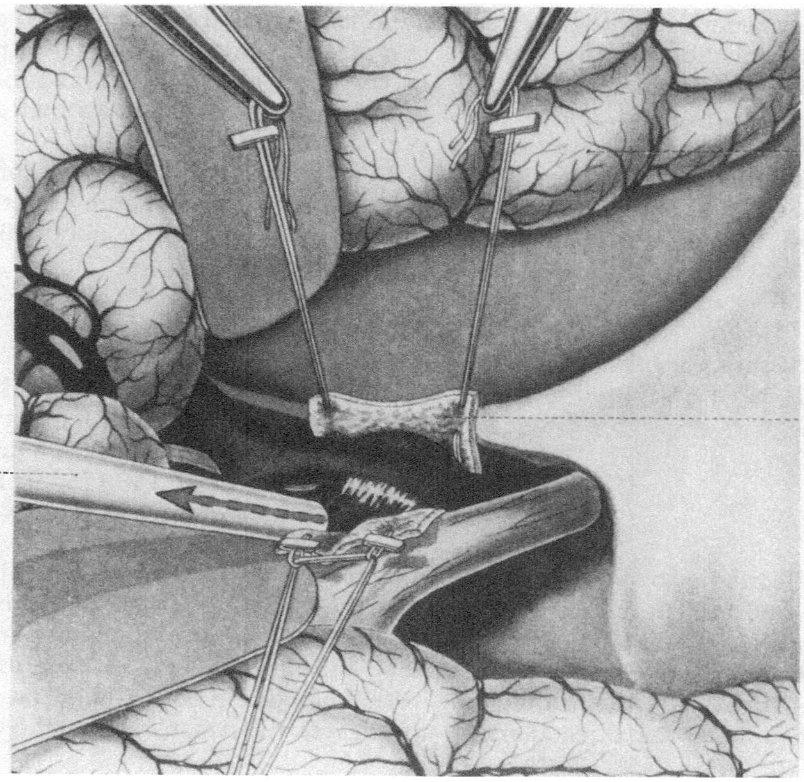

Fig. 28.1 H

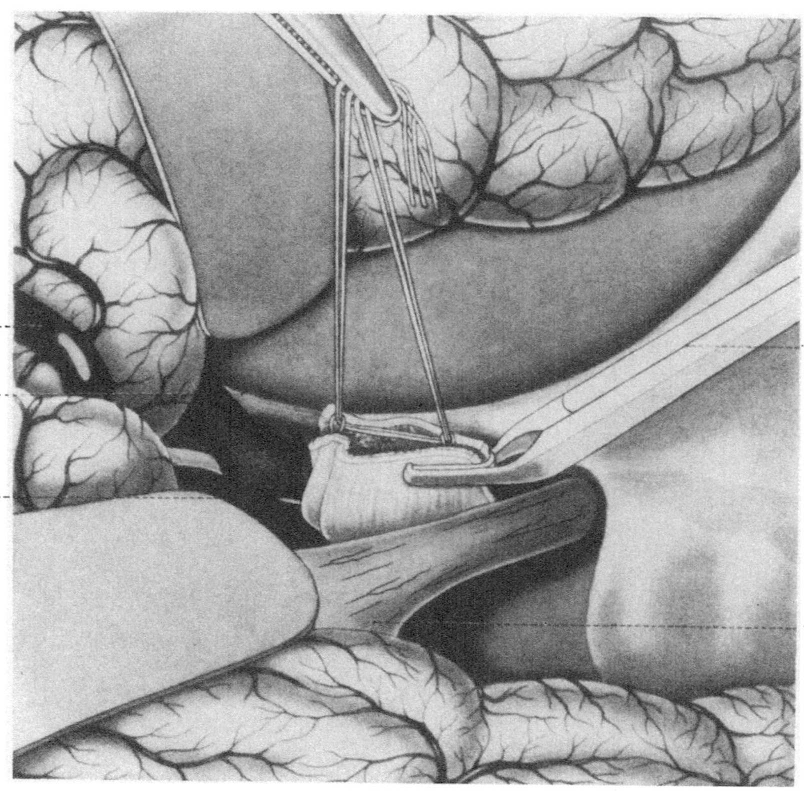

Fig. 28.1 I

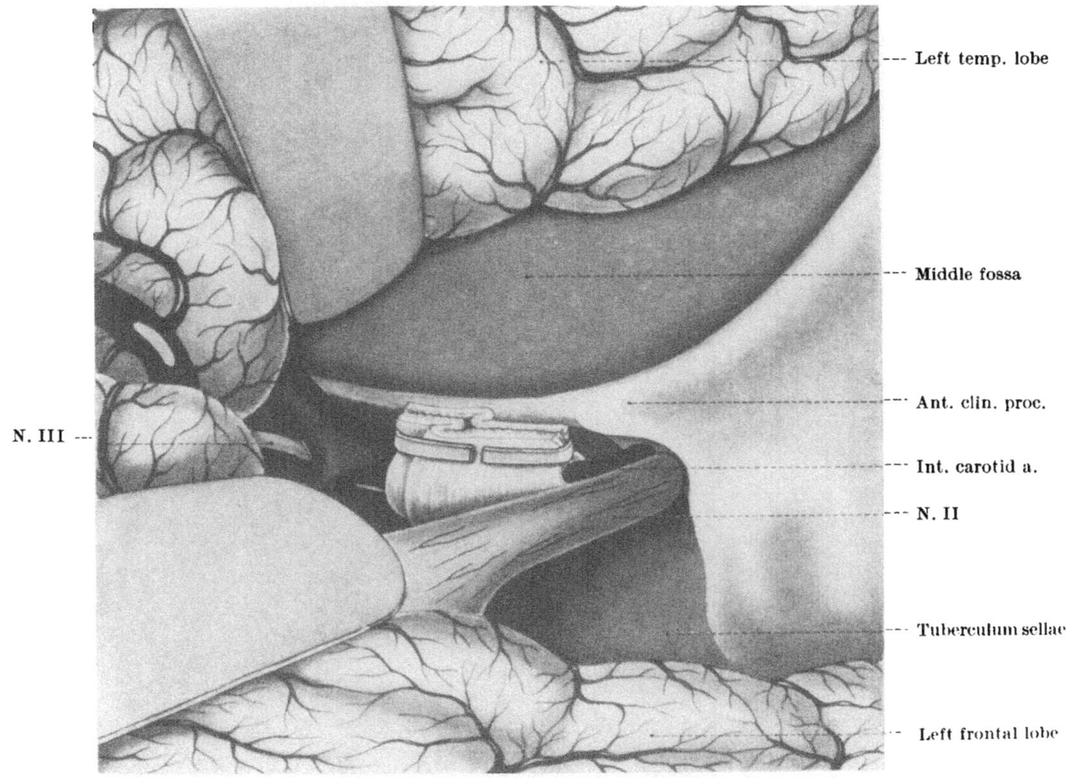

Fig. 28.1 J

rysms. Since then it has been applied, often with success, about aneurysms otherwise difficult to treat (4,18,26,29–31,45,50–52,61,70,74–76,91,95,96,104,106,110,111,115,116,124,127,131,132,134,141–143,147,157,157a,165–167,177,178,180,181).

The technique of application varies. Some apply wisps of cotton or stamps of muslin, whereas others secure the wall with a well-tailored cloth held about the aneurysm with malleable clips or sutures (Fig. 28.2) (91,106). Surgeons on occasion have added methyl methacrylate (91), thorium dioxide (123), gelfoam, muscle, and/or tissue adhesives. Gelfoam or muscle covering the cotton may protect adjacent tissues from involvement in the fibrous reaction. In spite of adequate technique, however, the aneurysm may continue to enlarge (31) or rebleed (18) later. When very small (less than 3 mm diameter) aneurysms are found incidentally at craniotomy, they may be well treated by covering with cotton fibers.

For individual case reports of aneurysms treated by cotton wrapping, see the *Surg* column (symbol *COT*) in Appendix 2.

Synthetic Coatings

In 1953 Woodhall and Golden (182) performed studies on canine arteries to determine the value of varnish, krylon, and latex as possible aneurysm-coating agents. All caused excess inflammation and eventual fragmentation of the coatings. In 1955 McCune et al. (109) investigated a latex and thorium dioxide mixture for possible use in aortic aneurysms, but these materials never got beyond the laboratory stage. In 1956 Dutton (36) was the first to report the use of a plastic material to coat human intracranial aneurysms; methyl methacrylate was used. Interest in other materials, e.g., cyanoacrylate tissue adhesives (66), synthetic resins (9,154), and silicone-rubber (169), soon developed. Reviews of the use of synthetic coatings are available elsewhere (16,61,66,68,107,112a).

Handa et al. (68) listed the following prerequisites for tissue adhesives:

1. Firm and rapid adhesion to the moist vessel wall
2. Rapid formation of a fairly strong, waterproof, flexible, and elastic film

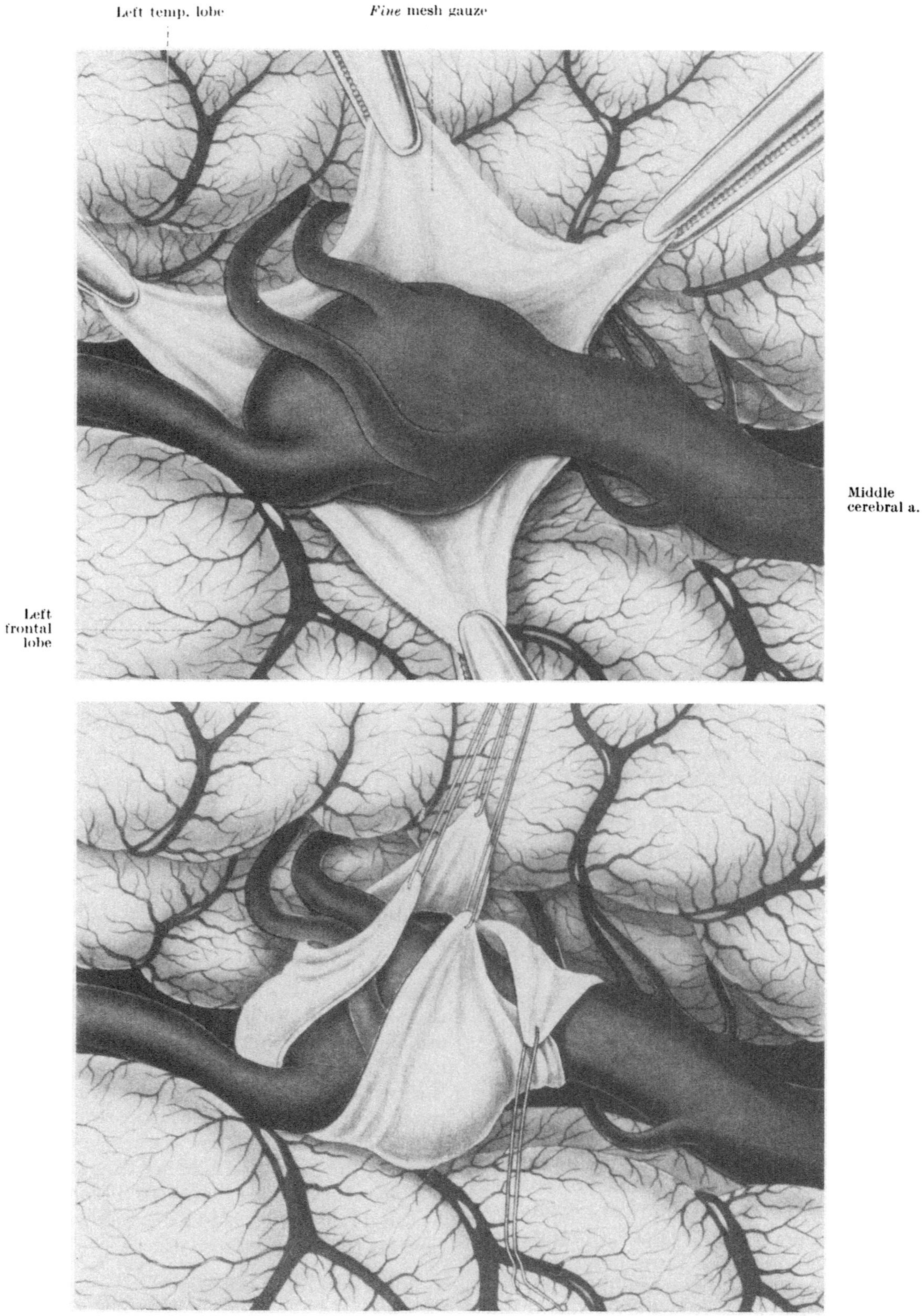

Fig. 28.2. Wrapping a large aneurysm with fine mesh cotton. From Kempe LG, ref. 91.

3. Absence of toxicity and tissue reaction
4. Absence of carcinogenic properties
5. Simple sterilization without changing properties
6. Storage without changing properties

Matsumoto et al. (107) studied various cyanoacrylate tissue adhesives. These adhesives are neither bacteriostatic nor bacteriocidal; the absence of bacteria in their presence is due to a lack of nutrients in the containers and due to the high manufacturing temperatures. Histotoxicity increases as the alkyl chain length decreases. Hence the methyl cyanoacrylate compound is the most toxic. The time needed for good bonding with tissue increases as the alkyl chain length increases. Matsumoto and co-workers (107) prefer *n*-butyl or isobutyl cyanoacrylates but noted some histotoxicity from their metabolites (formaldehyde and thiocyanate). It is likely that a minimal tissue reaction is helpful, for it would help bind the coat to the aneurysm and create protective adhesions.

For individual case reports of aneurysms treated by synthetic coatings (type not specified), see the *Surg* column (symbol *SYN*) in Appendix 2.

Methyl Methacrylate

Methyl methacrylate has been used extensively in clinical surgery for replacement of bony parts, e.g., cranioplasty. Dutton used this substance to coat aneurysms and first reported his technique in 1956 (36). Subsequently a number of surgeons have reported successful use of this material (Fig. 28.3), commercially sold as Aneuroplasty (3,23,34–36,64,65,72,91,117,137,181).

By 1968 a series of 102 aneurysm cases had been coated with methyl methacrylate at the Walter Reed Army Medical Center (64). There were two late rebleeds from aneurysms not completely encased, emphasizing the need for total encasement for adequate protection. There has been no clinical evidence of toxicity reported.

Methyl Cyanoacrylate

In 1962 Carton and his colleagues (12) used methyl cyanoacrylate (Eastman 910 polymer, Ad-Here, Mecrylate), a tissue adhesive or glue, to patch a hole in the internal carotid artery with a piece of dura. This was the site of an ICAA that ruptured at surgery. Postoperative angiography revealed marked constriction at the site of the graft. Carton et al. (13) later reported several patients in whom this adhesive was used to hold a clip in place or patch a hole in the artery. A few other cases of coating aneurysms with methyl cyanoacrylate were described (59,80,112,144,188). However, there have been reports of arterial occlusion (17) or aneurysm wall necrosis with rebleed (144).

Subsequently it became apparent that methyl cyanoacrylate was too toxic. Experiments confirmed the occurrence of severe inflammation, adhesions, necrosis, vascular occlusion, or aneurysm formation, as well as neuronal injury (80,92,144,174,175,188,189). This material has since been abandoned for aneurysm treatment except in conjunction with other synthetic materials, which presumably reduce its toxicity (see EDH Adhesive, below).

Ethyl Cyanoacrylate

Another tissue adhesive used for coating intracranial aneurysms is ethyl cyanoacrylate (Aron Alpha, Krazy Glue). Like the methyl series, this ethyl series polymerizes rapidly on contact with ionic solutions, e.g., the moist wall of aneurysms. A hard but poorly resilient coating develops about the aneurysm wall (or on other tissue or even instruments). Early reports on the application of ethyl cyanoacrylate to aneurysms came from Sano (146) and Lapras and Goutelle (100), and others followed (15,16, 108,114,145,162,183,185,186).

Chou and co-workers (16) used this material on 45 aneurysms and found no ill effects from its use. They described their technique:

> The surgical technique requires that the aneurysmal sac be dissected free from all the surrounding tissues. The [tissue adhesive] is drawn into a disposable syringe and is applied to the aneurysm by slowly and steadily injecting a uniform stream from a bent, disposable, 20-gauge, blunt spinal needle. The application should start from the depths and progress outward as a rule. If the dome or the small "tit" which is the usual bleeding spot can be exposed first, it is desirable to apply a small drop thereon to prevent rupture during the dissection. The agent, being viscous, "glazes" over the dome nicely. Extreme care should be taken to avoid applying excessive material at this time, for once polymerization takes place, the coated area becomes so rigid that further exposure of the remainder of the lesion may be difficult. It

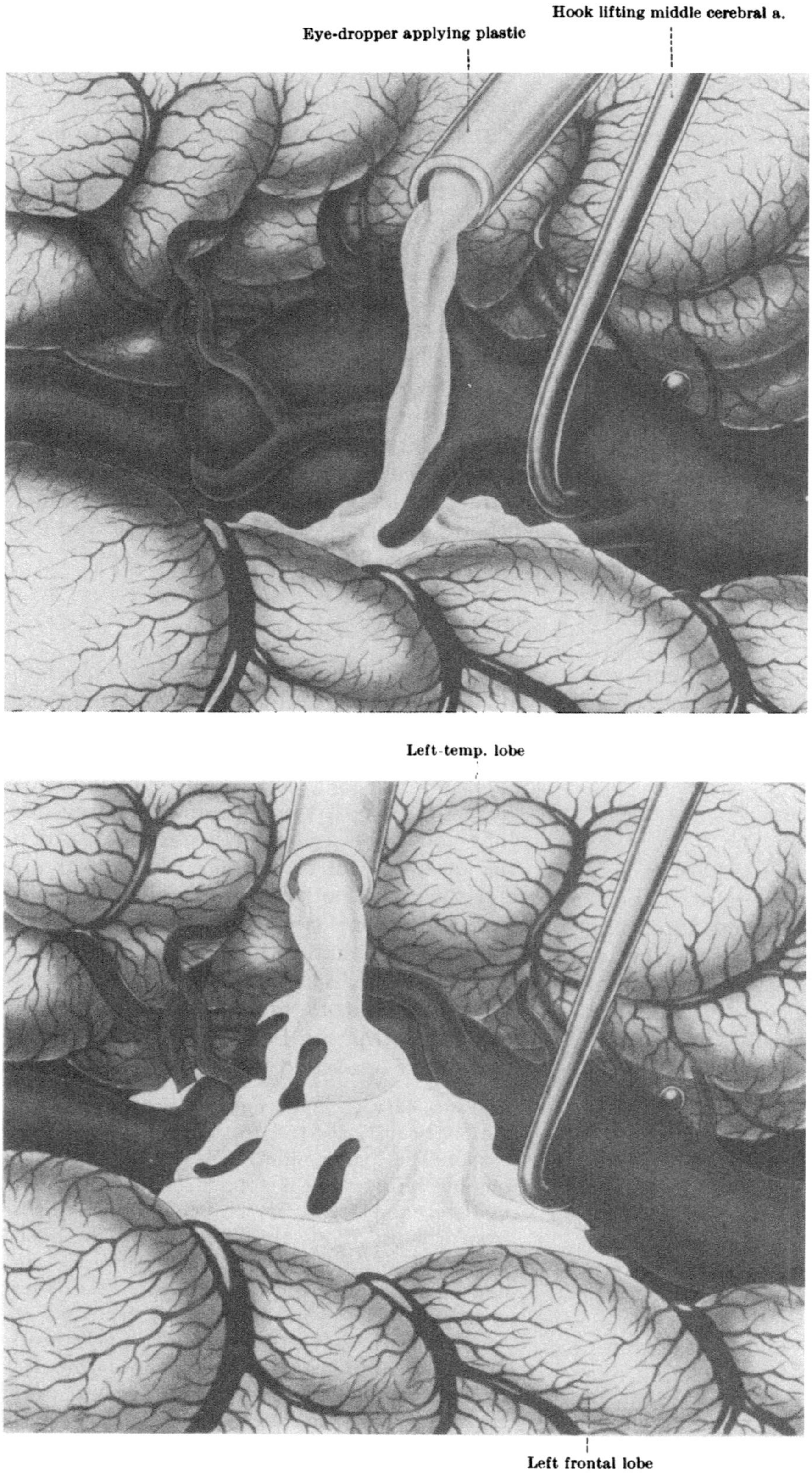

Fig. 28.3. Coating of a MCAA with methyl methacrylate. From Kempe LG, ref. 91.

is also important to remove such items as brain retractors, cottonoids, and suction tips from the area of coating so that they will not be "glued in."

Ethyl cyanoacrylate, although less toxic than its methyl analogue, possesses significant histotoxicity (22,189). The products that stand for long periods on the shelf between manufacture and usage create the greatest reactions (14,22). It appears inadvisable to use this cyanoacrylate compound as routine treatment for aneurysms; it should be reserved for selected cases where such treatment is lifesaving or at least obviously safer than other techniques.

Isobutyl Cyanoacrylate

Isobutyl cyanoacrylate (Bucrylate, Histoacryl Blue) contains the longer alkyl chain, which may be somewhat less toxic than its shorter-chain methyl and ethyl analogues (107). It has been used by a few surgeons to coat aneurysms or secure clips about aneurysms (33,184, 185,188).

EDH Adhesive

EDH adhesive (Biobond) was developed by Handa and his colleagues (6,66–68) as a physicochemical mixture of methyl cyanoacrylate (Eastman 910), a polyisocyanate (Desmodur T), and a nitrile rubber (Hycar No. 1041). The letters EDH are derived from the first letters of the above words (Eastman, Desmodur T, Hycar). The main tissue binding agent is methyl cyanoacrylate, but it is made more flexible and less toxic by the addition of the other two materials. This compound, painted on the wall of the aneurysm, takes a few hours to achieve its final tissue union and firm state.

EDH adhesive has been used by many surgeons to coat aneurysms (10,11,84,86,93, 94,118,125,128,160–164,173,181). However, it has some histotoxicity (175,189). Cases of rebleed after surgery have been reported (10). Complete exposure and encasement of the aneurysm without precipitating rupture is still required.

Synthetic Resins

Another coating material is the synthetic resin developed by Selverstone and Ronis in 1958 (148–154), which has been used by other surgeons as well (26,28,29,31,90,111,115,116, 136,137,159).

Selverstone described his method in 1977 (149). The field must be dry and adjacent areas covered with gelatin sponge. The wall of the aneurysm is dried with a helium air brush. The same instrument is then used to spray a fine layer of latex (vinylchloride–vinylidenedichloride copolymer) on the aneurysm four times. The two components of an epoxy resin (epoxy–polyamide) are mixed in a plastic syringe and extruded onto the aneurysm through a plastic cannula. This forms a hard outer coating. As with the other synthetic coatings, there is some histotoxicity and tissue reaction (175).

Other synthetic resins that have been used only in the laboratory are the polyurethane rubbers (9). Although a good seal formed about arteries with these materials, inflammation and thrombosis were excessive.

Silicone-Rubber

Todd et al. (168,169) used a special silicone-rubber (polydimethyl siloxane, Silastic) material as a protective jacket about aneurysms, but so far this method has not been widely used on a clinical basis. It causes some mild tissue reaction (175). Rand (140) has added iron (ferrosilicone) and used this combination to coat aneurysms.

Polyester Fiber Mesh

In 1979 Drake (27) described the application of a polyester fiber mesh known as Mersilene mesh. He wrapped a giant aneurysm in this material, which is also commonly used for vascular prostheses and hernia repair.

Summary

The use of protective coatings to prevent rupture and expansion of an intracranial aneurysm, although popular at one time, is not commonly used as routine therapy now. Aneurysms which cannot be clipped satisfactorily, however, may be treated by this technique. The several methods of coating aneurysms and their drawbacks have been reviewed. The principal disadvantages include: (a) the need for complete dissection, exposure, and encasement of the aneurysm, and (b) the histotoxic effects of many of the materials used.

Bibliography

1. af Björkesten G: Arterial aneurysms of the internal carotid artery and its bifurcation. An analysis of 69 aneurysms treated mainly by direct surgical attack. J Neurosurg 15:400–410, 1958
2. af Björkesten G. Troupp H: A controlled trial of delayed surgery for intracranial arterial aneurysms. First results. Prog Brain Res 30:353–356, 1968
3. Almeida GM, Bianco E, Shibata MK: Anterior communicating artery aneurysms. J. Neurosurg 33:53–57, 1976
4. Amias AG: Cerebral vascular disease in pregnancy. I. Haemorrhage. J Obstet Gynaecol Br Commonw 77:100–120, 1970
5. Antunes JL, Correll JW: Cerebral emboli from intracranial aneurysms. Surg Neurol 6:7–10, 1976
6. Araki C, Handa H, Ohta T: Coating and reinforcement of the intracranial aneurysm with synthetic resins and rubbers. Neurochirurgia (Stuttgt) 6:123–136, 1963
7. Arseni C, Ghitescu M, Cristescu A, et al.: Intrasellar aneurysms simulating hypophyseal tumors. Eur Neurol 3:321–329, 1970
8. Avman N, Fisher RG: Exposure of middle cerebral aneurysm after the use of urea. Surgery 48:491–494, 1960
9. Bernhard WF, Cummin AS, Harris PD, et al.: New flexible vascular adhesive for use in cardiovascular surgery. Circulation 27:739–341, 1963
10. Bohm E, Hugosson R: Experiences of surgical treatment of 400 consecutive ruptured cerebral arterial aneurysms. Acta Neurochir (Wien) 40:33–43, 1978
11. Bohm E, Hugosson R: Results of surgical treatment of 200 consecutive cerebral arterial aneurysms. Acta Neurol Scand 46:43–52, 1970
12. Carton CA, Heifetz MD, Kessler LA: Patching of intracranial internal carotid artery in man using a plastic adhesive (Eastman 910 adhesive). J Neurosurg 19:887–895, 1962
13. Carton CA, Kennady JC, Heifetz MD, et al.: The use of a plastic adhesive (methyl-2-cyanoacrylate monomer) in the management of intracranial aneurysms and leaking cerebral vessels: a report of 15 cases. In Fields WS, Sahs AL (eds.): Intracranial Aneurysms and Subarachnoid Hemorrhage. Springfield, Ill., Thomas, 1965, pp. 372–440
14. Chou SN: Use of cyanoacrylates [letter]. J Neurosurg 46:226, 1977
15. Chou SN, Ortiz-Suarez HJ: Surgical treatment of arterial aneurysms of the vertebrobasilar circulation. J Neurosurg 41:671–680, 1974
16. Chou SN, Ortiz-Surez HJ, Brown WE: Technique and material for coating aneurysms. Clin Neurosurg 21:182–193, 1974
17. Coe JE, Bondurant CP Jr: Late thrombosis following the use of autogenous fascia and a cyanoacrylate (Eastman 910 Monomer) for the wrapping of an intracranial aneurysm. J Neurosurg 21:884–886, 1964
18. Crompton MR: Recurrent haemorrhage from cerebral aneurysms and its prevention by surgery. J Neurol Neurosurg Psychiatry 29:164–170, 1966
19. Cushing H: The control of bleeding in operations for brain tumors. With the description of silver "clips" for the occlusion of vessels inaccessible to the ligature. Ann Surg 54:1–19, 1911
20. Davis RA: The results of delayed intracranial surgery in a series of 75 selected cerebral aneurysms. Q Bull Northwest Univ Med School 36:237–244, 1962
21. Dencker H, Flyger G: The histological reaction of hammered muscle applied to the brain. In experimental investigation in rabbits (with special reference to the "wrapping" of arterial cerebral aneurysms). Acta Chir Scand 118:178–183, 1960
22. Diaz FG, Mastri AR, Chou SN: Neural and vascular tissue reaction to aneurysm-coating adhesive (ethyl 2-cyanoacrylate). Neurosurgery 3:45–49, 1978
23. Dickmann GH, Ottino CA: Empaquetamiento de aneurismas del grupo silviano con un polimero del metil metacrilato. Prensa Med Argent 52:1306–1310, 1965
24. Dimsdale H, Logue V: Ruptured posterior fossa aneurysms and their surgical treatment. J Neurol Neurosurg Psychiatry 22:202–217, 1959
25. Dott NM: Intracranial aneurysms: cerebral arterio-radiography: surgical treatment. Edinburgh Med J 40:219–234, 1933
26. Drake CG: Further experience with surgical treatment of aneurysms of the basilar artery. J Neurosurg 29:372–392, 1968
27. Drake CG: Giant intracranial aneurysms: experience in 174 patients. Clin Neurosurg 26:12–95, 1979
28. Drake CG: Surgical treatment of rupture of aneurysms of the basilar artery. Experience with 14 cases. J Neurosurg 23:457–473, 1965
29. Drake CG: The surgical treatment of vertebral-basilar aneurysms. Clin Neurosurg 16:114–169, 1969
30. Drake CG, Jory TA: Spontaneous intracranial haemorrhage: "subarachnoid haemorrhage": a review of investigation and treatment of 189 cases. Can J Surg 4:4–11, 1960

31. Drake CG, Vanderlinden RG: The late consequences of incomplete surgical treatment of cerebral aneurysms. J Neurosurg 27:226–238, 1967
32. Duffy G: The surgical treatment of anterior communicating artery aneurysms. Aust NZ J Surg 44:257–260, 1974
33. Dujovny M, Kossovsky N, Kossowsky R, et al.: Heifetz clip failure. A metallurgical study. J Neurosurg 50:368–373, 1979
34. Dutton J: Acrylic investment of intracranial aneurysms. Br Med J 2:597–602, 1959
35. Dutton J: Acrylic investment of intracranial aneurysms. A report of 12 years' experience. J Neurosurg 31:652–657, 1969
36. Dutton JEM: Intracranial aneurysm. A new method of surgical treatment. Br Med J 2:585–586, 1956
37. Elvidge AR, Feindel WH: Surgical treatment of aneurysm of the anterior cerebral and the anterior communicating arteries diagnosed by angiography and electroencephalography. J Neurosurg 7:13–32, 1950
38. Fager CA, Poppen, JL: Observations on controlled ligation of the internal carotid artery. Surg Clin North Am 36:567–582, 1956
39. Falconer MA: Progress in the surgical treatment of spontaneous cerebral haemorrhage. Proc R Soc Med 49:166–169, 1956
40. Falconer MA: Surgical treatment of spontaneous intracranial haemorrhage. Br Med J 1:790–792, 1958
41. Falconer MA: Surgical treatment of spontaneous subarachnoid haemorrhage. Preliminary report. Br Med J 1:809–813, 1950
42. Falconer MA: The future of surgery in the treatment of spontaneous cerebral haemorrhage. Lancet 2:945–950, 1952
43. Falconer MA: The surgical treatment of bleeding intracranial aneurysms. J Neurol Neurosurg Psychiatry 14:153–186, 1951
44. Frantzen E, Krenchel NJ: Prognosen ved intracranielle sacculate aneurysmer en efterundersøgelse. Nord Med 51:130–134, 1954
45. French LA, Chou SN, Long DM: The direct approach to intracranial aneurysms. Clin Neurosurg 15:117–132, 1968
46. Froman C, Lipschitz R: Belated recurrent haemorrhage from an aneurysm of the posterior communicating artery after carotid ligation. S Afr J Surg 7:27–32, 1969
47. Gardner WJ: Cerebral angiomas and aneurysms. Surg Clin North Am 16:1019–1030, 1936
48. Ghosh BB, Bhattacharyya MK, Bagchi AK: Intracranial saccular aneurysms. A radiological review J Indian Med Assoc 55:57–60, 1970
49. Gillingham FJ: The management of ruptured intracranial aneurysm. Ann R Coll Surg 23:89–117, 1958
50. Gillingham FJ: The management of ruptured intracranial aneurysms. Scott Med J 12:377–383, 1967
51. Gillingham FJ: Twenty-five years' experience with middle cerebral aneurysms. J Neurol Neurosurg Psychiatry 38:405, 1975
52. Gillingham FJ: Twenty-five years' experience with middle cerebral aneurysms. Rev Inst Nacl Neurol (Mex) 10:16–21, 1976
53. Graf CJ: Results of direct attack on nonfistulous intracranial aneurysm with remarks on statistics. J Neurosurg 12:146–153, 1955
54. Groff RA: Experience with direct surgical treatment of intracranial aneurysms. Arch Neurol Psychiatry 72:782, 1954
55. Gros C, Vlahovitch B, Auteroche B: Réflexions sur une série de 46 anévrysmes supraclinoidiens rompus. Évaluation du traitement chirurgical. Neurochirurgie 3:253–258, 1957
56. Grote W, Bettag W: Multiple Hirnaneurysmen (Fallbericht). Zentralbl Neurochir 17:151–155, 1957
57. Grote W, Röttgen P, Wappenschmidt J: Erfahrungen mit Aneurysmen der Arteria communicans anterior. Neurochirurgie 6:63–71, 1960
58. Guidetti B: Surgical treatment of aneurysms of the anterior communicating artery. Prog Brain Res 30:303–307, 1968
59. Guidetti B, La Torre E: Carotid-ophthalmic aneurysms. A series of 16 cases treated by direct approach. Acta Neurochir (Wien) 22:289–304, 1970
60. Hamby WB: Intracranial Aneurysms. Springfield, Ill., Thomas, 1952
61. Hamby WB: Intracranial surgery for aneurysms. Prog Neurol Surg 3:1–65, 1969
62. Hamby WB: The modern treatment of intracranial aneurysms. NY State J Med 52:2497–2502, 1952
63. Hamilton JG, Falconer MA: Immediate and late results of surgery in cases of saccular intracranial aneurysms. J Neurosurg 16:514–541, 1959
64. Hammon WM: Intracranial aneurysm encasement. J Neurol Neurosurg Psychiatry 31:524–527, 1968
65. Hammon WM, Kempe LG: The posterior fossa approach to aneurysms of the vertebral and basilar arteries. J Neurosurg 37:339–347, 1972
66. Handa H: The neurosurgical treatment of intracranial vascular malformations, particularly with the use of plastics and polarographic measurements. Clin Neurosurg 9:223–244, 1963

67. Handa H, Ohta T, Ishikawa S, et al.: Coating and reinforcing of experimental cervical aneurysms with synthetic resins and rubbers. Neurol Med Chir (Tokyo) 2:158–186, 1960
68. Handa H, Ohta T, Kamijyo Y: Encasement of intracranial aneurysms with plastic compounds. Prog Neurol Surg 3:149–192, 1969
69. Handa J, Kamijyo Y, Handa H: Posttraumatisches Aneurysma der leptomeningealen Arterien (Bericht über einen Fall). Arch Psychiatr Nervenkr 221:357–364, 1968
70. Harris P: Aneurysms of the anterior communicating artery. Cincinnati J Med 42:1–7, 1961
71. Harris P, Udvarhelyi GB: Aneurysms arising at the internal carotid-posterior communicating artery junction. J Neurosurg 14:180–191, 1957
72. Hayes GJ, Leaver RC: Methyl methacrylate investment of intracranial aneurysms. A report of seven years experience. J Neurosurg 25:79–80, 1966
73. Hazouri LA: Five years experience with intracranial aneurysms. J Med Assoc Ga 57:62–64, 1968
74. Helme WB: Infrequent aneurysm surgery. Neurosurgery 3:210–212, 1978
75. Hockley A: Proximal occlusion of the anterior cerebral artery for anterior communicating aneurysm. J Neurol Neurosurg Psychiatry 37:1280, 1974
76. Hockley AD: Proximal occlusion of the anterior cerebral artery for anterior communicating aneurysm. J Neurosurg 43:426–431, 1975
77. Höök O, Norlén G: Aneurysms of the anterior communicating artery. Acta Neurol Scand 40:219–240, 1964
78. Höök O, Norlén G: Aneurysms of the internal carotid artery. Acta Neurol Scand 40:200–218, 1964
79. Höök O, Norlén G: Aneurysms of the middle cerebral artery. A report of 80 cases. Acta Chir Scand [Suppl] 235:1–39, 1958
80. Hoppenstein RD, Weissberg D, Goetz RH: Fusiform dilatation and thrombosis of arteries following the application of methyl-2-cyanoacrylate (Eastman 910 monomer). J Neurosurg 23:556–564, 1965
81. Horrax G: Discussion of Dandy WE: The surgical treatment of intracranial aneurysms of the internal carotid artery. Ann Surg 114:336–340, 1941
82. Horsley V: Note on haemostasis by application of living tissue. Br Med J 2:8, 1914
83. Hughes B: The treatment of intracranial aneurysm. Med Press 231:181–184, 1954
84. Hugosson R: The value of reinforcing intracranial aneurysms with plastic coating. Acta Chir Scand 141:182–186, 1975
85. Ingraham FD, Bailey OT, Nulsen FE: Studies of fibrin foam as a hemostatic agent in neurosurgery, with special reference to its comparison with muscle. J Neurosurg 1:171–181, 1944
86. Isamat F, Ullrich DP, Berglund G: Recubrimiento con resinas plasticos de los aneurismas intracraneales. Revision de un grupo de veintiseis aneurismas asi tratados. Rev Clin Esp 109:307–310, 1968
87. Jaeger R: Aneurysm of the intracranial carotid artery. Syndrome of frontal headache with oculomotor nerve paralysis. JAMA 142:304–309, 1950
88. Jefferson G: Compression of the chiasma, optic nerves, and optic tracts by intracranial aneurysms. Brain 60:444–497, 1937
89. Jefferson G: Further concerning compression of the optic pathways by intracranial aneurysms. Clin Neurosurg 1:55–103, 1955
90. Keith J: Intracranial aneurysm treated by plastic coating. J Ky Med Assoc 58:481–482, 1960
91. Kempe LG: Operative Neurosurgery, Vol 1: Cranial, Cerebral, and Intracranial Vascular Disease. Berlin, Springer-Verlag, 1968, pp. 1–75, 203–214
92. Kline DG, Hayes GJ: An experimental evaluation of the effect of a plastic adhesive, methyl-2-cyanoacrylate, on neural tissue. J Neurosurg 20:647–654, 1963
93. Krayenbühl H: Behandlung intracranieller Aneurysmen mit synthetischem Klebestoff. Munch Med Wochenschr 106:1370–1373, 1964
94. Krayenbühl HA, Yaşargil MG, Flamm, ES, et al.: Microsurgical treatment of intracranial saccular aneurysms. J Neurosurg 37:678–686, 1972
95. Kunc Z: [Aneurysm of the anterior communicating artery.] Cesk Neurol 33:169–177, 1970
96. Kunc Z: Aneurysms of carotid and posterior communicating artery. Prog Brain Res 30:309–315, 1968
97. Laine E: Traitement chirurgical des anévrysmes de l'artère communicante antérieure. In Krayenbühl H, et al. (eds.): L'Anévrysme de l'Artère Communicante Antérieure. Paris, Masson et Cie, 1959, pp. 131–182
98. Laitinen L, Troupp H: Reliability of partial ligation in the treatment of intracranial arterial aneurysm. Acta Neurol Scand 37:62–66, 1961
99. Lang EF, Poppen JL: Aneurysms of the anterior communicating artery: results of surgical treatment. Surg Clin North Am 42:793–805, 1962
100. Lapras C, Goutelle A: Le traitement des anévrismes intra-crâniens par enrobage plastique. Neurochirurgie 15:107–112, 1969

101. Le Beau J: Anévrismes de l'artère communicante antérieure. Ruptures et indications neurochirurgicales. neurochirurgia (Stuttgt) 5:38–57, 1962
102. Le Beau J: Indications opératories et traitement chirurgical des anévrismes artériels intra-craniens sus-tentoriels. Ann Chir 15:1153–1163, 1961
103. Light RU: Hemostasis in neurosurgery. J Neurosurg 2:414–434, 1945
104. Logue V: Posterior fossa aneurysms. Clin Neurosurg 11:183–207, 1964
105. Logue V: Surgery in spontaneous subarachnoid haemorrhage. Operative treatment of aneurysms on the anterior cerebral and anterior communicating artery. Br Med J 1:473–479, 1956
106. Lougheed WM, Botterell EH, Morley, TP: Results of the direct attack in the surgical management of internal carotid and middle cerebral aneurysms. Clin Neurosurg 9:193–200, 1963
107. Matsumoto T, Nemhauser GM, Soloway HB, et al.: Cyanoacrylate tissue adhesives: an experimental and clinical evaluation. Milit Med 134:247–252, 1969
108. Mazur JB, Salazar JL: Late thrombosis of middle cerebral artery following clipping and coating of aneurysms. Surg Neurol 10:131–133, 1978
109. McCune WS, Raad A, Blades B: Latex and thorium dioxide (Thorotrast) in treatment of aneurysms. Arch Surg 70:583–590, 1955
110. McKissock W, Richardson A, Walsh L: Middle-cerebral aneurysms. Further results in the controlled trial of conservative and surgical treatment of ruptured intracranial aneurysms. Lancet 2:417–421, 1962
111. McMurtry JG III, Housepian EM, Bowman FO Jr, et al.: Surgical treatment of basilar artery aneurysms. Elective circulatory arrest with thoracotomy in 12 cases. J Neurosurg 40:486–498, 1974
112. Messer HD, Strenger L, McVeety HJ: Use of plastic adhesive for reinforcement of a ruptured intracranial aneurysm. J Neurosurg 20:360–361, 1963
112a. Mickey BE, Samson D: Neurosurgical applications of the cyanoacrylate adhesives. Clin Neurosurg 28:429–444, 1981
113. Morello G: Remarks on the direct attack on intracranial aneurysms. Prog Brain Res 30:347–349, 1968
114. Mori K, Miyazaki H, Ono H: Aneurysm of the anterior inferior cerebellar artery at the internal auditory meatus. Surg Neurol 10:297–300, 1978
115. Mount LA, Antunes JL: Results of treatment of intracranial aneurysms by wrapping and coating. J Neurosurg 42:189–193, 1975
116. Mount LA, Brisman, R: Treatment of multiple aneurysms—symptomatic and asymptomatic. Clin Neurosurg 21:166–170, 1974
117. Moyes PD: Management and surgical treatment of ruptured intracranial aneurysms. Can Med Assoc J 94:13–18, 1966
118. New PFJ: Arterial stationary waves. Am J Roentgenol 97:488–499, 1966
119. Norlén G: Aneurysm of the anterior communicating artery. Prog Brain Res 30:295–302, 1968
120. Norlén G: The pathology, diagnosis and treatment of intracranial saccular aneurysms. Proc R Soc Med 45:291–302, 1952
121. Norlén G, Barnum AS: Surgical treatment of aneurysms of the anterior communicating artery. J Neurosurg 10:634–650, 1953
122. Norlén G, Olivecrona H: The treatment of aneurysms of the circle of Willis. J Neurosurg 10:404–415, 1953
123. Northfield DWC: Discussion. Proc R Soc Med 45:302, 1952
124. Northfield DWC: The Surgery of the Central Nervous System. Oxford, Blackwell, 1973, pp. 346–401
125. Nukui H, Aiba T: [Clinical features in cases with the ruptured aneurysm of the distal anterior cerebral artery.] Neurol Med Chir (Tokyo) 18:39–47, 1978
126. Obrador S, Rábago G, Córdoba A, et al.: Aneurismas arteriales multiples del cerebro operados bajo parado circulatoria. Rev Clin Esp 95:288–294, 1964
127. Overgaard J, Riishede J: Multiple cerebral saccular aneurysms. Acta Neurol Scand 41:363–371, 1965
128. Paillas JE, Bonnal J: Anévrysmes artériels. In Patel J, Leger L (eds.): Nouveau Traité de Technique Chirurgicale, Vol 6. Paris, Masson & Cie, 1975, pp. 237–277
129. Pertuiset B: Les anévrysmes sacculaires de la carotide interne supra-clinoidienne. Étude anatomo-clinique et thérapeutique d'après 16 cas. Neurochirurgie 5:183–206, 1959
130. Pool JL: Aneurysms of the anterior communicating artery. Bifrontal craniotomy and routine use of temporary clips. J Neurosurg 18:98–111, 1961
131. Pool JL: Bifrontal craniotomy for anterior communicating artery aneurysms. J Neurosurg 36:212–220, 1972
132. Pool JL: Muslin gauze in intracranial vascular surgery. Technical note. J Neurosurg 44:127–128, 1976
133. Pool JL: Timing and techniques in the intracranial surgery of ruptured aneurysms of the

anterior communicating artery. J Neurosurg 19:378–388, 1962
134. Pool JL, Potts DG: Aneurysms and Arteriovenous Anomalies of the Brain. Diagnosis and Treatment. New York, Harper & Row, 1965
135. Poppen JL: An Atlas of Neurosurgical Techniques. Philadelphia, Saunders, 1960, pp. 156–181
136. Poppen JL: Operative treatment for aneurysms of the anterior communicating artery. Clin Neurosurg 11:8–13, 1964
137. Poppen JL, Fager CA: Anterior communicating aneurysms: improved surgical mortality and morbidity. Lahey Clin Found Bull 19:1–7, 1970
138. Potondi A, Danka L: Basalaneurysma von ungewöhnlichem Ausmass. Zbl Neurochir 26:165–168, 1965
139. Puncernau R, Espuña J: Atrofia optica catalogada de congenita por voluminoso aneurisma de la communicante posterior. Angiologia 13:181–186, 1961
140. Rand RW: Microneurosurgery, 2nd ed. St Louis, Mosby, 1978, pp. 43–44, 311–324
141. Rhoton AL, Jackson FE, Gleave J, et al.: Congenital and traumatic intracranial aneurysms. Clin Symp 29:1–40, 1977
142. Robinson RG: Ruptured aneurysms of the middle cerebral artery. J Neurosurg 35:25–33, 1971
143. Sachs E Jr: The fate of muscle and cotton wrapped about intracranial carotid arteries and aneurysms. A laboratory and clinicopathological study. Acta Neurochir (Wien) 26:121–137, 1972
144. Sachs E Jr, Erbengi A, Margolis G, et al.: Fatality from ruptured intracranial aneurysm after coating with methyl-2-cyanoacrylate (Eastman 910 monomer, M2 C-L). Case report. J Neurosurg 24:889–891, 1966
145. Salazar JL: Treatment of ruptured and unruptured internal carotid artery aneurysms. Surg Neurol 11:451–455, 1979
146. Sano K: [Surgery of intracranial aneurysm.] Brain Nerve (Tokyo) 23:1252–1264, 1971
147. Sato O, Kanazawa I, Kokunai T, et al.: Seven intracranial aneurysms of the internal carotid arteries. Diagnosis by magnification angioautotomography. Neuroradiology 15:189–192, 1978
148. Selverstone B: Aneurysms at middle cerebral "trifurcation": treatment with adherent plastics. J Neurosurg 19:884–886, 1962
149. Selverstone B: Coating of intracranial aneurysms with nontoxic adherent plastics. In Schmidek HH, Sweet WH (eds.): Current Techniques in Operative Neurosurgery. New York, Grune & Stratton, 1977, pp. 31–40
150. Selverstone B: Reinforcement of intracranial aneurysms with adherent plastics. J Neurol Neurosurg Psychiatry 24:93, 1961
151. Selverstone B: Treatment of intracranial aneurysms with adherent plastics. N Engl J Med 265:100, 1961
152. Selverstone B: Treatment of intracranial aneurysms with adherent plastics. Clin Neurosurg 9:201–213, 1963
153. Selverstone B: Vascular reinforcement with adherent plastics. N Engl Vasc Soc Proc 19:37, 1960
154. Selverstone B, Ronis N: Coating and reinforcement of intracranial aneurysms with synthetic resins. Bull Tufts N Engl Med Center 4:8–12, 1958
155. Sharkey PC, Apostolou A: Intracranial aneurysms: a partial community study. South Med J 59:185–191, 1966
156. Sjöqvist O: Thread ligature of intracranial saccular aneurysms. In Proceedings of the 5th Congress of Neurology, Lisbon, Vol 3, 1953, pp. 108–115
157. Skultety FM, Nishioka H: Report on the cooperative study of intracranial aneurysms and subarachnoid hemorrhage. Section VIII, Part 2. The results of intracranial surgery in the treatment of aneurysms. J Neurosurg 25:683–704, 1966
157a. Skultety FM, Nishioka H: The results of intracranial surgery in the treatment of aneurysms. In Sahs AL, Perret GE, Locksley HB, et al. (eds.): Intracranial Aneurysms and Subarachnoid Hemorrhage. A Cooperative Study. Philadelphia, Lippincott, 1969, pp. 173–194
158. Steelman HF, Hayes GJ, Rizzoli HV: Surgical treatment of saccular intracranial aneurysms. J Neurosurg 10:564–576, 1953
159. Stepien L: Reinforcement of intracranial aneurysm with adherent plastics: Selverstone method. Prog Brain Res 30:361–365, 1968
160. Stöwsand D, Buhl K: Früh- und Spätbefunde nach Biobond-Beschichtung von intrakraniellen Aneurysmen. Acta Neurochir (Wien) 32:73–82, 1975
161. Stroobandt G, Cornelis G, Thauvoy C: Les anévrismes intracrâniens multiples. I. Evolution et orientation actuelle du traitement chirurgical. Acta Neurol Belg 73:298–310, 1973
162. Stroobandt G, Cornelis G, Thauvoy C: Les anévrismes intracrâniens multiples. II. Problèmes posés par les lésions de petite taille. Acta Neurol Belg 73:311–319, 1973
163. Stroobandt G, Cornelis G, Vermonden J: Le traitement chirurgical des anévrysmes sylviens. Acta Neurol Belg 69:661–680, 1969
164. Sugar O, Tsuchiya G: Plastic coating of intracranial aneurysms with "EDH-adhesive." J Neurosurg 21:114–117, 1964
165. Symon L: Subarachnoid haemorrhage from in-

tracranial aneurysm and angioma. In Russell RWR (ed.): Cerebral Arterial Disease. Edinburgh, Churchill Livingstone, 1976, pp. 231–261

166. Taylor JC, Choudhury AR: Reinforcement with gauze wrapping for ruptured aneurysms of the middle cerebral artery. J Neurosurg 47:828–832, 1977
167. Taylor JC, Choudhury AR, Shephard RH: Surgery of aneurysms of the middle cerebral artery: a comparison of results of "wrapping" and "clipping" procedures. J Neurol Neurosurg Psychiatry 40:200, 1977
168. Todd EM, Crue BL Jr: The coating of aneurysms with plastic materials. In Fields WS, Sahs AL (eds.): Intracranial Aneurysms and Subarachnoid Hemorrhage. Springfield, Ill., Thomas, 1965, pp. 357–371
169. Todd EM, Sheldon CH, Crue BL Jr, et al.: Plastic jackets for certain intracranial aneurysms. JAMA 179:935–939, 1962
170. Tönnis W: Erfolgreiche Behandlung eines Aneurysma der Art. commun. ant. cerebri. Zbl Neurochir 1:39–42, 1936
171. Tönnis W: Probleme und Ergebnisse der Behandlung intrakranieller Aneurysmen. Langenbecks Arch Klin Chir 287:634–639, 1957
172. Tönnis W: Zur Behandlung der intrakranieller Aneurysmen. Langenbecks Arch Klin Chir 189:474–476, 1937
173. Tovi D, Nilsson IM, Thulin C-A: Fibrinolytic activity of the cerebrospinal fluid after subarachnoid haemorrhage. Acta Neurol Scand 49:1–9, 1973
174. Troupp H, Rinne T: Methyl-2-cyanoacrylate (Eastman 910) in experimental vascular surgery with a note on experimental arterial arterial aneurysms. J Neurosurg 21:1067–1069, 1964
175. Tsuchiya G, Sugar O, Yashon D, et al.: Reactions of rabbit brain and peripheral vessels to plastics used in coating arterial aneurysms. J Neurosurg 28:409–416, 1968
176. Uihlein A, Thomas RL, Cleary J: Aneurysms of the anterior communicating artery complex. Proc Mayo Clin 42:73–87, 1967
177. Uttley AHC, Buckell M: Biochemical changes after spontaneous subarachnoid haemorrhage. Part III. Coagulation and lysis with special reference to recurrent haemorrhage. J Neurol Neurosurg Psychiatry 31:621–627, 1968
178. Vaishnoraite PY, Filatov YM: [Strengthening of the walls of saccular arterial aneurysms of the brain by means of gauze.] Vopr Neirokhir 32:44–48, 1968
179. Wilkins: Discussion of: Intracranial aneurysm: a surgical problem. Zbl Neurochir 3:352, 1938
180. Wilson CB, Christensen FK, Subrahmanian MV: Intracranial aneurysms at the pericallosol artery bifurcation. Am Surg 31:386–393, 1965
181. Wilson CB, U HS: Surgical treatment for aneurysms of the upper basilar artery. J Neurosurg 44:537–543, 1976
182. Woodhall B, Golden J: Fibroblastic stimulation of rabbit artery advantitia by marine varnish, "Krylon," and latex. Laboratory study related to the surgery of congenital cerebral aneurysm. Arch Surg 66:587–592, 1953
183. Yaşargil MG, Antic J. Laciga R, et al.: Microsurgical pterional approach to aneurysms of the basilar bifurcation. Surg Neurol 6:83–91, 1976
184. Yaşargil MG, Fox JL: The microsurgical approach to intracranial aneurysms. Surg Neurol 3:7–14, 1975
185. Yaşargil MG, Fox JL, Ray MW: The operative approach to aneurysms of the anterior communicating artery. In Krayenbühl H (ed.): Advances and Technical Standards in Neurosurgery, Vol 2. New York, Springer-Verlag, 1975, pp. 113–170
186. Yaşargil MG, Gasser JC, Hodosh RM, et al.: Carotid-ophthalmic aneurysms: direct microsurgical approach. Surg Neurol 8:155–165, 1977
187. Yashon D, Jane JA, Gordon MC, et al.: Effects of methyl 2-cyanoacrylate adhesives on the somatic vessels and the central nervous system of animals. J Neurosurg 24:883–888, 1966
188. Yashon D, White RJ, Arias, BA, et al.: Cyanocrylate encasement of intracranial aneurysms. Technical note. J Neurosurg 34:709–713, 1971
189. Yodh SB, Wright RL: Experimental evaluation of four synthetic adhesives for possible treatment of aneurysms. J Neurosurg 26:504–510, 1967

29

Craniotomy for Aneurysm

V. Cranial Approaches

The various cranial approaches to intracranial aneurysms are summarized in Tables 29.1–29.6 and illustrated in Figs. 29.1–29.60. It is impossible to strictly categorize all types of craniotomy flaps and approaches. There is enough overlap that a flap reported by any given surgeon probably could fit into either of two categories, especially when the illustration is not clear in its orientation or when the written description does not quite match the illustration. Nevertheless, it is instructive to review the history of such approaches. It is of interest that more exacting diagnostic techniques, better anesthetic methods, and the use of modern instrumentation and microsurgical techniques have resulted in a trend toward a smaller and more basal cranial opening for intracranial aneurysm.

The benefits of a small dural opening include a better cosmetic result, shorter operating time, and less brain injury from air exposure, the latter of which causes blood-brain barrier changes and brain edema (161,174). In 1970 Hamby (74) pointed out that

> brain tissue is splinted by its surroundings and becomes edematous when exposed to air and the heat of surgical illumination. Large craniotomies permit brain tissue to be displaced beyond dural borders, stretching deep vessels and producing localized relative ischemia.

Small bone flaps can have the disadvantages of providing inadequate exposure (not usually a problem with microsurgical technique), causing difficulty with placement of retractors (they require room to retract without striking the skull edge), and allowing insufficient surface area for temporalis muscle attachment (in small frontolateral flaps).

Some surgeons have standardized basic bone flaps for all anterior circle of Willis aneurysms, with minor modifications for specific aneurysm sites. The basic unilateral frontal flap has been advocated by a few (10,46,223), but the frontolateral (frontotemporal, frontosphenoidal, pterional) bone flap has been most commonly utilized (1, 3, 12, 14, 21, 25, 27, 49, 65, 66, 81, 103, 105, 106, 110, 112, 142, 150, 166, 167, 181, 206, 217, 221, 231, 235, 238). See Chapter 34 for additional details.

The advantages of using a standardized bone flap for all anterior circle of Willis aneurysms include better orientation of anatomy and the ability to comfortably treat multiple aneurysms at various sites during one operation. As early as 1944 Dandy was reporting on the routine use of the frontolateral "hypophyseal" flap (the "Dandy flap") for attacking all such aneurysms (Fig. 29.1) (21,102). His skin flap used a "concealed incision" (i.e., behind the hairline). This approach now is commonly utilized for multiple aneurysm cases. For attacking bilateral aneurysms at one sitting, some surgeons have used the bifrontal flap for bilateral MCAA (134), bilateral pcaICAA (227), and bilateral giant oaICAA (59). Suzuki and his co-workers (199, 201) reported several common and uncommon approaches to cases with multiple aneurysms (Fig. 29.2).

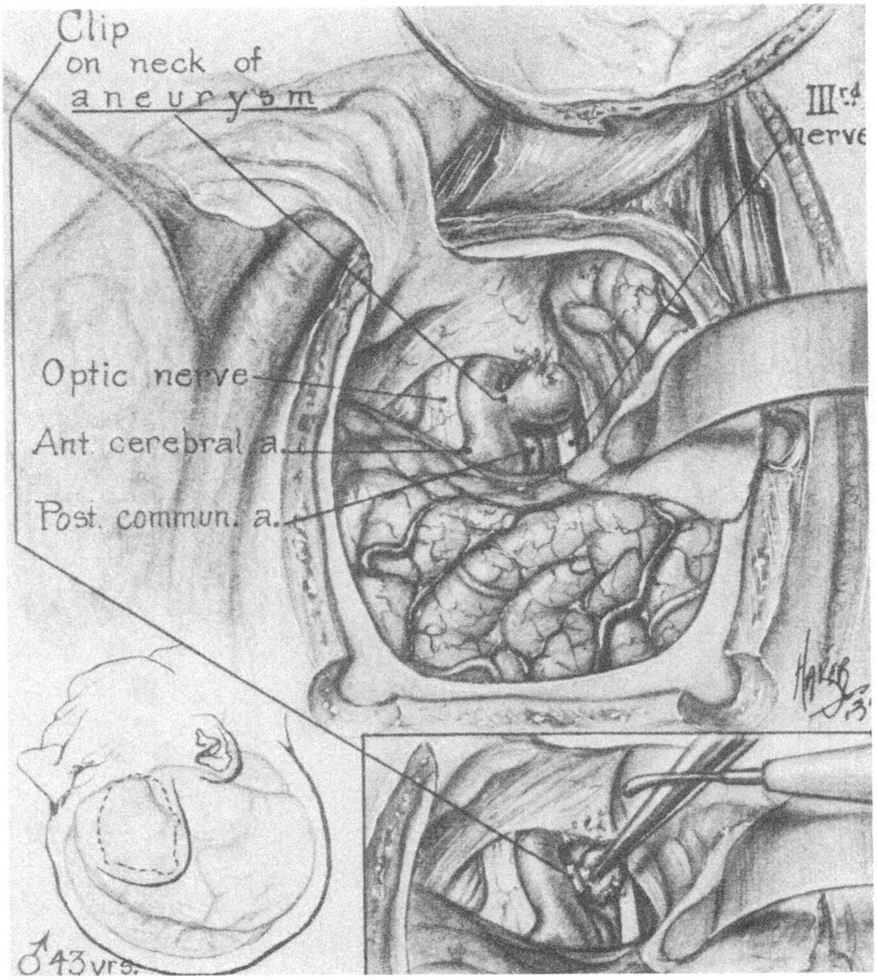

Fig. 29.1. ***Lower left*** Dandy's 1938 frontolateral flap under his incision concealed behind the hairline. ***Top*** pcaICAA seen between sylvian fissure and sphenoid wing. Note bone flap attached to temporalis muscle. ***Lower right*** Silver clip on neck of aneurysm; this is the first report of aneurysm clipping. Dome of aneurysm is being electrocoagulated. From Dandy WE, ref. 20.

Anterior Communicating Artery Aneurysms

Four basic approaches to the ACoAA have evolved (Table 29.1; Fig. 29.3): (a) subfrontal approach through a frontal unilateral bone flap; (b) transcallosal approach through a bifrontal bone flap; (c) interhemispheric subfrontal approach through a bifrontal bone flap; and (d) frontolateral (frontotemporal, frontosphenoidal, or pterional) approach between the sphenoid wing and sylvian fissure. Many modifications have been made on these basic patterns.

Unilateral Subfrontal Approach for ACoAA

Until the 1970s the subfrontal approach, usually right-sided, through a frontal unilateral bone flap was the most popular method for ACoAA. This flap originally was reported by Krause (108) in 1908 for exposure of sellar and suprasellar tumors. Cushing (18) in 1929 exposed these tumors by a similar approach, and in so doing he found two patients with large aneurysms of unknown origin under the optic chiasm (Fig. 29.4).

Since then there has been considerable variation in the sizes and configurations of the uni-

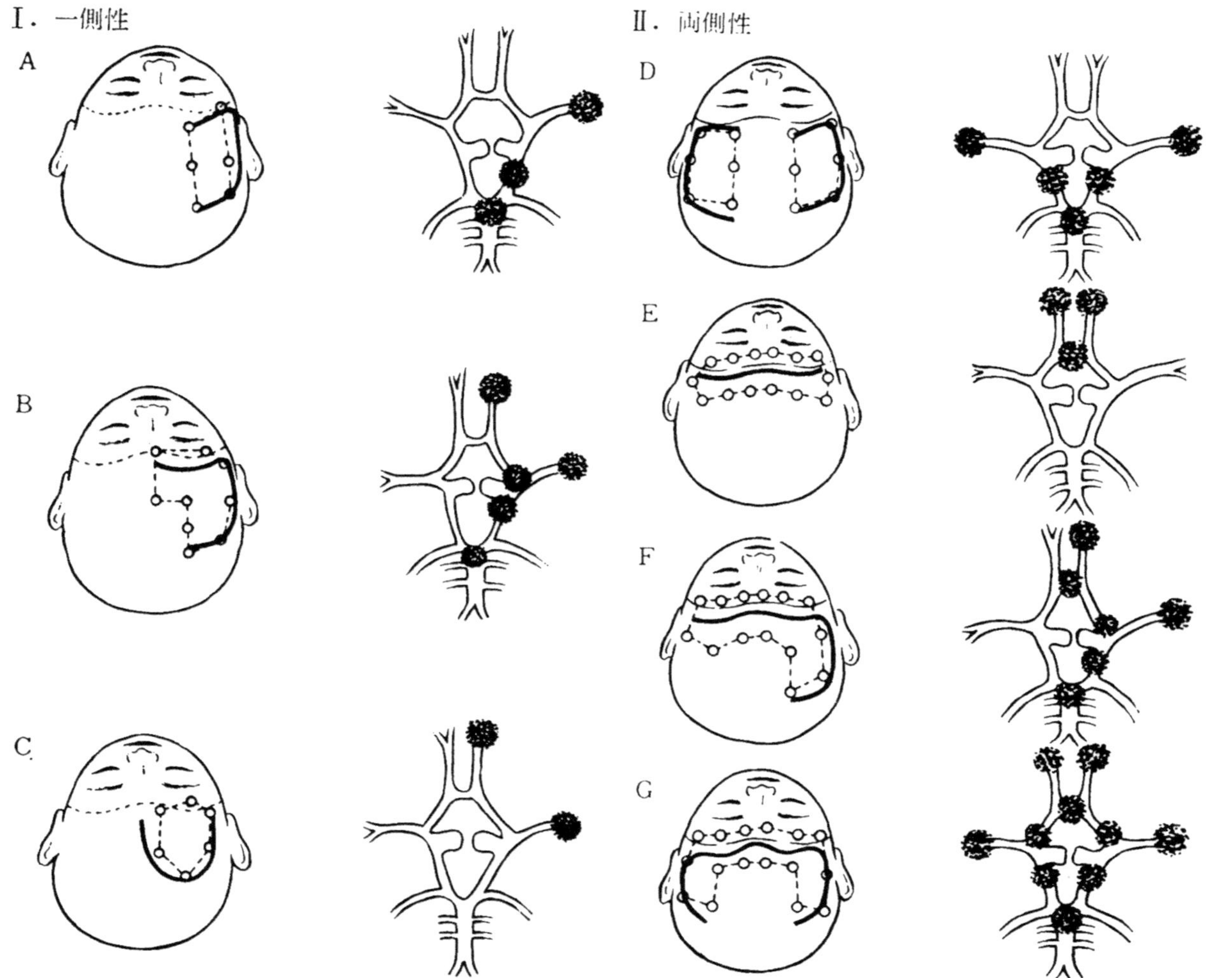

Fig. 29.2. Various cranial flaps used by Suzuki and colleagues to approach single, multiple, and bilateral aneurysms. From Suzuki J, Iwabuchi T, Takaku A, et al., ref. 199.

lateral frontal bone flap (Table 29.1; Figs. 29.5–29.10). Some had large extensions medially across the midline or laterally into the temporal bone. Others were very low, small frontal exposures (Fig. 29.9) (95,223). Gurdjian and Thomas (71) believed that with their flap extending across the midline (really a bifrontal flap) they could more easily choose either a subfrontal approach or an interhemispheric exposure with section of the falx as the situation warranted (see Fig. 29.15, below). Although many surgeons operated on the nondominant side, Poppen (159) believed that right-handed surgeons should use the right frontal approach and left-handed surgeons the left frontal approach. Martinez Coll and Del Corral (131) operated on the side from which the aneurysm filled at angiography. Skin incisions could be either unilateral or coronal for the unilateral frontal flap. Nearly all surgeons placed the patient in the standard supine position, often with the head extended to allow the frontal lobes to fall back. Sheldon et al. (183,184), however, preferred to have the patient in the prone, face-forward position (Fig. 29.10); this unusual approach was made with the retractor holding the frontal lobe vertically upward rather than horizontally toward the surgeon.

Transcallosal Approach for ACoAA

In 1944 Dandy (21) stated, "one [ACoAA] was exposed by the pineal approach and the hemorrhage was evacuated, but the aneurysm was

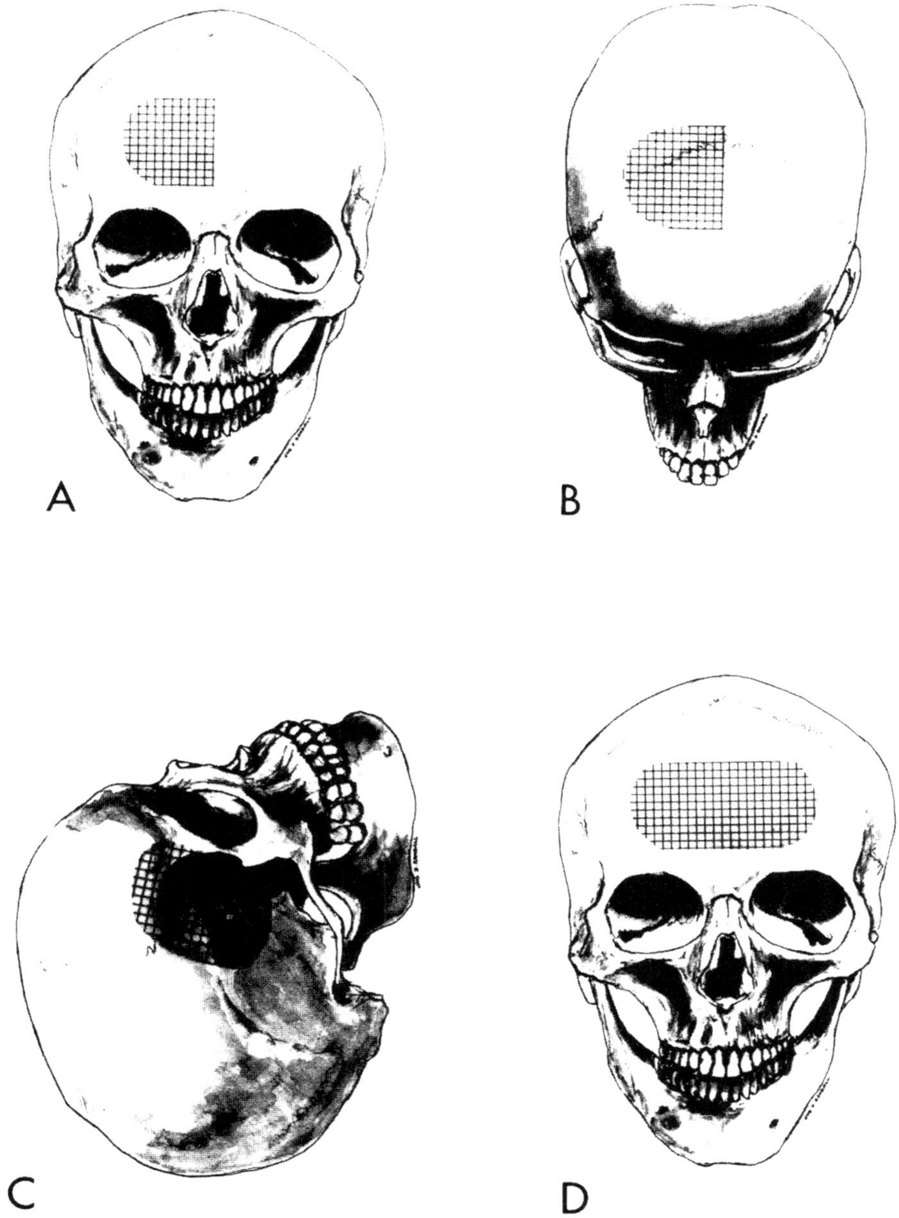

Fig. 29.3 Four basic cranial flap zones (*hatched lines*) used for approaching ACoAA. **A** Unilateral subfrontal. **B** Transcallosal. **C** Frontolateral. **D** Bifrontal. Drawings by Mr. Jno Randall, George Washington University, Washington, DC.

not seen." The ACoAA had bled into the third ventricle. This transcallosal approach, however, really originated in 1936 with Tönnis (210, 211,212) (Fig. 29.11). Basically this is a right unilateral frontal craniotomy, but the bone flap is more posterior and may include part of the parietal bone to allow access to the ACoAA through the anterior corpus callosum. This method also was used in a few patients at other clinics (Table 29.1; Fig. 29.12), but the investigators abandoned this approach for the unilateral subfrontal exposure. The technique of Tönnis required splitting the anterior corpus callosum after retracting the right frontal lobe laterally and the falx and left frontal lobe to the left.

Table 29.1. Surgical Approaches to Anterior Communicating Artery Aneurysms

Unilateral Subfrontal Approach			*Transcallosal Approach*		
Author	*Year*	*Fig.*	*Author*	*Year*	*Fig.*
Gardner (60)	1936		Tönnis (210)	1936	29.11
Jefferson (99)	1937		Hamby (75)	1952	29.12
Klemme & Woolsey (107)	1942		Norlén & Barnum (139)	1953	
Sheldon et al. (184)	1945	29.10	Norlén & Olivecrona (140)	1953	
Elvidge & Feindel (44)	1950		Hamby (76)	1954	
Sheldon et al. (183)	1950		Botterell et al. (13)	1956	
Falconer (46)	1951	29.5	Tönnis & Walter (212)	1960	
Bassett et al. (10)	1952		Harris (78)	1961	
Hamby (72)	1952		Norlén (137)	1963	
Norlén & Barnum (139)	1953	29.6	Höök & Norlén (90)	1964	
Norlén & Olivecrona (140)	1953		Tönnis & Walter (211)	1966	
Botterell et al. (13)	1956				
Asenjo & Donoso (7)	1957				
Gillingham (62)	1958				
Guidetti (64)	1958				
Krayenbühl & Yaşargil (110)	1958				
Laine (115)	1959				
Lepoire & Coxam (124)	1959				
Poppen (158)	1960	29.7			
Harris (78)	1961				
French et al. (57)	1962				
Frugoni & Conforti (58)	1962				
Lang & Poppen (121)	1962				
French et al. (54)	1963				
Norlén (137)	1963				
Höök & Norlén (90)	1964				
Poppen (159)	1964				
Thiry et al. (209)	1964				
Pool & Potts (156)	1965				
French et al. (55)	1968	29.8			
David et al. (23)	1968				
David et al. (24)	1968				
French et al. (53)	1968				
Guidetti (67)	1968				
Norlén (136)	1968				
Hamby (73)	1969				
Rand (163)	1969				
Bohm & Hugosson (11)	1970				
Drake (36)	1971				
Jamieson (98)	1971				
Pool (154)	1971				
Wilson (223)	1971	29.9			
Northfield (143)	1973				
French & Ortiz-Suarez (56)	1974				
Jain (95)	1974				
Martinez Coll & Del Corral (131)	1975				
Rand (164)	1978				

Bilateral Subfrontal Approach		
Author	*Year*	*Fig.*
Pool (153)	1959	
Pool et al. (157)	1959	
Lepoire & Coxam (124)	1959	
Pool (151)	1961	29.13
LeBeau (123)	1961	
LeBeau (122)	1962	
Pool (155)	1962	
Maspes & Marini (132)	1963	
Ranshoff (165)	1963	
Speakman & Barlass (188)	1963	29.14
Suzuki et al. (200)	1964	
Drake (34)	1965	
Pool & Potts (156)	1965	
Suzuki (196)	1966	
Suzuki et al. (199)	1967	
Guidetti (67)	1968	
Hamby (73)	1969	
Lougheed (127)	1969	
Lougheed & Marshall (130)	1969	
Gurdjian & Thomas (71)	1970	29.15
Drake (36)	1971	
Pool (154)	1971	
Pool (152)	1972	
Sundt (194)	1972	29.16
Corkill & Hodgson (17)	1973	
Lougheed & Marshall (129)	1973	29.17
Suzuki et al. (202)	1973	
Endo & Suzuki (45)	1974	
Almeida et al. (6)	1976	
Suzuki (197)	1976	
Ito (94)	1977	
Hori & Suzuki (92)	1979	

Frontolateral Approach		
Author	*Year*	*Fig.*
Dandy (19)	1942	29.18
Dandy (21)	1944	
Dandy (22)	1945	
Asenjo & Donoso (7)	1957	
Snellman et al. (187)	1959	
Laitinen (119)	1961	
Hayes & Slocum (82)	1962	
Kempe (103)	1968	29.19
Yaşargil (231)	1969	
Krayenbühl & Yaşargil (111)	1970	
VanderArk & Kempe (216)	1970	
Yaşargil (230)	1970	
Kempe & VanderArk (105)	1971	
Sano (177)	1971	29.21
De Grood (25)	1972	
Krayenbühl et al. (112)	1972	
Guidetti (66)	1973	
Bonnal et al. (12)	1974	
De Klerk & De Villiers (26)	1974	
VanderArk et al. (217)	1974	
Yaşargil & Fox (235)	1975	
Yaşargil et al. (236)	1975	
Aiba (3)	1976	
Deruty et al. (27)	1976	
Kikuchi (106)	1976	
Symon (206)	1976	
Rhoton et al. (166)	1977	
Selverstone (181)	1977	
Yaşargil & Smith (238)	1977	
Adams et al. (1)	1978	
Brock & Dietz (14)	1978	29.22
Guidetti (65)	1978	
Pia (150)	1978	
Drake (40)	1979	29.23
Fox (49)	1979	
Nornes & Wikeby (142)	1979	
Rhoton et al. (167)	1979	
Wilson & Spetzler (221)	1979	

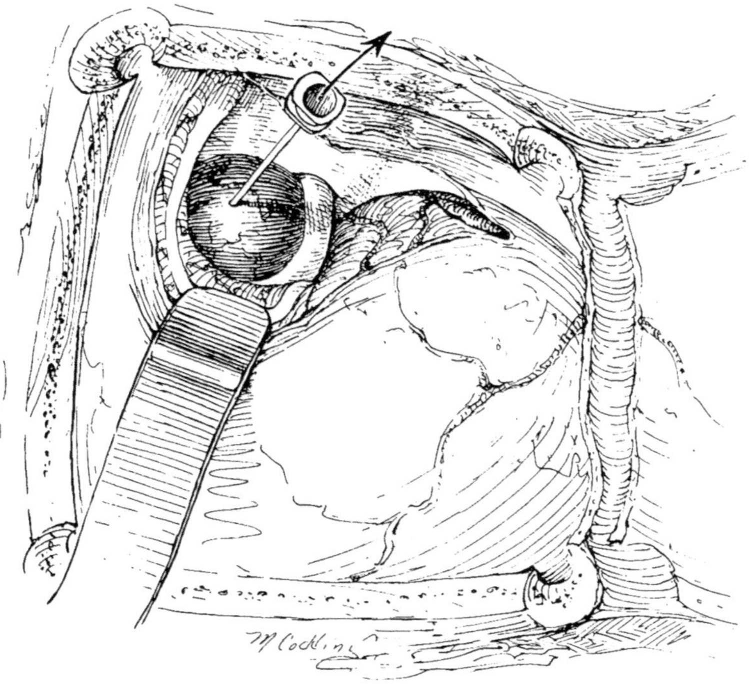

Fig. 29.4. Cushing's 1929 sketch of a large suprasellar aneurysm pushing up from under the optic chiasm and optic nerves. The preoperative diagnosis was pituitary adenoma, but needle puncture after the unilateral subfrontal craniotomy proved the tumor to be an aneurysm. Cushing said, "From just what branch of the circle the aneurysm actually took its origin is problematic, but in view of its position beneath the chiasm, it probably arose from the posterior communicating artery on the side of primary blindness." From Cushing H, ref. 18.

Bilateral Frontal Approach for ACoAA

In 1959 Pool et al. (153,157) and Lepoire and Coxam (124) separately reported a bifrontal approach to ACoAA. Pool subsequently popularized this technique (Fig. 29.13) in several publications (151,152,154–156). Using this technique the falx and anterior part of the superior sagittal sinus were sectioned, allowing lateral, superior, and posterior displacement of both frontal lobes. The aneurysm was exposed by the interhemispheric route, which usually required sacrificing both olfactory nerves. This method has been used by a number of other neurosurgeons (Table 29.1; Figs. 29.13–29.17). Pool himself used a fairly small bone flap with four burr holes. Others, such as Maspes and Marini (132), preferred a larger flap. Drake (34) and Sundt (194) often did not cut the falx, starting their approach under the right frontal lobe after removing the bifrontal bone flap. Rarely, resection of frontal lobe tissue was needed (156). Usually a free bone flap was turned. Variations included either leaving the bone attached to one temporalis muscle or splitting the bone flap, leaving half of it attached to each tempo-

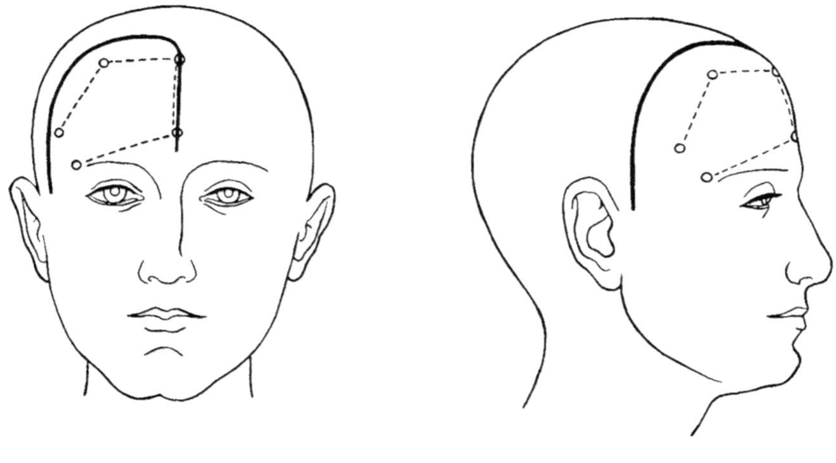

Fig. 29.5. Falconer's 1951 unilateral frontal approach to ACoAA. A minor modification of the same flap was used for ICAA and MCAA. The bone flap was frontal even though the skin incision extended into the temporal region. From Falconer MA, ref. 46.

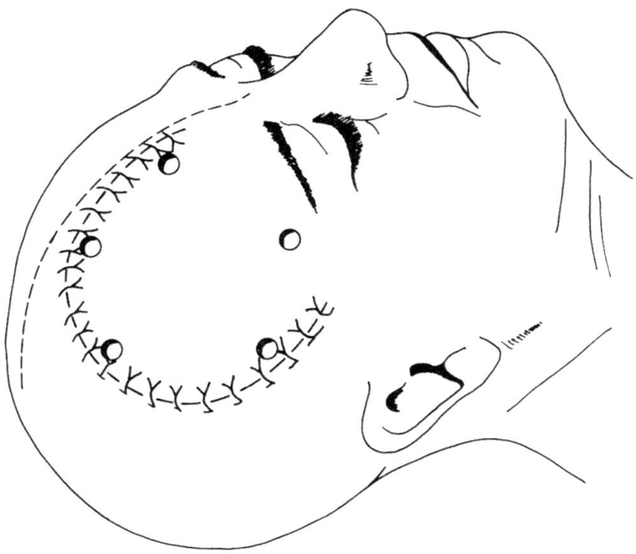

Fig. 29.6. Unilateral subfrontal flap used in 1953 by Norlén and Barnum for ACoAA. From Norlén G, Barnum AS, ref. 139.

ralis muscle. Sometimes the flap was centered a little toward the right. Suzuki et al. (202) stated that their approach avoided injury to either olfactory nerve while allowing a good exposure.

Frontolateral Approach for ACoAA

In 1942 Dandy (19), at The Johns Hopkins Hospital, reported his pterional, or frontotemporal, approach to a large ACoAA excised in 1941

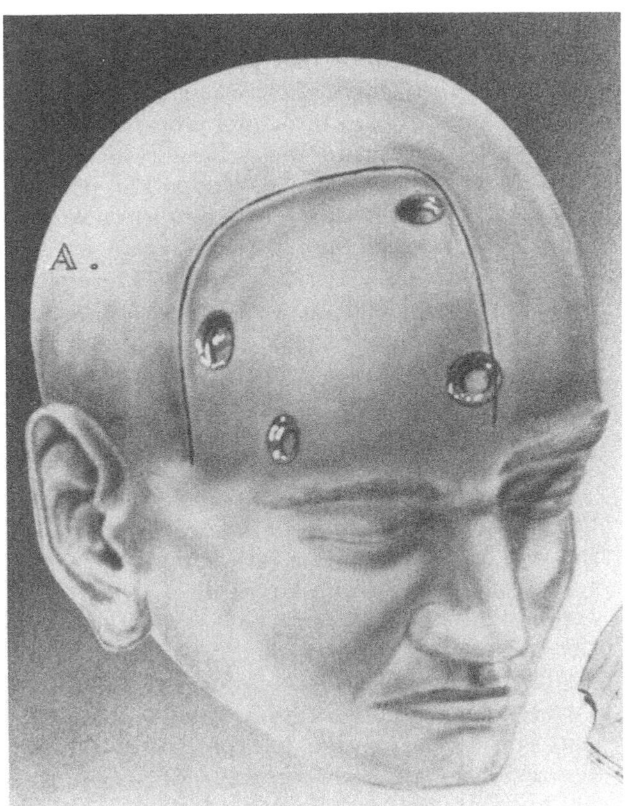

Fig. 29.7. Poppen's 1960 unilateral subfrontal approach to ACoAA. From Poppen JL, ref. 158.

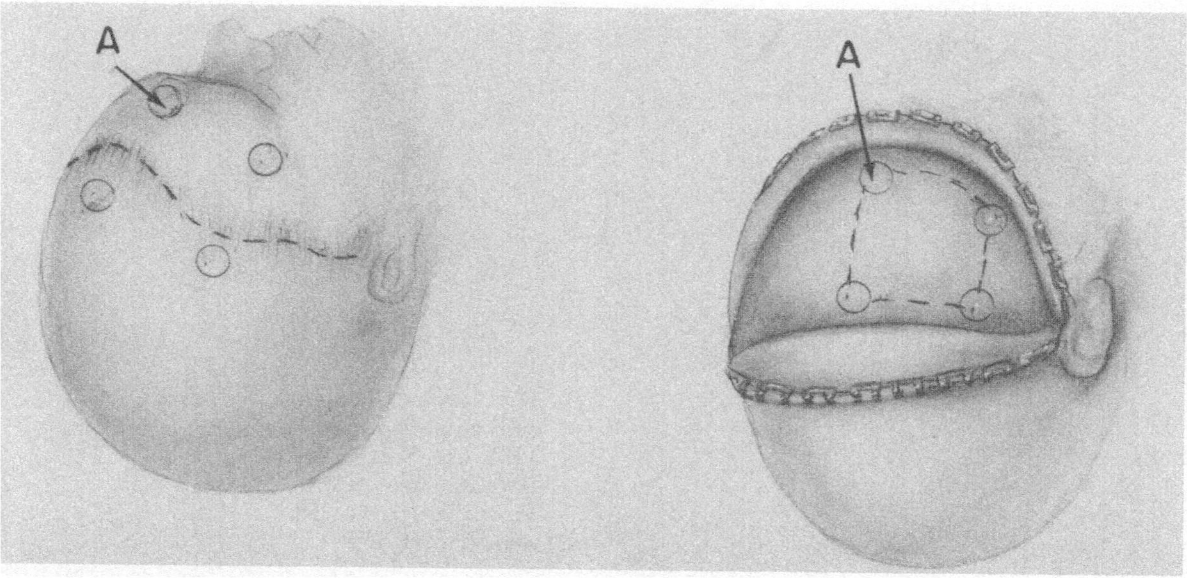

Fig. 29.8. Unilateral frontal flap turned by French and his colleagues for ACoAA in 1966. They used a coronal skin incision. From French LA, Chou SN, Story JL, et al., ref. 55.

(Fig. 29.18). This "Dandy flap" actually appears to be a modification of the approach suggested in 1918 by Heuer (85–87), one of Dandy's students. Heuer used the flap for sellar and suprasellar tumors. Dandy (19,21,22,102) continued to use this "hypophyseal" approach with the skin incision concealed behind the hairline. This approach, or its modification, has been utilized by others (Table 29.1; Figs. 29.19–29.23), especially Dandy's trainees and their students. Among Dandy's residents using the pterional approach are Woodhall (144,225), Rizzoli (49), and Hayes (81,82). Kempe (103,105,216,217), an associate of Hayes, described the commonly used modification of this pterional flap (Fig. 29.19). The critical burr hole was at the junction of the temporal line, the zygomatic process of the frontal bone, and the orbital ridge. This became known as the "psychopathic point" (105,217), probably in reference to the disposition of the surgeon should the assistant fail to place the burr hole correctly! Dandy's disciples routinely ronguered away the sphenoid wing to gain a low, basal exposure of the aneurysm. Fox (49) learned this frontolateral approach from Rizzoli, Hayes, and Kempe, and later added some of the microsurgical techniques of Yaşargil.

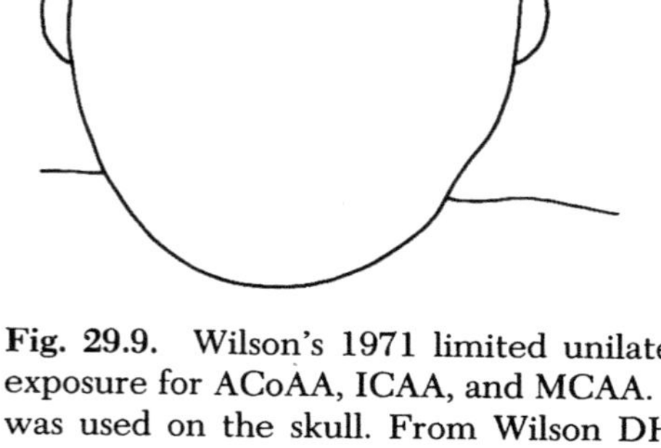

Fig. 29.9. Wilson's 1971 limited unilateral frontal exposure for ACoAA, ICAA, and MCAA. A trephine was used on the skull. From Wilson DH, ref. 223.

Yaşargil (111,112,230,231,235,236,238) further modified this pterional approach by making it a frontosphenoidal rather than a frontotemporal craniotomy. He drilled down the sphenoid bone and orbital roof projections under the operating microscope. A model of the frontosphenoidal flap is seen in Fig. 29.20. Yaşargil et al. (236) on occasion actually removed part of the orbital ridge and roof and retracted the orbital tissue if the orbital roof had a pronounced upward extension.

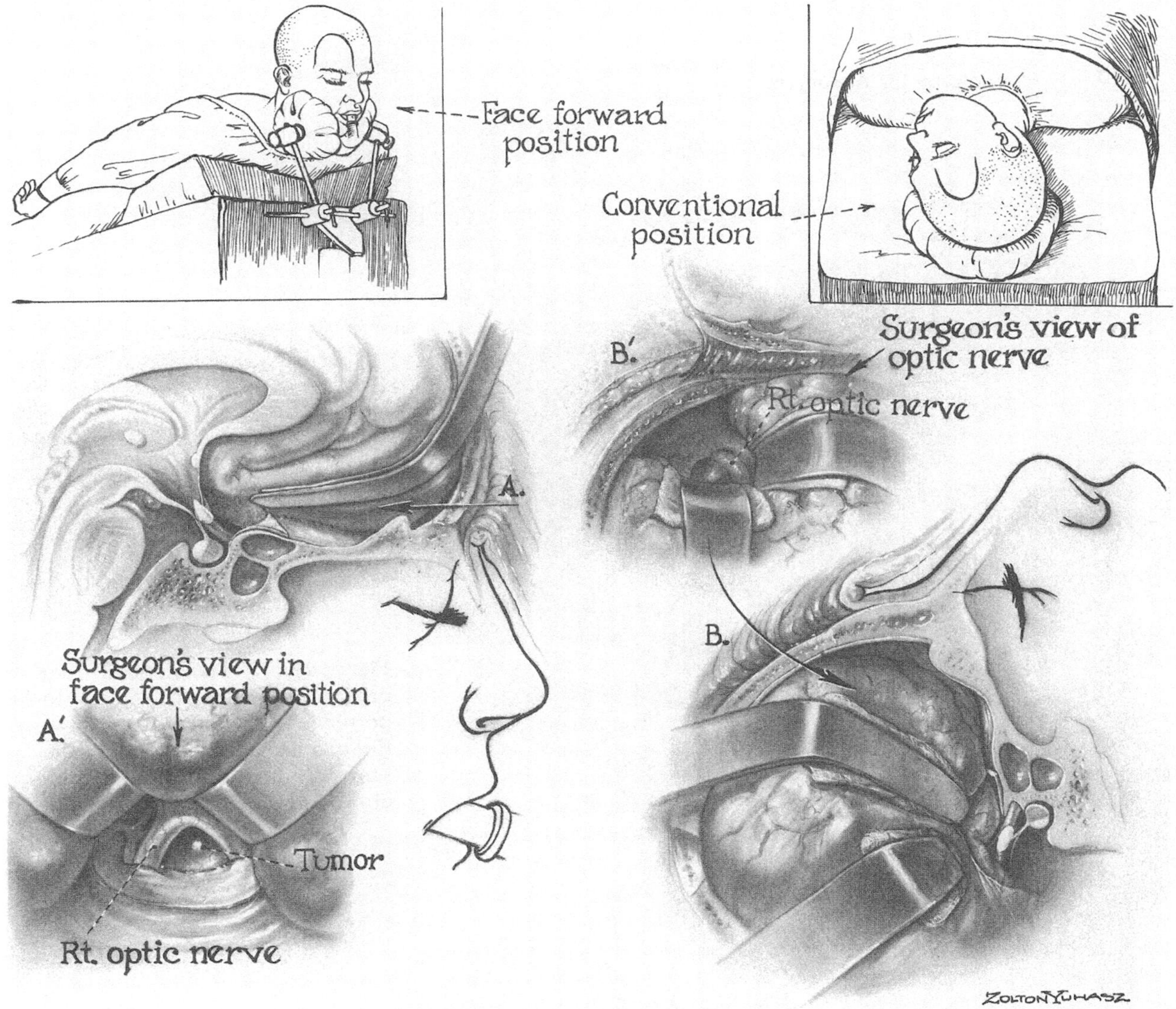

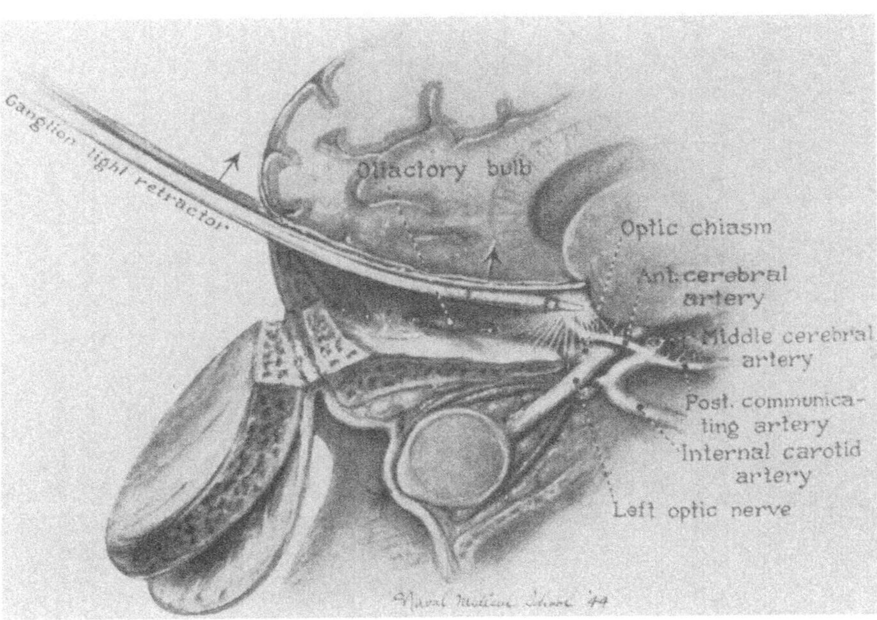

Fig. 29.10. *Left.* Above insert illustrates face-forward prone position and unilateral frontal craniotomy described by Sheldon and co-workers in 1945. **A** View as diagrammed from side projection. **A′** Diagram of surgeon's view. *Below.* Lighted retractor elevating frontal lobe. *Right.* Above insert illustrates conventional position of patient for right frontal craniotomy. **B′** Diagram of surgeon's view between frontal and temporal lobes. **B** Modified side projection of the same. Modified from Sheldon CH, Pudenz RH, Restarski JS, ref. 184. Courtesy of C. Hunter Sheldon, May 1982.

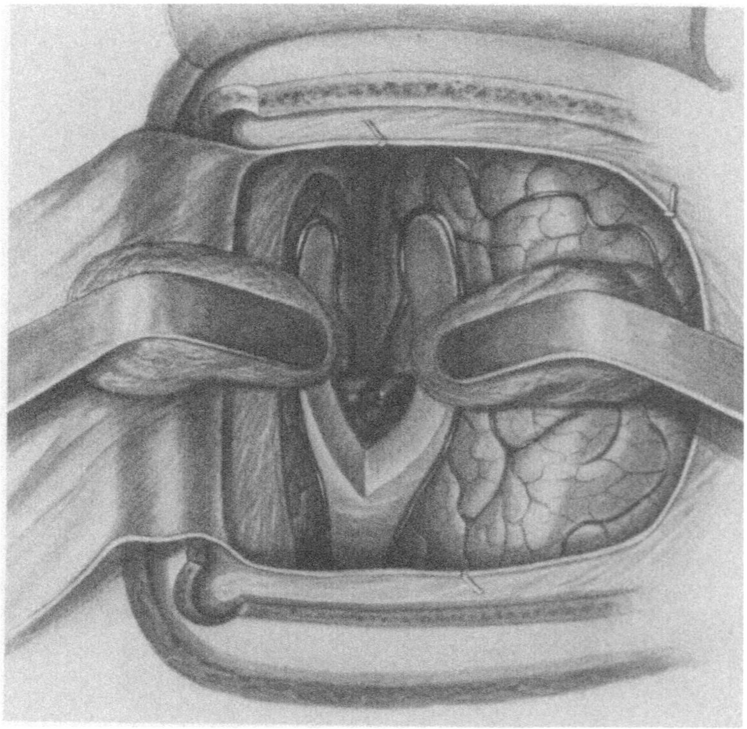

Fig. 29.11. Transcallosal approach of Tönnis to ACoAA reported in 1936. Retractors separate the two halves of the corpus callosum via a high right frontal craniotomy. From Tönnis W, ref. 210.

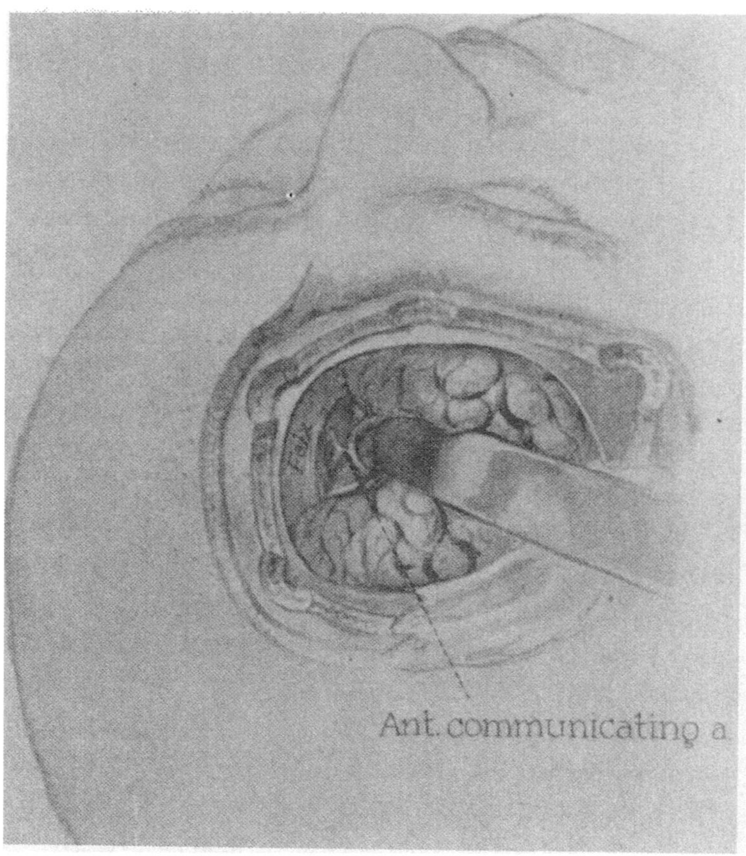

Fig. 29.12. Hamby's 1952 frontal transcallosal exposure for ACoAA. From Hamby WB, ref. 75.

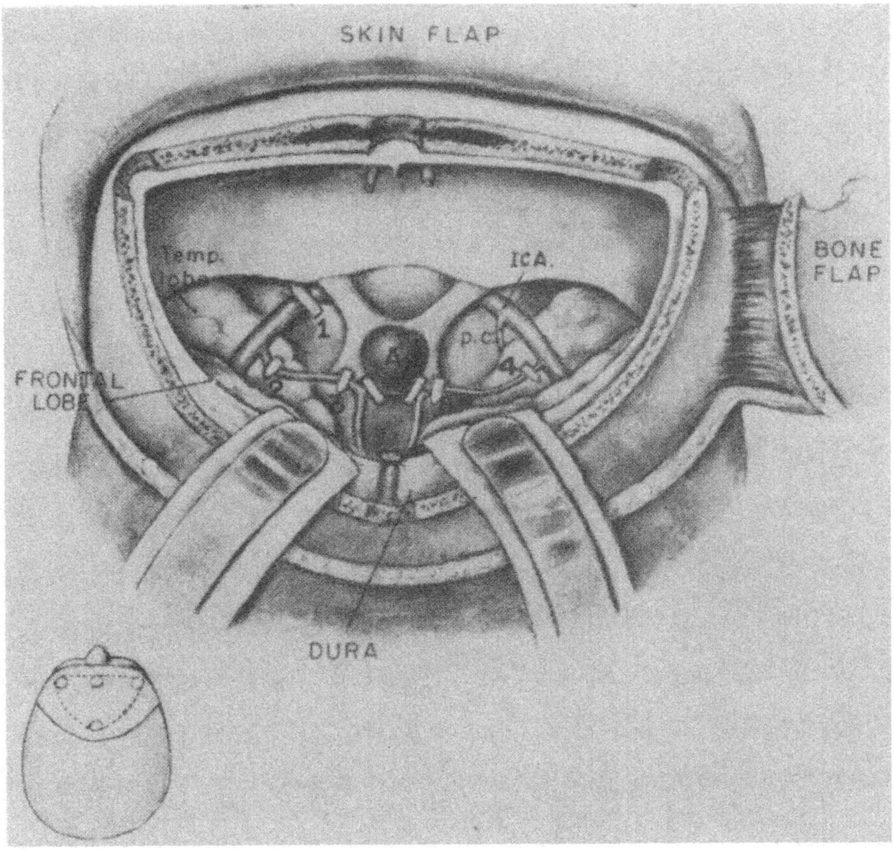

Fig. 29.13. Pool's 1961 bifrontal craniotomy for ACoAA. Note the wide exposure, use of temporary clips (*1–4*), and severance of the falx and both olfactory nerves. The bone flap is attached to the right temporalis muscle. From Pool JL, ref. 151.

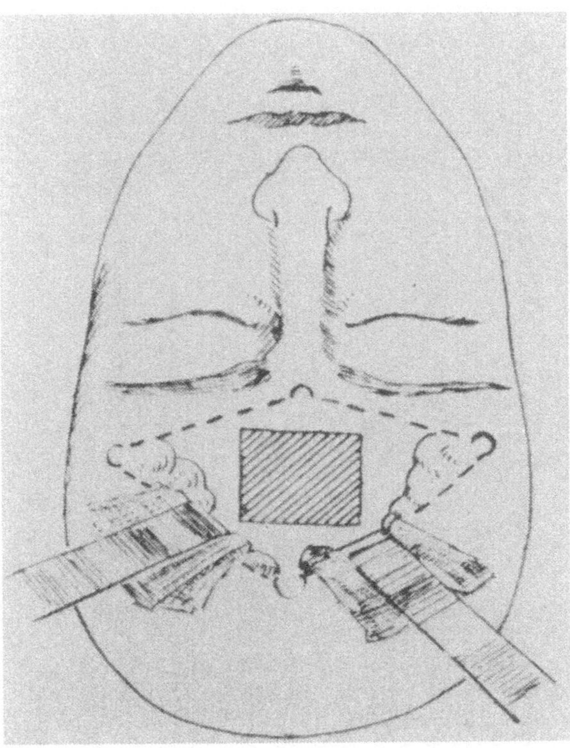

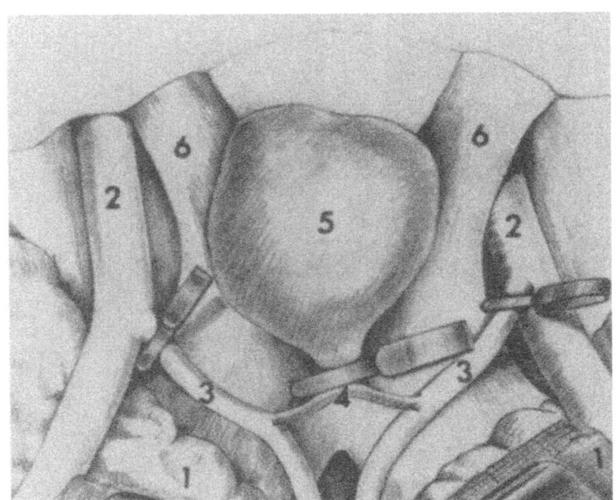

Fig. 29.14. Bifrontal approach of Speakman and Barlass for ACoAA in 1963. *1,* Frontal lobe. *2,* ICA. *3,* A-1 arteries. *4,* ACoA. *5,* ACoAA. *6,* Optic nerves. Note temporary Mayfield clips on the A-1 arteries and Mayfield clip on ACoAA neck. From Speakman TJ, Barlass JL, ref. 188.

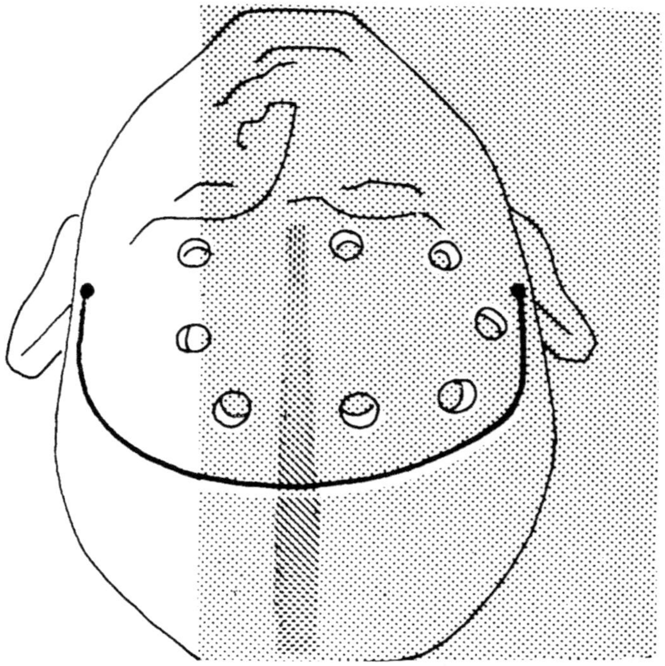

Fig. 29.15. Bifrontal approach of Gurdjian and Thomas for ACoAA. From Gurdjian ES, Thomas LM, ref. 71.

The frontolateral approach has gained popularity in recent years (Table 29.1). Some have made the flap smaller so that it is mainly a sphenoidal-temporal flap (Fig. 29.21) (177) or a lateral frontal flap (Fig. 29.22) (14). It has the advantage, if sphenoid bone is partially removed, of shortening the distance to the ACoAA by at least 1 cm compared with the frontal approach. Moreover, multiple aneurysms, including the bBAA, can be attacked by the same approach. See Chapter 35 for additional details.

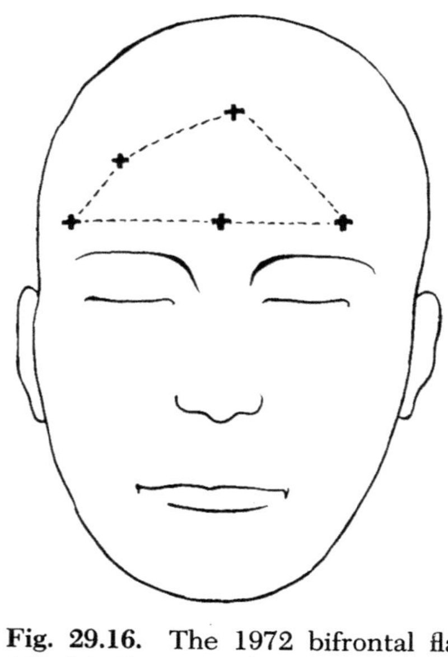

Fig. 29.16. The 1972 bifrontal flap of Sundt for ACoAA. From Sundt TM Jr, ref. 194.

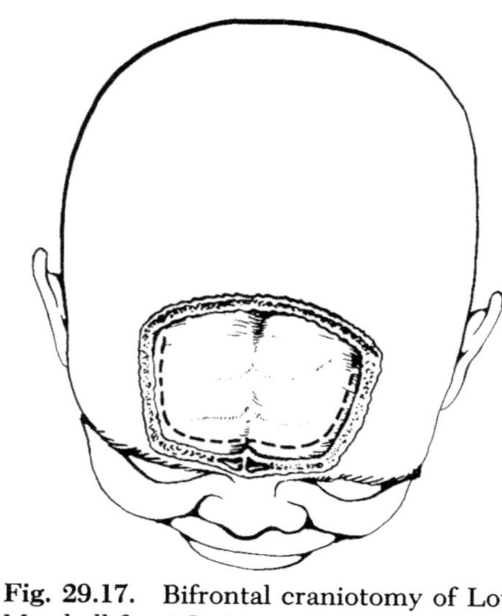

Fig. 29.17. Bifrontal craniotomy of Lougheed and Marshall for ACoAA in 1973. From Lougheed WM, Marshall BM, ref. 129.

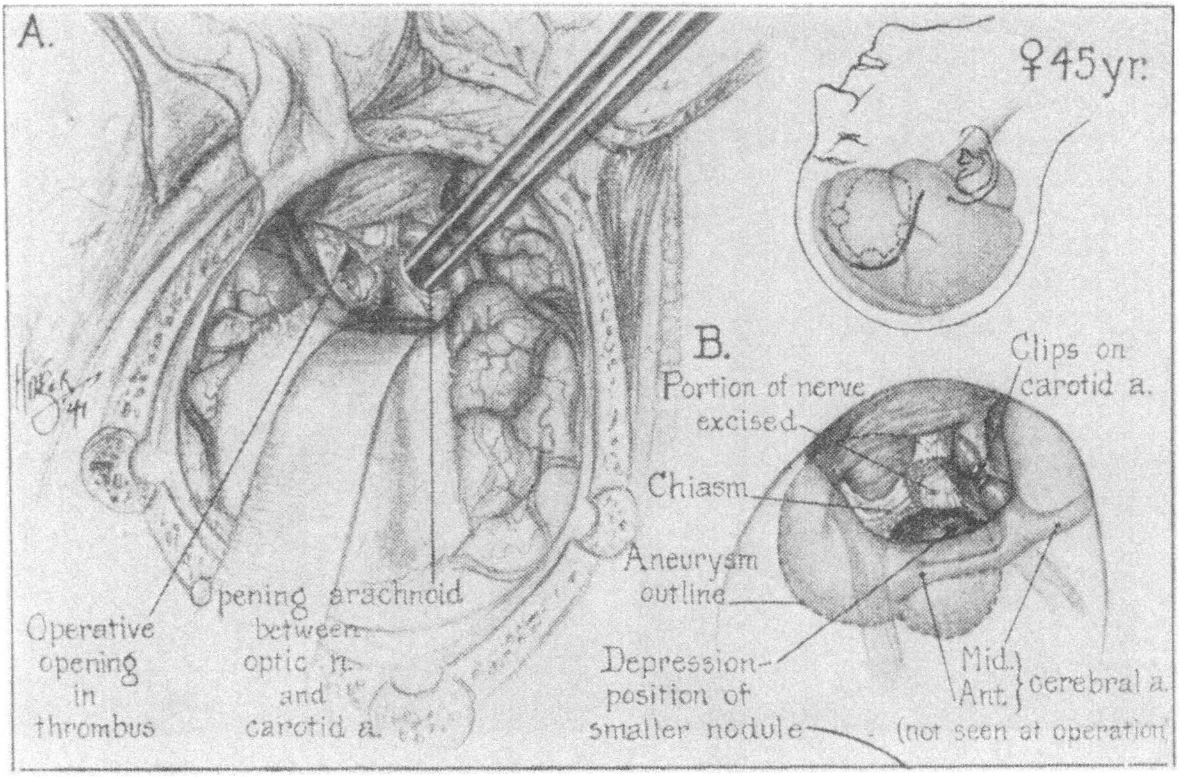

Fig. 29.18. A Dandy's forceps opening arachnoid in chiasmatic cistern. **B,** *top* Dandy's frontolateral (pterional) flap for a giant ACoAA in 1942. **B,** *bottom* Outline of aneurysm and environs. From Dandy WE, ref. 19.

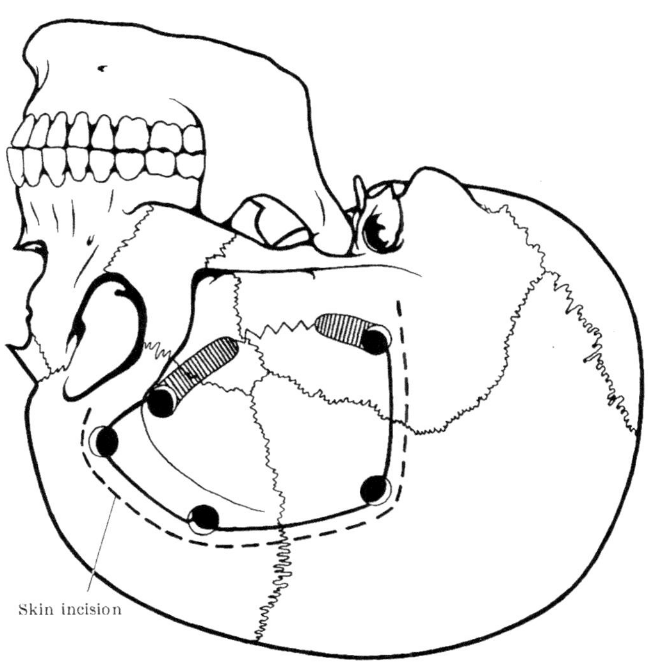

Fig. 29.19. Kempe's 1968 frontolateral (pterional) flap for ACoAA, ICAA, and MCAA. From Kempe LG, ref. 103.

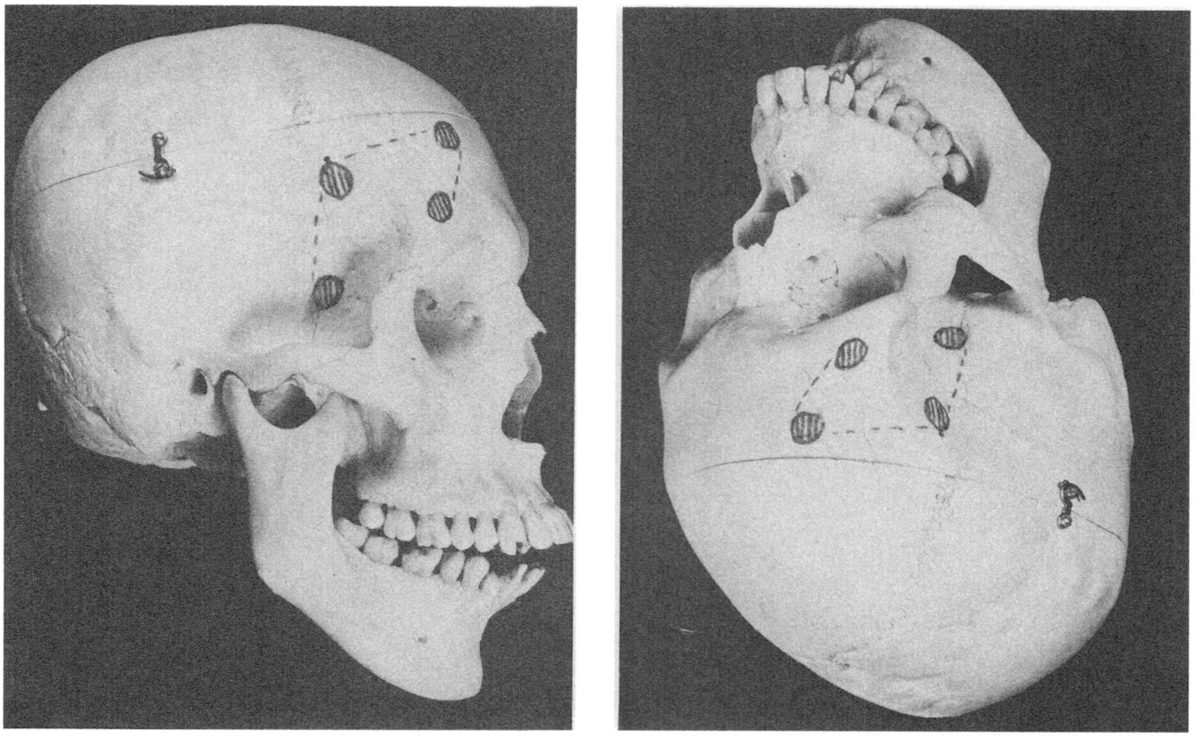

A B

Fig. 29.20. Model skull with outline of the frontosphenoidal type of frontolateral cranial opening for most aneurysms on the circle of Willis. **A** Lateral view. **B** Surgeon's view.

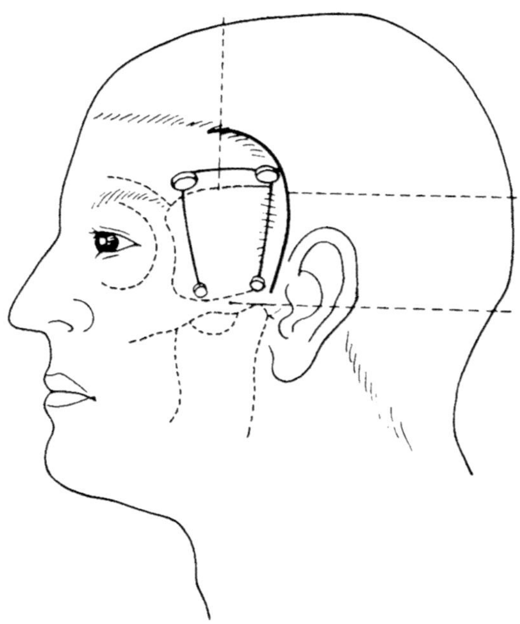

Fig. 29.21. Sano's 1971 frontolateral craniotomy for ACoAA, ICAA, and MCAA. From Sano K, ref. 177.

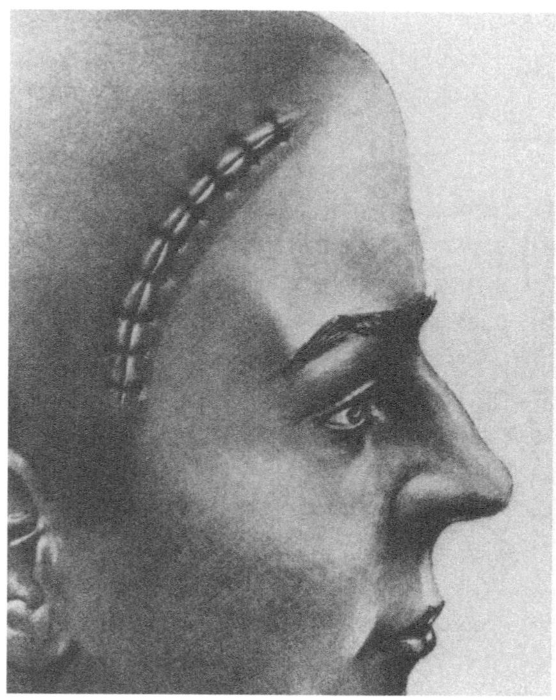

Fig. 29.22. The small frontolateral cranial exposure of Brock and Dietz in 1978 for ACoAA, ICAA, and MCAA. From Brock M, Dietz H, ref. 14.

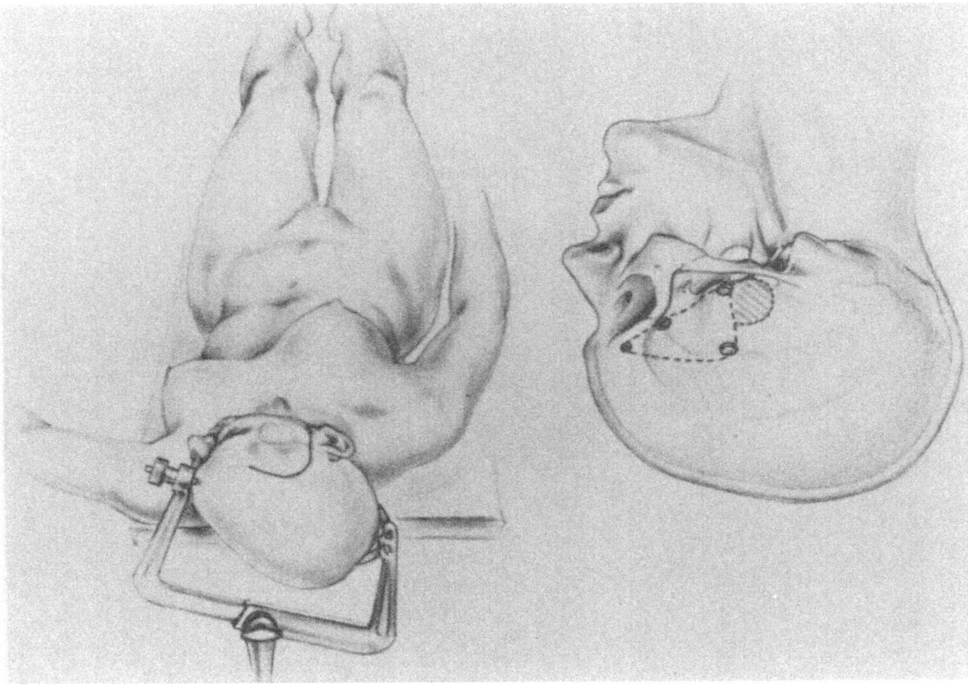

Fig. 29.23. Drake's 1979 frontolateral craniotomy for ACoAA, ICAA, and MCAA. It is sometimes used for BAA when multiple aneurysms are present, in which case the flap is extended posteriorly (*shaded zone*). From Drake CG, ref. 40.

Anterior Cerebral Artery Aneurysms

In 1949 Whalley (219) reported a case of ruptured ACeAA distal to the ACoA that was operated and trapped via a frontal craniotomy. Krayenbühl and Richter (109) reported on another ACeAA case operated and clipped by a similar approach. Subsequently a number of cases of direct surgery on these aneurysms appeared in the literature. The unilateral frontal, parasagittal bone flap (higher than that for the ACoAA, often including the parietal bone, and often extending across the midline) has become the standard approach (13,120,150,204,220, 221,234,240). Suzuki et al. (204) and Yoshimoto et al. (240) used this unilateral parasagittal craniotomy flap for aneurysms behind the genu of the corpus callosum; for those between the genu and the ACoA, they used the bifrontal flap. Figure 29.24 shows a parasagittal frontal flap for clipping ACeAA at the genu of the corpus callosum. A more posterior flap is needed for aneurysms behind the genu.

Internal Carotid Artery Aneurysms

There are three basic approaches to the ICAA (Table 29.2): (a) frontal; (b) temporal; and (c) frontolateral. Except for the temporal approach, these were discussed in the preceding section. An unusual exception is Finkemeyer's transethmoidal-transphenoidal attack to pack (with muscle) a traumatic csICAA (48).

Frontal Approach for ICAA

The first case of a ruptured intracranial aneurysm diagnosed before surgery was a patient with a bICAA at the M-1 take-off. This was operated by Dott (29) in 1931 and reported in 1933 as being done by a frontal approach. The approach is similar to that for the ACoAA except the line of attack is directed more laterally under the frontal lobe (Figs. 29.25, 29.26). Table 29.2 lists the authors who have mentioned using such an approach. Often the bone flap was large, becoming almost a frontotemporal flap.

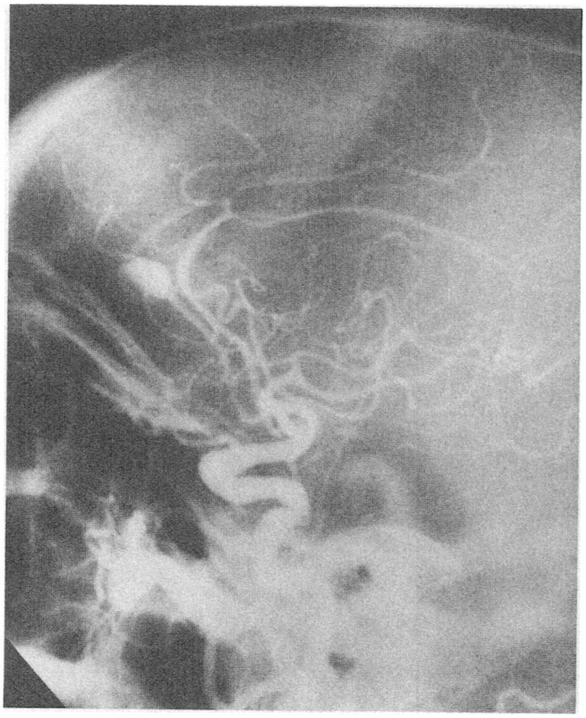

A

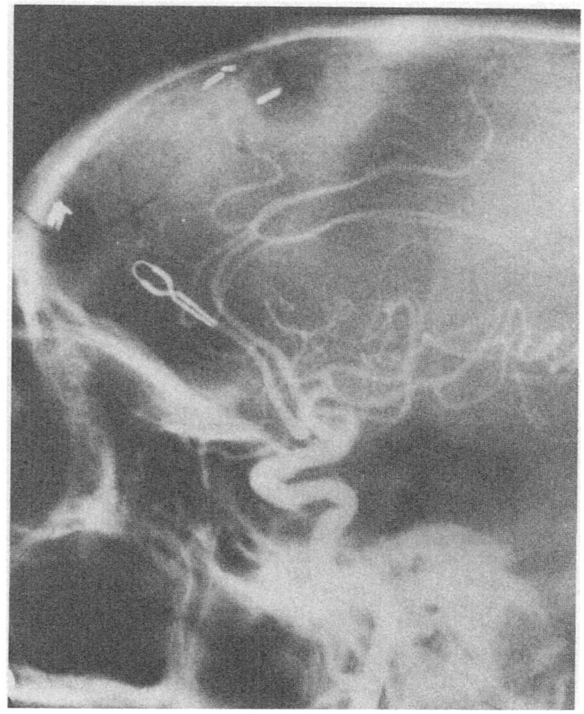

B

Fig. 29.24. **A** Angiogram showing ACeAA at or just below the genu of the corpus callosum. **B** Lateral view of bone flap (parasagittal, frontal) after clipping.

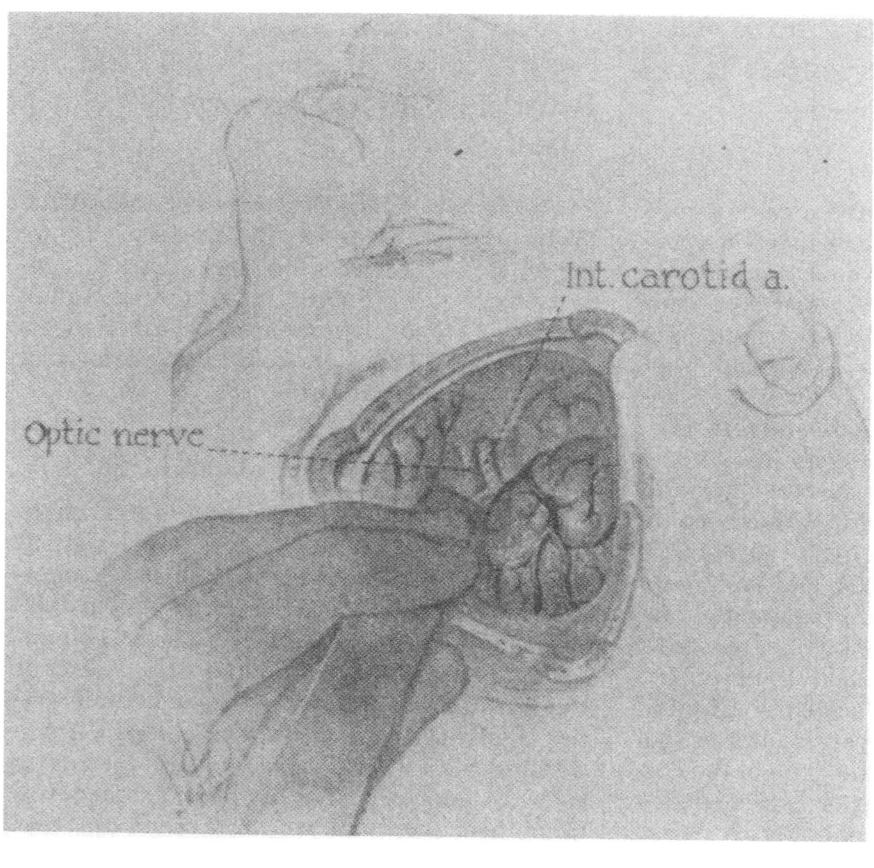

Fig. 29.25. Hamby's 1952 subfrontal approach to ICAA. From Hamby WB, ref. 75.

Table 29.2. Surgical Approaches to Internal Carotid Artery Aneurysms

Frontal Approach			*Temporal Approach*			*Frontolateral Approach*		
Author	*Year*	*Fig.*	*Author*	*Year*	*Fig.*	*Author*	*Year*	*Fig.*
Dott (29)	1933		Trevani (213)	1932		Dandy (20)	1938	29.1
Jefferson (99)	1937		Gardner (60)	1936		Dandy (21)	1944	
List & Hodges (125)	1946		Jefferson (99)	1937		Hamby (75)	1952	
Falconer (46)	1951	29.5	Norlén & Olivecrona (140)	1953		Steelman et al. (189)	1953	
Bassett et al. (10)	1952		Uihlein & Hughes (214)	1955	29.27	Hamby (76)	1954	
Hamby (72)	1952		Botterell et al. (13)	1956		af Björkesten (2)	1958	
Hamby (75)	1952	29.25	Harris & Udvarhelyi (79)	1957		Krayenbühl & Yaşargil (110)	1958	
Hamby (76)	1954		Gillingham (62)	1958		Tönnis & Walter (212)	1960	
Drake (34)	1965		Poppen (158)	1960	29.28	Pertuiset (148)	1962	
Rana (162)	1965		Suzuki et al. (198)	1965	29.30	Lougheed et al. (128)	1963	
Pertuiset et al. (149)	1966		Suzuki (196)	1966		Pool & Potts (156)	1965	
Drake et al. (42a)	1968		Suzuki et al. (199)	1967		Tönnis & Walter (211)	1966	
Drake et al. (42b)	1968		Kunc (113)	1968		Kempe (103)	1968	29.19
Hamby (73)	1969		Gurdjian & Thomas (71)	1970	29.29	Paterson (145)	1968	
Guidetti & La Torre (68)	1970		Suzuki et al. (203)	1970		Lougheed (127)	1969	
Drake (36)	1971	29.26				Sundt & Murphy (195)	1969	
Wilson (223)	1971	29.9				Yaşargil (231)	1969	
						Krayenbühl & Yaşargil (111)	1970	
						Yaşargil (230)	1970	
						Kempe & VanderArk (105)	1971	
						Paterson (146)	1971	
						Sano (177)	1971	29.21
						De Grood (25)	1972	
						Krayenbühl et al. (112)	1972	
						Corkill & Hodgson (17)	1973	
						Guidetti (66)	1973	
						Lougheed & Marshall (129)	1973	29.31
						Bonnal et al. (12)	1974	
						De Klerk & De Villiers (26)	1974	
						Peerless (147)	1974	
						VanderArk et al. (217)	1974	
						Guidetti & La Torre (69)	1975	
						Sengupta et al. (182)	1975	
						Yada & Owada (228)	1975	
						Yaşargil & Fox (235)	1975	
						Aiba (3)	1976	
						Deruty et al. (27)	1976	
						Kikuchi (106)	1976	
						Symon (206)	1976	
						Hollin & Decker (89)	1977	
						Rhoton et al. (166)	1977	
						Selverstone (181)	1977	
						Yaşargil et al. (237)	1977	
						Yaşargil & Smith (238)	1977	
						Adams et al. (1)	1978	
						Brock & Dietz (14)	1978	29.22
						Guidetti (65)	1978	
						Pia (150)	1978	
						Rand (164)	1978	
						Yaşargil et al. (233)	1978	
						Drake (40)	1979	29.23
						Fox (49)	1979	
						Nornes & Wikeby (142)	1979	
						Rhoton et al. (167)	1979	
						Salazar (173)	1979	
						Viale & Pau (218)	1979	
						Wilson & Spetzler (221)	1979	

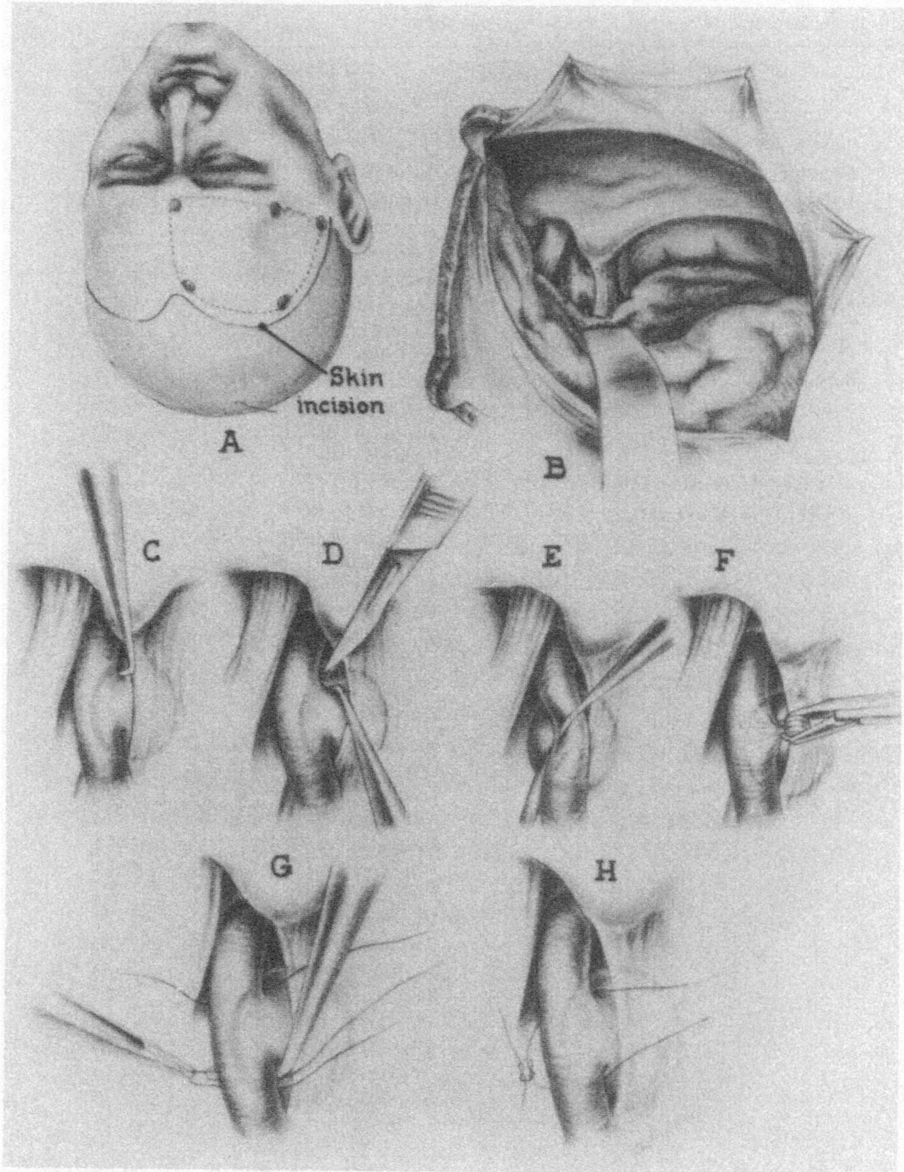

Fig. 29.26. Drake's 1971 subfrontal approach to ICAA. **A** Note temporal extension of frontal bone flap. **B** Elevation of frontal lobe. **C–E** Dissection ICAA. **F** Applying Scoville clip. **G–H** Applying ligature. From Drake CG, ref. 36.

Temporal Approach for ICAA

In 1932 Trevani (213) described a large temporal flap extending into the frontal and parietal regions. He was exploring the patient for a tumor and found a giant ICAA. In 1936 Gardner (60) reported on a case operated by the temporal route for a hypophyseal tumor that turned out to be an ICAA. The aneurysm ruptured and required packing with gauze, which became infected and was removed 2 years later. Similarly, in 1937 Jefferson (99) reported a case of a giant ICAA exposed during exploration for tumor. Others subsequently used the temporal route for planned operations on ICAA (Table 29.2; Figs. 29.27–29.30). Harris and Udvarhelyi (79) recommended a small subtemporal craniectomy instead of craniotomy. Suzuki et al. (196,198,199,203) described their unusual "temporal keel form incision" in which the base of the skin flap was superior rather than inferior (Fig. 29.30), resembling the keel of a boat.

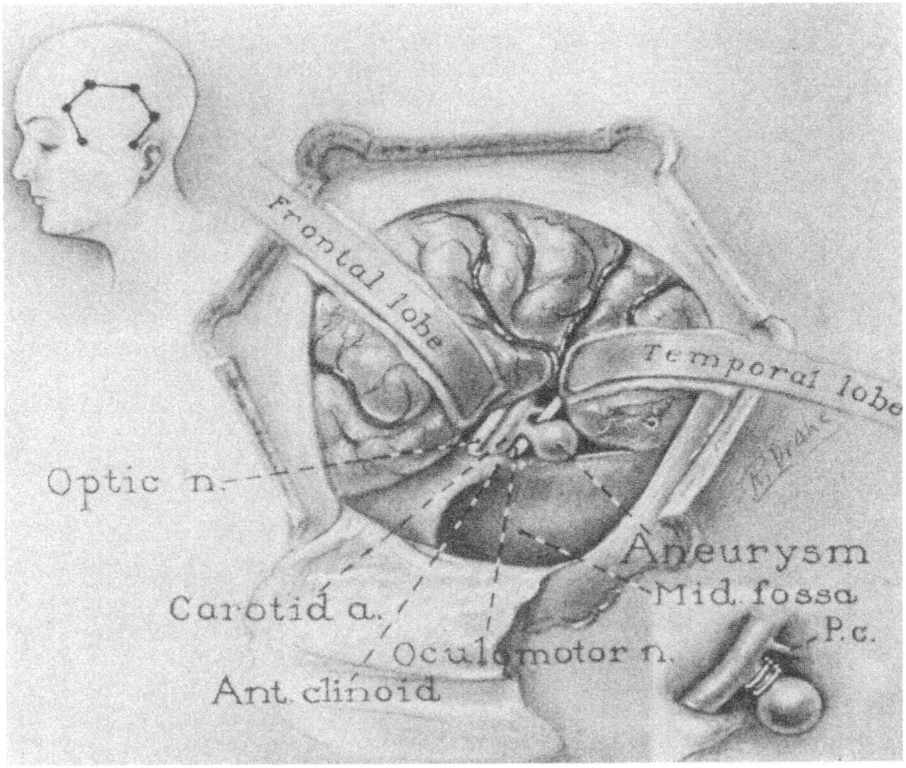

Fig. 29.27. Temporal craniotomy by Uihlein and Hughes for ICAA in 1955. From Uihlein A, Hughes RA, ref. 214.

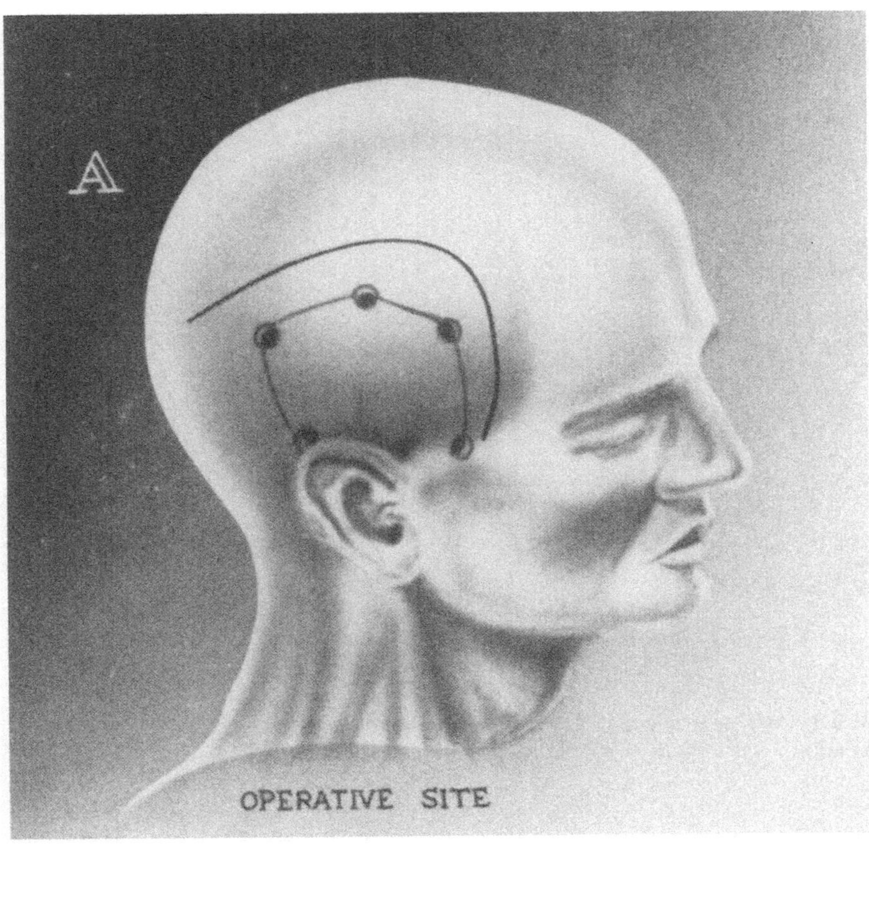

Fig. 29.28. Poppen's 1960 temporal craniotomy for ICAA and MCAA. From Poppen JL, ref. 158.

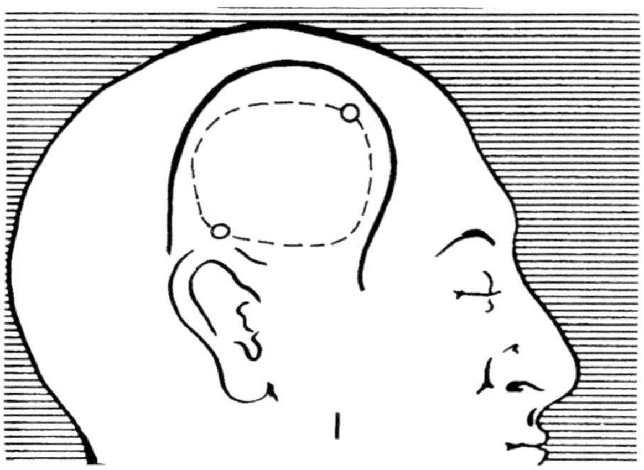

Fig. 29.29. Temporal flap used by Gurdjian and Thomas for ICAA. From Gurdjian ES, Thomas LM, ref. 71.

Frontolateral Approach for ICAA

In 1938 Dandy (20) reported his frontolateral "hypophyseal" approach to a pcaICAA (Fig. 29.1). This was the first aneurysm treated by application of a metallic (silver) clip to its neck. Since then the frontolateral approach to the ICAA has been the one most commonly used (Table 29.2). Most surgeons utilize an approach between the frontal and temporal lobes, opening the sylvian fissure to various degrees. Descriptions of the flap (Fig. 29.31) are given in the previous section for ACoAA. Also see Chapter 36 for additional details.

Middle Cerebral Artery Aneurysms

Direct attack on the MCAA was much less common in earlier days than the direct approach to ACoAA or ICAA. Craniotomy, if done, was

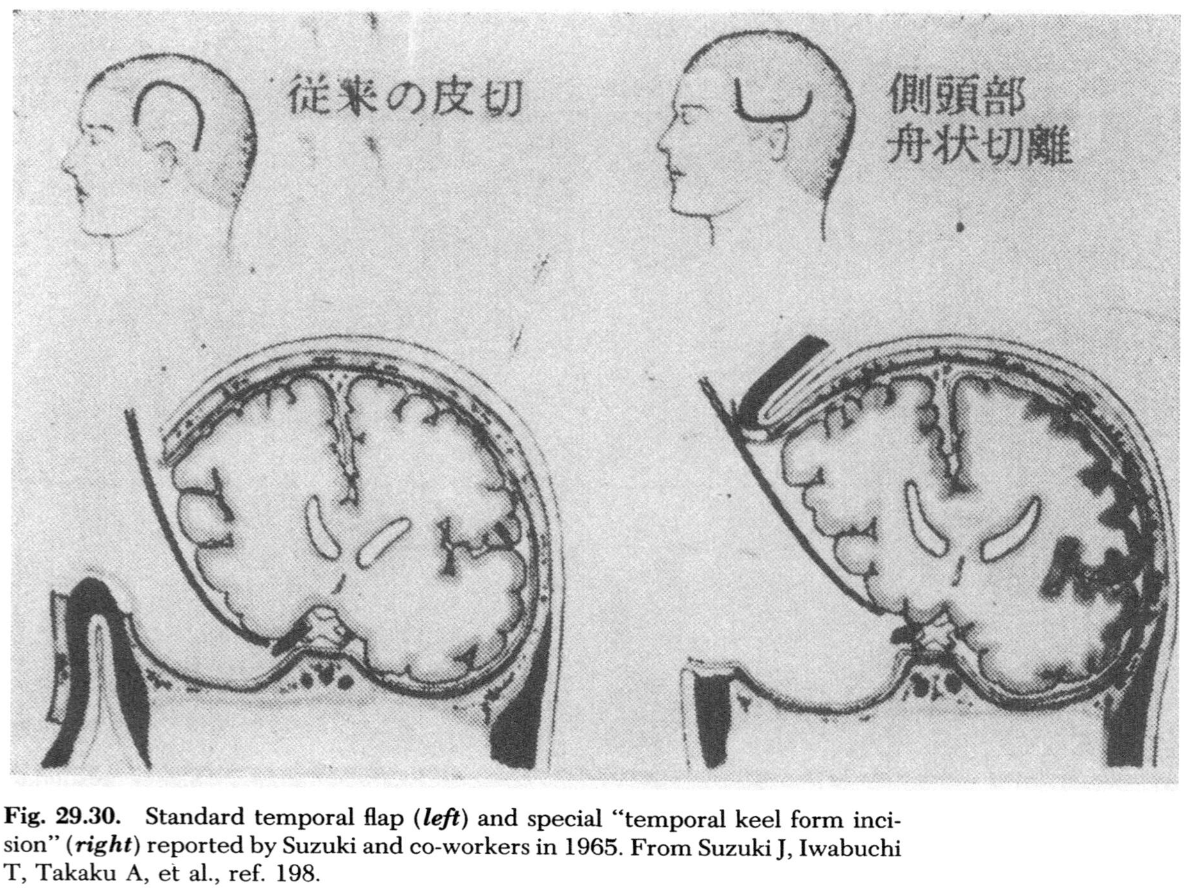

Fig. 29.30. Standard temporal flap (*left*) and special "temporal keel form incision" (*right*) reported by Suzuki and co-workers in 1965. From Suzuki J, Iwabuchi T, Takaku A, et al., ref. 198.

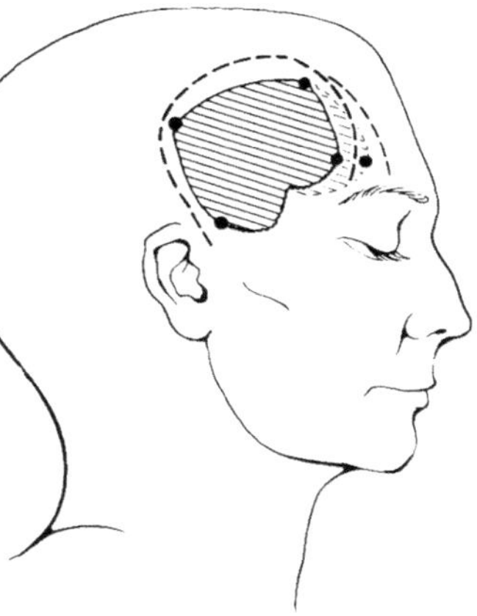

Fig. 29.31. Frontolateral flap used by Lougheed and Marshall for ICAA and MCAA in 1973. From Lougheed WM, Marshall BM, ref. 129.

usually performed to explore for a tumor or clot and for decompression (43,63,171). These aneurysms were mainly treated by cervical carotid artery ligation unless a hematoma forced a craniotomy. In 1944 Dandy (21) operated on four such cases with poor results (the patients had either a giant aneurysm or a hematoma). He did not detail his approach, although it is likely he used some modification of his standard frontotemporal flap. Reports of MCAA surgery were forthcoming after the 1940s (Table 29.3).

Frontal Approach for MCAA

The frontal approach for the MCAA is not commonly used. The unilateral subfrontal flap has already been described, in the previous section on ACoAA.

Temporal Approach for MCAA

In 1948 Swain (205) turned a large temporal flap extending into the parietal and frontal regions. Subsequently others used smaller temporal exposures (Table 29.3; Figs. 29.27–29.30, 29.32–29.34). Suzuki et al. (196,199,203) described three types of temporal approach (Fig. 14.32) including the "temporal keel form incision" mentioned in the section on approaches to ICAA. Surgeons varied on their technique of either following the MCA outward in the sylvian fissure from the ICA bifurcation or going inward along the sylvian fissure or through the superior temporal gyrus. Shephard (185) preferred a small linear incision with a small trephine for exposure (Fig. 29.34).

Frontolateral Approach for MCAA

In his 1944 monograph Dandy (21) did not make it clear that he used the frontotemporal approach in his MCAA cases; however, it is likely that he did use some modification of his standard "Dandy flap." Since Hamby's publication (75) (Fig. 29.35), the frontolateral approach has been the most popular cranial exposure for the MCAA (Table 29.3; Figs. 29.35–29.39) just as it was for the ICAA. Campbell and Burklund (15) (Fig. 29.36) and Gurdjian and Thomas (71) (Fig. 29.37) reported using enormous frontotemporal flaps, but most prefer the smaller exposures. See Chapter 37 for additional details.

Basilar Artery Aneurysms

Regarding exposure of a BAA, Dandy (21) said in 1944, "It would perhaps be possible to resect a temporal lobe and thus gain access to such an aneurysm, for the anterior tip of this vessel is usually in full view when performing a third ventriculostomy for strictures at the sylvian aqueduct." However, a deliberate, planned direct attack on a basilar artery aneurysm diagnosed prior to surgery was not reported until the publications of Gillingham in 1958 (62), Drake in 1961 (30), Logue in 1964 (126), and Jamieson in 1964 (97). It is noteworthy that in 1963 Höök et al. (91) presented two cases of bBAA operated by Olivecrona in 1946 (explored only) and 1954 (clipped), two cases of bBAA operated by Bohm in 1955 (clipped) and 1956 (no details), and a case of bBAA operated by Norlén in 1955 (clipped). Prior to this time BAA were exposed at surgical exploration for tumor, clot, or decompression (5,70,83,84,160,191,215). In addition, craniotomy had been performed by Dandy (21) to do a trigeminal rhizotomy for the relief of pain presumably caused by irritation of the trigeminal nerve by the giant BAA.

The difficulties of a direct attack on the most difficult and threatening of all aneurysms, a bBAA, is illustrated in Figs. 29.40–29.42. The aneurysm lies buried in the interpeduncular cistern between the cerebral peduncles and the oculomotor nerves. The aneurysm often is sur-

Table 29.3. Surgical Approaches to Middle Cerebral Artery Aneurysms

Frontal Approach			*Temporal Approach*			*Frontolateral Approach*		
Author	*Year*	*Fig.*	*Author*	*Year*	*Fig.*	*Author*	*Year*	*Fig.*
Falconer (46)	1951	29.5	Swain (205)	1948		Dandy (21)	1944	
Bassett et al. (10)	1952		Norlén & Olivecrona (140)	1953		Hamby (75)	1952	29.35
Pertuiset et al. (149)	1966		Botterell et al. (13)	1956		Campbell & Burklund (15)	1953	29.36
Robinson (172)	1971		Krayenbühl & Yaşargil (110)	1958		Hamby (76)	1954	
Wilson (223)	1971	29.9	Avman & Fisher (8)	1960	29.32	Botterell et al. (13)	1956	
			Poppen (158)	1960	29.28	Gass et al. (61)	1958	
			Suzuki (196)	1966		Tönnis & Walter (212)	1960	
			Suzuki et al. (199)	1967		Lougheed et al. (128)	1963	
			Suzuki et al. (203)	1970	29.33	Drake (34)	1965	
			Shephard (185)	1971	29.34	Tönnis & Walter (211)	1966	
			Yashon et al. (239)	1971		Kempe (103)	1968	29.19
						Hamby (73)	1969	
						Lougheed (127)	1969	
						Yaşargil (231)	1969	
						Gurdjian & Thomas (71)	1970	29.37
						Krayenbühl & Yaşargil (111)	1970	
						Laine et al. (117)	1970	
						Yaşargil (230)	1970	
						Drake (36)	1971	29.38
						Kempe & VanderArk (105)	1971	
						Sano (177)	1971	29.21
						De Grood (25)	1972	
						Krayenbühl et al. (112)	1972	
						Corkill & Hodgson (17)	1973	
						Guidetti (66)	1973	
						Lougheed & Marshall (129)	1973	29.31
						Bonnal et al. (12)	1974	
						De Klerk & De Villiers (26)	1974	
						Peerless (147)	1974	
						VanderArk et al. (217)	1974	
						Aiba (4)	1975	29.39
						Yaşargil & Fox (235)	1975	
						Aiba (3)	1976	
						Deruty et al. (27)	1976	
						Kikuchi (106)	1976	
						Symon (206)	1976	
						Rhoton et al. (166)	1977	
						Selverstone (181)	1977	
						Taylor & Choudhury (208)	1977	
						Yaşargil & Smith (238)	1977	
						Adams et al. (1)	1978	
						Brock & Dietz (14)	1978	29.22
						Guidetti (65)	1978	
						Pia (150)	1978	
						Rand (164)	1978	
						Drake (40)	1979	29.23
						Fox (49)	1979	
						Nornes & Wikeby (142)	1979	
						Rhoton et al. (167)	1979	
						Wilson & Spetzler (221)	1979	

rounded by a leash of vital posterior thalamic and midbrain perforators. It lies between the clivus and midbrain and the hypothalamus and pons. Access requires retraction of the temporal lobe and traversing the tentorium. Although the posterior clinoid process and PCoA may be obstacles when using the frontolateral approach (Fig. 29.42), these difficulties are being surmounted.

More than anyone else, Drake (30–42b) demonstrated the feasibility, with experience and teamwork, of direct attack on the BAA. Since

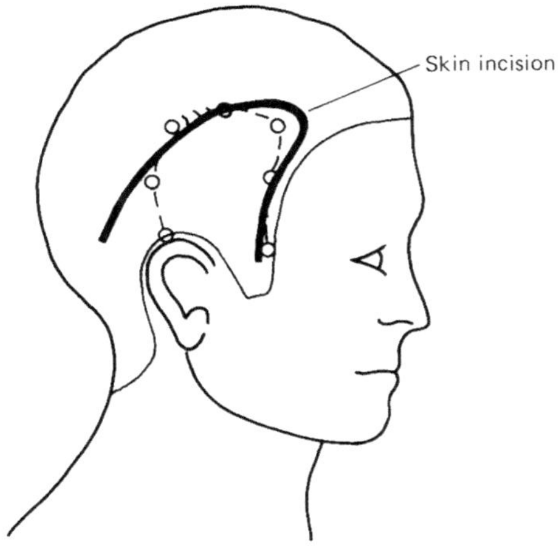

Fig. 29.32. Temporal flap reported by Avman and Fisher for MCAA in 1960. From Avman N, Fisher RG, ref. 8.

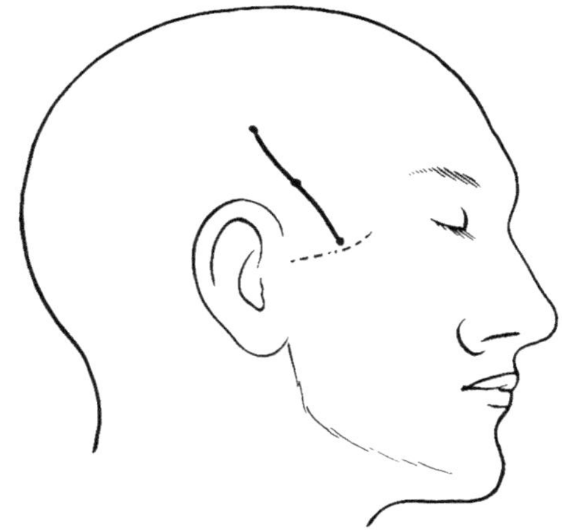

Fig. 29.34. Shephard's 1971 temporal incision and trephine craniotomy for MCAA. From Shepherd RH, ref. 185.

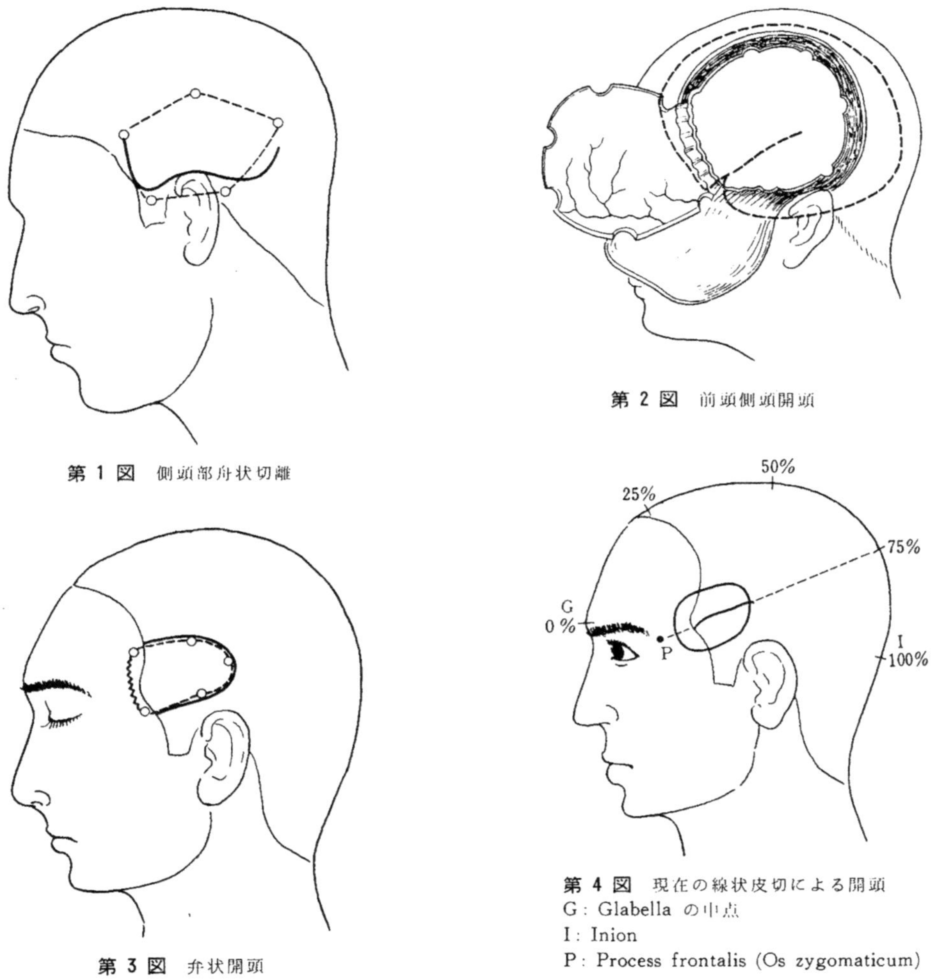

Fig. 29.33. Various types of temporal craniotomy flap diagrammed by Suzuki and colleagues for MCAA in 1970. From Suzuki J, Takaku A, Hori S, et al., ref. 203.

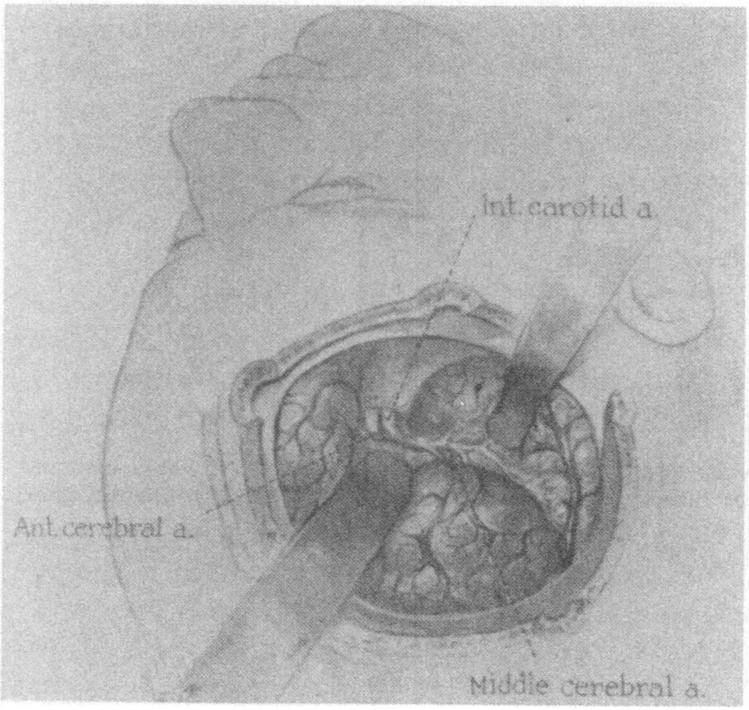

Fig. 29.35. Hamby's 1952 frontolateral exposure from MCAA. From Hamby WB, ref. 75.

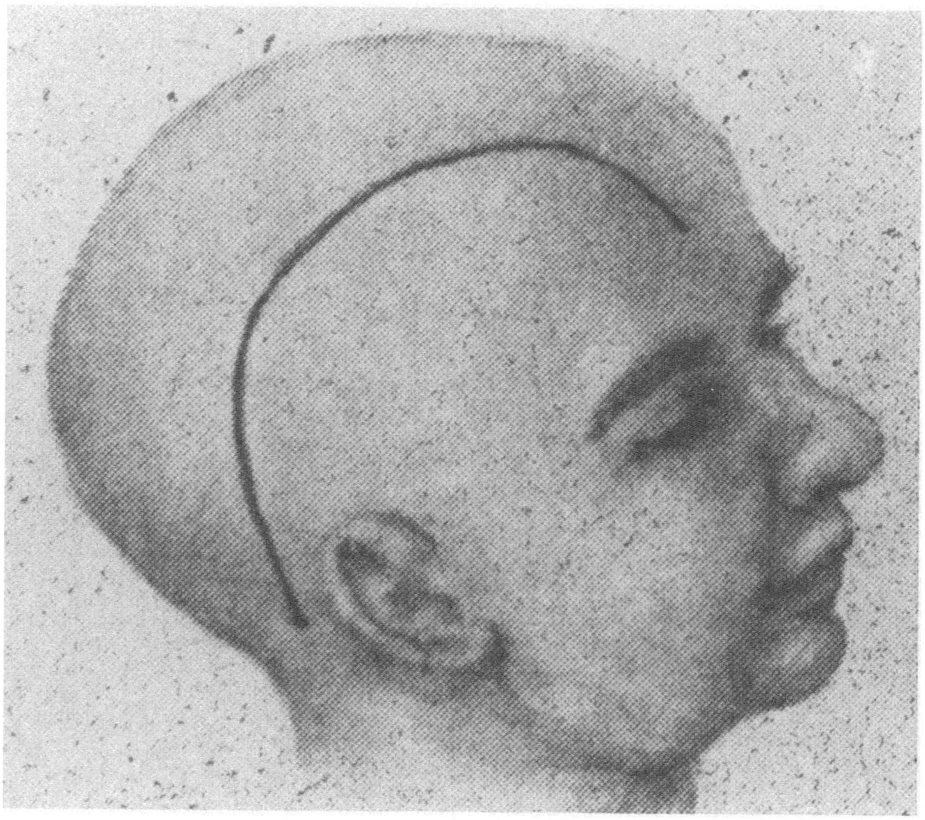

Fig. 29.36. Large frontotemporal flap reported by Campbell and Burklund for MCAA in 1953. From Campbell E, Burklund WC, ref. 15.

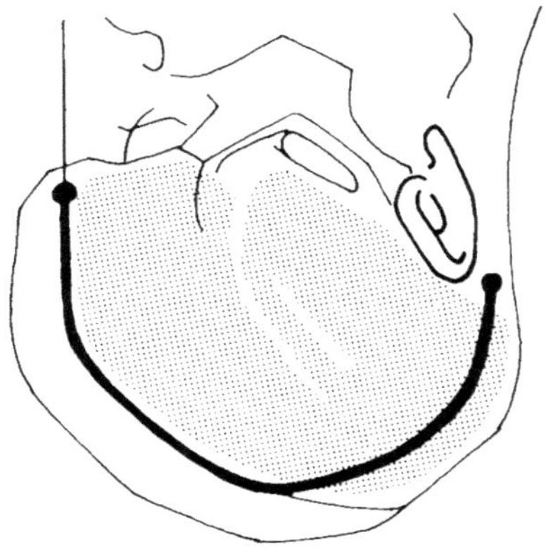

Fig. 29.37. Large frontotemporal flap designed by Gurdjian and Thomas for MCAA in 1970. From Gurdjian ES, Thomas LM, ref. 71.

then, a number of neurosurgeons have reported on intracranial surgery for BAA (Table 29.4).

Temporal Approach for BAA

In 1958 Gillingham (62) reported using the subtemporal route for a direct attack on four bBAA cases. Two were clipped, and two were wrapped with fascia. Jamieson (96,97) described using the temporal and frontotemporal routes. Drake (30–42b) for several years established the low temporal (subtemporal) route as the preferred one for most BAA on the trunk and at the bifurcation (Fig. 29.43). As time went by his flap became smaller and more anterior (Fig. 29.44). The more posterior temporal flaps

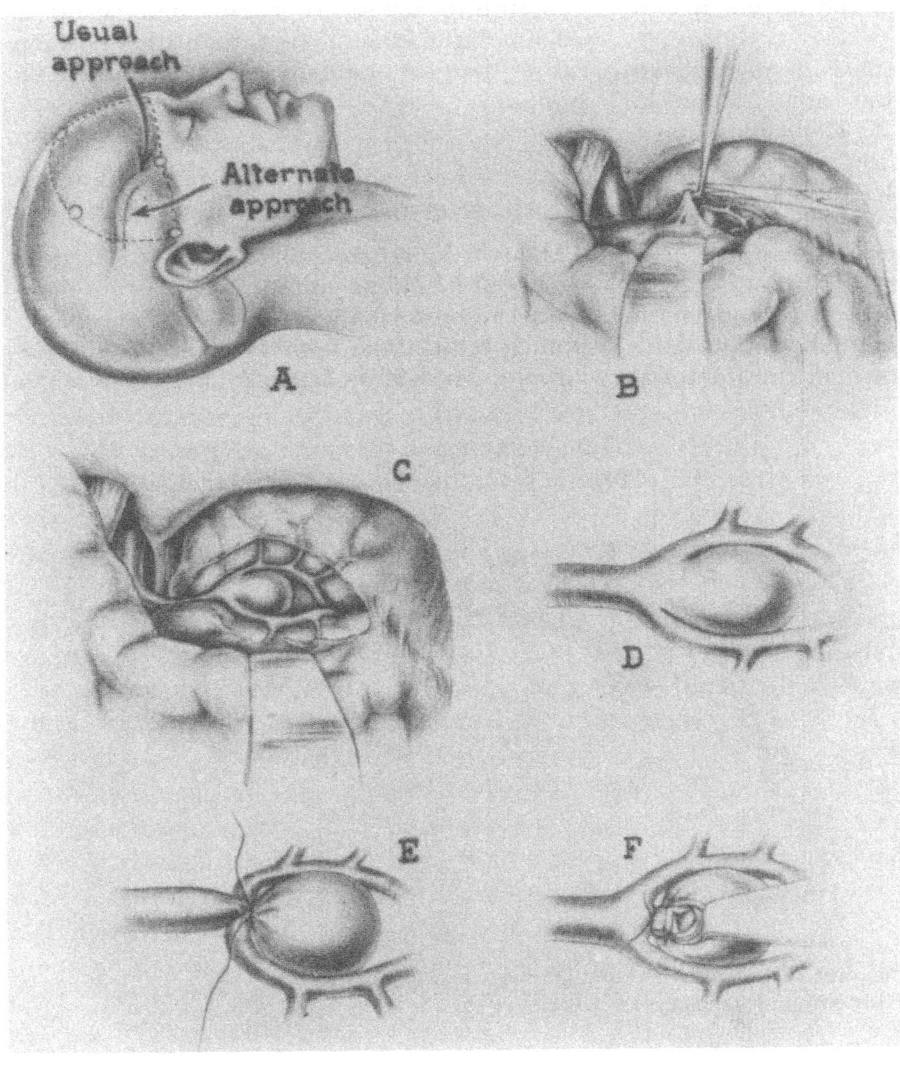

Fig. 29.38. Drake's 1971 frontolateral approach to MCAA. The bone flap (**A**) is similar to his flap for ICAA in Fig. 29.26 except that for MCAA he goes down the sylvian fissure (**A, B, C**) or into the superior temporal gyrus (**A**). **D–F** Exposing, ligating, or clipping MCAA. From Drake CG, ref. 36.

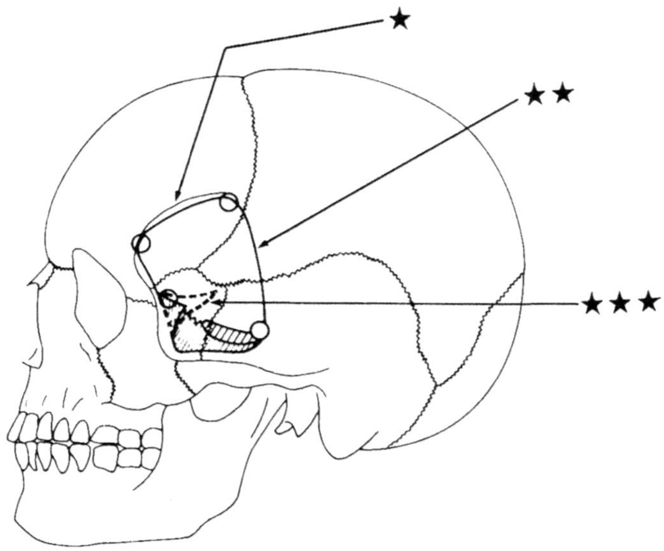

Fig. 29.39. Aiba's 1975 frontolateral craniotomy for MCAA. From Aiba T, ref. 4.

were used for exposure of the lower-situated BAA (Fig. 29.45).

A number of surgeons subsequently utilized the subtemporal route, often with variations in the flap (Table 29.4; Figs. 29.43–29.50). Kempe (103) also emphasized the low exposure and removed much of the basal temporal and sphenoid bones (Fig. 29.46). For low-lying BAA some preferred an occipitotemporal flap, usually with section of the tentorium (16,126, 163,226). Kasdon and Stein (101) turned a temporal flap and removed some suboccipital bone to give a combined supra- and infratentorial exposure for low-lying basilar aneurysms (Fig. 29.50). Bartal et al. (9) used the sitting position rather than the standard supine or semilateral position.

Frontolateral Approach for BAA

Although Jamieson (96,97) and Richardson (168,169) mentioned the use of a "frontotemporal exposure" to the BAA, they went subtemporally rather than via the sylvian fissure. Beginning in 1969 Yaşargil and co-workers

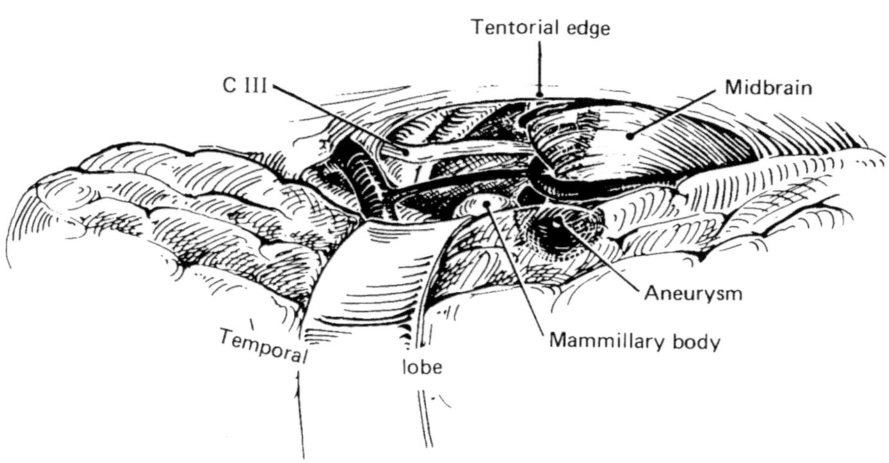

A

Fig. 29.40. Drake's 1965 diagram of the interpeduncular fossa and bBAA. **A** As seen by a standard right subtemporal exposure (*continued*).

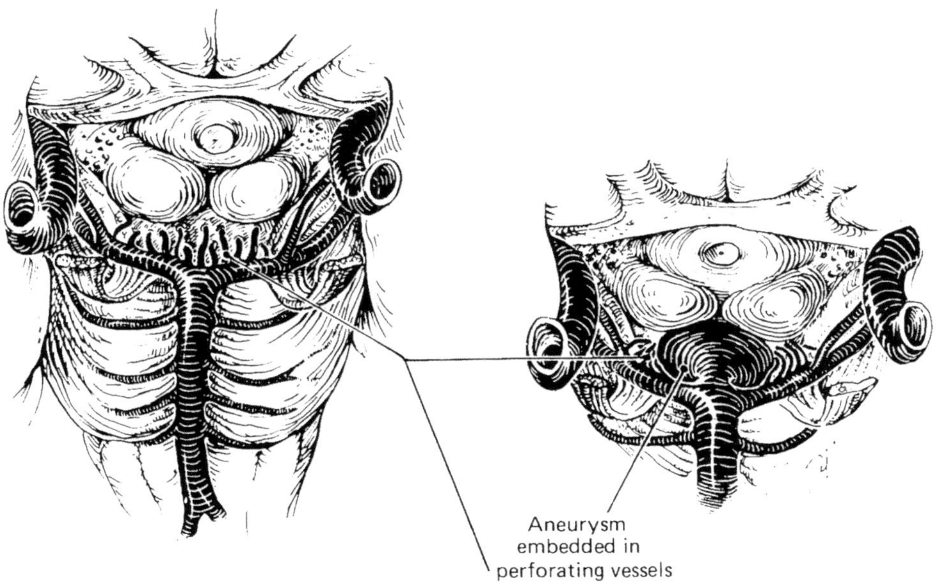

B Relation of bBAA to perforators, pons, midbrain, and hypothalmus. Note BA, P-1, PCoA, ICA, mammillary bodies, pituitary stalk, and optic chiasm in **B.** From Drake CG, ref. 35.

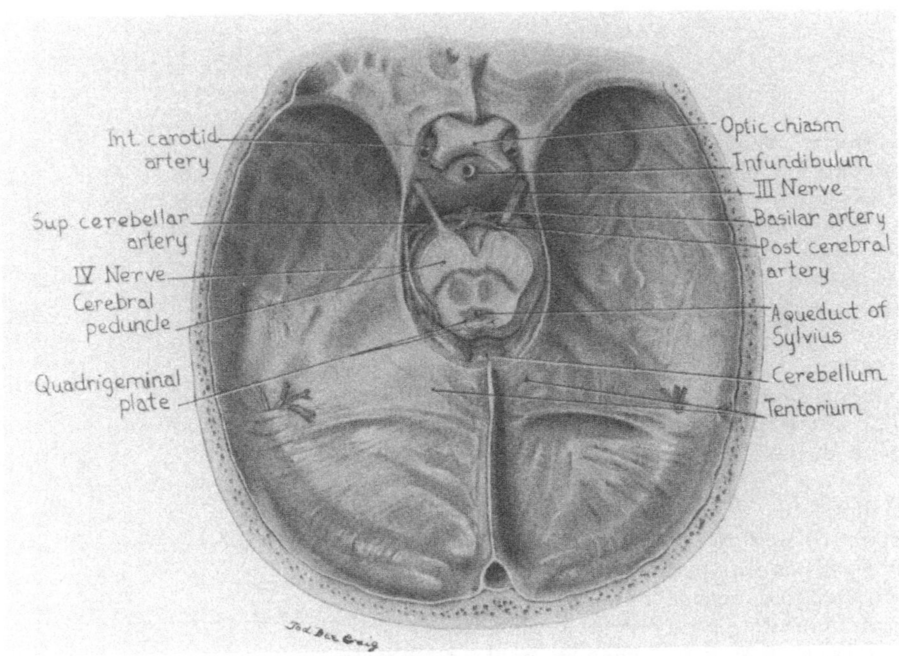

Fig. 29.41. Incisura of the tentorium. The midbrain was sectioned transversely, and the hemispheres have been removed. Note relation of the bifurcation of the basilar artery to the environs in terms of a temporal or a frontolateral approach to this region and in terms of structures compressed by a large bBAA. From Taveras, JM. The roentgen diagnosis of intracranial incisural space occupying lesions. Am. J. Roentgenol. 84:52–69. © 1960, American Roentgen Ray Society. Permission granted by publisher, ref. 207.

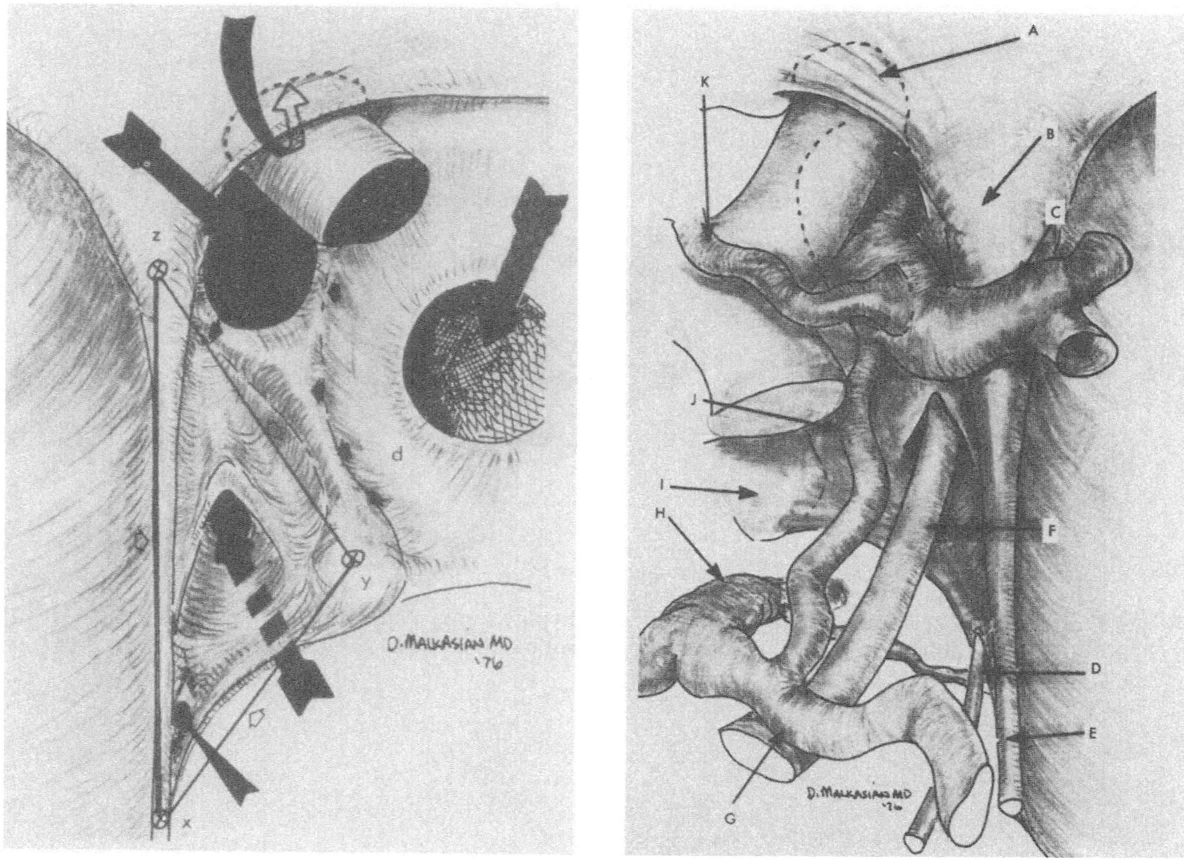

A **B**

Fig. 29.42. Relationship of posterior clinoid process on the left (**A**) and right (**B**) to the oculomotor nerve and circle of Willis. Note relation of posterior clinoid process, PCoA, P-1 artery, and CN-3 to tip of basilar artery in terms of a temporal or a frontolateral approach to a bBAA. From Malkasian DR, Rand RW, ref. 130a.

A Superior view of the left sellar and parasellar region demonstrating the dural reflections and the "oculomotor trigone." *Lines with adjacent open arrows:* Boundaries of the oculomotor trigone. *x* Medial reflections of the tentorium cerebelli. *y* Posterior clinoid process. *z* Anterior clinoid process. *d* Diaphragm sellae. *Straight arrow:* Ostium of the internal carotid artery. *Curved arrow:* Over optic nerve and under falciform ligament. *Dotted line:* Opening to the optic foramen. *Black checkered arrow:* Opening in the diaphragm sellae. *Broken arrow:* Oculomotor ostium. *Arrowhead:* Ostium for the fourth cranial nerve. *Small dark arrows:* "Y" dural fold.

B Superior view of the sella illustrating the relationship of the anterior clinoid process (*B*), middle cerebral artery (*C*), posterior communicating artery (*J*), oculomotor nerve (*F*), trochlear nerve (*D*), posterior cerebral artery (*G*), and tentorium cerebelli medial reflection (*E–I*). Note that the oculomotor nerve is slightly lateral and inferior to the posterior communicating artery at the oculomotor ostium as it penetrates the dura in the oculomotor trigone. However, as the oculomotor nerve passes inferior to the posterior communicating artery (proximal to the midbrain), it may be immediately inferior or slightly medial to the posterior cerebral artery–posterior communicating artery junction. The anterior choroidal artery has not been included. *A* Falciform ligament over the optic nerve as it enters the optic canal. *E* Free edge of the tentorium cerebelli and its medial reflection. *H* Basilar artery. *I* Posterior clinoid process. *K* Anterior cerebral artery.

Table 29.4. Surgical Approaches to Basilar Artery Aneurysms

Temporal Approach			*Frontolateral Approach*		
Author	*Year*	*Fig.*	*Author*	*Year*	*Fig.*
Gillingham (62)	1958		Yaşargil (231)	1969	
Drake (30)	1961		Yaşargil & Fox (235)	1975	
Jamieson (97)	1964		Yaşargil et al.	1976	
Logue (126)	1964		Rhoton et al. (166)	1977	
Drake (34)	1965		Sugita et al. (193)	1977	
Drake (35)	1965	29.40	Drake (31)	1978	
Fox & Leussenhop (52)	1967		Samson et al. (175)	1978	29.51, 29.52
Housepain et al. (93)	1967		Drake (40)	1979	29.23
Bartal et al. (9)	1968		Fox (49)	1979	
Drake (32)	1968		Sugita et al. (192)	1979	29.53
Drake (38)	1968	29.43	Wright & Wilson (226)	1979	
Fox (51)	1968				
French et al. (53)	1968				
Jamieson (96)	1968				
Kempe (103)	1968	29.46			
Laine (114)	1968				
Drake (39)	1969				
Hamby (73)	1969				
Lougheed & Marshall (130)	1969				
Rand (163)	1969				
Gurdjian & Thomas (71)	1970	29.47			
Richardson (169)	1971				
Sano (177)	1971	29.48			
Wilson (223)	1971	29.49			
Yashon et al. (239)	1971				
Richardson (168)	1972				
Laine et al. (116)	1972				
Drake (33)	1973				
Northfield (143)	1973				
Sano (176)	1973				
Chou & Ortiz-Suarez (16)	1974				
McMurtry et al. (133)	1974				
Drake (37)	1976				
Wilson & U (222)	1976				
Rhoton et al. (166)	1977				
Shields (186)	1977				
Sugita et al. (193)	1977				
Drake (31)	1978				
Rand (164)	1978				
Drake (40)	1979	29.44,29.45			
Kasdon & Stein (101)	1979	29.50			
Nornes & Wikeby (142)	1979				
Rhoton et al. (167)	1979				
Wilson & Spetzler (221)	1979				
Wright & Wilson (226)	1979				

(231,232,235) described a frontolateral, transylvian approach. Others have since utilized the same basic frontolateral exposure used for the previously described anterior circulation aneurysms (Table 29.4; Figs 29.51–29.53) for the bBAA. It is advisable to open the sylvian fissure widely. This transylvian approach passes between the depths of the sylvian fissure and the drilled-down sphenoid wing. It is often necessary to retract the ICA and/or the M-1 artery (Fig. 29.53) and sever either the PCoA or the P-1 artery (49,192). Details of this exposure are found elsewhere (Chapter 38).

Samson et al. (175) emphasized the importance of appreciating the relationship of the posterior clinoid process to the neck of the

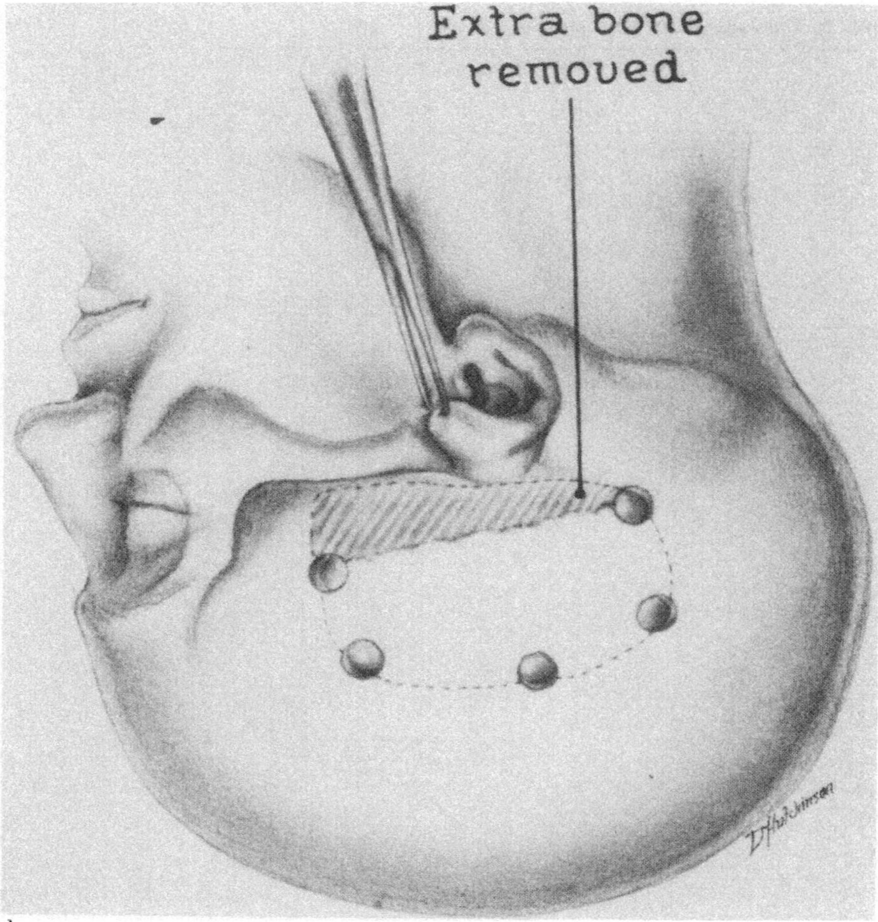

A

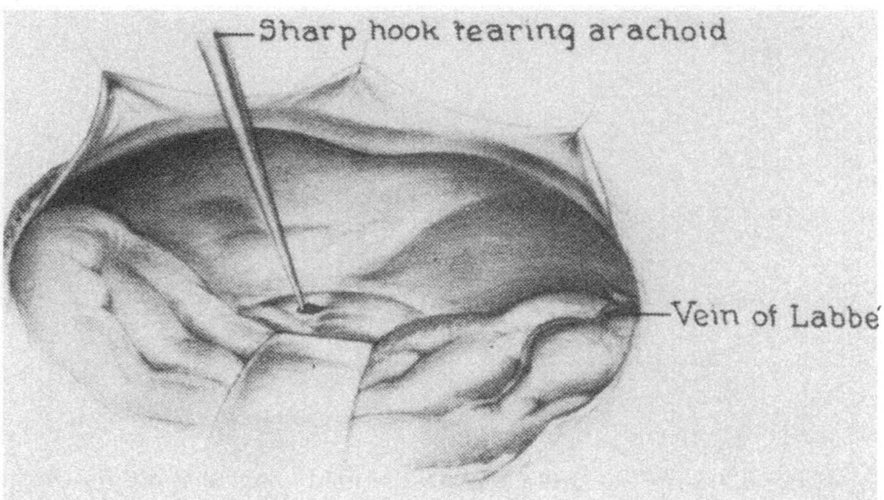

B

Fig. 29.43. Drake's 1968 right subtemporal approach to the bBAA. **A** The craniotomy flap with bone ronguered (*hatched lines*) to base of skull. **B** Retractor on right temporal lobe exposing arachnoid of interpeduncular cistern. **C** Clot in interpeduncular cistern. **D** Retractors on right temporal lobe and cerebral peduncle. Aneurysm shown in relation to BA, P-1, P-2, PCoA, and ICA. From Drake CG, ref. 38.

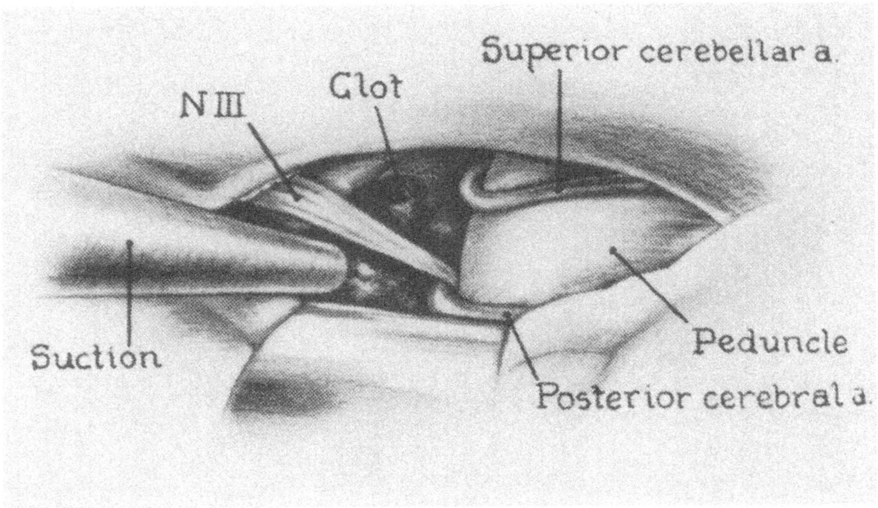

C

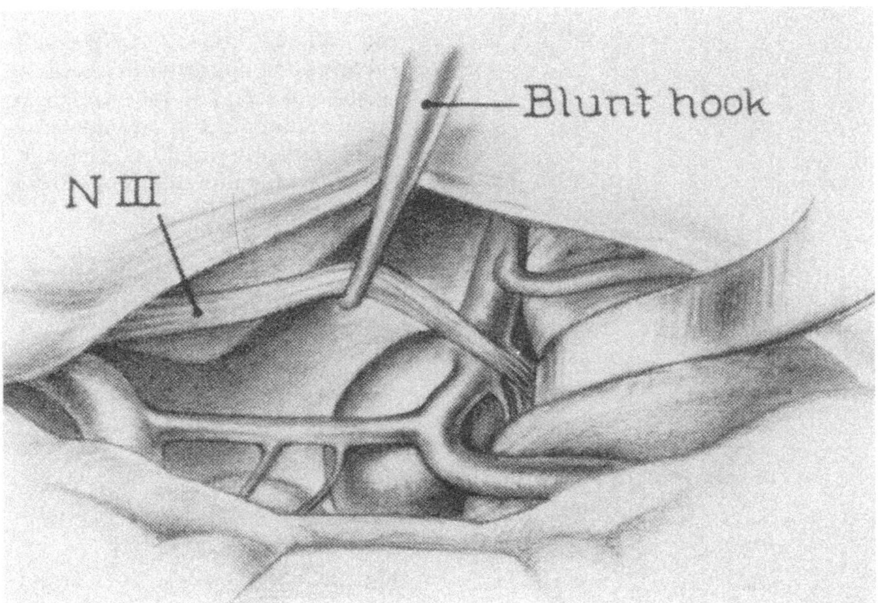

D

aneurysm on the lateral arteriogram. In Figure 29.54 they demonstrated the frequency with which the tip of the BA is found above, at, or below the posterior clinoid region. Samson et al. (175) and Wright and Wilson (226) concluded that the frontolateral approach is too difficult if the neck of the aneurysm lies below the level of the posterior clinoid process. However, with a wide opening of the sylvian fissure and excellent brain relaxation, we believe it is usually possible to deal with these low-lying bBAA (Fig. 29.55).

Yaşargil and colleagues (232) preferred the frontolateral to the subtemporal route because:

1. There is less retraction pressure on the temporal lobe.
2. The anatomy of the interpeduncular cistern is seen better (both P-1 arteries and perforators) with a view facing the bBAA more from in front.
3. The oculomotor and trochlear nerves are less disturbed.
4. The surgeon can better treat additional

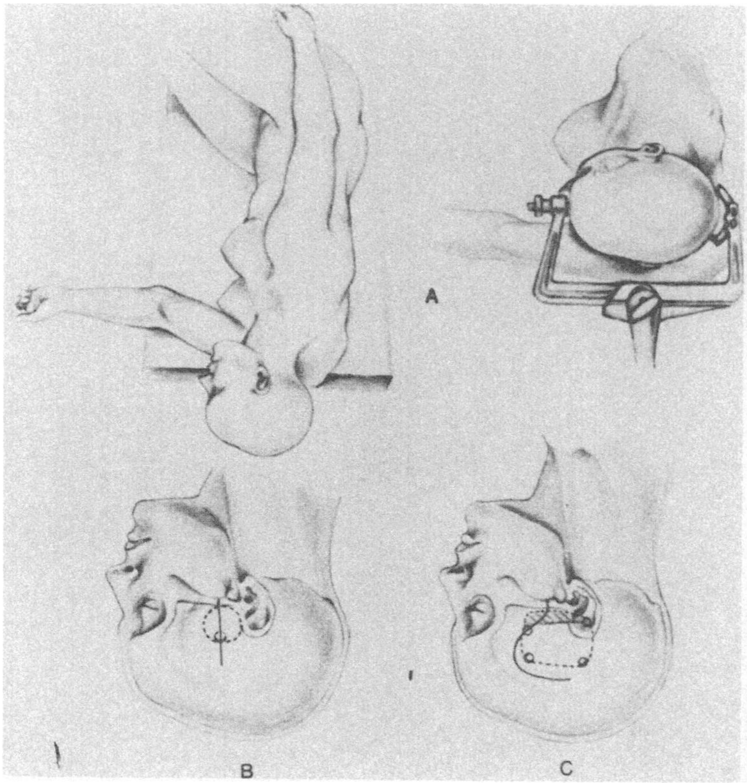

Fig. 29.44. Drake's 1979 right subtemporal approach to bBAA. **A** (*right and left*) Lateral position. **B** Small subtemporal craniectomy more recently used. **C** Conventional temporal craniotomy. From Drake CG, ref. 40.

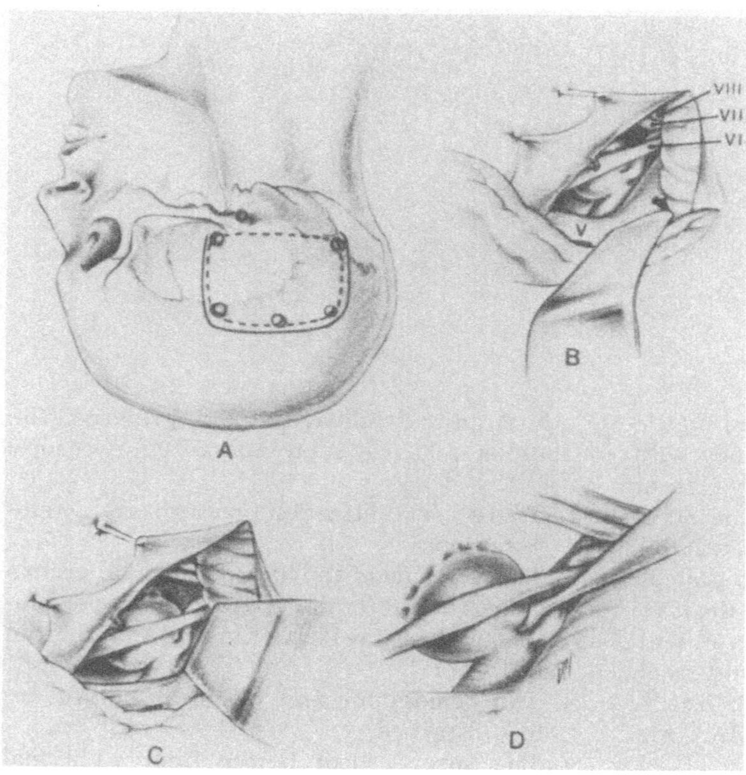

Fig. 29.45. Drake's 1979 right posterior subtemporal, transtentorial approach to lower BAA and vaBAA. **A** Posteriorly placed bone flap so as to allow posterior temporal retraction for line of vision down posterior slopes of petrous bone. **B** Tentorium divided 1–2 cm behind petrous ridge to near lateral sinus. Anterior leaflet of tentorium tied firmly forward to floor of middle fossa. Petrosal vein coagulated and divided. **C** aicaBAA exposed with CN-6 flattened over dome, which is adherent to clivus. **D** Careful separation of AICA from neck of aneurysm before clipping. From Drake CG, ref. 40.

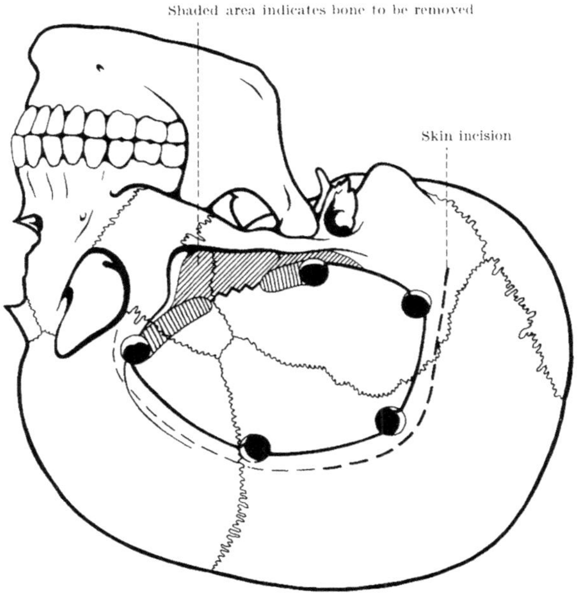

Fig. 29.46. Kempe's 1968 temporal flap for BAA. Note burr hole at "psychopathic point" (junction of temporal line, zygomatic process of frontal bone, and orbital ridge) and extent of base of sphenoid and temporal bone removal (*shaded area*). From Kempe LG, ref. 103.

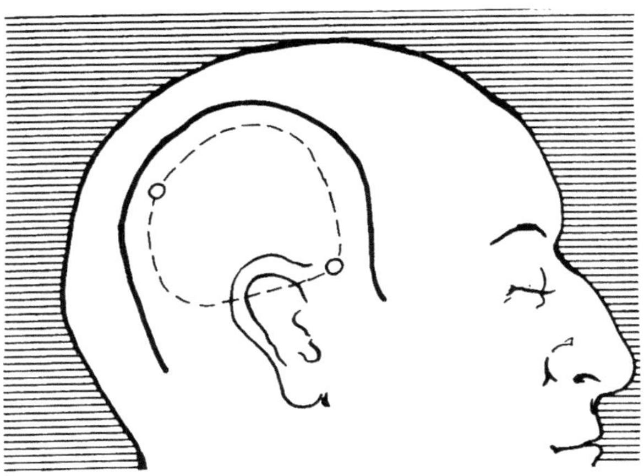

Fig. 29.47. Posterior temporal craniotomy used by Gurdjian and Thomas in 1970 for BAA. From Gurdjian ES, Thomas LM, ref. 71.

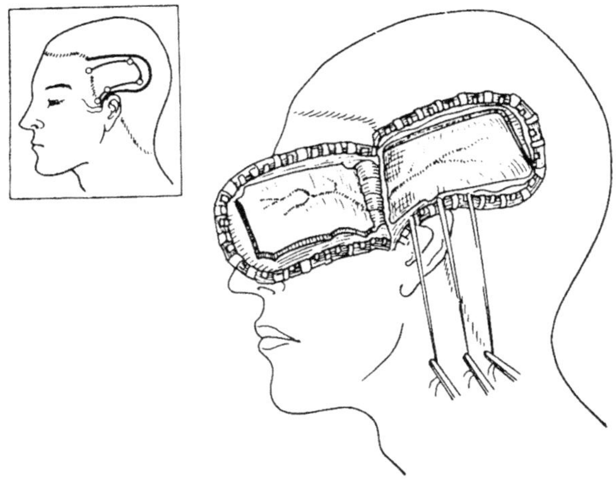

Fig. 29.48. Sano's 1971 temporal approach to BAA. From Sano K, ref. 177.

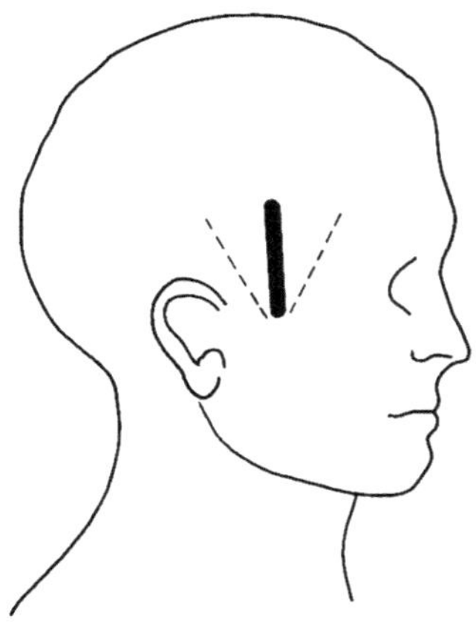

Fig. 29.49. Wilson's 1971 temporal exposure for BAA. A trephine is used. From Wilson DH, ref. 223.

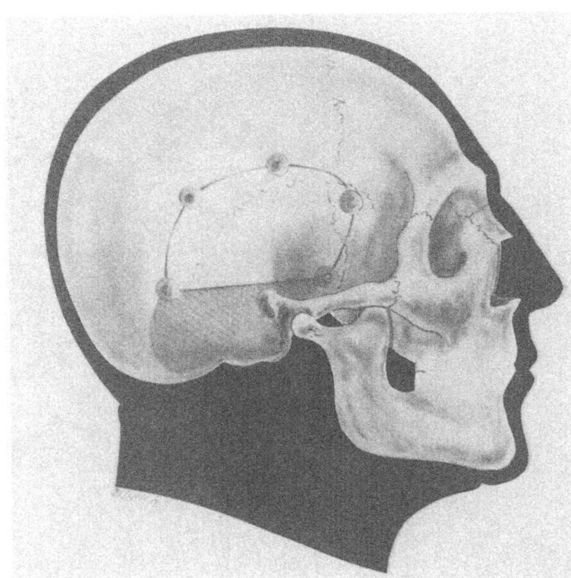

Fig. 29.50. The 1979 combined supratentorial and infratentorial exposure by Kasdon and Stein for low-lying BAA. Note the temporal craniotomy and the lateral suboccipital craniectomy (*shaded*). From Kasdon DL, Stein, BM, ref. 101.

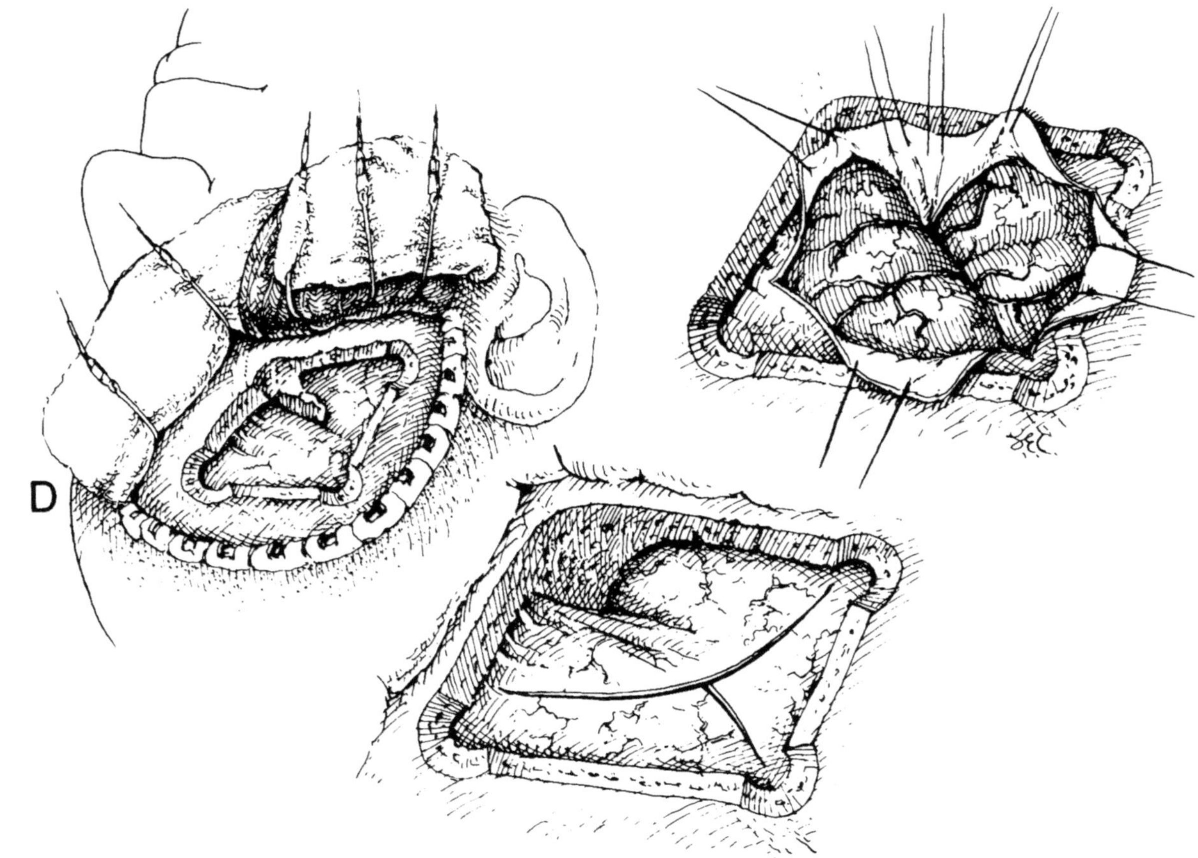

Fig. 29.51. Right frontolateral craniotomy of Samson and colleagues for bBAA in 1978 (used for anterior circulation aneurysms also.) They use a free bone flap rather than one attached to the temporalis muscle retracted here by fishhooks (*D*). From Samson DS, Hodosh RM, Clark WK, ref. 175.

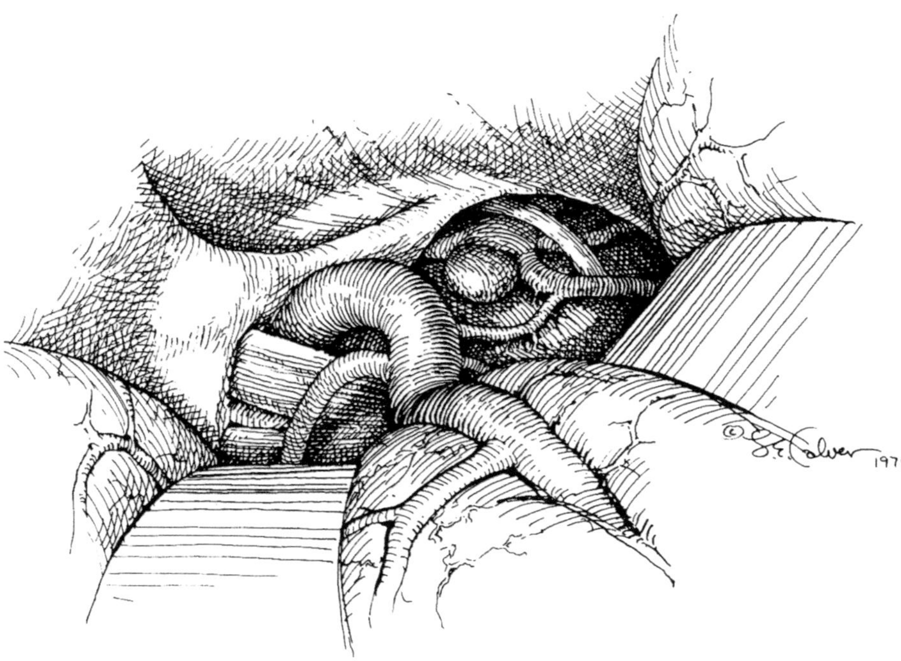

Fig. 29.52. Line of vision to the bBAA via the right frontolateral exposure. *Left to right:* CN-2 and A-1, ICA, PCoA, P-1 and P-2. CN-3, SCA. Retractors on right frontal lobe and right temporal lobe flanking M-1. From Samson DS, Hodosh RM, Clark WK, ref. 175.

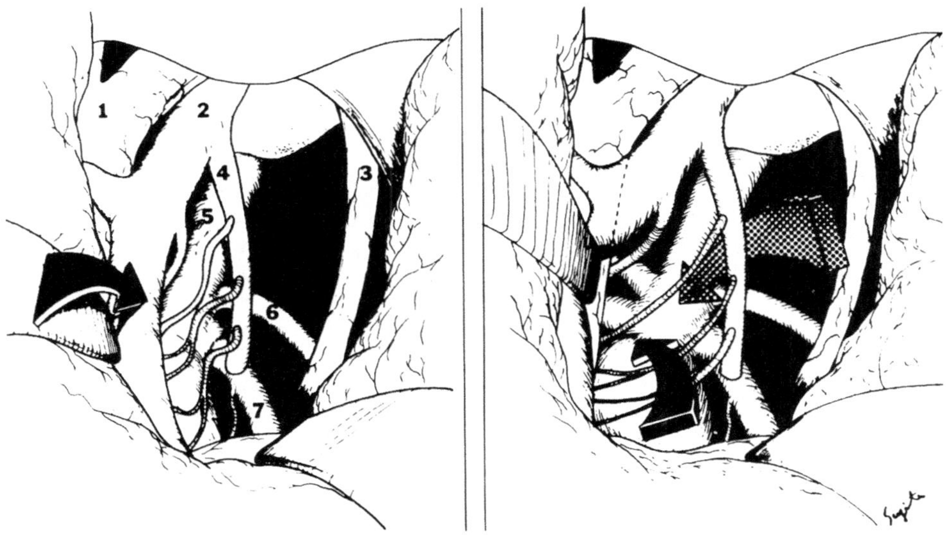

Fig. 29.53. Right frontolateral (transylvian) approach to bBAA. *Left* Initial step of the procedure. The tapered retractor on the frontal lobe (*solid arrow*) is shifted down to include the M-1 segment of the middle cerebral artery. *Right* After retraction of the M-1 segment (a part of the optic tract is seen laterally under M-1). The *dotted arrow* shows their routine approach. The *solid arrow* shows a route between the perforators for aneurysms of the high-placed bifurcation. *1,* Optic nerve. *2,* Carotid artery. *3,* Oculomotor nerve. *4,* Posterior communicating artery. *5,* Basilar artery. *6,* Superior cerebellar artery. *7,* Posterior cerebral artery. From Sugita K, Kobayashi S, Shintani A, et al., ref. 192.

aneurysms on the anterior circle of Willis at the same time.

Disadvantages of the frontolateral route may include:

1. Retraction of the ICA or M-1 artery is often needed (dangerous if it is atherosclerotic or if the blood pressure drops very low).

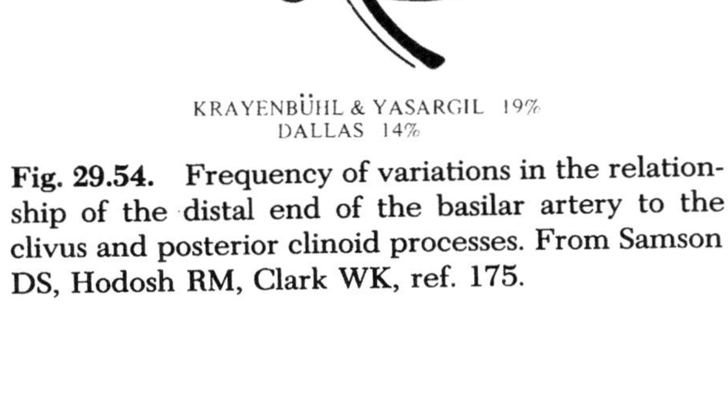

Fig. 29.54. Frequency of variations in the relationship of the distal end of the basilar artery to the clivus and posterior clinoid processes. From Samson DS, Hodosh RM, Clark WK, ref. 175.

2. Ligation and section of the PCoA or P-1 artery is often necessary.
3. The posterior clinoid process may be in the way of low-lying bBAA.
4. bBAA high up in the interpeduncular cistern or projecting backward are more difficult to visualize.
5. Perforators between the posterior aspect of the aneurysm and the brainstem is less easily seen in some cases.
6. The working space between the ICA and CN-3 or occasionally between the ICA and CN-2 is confining, requiring expert microtechnique.

Drake (31) concluded that

> [T]here will be a place for the sylvian approach to certain basilar aneurysms, particularly because of its familiarity for anterior aneurysms. While not refuting the authors' conclusions, the degree of brain retraction is only slightly less forceful and, although there may be better visualization of one aspect of these aneurysms, other problems with the sylvian approach, as noted above, should be known. The simpler, shallower, wider exposure subtemporally and the clearer visualization of the

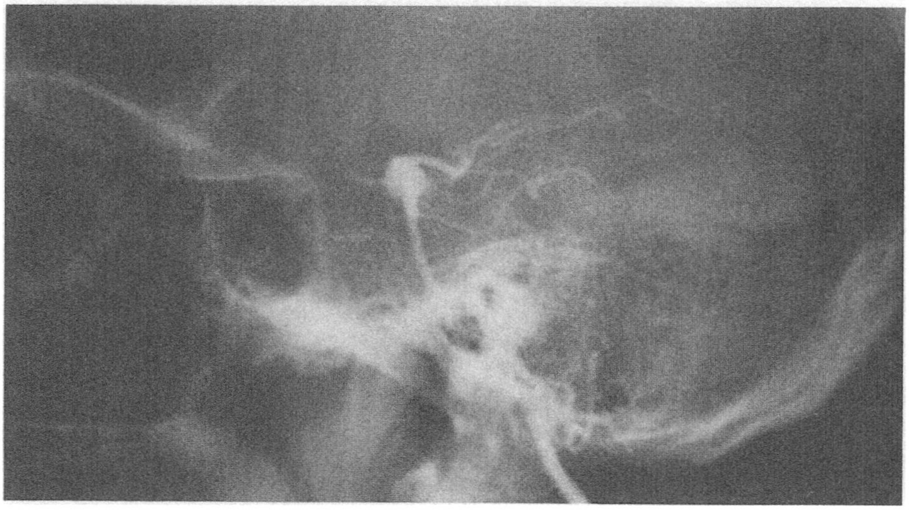

Fig. 29.55. Example of bBAA where neck of aneurysm lies well below the level of the posterior clinoid processes. This was exposed via a right frontolateral craniotomy with a transylvian approach. The aneurysm neck was well exposed and successfully clipped.

posterior aspect of these aneurysms, where the trouble is, as well as the ability to deal with all sacs in the region, has merit, too. Much of the merit of an approach is a matter of continued use and familiarity with the intimate anatomy of the region. Even so, when troubled with a sylvian paracarotid exposure, the surgeon should know he can fall back on the subtemporal or combined approach to deal with most situations in the region (Fig. 29.23).

Suboccipital Approach for BAA

The suboccipital approach is rarely used except for some inferiorly located BAA (163,226). It is quite difficult to reach aneurysms lying below

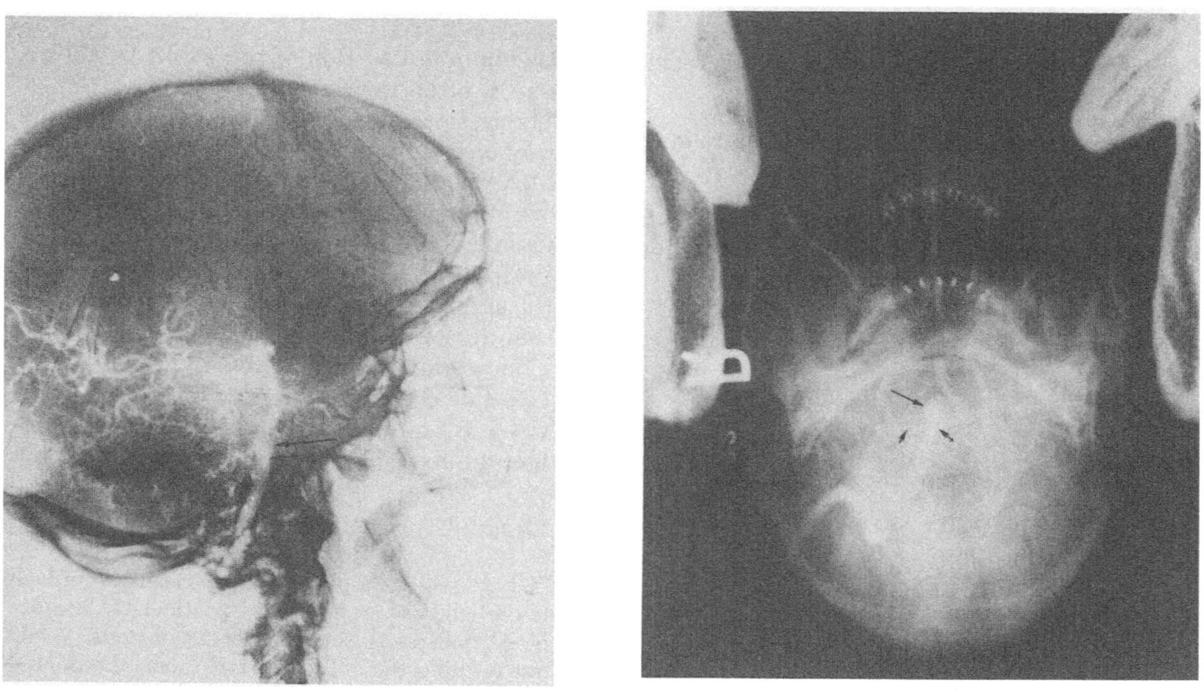

A **B**

Fig. 29.56. Example of midline picaVAA operated in 1966, by the submandibular, transclival approach. **A** Partially subtracted lateral angiogram. *Long arrow:* Aneurysm. *Short arrow:* PICA. **B** Submental view of vertebral angiogram. *Long arrow.* Aneurysm. *Short arrows:* PICA. From Fox JL, ref. 50.

the level of the jugular tubercle via the subtemporal, transtentorial route.

Transclival Approach for BAA

In the region of the vertebrobasilar junction at the midline is a zone difficult to reach by either the subtemporal or the suboccipital routes. The jugular tubercle obstructs vision from above. The midline aneurysms are surrounded by brainstem and cranial nerves, limiting the approach from below. Drake (33) called this "no man's land." In 1966, following the transoral route of Fang and Ong for upper cervical lesions (47), Sano et al. (176,178) operated and reported a vaBAA coated with muscle and Biobond adhesive via the transoral, transclival approach. In 1967 Fox (50) described the submandibular, transclival route to a midline picaVAA (Fig. 29.56). The aneurysm was clipped successfully via the same route Stevenson et al. (190) had utilized for a clivus chordoma. This approach, seen in Figure 29.57, has the advantage of having no risk of CSF contamina-

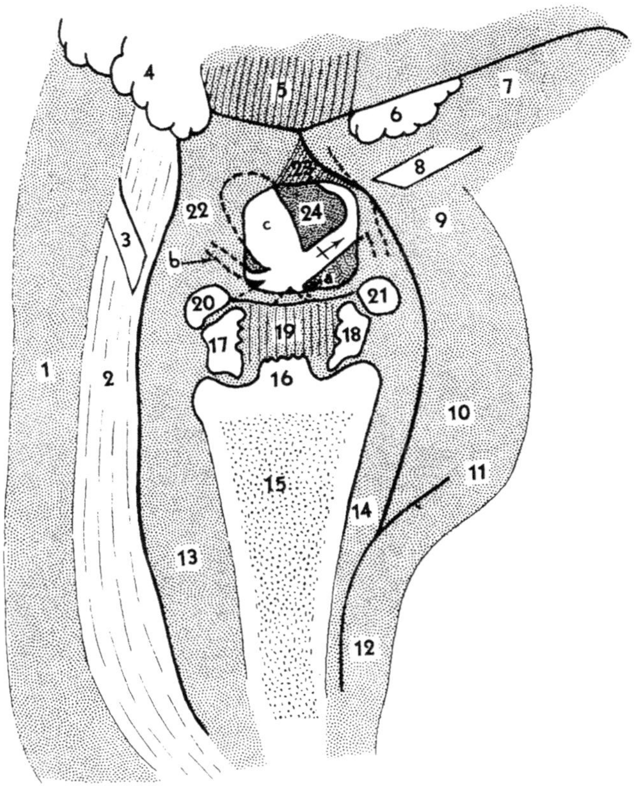

Fig. 29.57. Submandibular, transclival route to the same aneurysm shown in Fig. 29.56. The approach to the clivus lies between the right carotid sheath (*2*) and the pharynx (*9*). The numbers refer to the following: *1*, sternomastoid m.; *2*, carotid sheath; *3*, cephalic end of cut hypoglossal n.; *4*, parotid gland; *5*, masseter m. at angle of jaw; *6*, submaxillary gland; *7*, myelohyoid m.; *8*, distal end of cut hypoglossal n. lying on hyoglossus m.; *9*, superior constrictor m.; *10*, middle constrictor m.; *11*, soft tissue over hyoid bone; *12*, inferior constrictor m.; *13,14*, right and left longus capitis et cervicis m.; *15*, prevertebral fascia; *16*, axis with odontoid removed; *17,18*, atlas with anterior arch removed; *19*, transverse ligament and membrana tectoria: *20,21*, right and left occipital condyles; *22*, right longus capitis m. adjacent to clivus; *23*, portion of rectus capitis anterior m. remaining on clivus above opening through clivus; *24*, anterior surface of brainstem as seen through opening in clivus. The *crossed arrow* lies on the right vertebral artery and points to its union with a left vertebral artery; *a*, points to the right anterior spinal artery, *b*, the right PICA, and *c*, the fundus of the aneurysm as exposed surgically. From Fox JL, ref. 50.

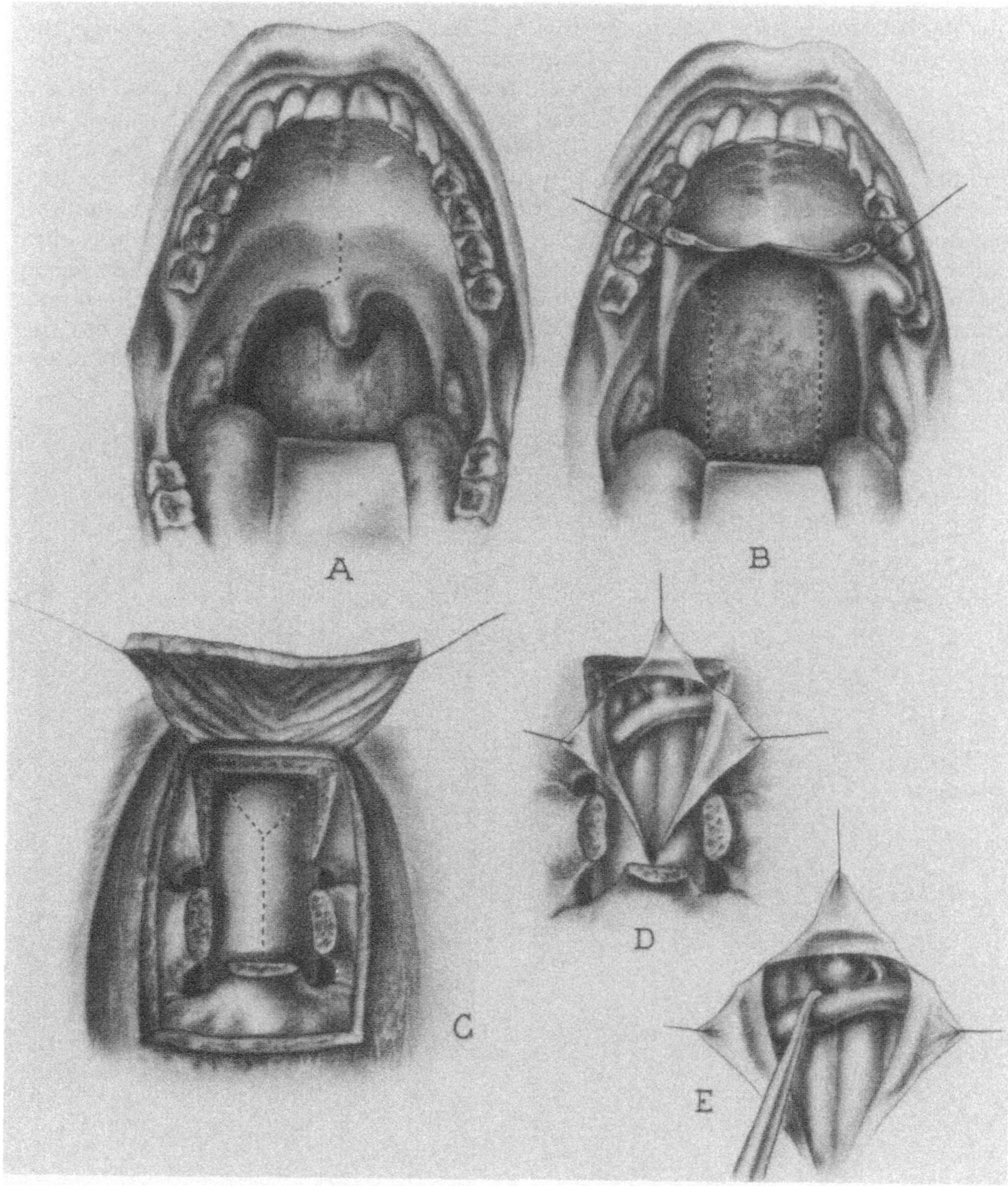

Fig. 29.58. Transoral, transclival route to some midline vertebrobasilar aneurysms. **A** Incision in soft palate. **B** Pharyngeal flap. **C** Removal of arch of atlas and odontoid and clival opening. **D** Dural opening to show vertebral artery and base of aneurysm. **E** Retraction of vertebral artery to expose neck of aneurysm. From Drake CG, ref. 33.

tion by oropharyngeal secretions. It has the disadvantage of being more difficult as well as interrupting CN-9 and CN-12 on one side, compared with the more direct transoral route.

Drake (33,39,41) stopped using the transoral route (Fig. 29.58) because of the risk of meningitis. Both approaches are difficult owing to working in a small space with little control of the parent circulation. The dura is adherent to the clivus; and if the aneurysm is adherent to the dura, premature rupture can occur. Using microsurgical techniques, most midline aneurysms can be handled by subtemporal or suboccipital approaches. Table 29.5 lists the studies reporting use of the transclival approach to vertebrobasilar aneurysms.

Table 29.5. Transclival Approach to Vertebrobasilar Aneurysms

Author	*Year*	*Fig.*	*Aneurysm*	*No. of Cases*	*Approach*
Sano et al. (178)	1966		vaBAA	1	Transoral
Fox (50)	1967	29.56, 29.57	picaVAA	1	Submandibular
Wissinger et al. (224)	1967		vaBAA	2	Submandibular
Drake (39)	1969		VAA	1	Transoral
Yaşargil (231)	1969		vaBAA	2	Transoral
Drake (41)	1971		VAA	1	Transoral
Jamieson (98)	1971		?	?	Submandibular
Drake (33)	1973	29.58	—	Reviewed approaches	
Sano (176)	1973		—	See Sano et al. (178)	
Chou & Ortiz-Suarez (16)	1974		—	See Wissinger et al. (224)	
Hashi et al. (80)	1976		vaBAA	1	Transoral
Laine & Jomin (118)	1977		vaBAA	1	Transoral
Yamaura et al. (229)	1979		trBAA	1	Transoral
Matricali & van Dulken (132a)	1981		vaBAA	2	Transoral
Hayakawa et al. (80a)	1981		aicaBAA	3	Transoral
Litvak et al. (125a)	1981		vaBAA	1	Transoral

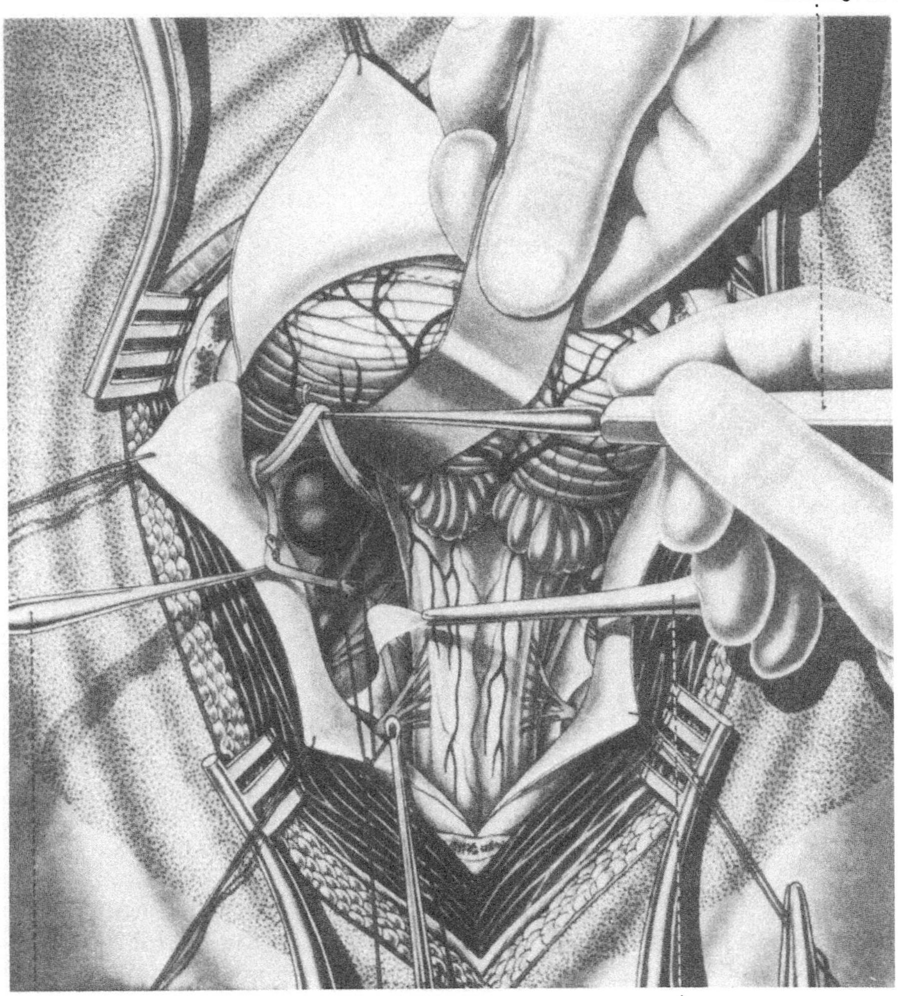

Fig. 29.59. Exposure of left VAA via a midline suboccipital craniectomy. From Kempe LG, ref. 104.

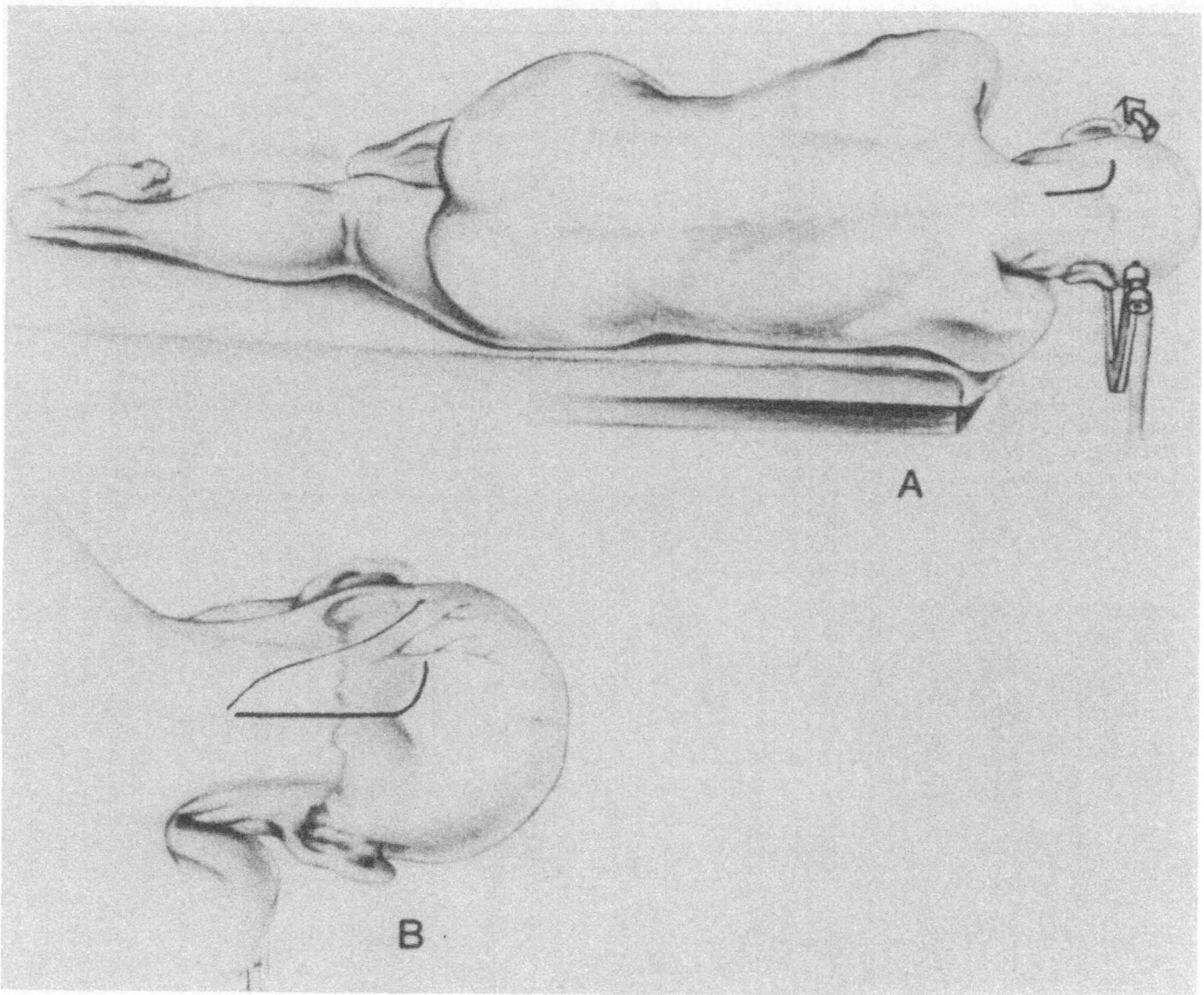

Fig. 29.60. Suboccipital exposure for VAA. **A** "Park bench" position with hockey stick incision just short of occipital nerves. **B** Alternate paramedian, or "S," incision. From Drake CG, ref. 40.

Vertebral Artery Aneurysms

Suboccipital Approach for VAA

The first deliberate operation on a berry aneurysm of the vertebral artery or its branches was performed by Schwartz (179) in 1946 (reported in 1948). It then remained a few years before such aneurysms were attacked directly (Table 29.6). The vast majority of cases were done by suboccipital craniectomy using the sitting position (Figs. 26.2, 29.59) or the lateral or semi-prone "park bench" position (Fig. 29.60). The exposure may be via a midline opening enlarged to one side (Fig. 29.59) or a unilateral

Table 29.6. Surgical Approach to the Vertebral Artery Aneurysm

Suboccipital Approach			*Temporal Approach*		
Author	*Year*	*Fig.*	*Author*	*Year*	*Fig.*
Schwartz (179)	1948		Drake (34)	1965	
Rizzoli & Hayes (170)	1953		Drake (32)	1968	
Steelman et al. (189)	1953		Drake (38)	1968	
Dimsdale & Logue (28)	1959		Drake (39)	1969	
Norlén & Paly (141)	1960		Drake (33)	1973	
Poppen (158)	1960		Drake (40)	1979	29.45
Höök et al. (91)	1963				
Sedzimir (180)	1963				
Jamieson (97)	1964				
Logue (126)	1964				
Drake (34)	1965				
Sano et al. (178)	1966				
Drake (39)	1969				
Hamby (73)	1969				
Rand (163)	1969				
Gurdjian & Thomas (71)	1970				
Kempe (104)	1970	29.59			
Jamieson (98)	1971				
Richardson (169)	1971				
Hammon & Kempe (77)	1972				
Drake (33)	1973				
Northfield (143)	1973				
Sano (176)	1973				
Yaşargil & Fox (235)	1975				
Karasawa et al. (100)	1977				
Rhoton et al. (166)	1977				
Pia (150)	1978				
Rand (164)	1978				
Drake (40)	1979	29.60			
Nornes & Wikeby (142)	1979				
Wilson & Spetzler (221)	1979				

opening similar to that used for a cerebellopontine angle tumor (Fig. 29.60). See Chapter 39.

Temporal Approach for VAA

In 1964 Logue (126) mentioned that VAA above the PICA take-off could be approached through a temperooccipital flap. Drake (Table 29.6) described some cases done by a subtemporal approach; he warned that VAA below the jugular tubercle should not be approached in this manner (32).

Transclival Approach for VAA

The transclival approach is described in the previous section of BAA and in Table 29.5.

Translabyrinthine Approach for VAA

In 1963 Hitselberger and Gardner (88) used the translabyrinthine approach to expose a "tumor." They found an AICAA in the acoustic canal. The exposure was extended more posteriorly and the aneurysm clipped.

Summary

Intracranial aneurysms now have been approached via nearly every corner of the cranium. A review of the many cranial routes for specific aneurysms is given. There is a trend toward using the low frontolateral approach and smaller exposures for most aneurysms.

Bibliography

1. Adams CBT, Chir M, Fearnside MR, et al.: An investigation with serial angiography into the evolution of cerebral arterial spasm following aneurysm. J Neurosurg 49:805–815, 1978
2. af Björkesten G: Arterial aneurysms of the internal carotid artery and its bifurcation. An analysis of 69 aneurysms treated mainly by direct surgical attack. J Neurosurg 15:400–410, 1958
3. Aiba T: [Operative indication and surgical technique of the cerebral aneurysm. 1.] Neurol Med Chir (Tokyo) 16 (6 Part 2):467–478, 1976
4. Aiba T: [Operative procedures of aneurysm of the middle cerebral artery.] Neurol Surg (Tokyo) 3:205–217, 1975
5. Alajouanine T, Le Beau J, Houdart R: La symptomatologie tumorale des volumineux anévrysmes des artères vertébrales et basilaires. Rev Neurol (Paris) 80:321–337, 1948
6. Almeida GM, Bianco E, Shibata MK: Anterior communicating artery aneurysms. J Neurosurg 33:53–57, 1976
7. Asenjo A, Donoso P: Aneurismas de la arteria comunicante anterior. Neurocirugia (Santiago) 15:9–14, 1957
8. Avman N, Fisher RG: Exposure of middle cerebral aneurysm after the use of urea. Surgery 48:491–494, 1960
9. Bartal A, Schiffer J, Weinstein M: A successful case of basilar bifurcation aneurysm surgery. Acta Neurochir (Wien) 19:163–170, 1968
10. Bassett RC, List CF, Lemmen LJ: Surgical treatment of intracranial aneurysm. Surg Gynecol Obstet 95:701–708, 1952
11. Bohm E, Hugosson R: Results of surgical treatment of 200 consecutive cerebral arterial aneurysms. Acta Neurol Scand 46:43–52, 1970
12. Bonnal J, Stevenaert A, Brotchi J, et al.: Bilan de neuf ans d'expérience de la chirurgie des anévrysmes artériels intracrâniens. Acta Neurol Belg 74:337–355, 1974
13. Botterell EH, Lougheed WM, Scott JW, et al.: Hypothermia, and interruption of carotid, or carotid and vertebral circulation, in the surgical management of intracranial aneurysms. J Neurosurg 13:1–42, 1956
14. Brock M, Dietz H: The small frontolateral approach for the microsurgical treatment of intracranial aneurysms. Neurochirurgia (Stuttg) 21:185–191, 1978
15. Campbell E, Burklund CW: Aneurysms of the middle cerebral artery. Ann Surg 137:18–28, 1953
16. Chou SN, Ortiz-Suarez HJ: Surgical treatment of arterial aneurysms of the vertebrobasilar circulation. J Neurosurg 41:671–680, 1974
17. Corkill G, Hodgson MJH: Hypotension with sodium nitroprusside in the surgery of cerebral aneurysms. Anaesthesia 28:191–194, 1973
18. Cushing H: The chiasmal syndrome of primary optic atrophy and bitemporal field defects in adult patients with a normal sella turcica. XIII Concilium Ophthalmologicum (Hollandia) 13(3):97–184, 1929
19. Dandy WE: Aneurysms of the anterior cerebral artery. JAMA 119:1253–1254, 1942
20. Dandy WE: Intracranial aneurysm of internal carotid artery, cured by operation. Ann Surg 107:654–659, 1938
21. Dandy WE: Intracranial Arterial Aneurysms. New York, Hafner, 1944, reprinted 1969
22. Dandy WE: Intracranial arterial aneurysms. In The Brain. New York, Harper & Row, 1969, pp. 395–412 (reprinted from Lewis Practice of Surgery, Hagerstown, Maryland, WF Prior Co, 1945)
23. David M, Pertuiset B, Guyot JF: La cure radicale des anévrysmes de la communicante antérieure sans résection cérébrale chez la malade conscient. Considérations cliniques post-opératoires. Rev Neurol (Paris) 118:150–151, 1968
24. David M, Pertuiset B, Guyot JF: La cure radicale des anévrysmes de la communicante antérieure sans résection cérébrale ni hypothermie chez le malade conscient. Considérations sur la mortalité et les troubles du comportement postopératoires. Press Med 76:1467–1470, 1968
25. de Grood MPAM: Neurosurgical technique in saccular aneurysms. Psychiatr Neurol Neurochir 75:425–428, 1972
26. De Klerk DJJ, De Villiers, JC: Microsurgery for aneurysms on the circle of Willis. S Afr Med J 48:825–830, 1974
27. Deruty R, Dechaume J-P, Lecuire J, et al.: Traitement microchirurgical d'une série d'anévrysmesartérielsintra-crânienssus-tentoriels. Neurochirurgie 22:227–238, 1976
28. Dimsdale H, Logue V: Ruptured posterior fossa aneurysms and their surgical treatment. J Neurol Neurosurg Psychiatry 22:202–217, 1959
29. Dott NM: Intracranial aneurysms: cerebral arterio-radiography: surgical treatment. Edinburgh Med J 40:219–234, 1933
30. Drake CG: Bleeding aneurysms of the basilar artery. Direct surgical management in four cases. J Neurosurg 18:230–238, 1961
31. Drake CG: Comment. Neurosurgery 3:140–141, 1978
32. Drake CG: Further experience with surgical

treatment of aneurysms of the basilar artery. J Neurosurg 29:372–392, 1968
33. Drake CG: Management of aneurysms of posterior circulation. In Youmans JR (ed.): Neurological Surgery, Vol 2. Philadelphia, Saunders, 1973, pp. 787–806
34. Drake CG: On the surgical treatment of ruptured intracranial aneurysms. Clin Neurosurg 13:122–155, 1965
35. Drake CG: Surgical treatment of rupture of aneurysms of the basilar artery. Experience with 14 cases. J Neurosurg 23:457–473, 1965
36. Drake CG: Surgical treatment of ruptured intracranial aneurysms. In Cooper P (ed.): The Craft of Surgery, Vol III, 2nd ed. Boston, Little, Brown, 1971, pp. 1765–1784
37. Drake CG: Surgical treatment of vertebrobasilar aneurysms. In Koos WT, Böck FW, Spetzler RF (eds.): Clinical Microneurosurgery. Stuttgart, Georg Thieme Verlag, 1976, pp. 213–219
38. Drake CG: The surgical treatment of aneurysms of the basilar artery. J Neurosurg 29:436–446, 1968
39. Drake CG: The surgical treatment of vertebral-basilar aneurysms. Clin Neurosurg 16:114–169, 1969
40. Drake CG: The treatment of aneurysms of the posterior circulation. Clin Neurosurg 26:96–144, 1979
41. Drake CG: Vertebral basilar aneurysms. A progress report. In Scientific Program Manuscript of the American Association of Neurological Surgeons, paper 61, 1971, pp. 1–8
42. Drake CG: Amacher AL: Aneurysms of the posterior cerebral artery. J Neurosurg 30:468–474, 1969
42a. Drake CG, Vanderlinden RG, Amacher AL: Carotid-choroidal aneurysms. J Neurosurg 29:32–36, 1968
42b. Drake CG, Vanderlinden RG, Amacher AL: Carotid-ophthalmic aneurysms. J Neurosurg 29:24–31, 1968
43. Elsberg CA: Ruptured aneurysm of the right middle cerebral artery. Bull NY Neurol Inst 1:210–212, 1918
44. Elvidge AR, Feindel WH: Surgical treatment of aneurysm of the anterior cerebral and the anterior communicating arteries diagnosed by angiography and electroencephalography. J Neurosurg 7:13–32, 1950
45. Endo S, Suzuki J: Anterior communicating artery aneurysm not visualized by angiography. Report of two successfully operated cases. Neurologia Med Chir 14(part I):69–73, 1974
46. Falconer MA: The surgical treatment of bleeding intracranial aneurysms. J Neurol Neurosurg Psychiatry 14:153–186, 1951
47. Fang HSY, Ong GB: Direct anterior approach to the upper cervical spine. J Bone Joint Surg 44A:1588–1604, 1962
48. Finkemyer H: Verletzungen der A. carotis interna in ihrem intrakraniellen extraduralen Abschnitt. Zbl Neurochir 15:65–73, 1955
49. Fox JL: Microsurgical exposure of intracranial aneurysms. J Microsurg 1:2–31, 1979
50. Fox JL: Obliteration of midline vertebral artery aneurysm via basilar craniectomy. J Neurosurg 26:406–412, 1967
51. Fox JL: Tentorial section for decompression of the brain stem and a large basilar aneurysm. Case report. J Neurosurg 28:74–77, 1968
52. Fox JL, Luessenhop AJ: Hydrocephalus secondary to hemorrhage from a basilar artery aneurysm. With a note on embolization technique. Acta Neurochir (Wien) 17:228–235, 1967
53. French LA, Chou SN, Long DM: The direct approach to intracranial aneurysms. Clin Neurosurg 15:117–132, 1968
54. French LA, Chou SN, Story JL: Aneurysms of the anterior communicating artery. Report of a method of surgical treatment and review of 40 cases. Postgrad Med 34:323–327, 1963
55. French LA, Chou SN, Story JL, et al.: Aneurysm of the anterior communicating artery. J Neurosurg 24:1058–1062, 1966
56. French LA, Ortiz-Suarez HJ: Anterior communicating artery aneurysms: technique of operation and results. Clin Neurosurg 21:115–119, 1974
57. French LA, Zarling ME, Schultz EA: Management of aneurysms of the anterior communicating artery. J Neurosurg 19:870–876, 1962
58. Frugoni P, Conforti P: Aneurismi sacculari di insolite dimensioni della cerebrale anteriore e del complesso cerebrale anteriore-comunicante anteriore. Minerva Neurochir 6:120–125, 1962
59. Garcia-Bengochea F, Deland FH: Bilateral giant carotid-ophthalmic aneurysms. Case report. J Neurosurg 42:589–592, 1975
60. Gardner WJ: Cerebral angiomas and aneurysms. Surg Clin North Am 16:1019–1030, 1936
61. Gass HH, McGuire JF, Simmons DR: Intracranial eradication of middle cerebral aneurysms. J Neurosurg 15:223–233, 1958
62. Gillingham FJ: The management of ruptured intracranial aneurysm. Ann R Coll Surg 23:89–117, 1958
63. Green FHK: "Congenital" aneurysm of the cerebral arteries. Q J Med 21:419–432, 1928
64. Guidetti B: Il trattamento chirurgico degli aneurismi della comunicante anteriore. Minerva Neurochir 2:4–14, 1958

65. Guidetti B: Microsurgical treatment of intracranial saccular aneurysms. Acta Neurochir (Wien) 43:153–162, 1978
66. Guidetti B: Results of 98 intracranial aneurysm operations performed with the aid of an operating microscope. Acta Neurochir (Wien) 29:65–71, 1973
67. Guidetti B: Surgical treatment of aneurysms of the anterior communicating artery. Prog Brain Res 30:303–307, 1968
68. Guidetti B, La Torre E: Carotid-ophthalmic aneurysms. A series of 16 cases treated by direct approach. Acta Neurochir (Wien) 22:289–304, 1970
69. Guidetti B, La Torre E: Management of carotid-ophthalmic aneurysms. J Neurosurg 42:438–442, 1975
70. Guillain G, Schmidt P, Bertrand I: Anévrysme du tronc basillaire ayant déterminé la symptomatologie d'une tumeur de l'angle pontocérébelleux. Rev Neurol (Paris) 5:795–802, 1930
71. Gurdjian ES, Thomas LM: Operative Neurosurgery, 3rd ed. Baltimore, Williams & Wilkins, 1970, pp. 324–333
72. Hamby WB: Intracranial Aneurysms. Springfield, Ill., Thomas, 1952
73. Hamby WB: Intracranial surgery for aneurysms. Prog Neurol Surg 3:1–65, 1969
74. Hamby WB: Remarks concerning intracranial aneurysm surgery. Clin Neurosurg 17:1–17, 1970
75. Hamby WB: The modern treatment of intracranial aneurysms. NY State J Med 52:2497–2502, 1952
76. Hamby WB: Treatment of ruptured intracranial aneurysms. Surg Clin North Am 34:1063–1075, 1954
77. Hammon WM, Kempe LG: The posterior fossa approach to aneurysms of the vertebral and basilar arteries. J Neurosurg 37:339–347, 1972
78. Harris P: Aneurysms of the anterior communicating artery. Cincinnati J Med 42:1–7, 1961
79. Harris P, Udvarhelyi GB: Aneurysms arising at the internal carotid-posterior communicating artery junction. J Neurosurg 14:180–191, 1957
80. Hashi K, Hakuba A, Ikuno H, et al.: [A midline vertebral artery aneurysm operated via transoral transclival approach.] Neurol Surg (Tokyo) 4:183–189, 1976
80a. Hayakawa T, Kamikawa K, Toshiteru O, et al.: Prevention of postoperative complications after a transoral transclival approach to basilar aneurysms. Technical note. J Neurosurg 54:699–703, 1981
81. Hayes GJ: Personal communication, 1974
82. Hayes GJ, Slocum HC: The achievement of optimal brain relaxation by hyperventilation technics of anesthesia. J Neurosurg 19:65–69, 1962
83. Hemmer R, Umbach W: Verlaufsformen intrakranieller sackförmiger Aneurysmen. Arch Psychiatr Nervenkr 200:612–625, 1960
84. Henderson JW: Intracranial arterial aneurysms. A study of 119 cases, with special reference to the ocular findings. Trans Am Ophthalmol Soc 53:349–462, 1955
89. Heuer GJ: Surgical experiences with an intracranial approach to chiasmal lesions. Arch Surg 1:368–381, 1920
86. Heuer GJ: The surgical approach and treatment of tumors and other lesions about the optic chiasm. Surg Gynecol Obstet 53:489–518, 1931
87. Heuer GJ, Dandy WE: A new hypophysis operation. Johns Hopkins Hosp Bull 29:154, 1918
88. Hitselberger WE, Gardner G Jr: Other tumors of the cerebellopontine angle. Arch Otolaryngol 88:712–714, 1968
89. Hollin SA, Decker RE: Microsurgical treatment of internal carotid artery aneurysms. J Neurosurg 47:142–149, 1977
90. Höök O, Norlén G: Aneurysms of the anterior communicating artery. Acta Neurol Scand 40:219–240, 1964
91. Höök O, Norlén G, Guzmán J: Saccular aneurysms of the vertebral-basilar arterial system. A report of 28 cases. Acta Neurol Scand 39:271–304, 1963
92. Hori S, Suzuki J: Early intracranial operations for ruptured aneurysms. Acta Neurochir (Wien) 46:93–104, 1979
93. Housepian EM, Bowman FO Jr, Gissen AJ: Elective circulatory arrest in intracranial surgery. Successful treatment of an aneurysm of the basilar artery with a method of open-chest circulatory arrest. J Neurosurg 26:594–597, 1967
94. Ito Z: Microsurgical interhemispheric approach for ruptured aneurysm of anterior communicating artery in acute stage. Excerpta Medica ICS No. 418:73, 1977
95. Jain KK: Surgery of anterior communicating aneurysms: experience with various techniques and evolution of a modified approach. Surg Neurol 2:31–33, 1974
96. Jamieson, KG: Aneurysms of the vertebrobasilar system. Further experience with nine cases. J Neurosurg 28:544–555, 1968
97. Jamieson KG: Aneurysms of the vertebrobasilar system. Surgical intervention in 19 cases. J Neurosurg 21:781–797, 1964
98. Jamieson KG: Direct operation for intracranial aneurysm: some technical problems and

attempts at their solution. Neurol Med Chir (Tokyo) 11:1–10, 1971
99. Jefferson G: Compression of the chiasma, optic nerves, and optic tracts by intracranial aneurysms. Brain 60:444–497, 1937
100. Karasawa J, Kikuchi H, Furuse S, et al.: [Surgery of vertebral aneurysms of the origin of PICA.] Neurol Surg (Tokyo) 4:1157–1164, 1977
101. Kasdon DL, Stein BM: Combined supratentorial and infratentorial exposure for low-lying basilar aneurysms. Neurosurgery 4:422–426, 1979
102. Kempe LG: Approach to circle of Willis. J Neurosurg 46:559, 1977
103. Kempe LG: Operative Neurosurgery, Vol 1: Cranial, Cerebral, and Intracranial Vascular Disease. Berlin, Springer-Verlag, 1968, pp. 1–75, 203–214
104. Kempe LG: Operative Neurosurgery, Vol 2: Posterior Fossa, Spinal Cord, and Peripheral Nerve Disease. Berlin, Springer-Verlag, 1970, pp. 66–71
105. Kempe LG, VanderArk GD: Anterior communicating artery aneurysms. Gyrus rectus approach. Neurochirurgia (Stuttg) 14:63–70, 1971
106. Kikuchi H: [Operative indication and surgical technique of the cerebral aneurysm.] Neurol Med Chir (Tokyo) 16 (6 Part 2):479–486, 1976
107. Klemme RM, Woolsey RD: Suprasellar aneurysm. Report of a case, with recovery. Arch Neurol Psychiatry 47:662–666, 1942
108. Krause F: Chirurgie des Gehirns und Rückenmarks nach eigenen Erfahrungen, Vol 1. Berlin, Urban & Schwarzenberg, 1908, p. 76, plate XVII, Fig a
109. Krayenbühl H, Richter HR: Die zerebrale Angiographie. Stuttgart, Georg Thieme Verlag, 1952
110. Krayenbühl H, Yaşargil MG: Das sackförmige Aneurysma der Hirnarterien. In Das Hirnaneurysma. Documenta Geigy. Series Chirurgica, No. 4. Basel, Geigy, 1958, pp. 10–65
111. Krayenbühl H, Yaşargil MG: Diagnosis and therapy of intracranial aneurysms. In Cooper P, Nyhus LM: Surgery Annual. New York, Appleton-Century-Crofts, 1970, pp. 327–343
112. Krayenbühl H, Yaşargil MG, Flamm ES, et al: Microsurgical treatment of intracranial saccular aneurysms. J Neurosurg 37:678–686, 1972
113. Kunc Z: Aneurysms of carotid and posterior communicating artery. Prog Brain Res 30:309–315, 1968
114. Laine E: Arterial vertebro-basilar aneurysms. Prog Brain Res 30:323–346, 1968
115. Laine E: Traitement chirurgical des anévrysmes de l'artère communicante antérieure. In Krayenbühl H, et al.: L'Anévrysme de l'Artère Communicante Antérieure. Paris, Masson et Cie, 1959, pp. 131–182
116. Laine E, Allègre GE, Goutelle A, et al.: Les anévrysmes vertébro-basilaires: choix de la voie d'abord. Problème de adjuvants per-opératoires. Neurochirurgie 18:317–332, 1972
117. Laine E, Andreussi L, Delandsheer J-M, et al.: Anévrysmes de l'artère cérébrale moyenne. Étude anatomique, clinique et thérapeutique. A propos d'une série de 116 cas dont 100 ont été opérés. Neurochirurgie 16:181–201, 1970
118. Laine E, Jomin M: Indications et possibilités de la voie trans-bucco-pharyngée en présence d'un anévrysme du confluent vertébro-basilaire. Neurochirurgie 23:307–314, 1977
119. Laitinen L: Aneurysms of the proximal portion of the anterior cerebral artery. Acta Psychiatr Scand 36:141–148, 1961
120. Laitinen L, Snellman A: Aneurysms of the pericallosal artery. A study of 14 cases verified angiographically and treated mainly by direct surgical attack. J Neurosurg 17:447–458, 1960
121. Lang EF, Poppen JL: Aneurysms of the anterior communicating artery: results of surgical treatment. Surg Clin North Am 42:793–805, 1962
122. Le Beau J: Anévrismes de l'artère communicante antérieure. Ruptures et indications neurochirurgicales. Neurochirurgia (Stuttg) 5:38–57, 1962
123. Le Beau J: Indications opératories et traitement chirurgical des anévrismes artériels intra-craniens sus-tentoriels. Ann Chir 15:1153–1163, 1961
124. Lepoire J, Coxam B: Les anévrismes de la communicante antérieure. Aspects anatomiques modalités opératoires. Neurochirurgie 5:162–182, 1959
125. List CF, Hodges FJ: Intracranial angiography. I. The diagnosis of vascular lesions. J Neurosurg 3:25–45, 1946
125a. Litvak J, Summers TC, Barron JL, et al.: A successful approach to vertebrobasilar aneurysms. Technical note. J Neurosurg 55:491–494, 1981
126. Logue V: Posterior fossa aneurysms. Clin Neurosurg 11:183–207, 1964
127. Lougheed WM: Selection, timing, and technique of aneurysm surgery of the anterior circle of Willis. Clin Neurosurg 16:95–113, 1969
128. Lougheed WM, Botterell EH, Morley TP: Results of the direct attack in the surgical management of internal carotid and middle cerebral aneurysms. Clin Neurosurg 9:193–200, 1963
129. Lougheed WM, Marshall BM: Management of aneurysms of the anterior circulation by intracranial procedures. In Youmans JR (ed.): Neu-

rological Surgery, Vol 2. Philadelphia, Saunders, 1973, pp. 731–767
130. Lougheed WM, Marshall BM: The diploscope in intracranial aneurysm surgery: results in 40 patients. Can J Surg 12:75–82, 1969
130a. Malkasian DR, Rand RW: Microsurgical anatomy. In Rand RW: Microneurosurgery, 2nd ed. St Louis, Mosby, 1978, pp. 37–70
131. Martinez Coll A, Del Corral JF: Experiences in intracranial surgery for aneurysms. Surg Neurol 3:191–193, 1975
132. Maspes PE, Marini G: Aneurysms of the anterior communicating artery. Result of direct surgical treatment. Acta Neurochir (Wien) 11:479–494, 1963
132a. Matricali B, van Dulken H: Aneurysm of fenestrated basilar artery. Surg Neurol 15:189–191, 1981
133. McMurtry JG III, Housepian EM, Bowman FO Jr, et al.: Surgical treatment of basilar artery aneurysms. Elective circulatory arrest with thoracotomy in 12 cases. J Neurosurg 40:486–498, 1974
134. Miyazaki Y: [Surgery of bilateral cerebral aneurysms with special reference to bilateral craniotomy and simultaneous direct surgery.] Shujutsu 24:17–28, 1970
135. Mraček Z: [Aneurysm of the superior cerebellar artery successfully treated by surgery.] Rozhl Chir 48:363–365, 1969
136. Norlén G: Aneurysm of the anterior communicating artery. Prog Brain Res 30:295–302, 1968
137. Norlén G: Some aspects of the surgical treatment of intracranial aneurysms. Clin Neurosurg 9:214–222, 1963
138. Norlén G: The pathology, diagnosis and treatment of intracranial saccular aneurysms. Proc R Soc Med 45:291–302, 1952
139. Norlén G, Barnum AS: Surgical treatment of aneurysms of the anterior communicating artery. J Neurosurg 10:634–650, 1953
140. Norlén G, Olivecrona H: The treatment of aneurysms of the circle of Willis. J Neurosurg 10:404–415, 1953
141. Norlén G, Paly SN: Aneurysms of the vertebral artery. Report of two operative cases. J Neurosurg 17:830–835, 1960
142. Nornes H, Wikeby P: Results of microsurgical management of intracranial aneurysms. J Neurosurg 51:608–614, 1979
143. Northfield DWC: The Surgery of the Central Nervous System. Oxford, Blackwell, 1973, pp. 346–401
144. Nugent GR: Personal communication, 1980
145. Paterson A: Direct surgery in the treatment of posterior communicating aneurysms. Lancet 2:808–811, 1968
146. Paterson A: Direct surgery of posterior communicating aneurysms. In Logue V (ed.): Operative Surgery, Vol 14: Neurosurgery, 2nd ed. Philadelphia, Lippincott, 1971, pp. 167–171
147. Peerless SJ: The surgical approach to middle cerebral and posterior communicating aneurysms. Clin Neurosurg 21:151–165, 1974
148. Pertuiset B: Les anévrysmes de l'artère communicante postérieure. Diagnostic et indications thérapeutiques (Sans la pathogénie). Presse Med 70:935–937, 1962
149. Pertuiset B, Vouyouklakis D, Guyot JF, et al.: Les résultats du traitement chirurgical des anévrysmes artériels sus-tentoriels rompus. D'après 81 cas personnels. Neurochirurgie 12:421–436, 1966
150. Pia HW: Microsurgical treatment of cerebral aneurysms. Neurosurg Rev 1:15–24, 1978
151. Pool JL: Aneurysms of the anterior communicating artery. Bifrontal craniotomy and routine use of temporary clips. J Neurosurg 18:98–111, 1961
152. Pool JL: Bifrontal craniotomy for anterior communicating artery aneurysms. J Neurosurg 36:212–220, 1972
153. Pool JL: Early treatment of ruptured intracranial aneurysms of the circle of Willis with special clip techniques. Bull NY Acad Med 35:357–369, 1959
154. Pool JL: Surgery of anterior cerebral and anterior communicating aneurysms. In Logue V (ed.): *Operative Surgery, Vol 14: Neurosurgery*, 2nd ed. Philadelphia, Lippincott, 1971, pp. 159–166
155. Pool JL: Timing and techniques in the intracranial surgery of ruptured aneurysms of the anterior communicating artery. J Neurosurg 19:378–388, 1962
156. Pool JL, Potts DG: Aneurysms and Arteriovenous Anomalies of the Brain. Diagnosis and Treatment. New York, Harper & Row, 1965
157. Pool JL, Ransohoff J, Yahr MD, et al.: Early surgical treatment of aneurysms of the circle of Willis. Neurology (NY) 9:478–486, 1959
158. Poppen JL: An Atlas of Neurosurgical Techniques. Philadelphia, Saunders, 1960, pp. 156–181
159. Poppen JL: Operative treatment for aneurysms of the anterior communicating artery. Clin Neurosurg 11:8–13, 1964
160. Poppen JL: Vascular surgery of the posterior fossa. Clin Neurosurg 6:198–209, 1959
161. Prados M, Strowger B, Feindel W: Studies on cerebral edema. II. Reaction of the brain to exposure to air; physiologic changes. Arch Neurol Psychiatry 54:290–300, 1945
162. Rana RS: Surgical management of internal ca-

rotid aneurysms. Results in 21 operated cases. Neurol India 13:59–61, 1965
163. Rand RW: Microneurosurgery. St. Louis, Mosby, 1969, pp. 198–209
164. Rand RW: Microneurosurgery, 2nd ed. St Louis, Mosby, 1978, pp. 43–44, 311–324
165. Ransohoff J: Treatment of subarachnoid hemorrhage. Current status. NY State J Med 63:2494–2501, 1963
166. Rhoton AL, Jackson FE, Gleave J, et al.: Congenital and traumatic intracranial aneurysms. Clin Symp 29:1–40, 1977
167. Rhoton AL, Saeki N, Pearlmutter D, et al.: Microsurgical anatomy of common aneurysm sites. Clin Neurosurg 26:248–306, 1979
168. Richardson AE: Surgery of basilar aneurysms. Psychiatr Neurol Neurochir 75:441–443, 1972
169. Richardson AE: Surgery of posterior circulation aneurysms. Vertebro-basilar system and branches. In Logue V (ed.): Operative Surgery, Vol 14: Neurosurgery, 2nd ed. Philadelphia, Lippincott, 1971, pp. 178–183
170. Rizzoli HV, Hayes GJ: Congenital berry aneurysm of the posterior fossa. Case report with successful operative excision. J Neurosurg 10:550–551, 1953
171. Robertson EG: Intracranial aneurysms, with special reference to surgical treatment. Aust NZ J Surg 8:132–144, 1938
172. Robinson RG: Ruptured aneurysms of the middle cerebral artery. J Neurosurg 35:25–33, 1971
173. Salazar JL: Treatment of ruptured and unruptured internal carotid artery aneurysms. Surg Neurol 11:451–455, 1979
174. Samorajski T, Moody RA: Changes in the blood-brain barrier after exposure of the brain. Arch Neurol Psychiatry 78:369–376, 1957
175. Samson DS, Hodosh RM, Clark WK: Microsurgical evaluation of the pterional approach to aneurysms of the distal basilar circulation. Neurosurgery 3:135–141, 1978
176. Sano K: Aneurysms of the vertebral and basilar arteries. Neurol Surg (Tokyo) 1:193–199, 1973
177. Sano K: [Surgery of intracranial aneurysm.] Brain Nerve (Tokyo) 23:1252–1264, 1971
178. Sano K, Jimbo M, Saito I: [Vertebro-basilar aneurysms—with special reference to the transpharyngeal transclival approach to the basilar artery aneurysm.] Brain Nerve (Tokyo) 18:1197–1203, 1966
179. Schwartz HG: Arterial aneurysm of the posterior fossa. J Neurosurg 5:312–316, 1948
180. Sedzimir CB: Surgical treatment of aneurysms of the vertebral artery. J Neurosurg 20:597–599, 1963
181. Selverstone B: Coating of intracranial aneurysms with nontoxic adherent plastics. In Schmidek HH, Sweet WH (eds.): Current Techniques in Operative Neurosurgery. New York, Grune & Stratton, 1977, pp. 31–40
182. Sengupta RP, Lassman LP, de Moraes AA, et al.: Treatment of internal carotid bifurcation aneurysms by direct surgery. J Neurosurg 43:343–351, 1975
183. Sheldon CH, Pundenz RH, Brannon LE: Intracranial aneurysms. Arch Surg 61:294–302, 1950
184. Sheldon CH, Pudenz RH, Restarski JS: A new position for frontal craniotomy. J Neurosurg 2:546–550, 1945
185. Shephard RH: Operation for aneurysms of the middle cerebral artery. In Logue V (ed.): Operative Surgery, Vol 14: Neurosurgery, 2nd ed. Philadelphia, Lippincott, 1971, pp. 172–177
186. Shields CB: Current trends in management of cerebral aneurysms. J Ky Med Assoc 75:529–535, 1977
187. Snellman A, Makela T, Nystrom S: Considérations sur les anéurysmes de la région située entre les artéries cérébrales antérieurs. (A propos d'une série de cinquante-deux cas opérés.) Neurochirurgie 5:143–161, 1959
188. Speakman TJ, Barlass JL: The bifrontal approach to aneurysms of the anterior communicating artery. Can J Surg 6:237–243, 1963
189. Steelman HF, Hayes GJ, Rizzoli HV: Surgical treatment of saccular intracranial aneurysms. J Neurosurg 10:564–576, 1953
190. Stevenson GC, Stoney RJ, Perkins RK, et al.: A transcervical transclival approach to the ventral surface of the brain stem for removal of a clivus chordoma. J Neurosurg 24:544–551, 1966
191. Strauss I, Globus JH, Ginsburg SW: Spontaneous subarachnoid hemorrhage. Its relation to aneurysms of cerebral blood vessels. Arch Neurol Psychiatry 27:1080–1132, 1932
192. Sugita K, Kobayashi S, Shintani A, et al.: Microneurosurgery for aneurysms of the basilar artery. J Neurosurg 51:615–620, 1979
193. Sugita K, Shintani A, Mutsuga N, et al.: [Microsurgery for vertebrobasilar aneurysms.] Neurol Med Chir (Tokyo) 17 (part 2):351–360, 1977
194. Sundt TM Jr: Clip-grafts for aneurysm and small vessel surgery. Part 4. Relative application to various aneurysms and repair of anterior communicating aneurysms using a right-angle clip holder. Technical note. J Neurosurg 37:753–758, 1972
195. Sundt TM Jr, Murphey F: Clip-grafts for aneurysm and small vessel surgery. Part 3. Clinical

experience in intracranial internal carotid artery aneurysm. J Neurosurg 31:59–71, 1969
196. Suzuki J: [Direct intracranial operative approach to cerebral aneurysms.] Brain Nerve (Tokyo) 18:478–487, 1966
197. Suzuki J: Operative indication and surgical technique of the cerebral aneurysm. 3. Neurol Med Chir (Tokyo) 16 (6 part 2):487–495, 1976
198. Suzuki J, Iwabuchi T, Takaku A, et al.: [Aneurysm arising at the junction of internal carotid and posterior communicating artery.] Brain Nerve (Tokyo) 17:1003–1008, 1965
199. Suzuki J, Iwabuchi T, Takaku A, et al.: [Management of intracranial aneurysms. Especially direct attack of 103 cases.] Brain Nerve (Tokyo) 19:815–824, 1967
200. Suzuki J, Kowada M, Asahi H, et al.: [Surgical treatment of aneurysms of the anterior communicating artery.] Brain Nerve (Tokyo) 16:391–397, 1964
201. Suzuki J, Miura Y: [Surgery for multiple cerebral aneurysms.] Shujutsu 21:67–76, 1967
202. Suzuki J, Takaku A, Hori S: New surgical techniques for direct intracranial surgery of anterior communicating artery aneurysm. Excerpta Medica Int Cong Series No. 293:96, 1973
203. Suzuki J, Takaku A, Hori S, et al.: [Direct operation for aneurysm of the middle cerebral artery. A new approach.] Brain Nerve (Tokyo) 22:445–454, 1970
204. Suzuki J, Yoshimoto T, Uchida K: [Surgical treatment of distal anterior cerebral artery aneurysms.] Neurol Surg (Tokyo) 5:29–33, 1977
205. Swain RD: The surgical treatment of certain intracranial arterial aneurysms. Surg Clin North Am 28:396–404, 1948
206. Symon L: Subarachnoid haemorrhage from intracranial aneurysm and angioma. In Russell RWR (ed.): Cerebral Arterial Disease. Edinburgh, Churchill Livingstone, 1976, pp. 231–261
207. Taveras JM: The roentgen diagnosis of intracranial incisural space occupying lesions. Am J Roentgenol 84:52–69, 1960
208. Taylor JC, Choudhury AR: Reinforcement with gauze wrapping for ruptured aneurysms of the middle cerebral artery. J Neurosurg 47:828–832, 1977
209. Thiry S, Hotermans JM, Brand H, et al.: Le traitement chirurgical des principaux anévrysmes arteriels intracrâniens supratentoriels. Acta Chir Belg 63:308–330, 1964
210. Tönnis W: Erfolgreiche Behandlung eines Aneurysma der Art. commun. ant. cerebri. Zbl Neurochir 1:39–42, 1936
211. Tönnis W, Walter W: Die Behandlung der sackförmigen intrakraniellen Aneurysmen. In Olivecrona H, Tönnis W (eds.): Klinik and Behandlung der raumbeengenden intrakraniellen Prozesse. Handbuch der Neurochirurgie, Vol 4, Part 2. Berlin, Springer-Verlag, 1966, pp. 212–363
212. Tönnis W, Walter W: Ein neuer operativer Zugang zu den sackförmigen Aneurysmen der basalen Hirngefässe. Wien Med Wochenschr 110:145–147, 1960
213. Trevani E: Ein als parasellarer Tumor operiertes Aneurysma der Arteria carotis interna. Dtsch Z Chir 237:534–535, 1932
214. Uihlein A, Hughes RA: The surgical treatment of intracranial vestigial aneurysms. Surg Clin North Am 35:1071–1083, 1955
215. Usbeck W: Über ein als Tumor imponierendes grosses Aneurysma der Arteria basialis. Zbl Neurochir 15:205–211, 1955
216. VanderArk GD, Kempe LC: Classification of anterior communicating aneurysms as a basis for surgical approach. J Neurosurg 32:300–303, 1970
217. VanderArk GD, Kempe LG, Smith DR: Anterior communicating aneurysms: the gyrus rectus approach. Clin Neurosurg 21:120–133, 1974
218. Viale GL, Pau A: Carotid-choroidal aneurysms: remarks on surgical treatment and outcome. Surg Neurol 11:141–145, 1979
219. Whalley N: Ruptured congenital aneurysm of anterior cerebral artery. J Neurol Neurosurg Psychiatry 12:322–324, 1949
220. Wilson CB, Christensen FK, Subrahmanian MV: Intracranial aneurysms at the pericallosal artery bifurcation. Am Surg 31:386–393, 1965
221. Wilson CB, Spetzler RF: Operative approaches to aneurysms. Clin Neurosurg 26:232–247, 1979
222. Wilson CB, U HS: Surgical treatment for aneurysms of the upper basilar artery. J Neurosurg 44:537–543, 1976
223. Wilson DH: Limited exposure in cerebral surgery. Technical note. J Neurosurg 34:102–106, 1971
224. Wissinger JP, Danoff D, Wisiol ES, et al.: Repair of an aneurysm of the basilar artery by a transclival approach. Case report. J Neurosurg 26:417–419, 1967
225. Woodhall B: Personal communication, 1980
226. Wright DC, Wilson CB: Surgical treatment of basilar aneurysms. Neurosurgery 5:325–333, 1979
227. Wright WH, Todd EM, Duemler LP, et al.: Simultaneous direct operations for bilateral internal carotid artery aneurysms. Surg Neurol 2:355–358, 1974
228. Yada K, Owada T: [Aneurysms of the internal carotid artery.] Neurol Surg (Tokyo) 3:459–465, 1975

229. Yamaura A, Makino H, Isobe K, et al.: Repair of cerebrospinal fluid fistula following transoral transclival approach to a basilar aneurysm. Technical note. J Neurosurg 50:834–836, 1979
230. Yaşargil MG: Intracranial microsurgery. Clin Neurosurg 17:250–255, 1970
231. Yaşargil MG: Microsurgery Applied to Neurosurgery. Stuttgart, Georg Thieme Verlag, 1969, pp. 119–143
232. Yaşargil MG, Antic J, Laciga R, et al.: Microsurgical pterional approach to aneurysms of the basilar bifurcation. Surg Neurol 6:83–91, 1976
233. Yaşargil MG, Boehm WB, Ho REM: Microsurgical treatment of cerebral aneurysms at the bifurcation of the internal carotid artery. Acta Neurochir (Wien) 41:61–72, 1978
234. Yaşargil MG, Carter LP: Saccular aneurysms of the distal anterior cerebral artery. J Neurosurg 39:218–223, 1974
235. Yaşargil MG, Fox JL: The microsurgical approach to intracranial aneurysms. Surg Neurol 3:7–14, 1975
236. Yaşargil MG, Fox JL, Ray MW: The operative approach to aneurysms of the anterior communicating artery. In Krayenbühl H (ed.): Advances and Technical Standards in Neurosurgery, Vol 2. New York, Springer-Verlag, 1975, pp. 113–170
237. Yaşargil MG, Gasser JC, Hodosh RM, et al.: Carotid-ophthalmic aneurysms: direct microsurgical approach. Surg Neurol 8:155–165, 1977
238. Yaşargil MG, Smith RD: Surgery on the carotid system in the treatment of hemorrhagic stroke. Adv Neurol 16:181–209, 1977
239. Yashon D, White RJ, Arias BA, et al.: Cyanocrylate encasement of intracranial aneurysms. Technical note. J Neurosurg 34:709–713, 1971
240. Yoshimoto T, Uchida K, Suzuki J: Surgical treatment of distal anterior cerebral artery aneurysms. J Neurosurg 50:40–44, 1979

30

Craniotomy for Aneurysm

VI. Tissue Section and Resection

Since the beginning of direct surgical intervention in the treatment of intracranial aneurysms, surgeons have been removing specific bony structures, dural separations, nerves, blood vessels, and brain tissue to expose the aneurysms or to provide symptomatic relief. As surgical techniques evolved there has been a reduced requirement to remove or section large amounts of functional brain tissue and nerves and an increased tendency to remove bone at the skull base to reduce the need for extensive brain retraction. Tissue incision/excision discussed here includes sphenoid bone, clinoid processes, tentorium and falx, cranial nerves (CN-1,2,5), vessels, and brain tissue.

Cranial Base

Sphenoid Wing

Except for the Tönnis (94) transcallosal approach to ACoAA and the parasagittal approach to ACeAA, nearly all types of cranial flaps to aneurysms on the circle of Willis provide for a low basal exposure, whether frontal, frontolateral, temporal, or suboccipital (Chapter 29). The frontolateral exposure originating with Dandy (10–12,45) and continued by his students evolved into a basal exposure with ronguering away of the sphenoid bone. We and others have continued with this technique since our early training in aneurysm surgery (see pp. 757–764) (21,37,46,99). Yaşargil et al. (49, 50,101,103,104,106) improved on this method by drilling down the sphenoid wing to the base of the anterior clinoid process as viewed under the operating microscope. Others also now use this technique (21,31,32,81). See Chapter 34 for details of the technique as used by us.

Anterior Clinoid Process

Removal of the anterior clinoid process after exposure of the optic nerve and ICA is commonly done in cases of oaICAA and vICCA (13,33,34,36,38,40,66,70,83,86,89,105). We also used this technique in one case of pcaICAA where there was remarkable overgrowth of the anterior clinoid that obscured the ICA–PCoA junction. In many instances actual bony removal is not necessary, for excision of the dura over the anterior clinoid with cutting current from the electrocautery unit and a small curette may be sufficient to expose the neck of the aneurysm. In some cases it is advisable to go so far as to unroof the optic canal (Fig. 30.1) and incise the dura propria to allow retraction of the optic nerve (36,38,40,86). Hauser and Gass (36) in 1952 removed the roof of the optic canal to decompress an optic nerve compromised by an unruptured oaICAA (aneurysm not clipped), with the result that there was considerable improvement in the patient's vision.

Although chisel and rongeur were used in earlier days, the high-speed diamond drill is utilized most often now for bony removal. A gentle touch is necessary, for the adjacent vital structures must not be injured. The reader is referred to some other articles for specialized techniques (66,105).

Posterior Clinoid Process

We are unable to find any references to removal of the posterior clinoid process. This may be considered in the frontolateral approach to BAA, but it is accompanied by great risk of injury to the oculomotor nerve and adjacent vessels.

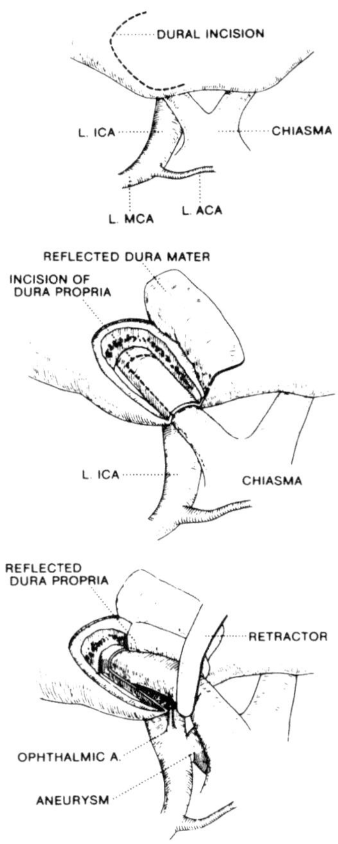

Fig. 30.1 Unroofing of the left optic canal to approach the neck of a difficult oaICCA. *Top* Dural incision (*dotted line*) over sphenoid bone above optic canal. *Middle* Optic canal unroofed; an incision (*dotted line*) is made in dura propria. *Bottom* Neck of medially located oaICAA is exposed under gently retracted optic nerve. From Iwabuchi T, Suzuki S, Sobata E, ref. 38.

Dural Structures

Falx

The anterior falx and its superior sagittal sinus are often incised during the bifrontal approach to ACoAA (see Fig. 29.13), causing no impairment (58,73).

Tentorium

Section of the tentorium to improve visualization of BAA, especially those lying inferiorly, is a well-documented technical adjunct (9,14–19,22,30,41,42,44,46,51,53,57,79,81,102). Figures 30.2 and 29.45 illustrate Drake's approach. Emphasis is placed on protecting the trochlear nerve. The incision is made well behind the superior petrosal sinus and the entrance of CN-4 under the tentorial leaf. Kasdon and Stein (44) cut the lateral sinus and tentorium (see Fig. 29.50) in a combined infratentorial–supratentorial exposure of a low basilar trunk aneurysm.

Pool and Potts (74) and French et al. (24) occasionally cut the anterior reflection of the tentorium for pcaICAA lying under the tentorium. Fox (22) cut the tentorium as the only treatment of a patient quadriparetic and mute from the pressure of a giant thrombosed bBAA (Fig. 30.3); complete recovery ensued. Using care and the microscope, one can easily cut the tentorium using the cutting current from the electrocautery unit.

Blood Vessels

Ligation and section of bridging veins (e.g., those between the temporal lobe and the sphenoparietal sinus or between the frontal lobe and superior sagittal sinus) is commonplace. However, this procedure should be limited if possible to avoid compromising local venous return.

Deliberate ligation and section of arterial channels is rarely done except with approaches to bBAA. In 1958 Gillingham (29) mentioned ligating and cutting the PCoA to gain exposure of bBAA. Since then deliberate severance of either the PCoA or the P-1 artery (whichever is smaller) has been done by the subtemporal and frontolateral transylvian approaches (9,15,16,21,29,41,102,103). In our experience no problems have arisen from clipping and severing either the PCoA or the P-1 if: (a) the clips do not compromise their perforating arteries; (b) the perforating arteries receive blood via the ICA and/or BA system; and (c) the clip on the aneurysm does not compromise the P-1 exits from the basilar tip.

Cranial Nerves

Olfactory Tract

The bifrontal approach to ACoAA has usually resulted in anosmia from bilateral olfactory tract severance. Suzuki et al. (90) preserve these nerves via their bifrontal technique. The unilateral approaches may cause an olfactory tract to tear apart from retraction or excess brain shrinkage.

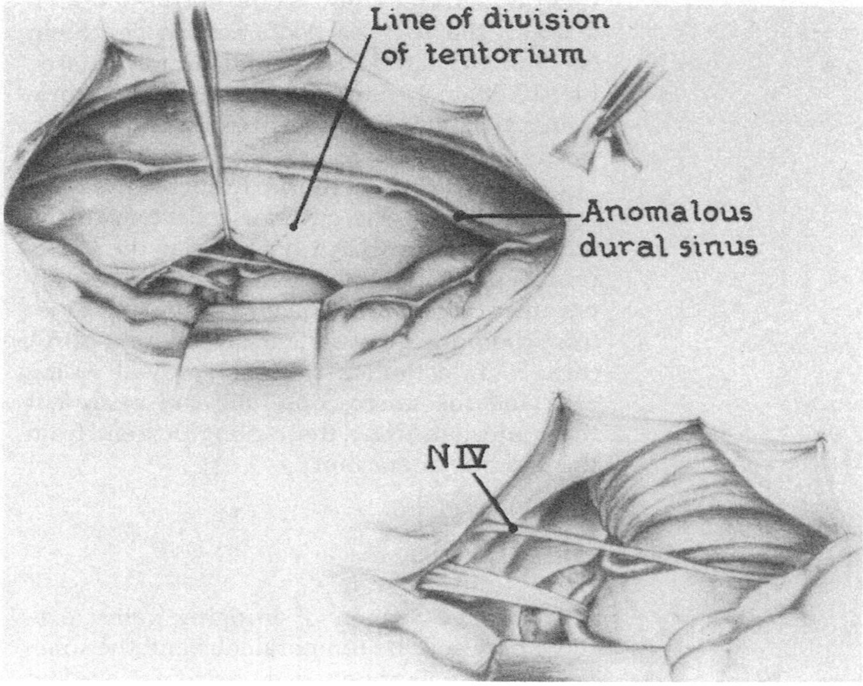

Fig. 30.2. Line of division of tentorium (*dotted line*) via a right subtemporal exposure, emphasizing protection of the trochlear nerve (*N IV*). Below (anterior) the trochlear nerve is the oculomotor nerve lateral to the bBAA and P-1. The SCA is seen medial to the trochlear nerve. From Drake CG, ref. 18.

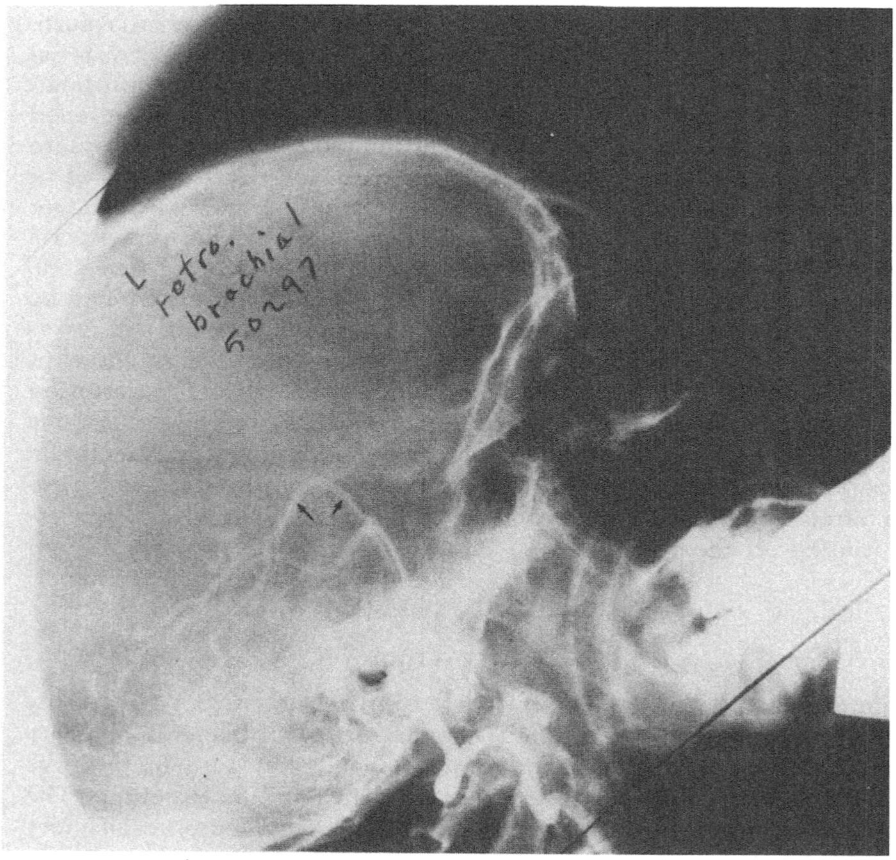

A

Fig. 30.3. A Vertebral angiogram of a patient with a giant thrombosed bBAA. Note stretching of the right P-1 and P-2 arteries (*arrows*).

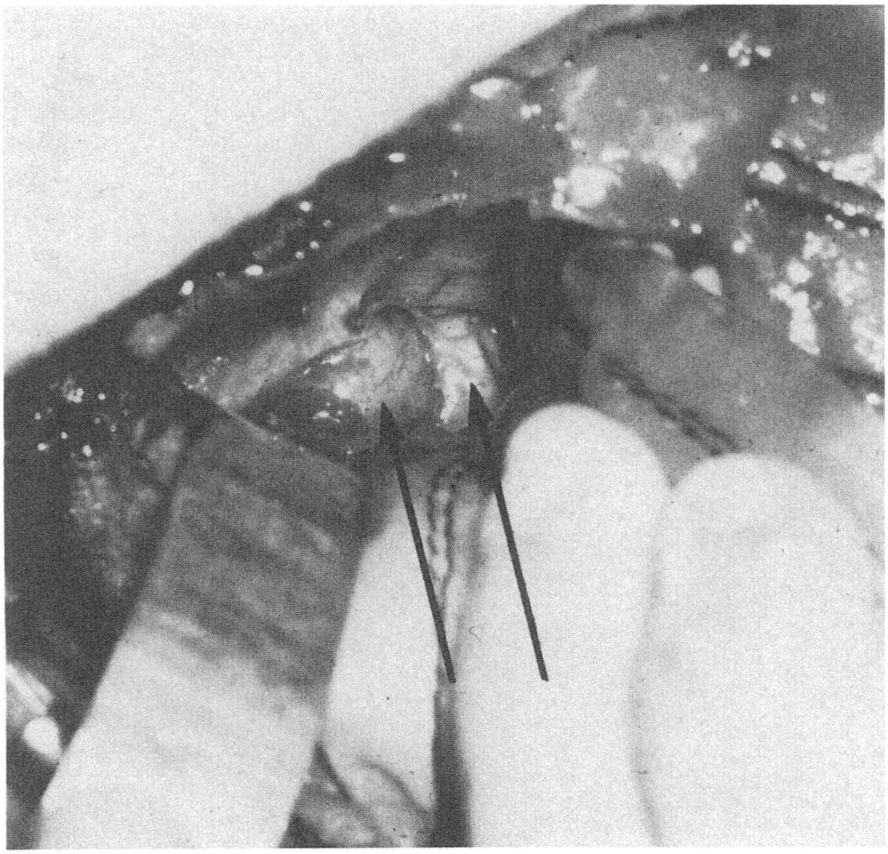

B

B Same patient. Right lateral view of subtemporal surgical exposure of a giant bBAA (*left long arrow*) compressing the brainstem (*right long arrow*). Below are the retractor, cottonoids, and the surgeon's gloved finger elevating the temporal lobe. Above the aneurysm and brainstem is the cut edge of the tentorium, with the superior surface of the cerebellum seen on the right. From Fox JL, ref. 22.

Optic Nerve

In 1942 Dandy (10) reported partially resecting the right optic nerve while excising a giant ACoAA. In 1949 Alpers and Ryan (2) described a case of a fusiform ICAA which was trapped after cutting CN-2. In 1957 Petit-Dutaillis and colleagues (72) cut the optic nerve to expose an ophthalmic artery aneurysm. Since then there have been additional reports of section of the optic nerve to surgically treat oaICAA or other ICAA (1a,3,5,48,74).

Trigeminal Nerve

In 1927 Magnus (60) cut a CN-5 for relief of pain secondary to a giant ic/csICAA, as did Jefferson (43) in 1938. Dandy (12) did the same for nine cases of giant BAA. Jaeger (39) and Marguth and Schiefer (61) also performed trigeminal rhizotomy for treatment of neuralgia secondary to large ICAA. All these cases had their CN-5 cut as the primary method of therapy rather than as a way to expose and treat the aneurysm itself. For individual case reports of aneurysms treated by trigeminal rhizotomy see the *Surg* column (symbol *TRI*) in Appendix 2.

Other Nerves

Exposure of an aneurysm adjacent to any cranial nerve, especially a giant aneurysm or one rupturing at surgery, risks injury and severance of that nerve. Exposure of VAA lying under the brainstem and surrounded by cranial nerves sometimes results in tearing or section of a rootlet or an entire nerve.

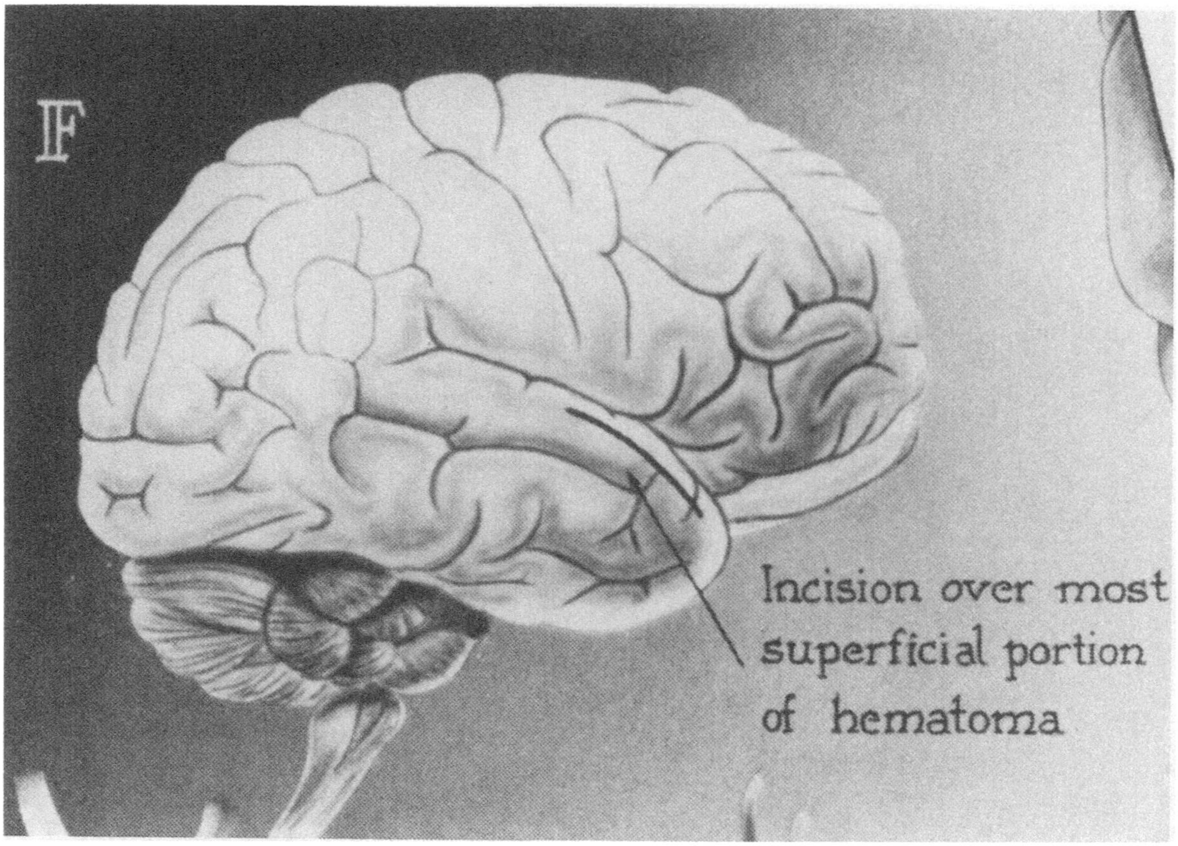

Fig. 30.4. Line of incision through superior temporal gyrus to reach underlying clot and MCAA. From Poppen JL, ref. 75.

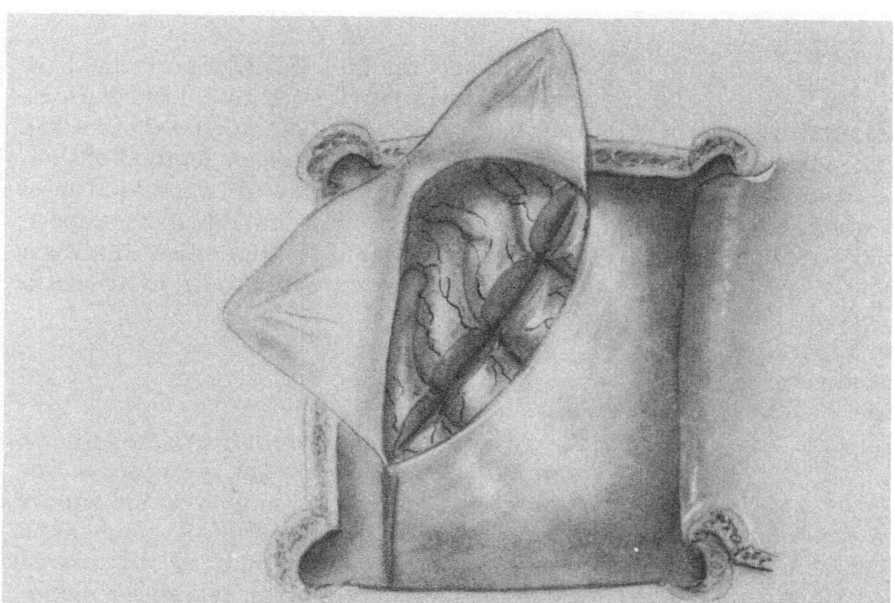

Fig. 30.5. After a unilateral frontal craniotomy the dura is opened and a medial wedge of right frontal lobe removed. At observer's upper left is most medial anterior burr hole. Note line of incision into the brain for exposure of ACoAA. From French LA, Chou SN, Story JL, et al., ref. 25.

Brain Tissue

Occipital Lobe

In 1938 German (28) reported performing an occipital lobectomy to remove a PCeAA.

Temporal Lobe

Bassett et al. (4) described removal of a temporal pole in the presence of edema and/or hematoma while attacking aneurysms. Wedges of inferior temporal gyrus, anterior temporal tip, or temporal lobe have been removed on occasion to gain access to BAA via subtemporal craniotomy (9,30,41,42,51,64,79). Some surgeons have removed portions of the temporal tip to reach an ICAA (59,65,69,74,88). Adjacent temporal and frontal lobe tissues have been removed on occasion in cases of bICAA (82,88). Frequently temporal lobe tissue, usually the superior temporal gyrus portion (Fig. 30.4), has been incised or excised to reach an MCAA (8,69,75,78,80,82,84,85,88,91,95). Some surgeons included the middle temporal gyrus as well.

Tönnis and Walter (96) recommended exposing all anterior circulation aneurysms through the superior temporal gyrus. Their approach opened into the sylvian fissure from which MCAA, ACoAA, and ICAA were attacked. This, in one sense, is the prelude to our technique of simply opening the sylvian fissure widely (transylvian approach) for all aneurysms of the circle of Willis via the frontolateral flap. The advantage is one of less brain retraction pressure on the frontal and temporal lobes.

Frontal Lobe

It was once routine among many neurosurgeons to resect a medial wedge (Fig. 30.5) of one frontal pole to gain adequate exposure of an ACoAA (1,4,6,7,23–27,35,52,54,55,59,63,65,67,69,71,73–77,82,85,87,92,93,97,100). This was often required in the presence of an edematous brain. With present-day methods of controlling ICP and patient selection, this amount of brain tissue removal is seldom necessary.

In 1953 Norlén and Olivecrona (68) wrote concerning the exposure of ACoAA: "Some brain tissue surrounding the aneurysm must usually be removed by suction in order to expose completely the aneurysm and its neck."

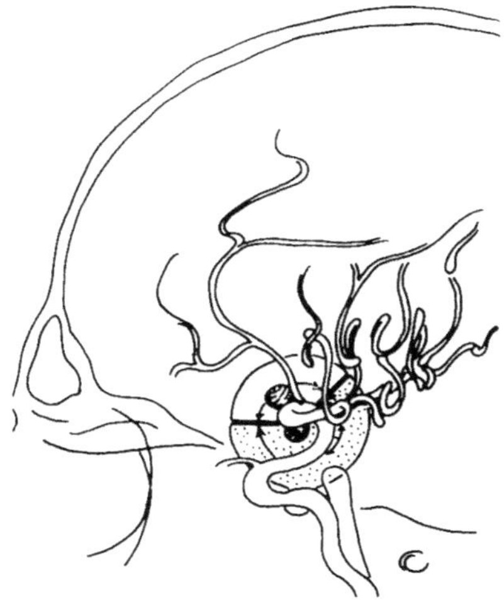

Fig. 30.6. Division of directions of the ACoAA on the basis of projection of the fundus. All aneurysms which project in any direction within the strippled arc of the circle are approached via the gyrus rectus incision, according to the authors. All aneurysms pointing in a direction within the clear arc of the circle are approached subfrontally via the pterional flap. From VanderArk GD, Kempe LG, ref. 98.

As the only tissue there that could be safely removed would be the gyrus rectus, this undoubtedly is one of the early descriptions of removal of portions of that tissue for ACoAA. In 1956 Ley (56) reported that he excised the posterior aspect of the gyrus rectus in a case of an ACoAA operated by a frontal approach. Kempe et al. (46,47,98,99) described the "gyrus rectus approach" to specific types of ACoAA via frontolateral craniotomy; others have also used it (20,21,50,62,103,104).

Kempe and co-workers (46,47,98,99) used the gyrus rectus approach mainly for ACoAA whose fundus pointed inferiorly (Fig. 30.6). This represented about 70% of their ACoAA cases. Figure 30.7 illustrates an ACoAA projecting upward and one projecting downward. The rationale for using the gyrus rectus approach for aneurysms pointing downward is to avoid lifting the frontal lobe and exposing the dome of the aneurysm before the neck is isolated. In cases where the fundus projects upward an approach directly through the longitudinal fissure by retraction of gyrus rectus will lead the surgeon to the neck before the dome is seen.

Figure 30.8 diagrams the gyrus rectus approach of Kempe and VanderArk (47). Basically a small incision is made in the gyrus rectus me-

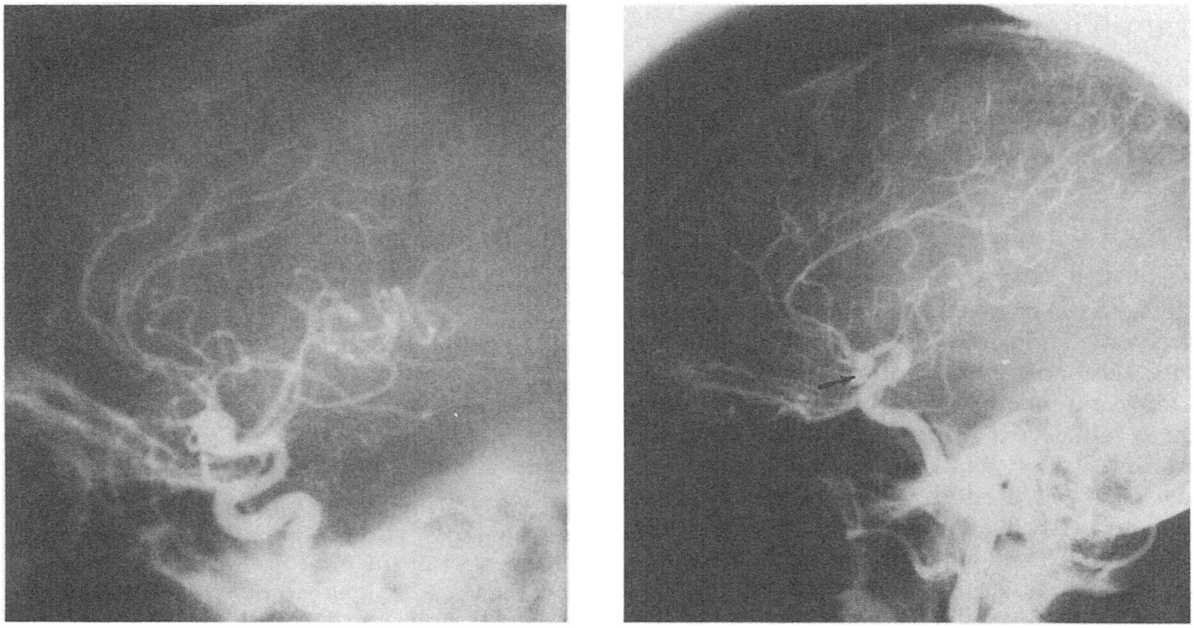

A B

Fig. 30.7. **A** Lateral view demonstrating upward projection of an ACoAA. **B** Lateral view demonstrating downward projection of an ACoAA.

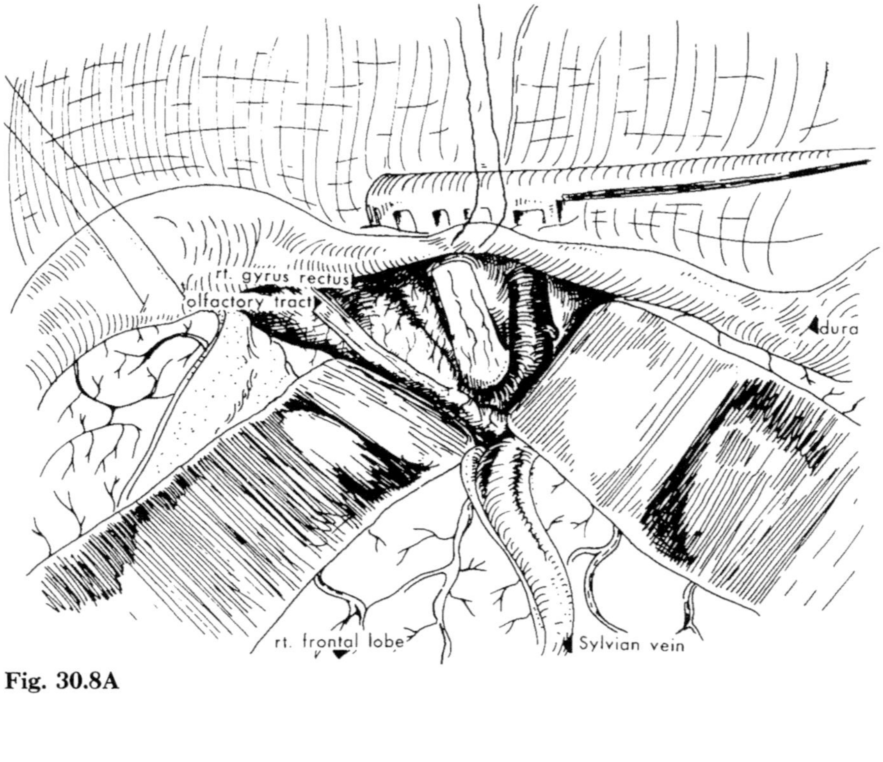

Fig. 30.8A

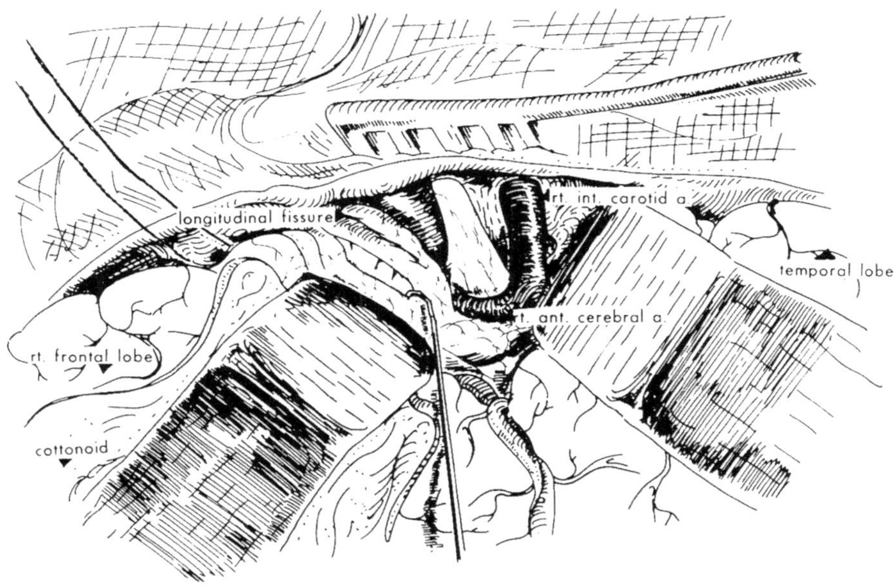

B

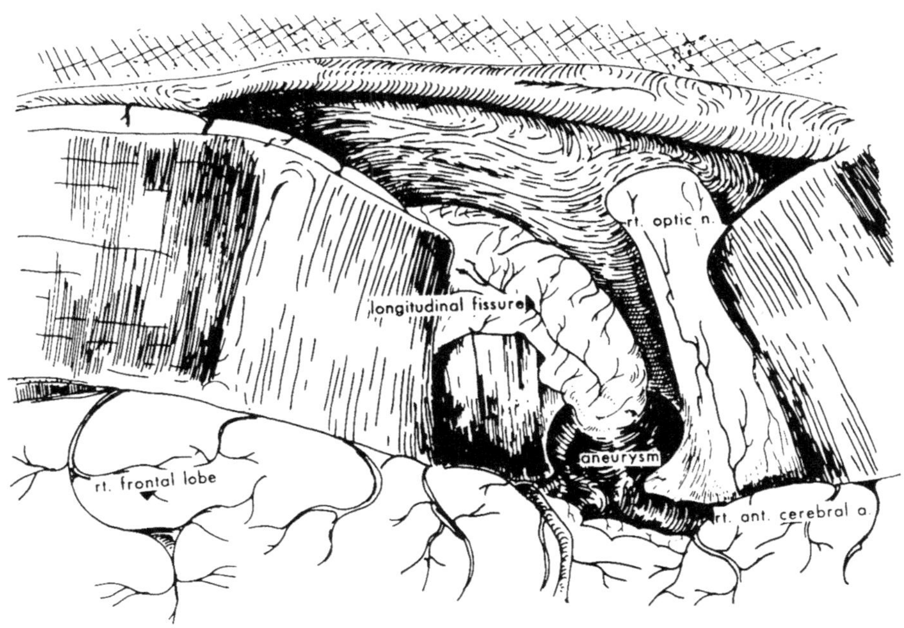

C

Fig. 30.8. Steps in the gyrus rectus approach to an ACoAA. From Kempe LG, VanderArk GD, ref. 47.

A Via the right pterional approach, the dissection is carried down the lesser wing of the sphenoid bone to expose the optic nerve and ICA. Retractors are on the frontal and temporal lobes. Sutures are retracting the dura over the sphenoid bone. The ICA has been followed to its bifurcation in this case. Between the optic nerve and olfactory tract is seen the gyrus rectus.

B An incision is made in the gyrus rectus just medial to and parallel with the olfactory tract.

C After removal of this portion of the gyrus rectus, the ACoAA is found without disturbance of the fundus.

dial to the olfactory tract. The ACoA region is reached within a depth of 1 cm or less. Further details are found in Chapter 35. Yaşargil et al. (103,104) and Fox (21) have used the gyrus rectus approach for most ACoAA cases, as there is less disturbance of the aneurysm even with the superiorily directed ACoAA.

Bibliography

1. Almeida GM, Bianco E, Shibata MK: Anterior communicating artery aneurysms. J Neurosurg 33:53–57, 1976

1a. Almeida GM, Shibata MK, Bianco E: Carotid-ophthalmic aneurysms. Surg Neurol 5:41–45, 1976

2. Alpers BJ, Ryan JJ: Verified cerebral aneurysms with negative arteriogram. J Nerv Ment Dis 109:220–225, 1949
3. Arseni C, Ghitescu M, Cristescu A, et al.: Intrasellar aneurysms simulating hypophyseal tumors. Eur Neurol 3:321–329, 1970
4. Bassett RC, List CF, Lemmen LJ: Surgical treatment of intracranial aneurysm. Surg Gynecol Obstet 95:701–708, 1952
5. Benedetti A, Curri D: Direct attack on carotid ophthalmic and large internal carotid aneurysms. Surg Neurol 8:49–54, 1977
6. Bohm E, Hugosson R: Results of surgical treatment of 200 consecutive cerebral arterial aneurysms. Acta Neurol Scand 46:43–52, 1970
7. Botterell EH, Lougheed WM, Scott JW, et al.: Hypothermia, and interruption of carotid, or carotid and vertebral circulation, in the surgical management of intracranial aneurysms. J Neurosurg 13:1–42, 1956
8. Campbell E, Burklund CW: Aneurysms of the middle cerebral artery. Ann Surg 137:18–28, 1953
9. Chou SN, Ortiz-Suarez HJ: Surgical treatment of arterial aneurysms of the vertebrobasilar circulation. J Neurosurg 41:671–680, 1974
10. Dandy WE: Aneurysms of the anterior cerebral artery. JAMA 119:1253–1254, 1942
11. Dandy WE: Intracranial aneurysm of internal carotid artery, cured by operation. Ann Surg 107:654–659, 1938
12. Dandy WE: Intracranial Arterial Aneurysms. New York, Hafner, 1944, reprinted 1969
13. Deruty R, Dechaume J-P, Lecuire J, et al.: Traitement microchirurgical d'une série d'anévrysmes artériels intra-crâniens sus-tentoriels. Neurochirurgie 22:227–238, 1976
14. Dimsdale H, Logue V: Ruptured posterior fossa aneurysms and their surgical treatment. J Neurol Neurosurg Psychiatry 22:202–217, 1959
15. Drake CG: Bleeding aneurysms of the basilar artery. Direct surgical management in four cases. J Neurosurg 18:230–238, 1961
16. Drake CG: Further experience with surgical treatment of aneurysms of the basilar artery. J Neurosurg 29:372–392, 1968
17. Drake CG: Surgical treatment of rupture of aneurysms of the basilar artery. Experience with 14 cases. J Neurosurg 23:457–473, 1965
18. Drake CG: The surgical treatment of aneurysms of the basilar artery. J Neurosurg 29: 436–446, 1968
19. Drake CG: The surgical treatment of vertebral-basilar aneurysms. Clin Neurosurg 16: 114–169, 1969
20. Duffy G: The surgical treatment of anterior communicating artery aneurysms. Aust NZ J Surg 44:257–260, 1974
21. Fox JL: Microsurgical exposure of intracranial aneurysms. J Microsurg 1:2–31, 1979
22. Fox JL: Tentorial section for decompression of the brain stem and a large basilar aneurysm. Case report. J Neurosurg 28:74–77, 1968
23. French LA: Discussion. Clin Neurosurg 11: 209–214, 1964
24. French LA, Chou SN, Long DM: The direct approach to intracranial aneurysms. Clin Neurosurg 15:117–132, 1968
25. French LA, Chou SN, Story JL, et al.: Aneurysm of the anterior communicating artery. J Neurosurg 24:1058–1062, 1966
26. French LA, Ortiz-Suarez HJ: Anterior communicating artery aneurysms: technique of operation and results. Clin Neurosurg 21:115–119, 1974
27. French LA, Zarling ME, Schultz EA: Management of aneurysms of the anterior communicating artery. J Neurosurg 19:870–876, 1962
28. German WJ: Intracranial aneurysm: a surgical problem. Zbl Neurochir 3:352–354, 1938
29. Gillingham FJ: The management of ruptured intracranial aneurysm. Ann R Coll Surg 23:89–117, 1958
30. Gissen AJ, Matteo RS, Housepian EM, et al.: Elective circulatory arrest during neurosurgery for basilar artery aneurysms. JAMA 207:1315–1318, 1969
31. Guidetti B: Microsurgical treatment of intracranial saccular aneurysms. Acta Neurochir (Wien) 43:153–162, 1978
32. Guidetti B: Results of 98 intracranial aneurysm operations performed with the aid of an operating microscope. Acta Neurochir (Wien) 29:65–71, 1973
33. Guidetti B, La Torre E: Carotid-ophthalmic aneurysms. A series of 16 cases treated by di-

rect approach. Acta Neurochir (Wien) 22:289–304, 1970
34. Guidetti B, La Torre E: Management of carotid-ophthalmic aneurysms. J Neurosurg 42: 438–442, 1975
35. Harris P: Aneurysms of the anterior communicating artery. Cincinnati J Med 42:1–7, 1961
36. Hauser MJ, Gass H: Optic nerve pressure by aneurysm relieved by decompression of optic nerve. Report of a case. Arch Ophthalmol 48:627–631, 1952
37. Hayes GJ: Personal communication, 1974
38. Iwabuchi T, Suzuki S, Sobata E: Intracranial direct operation for carotid-ophthalmic aneurysm by unroofing of the optic canal. Acta Neurochir (Wien) 43:163–169, 1978
39. Jaeger R: Aneurysm of the intracranial carotid artery. Syndrome of frontal headache with oculomotor nerve paralysis. JAMA 142:304–309, 1950
40. Jain, KK: Saccular aneurysm of the ophthalmic artery. Am J Ophthalmol 69:997–998, 1970
41. Jamieson, KG: Aneurysms of the vertebrobasilar system. Further experience with nine cases. J Neurosurg 28:544–555, 1968
42. Jamieson KG: Aneurysms of the vertebrobasilar system. Surgical intervention in 19 cases. J Neurosurg 21:781–797, 1964
43. Jefferson G: On the saccular aneurysms of the internal carotid artery in the cavernous sinus. Br J Surg 26:267–302, 1938
44. Kasdon DL, Stein BM: Combined supratentorial and infratentorial exposure for low-lying basilar aneurysms. Neurosurgery 4:422–426, 1979
45. Kempe LG: Approach to circle of Willis. J Neurosurg 46:559, 1977
46. Kempe LG: Operative Neurosurgery, Vol 1: Cranial, Cerebral, and Intracranial Vascular Disease. Berlin, Springer-Verlag, 1968, pp. 1–75, 203–214
47. Kempe LG, VanderArk GD: Anterior communicating artery aneurysms. Gyrus rectus approach. Neurochirurgia (Stuttg) 14:63–70, 1971
48. Kothandaram P, Dawson BH, Kruyt RC: Carotid-ophthalmic aneurysms. A study of 19 patients. J Neurosurg 34:544–548, 1971
49. Krayenbühl H, Yaşargil MG: Diagnosis and therapy of intracranial aneurysms. In Cooper P, Nyhus LM: *Surgery Annual.* New York, Appleton-Century-Crofts, 1970, pp. 327–343
50. Krayenbühl HA, Yaşargil MG, Flamm ES, et al.: Microsurgical treatment of intracranial saccular aneurysms. J Neurosurg 37:678–686, 1972
51. Laine E: Arterial vertebro-basilar aneurysms. Prog Brain Res 30:323–346, 1968
52. Laine E: Traitement chirurgical des anévrysmes de l'artère communicante antérieure. In Krayenbühl H, et al. (eds.): *L'Anévrysme de l'Artère Communicante Antérieure.* Paris, Masson et Cie, 1959, pp. 131–182
53. Laine E, Allègre GE, Goutelle A, et al.: Les anévrysmes vertébro-basilaires: choix de la voie d'abord. Problème de adjuvants peropératoires. Neurochirurgie 18:317–332, 1972
54. Lang EF, Poppen JL: Aneurysms of the anterior communicating artery: results of surgical treatment. Surg Clin North Am 42:793–805, 1962
55. Lapras C, Goutelle A, Dechaume J-P, et al.: Pronostic des anévrysmes de la communicante antérieure traités par abord direct. Neurochirurgie 15:369–378, 1969
56. Ley E Jr: Successful treatment of an aneurysm of the anterior communicating artery. J Neurosurg 13:294–298, 1956
57. Logue V: Posterior fossa aneurysms. Clin Neurosurg 11:183–207, 1964
58. Lougheed WM: Selection, timing, and technique of aneurysm surgery of the anterior circle of Willis. Clin Neurosurg 16:95–113, 1969
59. Lougheed WM, Marshall BM: Management of aneurysms of the anterior circulation by intracranial procedures. In Youmans JR (ed.): Neurological Surgery, Vol 2. Philadelphia, Saunders, 1973, pp. 731–767
60. Magnus V: Aneurysm of the internal carotid artery. JAMA 88:1712–1713, 1927
61. Marguth F, Schiefer W: Spontanheilung eines intrakraniellen Aneurysmas angiographisch nachgeweisen. Acta Neurochir (Wien) 5:38–45, 1957
62. Martinez Coll A, Del Corral JF: Experiences in intracranial surgery for aneurysms. Surg Neurol 3:191–193, 1975
63. Matson DD: Intracranial arterial aneurysms in childhood. J Neurosurg 23:578–583, 1965
64. McMurtry JG III, Housepian EM, Bowman FO Jr, et al.: Surgical treatment of basilar artery aneurysms. Elective circulatory arrest with thoracotomy in 12 cases. J Neurosurg 40:486–498, 1974
65. Morello G: Remarks on the direct attack on intracranial aneurysms. Prog Brain Res 30: 347–349, 1968
66. Morgan F: Removal of anterior clinoid process in the surgery of carotid aneurysm. With some notes on recurrent subarachnoid haemorrhage during craniotomy. Schwiez Arch Neurol Neurochir Psychiatr 111:363–368, 1972
67. Norlén G, Barnum AS: Surgical treatment of aneurysms of the anterior communicating artery. J Neurosurg 10:634–650, 1953

68. Norlén G, Olivecrona H: The treatment of aneurysms of the circle of Willis. J Neurosurg 10:404–415, 1953
69. Northfield DWC: The Surgery of the Central Nervous System. Oxford, Blackwell, 1973, pp. 346–401
70. Nutik S: Carotid paraclinoid aneurysms with intradural origin and intracavernous location. J Neurosurg 48:526–533, 1978
71. Patterson RH Jr, Ray BS: Profound hypothermia for intracranial surgery: laboratory and clinical experiences with extracorporeal circulation by peripheral cannulation. Ann Surg 156:377–393, 1962
72. Petit-Dutaillis D, Guillaumat L, Rougerie J: Syndrome de compression du nerf optique droit. Déconverte operatoire d'un anévrisme de l'artère ophtalmique. Traitement par la méthode du "trapping." Neurochirurgie 3:22–29, 1957
73. Pool JL: Aneurysms of the anterior communicating artery. Bifrontal craniotomy and routine use of temporary clips. J Neurosurg 18:98–111, 1961
74. Pool JL, Potts DG: Aneurysms and Arteriovenous Anomalies of the Brain. Diagnosis and Treatment. New York, Harper & Row, 1965
75. Poppen JL: An Atlas of Neurosurgical Techniques. Philadelphia, Saunders, 1960, pp. 156–181
76. Poppen JL: Discussion. Clin Neurosurg 11: 183–219, 1964
77. Poppen JL: Operative treatment for aneurysms of the anterior communicating artery. Clin Neurosurg 11:8–13, 1964
78. Posnikoff J: Cure of intracranial aneurysm without use of blood transfusion. Calif Med 106:124–127, 1967
79. Richardson AE: Surgery of basilar aneurysms. Psychiatr Neurol Neurochir 75:441–443, 1972
80. Robinson RG: Ruptured aneurysms of the middle cerebral artery. J Neurosurg 35:25–33, 1971
81. Samson DS, Hodosh RM, Clark WK: Microsurgical evaluation of the pterional approach to aneurysms of the distal basilar circulation. Neurosurgery 3:135–141, 1978
82. Selverstone B: Coating of intracranial aneurysms with nontoxic adherent plastics. In Schmidek HH, Sweet WH (eds.): Current Techniques in Operative Neurosurgery. New York, Grune & Stratton, 1977, pp. 31–40
83. Sengupta RP, Gryspeerdt GL, Hankinson J: Carotid-ophthalmic aneurysms. J Neurol Neurosurg Psychiatry 39:837–853, 1976
84. Shephard RH: Operation for aneurysms of the middle cerebral artery. In Logue V (ed.): Operative Surgery, Vol 14: Neurosurgery, 2nd ed. Philadelphia, Lippincott, 1971, pp. 172–177
85. Sjöqvist O: Thread ligature of intracranial saccular aneurysms. In Proceedings of the 5th Congress of Neurology, Lisbon, Vol 3, 1953, pp. 108–115
86. Stroobandt G, Cornelis G: Intrasellar carotid-ophthalmic aneurysm. Angiotomographic demonstration and surgical cure. Neurochirurgia (Stuttg) 14:220–224, 1971
87. Sugar O: Discussion. Arch Neurol Psychiatry 68:843–844, 1952
88. Sugar O, Tsuchiya G: Plastic coating of intracranial aneurysms with "EDH-adhesive." J Neurosurg 21:114–117, 1964
89. Sundt TM Jr, Piepgras DG: Surgical approach to giant intracranial aneurysms. Operative experience with 80 cases. J Neurosurg 51:731–742, 1979
90. Suzuki J, Takaku A, Hori S: New surgical techniques for direct intracranial surgery of anterior communicating artery aneurysm. Excerpta Medica Int Cong Series No. 293:96, 1973
91. Taylor JC, Choudhury AR, Shephard RH: Surgery of aneurysms of the middle cerebral artery: a comparison of results of "wrapping" and "clipping" procedures. J Neurol Neurosurg Psychiatry 40:200, 1977
92. Thiry S, Hotermans JM, Brand H, et al.: Le traitement chirurgical des principaux anévrysmes arteriels intracrâniens supratentoriels. Acta Chir Belg 63:308–330, 1964
93. Todd EM, Sheldon CH, Crue BL Jr, et al.: Plastic jackets for certain intracranial aneurysms. JAMA 179:935–939, 1962
94. Tönnis W: Erfolgreiche Behandlung eines Aneurysma der Art. commun. ant. cerebri. Zbl Neurochir 1:39–42, 1936
95. Tönnis W, Walter W: Die Behandlung der sackförmigen intrakraniellen Aneurysmen. In Olivecrona H, Tönnis W (eds.): Klinik and Behandlung der raumbeengenden intrakraniellen Prozesse. Handbuch der Neurochirurgie, Vol 4, Part 2. Berlin, Springer-Verlag, 1966, pp. 212–363
96. Tönnis W, Walter W: Ein neuer operativer Zugang zu den sackförmigen Aneurysmen der basalen Hirngefässe. Wien Med Wochenschr 110:145–147, 1960
97. Uihlein A, Thomas RL, Cleary J: Aneurysms of the anterior communicating artery complex. Proc Mayo Clin 42:73–87, 1967
98. VanderArk GD, Kempe LG: Classification of anterior communicating aneurysms as a basis for surgical approach. J Neurosurg 32:300–303, 1970
99. VanderArk GD, Kempe LG, Smith DR: Ante-

rior communicating aneurysms: the gyrus rectus approach. Clin Neurosurg 21:120–133, 1974
100. Williams BN, Turner EA: Report on 10 operations under local cerebral hypothermia, J Neurol Neurosurg Psychiatry 33:647–655, 1970
101. Yaşargil MG: Microsurgery Applied to Neurosurgery. Stuttgart, Georg Thieme Verlag, 1969, pp. 119–143
102. Yaşargil MG, Antic J, Laciga R, et al.: Microsurgical pterional approach to aneurysms of the basilar bifurcation. Surg Neurol 6:83–91, 1976
103. Yaşargil MG, Fox JL: The microsurgical approach to intracranial aneurysms. Surg Neurol 3:7–14, 1975
104. Yaşargil MG, Fox JL, Ray MW: The operative approach to aneurysms of the anterior communicating artery. In Krayenbühl H (ed.): Advances and Technical Standards in Neurosurgery, Vol 2. New York, Springer-Verlag, 1975, pp. 113–170
105. Yaşargil MG, Gasser JC, Hodosh RM, et al.: Carotid-ophthalmic aneurysms: direct microsurgical approach. Surg Neurol 8:155–165, 1977
106. Yaşargil MG, Smith RD: Surgery on the carotid system in the treatment of hemorrhagic stroke. Adv Neurol 16:181–209, 1977

31

Craniotomy for Aneurysm

VII. Special Methods of Treating the Aneurysm

Throughout the years a number of surgical methods of eliminating intracranial aneurysms, rendering them impotent, or at least defusing their explosive threat of expansion and/or rupture have been developed. As intracranial surgical techniques have improved, some "stop-gap" methods have been eliminated and more effective techniques of direct attack have evolved.

Decompression Craniectomy

In earlier days a decompression procedure commonly was done to reduce the effects of edema and clot after an SAH or to decompress an otherwise inoperable giant aneurysm. In most of these cases a "tumor" was suspected, and the true diagnosis was made at surgical exploration or autopsy. The following gives examples in chronological order.

In 1916 Dandy and Heuer (52,161) performed a subtemporal decompression for a giant ICAA, as did Elsberg (189) for a similar problem that same year. Again in 1918 Elsberg performed bilateral subtemporal decompressions for elevated ICP following rupture of a MCAA (249). In 1921 Foerster (105) treated two cases of ICAA by subtemporal decompression. Cushing performed a similar procedure on a patient who had ruptured a pcaICAA (317,329). By 1925 Borchardt (38) presented two cases treated by decompression craniotomy: In one the exact site of the ruptured aneurysm is not clear; in the other a giant ICAA was found. The same author reviewed 11 earlier similar cases in the literature.

In 1932 Howell (172) had performed cranial decompression for signs of a tumor (papilledema) only to find a ruptured ACoAA at autopsy. On the other hand Jefferson (180) in 1938 obtained improvement by decompressing a giant csICAA. Other such cases were reported subsequently (52,156,225,284,312,330,333).

In general the results were poor. For individual case reports of aneurysms treated by decompression see the *Surg* column (symbol *DEC*) in Appendix 2.

Cauterization of Aneurysms

Occasionally surgeons obliterated aneurysms (and often their adjoining parent artery) with a standard electrocautery unit (52,328). For additional details see pp. 816–818 regarding techniques of narrowing the neck of an aneurysm. For individual case reports of aneurysms treated by electrocautery see the *Surg* column (symbol *ELE*) in Appendix 2.

Ligation of Afferent Artery

Cervical Carotid Artery Ligation

See Chapter 33, for a detailed discussion of this subject.

Anterior Cerebral Artery (A-1) Ligation

In 1938 Poppen (272) discribed ligation of the anterior cerebral artery without ill effects in eight patients, but he gave no details of the site or reason for the ligation. In 1969 Dott (75) claimed he did the first A-1 ligation (clipping technique) for treating an ACoAA in 1944. During the 1950s further descriptions were given by Baumann and Bucy (31), Gillingham (130), Graf (132), Hamby (145), Hamilton and Falconer (151), Logue (208), and Rowbotham and Hay (290). The number of authors reporting this technique to treat ACoAA were considerable (5,31,43,44,48,74,75,88,130,132,137, 145,146,151,153,158,164,165,166,173,208,209, 247,290,304,314,338,339,344). For additional case reports of ACoAA treated by ligation or clipping of A-1, see the *Surg* columns (symbol *ANT*) of Appendix 2, under Adult, Pregnancy Related, Child, and Giant classifications—including single ACoAA cases and the "multiple" sections.

Tindall et al. (338,339) occluded one A-1 and the opposite cervical carotid artery under certain conditions (Chapter 33).

Opinions differ regarding whether to clip the A-1 close to the ACoAA (44) or close to the ICA (208,304,338). Those clipping near the ICA bifurcation believed there was less danger of ACoAA rupture at surgery and less chance of perforating artery injury. Others believed that clipping close to the ACoA allowed better protection from future rebleed and better feeding of ipsilateral perforators from the ICA system. Of course either technique risked ischemia of the brain and provided uncertain long-term protection of the aneurysm (268). Crompton (48) reported five later rebleeds in 13 ACoAA cases following A-1 clipping; on the other hand, Choudhury (43) claimed no rebleeds in 27 cases over a 2.0- to 4.5-year period. Other reports varied from these extremes, with operative mortality rates correlating positively with the patient's preoperative grade (74). Postoperative angiography revealed a wide range of results, varying from an absent, smaller, same size, or larger ACoAA compared to its preoperative size depending on the series reported (43,88,137,208).

The basic technique comprised applying a malleable or spring clip to the A-1 artery with minimal brain or aneurysm disturbance. Sometimes a ligature was gently applied. Smith (314) used a screw clamp but gave no details. See below for the Hamby-Drake tourniquet method. Cook et al. (44) included a second clip on the A-2 artery in some instances. The A-1 was usually clipped on the side that mainly filled the ACoAA during carotid angiography, with the reservation that both A-2 arteries filled during cross compression of the opposite cervical carotid artery during repeated injection of contrast medium into the ipsilateral carotid system (43,44,338). Kirgis et al. (194) and Lazorthes et al. (205), however, warned of the risks of ischemia (especially from insufficient flow into perforators) when the larger of the two A-1 arteries was occluded. At present A-1 ligation or clipping is less commonly used than it once was.

Other Anterior Circulation Arteries

For individual case reports of patients treated by proximal ligation of an artery afferent to the aneurysm, see the *Surg* column (symbol *PRO*) in Appendix 2. Ligation or clipping of an afferent artery to an aneurysm carries a real risk of ischemia if collateral circulation is not sufficient. However, a number of cases are reported in which intracranial aneurysms were so treated, often with success (76,78,123,193, 257,274,302,316). The aneurysms so treated included those on the MCA, ACeA, and PCoA or their branches.

In 1953 Campbell and Burklund (40) used a 00 silk noose to temporarily occlude a parent vessel. Laine (200) described a similar method in 1959. In 1969 Hamby (146,148) described the clever technique of placing a temporary "Hunterian ligature" on an artery proximal to the aneurysm. This became known as the "Hamby snare" and is illustrated in fig. 25.1. The suture was placed gently around the artery and the free ends passed through separate openings at the distal end of a polyethylene tube. A toothpick pushed into the proximal (surgeon's) end of the tube held the sutures in place and allowed occlusion of the vessel at the distal end of the tube.

Subsequently Drake and Allcock (15,76,78) extended Hamby's idea to allow a gradual, permanent occlusion of parent vessels in cases where the aneurysm (usually giant) was inoperable. The Drake tourniquet technique used a size 190 polyethylene tubing cut to appropriate length. The inner tip was marked with a small metal clip to denote its position next to the artery on subsequent radiographic films. Drake used 3-0 Prolene sutures instead of silk. He secured the suture at the proper tightness, or constriction, about the parent artery by using a clip tightened onto the distal end of the suture buried under the skin. Final closure of the artery then could be done under angiographic control hours or days after craniotomy. At that time the scalp wound was reopened to expose the buried distal end of the tourniquet. The artery would be closed slowly while watching for any evolving neurologic impairment. Drake and his colleagues have successfully treated some giant aneurysms in this manner, often with a concomitant extracranial–intracranial anastomosis to improve collateral circulation. Drake gave more details of technique and risks elsewhere (78). He also applied similar techniques to occlusion of vertebrobasilar arteries (see below).

Vertebrobasilar Artery Ligation

Ligation of one vertebral artery (VA) is a relatively safe procedure so long as the opposite vertebral artery is not atretic or absent, or already ligated, and so long as the patient has a good aneurysm grade status. This is an important reason for visualizing *both* vertebral arteries on angiography (or at surgery) before attacking an aneurysm of the vertebral system. If one must proximally ligate one VA or trap its aneurysm, the surgeon must be confident that the opposite VA is functioning well. Thereby came the famous warning issued by Dandy (54) in 1937. In a case of "Menieres syndrome" secondary to a left VAA, Dandy treated the patient by ligating the left VA in the neck. He subsequently exposed the right VA and "Momentarily compressed [it] between the blades of the forceps; death resulted apparently simultaneously and instantly—the quickest death I have ever seen." Additional deaths from single VA ligation for V-B aneurysms have been reported (79,94,116,143,255,307,313, 313a,348). Most of these are related to an atretic opposite VA, the presence of vasospasm with inadequate collateral flow, the presence of a giant aneurysm compressing brainstem vasculature, propagating thrombosis or embolism, and rupture of the aneurysm. Shintani and Zervas (311) reviewed 100 cases of VA ligation for various reasons and found an overall mortality rate of 12%. Transient elevation of the blood pressure or blood thinners may be considered in some instances.

Yet there is still a place for proximal ligation of the VA (low in the neck, at the occipital-cervical junction, or intracranially proximal to the aneurysm). Drake's tourniquet technique may prove to be a significant advance in therapeutic vertebrobasilar ligation (76,78). It is interesting that Bhushan et al. (33) were successful in ligating *both* vertebral arteries at the same operation for a giant vaBAA. When faced with this possibility, Amacher and Drake (17,79) have preferred to stage ligations to allow better collateral evolution (three cases). At least 50 cases of V-B aneurysms have been treated by ligation and clipping of a vertebral artery (2,17,25,26,33,52,54,69,79,93,94,96,97,116,143, 151,152,181,187,193,199,207,255,274,294,307, 311,313,313a,336,348).

Ligation of the basilar artery (BA) has rarely been done because of the obvious inherent risks. In 1962 Mount and Taveras (229) successfully treated a bBAA by clipping the BA between the take-offs of the SCA and P-1 arteries. Collateral circulation was maintained, for both posterior cerebral arteries were also fed by large posterior communicating arteries. The BA was ligated or clipped in at least 11 instances (27,79,229,292,360). Most were performed by Drake (79). Two deaths were reported.

For individual case reports of aneurysms treated by VA ligation or BA ligation, see the *Surg* column (symbols *VER* or *BAS*) in Appendix 2.

Trapping Procedures

Extracranial–Intracranial Trapping

Ligation of the cervical ICA and then the intracranial ICA to trap an ICAA has been commonplace in the past (29,30,52,53,55,56,59,66, 72,90,92,95,102,104,131,132,140,141,145,149–151,156,193,206,220,253,270,273,275,278,289, 295,305,306,320,358). One of the first of these procedures (Fig. 31.1) was done by Dandy (56) and reported in 1939. Many of the operations were performed for giant, broad-based, or cavernous sinus ICAA. Hamby (145), on reviewing the evidence, concluded that the ophthalmic artery had sufficient collateral circulation and rarely was placed in jeopardy by this procedure. However, one does lose the collateral cir-

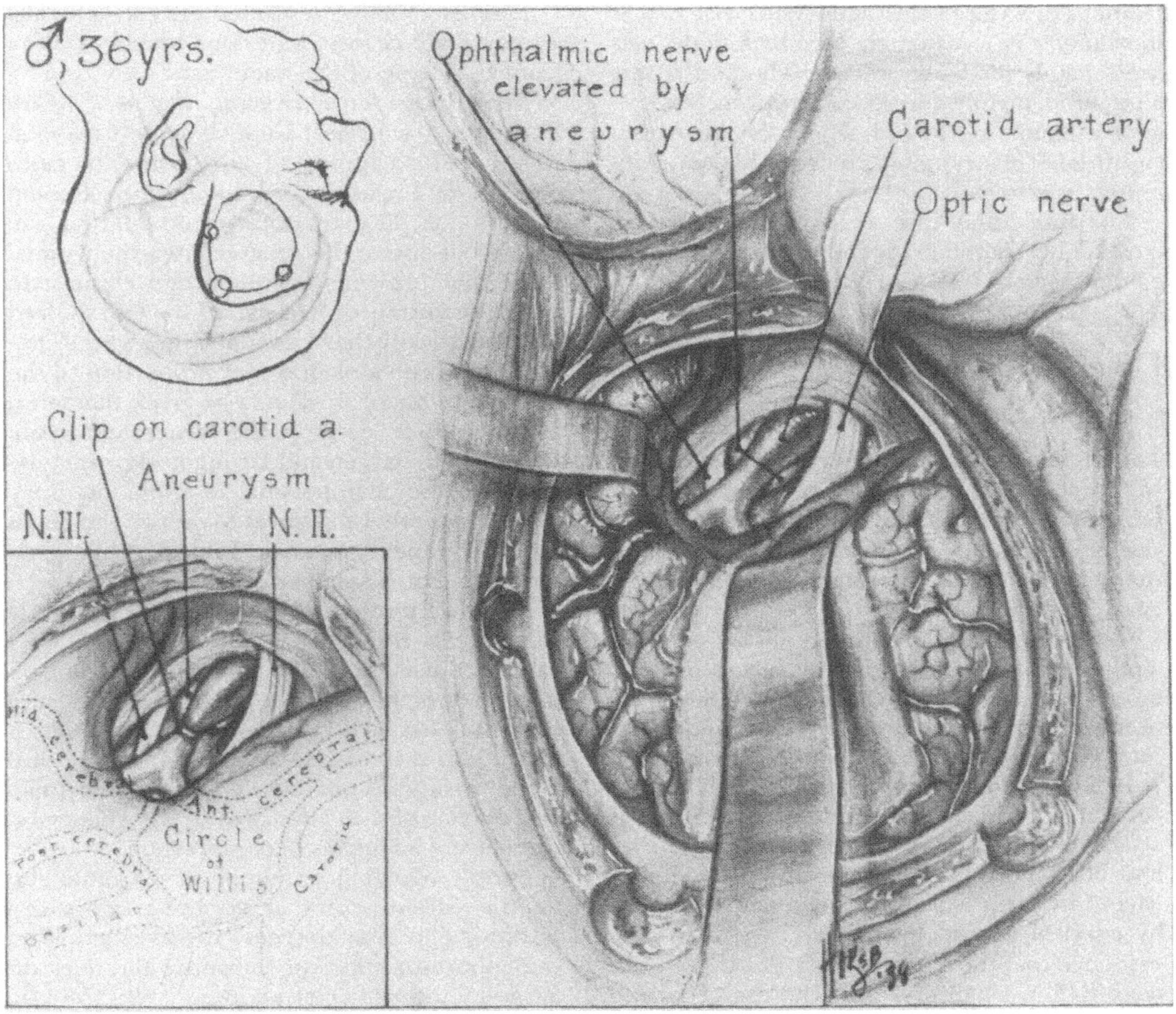

Fig. 31.1 In this case of extracranial–intracranial trapping of a right ICAA, Dandy first did the cranial clipping of the ICA (*inset*) and then tied off the cervical ICA in the neck 5 days later. This was not done in the usual reverse order due to the fact that Dandy had hoped he could deal with the aneurysm directly without trapping. From Dandy WE, ref. 56.

culation to the carotid artery via the external carotid artery to ophthalmic artery flow (retrograde flow).

Intracranial Trapping

Throughout the years, especially during the early history of aneurysm treatment, it was common to trap an intracranial aneurysm between clips or ligatures on the parent artery. Nearly every type of intracranial aneurysm which could be flanked by clips applied to the parent artery was trapped at one time or another (21,28,29,31,32,35,42,53,55,68,69,79,87, 111,118,125,131,132,134,135,139–141,145,146, 149, 150, 154, 156–159, 166–168, 175, 177, 179, 187, 188, 193, 200, 204, 226, 238, 240, 242, 244,250, 254, 273, 275, 283, 291, 293, 312, 313, 313a, 320, 322, 325, 342–344, 352, 357).

The success of such a procedure depends, of course, on adequate collateral perfusion, uncompromised perforators, and sufficient perfusion pressure. The mortality rates in many of these cases were quite high. For example,

Hamby (146) trapped 49 aneurysms with a 51% mortality rate. Although this technique was used mainly for ICAA in the early days, it was later used mainly for ACoAA. Often the surgeon's hand was forced when the aneurysm ruptured. This trapping procedure is not commonly used now.

For individual case reports of aneurysms treated by trapping procedures see the *Surg* column (symbol *TRA*) in Appendix 2.

Direct Obliteration of Aneurysms

Clipping the Aneurysm

The history and use of aneurysm clips is given in Chapter 27. Also see Chapters 34–39 for our technique of clipping aneurysms. Advances in the development of aneurysm clips is one of many important changes that have made aneurysm surgery safer.

We have not differentiated aneurysm neck ligation by a clip from that by suture ligature in our case reports in Appendix 2 (either ligation method is symbolized by *CLP* under the *Surg* column).

A few surgeons first ligated the cervical carotid artery and clipped the aneurysm by direct attack later (20,52,145,149), a technique that had little merit. It has since been abandoned except in cases where an aneurysm is treated by cervical carotid ligation and there is later evidence that the aneurysm is still a threat. See page 645 in Chapter 22 for the use of *partial* cervical carotid artery ligation while awaiting the proper time for craniotomy.

An interesting clip-applying technique for special circumstances is described by McFadden (Fig. 31.2) (222):

> Open the clip with the clip applier. Chock the legs open at the hub with a tiny roll of gauze, or other material, remove the appliers, and pass a fine silk suture through the chock posteriorly. Set the opened clip legs astride the aneurysm with forceps or nerve hooks, reapply the clip applier, and squeeze the clip spring to loosen the chock. Remove the chock with the attached suture, and release the clip.

This method allows the clip to be put in awkward positions that otherwise would make it difficult for the clip, when attached to the clip applier, to surround the neck of the aneurysm.

Parkinson (250a) described the use of an airgun to displace perforators or branches away from the dome of the aneurysm.

Techniques for narrowing the neck of an aneurysm are surgical adjuncts sometimes vital to successful clipping of aneurysms. In cases of large or broad-necked aneurysms, clipping is more difficult due not only to the larger size per se but also to the greater intra-aneurysmal force that prevents adequate clip closure. In such circumstances Early and Fink (89) showed mathematically that a stronger clip, whose closing force is greater in direct proportion to the relative increase in aneurysm neck diameter, is required to occlude the larger aneurysm. However, as larger and stronger clips may be cumbersome or impossible to apply, one may have to use other measures to reduce the diameter of the aneurysm neck. Table 31.1 lists some methods that have been reported.

Needle aspiration of the aneurysm sac (while temporarily trapped or while applying a clip) can be done (250). The needle can be connected directly to strong suction. Morley and Barr (227) warned that needling an aneurysm may cause it to disintegrate, especially if local blood pressure is not lowered. The needle may also enter a clot or atheroma in the aneurysm, preventing adequate decompression.

Simply applying a temporary proximal clip on the parent artery or applying temporary trapping clips may decrease the tension within the aneurysm sufficient to reduce the neck diameter and permit clipping (129,146,148, 250,285,362,363,365). In such circumstances it

Table 31.1. Methods to Narrow the Neck of an Aneurysm

1. Needle-aspirate the aneurysm while applying a clip or ligature.
2. Reduce intraaneurysmal tension with a temporary proximal clip or by trapping.
3. Deliberately rupture the aneurysm (usually used with item 2, above).
4. Partially close the neck by suture ligature.
5. Twist the aneurysm.
6. Temporarily place a clip, clamp, or forceps on the aneurysm until a permanent clip can be applied.
7. Place a large clip on the dome followed by a clip on the neck.
8. Compress the aneurysm dome with the suction tube against cotton while clipping the neck.
9. Electrocoagulate the aneurysm.

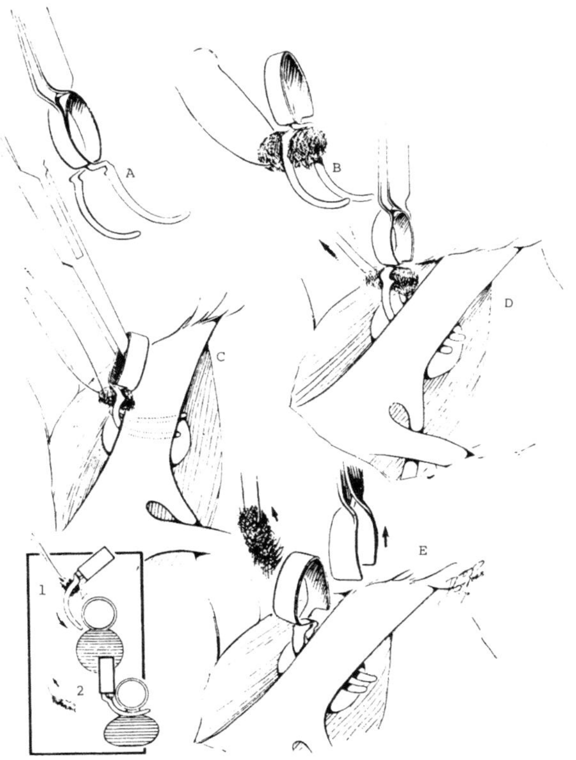

Fig. 31.2. McFadden's technique of chocked-clip aneurysmorrhaphy. **A** Crossed-action clip opened with applier. **B** Clip chocked open and stitch passed posteriorly. **C** Chocked-open clip set astride aneurysm neck with hemostat. **D** Applier compressing spring to loosen chock. **E** Chock removed and clip released. From McFadden JT, ref. 222.

usually is necessary to then open the sac of the aneurysm so as to collapse it and then apply the clip. Deliberate rupture of an aneurysm under prepared conditions has been an occasional, though hazardous, means of reducing the size of the waist of the aneurysm (112–115,117,139,155,178,201,270,271,362,363,365). Again, such a maneuver is best performed under local vascular hypotension, which is usually accomplished by temporarily clipping or trapping the proximal arterial. Laine et al. (201) had an assistant open the sac while the surgeon tied the suture ligature on the neck of the aneurysm.

A well-known method of narrowing the waist of a large aneurysm is application of a suture ligature (82,178,250,362,363,365). Such a ligature is tied down gently (see below for the technique of suture ligature of an aneurysm), enough to narrow the neck but not enough to distort or occlude the neck of the aneurysm. A clip is then applied.

Jamieson (178) stated that he has twisted an aneurysm, causing torsion and narrowing at its base. The dangers inherent in this procedure are obvious.

Yaşargil et al. (362,363,365) used special clips that opened widely in order to occlude a large aneurysm; this was followed by permanent application of a smaller, stronger clip at the neck. Drake (78) has suggested the possibility of crushing the waist of a giant aneurysm with a clamp or hemostat and then applying the clip. One also can close the aneurysm with a forceps and then apply the clip (82).

The use of electrocautery to reduce the size of an aneurysm, with or without clipping or trapping, has been used occasionally since the 1930s by Dandy (51,52,55), Greenwood (133), Swain (328), and Hazouri (155). In 1938 Dandy wrote (51): "A word may be added concerning the cauterization of the aneurysm by which it is shriveled to a small shred. . . ." He feared possible extension of an iatrogenic thrombus into the parent artery; hence he preferred to cauterize after applying a silver clip. After clipping the neck of an ICAA, Dandy (55) stated in 1941 that the "aneurysm is then shrunk by the electrocautery, in order to remove its contact with the third nerve. . . ." In 1944 Dandy (52) described inserting a needle into an ACoAA and cauterizing the aneurysm via this needle. In another ACoAA he packed the inside with muscle and then cauterized it. In these cases "monopolar" coagulating current was used. In some ICAA cases that ruptured at operation the aneurysm and its parent artery were electrocoagulated.

The use of *bipolar* electrocautery to shrink the neck of an aneurysm was first described by Yaşargil in 1969 (359). Although Nornes and Wikeby (243) made a point of stating that they never use bipolar electrocoagulation for this purpose, many surgeons have found this method of reducing the diameter of an aneurysm neck valuable in some circumstances (16, 37, 45, 46, 57, 106, 138, 141, 198, 250, 256, 261–263, 265, 346, 362, 363, 365). Yaşargil and co-workers (363) give an excellent description of the use of bipolar electrocautery to shrink the neck of an intracranial aneurysm.

For large, thick-walled aneurysms use the large-tip forceps. When changing to small-tip diameters (1.0–0.5 mm), lower the electrocautery output (usually use No. 25 on the Malis unit sold by Codman and Shurtleff). The current density increases as the forceps–aneurysm contact surface decreases. Place cotton microsponges between perforators (vessels) and the forceps. Be sure the forceps tips are completely across the aneurysm neck; otherwise the aneurysm may rupture at the point at which the tips touch the aneurysm. Avoid perforators or branches beyond the aneurysm. Close the forceps blades slowly around the aneurysm neck and keep the blades a short distance from the parent vessel wall. Use intermittent bursts of electricity (a few seconds at a time). Inspect and repeat the process as needed. Stop the current when the wall begins to desiccate, fry, and shrivel. Reinspect and repeat as needed. Keep the field wet as needed to avoid drying and cracking of the aneurysm wall and to avoid sticking of the forceps tips. Knead, or rapidly but minimally open and close, the forceps tips as the coagulation continues. It may help to evacuate some blood in the aneurysm by compressing the dome of the aneurysm with the suction tube against cotton on the aneurysm fundus. If the aneurysm ruptures during the process, insert the forcep blades deeper, close the forceps, and continue the electrocauterization.

In our experience (106) there has been no clinical evidence of harmful embolization as a result of using bipolar electrocautery on the aneurysm. We have not found the technique helpful for thick-walled, atherosclerotic aneurysms. The procedure does narrow the aneurysm neck and make it firmer and more cylindrical. This not only permits accurate clip placement but also allows the surgeon to see previously hidden perforators, vessels, and nerves to be avoided by the clip.

Suture Ligature of Aneurysms

In 1969 Dott (75) stated that he had been employing ligatures and ligature passers in 1942. In 1953 Campbell and Burklund (40), Norlén, Olivecrona, and Barnum (240,241), and Sjöqvist (312) described the use of a suture ligature to occlude the aneurysm neck. Silk was used most commonly, but linen, cotton, and nylon also were utilized by some (4,6,34,36,40,58,75, 77, 80–82, 136, 139, 144, 146, 147, 167–169, 188, 197, 200, 202, 204, 210, 211, 219, 240, 241, 245, 248, 250, 258–260, 264, 279, 297, 312, 326, 327, 337, 349, 353, 356, 359).

Sjöqvist (312), who began treating intracranial aneurysms by suture ligature in 1948, used paraffined silk thread. His publication in 1953 (312) gave an excellent description of his technique. Figures 31.3 and 31.4 illustrate Norlén's and Kempe's respective methods of ligating an intracranial aneurysm, assisted by ligature carriers. Some commonly used ligature carriers are shown in Fig. 31.5.

Drake (81,82) used wet 3-0 silk sutures. He also described his "figure-of-eight" suture for large bilobed aneurysms (80). Drake (82) preferred to use special knot-tying forceps with longitudinal grooves at the tip (rather than the usual horizontal groves). Hamby (147) used coarse linen or cotton sutures as a ligature so that the knot would hold better (compared to braided silk).

Hallac and Hamby (144) described a method of clamping the suture in place, rather than tying a knot (Fig. 31.6). A silk suture is passed around the aneurysm neck, and then both ends of the suture go through a hole in a 3 mm diameter lead disc. The disc is slid down until it

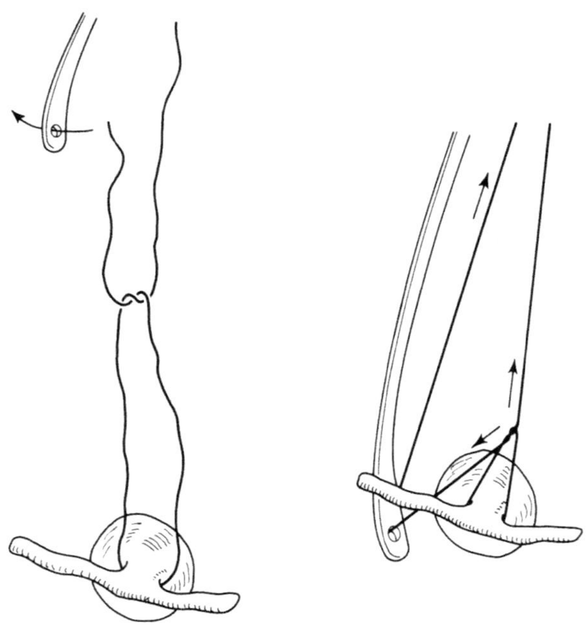

Fig. 31.3. Norlén's technique of ligating the neck of an aneurysm. The instrument and one end of the thread is held with the left hand, and the tying is then performed by pulling the other end of the thread with the right hand. From Norlén G, Barnum AS, ref. 240.

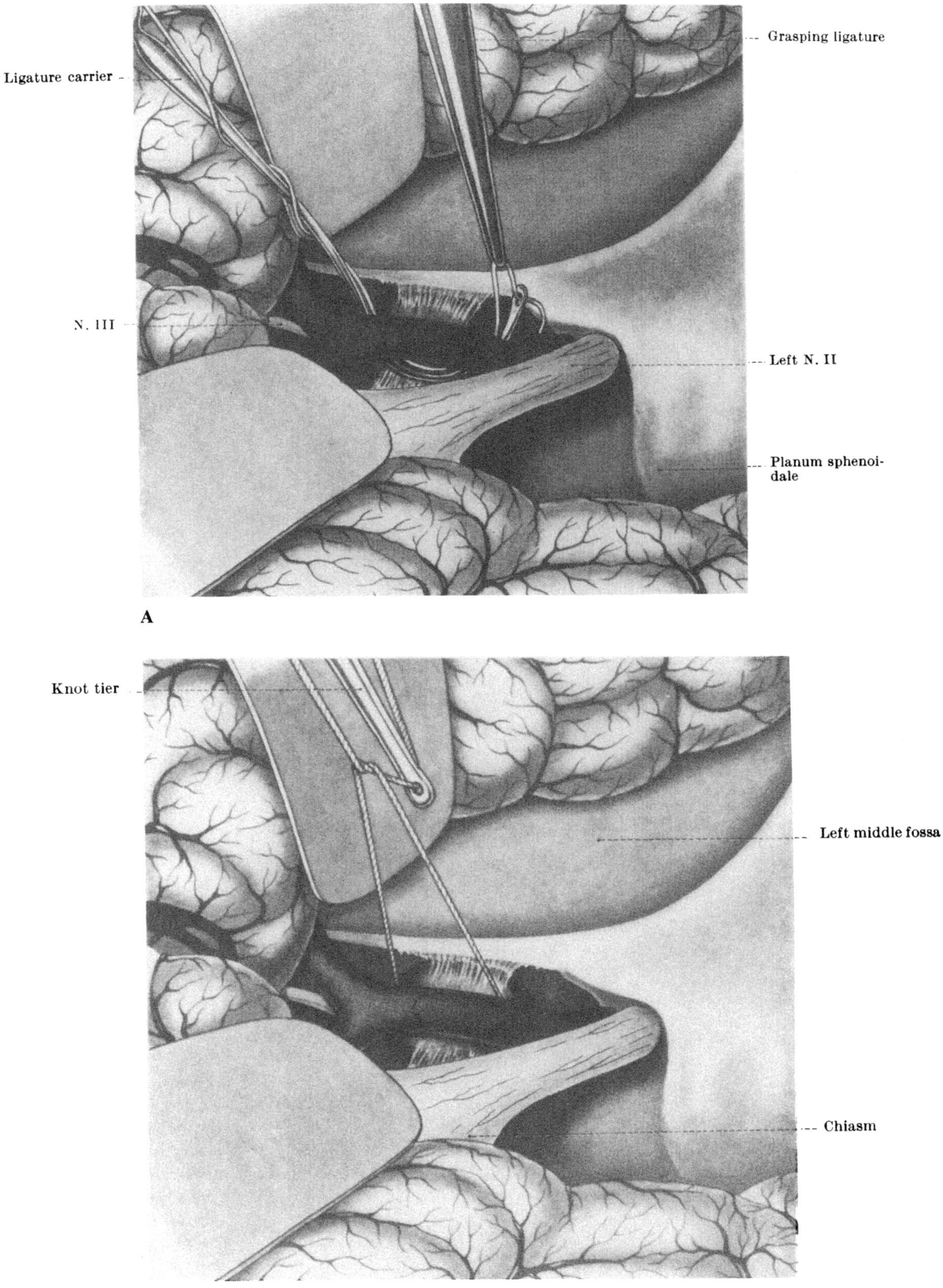

Fig. 31.4. Kempe's method of ligating an aneurysm with silk suture. **A** Passing ligature with instrument around left ICAA. **B** First an overhand knot is made high outside the cranial cavity and carried down by the knot tier (*continued*).

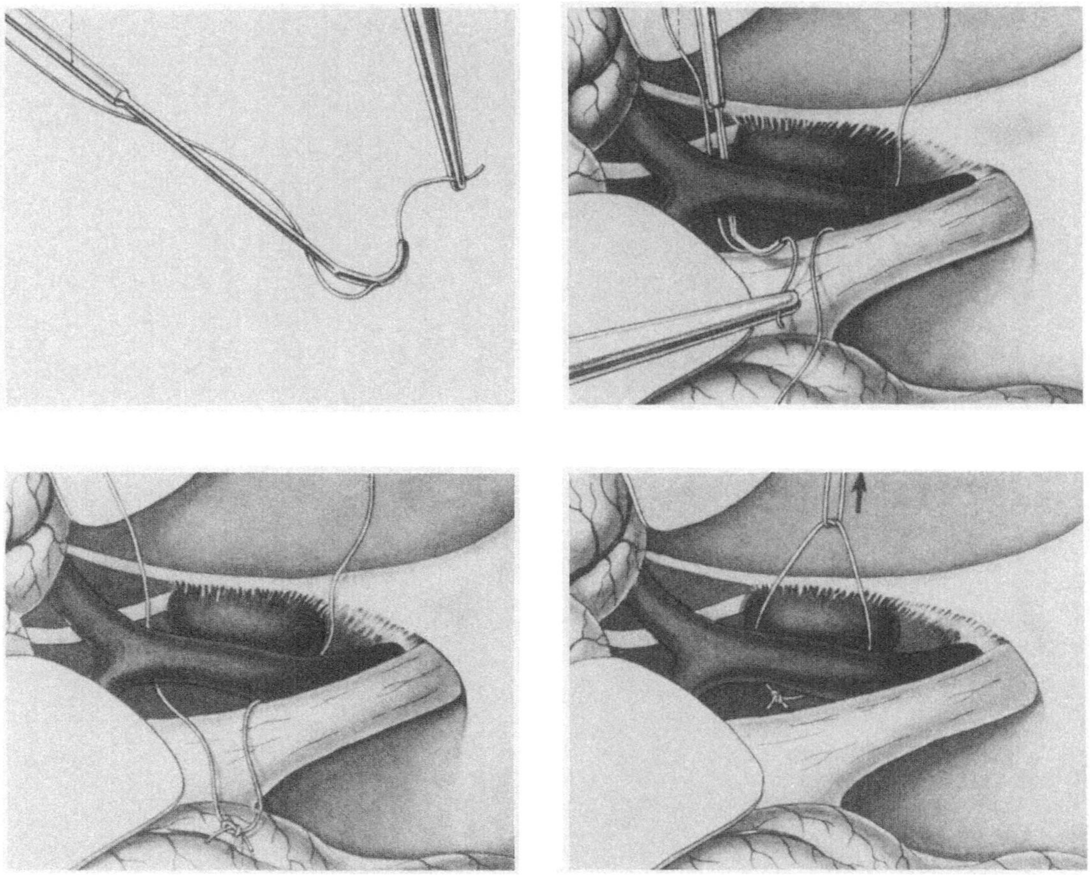

Fig. 31.4C-F Alternative method of ligature placement shown. From Kempe LG, ref. 188.

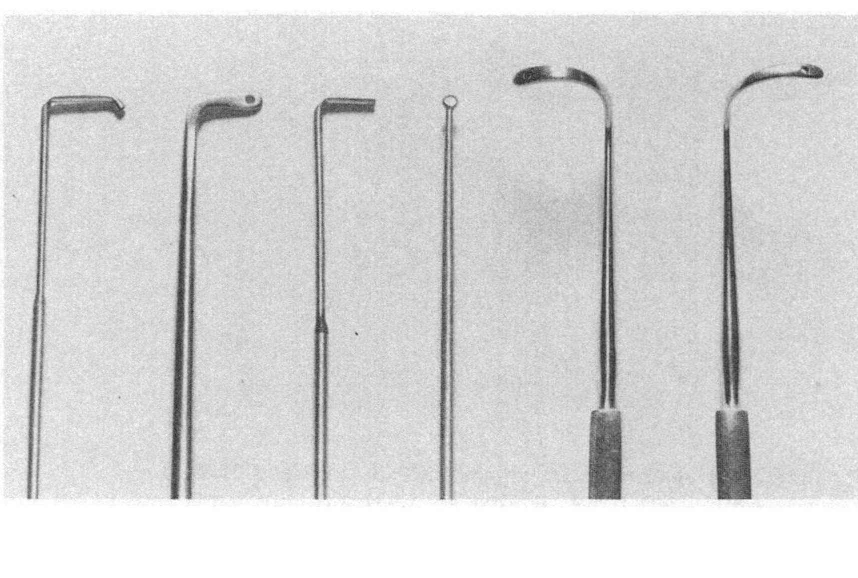

Fig. 31.5. Ligature passers. *Left to right:* Retter aneurysm needle No. 1, Adson aneurysm needle, Retter aneurysm needle No. 2, Shaw aneurysm needle, and a left and right curved Kronecker aneurysm needle. Courtesy of Codman & Shurtleff, Inc., Randolph, Massachusetts.

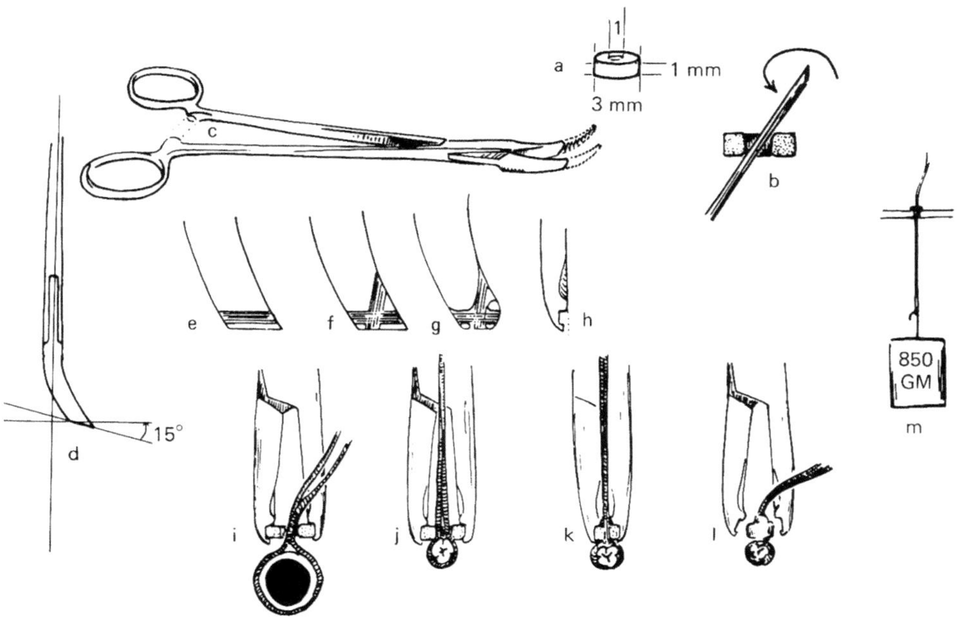

Fig. 31.6. Securing a suture ligating an aneurysm with a lead disc. See text for details. From Hallec I, Hamby WB, ref. 144.

forces the suture to occlude the aneurysm. The disc is then squeezed shut, gripping the suture just as a fisherman affixes a lead weight to his fishing line. A similar method was used by Weickmann and Buchholz (349).

Suzuki et al. (327) used a nylon suture attached to a steel ball. A platinum cobolt magnet at the end of a silver probe was used to pull the steel ball and its suture around the back side of the aneurysm. The suture then was grasped, pulled to an appropriate length, and tied around the aneurysm neck.

Lougheed and Marshall (211) preferred clips to sutures in most instances. They pointed out that the suture may kink the parent vessel along with the neck of the aneurysm and thus narrow the lumen of the vessel. Excess tying force may amputate the neck of the aneurysm [as Sjöqvist (312) originally warned in 1953]. As clips are easily manipulated by most surgeons, suture ligature is utilized less commonly now. However, suture ligature may *narrow* the neck of a large aneurysm sufficient to allow proper application of an aneurysm clip.

We have not differentiated aneurysm neck ligation by suture ligature from that by a clip in our case reports in Appendix 2. Either ligation method is symbolized by *CLP* under the *Surg* column.

Excision and Suture Repair of Aneurysms

There are some large and giant aneurysms with a broad base that may not be amenable to clipping or suture ligation, although they may cause pressure phenomena and so deserve excision. Many or even most of these contain some intraluminal clot and atherosclerotic thickening. Hence the procedure is usually one of: (a) temporary trapping; (b) opening the fundus of the aneurysm; (c) excising the clot, atherosclerotic material, and excess aneurysm wall; followed by (d) suture closure (oversewing) of sufficient aneurysm wall to allow reconstitution of the parent vessel lumen (Fig. 31.7). This is usually an endaneurysmorrhaphy. There are a number of descriptions of this procedure (2,24, 40, 50, 52, 83, 84, 86, 128, 146, 179, 188, 214, 223, 237, 253, 255, 282, 285, 298).

Unfortunately, in many of the early case reports it is difficult to determine whether, in fact,

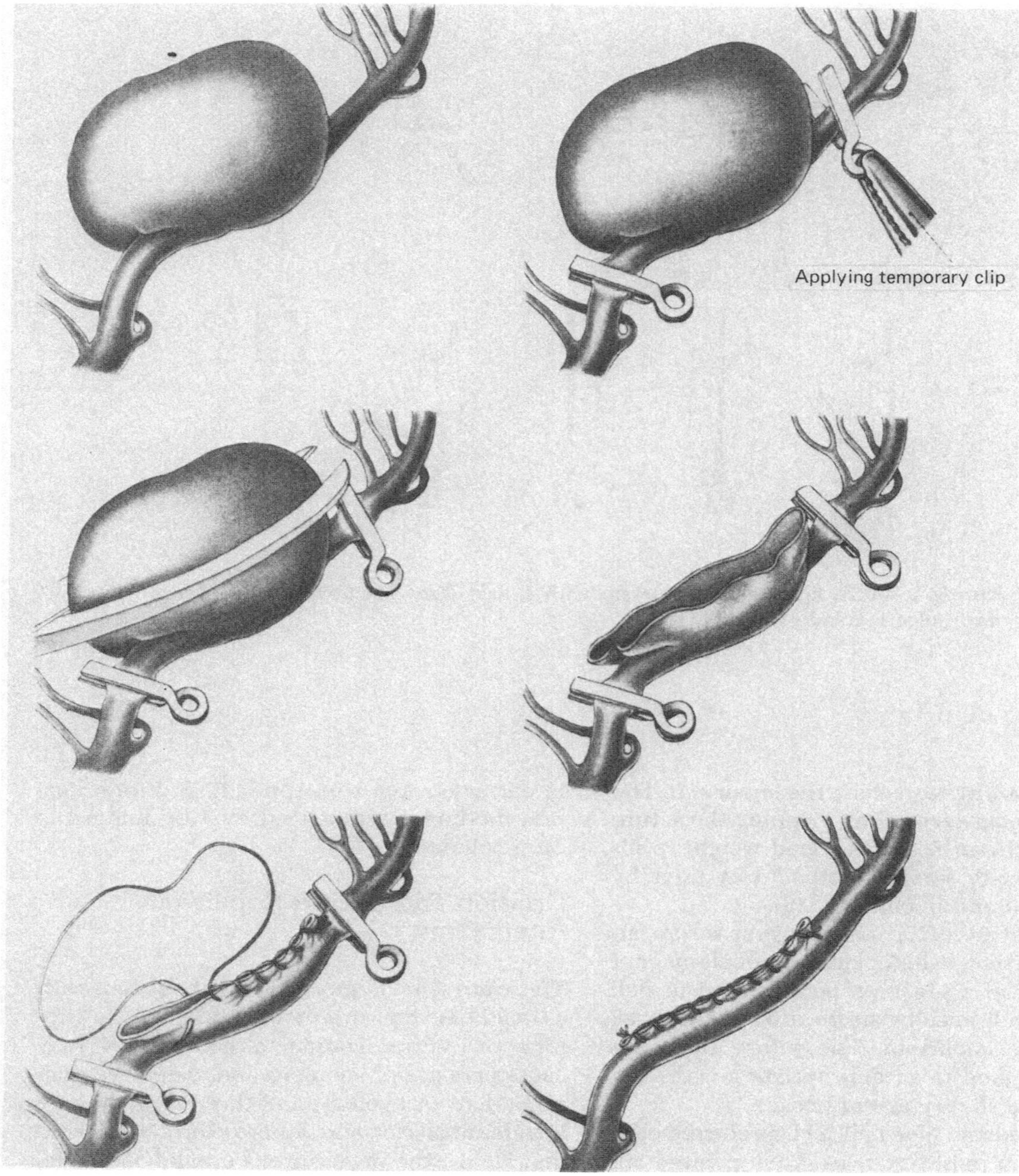

Fig. 31.7. Excision of a giant aneurysm followed by suture closure of the remaining wall to reconstitute the parent artery. From Kempe LG, ref. 188.

an aneurysm wall repair was carried out after excision of the aneurysm or a permanent trapping procedure was done. Case reports of aneurysm excision and definite reconstitution of the parent artery include those of Campbell and Burklund in 1953 (40), Abbott and colleagues in 1961 (2), Patterson and Ray in 1962 (253), Drake and Vanderlinden in 1967 (86), Kempe in 1968 (188), Drake and Amacher in 1969 (84), Nakahara et al. in 1975 (237), Santini and Gouazé in 1975 (298), and Rosenbaum and Sundt in 1978 (285). For individual case reports of aneurysms treated by excision see the *Surg* column (symbol *EXC*) in Appendix 2.

Coating of Aneurysms

See Chapter 28 for a detailed discussion of coating aneurysms.

Internal Occlusion of Aneurysms

A number of methods to internally occlude intracranial aneurysms have been described. Basically the internal cavity of the sac is filled with iatrogenically induced clot or other substance to prevent blood from entering the aneurysm. Such substances have been introduced both by stereotaxic procedures and after open craniotomy exposure.

Muscle Insertion

As opposed to muscle covering or wrapping of the aneurysm, the muscle fragment is introduced inside the aneurysm through a hole made in its wall. In some cases this was done perforce when a large aneurysm ruptured upon exposure. Several cases of internal muscle packing have been reported (20,49,52,85,86,111,145, 174,195,215,221,228,303,340). Many of these patients died because of the urgent circumstances.

There is a risk of muscle tissue occluding the parent vessel with this procedure. Drake and Vanderlinden (86), reported four cases; two of the patients subsequently developed false aneurysms (one rebled and died).

For individual case reports of aneurysms treated by muscle insertion see the *Surg* column (symbol *IMU*) in Appendix 2.

Oxycellulose Packing

Adams (3) reported one case of a giant csICAA which he opened, packed with oxycellulose gauze, and resutured the wall. For individual case reports of aneurysms treated by oxycellulose packing see the *Surg* column (symbol *IOX*) in Appendix 2.

Gelfoam Packing

Turner (341) reported a giant csICAA treated by cervical CCA ligation. The aneurysm was opened and packed inside with gelfoam, thrombin, and tantalum dust. The wall was then sutured.

Thrombin-Induced Thrombosis

Denecke and Hartert (67) reported a posttraumatic csICAA presenting with epistaxis. After ligating both cervical ECA and the left cervical ICA, they exposed the aneurysm via the sphenoid bone and injected a thrombin solution into it to promote clotting. This appeared to stop the patient's epistaxis.

Cryogenic Thrombosis

In 1968 Walder (347) suggested the possibility of using a cryoprobe to temporarily freeze the aneurysm. The resulting injury might induce intraaneurysmal thrombosis. Verbiest (345) did this to induce AVM thrombosis.

Laser-Induced Thrombosis

Maira and co-workers (216,217) used an argon laser unit on experimental aneurysms in animals. They were able to shrink the aneurysm to obliteration with this blue-green light. Studies with infrared laser irradiation suggested that this technique would not effectively obliterate intracranial aneurysms in many instances and would risk burning a hole through the wall of the aneurysm (107).

Cotton Gauze Packing

In 1936 Gardner (124) opened a giant ICAA believing it was a tumor and packed it with five cotton sponges. The patient did well, although the sponges had to be removed 2 years later due to infection.

For individual case reports of aneurysms treated by internal cotton packing see the *Surg* column (symbol *ICO*) in Appendix 2.

Other Synthetic Materials

Experimental aneurysms in animals have been occluded with methyl methacrylate (127) or ciacrine (192). See the section on iron materials (pp. 827–828) for the use of iron-impregnated methyl methacrylate in humans.

Experimental aneurysms in animals have been successfully occluded with intraaneurysmal injection of isobutyl cyanoacrylate (367). Excessive amounts caused embolization. In 1977 Sheptak et al. (310) treated some patients by intraaneurysmal injection of isobutyl cyanoacrylate directly at open operation (18 cases) and by stereotaxic injection (two cases). They noted a 25% expansion of the cyanoacrylate when it interspersed with blood in the aneurysm. The aneurysm was effectively and completely occluded in seven cases.

Ohta and co-workers (246) injected compressed polyurethane foam (size of a grain of rice) into a carotid-cavernous fistula. The foam expanded within a few minutes and obliterated the fistula. This may have theoretical application to intracranial aneurysms.

Luessenhop et al. (108,212,213) worked with Silastic beads, embolizing them to a bBAA, an MCAA, and an oaICAA. The results were equivocal. Kosary et al. (196) tried the same with a porcelain bead in a csICAA. For individual case reports of aneurysms treated by pellet embolization see the *Surg* column (symbol *PEL*) in Appendix 2.

We (J.L.F.) have had the following two cases of giant csICAA: a 46-year-old woman with a right CN-6 weakness, and a 64-year-old woman with total left ophthalmoplegia and CN-5 sensory loss. In both cases the aneurysm was exposed by craniotomy. The blood pressure was raised during temporary trapping between cervical carotid ligation and intracranial ICA clipping. The dura of the cavernous sinus and the juxtaposed aneurysm wall were incised. The cavity was filled with preformed polyvinyl alcohol foam (Ivalon) sponge, the wall sutured, and the temporary ligatures released. Both patients did well. Postoperative angiography showed occlusion of the aneurysm and ICA, but fortunately the intracranial ICA filled via the ophthalmic system, an advantage not permitted by trapping.

For individual case reports of aneurysms treated by internal synthetic packing (type not specified) see the *Surg* column (symbol *ISY*) in Appendix 2.

Balloon/Catheter Techniques

See pp. 829–832 for a discussion of balloon/catheter techniques.

Suture-Induced Thrombosis

During the early 1940s Dandy (52,53) attempted to induce thrombosis in a giant csICAA by passing eight silk sutures through the aneurysm walls, leaving the sutures dangling inside the aneurysm. He reoperated 5 days later, found the aneurysm pulsating, and then utilized a trapping procedure. For individual case reports of aneurysms treated by internal silk suture placement see the *Surg* column (symbol *ISI*) in Appendix 2.

Wire-Induced Thrombosis Without Electricity

In 1941 Werner et al. (351) described the case of a 15-year-old girl who had a giant right ICAA eroding the floor and orbital wall of the skull. She was initially treated by serial cervical carotid ligations: right ICA, right ECA, left ECA, and then left CCA. The mass continued to grow. Through a needle inserted into a defect in the right orbit, the surgeons passed 30 feet of No. 34 gauge wire (coin silver enameled wire) and then heated the wire for 40 s. The patient survived, and the tumorous aneurysm apparently stopped growing. The skull x-rays (Fig. 31.8) show the wire coiled inside the aneurysm.

Mullan (230), while using a wire with electrical current (see the next section), found that beryllium–copper wire and copper wire alone are sufficiently thrombogenic to induce occlusion of large intracranial aneurysms. The aneurysm is exposed by open craniotomy and 0.002-inch diameter wire is inserted into the aneurysm through a 33-gauge needle. The wire, pumped (Fig. 31.9) into the aneurysm via 22-gauge steel tubing fitting over the needle, coils inside the aneurysm. Mullan obtained adequate thrombosis in 12 of the 15 cases reported. Others have described similar procedures (47,171).

For individual case reports of aneurysms treated by internal insertion of wire (with or without electrical current application) see the *Surg* column (symbol *IWI* if via open craniotomy and *SWI* if via a stereotaxic procedure) in Appendix 2.

Wire-Induced Thrombosis With Electricity

In 1953 Sawyer and Pate (301) discovered that when electrical direct current (DC current) was passed through blood, clotting tended to occur at the positive electrode. They theorized that blood cells, which have a negative surface charge, were attracted to this positive pole. This work provided the impetus for later use

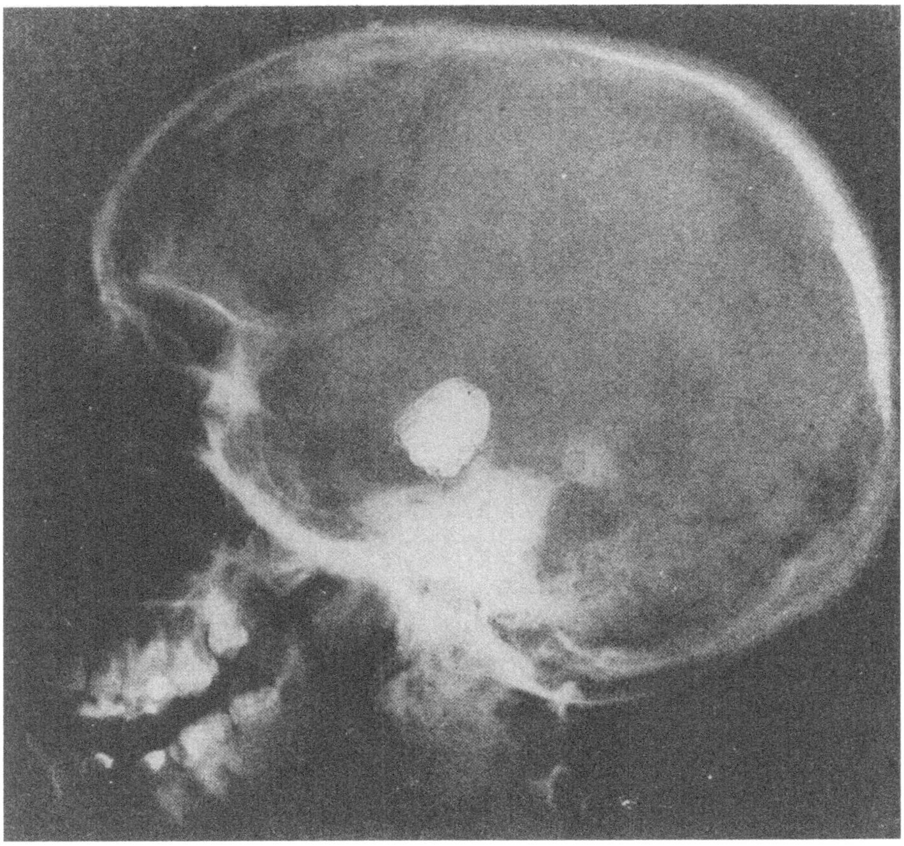

Fig. 31.8. Skull x-rays showing the density of a therapeutic wire coiled inside a giant aneurysm. From Werner SC, Blakemore AH, King BG. Aneurysm of internal carotid artery within the skull. Wiring and electrothermic coagulation. JAMA 116:578–582. © 1941, American Medical Association. Permission granted by publisher, ref. 351.

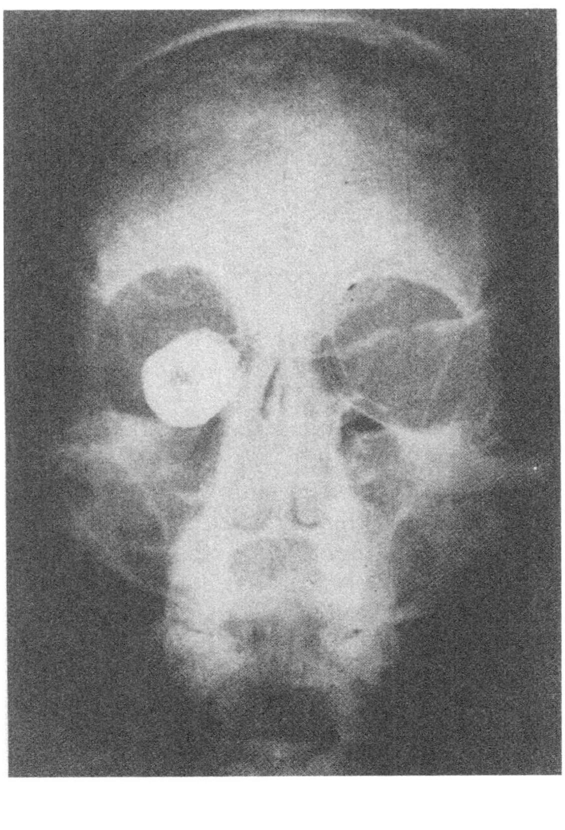

of DC current in an attempt to induce internal thrombosis of intracranial aneurysms.

Actually the treatment of systemic arterial aneurysms by galvanopuncture probably began in Lyons, France, during the nineteenth century (39). Bouchet reviewed the early history of this procedure in 1972 (39).

In 1957 Guillaume and colleagues (142) exposed an A-1 aneurysm and placed two electrodes inside the aneurysm and one on its surface. After applying electrical "bipolar" current (type?), partial thrombosis was induced inside the aneurysm.

It has been found that experimental aneurysms in animals could be thrombosed at the site at which anodal DC current was applied (224,233), and that an internal anode was more effective than an external anode. As a result of such studies Mullan et al. (231,235) in 1965 reported on stereotaxic insertion of wire into the aneurysm for induction of thrombosis by galvanic (DC) current. This form of treatment was continued in some centers (19,171,230–232,234–236,296).

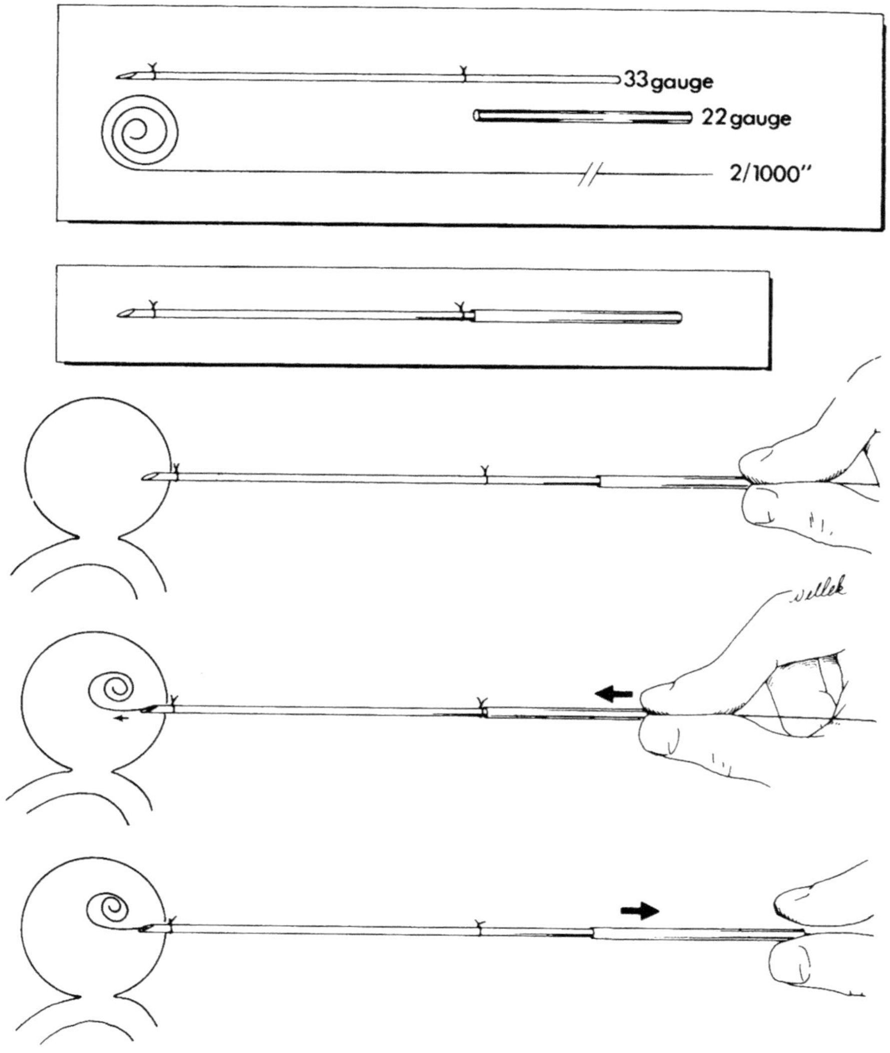

Fig. 31.9. Mullan's method of using a pumping action of a segment of 22-gauge steel tubing to insert wire into an aneurysm. This technique prevents kinking of the wire during insertion. From Mullan S, ref. 230.

Mullan (230) perfected his stereotaxic method of inserting fine copper-plated steel wire (0.2 mm diameter) across the neck of the aneurysm at 1.0-mm intervals (Fig. 31.10). DC anodal current (0.5–1.0 m-amp) for at least 5 min was passed through each needle (wire). In 1974 he reported his results in 61 patients (230). Mullan concluded that this technique was not significantly better than modern medical therapy followed by direct operation. The main problems included aggravation of vasospasm, injury to overlying arterial branches, incomplete thrombosis, and excessive thrombosis (236).

A unique procedure was reported by Hilal et al. (163) in which they guided an electrode by intravascular technique into a BAA. The other pole of the electrode was placed on the skin closest to the dome of the aneurysm. Partial occlusion was achieved, but recanalization followed.

We have some doubt about the added value of electrical current (as opposed to wire-induced thrombosis without electrical current).

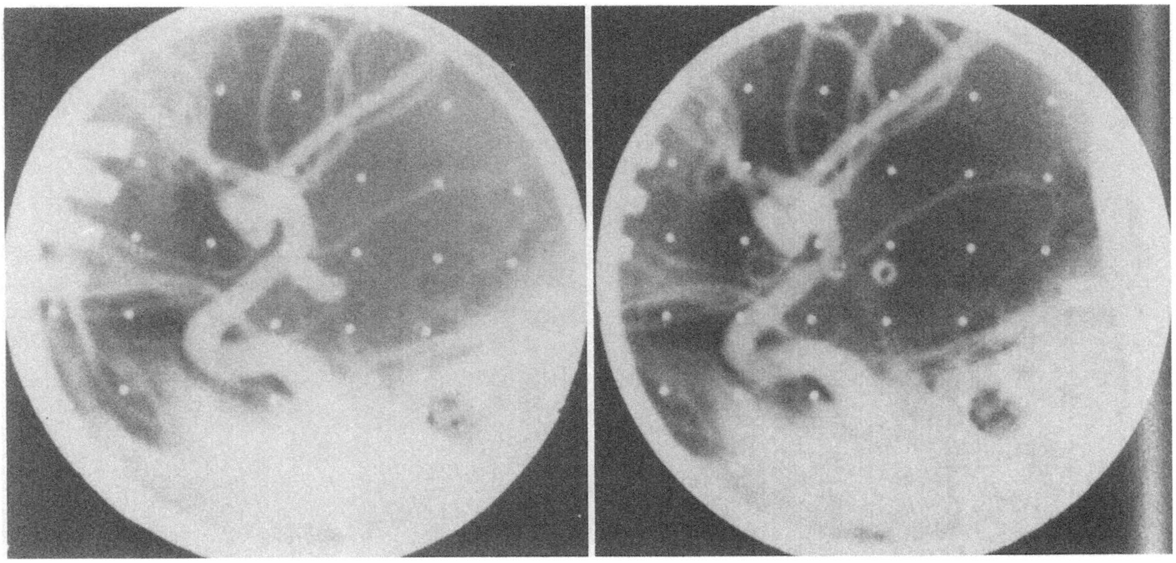

Fig. 31.10. Mullan's method of stereotaxic electrical wire thrombosis of intracranial aneurysms. Using a special stereotaxic device combined with angiography, the surgeon places the target circle (*left*) on the neck of the aneurysm. *Right* Three needles across the neck of the aneurysm have obliterated it. From Mullan S, ref. 230.

Fox and Yaşargil (109,110) found no thrombosis (unless injury occurred) when DC current was applied to arteries of experimental animals. There was an electrochemical reaction causing acidic or alkaline hematin formation and protein denaturization of the blood, with clumps of such material embolizing distally. This suggested that such dangerous embolic phenomena also would occur in the intracranial arteries during the electrical thrombosis treatment.

Pilojection-Induced Thrombosis

In 1962 Gallagher (119) described a technique of injecting horse or hog hairs into intracranial aneurysms exposed at surgery. He continued his work for a few years (77,119–122), but the method never became popular.

The technique involved placing the nozzle of a specially made airgun against the wall of the aneurysm. Horse hairs 6 mm long were usually used; they were fired under pneumatic power into the wall of the aneurysm so as to project from the wall into the lumen of the aneurysm. Up to several dozen hairs were used in large aneurysms, although six hairs were used for the average aneurysm. Gallagher (122) reported on 17 such cases in 1965. He opined that injury currents or natural electrical charges on the hairs contributed to the thrombosis. Unfortunately, the thrombosis was inadequate in many of the cases.

For individual case reports of aneurysms treated by pilojection see the *Surg* column (symbol *PIL*) in Appendix 2.

Iron-Induced Thrombosis

Alksne and Fingerhut (7,10,103), using experimental glass "aneurysms" and experimental aneurysms in animals, found that carbonyl iron suspension could be held inside the aneurysm by a magnet until clotting developed. Subsequently Alksne et al. (11) and Rosomoff (286) injected iron particulate suspensions into the cervical ICA of patients with aneurysms while a stereotaxically placed pencil-shaped magnet was held against the aneurysm. Although there was some iron-induced thrombosis of aneurysms, the risk of embolic phenomena was too great.

Thereafter Alksne and colleagues (8,9,11–14,98) evolved a method of inserting the iron suspension directly into the aneurysm stereotaxically via a needle passed through the stereotaxic probe (the magnetic Alnico No. 5 0.25-inch magnet). Figures 31.11 and 31.12 detail the technique. More recently iron particles

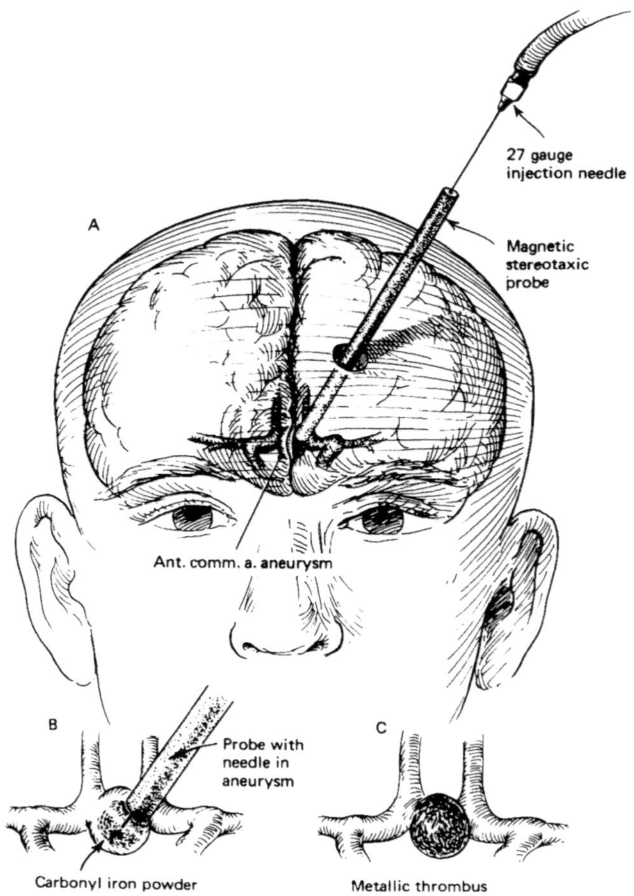

Fig. 31.11. Alksne's technique of magnetically controlled magnetic thrombosis of an intracranial aneurysm.

A The magnetic probe is shown passing through a small burr hole to abut against an aneurysm of the anterior communicating artery. The 27-gauge needle for injection is in place. In an actual case the probe would be held by a stereotaxic instrument and guided to its location under x-ray control. No retraction of brain or manipulation of blood vessels is required.

B A close-up view of the magnet against the aneurysm. The aneurysm has been penetrated by the 27-gauge needle, which was passed down the probe. Iron suspension has been injected through the needle, and the iron powder is being held within the aneurysm by the magnetic field.

C The aneurysm is completely filled with a mixture of iron powder and clotted blood. Eventually the metallic thrombus will organize, and the aneurysm will be replaced by scar tissue. From Alksne JF, ref. 8.

have been mixed with methyl methacrylate (14,315) or silicone rubber (ferrosilicone) (280) and stereotaxically injected into the aneurysm. The magnet holds the material in place until hardening occurs and the aneurysm is occluded.

For individual case reports of aneurysms treated by stereotaxic insertion of iron mixtures see the *Surg* column (symbol *SIR*) in Appendix 2.

Stereotaxic Techniques

Most of the work done on stereotaxic techniques regarding intracranial aneurysms was reviewed in the previous section on internal occlusion of aneurysms. Rather sophisticated electronic radiographic methods utilizing television (fluoroscopic units and disc recording devices to store images are being developed

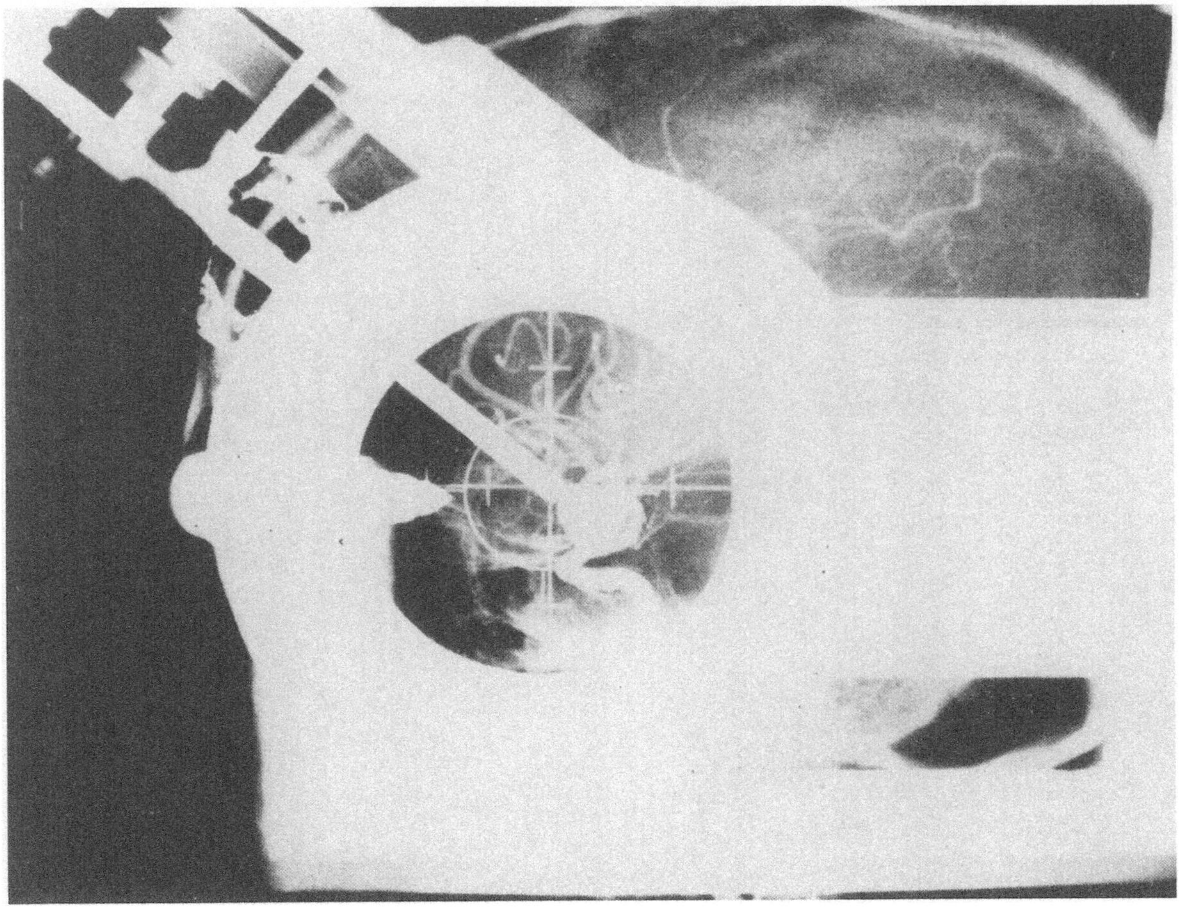

Fig. 31.12. Lateral x-ray film of a patient with the Rand-Wells stereotaxic guide in place. The magnetic probe has been positioned against an intracranial aneurysm. The circle and cross hairs are part of the apparatus used to align the guide for accurate placement of the probe. From Alksne JF, Fingerhut A, Rand R, ref. 11.

(218,299,300,315). In this way the probe can be inserted toward the stored image of the aneurysm so that fewer angiographic contrast injections are needed during the stereotaxic procedure.

Steiner et al. (321) have used stereotaxic radiosurgery with cobalt-60 irradiation to obliterate some arteriovenous malformations. They stated that anticipated problems of such therapy with aneurysms would be: (a) the length of the latent period (weeks) before obliteration; and (b) the risk of incomplete or excessive obliteration.

Kikut (191) claimed to have induced thrombosis in nine aneurysms stereotaxically placed in a strong magnetic field. It was stated that bioelectrical phenomena are induced, leading to thrombosis when the magnetic field passes perpendicular to the flow of blood.

Kandel and Peresedov (182–185) described a method wherein a clip is applied on a parent vessel or the neck of an aneurysm via a cylinder stereotaxically placed next to the aneurysm (Fig. 31.13). Kandel (182) reported they had treated 34 cases of aneurysm and AVM by this method. For individual case reports of aneurysms treated by stereotaxic clipping see the *Surg* column (symbol *SCL*) in Appendix 2.

Intravascular Catheter and Balloon Methods

Intravascular catheter techniques of diagnosis and therapy ("angiotaxic surgery") are advancing rapidly. In 1962 Rothenberg et al. (287) worked with experimental animals and described an intravascular catheter that released

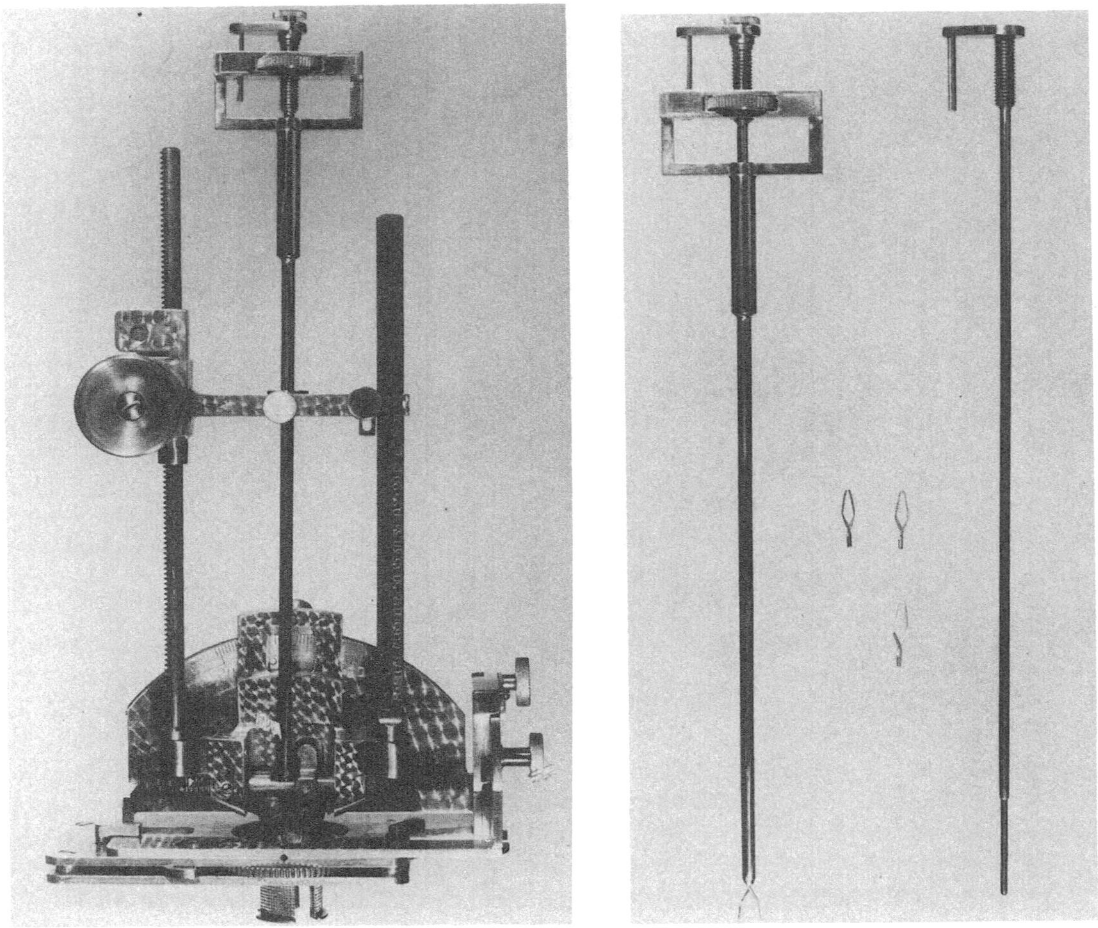

A

Fig. 31.13. **A** *Left:* Stereotaxic clipping device of Kandel and Peresedov in assembly with stereotaxic apparatus. *Right:* The clipping device is shown unassembled (*right*) and with open clip on the tip and first pivot (*left*). Three clips of different sizes are shown (*center*).

B *Top:* Angiograms during stereotaxic clipping of ICAA. *Bottom:* Angiograms after aneurysm clipped. From Kandel EI, Peresedov VV, ref. 184.

an expandable sleeve to occlude an experimental aneurysm (Fig. 31.14). In 1964 Luessenhop and Velasquez (213) studied two cases of AVM and one case of aneurysm in their evaluation of pellet embolization techniques. They noted that withdrawal of the catheter from intracranial vessels may aggravate vasospasm. More recently special catheters with magnetic tips that can be partially guided by magnetic fields have evolved (41,163,335,366). Some of these vibrate at their tips, an effect which seems to allow easier guidance around bends. Finally the sophisticated electronic television imaging and disc recording used for stereotaxic surgery is applicable here too (218,299,300,315).

Taren and Gabrielsen (334,335) have described an intravascular catheter with a tiny magnet at its tip. Not only do the magnetic fields assist in guidance but the tip can be heated. They suggested that this apparatus could be used to induce thrombosis inside intracranial aneurysms. Hilal et al. (163), using DC electrical current at the tip of the catheter, tried to induce thrombosis inside a BAA, but only partial occlusion occurred. See pages 824–827 regarding the problems of such attempts.

There is considerable investigation into the use of some substances, e.g., a Silastic liquid material impregnated with tantalum dust, to

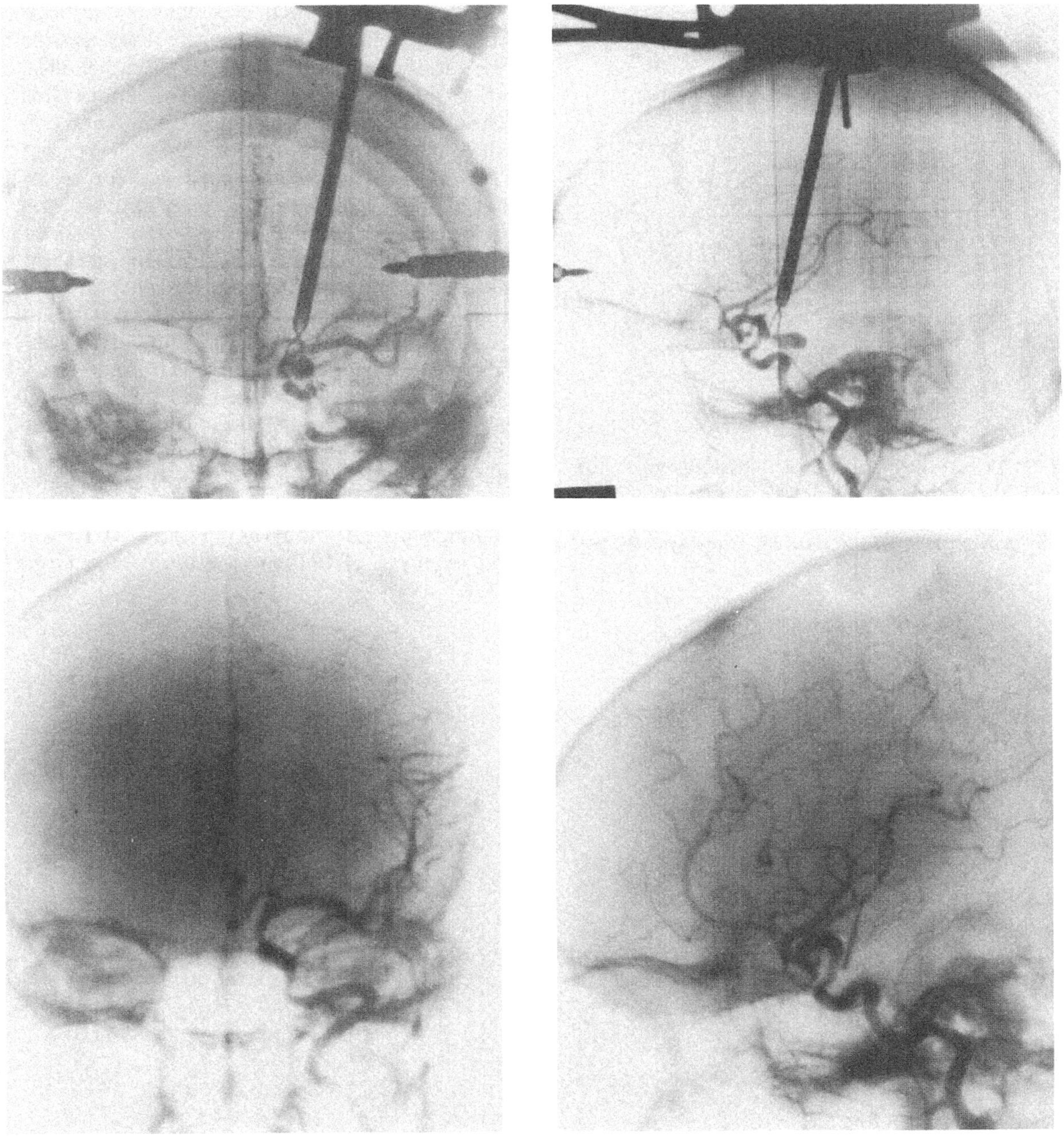

B

fill AVM vessels and vascular tumors (162). This technique may have application to aneurysms in the future.

Balloon–Catheter Techniques

Of particular interest are the catheters with a balloon attachment (Fig. 31.15); with some types of catheter this balloon can be released selectively to occlude vessels and aneurysms. There are several descriptions of nonreleasable and releasable balloons for theoretical use in aneurysms and for actual use in animal experimental aneurysms (41,64,70,71,190,203, 332,354,355). Debrun et al. (63) and Taki et al. (331) gave a good review and descriptions of the types of detachable balloon systems.

Most balloon catheter systems were first used to treat carotid-cavernous fistulas (65,101, 160,266,276,277,288). Subsequently, however,

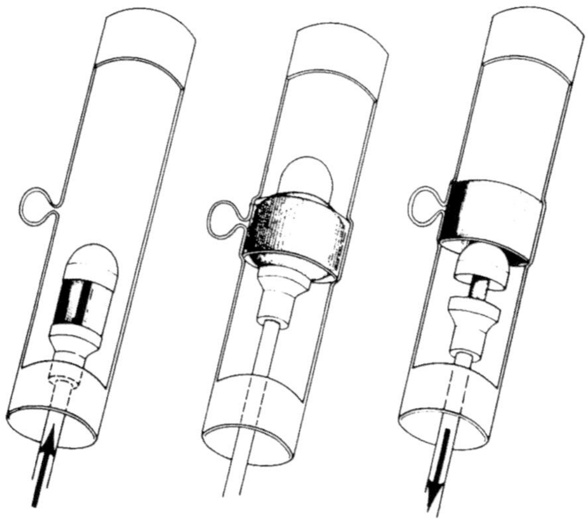

Fig. 31.14. Introduction of a folded sleeve at the end of the catheter. The sleeve is expanded after placement, occluding the mouth of the aneurysm. From Rothenberg SF, Penka EJ, Conway LW, ref. 287.

there have been reports of successful and unsuccessful occlusion of intracranial aneurysms by releasable balloons (60–63,160,308,309,331). For individual case reports of aneurysms treated by balloon occlusion see the *Surg* column (symbol *BAL*) in Appendix 2.

The use of "angiotaxic surgery" for treatment of aneurysms is in the investigative stage. Some of the problems, reviewed by Debrun and colleagues (63), are: (a) The balloon is not sucked into the aneurysm as it is into an A-V fistula. (b) After several days of balloon inflation it may leak, causing deflation and, in the absence of a fibrotic or clotting reaction, reentry of blood into the aneurysm. These authors suggest that a permanent silicone-rubber or tissue adhesive substance may be needed to maintain inflation of the balloon. (c) There is a definite risk of rupture unless the balloon perfectly fits the shape of the aneurysm. Figure 31.16 is a good example of balloon occlusion of a large bBAA.

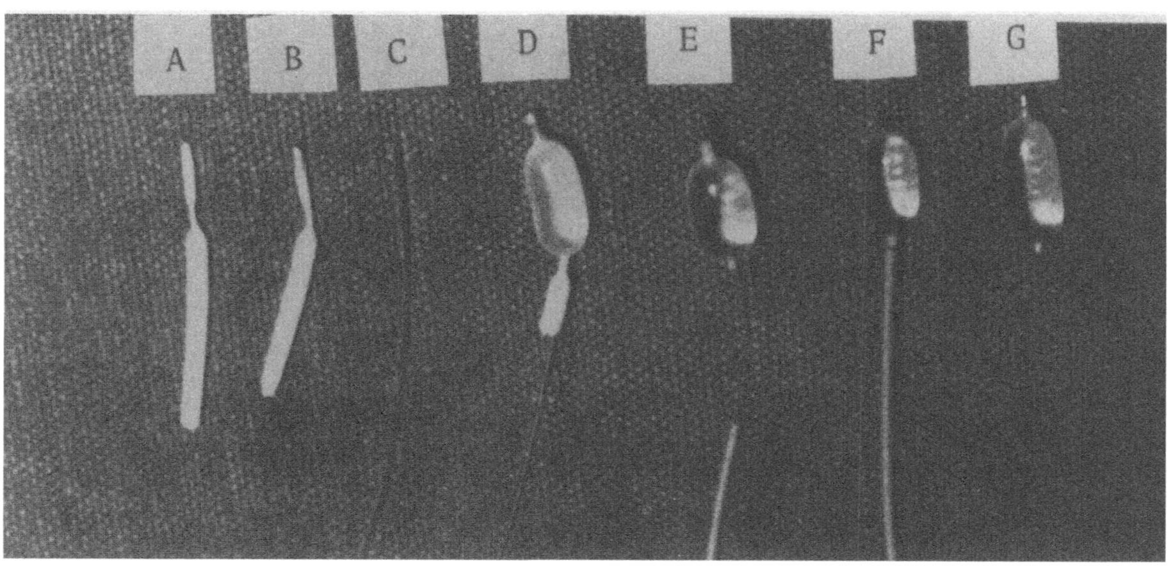

Fig. 31.15. Self-sealing intravascular balloons with elastic ligature. **A, B** Latex sleeves. **C** Teflon catheter. **D** Catheter in position in sleeve, which is then inflated. **E** Sleeve is ligated over the catheter with latex thread, and the proximal part of the sleeve is cut away; a polyethylene coaxial catheter is being slipped over the Teflon tube. **F** To detach the balloon, the polyethylene catheter is slid up over the inner Teflon catheter into contact with the base of the balloon; the outer polyethylene catheter is held in place while the inside tube is pulled back out of the balloon to detach the balloon. **G** The latex ligature immediately closes the aperture of the balloon, thus keeping the balloon expanded. From Debrun G, Lacour P, Caron J-P, et al., ref. 63.

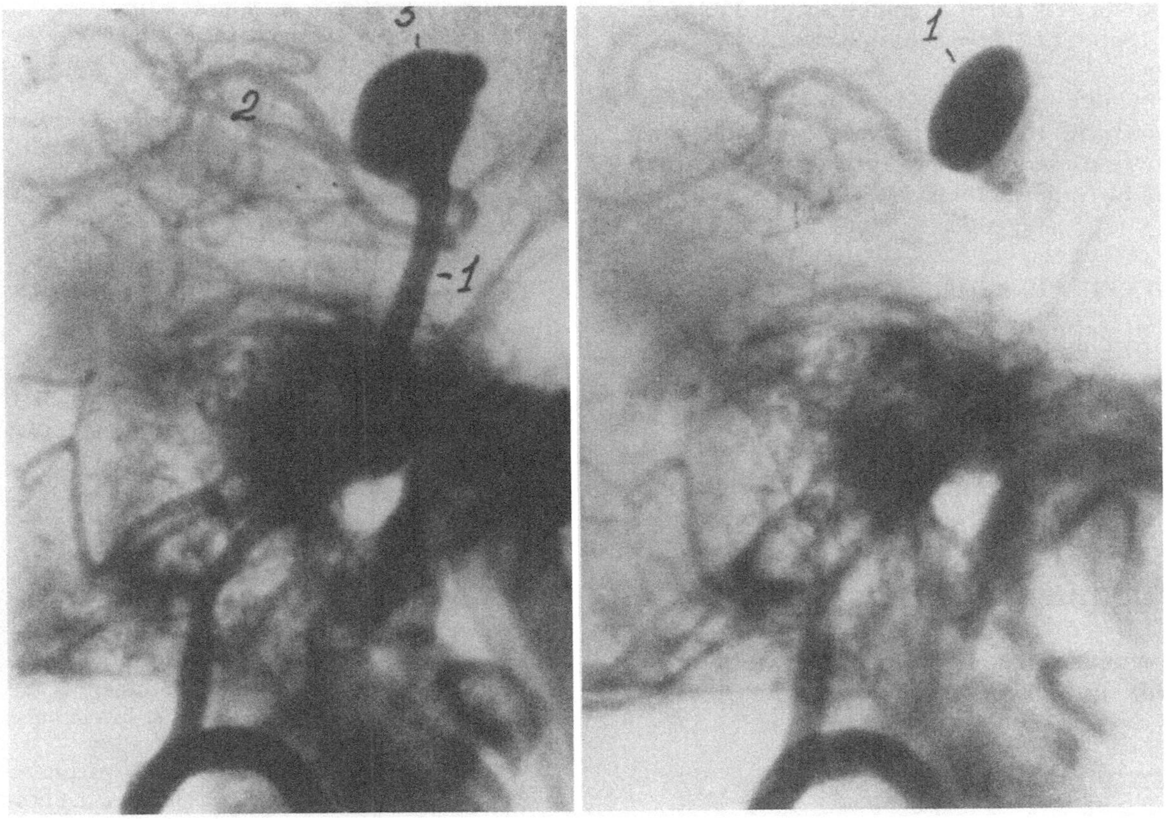

Fig. 31.16. Angiogram of bBAA illustrating occlusion of the aneurysm by a balloon. *Left* Preoperative angiogram showing basilar artery (*1*), posterior cerebral arteries (*2*), and aneurysm (*3*). ***Right*** Postoperative angiogram showing the balloon filled with contrast material in the aneurysmal cavity (*1*). From Serbinenko FA, ref. 308.

Extracranial–Intracranial Bypass

In 1951 Pool (267,269) placed a plastic tube from the left superficial temporal artery to the anterior cerebral artery distal to an ACeAA treated by proximal ligation of the parent artery. The tube was left in, and angiography 12 years later showed an absence of blood flow in the tube.

Subsequent to the evolution of microvascular anastomosis techniques, e.g., superficial temporal artery to middle cerebral artery (STA-MCA) anastomosis, came a new adjunctive technique for handling large or giant aneurysms and csICAA previously believed to be inoperable. Thus a number of cases have been reported where the aneurysm was trapped or its feeding artery ligated in association with an extracranial–intracranial anastomotic procedure (18,78, 100, 126, 170, 176, 186, 281, 295, 318, 323, 324,361). Some surgeons have used cerebral blood studies intraoperatively to determine if such anastomoses are needed (126,323). In cases of MCAA the proximal clip should be distal to the lenticulostriate arteries. Hopkins and Grand (170) believed that the anastomosis should not precede the trapping by days because the anastomosis may fail in the absence of the pressure drop which the trapping or proximal clipping provides. However, Ferguson (99) did not agree and believed that the anastomosis can precede the aneurysm operation. However, they recommended the Drake tourniquet method (pp. 813–814) for the proximal feeder ligation.

Dolenc (73) excised small fusiform MCAA in two patients. He reanastomosed the MCA branches.

For individual case reports of aneurysms treated with the extracranial–intracranial anastomosis adjunct see the *Surg* column (symbol *AEI*) in Appendix 2.

Cavernous Sinus Repair

In 1973 Parkinson (251) described his direct surgical approach to carotid-cavernous fistulas inside the cavernous sinus. In 1978 the same author (252) reported on opening the cavernous sinus and repairing csICAA in three patients.

Trigeminal Rhizotomy

Trigeminal rhizotomy is a form of symptomatic treatment. It is reviewed in Chapter 30.

Summary

This chapter details the many and varied operative treatments that have been attempted by surgeons, successfully and unsuccessfully, to cure the patient afflicted with an intracranial aneurysm. Although clipping the aneurysm with a microvascular technique remains the treatment of choice for preventing future rupture, other methods under investigation may prove to be safer and more effective.

Bibliography

1. Aarobi B, Chambers J: Giant thrombosed aneurysm associated with an arteriovenous malformation. Case report. J Neurosurg 49:278–282, 1978
2. Abbott KH, Hubbell DV, Vogel PJ: The surgical treatment of vertebral aneurysms. Report of a case. Bull Los Angeles Neurol Soc 26:79–85, 1961
3. Adams JE: Clinical experiences with hypothermia. In Fields WS, Sahs AL (eds.): Intracranial Aneurysms and Subarachnoid Hemorrhage. Springfield, Ill., Thomas, 1965, pp 275–294
4. Af Björkesten G: Arterial aneurysms of the internal carotid artery and its bifurcation. An analysis of 69 aneurysms treated mainly by direct surgical attack. J Neurosurg 15:400–410, 1958
5. Ahmed RH, Sedzimir CB: Ruptured anterior communicating aneurysms. A comparison of medical and specific surgical treatment. J Neurosurg 26:213–217, 1967
6. Aiba T: [Operative indication and surgical technique of the cerebral aneurysm. 1.] Neurol Med Chir (Tokyo) 16 (6 Part 2):467–478, 1976
7. Alksne JF: Magnetically controlled intravascular catheter. Surgery 64:339–345, 1968
8. Alksne JF: Stereotactic thrombosis of intracranial aneurysms. N Engl J Med 284:171–174, 1971
9. Alksne JF: Stereotactic thrombosis of intracranial aneurysms using a magnetic probe. Confin Neurol 31:95–98, 1969
10. Alksne JF, Fingerhut AG: Magnetically controlled metallic thrombosis of intracranial aneurysms. A preliminary report. Bull Los Angeles Neurol Soc 30:153–155, 1965
11. Alksne JF, Fingerhut A, Rand R: Magnetically controlled metallic thrombosis of intracranial aneurysms. Surgery 60:212–218, 1966
12. Alksne JF, Fingerhut AG, Rand RW: Magnetic probe for the stereotactic thrombosis of intracranial aneurysms. J Neurol Neurosurg Psychiatry 30:159–162, 1967
13. Alksne JF, Rand RW: Current status of metallic thrombosis of intracranial aneurysms. Prog Neurol Surg 3:212–229, 1969
14. Alksne JF, Smith RW: Iron-acrylic compound for stereotaxic aneurysm thrombosis. J Neurosurg 47:137–141, 1977
15. Allcock JM, Drake CG: New approaches to the treatment of intracranial aneurysms. Neuroradiology 12:46, 1976
16. Almeida GM, Bianco E, Shibata MK: Anterior communicating artery aneurysms. J Neurosurg 33:53–57, 1976
17. Amacher AL, Drake CG: Cerebral artery aneurysms in infancy, childhood and adolescence. Childs Brain 1:72–80, 1975
18. Ammerman BJ, Smith DR: Giant fusiform middle cerebral aneurysm: successful treatment utilizing microvascular bypass. Surg Neurol 7:255–257, 1977
19. Araki C, Handa H, Yoshida K, et al.: Electrically induced thrombosis for the treatment of intracranial aneurysms and angiomas. Excerpta Med ICS No. 110:651–653, 1966
20. Arseni C, Ghitescu M, Cristescu A, et al.: Intrasellar aneurysms simulating hypophyseal tumors. Eur Neurol 3:321–329, 1970
21. Arseni C, Nash F: Anévrysme intracrânien rompu de l'artere vertébrale gauche traité par

abord chirurgical direct. Neurochirurgia 10:293–296, 1964
22. Atkinson WJ: New approach to management of intracranial aneurysms. Lancet 1:5–9, 1975
23. Atkinson WJ: The "A" principle—a new approach to the management of intracranial aneurysms. J Neurol Neurosurg Psychiatry 38:405–406, 1975
24. Auld AW, Shafey S: Transient ischemia attacks not produced by extracranial vascular disease: a plea for complete and early angiographic investigation. South Med J 69:722–724, 1976
25. Bakay L, Sweet WH: Intra-arterial pressures in the neck and brain. Late changes after carotid closure, acute measurements after vertebral closure. J Neurosurg 10:353–359, 1953
26. Bank WO, Nelson PB, Drayer BP, et al.: Traumatic aneurysm of the basilar artery. Am J Roentgenol 130:975–977, 1978
27. Bartal A, Schiffer J, Weinstein M: A successful case of basilar bifurcation aneurysm surgery. Acta Neurochir (Wien) 19:163–170, 1968
28. Bassett RC: Multiple cerebral aneurysm. Report of a case. J Neurosurg 8:132–133, 1951
29. Bassett RC, Lemmen LJ: Subdural hematoma associated with bleeding intracranial aneurysm. J Neurosurg 9:443–450, 1952
30. Bassett RC, List CF, Lemmen LJ: Surgical treatment of intracranial aneurysm. Surg Gynecol Obstet 95:701–708, 1952
31. Baumann CHH, Bucy PC: Aneurysms of the anterior cerebral artery. Evaluation of surgical and "conservative" treatments. JAMA 163: 1448–1454, 1957
32. Bell WE, Butler C: Cerebral mycotic aneurysms in children. Two case reports. Neurology (NY) 18:81–86, 1968
33. Bhushan C, Hodges FJ, Posey J: Successful surgical treatment of giant aneurysm of the basilar artery. Case report. J Neurosurg 49:124–128, 1978
34. Bohm E, Hugosson R: Results of surgical treatment of 200 consecutive cerebral arterial aneurysms. Acta Neurol Scand 46:43–52, 1970
35. Bonnal J, Navarrane R, Aymard J: Peut-on lier l'artère cérébrale antérieure au cours de la cure chirurgicale des anévrysmes situés à la jonction de cette artère et de l'artere communicante antérieure? Neurochirurgie 1:168–176, 1955
36. Bonnal J, Stevenaert A: Indications actuelles de l'abord direct des anévrysmes artériels du polygone de Willis. Acta Neurol Belg 70:240–268, 1970
37. Bonnal J, Stevenaert A, Brotchi J, et al.: Bilan de neuf ans d'expérience de la chirurgie des anévrysmes artériels intracrâniens. Acta Neurol Belg 74:337–355, 1974
38. Borchardt M: Die chirurgische Bedeutung der Gehirnaneurysmen. Bruns Beitr Klin Chir 133:429–451, 1925
39. Bouchet A: Une ingénieuse découverte Lyonnaise au XIXe siècle: le traitement des anévrysmes artériels par la galvono-puncture. Lyon Med 227:67–77, 1972
40. Campbell E, Burklund CW: Aneurysms of the middle cerebral artery. Ann Surg 137:18–28, 1953
41. Cares HL, Hale JR, Montgomery DB, et al.: Laboratory experience with the magnetically guided intravascular catheter system. J Neurosurg 38:145–154, 1973
42. Chou SN, Ortiz-Suarez HJ: Surgical treatment of arterial aneurysms of the vertebrobasilar circulation. J Neurosurg 41:671–680, 1974
43. Choudhury AR: Proximal occlusion of the dominant anterior cerebral artery for anterior communicating aneurysm. J Neurosurg 45:484–490, 1976
44. Cook AW, Dooley DM, Browder EJ: Anterior communicating aneurysms: treatment by ligation of an anterior cerebral artery. J Neurosurg 23:371–374, 1965
45. Cophignon J, Rey A, Thurel C, et al.: Microchirurgie des anévrysmes artériels de la partie antérieure du polygone de Willis. Étude d'une série consécutive de 48 cas. Neurochirurgie 19:519–530, 1973
46. Cophignon J, Rey A, Thurel C, et al.: Microchirurgie des anévrysmes intracrâniens. Etude d'une série consécutive de 50 cas. Nouv Presse Med 2:2935–2938, 1973
47. Crockard HA, Gordon DA: Treatment of giant aneurysms by intra-aneurysmal cuprous wiring. Acta Neurochir (Wiens) 46:173, 1979
48. Crompton MR: Recurrent haemorrhage from cerebral aneurysms and its prevention by surgery. J Neurol Neurosurg Psychiatry 29:164–170, 1966
49. Cushing H: The chiasmal syndrome of primary optic atrophy and bitemporal field defects in adult patients with a normal sella turcica. XIII Concilium Ophthalmologicum (Hollandia) 13(3):97–184, 1929
50. Dandy WE: Aneurysms of the anterior cerebral artery. JAMA 119:1253–1254, 1942
51. Dandy WE: Intracranial aneurysm of internal carotid artery, cured by operation. Ann Surg 107:654–659, 1938
52. Dandy WE: Intracranial Arterial Aneurysms. New York, Hafner, 1944, reprinted 1969
53. Dandy WE: Intracranial arterial aneurysms in the carotid canal. Diagnosis and treatment. Arch Surg 45:335–350, 1942
54. Dandy WE: Pathologic changes in Ménière's disease. JAMA 108:931–937, 1937
55. Dandy WE: The surgical treatment of intra-

cranial aneurysms of the internal carotid artery. Ann Surg 114:336–340, 1941
56. Dandy WE: The treatment of internal carotid aneurysms within the cavernous sinus and the cranial chamber. Report of three cases. Ann Surg 109:689–711, 1939
57. Di Pian R, Pasqualin A, Scienza R: Direct microsurgical approach to aneurysms of the internal carotid bifurcation. Surg Neurol 13:27–37, 1980
58. David M, Sachs M: Les anéurysmes de la bifurcation de la carotide interne. Neurochirugia (Stuttgt) 10:96–105, 1967
59. Davis RA: The results of delayed intracranial surgery in a series of 75 selected cerebral aneurysms. Bull Northwest Univ Med Sch 36:237–244, 1962
60. Debrun G: Treatment of certain intracerebral vascular lesions with releasable balloon catheter. In Schmidek HH, Sweet WH (eds.): Current Techniques in Operative Neurosurgery. New York, Grune & Stratton, 1977, pp. 41–55.
60a. Debrun G, Fox A, Drake C, et al.: Giant unclippable aneurysms: treatment with detachable balloons. Am J Neuroradiol 2:167–173, 1981
61. Debrun G, Lacour P, Caron JP: Balloon arterial catheter techniques in the treatment of arterial intracranial diseases. In: Krayenbühl H (ed.): Advances and Technical Standards in Neurosurgery, Vol 4. Wien, Springer-Verlag, 1977, pp 132–145.
62. Debrun G, Lacour P, Caron JP: Treatment of cerebral aneurysms with a detachable balloon. Neuroradiology 15:53, 1978
63. Debrun G, Lacour P, Caron J-P, et al.: Detachable balloon and calibrated-leak balloon techniques in the treatment of cerebral vascular lesions. J Neurosurg 49:635–649, 1978
64. Debrun G, Lacour P, Caron JP, et al.: Inflatable and released balloon technique experimentation in dog—application in man. Neuroradiology 9:267–271, 1975
65. Debrun G, Lacour P, Caron JP, et al.: Technique du ballon gonflable et largable en neurologie. Étude experimentale. Application chez l'homme. Rev Neurol (Paris) 132:23–31, 1976
66. Decker A, Rowe EC: Subarachnoid hemorrhage complicating pregnancy. Am J Surg 85:561–563, 1953
67. Denecke HJ, Hartert H: Carotis interna-Verletzung unt unstillbarem Nasenbluten, geheilt durch intraarterielle Thrombininjektion. Mit einem experimentellen Beitrag. Chirurg 25:470–472, 1954
68. DeSaussure RL, Hunter SE, Robertson JT: Saccular aneurysms of the posterior fossa. J Neurosurg 15:385–391, 1958
69. Dimsdale H, Logue V: Ruptured posterior fossa aneurysms and their surgical treatment. J Neurol Neurosurg Psychiatry 22:202–217, 1959
70. DiTullio MV Jr, Rand RW, Frisch E: Detachable balloon catheter. Its application in experimental arteriovenous fistulae. J Neurosurg 48:717–723, 1978
71. DiTullio MV Jr, Rand RW, Frisch E: Development of a detachable vascular balloon catheter. A preliminary report. Bull Los Angeles Neurol Soc 41:2–5, 1976
72. Dixon JM: Angioid streaks and pseudoxanthoma elasticum with aneurysm of the internal carotid artery. Am J Ophthalmol 34:1322–1323, 1951
73. Dolenc V: Treatment of fusiform aneurysms of the peripheral cerebral arteries. Report of two cases. J Neurosurg 49:272–277, 1978
74. Dooley DM, Cook AW, Browder EJ: Surgical occlusion of anterior cerebral artery. NY J Med 69:2786–2789, 1969
75. Dott NM: Intracranial aneurysmal formations. Clin Neurosurg 16:1–15, 1969
76. Drake CG: Advances in the neurosurgical treatment of aneurysms, arteriovenous malformations, and hematomas of the vertebral circulation. Adv Neurol 16:211–225, 1977
77. Drake CG: Further experience with surgical treatment of aneurysms of the basilar artery. J Neurosurg 29:372–392, 1968
78. Drake CG: Giant intracranial aneurysms: experience in 174 patients. Clin Neurosurg 26:12–95, 1979
79. Drake CG: Ligation of the vertebral (unilateral or bilateral) or basilar artery in the treatment of large intracranial aneurysms. J Neurosurg 43:255–274, 1975
80. Drake CG: On the surgical treatment of ruptured intracranial aneurysms. Clin Neurosurg 13:122–155, 1965
81. Drake CG: The surgical treatment of aneurysms of the basilar artery. J Neurosurg 29: 436–446, 1968
82. Drake CG: The surgical treatment of vertebral-basilar aneurysms. Clin Neurosurg 16: 114–169, 1969
83. Drake CG, Allcock JM: Postoperative angiography and the "slipped" clip. J Neurosurg 39:683–689, 1973
84. Drake CG, Amacher AL: Aneurysms of the posterior cerebral artery. J Neurosurg 30:468–474, 1969
85. Drake CG, Jory TA: Spontaneous intracranial haemorrhage: "subarachnoid haemorrhage": a review of investigation and treatment in 189

cases. Can J Surg 4:4–11, 1960
86. Drake CG, Vanderlinden RG: The late consequences of incomplete surgical treatment of cerebral aneurysms. J Neurosurg 27:226–238, 1967
87. Dueker HW: Surgical treatment of intracranial aneurysms. Bull Los Angeles Neurol Soc 16:150–161, 1951
88. Durity F, Logue V: The effect of proximal anterior cerebral occlusion on anterior communicating artery aneurysms. Postoperative radiological survey of 43 cases. J Neurosurg 35:16–19, 1971
89. Early CB, Fink LH: Some fundamental applications of the law of La Place in neurosurgery. Surg Neurol 6:185–189, 1976
90. Einspruch BC, Clark K: Clinical experiences with intravenous urea used to lower intracranial pressure. Texas Rep Biol Med 20:176–179, 1962
91. Elsberg CA: Ruptured aneurysm of the right middle cerebral artery. Bull NY Neurol Inst 1:210–212, 1918
92. Fager CA, Poppen JL: Observations on controlled ligation of the internal carotid artery. Surg Clin North Am 36:567–582, 1956
93. Falconer MA: Progress in the surgical treatment of spontaneous cerebral haemorrhage. Proc R Soc Med 49:166–169, 1956
94. Falconer MA: Surgical treatment of spontaneous intracranial haemorrhage. Br Med J 1:790–792, 1958
95. Falconer MA: Surgical treatment of spontaneous subarachnoid haemorrhage. Preliminary report. Br Med J 1:809–813, 1950
96. Falconer MA: The future of surgery in the treatment of spontaneous cerebral haemorrhage. Lancet 2:945–950, 1952
97. Falconer MA: The surgical treatment of bleeding intracranial aneurysms. J Neurol Neurosurg Psychiatry 14:153–186, 1951
98. Feigenbaum J, Alksne J: The stereotaxic obliteration of intracranial aneurysms. Bull Los Angeles Neurol Soc 32:77–85, 1967
99. Ferguson GG: Comments. Neurosurgery 5:29–30, 1979
100. Ferguson GG, Drake CG, Peerless SJ: Extracranial-intracranial arterial bypass in the treatment of "giant" intracranial aneurysms. Stroke 8:11, 1977
101. Fierstien SB, DeFes D, Nutkiewicz A: Complete obliteration of a carotid cavernous fistula with sparing of the carotid blood flow using a detachable balloon catheter. Surg Neurol 9:227–280, 1978
102. Fincher EF: An aneurysm of the intracranial carotid artery treated surgically. Yale J Biol Med 11:423–424, 1939
103. Fingerhut AG, Alksne JF: Thrombosis of intracranial aneurysms. An experimental approach utilizing magnetically controlled iron particles. Radiology 86:342–343, 1966
104. Fodstad H, Liliequist B, Wirell S, et al.: Giant serpentine intracranial aneurysm after carotid ligation. Case report. J Neurosurg 49:903–909, 1978
105. Foerster O: Aneurysma der Carotis interna. Berl Klin Wochenschr 58:1057–1058, 1921
106. Fox JL: Microsurgical exposure of intracranial aneurysms. J Microsurg 1:2–31, 1979
107. Fox JL: The use of laser radiation as a surgical "light knife." J Surg Res 9:199–205, 1969
108. Fox JL, Luessenhop AJ: Hydrocephalus secondary to hemorrhage from a basilar artery aneurysm. With a note on embolization technique. Acta Neurochir (Wien) 17:228–235, 1967
109. Fox JL, Yaşargil MG: The effect of DC electrical current on the rodent artery. Surg Neurol 2:13–16, 1974
110. Fox JL, Yaşargil MG: The experimental effect of direct electrical current on intracranial arteries and the blood-brain barrier. J Neurosurg 41:582–589, 1974
111. Frantzen E, Krenchel NJ: Prognosen ved intracranielle sacculate aneurysmer en efterundersøgelse. Nord Med 51:130–134, 1954
112. French LA: Discussion. Clin Neurosurg 11:209–214, 1964
113. French LA, Chou SN, Long DM: The direct approach to intracranial aneurysms. Clin Neurosurg 15:117–132, 1968
114. French LA, Chou SN, Story JL: Aneurysms of the anterior communicating artery. Report of a method of surgical treatment and review of 40 cases. Postgrad Med 34:323–327, 1963
115. French LA, Chou SN, Story JL, et al.: Aneurysm of the anterior communicating artery. J Neurosurg 24:1058–1062, 1966
116. French LA, Haines GL: Unilateral vertebral artery ligation. Report of a case ending fatally with thrombosis of the basilar artery. J Neurosurg 7:156–158, 1950
117. French LA, Zarling ME, Schultz EA: Management of aneurysms of the anterior communicating artery. J Neurosurg 19:870–876, 1962
118. Gage EL: Treatment of berry aneurysms of the carotids and their branches. W Va Med J 60:29–34, 1964
119. Gallagher JP: A new method for obliterating dangerous aneurysms of the brain. Mammalian hairs "shot" into lesions with navy-developed gun. Naval Res Rev (Wash), August 1962, pp. 1–6
120. Gallagher JP: Obliteration of intracranial

aneurysms by pilojection. JAMA 183:231–236, 1963
121. Gallagher JP: Pilojection for intracranial aneurysms. Report of progress. J Neurosurg 21:129–134, 1964
122. Gallagher JP: The closure of intracranial aneurysms by pilojection. In Fields WS, Sahs AL (eds.): Intracranial Aneurysms and Subarachnoid Hemorrhage. Springfield Ill., Thomas, 1965, pp. 444–458
123. Garcia-Bengochea F: Giant aneurysms and the juxta-aneurysmatic ligation of their parent arteries without neurological sequelae. Neurosurgery 1:155–156, 1977
124. Gardner WJ: Cerebral angiomas and aneurysms. Surg Clin North Am 16:1019–1030, 1936
125. Gass HH, McGuire JF, Simmons DR: Intracranial eradication of middle cerebral aneurysms. J Neurosurg 15:223–233, 1958
126. Gelber BR, Sundt TM Jr: Treatment of intracavernous and giant carotid aneurysms by combined internal carotid ligation and extra- to intracranial bypass. J Neurosurg 52:1–10, 1980
127. Genest AS: Experimental use of intraluminal plastic in the treatment of carotid aneurysms. Preliminary report. J Neurosurg 22:136–141, 1965
128. German WJ: Intracranial aneurysm: a surgical problem. Zbl Neurochir 3:352–354, 1938
129. Gibbs JR: On the advantages of opening certain intracranial aneurysms. J Neurol Neurosurg Psychiatry 20:165–171, 1957
130. Gillingham FJ: The management of ruptured intracranial aneurysm. Ann R Coll Surg 23:89–117, 1958
131. Glaser HT: The diagnosis and treatment of intracranial aneurysms. Ohio State Med J 54:325–328, 1958
132. Graf CJ: Results of direct attack on nonfistulous intracranial aneurysm with remarks on statistics. J Neurosurg 12:146–153, 1955
133. Greenwood J Jr: The surgery of intracranial aneurysms. Texas State J Med 40:423–426, 1944
134. Groff RA: Experience with direct surgical treatment of intracranial aneurysms. Arch Neurol Psychiatry 72:782, 1954
135. Gros C, Vlahovitch B, Auteroche B: Réflexions sur une série de 46 anévrysmes supraclinoidiens rompus. Évaluation du traitement chirurgical. Neurochirurgie 3:253–258, 1957
136. Grote W, Röttgen P, Wappenschmidt J: Erfahrungen mit Aneurysmen der Arteria communicans anterior. Neurochirurgie 6:63–71, 1960
137. Gryspeerdt GL: Angiographic studies of the blood flow in the circle of Willis. The value of various arterial compression tests. Acta Radiol [Diagn] (Stockh) 1 (Part 1): 298–313, 1963
138. Guidetti B: Microsurgical treatment of intracranial saccular aneurysms. Acta Neurochir (Wien) 43:153–162, 1978
139. Guidetti B: Surgical treatment of aneurysms of the anterior communicating artery. Prog Brain Res 30:303–307, 1968
140. Guidetti B, LaTorre E: Carotid-ophthalmic aneurysms. A series of 16 cases treated by direct approach. Acta Neurochir (Wien) 22:289–304, 1970
141. Guidetti B, La Torre E: Management of carotid-ophthalmic aneurysms. J Neurosurg 42:438–442, 1975
142. Guillaume J, Mazars G, Pansini A: Essais de coagulation intra-cavitaire des anévrysmes endocraniens. Neurochirurgie 3:226–228, 1957
143. Guthkelch AN: Large saccular aneurysm of intracranial part of vertebral artery. Br J Surg 37:107–108, 1949
144. Hallac I, Hamby WB: A metallic fastener for intracranial vascular ligation. J Neurosurg 18:261–262, 1961
145. Hamby WB: Intracranial Aneurysms. Springfield, Ill., Thomas, 1952
146. Hamby WB: Intracranial surgery for aneurysms. Prog Neurol Surg 3:1–65, 1969
147. Hamby WB: Intracranial surgical procedures in subarachnoid hemorrhage and intracranial aneurysms. In Fields WS (ed.): Pathogenesis and Treatment of Cerebrovascular Disease. Springfield, Ill., Thomas, 1961, pp 496–507
148. Hamby WB: Remarks concerning intracranial aneurysm surgery. Clin Neurosurg 17:1–17, 1970
149. Hamby WB: The modern treatment of intracranial aneurysms. NY State J Med 52:2497–2502, 1952
150. Hamby WB: The surgical management of intracranial aneurysms. Acta Neurol Latinoam 4:341–346, 1956
151. Hamilton JG, Falconer MA: Immediate and late results of surgery in cases of saccular intracranial aneurysms. J Neurosurg 16:514–541, 1959
152. Hann EC, Luros JT, Lang EK: Aneurysm of the left posterior inferior cerebellar artery with repeated bleeding episodes. J Indiana Med Assoc 57:970–972, 1964
153. Harris P: Aneurysms of the anterior communicating artery. Cincinnati J Med 42:1–7, 1961
154. Hashi K, Hakuba A, Ikuno H, et al.: [A midline vertebral artery aneurysm operated via transoral transclival approach.] Neurol Surg (Tokyo) 4:183–189, 1976

155. Hazouri LA: Five year experience with intracranial aneurysms. J Med Assoc Ga 57:62–64, 1968
156. Henderson JW: Intracranial arterial aneurysms. A study of 119 cases, with special reference to the ocular findings. Trans Am Ophthalmol Soc 53:349–462, 1955
157. Heppner F: Das Aneurysma der vorderen kommunizierenden Hirnarterie als neurochirurgisches Problem. Wien Med Wochenschr 120:849–851, 1970
158. Heppner F: Réflexions sur le traitement des anévrysmes de l'artère communicante antérieure. Neurochirurgie 6:56–57, 1960
159. Hermann K, Obrador S, Dott NM: Intracranial aneurysms and allied clinical syndromes: cerebral arteriography in their management. Lisboa Med 14:782–814, 1937
160. Herrmann H-D, Fischer D, Loew F: Experiences with intraluminal occlusion with the Fogarty catheter in the treatment of carotid-cavernous sinus fistulas and other lesions at the base of the skull. Acta Neurochir (Wien) 32:35–54, 1975
161. Heuer GJ, Dandy WE: Roentgenography in the localization of brain tumor, based upon a series of one hundred consecutive cases. Bull Johns Hopkins Hosp 26:311–322, 1916
162. Hilal SK, Michelsen JW: Therapeutic percutaneous embolization for extra-axial vascular lesions of the head, neck and spine. J Neurosurg 43:275–287, 1975
163. Hilal SK, Michelsen WJ, Driller J, et al.: Magnetically guided devices for vascular exploration and treatment. Laboratory and clinical investigations. Radiology 113:529–540, 1974
164. Hockley A: Proximal occlusion of the anterior cerebral artery for anterior communicating aneurysm. J Neurol Neurosurg Psychiatry 37:1280, 1974
165. Hockley A: Proximal occlusion of the anterior cerebral artery for anterior communicating aneurysm. J Neurosurg 43:426–431, 1975
166. Hoffman GR, Derom F, Meirsman G, et al.: Traitement neurochirurgical de l'anévrysme de l'artère communicante anterieure. Acta Chir Belg 59:610–630, 1960
167. Höök O, Norlén G: Aneurysms of the anterior communicating artery. Acta Neurol Scand 40:219–240, 1964
168. Höök O, Norlén G: Aneurysms of the internal carotid artery. Acta Neurol Scand 40:200–218, 1964
169. Höök O, Norlén G: Aneurysms of the middle cerebral artery. A report of 80 cases. Acta Chir Scand [Suppl] 235:1–39, 1958
170. Hopkins LN, Grand W: Extracranial-intracranial arterial bypass in the treatment of aneurysms of the carotid and middle cerebral arteries. Neurosurgery 5:21–31, 1979
171. Hosobuchi Y: Direct surgical treatment of giant intracranial aneurysms. J Neurosurg 51:743–756, 1979
172. Howell CMH: Some notes on cerebral aneurysms. Barth Hosp J 39:130–133, 1932
173. Hugenholtz H, Morley TP: The results of proximal anterior cerebral artery occlusion for anterior communicating aneurysms. J Neurosurg 37:65–70, 1972
174. Hughes B: The treatment of intracranial aneurysm. Med Press 231:181–184, 1954
175. Hunt WE, Hess RM: Aneurysm of the posterior cerebral artery with unexpected postoperative neurological deficit. Case report. J Neurosurg 26:633–635, 1967
176. Iwabuchi T, Kudo T, Hatanaka M, et al.: Vein graft bypass in treatment of giant aneurysm. Surg Neurol 12:463–466, 1979
177. Jaeger R: Aneurysm of the intracranial carotid artery. Syndrome of frontal headache with oculomotor nerve paralysis. JAMA 142:304–309, 1950
178. Jamieson KG: Direct operation for intracranial aneurysm: some technical problems and attempts at their solution. Neurol Med Chir (Tokyo) 11:1–10, 1971
179. Jefferson G: Further concerning compression of the optic pathways by intracranial aneurysms. Clin Neurosurg 1:55–103, 1955
180. Jefferson G: On the saccular aneurysms of the internal carotid artery in the cavernous sinus. Br J Surg 26:267–302, 1938
181. Kamano S, Hanamura T, Amano K: [Ligation of the vertebral artery as a treatment of a large basilar aneurysm.] Neurol Surg (Tokyo) 5:883–887, 1977
182. Kandel EI: Personal communication, 22 November 1978
183. Kandel EI, Peresedov VV: [Device for stereotaxic clipping of arterial and arteriovenous aneurysms in the brain.] Vopr Neurokhir, Mar-Apr 1977, pp 53–55
184. Kandel EI, Peresedov VV: Stereotaxic clipping of arterial aneurysms and arteriovenous malformations. J Neurosurg 46:12–23, 1977
185. Kandel EI, Peresedov VV: [Stereotaxic clipping of cerebral arterial aneurysms.] Vopr Neirokhir, Jan-Feb 1975, pp 13–15
186. Kapp JP: Hyperbaric oxygen as an adjunct to acute revascularization of the brain. Surg Neurol 12:457–461, 1979
187. Karasawa J, Kikuchi H, Furuse S, et al.: [Surgery of vertebral aneurysms of the origin of PICA.] Neurol Surg (Tokyo) 4:1157–1164, 1977
188. Kempe LG: Operative Neurosurgery, Vol 1:

Cranial, Cerebral, and Intracranial Vascular Disease. Berlin, Springer-Verlag, 1968, pp. 1–75, 203–214

189. Kennedy F: A further note on the diagnostic value in expanding lesions of the frontal lobes with a report of this syndrome in a case of aneurysm of the right internal carotid artery. JAMA 67:1361–1363, 1916
190. Kerber C: Balloon catheter with a graduated leak. A new system for superselective angiography and occlusive catheter therapy. Radiology 120:547–550, 1976
191. Kikut RP: [Treatment of aneurysms of the cerebral arteries using stereotaxically oriented external uniform magnetic fields.] Vopr Neirokhir, Jan-Feb 1976, pp. 3–7
192. Kikut RP: [Treatment of experimental aneurysms by filling with rapidly-hardening plastics.] Vopr Neirokhir 30:28–31, 1966
193. Kirgis HD, Echols DH: Management of intracranial arterial aneurysms. Surg Clin North Am 33:1003–1021, 1953
194. Kirgis HD, Fisher WL, Llewellyn RC, et al.: Aneurysms of the anterior communicating artery and gross anomalies of the circle of Willis. J Neurosurg 25:73–78, 1966
195. Klemme RM, Woolsey RD: Suprasellar aneurysm. Report of a case, with recovery. Arch Neurol Psychiatry 47:662–666, 1942
196. Kosary IZ, Shacked IJ, Tadmor R, et al.: Cavernous sinus carotid aneurysm treated by artificial embolization. Neurochirurgia (Stuttg) 14:98–101, 1971
197. Krayenbühl H, Yaşargil MG: Diagnosis and therapy of intracranial aneurysms. In Cooper P, Nyhus LM (eds.): Surgery Annual. New York, Appleton-Century-Crofts, 1970, pp. 327–343
198. Krayenbühl HA, Yaşargil MG, Flamm ES, et al.: Microsurgical treatment of intracranial saccular aneurysms. J Neurosurg 37:678–686, 1972
199. Kusaka K, Yamashita S, Kashihara M, et al.: [Occlusion of the intracranial vertebral artery for treatment of vertebral aneurysm at the origin of the posterior inferior cerebellar artery—report of two cases and hydrodynamic experimental study.] No Shinkei Geka 6:135–142, 1978
200. Laine E: Traitement chirurgical des anévrysmes de l'artère communicante antérieure. In Krayenbühl H, et al. (eds.): L'Anévrysme de l'Artère Communicante Antérieure. Paris, Masson et Cie, 1959, pp. 131–182
201. Laine E, Andreussi L, Delandsheer J-M, et al.: Anévrysmes de l'artère cérébrale moyenne. Étude anatomique, clinique et thérapeutique. A propos d'une série de 116 cas dont 100 ont été opérés. Neurochirurgie 16:181–201, 1970
202. Laitinen L: [Arterial aneurysm with subarachnoid hemorrhage in children.] Nord Med 71:329–333, 1964
203. Laitinen L, Servo A: Embolization of cerebral vessels with inflatable and detachable balloons. Technical note. J Neurosurg 48:307–308, 1978
204. Laitinen L, Troupp H: Reliability of partial ligation in the treatment of intracranial arterial aneurysm. Acta Neurol Scand 37:62–66, 1961
205. Lazorthes G, Gaubert J, Poulhes J: La distribution centrale et corticale de l'artère cérébrale antérieure. Étude anatomique et incidences neurochirurgicales. Neurochirurgie 2:237–253, 1956
206. List CF: Diagnosis and treatment of intracranial aneurysms. Arch Neurol Psychiatry 68: 842–845, 1952
207. Logue V: Posterior fossa aneurysms. Clin Neurosurg 11:183–207, 1964
208. Logue V: Surgery in spontaneous subarachnoid haemorrhage. Operative treatment of aneurysms on the anterior cerebral and anterior communicating artery. Br Med J 1:473–479, 1956
209. Lougheed WM: Selection, timing, and technique of aneurysm surgery of the anterior circle of Willis. Clin Neurosurg 16:95–113, 1969
210. Lougheed WM, Botterell EH, Morley TP: Results of the direct attack in the surgical management of internal carotid and middle cerebral aneurysms. Clin Neurosurg 9:193–200, 1963
211. Lougheed WM, Marshall BM: Management of aneurysms of the anterior circulation by intracranial procedures. In Youmans JR (ed.): Neurological Surgery, Vol 2. Philadelphia, Saunders, 1973, pp. 731–767
212. Luessenhop AJ: Artificial embolization for cerebral arteriovenous malformations. Prog Neurol Surg 3:320–362, 1969
213. Luessenhop AJ, Velasquez AC: Observations on the tolerance of intracranial arteries to catheterization. J Neurosurg 21:85–91, 1964
214. Lyerly: Discussion of intracranial aneurysm: a surgical problem. Zentralbl Neurochir 3:353, 1938
215. Magner W: Multiple intracranial aneurysms. Can Med Assoc J 33:401–403, 1935
216. Maira G, Hardy J: Experimental approach to the treatment of aneurysms with photocoagulation by laser beam. Acta Neurochir (Wien) 42:146, 1978
217. Maira G, Mohr G, Panisset A, et al.: Laser photocoagulation for treatment of experimental aneurysms. J Microsurg 1:137–147, 1979
218. Maroon JC, Sashin D: Electronic radiography

in neurosurgery. Surg Neurol 8:187–190, 1977
219. Martinez Coll A, Del Corral JF: Experiences in intracranial surgery for aneurysms. Surg Neurol 3:191–193, 1975
220. Matson DD, Woodhall B: Intracranial and cervical trap ligation of the carotid artery complicated by blindness of the homolateral eye. J Neurosurg 5:567–571, 1948
221. McConnell AA: Subchiasmal aneurysmal treated by implantation of muscle. Zbl Neurochir 2:269–274, 1937
222. McFadden JT: Chocked-clip aneurysmorrhaphy. Surg Gynecol Obstet 132:898, 1971
223. McKenzie KG: Discussion of intracranial aneurysm: a surgical problem. Zbl Neurochir 3:352, 1938
224. Miyazaki M, Ishikawa S, Hibino H, et al.: [Electric thrombosis of the experimental aneurysm. Effect of alteration in intra-aneurysmal hemodynamics on thrombosis.] Neurol Surg (Tokyo) 3:655–662, 1975
225. Moolten SE: Cerebral aneurysm as a cause of hemiplegia and massive cerebral hemorrhage. J Mt Sinai Hosp 12:516–522, 1945
226. Morello G: Remarks on the direct attack on intracranial aneurysms. Prog Brain Res 30: 347–349, 1968
227. Morley TP, Barr HWK: Giant intracranial aneurysms: diagnosis, course, and management. Clin Neurosurg 16:73–93, 1969
228. Mount LA: Treatment of spontaneous subarachnoid hemorrhage. JAMA 146:693–698, 1951
229. Mount LA, Taveras JM: Ligation of basilar artery in treatment of an aneurysm at the basilar-artery bifurcation. J Neurosurg 19:167–170, 1962
230. Mullan S: Experiences with surgical thrombosis of intracranial berry aneurysms and carotid cavernous fistulas. J Neurosurg 41:657–670, 1974
231. Mullan S: New techniques in neurosurgery. Postgrad Med 37:636–641, 1965
232. Mullan S: Stereotactic thrombosis of intracranial aneurysms. Confin Neurol 31:94, 1969
233. Mullan S, Beckman F, Vailati G, et al.: An experimental approach to the problem of cerebral aneurysm. J Neurosurg 21:838–845, 1964
234. Mullan S, Dobben G, Vailati G, et al.: Copper electric thrombosis of intracranial aneurysms. Excerpta Med ICS No. 110:655–661, 1966
235. Mullan S, Raimondi AJ, Dobben G, et al.: Electrically induced thrombosis in intracranial aneurysms. J Neurosurg 22:539–547, 1965
236. Mullan S, Reyes C, Dawley J, et al.: Stereotactic copper electric thrombosis of intracranial aneurysms. Prog Neurol Surg 3:193–211, 1969
237. Nakahara A, Asakura T, Kawabatake H, et al.: [A giant aneurysm of the internal carotid artery treated by indirect surgery. With a special reference to the anatomical relationship between the cavernous sinus and the internal carotid artery.] Neurol Surg (Tokyo) 3:783–789, 1975
238. Norlén G: Aneurysm of the anterior communicating artery. Prog Brain Res 30:295–302, 1968
239. Norlén G: The pathology, diagnosis and treatment of intracranial saccular aneurysms. Proc R Soc Med 45:291–302, 1952
240. Norlén G, Barnum AS: Surgical treatment of aneurysms of the anterior communicating artery. J Neurosurg 10:634–650, 1953
241. Norlén G, Olivecrona H: The treatment of aneurysms of the circle of Willis. J Neurosurg 10:404–415, 1953
242. Nornes H, Wikeby P: Cerebral arterial blood flow and aneurysm surgery. Part 1. Local arterial flow dynamics. J Neurosurg 47:810–818, 1977
243. Nornes H, Wikeby P: Results of microsurgical management of intracranial aneurysms. J Neurosurg 51:608–614, 1979
244. Nukui H, Aiba T: [Clinical features in cases with the ruptured aneurysm of the distal anterior cerebral artery.] Neurol Med Chir (Tokyo) 18:39–47, 1978
245. Nyström S, Snellman A, Mäkelä T: Sur le traitement des anévrysmes de la "communicante anterieure." A propos d'une série de cent quarante-sept cas opérés. Neurochirurgie 8:414–422, 1962
246. Ohta T, Nishimura S, Kikuchi H, et al.: Closure of carotid-cavernous fistula with polyurethane foam embolus. Technical note. J Neurosurg 38:107–112, 1973
247. Okawara S: [Ligation of the proximal anterior cerebral artery for anterior communicating aneurysm.] Brain Nerve (Tokyo) 20:1253–1258, 1968
248. Overgaard J, Riishede J: Multiple cerebral saccular aneurysms. Acta Neurol Scand 41:363–371, 1965
249. Packard M, Zabriskie EG: Basal cerebral hemorrhages. JAMA 85:1633–1637, 1925
250. Paillas JE, Bonnal J: Anévrysmes artériels. In Patel J, Leger L (eds.): Nouveau Traité de Technique Chirurgicale, Vol 6. Paris, Masson & Cie, 1975, pp. 237–277
250a. Parkinson D: "Airgun retraction" for major bifurcation saccular aneurysms. Technical note. J Neurosurg 54:844, 1981
251. Parkinson D: Carotid cavernous fistula: direct repair with preservation of the carotid artery. Technical note. J Neurosurg 38:99–106, 1973
252. Parkinson D: Neurosurgical aspects of cavern-

ous sinus lesions. Presented at the American Association of Neurological Surgeons, New Orleans, 26 April 1978
253. Patterson RH Jr, Ray BS: Profound hypothermia for intracranial surgery: laboratory and clinical experience with extracorporeal circulation by peripheral cannulation. Ann Surg 156:377–393, 1962
254. Paul RL, Arnold JG Jr: Operative factors influencing mortality in intracranial aneurysm surgery: analysis of 186 consecutive cases. J Neurosurg 32:289–294, 1970
255. Paulson G, Nashold BS Jr, Margolis G: Aneurysms of the vertebral artery. Report of 5 cases. Neurology 9:590–598, 1959
256. Peerless SJ: The surgical approach to middle cerebral and posterior communicating aneurysms. Clin Neurosurg 21:151–165, 1974
257. Peet MM, Isberg EM, Bassett RC: Hypertension complicated spontaneous subarachnoid hemorrhage. Am J Surg 78:912–917, 1949
258. Perria L, Rivano C, Rossi GF, et al.: Aneurysms of the bifurcation of the internal carotid artery. Acta Neurochir (Wien) 19:51–68, 1968
259. Perria L, Viale GL, Rivano C: Anévrysmes de la jonction carotide interne—choroidienne antérieure. Acta Neurochir (Wien) 21:153–166, 1969
260. Pertuiset B: Les anévrysmes sacculaires de la carotide interne supra-clinoidienne. Étude anatomo-clinique et thérapeutique d'après 16 cas. Neurochirurgie 5:183–206, 1959
261. Pertuiset B, Houtteville J-P, van Effenterre R, et al.: Chirurgie des anévrysmes artériels sus-tentoriels. Réduction par coagulation bipolaire sous hypotension profonde et exclusion par clip autobloquant: (52 cas opérés sous microscope). Nouv Presse Med 3:1649–1652, 1974
262. Pertuiset B, van Effenterre R, Caruel N, et al.: Les résultats de l'abord direct des anévrysmes intra-crâniens sus-tentoriels en fonction de l'hypotension contrôlée, de la coagulation bipolaire et de la magnification optique. Rev Neurol (Paris) 129:57–59, 1973
263. Pertuiset B, van Effenterre R, Goutorbe J, et al.: Management of aneurysmal rupture during surgery, using bipolar coagulation, deep hypotension, and the operating microscope. Acta Neurochir (Wien) 30:195–205, 1974
264. Petit-Dutaillis D, Pittman HW: Aneurysms of the middle cerebral artery. Report of seven operative cases; review of literature; evaluation of surgical therapy. J Neurosurg 12:1–12, 1955
265. Pia HW: Microsurgical treatment of cerebral aneurysms. Neurosurg Rev 1:15–24, 1978
266. Picard L, Lepoire J, Montaut J, et al.: Endarterial occlusion of carotid-cavernous sinus fistulas using a balloon tipped catheter. Neuroradiology 8:5–11, 1974
267. Pool JL: The development of modern intracranial aneurysm surgery. Neurosurgery 1:233–237, 1977
268. Pool JL: Timing and techniques in the intracranial surgery of ruptured aneurysms of the anterior communicating artery. J Neurosurg 19:378–388, 1962
269. Pool JL, Potts DG: Aneurysms and Arteriovenous Anomalies of the Brain. Diagnosis and Treatment. New York, Harper & Row, 1965
270. Poppen JL: An Atlas of Neurosurgical Techniques. Philadelphia, Saunders, 1960, pp 156–181
271. Poppen JL: Discussion. Clin Neurosurg 11:183–219, 1964
272. Poppen JL: Experiences with ligation of the left anterior cerebral artery. Zbl Neurochir 3:355, 1938
273. Poppen JL: Specific treatment of intracranial aneurysms. Experience with 143 surgically treated patients. J Neurosurg 8:75–102, 1951
274. Poppen JL: Vascular surgery of the posterior fossa. Clin Neurosurg 6:198–209, 1959
275. Poppen JL, Fager CA: Intracranial aneurysms. Results of surgical treatment. J Neurosurg 17:283–296, 1960
276. Prolo DJ, Burres KP, Hanbery JW: Balloon occlusion of carotid-cavernous fistula: introduction of a new catheter. Surg Neurol 7:209–214, 1977
277. Prolo DJ, Hanbery JW: Intraluminal occlusion of a carotid-cavernous sinus fistula with a balloon catheter. Technical note. J Neurosurg 35:237–242, 1971
278. Rana RS: Surgical management of internal carotid aneurysms. Results in 21 operated cases. Neurol India 13:59–61, 1965
279. Rand RW: Microneurosurgery, 2nd ed. St Louis, Mosby, 1978, pp. 43–44, 311–324
280. Rand RW, Mosso JA: Treatment of cerebral aneurysms by stereotaxic ferromagnetic silicone thrombosis. Case report. Bull Los Angeles Neurol Soc 38:21–23, 1973
281. Reichman OH: Complications of cerebral revascularization. Clin Neurosurg 23:318–335, 1976
282. Rhoton AL, Jackson FE, Gleave J, et al.: Congenital and traumatic intracranial aneurysms. Clin Symp 29:1–40, 1977
283. Rizzoli HV, Hayes GJ: Congenital berry aneurysm of the posterior fossa. Case report with successful operative excision. J Neurosurg 10:550–551, 1953
284. Robertson EG: Intracranial aneurysms, with special reference to surgical treatment. Aust NZ J Surg 8:132–144, 1938
285. Rosenbaum TJ, Sundt TM Jr: Interrelationship

of aneurysm clips and vascular tissue. J Neurosurg 48:929–934, 1978
286. Rosomoff HL: Stereomagnetic occlusion of intracranial aneurysm: principle and application. Trans Am Neurol Assoc 91:330–331, 1966
287. Rothenberg SF, Penka EJ, Conway LW: Angiotactic surgery. Preliminary studies. J Neurosurg 19:877–883, 1962
288. Rougerie J, Guilmet D, Bamberger-Bozo C: Anévrysme carotido-caverneux. A propos d'une orientation thérapeutique nouvelle. Neurochirurgie 19:649–654, 1973
289. Rousseaux R, Lepoire J: Anévrismes vestigiaux du segment supraclinoidien de la carotide. Neurochirurgie 2:254–270, 1956
290. Rowbotham GF, Hay RK: Leaking aneurysms of the brain. Newcastle Med J 24:319–331, 1955
291. Rowe SN, Grunnagle JF, Susen AF, et al.: Results of direct attack on intracranial aneurysm. J Neurosurg 12:475–486, 1955
292. Rozario RA, Stein BM: Ligation of the basilar artery as the definitive treatment for a giant aneurysm of the basilar artery apex: case report. Neurosurgery 6:87–91, 1980
293. Russel CK: Spontaneous subarachnoid haemorrhage following rupture of congenital aneurysm of the anterior communicating artery of the circle of Willis. Report of a case in which the aneurysm was excised. Trans Am Neurol Assoc 65:130–133, 1939
294. Sakaki S, Zenke M, Shishido T, et al.: [A case of ruptured vertebral aneurysm in association with bilateral abducens palsy and sleep induced dyspnea.] No Shinkei Geka 6:269–273, 1978
295. Sakaki T, Kikuchi H, Furuse S, et al.: [The usefulness of STA-MCA anastomosis in trapping vascular disorder.] Neurol Surg (Tokyo) 5:253–259, 1977
296. Samotokin BA, Hilko VA: [Aneurysms and Arteriovenous Fistulas of the Brain.] Lenigrad, Meditsina, 1973
297. Sano K: [Surgery of intracranial aneurysm.] Brain Nerve (Tokyo) 23:1252–1264, 1971
298. Santini J-J, Gouazé A: L'endo-anévrysmorraphe. A propos de 2 cas d'anévrysme sylvien géant. Rev Otoneuroophtalmol 47:9–13, 1975
299. Sashin D, Goldman RL, Zanetti P, et al.: Electronic radiography in stereotaxic thrombosis of intracranial aneurysms and catheter embolization of cerebral arteriovenous malformations. Radiology 105:359–363, 1972
300. Sashin D, Hoy RJ: Some applications of electronic radiography. Australas Radiol 18:215–222, 1974
301. Sawyer PN, Pate JW: Bio-electric phenomena as an etiologic factor in intravascular thrombosis. Am J Physiol 175:103–107, 1953
302. Schaeffer HR: Aneurysms of the posterior cerebral artery. Med J Aust 1:632–633, 1964
303. Schlosshauer B, Vosteen K-H: Zur Diagnostik und Therapie der Carotisblutung nach Keilbeinhöhlenfrakturen. Arch Ohr Nas Kehlheilk 165:270–277, 1954
304. Scott M: Ligation of an anterior cerebral artery for aneurysms of the anterior communicating artery complex. J Neurosurg 38:481–487, 1973
305. Scott M, Skwarok E: The treatment of cerebral aneurysms by ligation of the common carotid artery. Surg Gynecol Obstet 113:54–61, 1961
306. Seltzer J, Hurteau EF: Bilateral symmetrical aneurysms of the internal carotid artery within the cavernous sinus. Case report. J Neurosurg 14:448–451, 1957
307. Sencer W: A study of subarachnoid hemorrhage and intracranial aneurysm. J Mount Sinai Hosp (NY) 30:302–323, 1963
308. Serbinenko FA: Balloon catheterization and occlusion of major cerebral vessels. J Neurosurg 41:125–145, 1974
309. Serbinenko FA: [Balloon occlusion of saccular aneurysms of the cerebral arteries.] Vopr Neirokhir :8–15, July–Aug, 1974
310. Sheptak PE, Zanetti PH, Susen AF: The treatment of intracranial aneurysms by injection with a tissue adhesive. Neurosurgery 1:25–29, 1977
311. Shintani A, Zervas NT: Consequence of ligation of the vertebral artery. J Neurosurg 36:447–450, 1972
312. Sjöqvist O: Thread ligature of intracranial saccular aneurysms. In Proceedings of the 5th Congress of Neurology, Lisbon, Vol 3, 1953, pp. 108–115
313. Skultety FM, Nishioka H: The results of intracranial surgery in the treatment of aneurysms. In Sahs AL, Perret GE, Locksley HB, et al. (eds.): Intracranial Aneurysms and Subarachnoid Hemorrhage. A Cooperative Study. Philadelphia, Lippincott, 1969, pp. 173–194
313a. Skultety FM, Nishioka H: Report on the cooperative study of intracranial aneurysms and subarachnoid hemorrhage. Section VIII, Part 2. The results of intracranial surgery in the treatment of aneurysms. J Neurosurg 25:683–704, 1966
314. Smith B: Cerebral pathology in subarachnoid haemorrhage. J Neurol Neurosurg Psychiatry 26:535–539, 1963
315. Smith RW, Alksne JF: Stereotoxic thrombosis of inaccessible intracranial aneurysms. J Neurosurg 47:833–839, 1977
316. Snyckers FD, Drake CG: Aneurysms of the distal anterior cerebral artery. A report on 24 verified cases. S Afr Med J 47:1787–1791, 1973

317. Sosman MC, Vogt EC: Aneurysms of the internal carotid artery and the circle of Willis, from a roentgenological viewpoint. Am J Roentgenol 15:122–134, 1926
318. Spetzler RF, Owen MP: Extracranial-intracranial arterial bypass to a single branch of the middle cerebral artery in the management of a traumatic aneurysm. Neurosurgery 4:334–337, 1979
319. Stallings JO, McCabe BF: Congenital middle ear aneurysm of internal carotid. Arch Otolaryngol 90:65–69, 1969
320. Steelman HF, Hayes GJ, Rizzoli HV: Surgical treatment of saccular intracranial aneurysms. J Neurosurg 10:564–576, 1953
321. Steiner L, Leksell L, Forster DMC, et al.: Stereotactic radiosurgery in intracranial arterio-venous malformations. Acta Neurochir [Suppl] 21:195–209, 1974
322. Sugar O: Discussion. Arch Neurol Psychiatry 68:843–844, 1952
323. Sundt TM Jr, Piepgras DG: Surgical approach to giant intracranial aneurysms. Operative experience with 80 cases. J Neurosurg 51:731–742, 1979
324. Sundt TM Jr, Sickert RG, Piepgras DG, et al.: Bypass surgery of the vascular disease of the carotid system. Mayo Clinic Proc 51:677–692, 1976
325. Suzuki J, Harada N: [Surgery of intra-and/or supra-sellar aneurysms associated with defects of the visual field.] Brain Nerve (Tokyo) 20:121–130, 1968
326. Suzuki J, Iwabuchi T, Takaku A, et al.: [Management of intracranial aneurysms. Especially direct attack of 103 cases.] Brain Nerve (Tokyo) 19:815–824, 1967
327. Suzuki J, Kaneko H, Homma M: A magnetic suture guide for ligation of intracranial aneurysms. J Neurosurg 25:319–320, 1966
328. Swain RD: The surgical treatment of certain intracranial arterial aneurysms. Surg Clin North Am 28:396–404, 1948
329. Symonds CP: Contributions to the clinical study of intracranial aneurysms. Guys Hosp Rep (Lond) 72:139–158, 1923
330. Taeffner JH: Intracranial aneurysms involving carotid artery and its branches. Arch Neurol Psychiatry 43:184–187, 1940
331. Taki W, Handa H, Yamagata S, et al.: Balloon embolization of a giant aneurysm using a newly developed catheter. Surg Neurol 12:363–365, 1979
332. Taki W, Handa H, Yamagata S, et al.: Embolization and superselective angiography by means of balloon catheters. Surg Neurol 12:7–14, 1979
333. Tangchai P, Khaoborisut V: Agenesis of internal carotid artery associated with aneurysm of contralateral middle cerebral artery. Neurology 20:809–812, 1970
334. Taren JA: Transarterial treatment of cranial arteriovenous malformations. In Fusek I, Kunc Z (eds.): Proceedings of the Fourth European Congress of Neurosurgery. Present Limits of Neurosurgery. Prague, Avicenum, Czechoslovak Medical Press, 1972, pp. 309–312
335. Taren JA, Gabrielsen TO: Radio-frequency thrombosis of vascular malformations with a transvascular magnetic catheter. Science 168: 138–141, 1970
336. Taylor AR, Kak VK: Cerebral circulation times in subarachnoid haemorrhage. Prog Brain Res 30:289–294, 1968
337. Thiry S, Hotermans JM, Brand H, et al.: Le traitement chirurgical des principaux anévrysmes arteriels intracrâniens supratentoriels. Acta Chir Belg 63:308–330, 1964
338. Tindall GT: The treatment of anterior communicating aneurysms by proximal anterior cerebral artery ligation. Clin Neurosurg 21:134–150, 1974
339. Tindall GT, Kapp J, Odom GL, et al.: A combined technique for treating certain aneurysms of the anterior communicating artery. J Neurosurg 33:41–47, 1970
340. Tönnis W: Zur Behandlung der intrakranieller Aneurysmen. Langenbecks Arch Klin Chir 189:474–476, 1937
341. Turner OA: Intracranial aneurysm. Report of a case with 17-year survival after treatment by carotid ligation and obliteration by packing. Ohio Med J 64:1030–1032, 1968
342. Tytus JS, Haven H: Present day concepts in the management of intracranial aneurysms. Rev Surg 20:230–240, 1963
343. Uihlein A, Hughes RA: The surgical treatment of intracranial vestigial aneurysms. Surg Clin North Am 35:1071–1083, 1955
344. Uihlein A, Thomas RL, Cleary J: Aneurysms of the anterior communicating artery complex. Proc Mayo Clin 42:73–87, 1967
345. Verbiest H: Arterio-venous malformations. In Logue V, Rob C, Smith R (eds.): Operative Surgery—14. Neurosurgery, 2nd ed. Philadelphia, Lippincott, 1971, pp. 130–141
346. Viale GL, Pau A: Carotid-choroidal aneurysms: remarks on surgical treatment and outcome. Surg Neurol 11:141–145, 1979
347. Walder HAD: Applications of cryosurgery. An experimental and clinical study of its effects on the blood vessels. J Cryosurg 1:306–313, 1968
348. Weibel J, Fields WS, Campos RJ: Aneurysms of the posterior cervicocranial circulation: clinical and angiographic considerations. J Neurosurg 26:223–234, 1967

349. Weickmann F, Buchholz W: Aneurysma-Ligatur durch Plombierung statt Knüpfung des Fadens. Zbl Neurochir 27:155–158, 1966
350. Wennerstrand JR, Galera R, Del Corral JF: An experimental method for the intraluminal occlusion of arterial aneurysms. Technical note. Eur Surg Res 1:309–313, 1969
351. Werner SC, Blakemore AH, King BG: Aneurysm of internal carotid artery within the skull. Wiring and electrothermic coagulation. JAMA 116:578–582, 1941
352. Whalley N: Ruptured congenital aneurysm of anterior cerebral artery. J Neurol Neurosurg Psychiatry 12:322–324, 1949
353. White R, Yashon D, Olbin M: [The treatment of cerebral aneurysms employing temporary parent vessel isolation.] Vopr Neurokhir, Jan–Feb 1975, pp. 3–7
354. Wholey MH, Kessler L, Boehnke M: A percutaneous balloon catheter technique for the treatment of intracranial aneurysms. Acta Radiol [Diagn] (Stockh) 13:286–292, 1972
355. Wholey MH, Stockdale R, Hung TK: A percutaneous balloon catheter for the immediate control of hemorrhage. Radiology 95:65–71, 1970
356. Wilson CB, Christensen FK, Subrahmanian MV: Intracranial aneurysms at the pericallosol artery bifurcation. Am Surg 31:386–393, 1965
357. Woodhall B, Lowenbach H: Congenital cerebral aneurysms lateralized by electroencephalography. South Med J 36:580–587, 1943
358. Woodhall B, Odom GL, Bloor BM, et al.: Direct measurement of intravascular pressure in components of the circle of Willis. A contribution to the surgery of congenital cerebral aneurysms and vascular anomalies of the brain. Ann Surg 135:911–921, 1952
359. Yaşargil MG: Microsurgery Applied to Neurosurgery. Stuttgart, Georg Thieme Verlag, 1969, pp. 119–143
360. Yaşargil MG, Antic J, Laciga R, et al.: Microsurgical pterional approach to aneurysms of the basilar bifurcation. Surg Neurol 6:83–91, 1976
361. Yaşargil MG, Boehm WB, Ho REM: Microsurgical treatment of cerebral aneurysms at the bifurcation of the internal carotid artery. Acta Neurochir (Wien) 41:61–72, 197
362. Yaşargil MG, Fox JL: The microsurgical approach to intracranial aneurysms. Surg Neurol 3:7–14, 1975
363. Yaşargil MG, Fox JL, Ray MW: The operative approach to aneurysms of the anterior communicating artery. In Krayenbühl H (ed.): Advances and Technical Standards in Neurosurgery, Vol 2. New York, Springer-Verlag, 1975, pp. 113–170
364. Yaşargil MG, Gasser JC, Hodosh RM, et al.: Carotid-ophthalmic aneurysms: direct microsurgical approach. Surg Neurol 8:155–165, 1977
365. Yaşargil MG, Smith RD: Surgery on the carotid system in the treatment of hemorrhagic stroke. Adv Neurol 16:181–209, 1977
366. Yodh SB, Pierce NT, Weggel RJ, et al.: A new system for "intravascular navigation." Med Biol Eng 6:143–147, 1968
367. Zanetti PH, Sherman FE: Experimental evaluation of a tissue adhesive as an agent for the treatment of aneurysms and arteriovenous anomalies. Neurosurgery 36:72–79, 1972

32

Craniotomy for Aneurysm

VIII. Operative Complications and Postoperative Care

A major aspect of postoperative care following craniotomy for aneurysm is the monitoring, avoidance, and treatment of complications. The latter include complications of: (a) any surgical procedure under anesthesia; (b) craniotomy in general; and (c) direct attack on intracranial aneurysms. The morbidity and mortality rates are related to many factors including: (a) the patient's grade at surgery; (b) the time elapsed since SAH; (c) the complexity and location of the aneurysm; (d) the age and medical condition of the patient; and (e) the experience and sophistication of the surgeon and his team. The reader is referred to Chapter 8 for a discussion of the secondary complications of SAH and Chapter 21 for a discussion on prognosis and timing.

Aneurysm Rupture at Surgery

In their review of the literature regarding complications of aneurysm surgery, Horwitz and Rizzoli (82) found a direct correlation between the rate of postoperative complications and the occurrence of intraoperative rupture of the aneurysm. In 1952 Hamby opined (74): "The greatest surgical hazard seems to lie in rupture of the aneurysm during its exposure. This often leads to the clipping of vessels that have not been properly identified." Hamby (74) concluded that the surgeon "was much in the position of the hunter arousing a tiger when stalking a deer." The phenomenon of aneurysm rupture at some point during the surgical procedure is well known and attested to by a multitude of surgeons (2, 6, 10, 15, 16, 18, 26, 27, 30, 31, 36–41, 44, 48, 52, 53, 55, 57, 58, 72, 74, 76–81, 84, 92, 95, 97, 113, 116, 118, 123, 126, 129–131, 133, 136, 140, 150, 151, 153, 155, 157–159, 163–166, 168–170, 172, 173, 175, 177, 178).

The incidence of such intraoperative rupture approached 50% before the days of routine use of the operating microscope, hypotensive anesthesia, and improved clips (15,26,37,74, 77,126). The variability in the present-day incidence of intraoperative rupture may relate to several factors, including the timing of surgery and the use of hypotension. Some reports have shown a reduced incidence of intraoperative rupture (41,72,80,95,118,175,178), whereas others have indicated a continued high incidence of rupture (27,58,92,129,130).

There are several critical periods during surgery when intraoperative rupture may occur (62,95,113,122): (a) Any elevation of BP or rapid changes in ICP during induction of anesthesia may change the differential transmural pressure of the aneurysm wall sufficient to rupture the aneurysm. (b) During skull fixation with pinions through the scalp, the patient must be well anesthetized so that his BP does not suddenly rise. (c) When the bone flap is turned, there may be a sudden reduction in ICP. This, combined with the vibrations (especially if the aneurysm is adherent to the skull base) due to the drilling, sawing, and cracking, may precipitate rupture. Hence before this point it may be wise to start lowering the BP. (d) Upon opening the dura the tamponading ICP is reduced to near-atmospheric pressure. (e) Upon release of a hematoma surrounding the aneurysm, the aneurysm is no longer tamponaded and may bleed. (f) The aneurysm may be disturbed and rupture during elevation of a frontal or temporal lobe or the cerebellum. (g) Gentle technique and controlled BP are advisable during dissection of the aneurysm, for this is the point at which most such ruptures occur. (h) Rupture may occur during the use of methods to reduce the diameter of the neck of the aneurysm (see Chapter 31). (i) During clipping of the aneurysm a weak spot in the neck–artery junction may give way (especially if it is atherosclerotic), the clip may not be fully across the aneurysm neck, the clip may be too weak or defective, the neck may be stretched between a rigid artery and an unyielding tentorium or brain tissue, or the surgeon's hand may be too tremorous. (j) The clip applier may fail to be withdrawn smoothly during its removal. (k) The clip may slip off the aneurysm during closure of the wound.

When an aneurysm ruptures at surgery before the dura is opened, the surgeon must use his own judgment regarding continuation of the operation. It has been our practice (J.L.F.) to reduce the BP rapidly, open the dura, and (using past experience for direction) directly attack the aneurysm. On the basis of our clinical experience (two cases), an acute rupture in this circumstance causes acute vasospasm of the circle of Willis and sudden loss of vascular autoregulation with elevation in ICP due to acute small-vessel vasodilation (similar to the events of acute head injury as seen with contrast enhancement on CT scanning). An acutely developing hematoma at the site of the aneurysm will contribute to the rise in ICP. We emphasize the lowering of BP here because it assists in acutely combating elevated ICP from loss of autoregulation and reduces the aneurysm wall transmural pressure.

When the aneurysm ruptures during its exposure or dissection, the operating microscope is of great assistance in providing light and visualization so that the dissection can continue while the suction tube clears the field of blood. This procedure is much more easily done if the patient is under controlled hypotension. More often than not, if the aneurysm is already exposed before rupture, the surgeon will see the start of the leak before it gets out of control. Pressure of the suction apparatus against a cottonoid on the aneurysm allows effective tamponading while the surgeon isolates the neck for clipping.

A number of authors have discussed techniques of controlling intraoperative aneurysm rupture (36,39,74,92,95,100,135,157,174). Producing local vascular hypotension by the use of a temporary clip on the proximal artery may be of significant assistance. (See Chapter 25, pp. 671–672, regarding control of circulation.) Some have advised compressing (or temporarily ligating if already exposed) the ipsilateral cervical carotid artery. However, external compression of the cervical ICA also causes compression of the jugular vein, and the net result may be a negative one. If a temporary clip (or trapping procedure) is applied to the parent vessel for a prolonged period, *elevation* of the blood pressure should be considered to permit good collateral cerebral perfusion. Bipolar forceps can be used to continue the dissection, close the neck of the aneurysm, and arrest the bleeding by closure and electrocoagulation. Readjustment of the clip or a second clip may be effective. Of paramount importance is the calm and deliberate attitude of the surgeon. In these difficult circumstances the rest of the team will function better if the surgeon sets a good example in his approach.

In earlier days surgeons often packed the bleeding aneurysm with muscle. Kempe (91) illustrated wrapping the aneurysm in a fascial sling (Fig. 28.1), and Sundt and Nofzinger (157) used an encircling clip-graft (Fig. 27.32). Carton et al. (36) used a dural graft held by tissue adhesive. Microsurgical suture repair of the parent artery may be needed (174).

Intraoperative rupture of an intracranial aneurysm, especially a BAA, increases the postoperative morbidity and mortality (38–40, 82,126,131). Such a rupture not only makes the surgery more difficult and risks damage to vital structures, it also causes a reversal of the perfusion gradient, with blood destined for brain tissue instead being drained by suction. The result may be temporary or permanent ischemic changes in brain tissue.

Postoperative Complications

There are a few good reviews on the complications following craniotomy for a direct attack on an aneurysm (5,39,82,162,176). The following summarizes many of the postoperative problems seen by neurosurgeons.

Recurrent Subarachnoid Hemorrhage

In 1965 Lougheed et al. (102) stated that the second most common cause of postoperative death was recurrent bleeding from inadequate aneurysm clipping (brain infarction being the most common cause). Bohm and Hugosson (21) reported a 4% incidence of death from rebleed: two from unrecognized aneurysms and three from aneurysms to which a synthetic coat had been applied. In their review of the literature Horwitz and Rizzoli (82) noted cases of rebleeding from the same or another aneurysm. This observation stresses the need for complete cerebral angiography prior to surgery.

Inadequate Clipping

Recurrent hemorrhage, routine postoperative angiography, repeat surgical exposure, and/or autopsy examinations have documented many incidences of either inadequate clipping where part of the aneurysm remains at risk or actual slippage of the clip from the aneurysm (4,8, 18,20,21,23,24,28,42,48,51,54,68,71,82,102,109, 118,124,142,143,156). See Chapter 27 for a further discussion of clip slippage and fracture.

Drake and Allcock (51) found a 13% incidence of inadequate clip placement in 329 aneurysm patients who underwent postoperative angiography. Paterson (124) reported an 8% incidence in 77 cases of ICAA. Sato et al. (142,143) claimed a 3% incidence in 369 cases. Steven (156) reported an 18% incidence (especially for ACoAA cases) in 250 cases studied. Bohm and Hugosson (20) had a 22% incidence where the aneurysm could not be adequately clipped at surgery, but this statistic is not comparable to those cited above: These authors (20) considered aneurysms which they *knew* at surgery could not be clipped, whereas the others included only aneurysms that were clipped but which proved at angiography that they were not adequately occluded.

Cerebral Infarction

Lougheed et al. (102) in 1965 considered cerebral infarction to be the most common cause of death after intracranial surgery for aneurysm. Adams et al. (1) reported two cases of cerebral thrombosis remote from the surgical site. Evidence for suture ligature or clips stenosing or occluding a parent artery on postoperative angiography has been presented (48, 53,68,82,146,156). Stevens (156) found angiographic evidence of occlusion by clip in 24% of 250 cases, but two-thirds of these were deliberate. Of these, 57% had postoperative clinical deterioration, compared to 37% who had no obvious vessel occlusion.

There are a number of other causes of cerebral infarction after this type of surgery (82), including vasospasm, thrombosis, embolic phenomena from the surgical zone, encroaching atherosclerotic plaques, blood hypercoagulability, excess brain retraction, prolonged temporary clip on a vessel, occlusion of venous drainage, trapping procedures, local inflammation, and vascular hypotension.

Robinson and Roberts (141) presented theoretical evidence that slight distortion of the parent vessel wall by an aneurysm clip may redirect the flow of blood sufficient to cause some neurologic symptoms. This is called the Coanda effect, whereby the jet flow of fluids caused by vessel distortion pulls blood into the direction of the lower pressure jet flow and away from a branch vessel.

Intracranial Pressure Changes

Patricolo (125) reported two patients suffering from the effects of low CSF pressure after aneurysm surgery, but this is quite unusual. The many causes of increased ICP, including cerebral edema, need not be repeated here (see Chapter 8), but they are well known to neurosurgeons (82,161).

Vasospasm

Worsening of preoperative vasospasm or development of new vasospasm after craniotomy for aneurysm is well known. Stevens (156) found that the spasm was made worse in 60% of patients who had postoperative angiography within 2 weeks of surgery. Hunt and Miller (83) saw vasospasm in nearly every case of postoperative angiography following aneurysm surgery. Ferguson et al. (60) demonstrated that a reduction in cerebral blood flow following surgery portended a poor result. See Chapters 9 and 10 for other aspects of vasospasm.

Hematoma

As with any craniotomy procedure, intracerebral, subdural, or extradural hematoma may evolve after clipping of an aneurysm (5,68, 82,95,176).

Infection

Abscess, meningitis, or local wound infection is now a rare complication of intracranial aneurysm surgery (5,39,176). This is true in spite of the fact that a foreign body (clip, cotton fibers, synthetic coating, etc.) is nearly always left at the aneurysm site.

Hydrocephalus

Hydrocephalus, usually subacute or chronic, is a well-known phenomenon after aneurysm surgery (5,39,68,95,118,176). However, it is likely that the original SAH also plays a significant role as an etiologic factor. Possibly the surgery hastens the evolution of the hydrocephalus. It appears that 5–10% of the patients develop significant hydrocephalus at some time following their surgery (95,118). See Chapter 8 for other aspects of hydrocephalus.

Epilepsy

Several cases of EEG abnormalities and epilepsy developing after craniotomy for aneurysm have been reported (3,14,33–35,70, 95,118,176). The reported incidence varied between 5% and 40%; the highest incidence was after surgery on MCAA. Again, the original hemorrhage also may play a role, but excess brain retraction pressure, cerebral incisions and excisions, and ischemia are also significant causes of brain injury and scarring and consequent epilepsy. See Chapter 8 for other aspects of epilepsy.

Fluid, Electrolyte, and Pituitary Disturbances

Kuwayama and colleagues (96) found a close correlation between the preoperative grade of the ACoAA patient and the incidence of defective postoperative hypophyseal endocrine function. Landolt and co-workers (98) analyzed 126 operated cases. One ACoAA patient developed inappropriate secretion of antidiuretic hormone (ISADH), five (four were ACoAA cases) had diabetes insipidus, and two ACoAA patients had disturbance of the hypothalamic thirst center (no thirst and consequent elevation of the serum sodium concentration). Forty-two patients developed mild to severe low serum sodium concentrations. We wonder if these were additional cases of ISADH. Takaku et al. (162) discovered only a 2% incidence of fluid and electrolyte imbalance, and most of these were in ACoAA patients. The proximity of the ACoAA to the hypothalmus and its perforators cannot escape notice here (Fig. 32.1).

Psychiatric Problems

A number of authors demonstrated psychiatric disturbances (transient and permanent) in patients who had undergone craniotomy for aneurysm (especially ACoAA) (5,19,29,93,98,99, 101,107,112,115,119–121,146,162,176). Many of these patients exhibited the Korsakoff syndrome (hallucinations, confusion, amnesia, and confabulation). Loss of initiative, personality changes, emotional lability, and memory and intellectual deficits were seen. In many instances, especially since the advent of the operating microscope, these deficits were transient. Improvement could be seen as long as 2 years after surgery, especially in the sphere of intellectual function.

As mentioned, most reported cases of the frontal lobe syndrome and Korsakoff's psychosis were ACoAA patients, and many of these had deficits prior to surgery (see Chapter 6). In 1966 Lindqvist and Norlén reported Korsakoff's syndrome in 17 of 33 cases operated for ACoAA (99). More recent evaluations have revealed a considerable reduction in the incidence of this complication (119–121,162).

Cranial Nerve Palsy

Depending on the location of the aneurysm, any of the cranial nerves may be injured (5, 39,46,47,49,50,73,82,106). The bifrontal approach to ACoAA or excess frontal lobe retraction or shrinkage may cause the olfactory tract or nerve to tear. The optic nerve is especially vulnerable during oaICAA surgery. The oculomotor nerve may be injured during nearby ICAA, PCoAA, P_1AA, or bBAA surgery as well as midbrain ischemia or temporal lobe herniation. The trochlear nerve is easily damaged during approaches to the upper basilar artery.

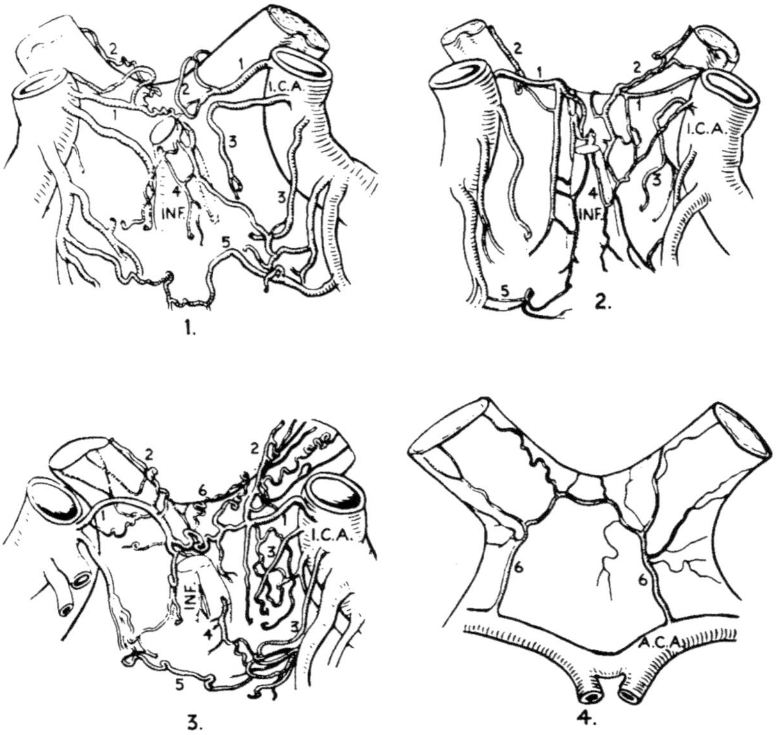

Fig. 32.1. **1,2,3** Variations in relationships of the arteries of the inferior chiasmal, infundibular, and hypothalamic areas. **4** Arterial network on the superior aspect of the optic chiasm. *I.C.A.*, Internal carotid artery. *A.C.A.*, Anterior communicating artery. *INF.*, Infundibulum of pituitary gland. *1–6*, Anterior thalamic, hypothalamic, and chiasmatic perforating arteries. From Dawson BH, ref. 45.

The lower cranial nerves of the brainstem are susceptible during surgical exposure of vertebrobasilar aneurysms. Of particular importance are the vagal and glossopharyngeal nerves, whose irritation or injury could precipitate serious cardiovascular (especially blood pressure or cardiac rhythm), respiratory (respiratory feedback and vocal cord control), and swallowing problems.

A common but comparatively minor nerve injury is that to the frontalis branch of the facial nerve, which is often stretched or incised while turning a frontolateral flap. These branches run between the galea and temporalis muscle anteriorly. If injured, function usually returns within 6 months.

Rhinorrhea and Otorrhea

A low frontal bone flap may enter the frontal sinuses, or a lateral suboccipital craniotomy may interrupt mastoid air cells (132,176). This may lead to signs of rhinorrhea or otorrhea after surgery and possible meningitis.

Gastrointestinal Hemorrhage

In an autopsy study Karch (90) noted that the incidence of gastrointestinal bleeding in patients dying of neurologic disorders was twice that of those dying from other causes. The bleeding usually was secondary to esophageal and/or duodenal ulceration. The occurrence of this complication after aneurysm surgery, though uncommon, is well known (5,39,89, 139,162,176). This seems particularly true of ACoAA cases (139). Takahu and colleagues (162) reported a 2% incidence of gastrointestinal bleeding among 1000 operated aneurysm cases. The role of the preexisting lesion (ruptured aneurysm) and prescribed corticosteroids is not clear.

Pulmonary Complications

The most serious pulmonary complication following aneurysm surgery is pulmonary embolism. As after any surgical procedure, this phenomenon can be lethal. The incidence of fatal pulmonary emboli in surgical patients has been reported to be 0.073–0.54% (149). Its occurrence after intracranial aneurysm surgery is documented (1,39,41,176). Using ^{125}I-fibrinogen and Doppler ultrasound tests, Joffe (85) and Valladares and Hankinson (167) discovered a 30–40% incidence of deep vein thrombosis in the legs of various neurosurgical patients, including those with aneurysm. The vast majority of these patients were asymptomatic.

Stein et al. (154) clearly demonstrated that the incidence of postoperative pulmonary complications rises in direct correlation with the presence of abnormal preoperative pulmonary function tests. For an excellent review of pulmonary function as related to neurosurgical patients the reader is referred to a publication by Frost in 1977 (65). See Chapter 8 for further details.

Cardiovascular Changes

Mauney et al. (108) found a close correlation between a history of preoperative abnormal ECG signs, the duration of intraoperative surgery and hypotension, and the presence of postoperative myocardial ischemia. Such patients are at particular risk for the stress of anesthesia and surgery, especially induced vascular hypotension.

The occurrence of postoperative hypotension may be related to excess fluid loss from osmotic agents or diuretics, blood loss at surgery, complicating postoperative cardiorespiratory problems such as myocardial infarction or pulmonary embolism, or overdosage with antihypertensive drugs. On the other hand, early acute elevations in BP can occur, especially if the patient is a known hypertensive and still has a high catecholamine level following the original SAH. The risk is great if the patient has one or more further aneurysms which have not been ligated.

Acute Fibrinolysis

Berger et al. (17) reported a case of acute fibrinolysis with diffuse bleeding during aneurysm surgery. The problem resolved with treatment by epsilon-aminocaproic acid (EACA) and fibrinogen administration. We (J.L.F.) treated a case of disseminated intravascular coagulopathy (DIC) following rupture of an ACoAA just as the temporal base of the bone flap was cracked. A massive right frontal hematoma was evacuated immediately and the aneurysm clipped. However, the patient developed DIC unresponsive to treatment and required two more frontal clot evacuations before he died.

Poikilothermia

Kahn (86) in 1958 described an interesting case of poikilothermia following ICA ligation and excision of a giant ICAA. He discussed the anatomic pathways (Fig. 32.2).

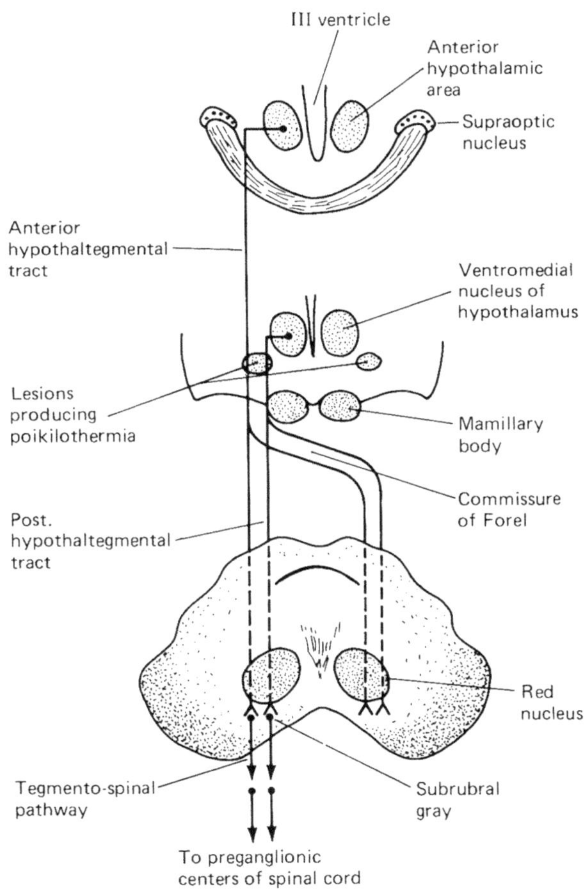

Fig. 32.2. Anatomic pathways showing the location of lesions that can produce disturbances of central temperature regulation. The anterior hypothalamic-tegmental tract from the heat-releasing center (stimulation causes skin vasodilation) is joined by the posterior hypothalamic-tegmental tract from the heat conservation center (stimulation causes skin vasoconstriction). From Kahn EA, ref. 86.

Postoperative Care

In 1965 Pool and Potts (134) kept patients at bedrest for 2 weeks after surgery. Now patients are activated much sooner, usually within a few days, although too early ambulation may compromise cerebral perfusion pressure in the presence of vasospasm or an unstable cardiovascular system. Respiratory care is mandatory, especially in patients with chronic lung disease. Details of such care can be obtained elsewhere (65,149). Carbon dioxide is one of the most potent agents to increase ICP; hence strict attention to airway measures is essential. We have found that if the patient is drowsy upon termination of anesthesia it is beneficial to leave the endotracheal tube in—even if the patient is awake. The patient's ventilation is assisted until the next day without any significant discomfort. Although hyperbaric oxygen benefited one patient with cerebral ischemia postoperatively (87), few centers have such facilities available.

In 1965 Bakay and Lee (13) made a cogent point: "Dehydration of the patient by withholding fluids or severely limiting fluid intake is pointless in the presence of cerebral edema. Such measures completely fail to have any effect on the edema of the brain while on the other hand they would have disastrous effects on the homeostasis of these already critically ill patients." There has been a tendency to restrict fluids in craniotomy patients, or at least to avoid high fluid intake (12,61,147,171). Mild fluid restriction does not disrupt body fluid homeostasis but does combat the effects of the commonly present mild inappropriate secretion of antidiuretic hormone (64). ISADH, by increasing body water content, also increases brain water content with consequent adverse effects on intracranial pressure.

One of the serious problems faced in aneurysm surgery is reduced cerebral perfusion secondary to vasospasm, clip encroachment, thrombosis, etc. Consequently, there now are those who advocate giving more than the usual amount of crystalloid solutions, plasma substitutes, and/or blood (with or without vasopressors) to expand intravascular volume and improve cerebral perfusion (68,94,103,104, 137,160). Hence the surgeon is in a dilemma: Should he give a restricted fluid intake to avoid edema or a high fluid intake to improve cerebrovascular perfusion? For adult patients our policy is to give 80 ml of 5% dextrose in half-normal saline solution per hour (about 2000 ml/day) unless circumstances dictate otherwise. All intraoperative blood loss is replaced, and we do not hesitate to give an extra unit of blood or plasma substitute.

Some surgeons have advocated the use of low-molecular-weight dextran (LMWD or Rheomacrodex) (32,50,88,110,111,160) based on studies indicating that LMWD: (a) reduces the hematocrit and blood viscosity; (b) retards intravascular sludging, stasis, and aggregation; and (c) improves blood flow (25,43,66). Drake (50) warned of accelerating or precipitating intracranial bleeding with the use of postoperative dextran infusions. Such substances are not commonly used, for they are osmotic diuretics and tend to have the net result of causing eventual dehydration and electrolyte disturbances unless corrective measures are taken. Instead, Pecker et al. (127) suggested the use of platelet antiaggregation agents such as aspirin to reduce the tendency toward sludging and platelet thrombosis in injured cerebral vessels (56,67).

Other measures include ICP monitoring as advocated by Nornes (117). Many surgeons use drains in the ventricular, cisternal, and/or subgaleal spaces to help eliminate the irritating by-products of surgery in the CSF (114,148). The value of steroids is controversial, but they are still commonly used to combat edema and inflammation as well as to retard the development of subarachnoid adhesions, which cause hydrocephalus.

The following valuable report summarizes the conclusions of a study group regarding postoperative evaluation and care of the intracranial aneurysm patient (63):

> Observation of the patient overnight in the recovery room or intensive care unit is advisable. Strict attention to the airway, appropriate intravenous fluid regulation (i.e., averaging 1500 to 2500 ml 5% dextrose in half-normal saline solution per day in the adult patient), and elevation of the head are standard precautions. Only uncommonly are more vigorous measures needed to reduce ICP after microsurgery. Subgaleal drains are advocated by some surgeons. Many neurosurgeons use prophylactic anticonvulsants that can be discontinued within 2 years if the patient remains free of seizures.
>
> Although still debated, continuing to give prophylactic antibiotics started before operation may

have some merit. Maintenance of normal BP is advisable. Inducing vascular hypertension may aid in cases of vascular insufficiency. If steroids are used for any prolonged period, they should be tapered in dosage when being discontinued. The routine use of prophylactic heparinization (5000 units every 12 hours) to prevent pulmonary embolism has not been accepted by many neurosurgeons, nor has the routine use of dextran (normal or low molecular weight) to prevent sludging of blood been proved useful. Effective methods of treating intracranial vasospasm are still under study. Ambulation for the alert, intact patient should be delayed until complete recovery of proper cardiovascular and cerebrovascular stability has occurred. This will avoid a drop in intracranial blood pressure (and consequent vascular insufficiency) caused by vasospasm and edema. The need for postoperative ICP monitoring in these cases has declined; the merits of such monitoring before, during, and after surgery must be individually assessed.

Although complications are definitely reduced when microtechnique is used by an experienced surgeon, such events still occur. . . . These conditions must be recognized and dealt with appropriately. Deterioration of the patient due to increased ICP often is managed by reopening the craniotomy flap. If a clot is present, it should be removed. A remote hematoma can be overlooked unless angiography or CT scanning is used. The surgeon should remember that another aneurysm can also bleed whether or not it is visualized on angiography. Pulmonary embolism and infection are dangers common to all operations. Steroids may suppress signs of infection and septic meningitis. The surgeon should watch for gastrointestinal bleeding and neurogenic stress ulcers. Patients may have other medical problems that, quiescent before surgery, are ostensibly aggravated by the operation. Although postoperative angiography has been considered unnecessary when the microscope is used for surgery, many surgeons still find it useful in confirming placement of the clip and preservation of vessels. The procedure may reveal evidence of subsequent hydrocephalus, hematoma, or vasospasm. Sometimes it will show that the clip has become dislodged. Also, angiography may bring to light another aneurysm unobserved on the preoperative angiogram.

Additional viewpoints on the treatment of vasospasm are given in Chapters 9 and 10. See Chapters 23 and 24 for aspects of monitoring and therapy from the anesthesiologist's standpoint.

Summary

The incidence of postoperative complications has markedly decreased with modern techniques of aneurysm surgery, an experienced team, and proper patient selection (see Chapter 21 on Prognosis and Timing). Yet careful observation and monitoring of the patient are still essential to a successful outcome. We have reviewed possible postoperative complications and care from the surgeon's viewpoint. Details of such care obviously depend on the presence and type of postoperative problems as well as the patient's preoperative medical and neurologic status. The actual extent of operation-induced brain damage often has been difficult to assess in the past. Postoperative CT scanning now is providing us with a faster, safer, and more accurate assessment of the situation. Chemical tests may be helpful in the future. For example, Rabow and Tibbling (138) found a close correlation between elevated venous blood hydroxybutyric dehydrogenase and/or lactate dehydrogenase and the extent of brain damage caused by aneurysm surgery.

The postoperative care from the surgeon's standpoint is discussed. More details on anesthesiology are found in Chapters 23 and 24.

Bibliography

1. Adams CBT, Loach AB, O'Laoire SA: Intracranial aneurysms: analysis of results of microneurosurgery. Br Med J 2:607–609, 1976
2. Af Björkesten G: Arterial aneurysms of the internal carotid artery and its bifurcation. An analysis of 69 aneurysms treated mainly by direct surgical attack. J Neurosurg 15:400–410, 1958
3. Af Björkesten G, Troupp H: Aneurysms of the middle cerebral artery. A report on 52 cases. Acta Chir Scand 115:153–159, 1958
4. Af Björkesten G, Troupp H: Changes in the size of intracranial arterial aneurysms. J Neurosurg 19:583–588, 1962
5. Aiba T, Kumagai N, Kawabuchi J: [Complications following direct surgery of cerebral arterial aneurysms (postoperative syndrome of direct intracranial surgery of cerebral arterial aneurysms).] Surg Ther (Osaka) 25:321–333, 1971
6. Aitken RR, Drake CG: A technique of anesthesia with induced hypotension for surgical

correction of intracranial aneurysms. Clin Neurosurg 21:107–114, 1974
7. Alexander E Jr, Adams JE, Davis CH Jr: Complications in the use of temporary intracranial arterial clip. J Neurosurg 20:810–811, 1963
8. Allcock JM, Drake CG: Postoperative angiography in cases of ruptured intracranial aneurysm. J Neurosurg 20:752–759, 1963
9. Allcock JM, Drake CG: Ruptured intracranial aneurysms—the role of arterial spasm. J Neurosurg 22:21–29, 1965
10. Almeida GM, Pindaro J, Plese P, et al.: Intracranial arterial aneurysms in infancy and childhood. Childs Brain 3:193–199, 1977
11. Antunes JL, Correll JW: Cerebral emboli from intracranial aneurysms. Surg Neurol 6:7–10, 1976
12. Bakay L, Crawford JD, White JC: The effects of intravenous fluids on cerebrospinal fluid pressure. Surg Gynecol Obstet 99:48–52, 1954
13. Bakay L, Lee JC: Cerebral Edema. Springfield, Ill., Thomas, 1965, p 128
14. Bartal A, Schiffer J, Weinstein M: A successful case of basilar bifurcation aneurysm surgery. Acta Neurochir (Wien) 19:163–170, 1968
15. Bassett RC, List CF, Lemmen LJ: Surgical treatment of intracranial aneurysm. Surg Gynecol Obstet 95:701–708, 1952
16. Benedetti A, Curri D: Direct attack on carotid ophthalmic and large internal carotid aneurysms. Surg Neurol 8:49–54, 1977
17. Berger E, Duval C, Kyriazidou M: Intracranial aneurysm surgery using the surgical microscope and hypotensive technique. In Koos TH, Böck FW, Spetzler RF (eds.): Clinical Microneurosurgery. Stuttgart, Georg Thieme Verlag, 1976, pp. 204–209
18. Boba A: Hypothermia. Appraisal of risk in 110 consecutive patients. J Neurosurg 19:924–933, 1962
19. Bohard F, Saillant C: Syndrome de Korsakoff post-opératoire symptomatatique d'un anévrisme de l'artère communicante antérieure (étude clinique et chimiotherapique). Evol Psychiatr (Paris) 34:109–132, 1969
20. Bohm E, Hugosson R: Experiences of surgical treatment of 400 consecutive ruptured cerebral arterial aneurysms. Acta Neurochir (Wien) 40:33–43, 1978
21. Bohm E, Hugosson R: Results of surgical treatment of 200 consecutive cerebral arterial aneurysms. Acta Neurol Scand 46:45–52, 1970
22. Bonnal J, Bérard-Badier M, Sedan R, et al.: La mort par ramollissement cérébral à la suite de l'attaque directe de deux anévrysmes de l'artère communicante antérieure. Étude anatomique. Neurochirurgie 6:37–42, 1960
23. Bonnal J, Stevenaert A: Evolution angiographique des anévrysmes artériels du polygone antérieur après intervention directe incomplète. Schweiz Arch Neurol Neurochir Psychiatr 104:11–29, 1969
24. Bonnal J, Stevenaert A: Thrombosis of intracranial aneurysms of the circle of Willis after incomplete obliteration by clip or ligature across the neck. J Neurosurg 30:158–164, 1969
25. Boschenstein FK, Reilly JA, Yahr MD, et al.: Effect of low molecular weight dextran on cortical blood flow. Arch Neurol 14:288–293, 1966
26. Botterell EH, Lougheed WM, Scott JW, et al.: Hypothermia, and interruption of carotid, or carotid and vertebral circulation, in the surgical management of intracranial aneurysms. J Neurosurg 13:1–42, 1956
27. Brenner H, Böck FW: Prognosis of aneurysms after microsurgery. In Koos TH, Böck FW, Spetzler RF (eds.): Clinical Microneurosurgery. Stuttgart, Georg Thieme Verlag, 1976, pp. 183–191
28. Brihaye J, Mouawad E, Jeanmart L: L'anévrysme de la bifurcation carotidienne intracrânienne. Acta Neurol Belg 76:129–141, 1976
29. Brion S, Derome P, Guiot G, et al.: Syndrome de Korsakoff par anévrysme de l'artère communicante antérieure; le problème des syndromes de Korsakoff par hémorragie méningée. Rev Neurol (Paris) 118:293–299, 1968
30. Brown AS, Horton JM: Elective hypotension with intracardiac pacemaking in the operative management of ruptured intracranial aneurysms. Acta Anaesth Scand [Suppl] 23:665–670, 1966
31. Browne L: Hypotensive anaesthesia for direct attack of intracranial aneurysms. J Irish Med Assoc 66:65–72, 1973
32. Burke AM, Chien S, McMurtry JG III, et al.: Effects of low molecular weight dextran on blood viscosity after craniotomy for intracranial aneurysms. Surg Gynecol Obstet 148:9–15, 1979
33. Cabral RJ, King TT, Scott DF: Epilepsy after two different neurosurgical approaches to the treatment of ruptured intracranial aneurysm. J Neurol Neurosurg Psychiatry 39:1052–1056, 1976
34. Cabral RJ, Scott DF: A possible association between migraine and post-operative epilepsy in patients with intracranial aneurysm. Acta Neurol Scand 54:204–206, 1976
35. Cabral RJ, Scott DF: EEG features associated with the occurrence of epilepsy after surgery for intracranial aneurysm and acoustic neuroma. J Neurol Neurosurg Psychiatry 40:97–99, 1977
36. Carton CA, Heifetz MD, Kessler LA: Patching of intracranial internal carotid artery in man

using a plastic adhesive (Eastman 910 adhesive). J Neurosurg 19:887–895, 1962
37. Carton CA, Kennady JC, Heifetz MD, et al.: The use of a plastic adhesive (methyl-2-cyanoacrylate monomer) in the management of intracranial aneurysms and leaking cerebral vessels: a report of 15 cases. In Fields WS, Sahs AL (eds.): Intracranial Aneurysms and Subarachnoid Hemorrhage. Springfield, Ill., Thomas, 1965, pp. 372–440
38. Chou SN, Ortiz-Suarez HJ: Surgical treatment of arterial aneurysms of the vertebrobasilar circulation. J Neurosur 41:671–680, 1974
39. Clark K: Complications of aneurysm surgery. Clin Neurosurg 23:342–356, 1976
40. Connolly RC: Cerebral ischaemia in spontaneous subarachnoid haemorrhage. Ann R Coll Surg Engl 30:102–116, 1962
41. Corkill G: Earlier operation and antifibrinolytic therapy in the management of aneurysmal subarachnoid haemorrhage. Review of recent experience in Tasmania. Med J Aust 1:468–470, 1974
42. Crompton MR: Recurrent haemorrhage from cerebral aneurysms and its prevention by surgery. J Neurol Neurosurg Psychiatry 29:164–170, 1966
43. Cyrus AE Jr, Close AS, Foster LL, et al.: Effect of low moleular weight dextran on infarction alter experimental occlusion of the middle cerebral artery. Surgery 52:25–31, 1962
44. Dandy WE: Intracranial Arterial Aneurysms. New York, Hafner, 1944, reprinted 1969
45. Dawson BH: The blood vessels of the human optic chiasma and their relation to those of the hypophysis and hypothalamus. Brain 81:207–217, 1958
46. Drake CG: Bleeding aneurysm of the basilar artery. Direct surgical management in four cases. J Neurosurg 18:230–238, 1961
47. Drake CG: Further experience with surgical treatment of aneurysms of the basilar artery. J Neurosurg 29:372–392, 1968
48. Drake CG: On the surgical treatment of ruptured intracranial aneurysms. Clin Neurosurg 13:122–155, 1965
49. Drake CG: Surgical treatment of rupture of aneurysms of the basilar artery. Experience with 14 cases. J Neurosurg 23:457–473, 1965
50. Drake CG: The surgical treatment of vertebral-basilar aneurysms. J Neurosurg 16:114–169, 1969
51. Drake CG, Allcock JM: Postoperative angiography and the "slipped" clip. J Neurosurg 39:683–689, 1973
52. Drake CG, Amacher AL: Aneurysms of the posterior cerebral artery. J Neurosurg 30:468–474, 1969
53. Drake CG, Jory TA: Spontaneous intracranial haemorrhage: "subarachnoid haemorrhage": a review of investigation and treatment in 189 cases. Can J Surg 4:4–11, 1960
54. Drake CG, Vanderlinden RG: The late consequences of incomplete surgical treatment of cerebral aneurysms. J Neurosurg 27:226–238, 1967
55. Drake CG, Vanderlinden RG, Amacher AL: Carotid-choroidal aneurysms. J Neurosurg 29:32–36, 1968
56. Dujovny M, Osgood, CP, Barrionuevo PJ, et al.: SEM evaluation of endothelial damage following temporary middle cerebral artery occlusion in dogs. J Neurosurg 48:42–48, 1978
57. Elvidge AR, Feindel WH: Surgical treatment of aneurysm of the anterior cerebral and the anterior communicating arteries diagnosed by angiography and electroencephalography. J Neurosurg 7:13–32, 1950
58. Fein JM, Weinstein J, McVeety H, et al.: Pacemaker-induced hypotension for intracranial aneurysm surgery. Arch Surg 107:374–378, 1973
59. Feldman S, Behar AJ, Sameuloff M: Effect of cortisone and hydrocortisone on pia arachnoid adhesions. Arch Neurol Psychiatry 74:681–688, 1955
60. Ferguson GG, Harper AM, Fitch W, et al.: Cerebral blood flow measurements after spontaneous subarachnoid haemorrhage. Eur Neurol 8:15–23, 1972
61. Fox JL: Development of recent thoughts on intracranial pressure and the blood-brain barrier. J Neurosurg 21:909–967, 1964
62. Fox, JL: Personal experience, 1979
63. Fox, JL, Albin MS, Bader DCH, et al.: Microsurgical treatment of neurovascular disease. Neurosurgery 3:285–337, 1978
64. Fox JL, Falik JL, Shalhoub RJ: Neurosurgical hyponatremia: the role of inappropriate antidiuresis. J Neurosurg 34:506–514, 1971
65. Frost EAM: Respiratory problems associated with head trauma. Neurosurgery 1:300–306, 1977
66. Gelin L-E, Ingelman B: Rheomacrodex—a new dextran solution for rheological treatment of impaired capillary flow. Acta Chir Scand 122:294–302, 1961
67. Gertz SD, Kurgan H, Wajnberg RS, et al.: Endothelial cell damage and thrombus formation following temporary arterial occlusion. J Neurosurg 50:578–586, 1979
68. Giannotta SL, McGillicuddy JE, Kindt GW: Diagnosis and treatment of postoperative cerebral vasospasm. Surg Neurol 8:286–290, 1977
69. Gillingham FJ: The management of ruptured intracranial aneurysm. Ann R Coll Surg 23:89–117, 1958

70. Gillingham FJ: Twenty-five years' experience with middle cerebral aneurysms. J Neurol Neurosurg Psychiatry 38:405, 1975
71. Grossart KWM, Turner JW: Pre-operative angiography in cerebral vascular surgery. Clin Radiol 25:279–292, 1974
72. Guidetti B: Microsurgical treatment of intracranial saccular aneurysms. Acta Neurochir (Wien) 43:153–162, 1978
73. Guidetti B, La Torre E: Management of carotid-ophthalmic aneurysms. J Neurosurg 42:438–442, 1975
74. Hamby WB: Intracranial Aneurysms. Springfield, Ill., Thomas, 1952.
75. Hamby WB: Remarks concerning intracranial aneurysm surgery. Clin Neurosurg 17:1–17, 1970
76. Hanafee W, Jannetta PJ: Aneurysm as a cause of stroke. Am J Roentgenol 98:647–652, 1966
77. Harris P: Aneurysms of the anterior communicating artery. Cincinnati J Med 42:1–7, 1961
78. Heiskanen O: Cerebral circulatory arrest caused by acute increase of intracranial pressure. A clinical and roentgenological study of 25 cases. Acta Neurol Scand [Suppl 7] 40:1–57, 1964
79. Heiskanen O, Marttila I: Risk of rupture of a second aneurysm in patients with multiple aneurysms. J Neurosurg 32:295–299, 1970
80. Hollin SA, Decker RE: Microsurgical treatment of internal carotid artery aneurysms. J Neurosurg 47:142–149, 1977
81. Hollin SA, Gross SW: Changing size of an aneurysm. Report of a case. J Neurosurg 24:573–575, 1966
82. Horwitz NH, Rizzoli HV: Aneurysms and arteriovenous fistulas. In Postoperative Complications in Neurosurgical Practice. Recognition, Prevention, and Management. Baltimore, Williams & Wilkins, 1967, pp. 83–129
83. Hunt WE, Miller, CA: The results of early operation for aneurysm. Clin Neurosurg 24:208–215, 1977
84. Jamieson, KG: Aneurysms of the vertebrobasilar system. Further experience with nine cases. J Neurosurg 28:544–555, 1968
85. Joffe SN: Incidence of postoperative deep vein thrombosis in neurosurgical patients. J Neurosurg 42:201–203, 1975
86. Kahn EA: Postoperative loss of temperature control—poikilothermia. J Neurosurg 15:329–337, 1958
87. Kapp, JP: Hyperbaric oxygen as an adjunct to acute revascularization of the brain. Surg Neurol 12:457–461, 1979
88. Karasawa J, Kikuchi H, Furuse S, et al.: [Surgery of multiple intracranial aneurysms.] Neurol Surg (Tokyo) 2:763–769, 1974
89. Karasawa J, Kikuchi H, Furuse S, et al.: [Surgery of vertebral aneurysms of the origin of PICA.] Neurol Surg (Tokyo) 4:1157–1164, 1977
90. Karch SB: Upper gastrointestinal bleeding as a complication of intracranial disease. J Neurosurg 37:27–29, 1972
91. Kempe LG: Operative Neurosurgery, Vol 1: Cranial, Cerebral, and Intracranial Vascular Disease. Berlin, Springer-Verlag, 1968, pp. 1–75, 203–214
92. Kikuchi H, Furuse S, Karasawa J: Microsurgery of cerebral aneurysm in acute phase (within 1 week after subarachnoid hemorrhage). In Koos TH, Böck FW, Spetzler RF (eds): Clinical Microneurosurgery. Stuttgart, Georg Thieme Verlag, 1976, pp. 202–203
93. Kodama T, Uemura S, Nonaka N, et al.: [The quantative analysis of psychiatric sequelae after direct surgery of anterior communicating aneurysms. Follow-up study.] Neurol Med Chir (Tokyo) 17 (Part 2):237–333, 1977
94. Kosnik EJ, Hunt WE: Postoperative hypertension in the management of patients with intracranial aneurysms. J Neurosurg 45:148–154, 1976
95. Krayenbühl HA, Yaşargil MG, Flamm ES, et al.: Microsurgical treatment of intracranial saccular aneurysms. J Neurosurg 37:678–686, 1972
96. Kuwayama A, Okada C, Takanohashi M, et al.: [Endocrine function in postoperative patients with anterior communicating aneurysm.] Neurol Med Chir (Tokyo) 17 (Part 2):209–217, 1977
97. Laitinen L: [Arterial aneurysm with subarachnoid hemorrhage in children.] Nord Med 71:329–333, 1964
98. Landolt AM, Yaşargil MG, Krayenbühl H: Disturbances of the serum electrolytes after surgery of intracranial arterial aneurysms. J Neurosurg 37:210–217, 1972
99. Lindqvist G, Norlén G: Korsakoff's syndrome after operation on ruptured aneurysm of the anterior communicating artery. Acta Psychiatr Scand 42:24–34, 1966
100. Logue V: Posterior fossa aneurysms. Clin Neurosurg 11:183–207, 1964
101. Logue V, Durward M, Pratt RTC, et al.: The quality of survival after rupture of an anterior cerebral aneurysm. Br J Psychiatry 114:137–160, 1968
102. Lougheed W, Morley T, Tasker R, et al.: The results of surgical treatment of ruptured berry aneurysms. In Fields WS, Sahs AL (eds.): Intracranial Aneurysms and Subarachnoid Hemorrhage. Springfield, Ill., Thomas, 1965, pp 295–307

103. Maroon JC: Comment. Neurosurgery 4:128, 1979
104. Maroon JC, Nelson PB: Hypovolemia in patients with subarachnoid hemorrhage: therapeutic implications. Neurosurgery 4:223–226, 1979
105. Martinez Coll A, Del Corral JF: Experiences in intracranial surgery for aneurysms. Surg Neurol 3:191–193, 1975
106. Maspes PE, Marini G: Aneurysms of the anterior communicating artery. Result of direct surgical treatment. Acta Neurochir (Wien) 11:479–494, 1963
107. Matsukado Y, Kitamura K, Shida K, et al.: [Psychiatric disorders after surgery of anterior communicating and internal carotid aneurysms.] Brain Nerve (Tokyo) 20:557–564, 1968
108. Mauney FM Jr, Ebert PA, Sabiston DC Jr: Postoperative myocardial infarction: a study of predisposing factors, diagnosis and mortality in a high risk group of surgical patients. Ann Surg 172:494–502, 1970
109. McKissock W: Recurrence of an intracranial aneurysm after excision. Report of a case. J Neurosurg 23:547–548, 1965
110. McMurtry JG III, Housepian EM, Bowman FO Jr, et al.: Surgical treatment of basilar artery aneurysms. Elective circulatory arrest with thoracotomy in 12 cases. J Neurosurg 40:486–498, 1974
111. McMurtry JG III, Pool JL, Nova HR: The use of Rheomacrodex in the surgery of intracranial aneurysms. J Neurosurg 26:218–222, 1967
112. Mihara T, Asakura T, Kawamura H, et al.: Postoperative psychiatric symptoms and electrocardiographic changes in aneurysm of the anterior communicating artery. Brain Nerve (Tokyo) 23:1271–1280, 1971
113. Morgan F: Removal of anterior clinoid process in the surgery of carotid aneurysm. With some notes on recurrent subarachnoid haemorrhage during craniotomy. Schwiez Arch Neurol Neurochir Psychiatr 111:363–368, 1972
114. Mullan S, Hanlon K, Brown F: Management of 136 consecutive supratentorial berry aneurysms. J Neurosurg 49:794–804, 1978
115. Norlén G: Aneurysm of the anterior communicating artery. Prog Brain Res 30:295–302, 1968
116. Nornes H: Cerebral arterial flow dynamics during aneurysm haemorrhage. Acta Neurochir (Wien) 41:39–48, 1978
117. Nornes H: Monitoring of patients with intracranial aneurysms. Clin Neurosurg 22:321–331, 1975
118. Nornes H, Wikeby P: Results of microsurgical management of intracranial aneurysms. J Neurosurg 52:608–614, 1979
119. Nukui H, Imai S, Fukamachi A, et al.: [Bilaterally symmetrical giant aneurysms of the internal carotid artery within the cavernous sinus, associated with an aneurysm of the basilar artery.] Neurol Surg (Tokyo) 5:479–484, 1977
120. Nukui H, Miyagi O, Nojiri K, et al.: [Psychiatric symptoms in cases with ruptured anterior communicating aneurysms before and after surgery.] Neurol Med Chir (Tokyo) 17 (Part 2):335–341, 1977
121. Nukui H, Tanaka S, Miyagi O, et al.: Psychiatric symptoms of ruptured anterior communicating aneurysms before and after operation. Excerpta Medica ICS No. 418:206, 1977
122. Nyström SHM: On factors related to growth and rupture of intracranial aneurysms. Acta Neuropathol (Berl), 16:64–72, 1970
123. Odom, GL: Cerebral vasospasm. Clin Neurosurg 22:29–58, 1975
124. Paterson A: Direct surgery in the treatment of posterior communicating aneurysms. Lancet 2:808–811, 1968
125. Patricolo A: Una rara complicanza nella chirurgia degli aneurismi arteriosi endocranici: l'ipotensione liquorale (osservazioni su due casi). Minerva Neurochir 15:151–155, 1971
126. Paul RL, Arnold JG Jr: Operative factors influencing mortality in intracranial aneurysm surgery: analysis of 186 consecutive cases. J Neurosurg 32:289–294, 1970
127. Pecker, J, Guy G, Fardoun R: La place des anti-agrégants et des macromolécules dans le traitement des anévrismes arteriels cérébraux. Anesth Analg (Paris) 3:653–658, 1976
128. Peerless SJ, Drake CG, Kassell NF: Neurological deterioration following subarachnoid hemorrhage: prevention, diagnosis and treatment. Neurosurgery 1:65, 1977
129. Pertuiset B, Houtteville J-P, van Effenterre R, et al.: Chirurgie des anévrysmes artériels sus-tentoriels. Réduction par coagulation bipolaire sous hypotension profonde et exclusion par clip autobloquant: (52 cas opérés sous microscope). Nouv Presse Med 3:1649–1652, 1974
130. Pertuiset B, van Effenterre R, Goutorbe J, et al.: Management of aneurysmal rupture during surgery, using bipolar coagulation, deep hypotension, and the operating microscope. Acta Neurochir (Wien) 30:195–205, 1974
131. Pool JL: Aneurysms of the anterior communicating artery. Bifrontal craniotomy and routine use of temporary clips. J Neurosurg 18:98–111, 1961
132. Pool JL: Bifrontal craniotomy for anterior communicating artery aneurysms. J Neurosurg 36:212–220, 1972
133. Pool JL: Timing and techniques in the intra-

cranial surgery of ruptured aneurysms of the anterior communicating artery. J Neurosurg 19:378–388, 1962
134. Pool JL, Potts DG: Aneurysms and Arteriovenous Anomalies of the Brain. Diagnosis and Treatment. New York, Harper & Row, 1965
135. Poppin JL: Discussion. Clin Neurosurg 11:183–219, 1964
136. Portnoy HD, Avellanosa A: Carotid aneurysm and contralateral carotid stenosis with successful surgical treatment of both lesions. Case report. J Neurosurg 32:476–482, 1970
137. Pritz MB, Giannotta SL, Kindt GW, et al.: Treatment of patients with neurological deficits associated with cerebral vasospasm by intravascular volume expansion. Neurosurgery 3:364–368, 1978
138. Rabow L, Tibbling G: Serum enzyme activity of hydroxybutyric dehydrogenase (HBD) and heat inactivated lactate dehydrogenase (LD) after operations on intracranial aneurysms. Acta Neurochir (Wien) 32:199–207, 1975
139. Redondo A, Hanau J, Creissard P, et al.: Complications gastro-duodénales des ruptures anévrismales du système communicant antérieur. Neurochirurgie 16:471–488, 1970
140. Rivano C, Rossi GF, Zattoni J: Variations of intraventricular and local brain pressures during neurosurgical procedures. In Brock M, Dietz H (eds.): Intracranial Pressure. Berlin, Springer-Verlag, 1972, pp. 343–347
141. Robinson JL, Roberts A: Operative treatment of aneurysms and Coanda effect: a working hypothesis. J Neurol Neurosurg Psychiatry 35:804–809, 1972
142. Sato S, Onuma T, Suzuki J: [A consideration of incomplete surgical treatment of intracranial aneurysm.] Brain Nerve (Tokyo) 23:157–162, 1971
143. Sato S, Suzuki J: Prognosis in cases of intracranial aneurysm after incomplete direct operations. Acta Neurochir (Wien) 24:245–252, 1971
144. Selverstone B: Coating of intracranial aneurysms with nontoxic adherent plastics. In Schmidek HH, Sweet WH (eds.): Current Techniques in Operative Neurosurgery. New York, Grune & Stratton, 1977, pp. 31–40
145. Sengupta RP: Anatomical varations in the origin of the posterior cerebral artery demonstrated by carotid angiography, and their significance in the direct surgical treatment of posterior communicating aneurysms. Neurochirurgia (Stuttgt) 18:33–42, 1975
146. Sengupta RP, Chiu JSP, Brierley H: Quality of survival following direct surgery for anterior communicating artery aneurysms. J Neurosurg 43:58–64, 1975
147. Shenkin HA, Bezier HS, Bouzarth WF: Restricted fluid intake. Rational management of the neurosurgical patient. J Neurosurg 45: 432–436, 1976
148. Shiobara R, Toya S, Iisaka Y, et al.: [An evaluation of the continuous ventricular drainage for ruptured cerebral aneurysms.] Neurol Med Chir (Tokyo) 17 (Part 2):145–152, 1977
149. Silver D: Pulmonary embolism: prevention, detection, and nonoperative management. Surg Clin North Am 54:1089–1095, 1974
150. Simeone FA, Trepper P: Cerebral vasospasm with infarction: Stroke 3:449–455, 1972
151. Simmons DR, Portnoy HD, Gurdjian ES: Packing with muscle of internal carotid artery for aneurysm with immediate occlusion and subsequent establishment of flow. J Neurosurg 20:1000–1004, 1963
152. Skultery FM, Nishioka H: The results of intracranial surgery in the treatment of aneurysms. In Sahs AL, Perret GE, Locksley HB, et al. (eds.): Intracranial Aneurysms and Subarachnoid Hemorrhage. A Cooperative Study. Philadelphia, Lippincott, 1969, pp. 173–194
152a. Skultety FM, Nishioka H: Report on the cooperative study of intracranial aneurysms and subarachnoid hemorrhage. Section VIII, Part 2. The results of intracranial surgery in the treatment of aneurysms. J Neurosurg 25:683–704, 1966
153. Somach FM, Shenkin HA: Bilateral intracranial carotid aneurysm. Report of a case successfully treated. Neurochirurgia (Stuttgt) 8:188–195, 1965
154. Stein M, Koota GM, Simon M, et al.: Pulmonary evaluation of surgical patients. JAMA 181:765–770, 1962
155. Stern WE: Mechanisms in the production of hemiparesis associated with intracranial aneurysm. Brain 78:503–513, 1955
156. Steven JL: Postoperative angiography in treatment of intracranial aneurysms. Acta Radiol [Diagn] (Stockh) 5:536–548, 1966
157. Sundt TM Jr, Nofzinger JD: Clip-grafts for aneurysm and small vessel surgery. Part 1. Repair of segmental defects with clip-grafts; laboratory studies and clinical correlations. Part 2. Clinical application of clip-grafts to aneurysms; technical considerations. J Neurosurg 27:477–489, 1967
158. Suzuki J, Yoshimoto T, Hori S: Continuous ventricular drainage to lessen surgical risk in ruptured intracranial aneurysm. Surg Neurol 2:87–90, 1974
159. Swain RD: The surgical treatment of certain intracranial arterial aneurysms. Surg Clin North Am 28:396–404, 1948

160. Symon L: Disordered cerebro-vascular physiology in aneurysmal subarachnoid haemorrhage. Acta Neurochir (Wien) 41:7–22, 1978
161. Takagi H, Miyasaka Y, Saito T, et al.: An analysis of postoperative time course of ICP in cases with ruptured aneurysms. Neurol Med Chir (Tokyo) 17 (Part II):517–523, 1977
162. Takaku A, Tanaka S, Mori T, et al.: Postoperative complications in 1,000 cases of intracranial aneurysms. Surg Neurol 12:137–144, 1979
163. Tönnis W: Zur Behandlung der intrakranieller Aneurysmen. Langenbecks Arch Klin Chir 189:474–476, 1937
169. Troupp H, Koshinen K, af Björkesten G: Ophthalmoplegia caused by intracranial aneurysm. Prognosis after intracranial surgery. Acta Ophthalmol (Copenh) 36:79–86, 1958
165. Troupp H, Laitinen L: Reliability of partial ligation in the treatment of intracranial arterial aneurysms. II. Acta Neurol Scand 40:369–374, 1964
166. Uihlein A, Thomas RL, Cleary J: Aneurysms of the anterior communicating artery complex. Proc Mayo Clin 42:73–87, 1967
167. Valladares JB, Hankinson J: Incidence of lower extremity deep vein thrombosis in neurosurgical patients. Neurosurgery 6:138–141, 1980
168. Weaver EN: Intracranial aneurysms, congenital and acquired: diagnosis, treatment and prognosis. J Int Coll Surg 27:576–589, 1957
169. Williamson WP, Brackett CE Jr: Management of intracranial aneurysms of the anterior communicating artery. Am Surg 22:100–107, 1956
170. Wilson CB, Christensen FK, Subrahmanian MV: Intracranial aneurysms at the pericallosol artery bifurcation. Am Surg 31:386–393, 1965
171. Wise BL: Fluid and Electrolytes in Neurological Surgery. Springfield, Ill., Thomas, 1965, pp 15–24
172. Woodhall B, Odom GL, Bloor BM, et al.: Direct measurement of intravascular pressure in components of the circle of Willis. A contribution to the surgery of congenital cerebral aneurysms and vascular anomalies of the brain. Ann Surg 135:911–921, 1952
173. Wright WH, Todd EM, Duemler LP, et al.: Simultaneous direct operations for bilateral internal carotid artery aneurysms. Surg Neurol 2:355–358, 1974
174. Yaşargil MG, Fox JL, Ray MW: The operative approach to aneurysms of the anterior communicating artery. In Krayenbühl H (ed.): Advances and Technical Standards in Neurosurgery, Vol 2. New York, Springer-Verlag, 1975, pp. 113–170
179. Yaşargil MG, Gasser JC, Hodosh RM, et al.: Carotid—ophthalmic aneurysms: direct microsurgical approach. Surg Neurol 8:155–165, 1977
176. Yaşargil MG, Smith RD: Surgery on the carotid system in the treatment of hemorrhagic stroke. Adv Neurol 16:181–209, 1977
177. Young B, Meacham WF, Allen JH: Documented enlargement and rupture of a small arterial sacculation. Case report. J Neurosurg 34:814–817, 1971
178. Zlotnik EI, Oleshkevich FV, Stolkarts JZ: Microsurgical technique in the treatment of intracranial aneurysms. J Neurosurg 46:591–595, 1977

33
Carotid Artery Ligation in the Neck

Deliberate occlusion of the cervical portion of the carotid artery for intracranial aneurysms has been a popular method of treatment. Commonly used methods have been ligation of the common carotid artery (CCA); the internal carotid artery (ICA); the internal and common carotid arteries; the internal and external carotid arteries (ECA); the common and external carotid arteries; or the common, internal, and external carotid arteries (simultaneously or staged).

Rogers stated (146): "The first account of the use of ligatures is given by Celcius, who lived in the time of Tiberius Caesar (25–30 B.C.–A.D. 45–50) and whose writings constitute the oldest medical document after the Hippocratic writings . . ." The technique thus became know as the "Celsian operation" and specifically referred to the type of procedure in which the vessel is severed between ligatures. Rogers (146) opined that the Celsian operation had the advantages of: (a) no recanalization; (b) simultaneous sympathetic fiber interruption to reduce vasospasm; (c) retraction and contraction of the divided ends, thereby reducing the risk of fatal hemorrhage from ulceration or infection; and (d) retraction and constriction of the arterial ends, thereby reducing the risk of embolism from the site of ligature.

Beekman (13) noted that ligation of an artery above and below a systemic aneurysm was performed as early as the third century A.D. by Antyllus, creator of arterial surgery. Advances in this type of surgery progressed with the work of the Hunter brothers—hence the origin of the "Hunterian ligature," or simple ligation of the artery proximal to the arterial lesion (13, 39a,78,130–132). John Hunter studied peripheral vascular concepts under his brother, William Hunter, and then developed use of the proximal arterial ligature during the 1780s to treat lesions such as popliteal artery aneurysms.

The reader should consult several excellent writings on the early history of cervical carotid artery ligation (13,29,31,36,66,90,107,141, 146,150,184,185). Such surgery was first performed by Hebenstreit in 1793, John Abernethy (a pupil of John Hunter) in 1798, David Fleming in 1803, Amos Twitchell in 1804, Astley Cooper in 1805, and Benjamin Travers in 1809 (146,150,184). At that time cervical carotid artery ligation was done for traumatic hemorrhage or aneurysm of the cervical internal carotid artery or for signs of a carotid-cavernous fistula. Large numbers of patients were so treated, often with high mortality rates. Such mortality correlated closely with the patient's general state of health and his or her age.

In 1865 Nunneley (122) reported on a woman who had had her right carotid artery ligated in 1864 for signs of ocular protrusion and congestion. She died of "apoplexy" (no subarachnoid hemorrhage) that same year and was autopsied, at which time a large thrombosed right oaICAA was discovered. In 1890 W. W. Keen (92) told of a large intracranial aneurysm (site?) exposed by Sir Victor Horsley (probably during the year 1885) and treated by bilateral cervical carotid artery ligation. Beadles (12) and Rogers (146) stated that in 1902 Horsley also ligated the common carotid artery of a woman whose giant ICAA was found by craniotomy. Schorstein (150) reported that Wilfred Trotter was the first to ligate the cervical carotid artery in 1924 as treatment of an unexposed intracranial aneurysm. There were other similar descriptions, but proof that an intracranial aneurysm was the etiology of symptoms was lacking. In 1929 Albright (1) described a 33-year-old man who had an SAH and left oculomotor palsy in 1928. Twelve days later Walter Dandy partially ligated the cervical internal carotid artery. Bilateral internal carotid artery aneurysms were seen at autopsy. In 1933 Norman Dott (38) reported on carotid ligation for a bICAA. In 1941 Schorstein (150) summarized 60 case reports of intracranial aneurysms during the 1930s beginning with those of Dott. It seemed that Oppenheim's 1913 prophecy that the only surgical treatment for internal carotid artery aneurysms would be cervical carotid artery ligation was being fulfilled (129).

Physiological Studies

In 1953 Black and German (16) believed that cervical carotid artery ligation served to reduce all those factors which tend to encourage expansion and rupture of an intracranial aneurysm—at least aneurysms on the internal carotid artery. These factors included local blood pressure and hence transmural hydrostatic pressure, pulsatile flow (pulse pressure or systolic thrust), turbulence in the bloodstream, and jet action in the neck of the aneurysm.

There seems to be little doubt that ICA or CCA oclusion in the neck reduces (at least temporarily) both the blood pressure and the pulse pressure above the point of ligation. The change is greater with ICA ligation than with CAA ligation. A number of pressure measurements in the carotid artery, intracranial arteries or aneurysms, and retinal arteries have confirmed this (8,52,77,89,106,162,163,165,166, 169,173,191–193). However, there was marked variation in the extent of pressure drop from person to person (166). Stern (162) found no correlation between the amount of pressure drop and the angiographic patterns of the circle of Willis. Normally there is a slight decrement in intraarterial pressure as one proceeds distally into the smaller arteries of the brain; upon carotid ligation the percentage drop in intraarterial pressure of the smaller and more distal arteries is equal to (163) or greater than (8) that in the carotid artery just above the ligature. Tindall et al. (173) studied 18 patients undergoing CCA occlusion in the neck and noted that there was no significant reduction in blood flow or pressure above the ligature until the cross-sectional area of the CCA was reduced by 70–90%. Jain's work in dogs suggested that partial carotid ligation reduced the pulsatile force of the bloodstream distally (81).

These investigations strongly suggest that the ICAA and possible the MCAA are better protected from rupture by ICA or CCA ligation. However, such protection may be only temporary. Holmes and co-workers (77) studied 11 patients and discovered that the carotid pressure above the ligature had partially recovered and the cerebral blood flow had returned nearly to normal by 30 min. Svien and Hollenhorst (165) noted that retinal artery pressures tended to return to normal over a period of months and years. These findings tend to support the concept that adequate collateral circulation eventually evolves or enlarges to bring blood-flow-compromised areas of the brain (and aneurysm) back to normal or to the original blood pressure and flow values. Winn and colleagues (189) concluded in their study of 34 cases of pcaICAA treated by CCA ligation that these patients are no longer protected from rebleed 6 months or more after the ligation.

Of interest are the flow patterns within the cervical ICA and ECA after CCA ligation. Tindall et al. (167,174) and Hardesty et al. (72) found that after CCA occlusion the blood flow was from ICA to ECA in about half of the cases and from ECA to ICA in the other half. ECA to ICA flow suggests that at the time of measurement there was poor intracranial collateral circulation, whereas ICA to ECA flow indicates excellent intracranial collateral circulation to that ICA. Youmans and co-workers (196) followed these measurements for a few hours and found that all of their patients who had initial ICA to ECA direction of flow eventually changed to ECA to ICA flow.

Ligation of the ICA may tend to lower systemic blood pressure as the carotid sinus receives the brunt of the CCA pulse wave. Ligation of the CCA may tend to raise systemic blood pressure by excluding the carotid sinus from the CCA blood pressure, for a higher blood pressure in the carotid sinus stimulates a reflex via the vagus and glossopharyngeal branches resulting in a lowering of systemic blood pressure and vice versa (25,155,189).

Indications

Over the years a number of physicians have proved the value of cervical carotid artery ligation in selected cases. Unfortunately, the procedure may have been used rather indiscriminately in earlier years. (Refer to the symbol *CER* for cervical carotid artery ligation in the Surgery column in Appendix 2, for case reports and references of aneurysms treated by carotid ligation.) The literature indicates that carotid ligature has been quite popular as treatment for certain intracranial aneurysms (1, 2, 5, 6, 9–12, 14–19, 23–35, 37–51, 54–58, 60–62, 64, 66–71, 73, 75–77, 79, 83–89, 91, 92, 94, 95, 99–105, 109–117, 119, 125, 127, 128, 133, 135–149, 151–156, 158–161, 163, 164, 166, 167, 169, 171–174, 176–181, 187, 188, 190, 194, 196).

Over the past few decades the indications for carotid artery ligation in the treatment of aneurysms have become fewer as techniques of direct attack on the aneurysm have improved (53). In 1953 Norlén (120) questioned the value of the ligature in these cases, but the results of direct attack on aneurysms at that time were disappointing. Jefferson (85) believed that carotid occlusion by the Hunterian ligature was especially apropos for the csICAA. More recently Galbraith and Clark (55) agreed and also included oaICAA, bICAA, other broad-based ICAA, giant ICAA, and other ICAA that cannot be satisfactorily attacked directly.

Tindall and Odom (167,171,172) summarized the indications for carotid ligation that they used up through the 1960s. They included: (a) ICAA at any site; (b) ACoAA filling from one side only (about 10% of ACoAA cases); and (c) MCAA in older (over 60 years of age) patients or with a broad base. They recommended direct attack on the other types of MCAA. If the ACoAA filled from both right and left carotid pathways without cross compression of carotid artery, they ligated one A-1 intracranially and later gradually occluded the opposite CCA (41,125,167,168,170–172). If the ACoAA filled from one carotid artery only and there was no cross filling via the anterior communicating artery during cross compression of the opposite carotid artery during angiography, the carotid artery was not ligated. This circumstance risks cerebral ischemia due to inadequate collateral circulation around the circle of Willis.

Large or giant aneurysms of the ICA inoperable by the direct approach have been considered good candidates for carotid ligation either as the definitive procedure or as a first step prior to trapping, excision, or other methods of obliteration (22,39a,55,59). Refer to the symbol *CER* for cervical carotid artery ligation or *TRA* for trapping procedure in the Surgery column in Appendix 2, file on giant aneurysms, for case reports and references on giant aneurysms treated by carotid ligation.

Evaluation of Collateral Cerebral Circulation

Matas Test

Temporary occlusion of the carotid artery in the neck prior to permanent ligation has become known as the Matas test. The physician may use a finger (his or the patient's) or a metallic neck band, the latter being less painful to the physician and perhaps more painful to the patient. The occlusion time may last only a few minutes or less if adverse symptoms of cerebrovascular insufficiency develop, or longer if no symptoms develop; the plan (theoretically) is to stimulate collateral circulation.

Matas (107,108) developed this test and reported it in 1911. At that time it was used prior to arterial ligation for peripheral vascular aneurysms and later prior to ligation for intracranial arteriovenous fistulas or aneurysms. However, it is quite clear that the test was used earlier by C. H. Parry in 1789 and T. Vanzetti in 1856 for various neurologic symptoms (185). See Webster and Gurdjian (185) for additional history.

A number of authors indicated they used the Matas test prior to carotid ligation (29,30,31, 51,68,69,74,107,108,140,151,181). If the Matas test led to signs of cerebral ischemia, Dandy (30) only partially ligated the carotid artery with fascia lata for 7–10 days to allow collateral circulation to build up before total ligation. Rand (140) suggested measuring retinal artery pressures by ophthalmodynomometry to determine the effectiveness of the planned carotid ligation.

Tindall and Odom (167,172) considered the Matas test to be unreliable as a predictor of the value of gradual carotid occlusion, for the test uses acute and total occlusion. Furthermore, by the Matas maneuver one cannot selectively occlude either the common or the internal carotid artery with preservation of jugular vein flow or without nerve or sympathetic plexus irritation.

Intraoperative Carotid Occlusion

Rather than rely entirely on the Matas test, some surgeons observed the effects of temporary carotid artery occlusion in the awake patient (17,56,75,80,83,167,171,172). They maintained occlusion for 30–60 min and proceeded with either acute or gradual occlusion if no neurologic symptoms evolved. Harris and Udvarhelyi (75) at the same time would drop the patient's systemic blood pressure 50 mm Hg below preoperative levels and watch for signs of cerebral ischemia.

Distal ICA Pressure

A number of authors have used measurements of carotid artery stump pressures (internal carotid artery pressures above temporary ligature) to estimate the danger or effectiveness of permanent carotid ligature (20,80,89,163, 166,167,169,171,172,188,194). Systolic blood pressure drops of greater than 50–70% of control values have been considered indicative of poor collateral circulation and the risk of cerebral ischemia. On the other hand, a systolic pressure that remains above 100 mm Hg risks inadequate aneurysm protection from a future rebleed (194). Horwitz and Rizzoli (80) recommended ICA pressures between 80 and 100 mm Hg as ideal. If the pressure is still high after CCA ligation, Brackett and Mount (20) considered additional ECA ligation—rather than ICA ligation, which risks intimal injury and spasm of the ICA.

Electroencephalography

A few authors have used electroencephalography (EEG) recordings during preliminary carotid occlusion to assist in the evaluation of this treatment (83,144,145). Rogers (144) was one of the first to do this in 1944. EEG slowing was said to predict an inability of the brain to tolerate permanent carotid occlusion; few or no EEG changes suggested that carotid occlusion would not cause future cerebral ischemia. However, more recent studies strongly suggest that there is no correlation between these EEG changes and the effects of gradual carotid occlusion (110,137,167,171,172,190).

Jugular Vein Blood Gases

Galbraith (54) found that if the jugular venous oxygen saturation was 60% or more after carotid ligation this therapy was well tolerated. Jawad et al. (82) and Miller et al. (110) found such monitoring to be of no predictive value.

Angiographic Findings

Whereas evidence of cross filling during carotid arteriography with compression of the opposite carotid artery suggested tolerance of occlusion to some authors (188), it appeared to be of no predictive value to others (110,137).

Cerebral Blood Flow

Cerebral blood flow (CBF) changes during temporary carotid ligation have been investigated (55,83,87,88,100,110). The conclusions were summarized by Jawad et al. (83):

1. If CBF $\geqslant$ 40 ml/100 g/min, it is safe to ligate the carotid artery.
2. If CBF $<$ 20 ml/100 g/min, do not ligate the carotid artery.
3. If CBF lies between the above two values, ligate only if the CBF drop is less than 25% of control CBF.
4. If the CBF drop is less than 35% of the control CBF, one can still ligate if the ICA pressure is more than 60 mm Hg above the occlusion site.

Methodology

Gradual Versus Acute Closure

Although most surgeons now agree that gradual and controlled closure of the cervical carotid artery is the least dangerous procedure for the patient, there has been and still remains considerable controversy about this. In earlier days acute closure was standard treatment if the patient tolerated the Matas test or any of the other tests meant to predict tolerance of carotid occlusion. Dandy (30) only partially closed the carotid artery with fascia lata in many cases and then completed closure 7–10 days later. Alexander et al (2) and Kak et al. (91) found no difference between the results of acute versus gradual ligation. Nishoka (118,118a) in the 1966 Cooperative Study concluded that there was little difference in ischemic complications between acute versus gradual carotid ligation if all variables were considered (even though acute occlusion caused greater morbidity overall). In 1970 Landolt and Millikan (98) reported a lower incidence of cerebral ischemia in patients undergoing acute occlusion, thus indicating that the controversy was still unsettled.

However, in 1909 Halsted (65) recommended gradual occlusion after his investigation with dogs. In later years proper clamps for gradual occlusion evolved, and many surgeons subsequently concluded that gradual occlusion was less hazardous (45,134,136).

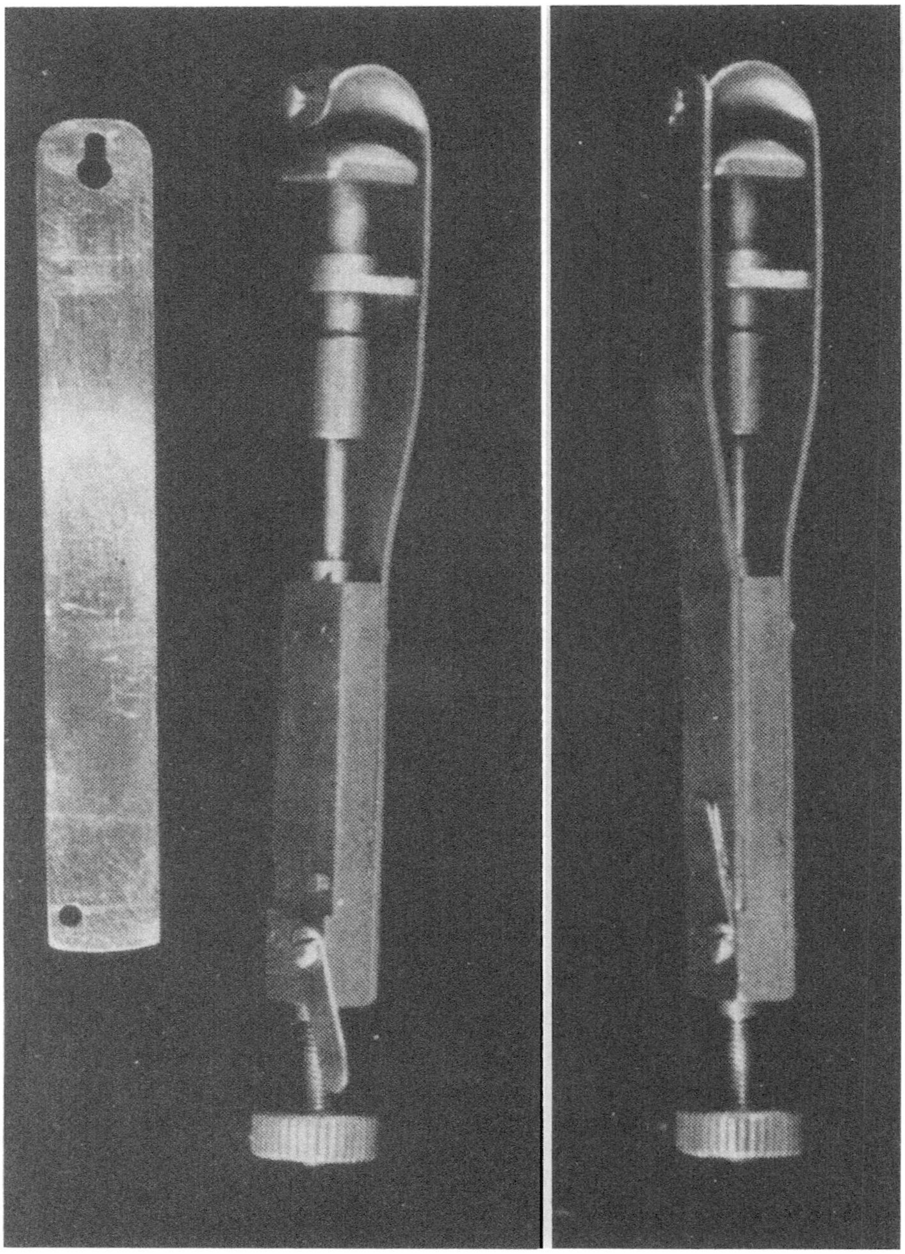

Fig. 33.1. Carotid artery clamp used by Dott since 1938. From Dott NM, ref. 37.

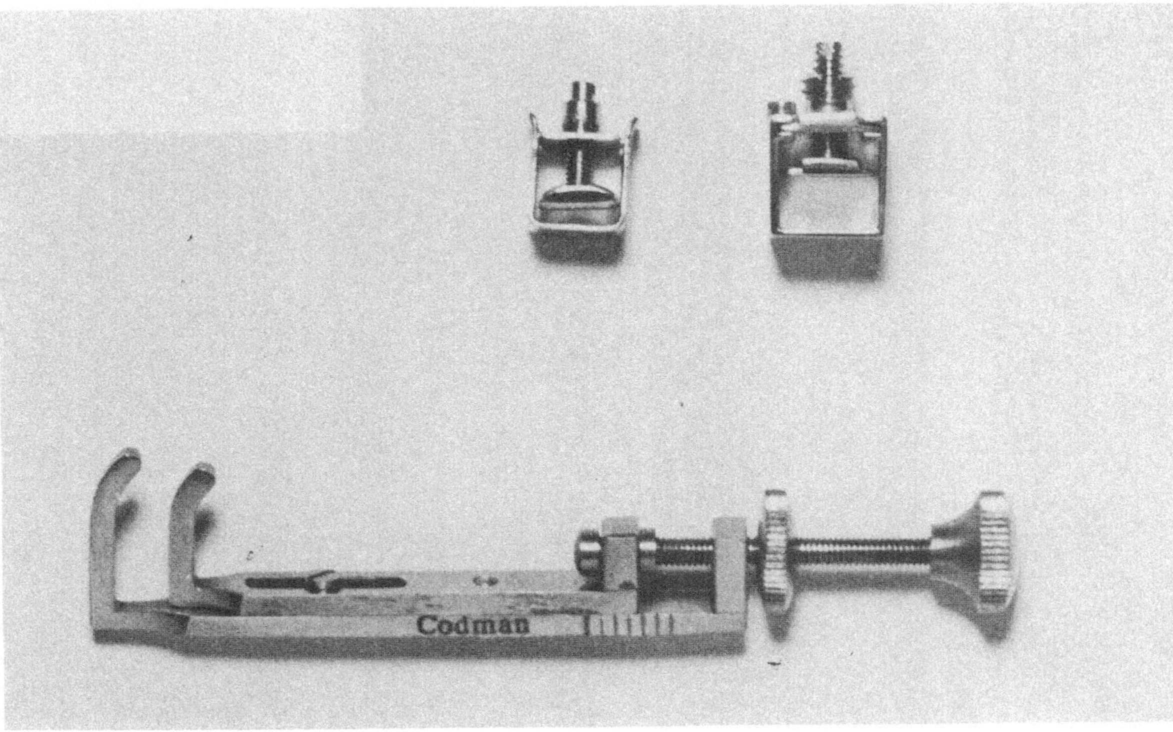

Fig. 33.2. Three commonly used carotid artery clamps. *Upper left* Crutchfield clamp (27). *Upper right* Selverstone clamp (152, 153). *Bottom* Poppen–Blaylock clamp (46, 136). Courtesy of Codman & Shurtleff, Inc., Randolph, Massachusetts.

Clamps for Gradual Occlusion

One of the earliest screw clamps used for gradual occlusion of the cervical carotid arteries was the Dott clamp (Fig. 33.1) used by Dott since 1938 (37). In 1959 Crutchfield (27) described his clamp (Fig. 33.2), which was later modified by Salibi (141) and Selverstone (152,153) (Figs. 33.2 and 33.3). Two other clamps, very similar to each other, are the Poppen–Blaylock clamp (46,136) (Fig. 33.2) and the Pertuiset clamp (133) (Fig. 33.4). These latter two clamps, like the Dott clamp, require removal of the entire clamp after ligating the artery following total occlusion. More recently the Kindt clamp (59) (Fig. 33.3), a modification of the Selverstone clamp, was described. The Crutchfield, Selverstone, Salibi, and Kindt clamps can be left in situ after the turning pole has been disconnected following completion of the gradual occlusion.

Other unusual methods for gradual occlusion have been described. Dandy (29–31) often partially ligated the artery with fascia lata and totally ligated it 7–10 days later. Hamby (67) once used a three-staged ligation: partial CCA ligation followed by total CCA ligation followed by total ICA ligation with fascia. Strobos and Mount (163) discussed the use of Cellophane wrapped about the internal carotid artery to promote scarring and gradual occlusion by the adhesions binding the artery. Gibbs (61) illustrated a method of twisting the carotid artery with a torsion device to occlude the artery.

Other Methods of Occlusion

Silk, linen, or synthetic ties have been commonly used for acute occlusion of the carotid artery or for final occlusion after gradual closure. Other materials have included fascia lata (30), strips of dura (30), strips of temporalis fascia (30), smooth-edged Michel clips (94), tantalum or aluminum bands or clips (19,105,115), and umbilical tape (115). Kessler and Wholey (93) used an intraluminal balloon catheter, expanding the balloon to occlude the ICA.

Closure may be complete or partial, with or without additional trapping by intracranial ca-

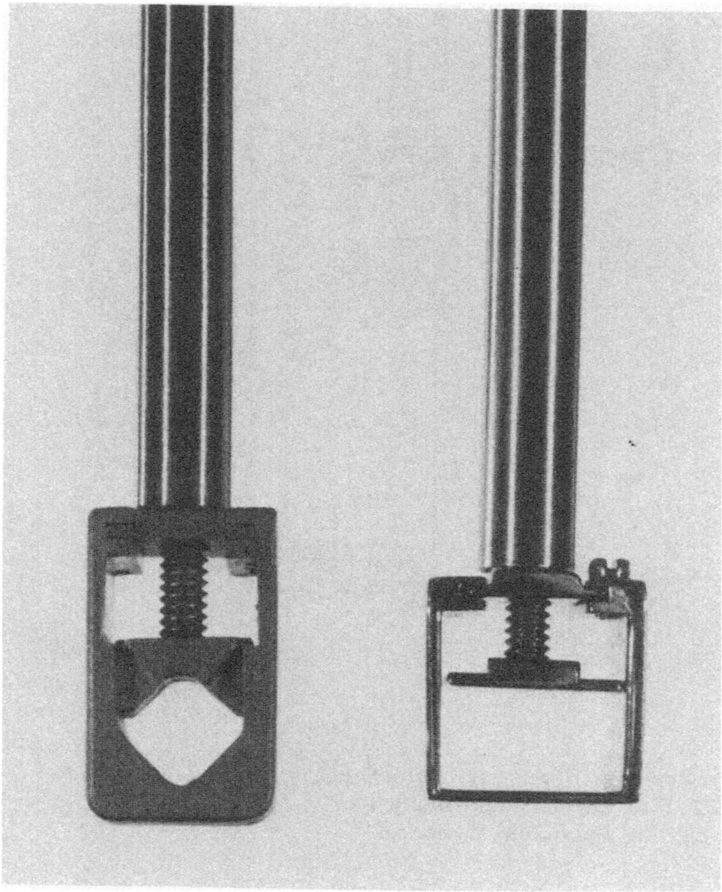

Fig. 33.3. *Left* Kindt carotid artery clamp. *Right* Selverstone carotid artery clamp. The Kindt clamp gradually reduces the circumference of the vessel, whereas the other types tend to deform the vessel into a rectangle. From Giannotta SL, McGillicuddy JE, Kindt GW, ref. 59.

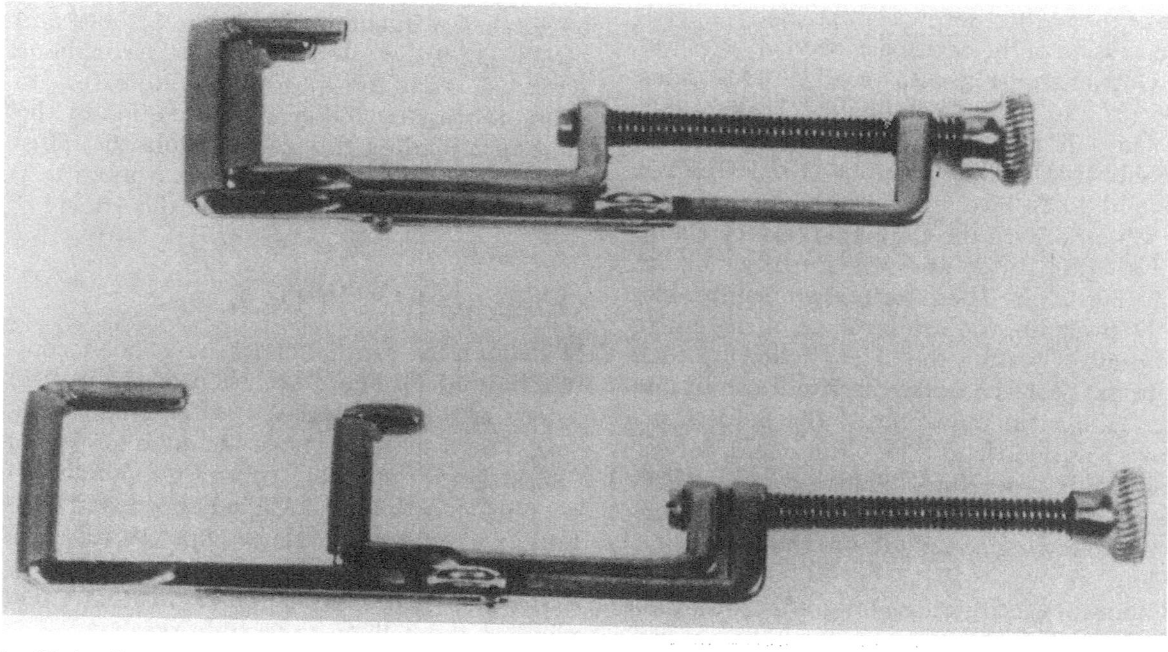

Fig. 33.4. Pertuiset carotid artery clamp. From Pertuiset B, ref. 133.

rotid ligation, with or without additional intracranial clipping or wrapping of the aneurysm, and with or without additional A-1 ligature (the latter for ACoAA).

Site of Ligature

Regardless of the method and speed of occlusion, the cervical carotid arteries can be ligated at one or more of several sites: ICA only; CCA only; CCA and ECA; CCA and ICA; ICA and ECA; or CCA, ICA, and ECA. Multiple sites may be ligated simultaneously or in stages. In earlier days the ICA was usually used, but more recently the CCA has been the preferred site in the belief that ischemic complications are less frequent. The 1966 Cooperative Study reported a lower incidence of ischemic complications from CCA ligation than with ICA ligation (118,118a). However, with CCA ligation collateral circulation via the ipsilateral CCA, ECA, and retrograde ophthalmic artery route is prevented.

One may wish to ligate the CCA and then the ECA later if the ICA systolic pressure exceeds 100 mm Hg. This procedure avoids injury to the ICA itself. If a trapping procedure is planned, occlusion of the ICA or the ICA (or CCA) and ECA may be preferred.

Occasionally bilateral carotid artery ligation has been reported. In 1890 Keen (92) described a case of Horsley's in which a large intracranial aneurysm was treated with exploration and bilateral cervical carotid artery ligation. In 1965 Nofzinger et al. (119) discussed a case of bilateral ICAA in which the left CCA was ligated. Nine years later the newly discovered right ICAA was treated by a left subclavian to CCA bypass (using a saphenous vein graft) followed by a successful right CCA ligation. In 1978 de Morais and Lana-Peixoto (35) described a patient who had bilateral csICAA. The left CCA was ligated in 1973 and the right CCA partially ligated in 1976.

Surgical Technique

The Dandy (29–31) technique with fascia has already been mentioned. Rogers (145,146) tied and cut the CCA acutely between ligatures to sever the sympathetic fibers (to reduce spasm), prevent recanalization, and reduce the chance of embolism. Cutting the ICA allowed it to retract and constrict about any contained clot, thus preventing that clot from embolizing to the brain. Poppen (135) described his imbrication technique of folding the wall in on itself. Harris and Udvarhelyi (75) occluded the carotid artery acutely and performed simultaneous periarterial sympathectomy. Boldrey (17) occluded the CCA by tying a heavy silk suture around a strip of fascia lata that surrounded the artery. He often followed this with ICA or ECA occlusion 7–10 days later.

Tindall and Odom (167,171,172) summarized their surgical technique of gradual closure with a Crutchfield clamp. They preferred local anesthesia if the patient was cooperative. The clamp is turned down to occlude the CCA 2 cm below its bifurcation. Appropriate pressure measurements are made (see above). The clamp is then opened enough to allow only a 10% reduction in blood pressure above the clamp (in the ICA). The wound is closed and the clamp left alone until the following day. This next day the screw is turned by half turns until the retinal artery pressure is reduced by 10%. [This technique using ophthalmodynamometry was suggested in 1953 by Lobstein et al. (103).] This is repeated once daily. Near termination, a quarter of a turn will reduce the pressure 10%. When the artery is closed (confirmed by an x-ray film of the clamp in the neck), the external screw part is detached 24 h later. Only then may gradual ambulation be started.

If signs of cerebral ischemia occur, open the clamp immediately and measure the retinal artery pressure to see if the artery is clotted (167,171,172). If it is clotted, close the clamp, open the wound, remove the clots, and then open the clamp. If it is not clotted according to the retinal artery pressures, just observe the patient with the clamp left open. If sufficient improvement occurs, then resume gradual closure of the clamp. If there is no improvement, elevate the blood pressure. Murphy (115) opposed opening the artery if it had been closed more than 30 min, as there may be a greater risk of an embolizing clot to the brain. He performed lumbar puncture to rule out rebleed and if this was negative proceeded to the operating room. He then needle-aspirated the carotid artery above and below the clamp. If a clot was present, he opened the artery and removed the clot. If a clot was not present, he clamped the ICA and opened the CCA clamp to allow small clots to escape into the ECA.

Postoperatively, the following adjuncts have been used: Trendelenberg position (17,135), oxygen inhalation with or without carbon dioxide (17,135), anticoagulation (135,181), low-molecular-weight dextran (139), and sympathetic block with procaine (181). Close observation and monitoring by nursing personnel is essential.

Results

Early Mortality

In 1966 Tönnis and Walter (175) reviewed the world literature from 1933 to 1960 and found a 3–41% mortality rate following carotid ligation for aneurysm in various series. As in any treatment of this problem, the highest mortality rates occurred in patients operated early and those with vasospasm or other causes of deficient cerebral perfusion. McKissock et al. and Walsh (109,182,183) in a controlled study found that CCA ligation for pcaICAA provided better results than bedrest alone. They found 100% mortality if the patient was in a poor condition (grade) and 8% mortality if the patient was in good condition.

Bakay (7) summarized the early work of Sweet et al. and concluded that carotid ligature carries a 10–20% risk of morbidity and mortality; he believes that present-day craniotomy techniques for aneurysm can do better. In more recent times some surgeons have obtained very low early mortality rates with carotid ligation: Chadduck et al. (24) 4%, Jeffreys and Holmes (86) 0%, Kak et al. (91) 6%, Miller et al (110) 0%. Dandy (31) reported only 5% mortality among 88 cases in 1942. As with cases selected for direct operation on the aneurysm, these good results are due in part to careful case selection.

Distal ICA Pressures

A number of workers have investigated late (months and years later) internal carotid artery and retinal artery pressures (8,26,76,125, 126,169,178). The majority of patients showed persistence of low pressures, although the pressures were not as low as they were immediately after ligation. Cristiansson (26) found an average of 20–25% reduction in ipsilateral retinal artery pressures 1–13 years later. Odom, Tindall, and colleagues (125,126,169) reported similar results with ICA and retinal artery pressures. They found a good correlation between low retinal artery pressures and a reduction in aneurysm size on late postoperative angiography (169). Tytus and co-workers (178) discovered a similar correlation, but only half of their cases had maintained any reductions in retinal artery pressures 4 months to 9 years after carotid ligation. In 1955 Bucy (21) suggested that whereas carotid ligation may not maintain a reduced ICA pressure in the long run it still may protect the aneurysm from rupture by: (a) redirection of blood flow, and (b) reduction of the systolic thrust inside the aneurysm.

Aneurysm Size

Several investigators have obtained late postoperative arteriograms to determine the incidence of reduction in aneurysm size (42, 55, 60,97,105,111–114,118,118a,125,126,147,160, 169, 176, 178). The majority of cases studied demonstrated a reduction in aneurysm size or disappearance of the aneurysm. Visualization of the aneurysm was by contrast media injection into: (a) the ipsilateral carotid artery above the clamp (often thrombosed); (b) the opposite carotid artery with cross filling; or (c) the vertebrobasilar circulation with forward filling through the posterior communicating artery. The latter method is usually the best technique. ACoAA and MCAA cases had the lowest incidence of size reduction. ICAA cases had the best protection from cervical carotid ligation as evidenced by the high incidence of reduction in aneurysm size in these cases.

Nishioka (118,118a) reported that two-thirds of the ICAA cases in the 1966 Cooperative Study showed a reduction in aneurysm size. Similarly, Odom and Tindall (125) demonstrated that in 77% of their ICAA cases the aneurysm was smaller or absent. Tuerk et al. (176) correlated maximal reduction in aneurysm size with a narrow aneurysm neck and long aneurysm sac causing stasis in the aneurysm.

Rebleed Incidence

Whereas the ICA or retinal artery pressure evaluations and the angiographic studies on aneurysm size suggest protection for the aneurysm, the final common denominator is the incidence of rebleed after completion of the ligation. Tindall (167) stated that "carotid ligation should result in permanent reduction in distal intravascular pressure for lasting benefit in treatment of intracranial aneurysms." However, does it result in *lasting* benefit?

Late recurrent bleeding following carotid ligature has been reported by various authors (2, 55, 79, 84, 86, 91, 105, 112, 125, 138, 149, 194). Their statistics are not very helpful due to failure to give an annual rebleeding rate (i.e., annual risk of rebleed per surviving patient). Furthermore, as Nishioka (118,118a) noted, some rebleeds may be SAH from another aneurysm or from another cause. Nishioka (118,118a) reviewed the 1966 Cooperative Study statistics, and the report of an 8% incidence of rebleed in 577 cases suffers from the same criticism. Only 462 of these cases were ligated for a single ICAA. The incidence of rebleeding for MCAA and ACoAA after carotid ligation was significantly higher than for ICAA.

In 1977 Winn et al. (189) reported on their long-term study of 34 cases of pcaICAA treated by CCA ligation. The study began 6 months after the ligation. They found no difference in rebleed rate (3% per year) between the treated cases and the nonoperated control group (pp. 608–609).

Complications

Table 33.1 summarizes the reported complications of cervical carotid artery ligation when used as treatment for intracranial aneurysm. Their incidence varies considerably, depending on the author (3, 5, 6, 14, 16, 17, 19, 25, 28, 36, 40, 45, 55, 56, 63, 64, 66, 79, 80, 84, 86, 91, 95, 98, 99, 104, 105, 112, 115, 116, 118, 118a, 124, 125, 127, 138, 147, 149–151, 155, 156, 164–167, 171, 172, 181, 184, 189, 194, 195). Good reviews are given by Dorrance (36), Hamby (66), Murphy (116), Walton (184), Luessenhop et al. (105), Nishioka (118,118a), Horwitz and Rizzoli (80), and Odom (124). Also see Chapter 11 for more details.

The most common complication is cerebral ischemia either from carotid occlusion in the presence of inadequate collateral circulation or from embolic phenomenon. Often it is impossible to determine which is responsible. These situations lead to hemispheric signs and occasional ipsilateral blindness. Sudden deterioration may be due to rebleed from the same or another aneurysm. Rarely the change in flow patterns encourages later formation of a new aneurysm on the other side (164). Occasionally there are cardiac arrhythmias from carotid sinus irritation, vascular hypertension from CCA ligation below the carotid sinus, or vascular hypotension from ICA ligation above the carotid sinus (25,155,189). Local complications in the cervical carotid artery (infection, hemorrhage, recanalization, poststenotic aneurysm formation) are uncommon. Often the patient deteriorates as a result of the natural course of the original SAH and its complications. Carotid ligation aggravates already reduced cerebral perfusion from increased intracranial pressure, hematoma, hydrocephalus, edema, and vasospasm.

Table 33.1. Complications of Carotid Ligation

Inadequate cerebral perfusion
Propagating thrombus
From internal carotid artery
From aneurysm sac
Embolization from ICA
Recurrent subarachnoid hemorrhage
From treated aneurysm
From another aneurysm
Development of new contralateral aneurysm
Carotid sinus malfunction
Cardiac arrhythmias
Blood pressure changes
Cervical carotid artery changes
Infection
Hemorrhage
Recanalization
Aneurysm of cervical carotid artery
Aggravation of SAH complication

There is an increased incidence of ischemic complications associated with increased CSF blood, increased CSF pressure, short time between SAH and ligation, poor grade status, poor medical condition, old age, stenosis of the opposite ICA, vascular hypotension or severe vascular hypertension, and the presence of bilateral intracranial aneurysms. Ischemic signs may appear as late as 15 days after ligation (17). However, 80% occur within the first 2 days and 90% within the first 4 days of completion of the ligation (118,118a). The incidence of these complications is greater with ICA ligation than with CCA ligation in most series. Whereas ICA ligation permits retrograde flow from the ECA through the ophthalmic artery, it unfortunately prevents ECA–ICA flow; this flow precludes thrombosis and embolic phenomena within the ICA system, a factor responsible for the greater safety of CCA ligation. Most workers prefer gradual occlusion, but there is still discussion as to whether acute occlusion causes more complications than does gradual occlusion of the cervical carotid artery.

Tindall (167) listed six contraindications to carotid ligation for aneurysm treatment:

1. Grade 3–5 status
2. Intracerebral clot
3. Vasospasm
4. Intolerance to test occlusion
5. Contralateral carotid stenosis
6. Serious systemic disease

Summary

Ligation of arteries proximal to the aneurysm (see pp. 670–672 and 812–816 for other arteries) has been common treatment in the past. Ligation of the cervical carotid artery is uncommonly used now as standard treatment for an intracranial aneurysm, although it still finds a place in some cases with inoperable ICAA due to aneurysmal size, position, or configuration. Even in 1953 Sjöqvist opined (157):

> The physiological function of the circle of Willis will make it evident that ligature of one carotid artery cannot occlude a basal aneurysm provided the communicating arteries are still patent, and if this is not the case grave circulatory disturbances of one cerebral hemisphere will result from the ligature. The ideal method would be a direct intracranial attack on the aneurysm itself occluding it in one way or another.

Bibliography

1. Albright F: The syndrome produced by aneurysm at or near the junction of the internal carotid artery and the circle of Willis. Johns Hopkins Hosp Bull 44:215–245, 1929
2. Alexander E Jr, David CH Jr, Kester NC: Intracranial aneurysms. Methods of treatment; value of hypothermia in the surgical approach. Arch Neurol Psychiatry 81:684–692, 1959
3. Allen MB Jr, Meeks WH: A review of current concepts regarding intracranial saccular aneurysms. Part I. Introduction and etiology. J Med Assoc G 56:355–360, 1967
4. Amias GA: Cerebral vascular disease in pregnancy. I. Haemorrhage. J Obstet Gynaecol Br Commonw 77:100–120, 1970
5. Arseni C, Nash F: Cerebral ischemia in the course of ruptured aneurysms. Eur Neurol 1:308–323, 1968
6. Austin DC: A review of intracranial aneurysms. Henry Ford Hosp Med Bull 12:251–271, 1964
7. Bakay L: Pressure in intracranial arteries and flow in aneurysms. NY State J Med 74: 1779–1781, 1974
8. Bakay L, Sweet WH: Cervical and intracranial intra-arterial pressures with and without vascular occlusion. Surg Gynecol Obstet 95:67–75, 1952
9. Bakay L, Sweet WH: Intra-arterial pressures in the neck and brain. Late changes after carotid closure, acute measurements after vertebral closure. J Neurosurg 10:353–359, 1953
10. Bassett RC, Gass HH: Ligation of internal carotid artery for aneurysmal lesions of circle of Willis. JAMA 177:842–846, 1951
11. Bassett RC, List CF, Lemmen LJ: Surgical treatment of intracranial aneurysm. Surg Gynecol Obstet 95:701–708, 1952
12. Beadles CF: Aneurysms of the larger cerebral arteries. Brain 30:285–336, 1907
13. Beekman F: Studies in aneurysm by William and John Hunter. Ann Med Hist 8:124–127, 1936
14. Bird AC, Nolan B, Gargano FP, et al.: Unruptured aneurysm of the supraclinoid carotid artery. A treatable cause of blindness. Neurology 20:445–454, 1970
15. Blaauw G, Braakman R: Carotid ligation for carotid aneurysms. Clin Neurol Neurosurg 79:187–202, 1976
16. Black SPW, German WJ: The treatment of internal carotid artery aneurysms by proximal arterial ligation. A follow-up study. J Neurosurg 10:590–601, 1953
17. Boldrey E: Long-term follow-up of aneurysms of the internal carotid-middle cerebral system. West J Surg 72:126–129, 1964
18. Bornstein MB, Bender MB: Subarachnoid hematoma complicating ruptured intracranial arterial aneurysm. Arch Intern Med 100:50–58, 1957
19. Brackett CE Jr: The complications of carotid artery ligation in the neck. J Neurosurg 10:91–106, 1953
20. Brackett CE Jr, Mount LA: Some observations on intra-carotid blood pressure made during carotid ligation for intracranial aneurysms. Surg Forum 48:344–350, 1950
21. Bucy PC: Cerebral vascular diseases. Neurosurgical aspects and therapeutic approach. In

Wright IS, Luckey EH: Cerebral Vascular Diseases. New York, Grune & Stratton, 1955, pp 133–144
22. Bull JWD: Massive aneurysms at the base of the brain. Brain 92:535–570, 1969
23. Cantu RC: Oculomotor palsy with posterior communicating artery aneurysm. Outcome with carotid ligation versus medical therapy. Int Surg 52:144–150, 1969
24. Chadduck WM, Crutchfield WG, Keswani RK: Clinical and experimental studies on gradual occlusion of the internal carotid artery. Surg Gynecol Obstet 121:1–9, 1965
25. Cook AW: Cartoid ligation for aneurysms [letter]. J. Neurosurg 42:118,1975.
26. Cristiansson J: On the late effect of carotid ligation upon the human eye. Acta Ophthalmol (Copenh) 40:271–280, 1962
27. Crutchfield WG: Instruments for use in the treatment of certain intracranial vascular lesions. J Neurosurg 16:471–475, 1959
28. Czernobilsky B, Bouzarth WF: Vascular malformations in the brain in a patient with multiple telangiectasia of the intestine and lungs. J Am Med Wom Assoc 20:337–340, 1965
29. Dandy WE: Intercranial Arterial Aneurysms. New York, Hafner, 1944, reprinted 1969.
30. Dandy WE: Results following bands and ligatures on human internal carotid artery. Ann Surg 123:384–396, 1946
31. Dandy WE: Results following ligation of the internal carotid artery. Arch Surg 45:521–533, 1942
32. Dandy WE: The surgical treatment of intracranial aneurysms of the internal carotid artery. Ann Surg 114:336–340, 1941
33. Davis CH Jr, Alexander E Jr: Intracranial aneurysms: an evaluation of methods of treatment. South Med J 52:357–360, 1959
34. Davis RA, Wetzel N, Davis L: An analysis of the results of treatment of intracranial vascular lesions by carotid artery ligation. Ann Surg 143:641–648, 1956
35. De Morais JV, Lana-Peixoto MT: Bilateral intracavernous carotid aneurysms: treatment by bilateral carotid ligation. Surg Neurol 9:379–381, 1978
36. Dorrance GM: Ligation of the great vessels of the neck. Ann Surg 99:721–742, 1934
37. Dott NM: Intracranial aneurysmal formations. Clin Neurosurg 16:1–15, 1969
38. Dott NM: Intracranial aneurysms: cerebral arterio-radiography: surgical treatment. Edinburgh Med J 40:(section on Trans Med-Chir Soc Edinburgh):219–234, 1933
39. Dowling JL: Surgical treatment of spontaneous subarachnoid haemorrhage. Med J Aust 2:130–135, 1953
39a. Drake CG: Giant intracranial aneurysms: experience with surgical treatment in 174 patients. Clin Neurosurg 26:12–95, 1979
40. Drew JH, Sweet WH: Complications of ligation of carotid artery in young people for treatment of intracranial aneurysm. J Nerv Ment Dis 112:79–82, 1950
41. Dukes HT, Odom GL, Woodhall B: The unilateral anterior cerebral circulation. Its importance in the management of aneurysms of the anterior communicating artery. J Neurosurg 22:40–46, 1965
42. Ecker A, Riemenschneider PA: Arteriographic demonstration of spasm of the intracranial arteries with special reference to saccular arterial aneurysms. J Neurosurg 8:660–667, 1951
43. Ectors L: La ligature de la carotide commune. Neurochirurgie 3:262–267, 1957
44. Ectors L: Traitement des anévrismes intracrâniens. Acta Neurol Belg 50:442–456, 1950
45. Fager CA: The effectiveness and risk of carotid ligation in the treatment of intracranial aneurysms. Lahey Clin Bull 10:226–233, 1958
46. Fager CA, Poppen JL: Observations on controlled ligation of the internal carotid artery. Surg Clin North Am 36:567–582, 1956
47. Falconer MA: Progress in the surgical treatment of spontaneous cerebral haemorrhage. Proc R Soc Med 49:166–169, 1956
48. Falconer MA: Surgical treatment of spontaneous intracranial haemorrhage. Br Med J 1:790–792, 1958
49. Falconer MA: Surgical treatment of spontaneous subarachnoid haemorrhage. Preliminary report. Br Med J 1:809–813, 1950
50. Falconer MA: The future of surgery in the treatment of spontaneous cerebral haemorrhage. Lancet 2:945–950, 1952
51. Falconer MA: The surgical treatment of bleeding intracranial aneurysms. J Neurol Neurosurg Psychiatry 14:153–186, 1951
52. Ferguson GG: Direct measurement of mean and pulsatile blood pressure of operation in human intracranial saccular aneurysms. J Neurosurg 36:560–563, 1972
53. Fox JL, Albin MS, Bader DCH, et al.: Microsurgical treatment of neurovascular disease. Neurosurgery 3:285–337, 1978
54. Galbraith JG: Monitoring of brain oxygenation during carotid ligation. J Neurosurg 27:102–104, 1967
55. Galbraith JG, Clark RM: Role of carotid ligation in the management of intracranial carotid aneurysms. Clin Neurosurg 21:171–181, 1974
56. German WJ: Intracranial aneurysms. J Maine Med Assoc 38:190, 1947

57. German WJ, Black SPW: Cervical ligation for internal carotid aneurysms. An extended follow-up. J Neurosurg 23:572–577, 1965
58. Giannotta SL, Kindt GW: Total morbidity and mortality rates of patients with surgically treated intracranial aneurysms. Neurosurgery 4:125–128, 1979
59. Giannotta SL, McGillicuddy JE, Kindt GW: Gradual carotid artery occlusion in the treatment of inaccessible internal carotid artery aneurysms. Neurosurgery 5:417–421, 1979
60. Gibbs JR: Effects of carotid ligation on the size of internal carotid aneurysms. J Neurol Neurosurg Psychiatry 28:383–394, 1965
61. Gibbs JR: Torsion: a new technique for closure of the cervical carotid artery. Br J Surg 52:947–952, 1965
62. Gillingham FJ: The management of ruptured intracranial aneurysm. Ann R Coll Surg 23:89–117, 1958
63. Gross SW, Holzman A: Aneurysm of common carotid artery in the neck following partial ligation for an intracranial aneurysm. J Neurosurg 11:209–212, 1954
64. Gurdjian ES, Thomas LM, Herman LH, et al.: Angiographic findings in 300 cases of aneurysm, arteriovenous malformation, and subarachnoid hemorrhage. In Fields WS, Sahs AL (eds.): Intracranial Aneurysms and Subarachnoid Hemorrhage. Springfield, Ill., Thomas, 1965, pp. 143–183
65. Halsted WS: Partial, progressive and complete occlusion of the aorta and other large arteries in the dog by means of the metal band. J Exp Med 11:373–391, 1909
66. Hamby WB: Intracranial Aneurysms. Springfield, Ill., Thomas, 1952
67. Hamby WB: The modern treatment of intracranial aneurysms. NY State J Med 52:2497–2502, 1952
68. Hamby WB, Gardner WJ: Treatment of pulsating exophthalmos with report of two cases. Arch Surg 27:676–685, 1933
69. Hamilton JG, Falconer MA: Immediate and late results of surgery in cases of saccular intracranial aneurysms. J Neurosurg 16:514–541, 1959
70. Hanbery JW: Pathology, diagnosis, and treatment of intracranial aneurysms. Stanford Med Bull 13:317–341, 1955
71. Handel SF, Perpetuo FOL, Handel CH: Subdural hematomas due to ruptured cerebral aneurysms: angiographic diagnosis and potential pitfall for CT. Am J Roentgenol 130:507–509, 1978
72. Hardesty WH, Roberts B, Toole JF, et al.: Studies on carotid artery flow. Surgery 49:251–256, 1961
73. Hardy WG, Thomas LM, Webster JE, et al.: Carotid ligation for intracranial aneurysm. A follow-up study of 54 patients. J Neurosurg 15:281–289, 1958
74. Harkness GF: Intracranial arterio-venous aneurysm: pulsating exophthalmos. Int J Med Surg 43:243–249, 1930
75. Harris P, Udvarhelyi GB: Aneurysms arising at the internal carotid-posterior communicating artery junction. J Neurosurg 14:180–191, 1957
76. Heyman A, Tindall GT, Finney WHM, et al.: Measurement of retinal artery and intracarotid pressures following carotid artery occlusion with the Crutchfield clamp. J Neurosurg 17:297–305, 1960
77. Holmes AE, James IM, Wise CC: Observations on distal intravascular pressure changes and cerebral blood flow after common carotid artery ligation in man. J Neurol Neurosurg Psychiatry 34:78–81, 1971
78. Home E: An account of Mr. Hunter's method of performing the operation for the cure of the popliteal aneurysm. Trans Soc Improvement Med Chir Knowledge 1:138–181, 1793
79. Höök O, Norlén G: Aneurysms of the internal carotid artery. Acta Neurol Scand 40:200–218, 1964
80. Horwitz NH, Rizzoli HV: Aneurysms and arteriovenous fistulas. In Postoperative Complications in Neurosurgical Practice. Recognition, Prevention, and Management. Baltimore, Williams & Wilkins, 1967, pp. 83–129
81. Jain KK: Partial carotid occlusion as treatment for intracranial internal carotid aneurysms. Can Med Assoc J 88:247–251, 1963
82. Jawad K, Miller JD, Fitch W, et al.: Measurement of jugular venous blood gases for prediction of brain ischaemia following carotid ligation. Eur Neurol 14:43–52, 1976
83. Jawad K, Miller JD, Wyper DJ, et al.: Measurement of CBF and carotid artery pressure compared with cerebral angiography in assessing collateral blood supply after carotid ligation. J Neurosurg 46:185–196, 1977
84. Jefferson G: Discussion. Proc R Soc Med 45: 301–303, 1952
85. Jefferson G: On the saccular aneurysms of the internal carotid artery in the cavernous sinus. Br J Surg 26:267–302, 1938
86. Jeffreys RV, Holmes AE: Common carotid ligation for the treatment of ruptured posterior communicating aneurysms. J Neurol Neurosurg Psychiatry 34:576–579, 1971
87. Jennett B, Miller JD, Harper AM: Effect of Carotid Artery Surgery on Cerebral Blood Flow. Amsterdam, Excerpta Medica, 1976
88. Jennett WB, Harper AM, Gillespie FC: Measurement of regional cerebral blood-flow during carotid ligation. Lancet 2:1162–1163, 1966

89. Johnson HC: Cervical intracarotid pressure studies: their significance in the management of intracranial aneurysms. Surgery 33:537–543, 1953
90. Johnson HC: Surgery of cerebral vascular anomalies. In Walker AE (ed.): A History of Neurological Surgery. Baltimore, Williams & Wilkins, 1951, pp. 250–269; reprinted: New York, Hafner, 1967
91. Kak VK, Taylor AR, Gordon DS: Proximal carotid ligation for internal carotid aneurysms. A long-term follow-up study. J Neurosurg 39:503–513, 1973
92. Keen WW: Intracranial lesions. Med News (NY) 57:439–449, 1890
93. Kessler LA, Wholey MH: Internal carotid occlusion for treatment of intracranial aneurysms. A new percutaneous technique. Radiology 95:581–583, 1970
94. King JEJ: Discussion of Davis RA, Wetzel N, Davis L: An analysis of the results of treatment of intracranial vascular lesions by carotid artery ligation. Ann Surg 143:649–650, 1956
95. Klemme WM: Hemorrhage from a previously undemonstrated intracranial aneurysm as a late complication of carotid artery ligation. Case report. J Neurosurg 46:654–658, 1977
96. Krayenbühl H, Yaşargil MG: Diagnosis and therapy of intracranial aneurysms. In Cooper P, Nyhus LM (eds.): Surgery Annual. New York, Appleton-Century-Crofts, 1970, pp. 327–343
97. Kricheff II, Chase NE, Lin JP, et al.: Brachial angiography for the evaluation of carotid artery occlusion in the treatment of "posterior communicating" aneurysm. Radiology 91: 1140–1146, 1968
98. Landolt AM, Millikan CH: Pathogenesis of cerebral infarction secondary to mechanical carotid artery occlusion. Stroke 1:52–62, 1970
99. Lee JF, Tindall GT: Arterial erosion and hemorrhage during graded carotid ligation with the Crutchfield clamp. J Neurosurg 27:52–55, 1967
100. Leech PJ, Miller JD, Fitch W, et al.: Cerebral blood flow, internal carotid artery pressure, and the EEG as a guide to the safety of carotid ligation. J Neurol Neurosurg Psychiatry 37: 854–862, 1974
101. Lipovšek M: Ruptured aneurysms of the proximal middle cerebral artery. J Neurosurg 39:498–502, 1973
102. List CF: Diagnosis and treatment of intracranial aneurysms. Arch Neurol Psychiatry 68:842–845, 1952
103. Lobstein A, Phillippidès D, Montrieul B: La mesure des pressions artérielles rétinienne et intracarotidienne au cours de la ligature de la carotide. Rev Otoneuroophthalmol 25:216–226, 1953
104. Love JG, Dart LH: Results of carotid ligation with particular reference to intracranial aneurysms. J Neurosurg 27:89–93, 1967
105. Luessenhop AJ, Mora F, Sweet WH: Subarachnoid hemorrhage, intracranial aneurysms and arterio-venous anomalies; treatment by cervical carotid occlusion. In Fields WS (ed.): Pathogenesis and Treatment of Cerebrovascular Disease. Springfield, Ill., Thomas, 1961, pp. 516–553
106. Martinez Coll A, Del Corral JF, Yazawa S, et al.: Intra-aneurysmal pressure differences in human saccular aneurysms. Surg Neurol 6:93–96, 1976
107. Matas R: Aneurysms of the circle of Willis. A discussion of Dr. Dandy's intracranial occlusion of the internal carotid for aneurysms of the circle of Willis, with supplementary remarks. Ann Surg 107:660–680, 1938
108. Matas R: Testing the efficiency of the collateral circulation as a preliminary to the occlusion of the great surgical arteries. Ann Surg 53:1–43, 1911
109. McKissock W, Richardson A, Walsh L: "Posterior-communicating" aneurysms. A controlled trial of conservative and surgical treatment of ruptured aneurysms of the internal carotid artery at or near the point of origin of the posterior communicating artery. Lancet 1:1203–1206, 1960
110. Miller JD, Jawad K, Jennett B: Safety of carotid ligation and its role in the management of intracranial aneurysms. J Neurol Neurosurg Psychiatry 40:64–72, 1977
111. Morris L: Arteriographic studies in aneurysm of the internal carotid artery treated by carotid occlusion. Acta Radio[Diagn] (Stockh) 1:367–372, 1963
112. Mount LA: Results of treatment of intracranial aneurysms using the Selverstone clamp. J Neurosurg 16:611–618, 1959
113. Mount LA, Taveras JM: Cerebral angiographic studies following surgical treatment of intracranial aneurysms. Angiographic evaluation of results. Acta Radiol 46:333–341, 1956
114. Mount LA, Taveras JM: The results of surgical treatment of intracranial aneurysms as demonstrated by progress arteriography. J Neurosurg 13:618–626, 1956
115. Murphy F: Extracranial carotid ligation: technical aspects. In Fields WS, Sahs AL (eds.): Intracranial Aneurysms and Subarachnoid Hemorrhage. Springfield, Ill., Thomas, 1965, pp. 315–323
116. Murphy JP: Subarachnoid hemorrhage; intracranial aneurysm. In Cerebrovascular Disease. Chicago, Year Book, 1954, pp. 199–241

117. Nicholds P: Screw-clamp stenosis for internal carotid aneurysms [letter]. J Neurosurg 43:122, 1975
118. Nishioka H: Evaluation of the conservative management of ruptured intracranial aneurysms. In Sahs AL, Perret GE, Locksley HB, et al. (eds.): Intracranial Aneurysms and Subarachnoid Hemorrhage. A Cooperative Study. Philadelphia, Lippincott, 1969, pp. 125–142
118a. Nishioka H: Report on the cooperative study of intracranial aneurysms and subarachnoid hemorrhage. Section VII, Part I. Evaluation of the conservative management of ruptured intracranial aneurysms. J Neurosurg 25:574–592, 1966
119. Nofzinger JD, Britt LG, Murphy F, et al.: Unusual treatment of an intracranial aneurysm contralateral to a previous common carotid ligation. A case report. J Neurosurg 22:182–184, 1965
120. Norlén G: Klinik und chirurgische Behandlung der sackförmigen Hirnaneurysmen. Dtsch Z Nervenheilk 170:446–459, 1953
121. Northfield DWC: The Surgery of the Central Nervous System. Oxford, Blackwell, 1973, pp. 346–401
122. Nunneley T: On vascular protrusion of the eyeball. Trans Med Chir Soc 48:15–37, 1865
123. O'Conner PS, Smith JL, Yates BM: Crossed external carotid ligation for giant aneurysms. Surg Neurol 9:382–385, 1978
124. Odom GL: Carotid ligation in the treatment of intracranial aneurysms. In Morley TP (ed.): Current Controversies in Neurosurgery. Philadelphia, 1976, pp. 270–273
125. Odom GL, Tindall GT: Carotid ligation in the treatment of certain intracranial aneurysms. Clin Neurosurg 15:101–116, 1968
126. Odom GL, Woodhall B, Tindall GT, et al.: Changes in distal intravascular pressure and size of intracranial aneurysm following common carotid ligation. J Neurosurg 19:41–50, 1962
127. Oldershaw JB, Voris HC: Internal carotid artery ligation. A follow-up study. Neurology (NY) 16:937–938, 1966
128. Olivecrona H: Ligature of the carotid artery in intracranial aneurysms. Acta Chir Scand 91:353–368, 1944
129. Oppenheim H: Lehrbuch der Nervenkrankheiten für Ärzte und Studierende, Vol 2. Berlin, Karger, 1913, pp. 1226–1231
130. Palmer JF (ed.): Hunter's Principles of Surgery. Philadelphia, Haswell, Barrington & Haswell, 1839, pp. 309–316
131. Palmer JF (ed.): The Works of John Hunter, F.R.S., with Notes, Vol 1. London, Longman, Rees, Orme, Brown, Green, and Longman, 1835, pp. 96–101, 536–551
132. Palmer JF (ed.): The Works of John Hunter, F.R.S., with Notes, Vol 3. London, Longman, Rees, Orme, Brown, Green, and Longman, 1837, pp. 159–173
133. Pertuiset B: La ligature progressive de la carotide interne dans le cou technique personnelle d'après 14 cas. Neurochirurgia (Stuttg) 6:103–107, 1963
134. Pool JL, Potts DG: Aneurysms and Arteriovenous Anomalies of the Brain. Diagnosis and Treatment. New York, Harper & Row, 1965
135. Poppen JL: Ligation of the internal carotid artery in the neck. Prevention of certain complications. J Neurosurg 7:532–538, 1950
136. Poppen JL, Fager CA: Intracranial aneurysms. Results of surgical treatment. J Neurosurg 17:283–296, 1960
137. Potter JM, Taylor FM: Electroencephalography during carotid occlusion. Arch Neurol Psychiatry 74:414–423, 1955
138. Raja IA: Common carotid ligation for intracranial aneurysm. Follow-up study of 144 patients. Vasc Surg 4:95–100, 1970
139. Raja, IA, Marshall M, Hankinson J: Effects of low-molecular-weight dextran and other factors in common carotid ligation. Angiology 21:151–160, 1970
140. Rand RW: Retinal arterial pressure studies associated with cervical carotid artery occlusion in the treatment of cerebral aneurysms. Bull Los Angeles Neurol Soc 21:175–187, 1956
141. Raskind R: Carotid artery ligation for intracranial aneurysm. Angiology 17:46–55, 1966
142. Raskind R, Doria A: Long term follow-up of intracranial aneurysms treated by cervical carotid artery ligation. Angiology 19:326–331, 1968
143. Raskind R, Weiss SR, Doria A: Common carotid artery ligation for intracranial aneurysm in patients over 50. Geriatrics 27:87–93, 1972
144. Rogers L: Carotid ligation for intracranial aneurysm. Report of a case studied by electroencephalography. Br J Surg 32:309–311, 1944
145. Rogers L: Ligation of the common carotid artery. Report of 19 personal cases. Lancet 1:949–950, 1949
146. Rogers L: Ligature of arteries, with particular reference to carotid occlusion and the circle of Willis. Br J Surg 35:43–50, 1947
147. Rossi P, Rosenblum AE, Zingesser LH: The fate of the carotid artery after occlusion for treatment of aneurysm. Radiology 95:567–575, 1970
148. Ruberti R: La legatura della carotide cervical nel trattamento chirurgico degli aneurismi sacculari intracranici. Acta Chir Ital 16:405–411, 1960
149. Salar G, Mingrino S: Ligature of the cervical carotid artery for the treatment of intracranial

carotid aneurysms. Complications and late results. Acta Neurochir (Wien) 36:152, 1977
150. Schorstein J: Carotid ligation in saccular intracranial aneurysms. Br J Surg 28:50–70, 1940
151. Scott M, Skwarok E: The treatment of cerebral aneurysms by ligation of the common carotid artery. Surg Gynecol Obstet 113:54–61, 1961
152. Selverstone B, White JC: A method for gradual occlusion of the internal carotid artery in the treatment of aneurysm. Proc N Engl Cardiovasc Soc 9:24–25, 1952
153. Selverstone B, White JC: A new technique for gradual occlusion of the carotid artery. Arch Neurol Psychiatry 66:246, 1951
154. Sharkey PC, Apostolcu A: Intracranial aneurysms: a partial community study. South Med J 59:185–191, 1966
155. Shenkin HA, Cabieses F, van den Noordt G, et al.: The hemodynamic effect of unilateral carotid ligation on the cerebral circulation of man. J Neurosurg 8:38–45, 1951
156. Shenkin HA, Polakoff P, Finneson BE: Intracranial internal carotid artery aneurysms. Results of treatment by cervical carotid artery ligation. J Neurosurg 15:183–191, 1958
157. Sjöqvist O: Thread ligature of intracranial saccular aneurysms. In Proceedings of the 5th Congress of Neurology, Lisbon, Vol 3, 1953, pp. 108–115
158. Smith FP: Differential carotid ligation for supraclinoid arterial cerebral aneurysms. J Neurosurg 19:787–792, 1962
159. Smolik EA, Nash FP: Intracranial aneurysm in the geriatric patient. Report of three surgically treated patients. JAMA 167:931–935, 1958
160. Somach FM, Shenkin HA: Angiographic end-results of carotid ligation in the treatment of carotid aneurysm. J Neurosurg 24:966–974, 1966
161. Steelman HF, Hayes GJ, Rizzoli HV: Surgical treatment of saccular intracranial aneurysms. J Neurosurg 10:564–576, 1953
162. Stern WE: Studies of pressures in the carotid artery of patients undergoing cerebral angiography. J Neurosurg 10:577–582, 1953
163. Strobos RRJ, Mount LA: Problems related to treatment of intracranial aneurysms by carotid ligation. Arch Neurol Psychiatry 69:118–128, 1953
164. Stuntz JT, Ojemann GA, Alvord EC Jr: Radiographic and histologic demonstration of an aneurysm developing on the infundibulum of the posterior communicating artery. Case report. J Neurosurg 33:591–595, 1970
165. Svien JH, Hollenhorst RW: Pressure in retinal arteries after ligation or occlusion of the carotid artery. Proc Mayo Clin 31:684–692, 1956
166. Sweet WH, Sarnoff SJ, Bakay L: A clinical method for recording internal carotid pressure. Significance of changes during carotid occlusion. Surg Gynecol Obstet 90:327–334, 1950
167. Tindall GT: Management of aneurysms of anterior circulation by carotid artery occlusion. In Youmans JR (ed.): Neurological Surgery, vol 2. Philadelphia, Saunders, 1973, pp. 768–786
168. Tindall GT: The treatment of anterior communicating aneurysms by proximal anterior cerebral artery ligation. Clin Neurosurg 21:134–150, 1974
169. Tindall GT, Goree JA, Lee JF, et al.: Effect of common carotid ligation on size of internal carotid aneurysms and distal intracarotid and retinal artery pressures. J Neurosurg 25:503–511, 1966
170. Tindall GT, Kapp J, Odom GL, et al.: A combined technique for treating certain aneurysms of the anterior communicating artery. J Neurosurg 33:41–47, 1970
171. Tindall GT, Odom GL: Saccular aneurysms of the brain. Surgical treatment. In Vinken PJ, Bruyn GW (eds.): Handbook of Clinical Neurology, Vol 12: Vascular Diseases of the Nervous System, Part II. Amsterdam, North Holland, 1972, pp. 205–226
172. Tindall GT, Odom GL: Treatment of intracranial aneurysms by proximal carotid ligation. Prog Neurol Surg 3:66–114, 1969
173. Tindall GT, Odom GL, Cupp HB Jr, et al.: Studies on carotid artery flow and pressure. Observations in 18 patients during graded occlusion of proximal carotid artery. J Neurosurg 19:917–923, 1962
174. Tindall GT, Odom GL, Dillon MG, et al.: Direction of blood flow in the internal and external carotid arteries following occlusion of the ipsilateral common carotid artery. Observations in 19 patients. J Neurosurg 20:985–994, 1963
175. Tönnis W, Walter W: Die Behandlung der sackförmigen intrakraniellen Aneurysmen. In Olivecrona H, Tönnis W (eds.): Klinik and Behandlung der raumbeengenden intrakraniellen Prozesse. Handbuch der Neurochirurgie, Vol 4, Part 2. Berlin, Springer-Verlag, 1966, pp. 212–363
176. Tuerk K, Chase NE, Kricheff II, et al.: Relation of preoperative angiographic characteristics of the posterior communicating artery to the results of common carotid ligation. J Neurosurg 36:564–568, 1972
177. Tytus JS, Haven H: Present day concepts in the management of intracranial aneurysms. Rev Surg 20:230–240, 1963
178. Tytus JS, Reifel E, Spencer MP, et al.: Common carotid ligation for intracranial aneu-

rysms. Results in 26 cases. J Neurosurg 32:63–73, 1970
179. Uihlein A, Lippert RG: Surgical treatment of verified intracranial aneurysms. Arch Surg 81:1005–1012, 1960
180. Van Meegroot WO: Carotid ligation in the treatment of ruptured intracranial aneurysms. Vasc Surg 1:184–189, 1967
181. Voris HC: Complications of ligation of the internal carotid artery. J Neurosurg 8:119–131, 1951
182. Walsh L: Experience in the conservative and surgical treatment of ruptured intracranial aneurysms. Res Publ Assoc Res Nerv Ment Dis 41:169–178, 1966
183. Walsh LS: Posterior communicating aneurysms. Neurology 11:158–161, 1961
184. Walton JN: Subarachnoid Haemorrhage. Edinburgh, Livingstone, 1956
185. Webster JE, Gurdjian ES: Carotid artery compression as employed both in the past and in the present. J Neurosurg 15:372–384, 1958
186. Werner SC, Blakemore AH, King BG: Aneurysm of internal carotid artery within the skull. Wiring and electrothermic coagulation. JAMA 116:578–582, 1941
187. Wetzel N, Davis RA: An analysis of the results of treatment of intracranial aneurysms by common carotid artery ligation. Surg Forum 6:510–514, 1956
188. Wilkinson HA, Wright RL, Sweet WH: Correlation of reduction in pressure and angiographic cross-filling with tolerance of carotid occlusion. J Neurosurg 22:241–245, 1965
189. Winn HR, Richardson AE, Jane JA: Late morbidity and mortality of common carotid ligation for posterior communicating aneurysms. A comparison to conservative treatment. J Neurosurg 47:727–736, 1977
190. Wise BL, Boldrey E, Aird RB: The value of electroencephalography in studying the effects of ligation of the carotid arteries. Electroencephalogr Clin Neurophysiol 6:261–268, 1954
191. Woodhall B, Odom GL, Bloor BM, et al.: Direct measurement of intravascular pressure in components of the circle of Willis. A contribution to the surgery of congenital cerebral aneurysms and vascular anomalies of the brain. Ann Surg 135:911–921, 1952
192. Woodhall B, Odom GL, Bloor BM, et al.: Studies on cerebral intravascular pressure. Further data concerning residual pressure in components of the circle of Willis and in blind arterial segments. J Neurosurg 10:28–34, 1953
193. Wright RL: Intraaneurysmal pressure reduction with carotid occlusion. Observations in three cases of middle cerebral aneurysms. J Neurosurg 29:139–142, 1968
194. Wright RL, Sweet WH: Carotid or vertebral occlusion in the treatment of intracranial aneurysms; value of early and late readings of carotid and retinal pressures. Clin Neurosurg 9:163–190, 1961
195. Wright R, Sweet WH: Intraarterial pressure determinations at the time of carotid occlusion. In Fields WS, Sahs AL (eds.): Intracranial Aneurysms and Subarachnoid Hemorrhage. Springfield, Ill., Thomas, 1965, pp. 324–346
196. Youmans JR, Kindt GW, Mitchell OC: Extended studies of direction of flow and pressure in the internal carotid artery following common carotid artery ligation. J Neurosurg 27:250–254, 1967

34

Technique of Aneurysm Surgery

I. Frontotemporal Approach

The surgical approach utilized by the author (J.L.F.) for all anterior circulation aneurysms and for aneurysms at or near the bifurcation of the basilar artery is the frontotemporal (also called frontolateral or pterional) approach. All aneurysms on or near the circle of Willis are accessible by this standard approach. The author is indebted to his teachers, including Hugo V. Rizzoli, George J. Hayes, Ludwig G. Kempe, and M. Gazi Yaşargil, whose techniques for the pterional approach were studied and applied. As described elsewhere (Chapter 1 on history and Chapter 29 on cranial approaches) this pterional approach for aneurysms began with Dandy (1), who in 1944 was the first to report on a series of surgically treated aneurysm patients.

The purpose of this and the following chapters on microtechnique is to illustrate the surgical approach to cerebral aneurysms and the surrounding anatomy as seen through an operating microscope. To date, there have been few published comprehensive color illustrations of the surgical anatomy of intracranial aneurysms as seen during a surgical procedure. [The reader is referred to the excellent artistic illustrations of Kempe's atlas (17) as well as the surgical photographs of Yaşargil (31) and Fox (5).] Several of the illustrations found in Chapters 34–39 were reproduced earlier (5). Unless otherwise indicated, all color photographs taken through the operating microscope were made with the original Zeiss magnification dial set at 16 (third setting), providing a true 6× magnification. See page 690 of Chapter 26 for the photographic details about these pictures.

For purposes of reference, Table 34.1 gives abbreviations symbolizing specific aneurysms. Table 34.2 compares the operative results of the author (J.L.F.) during 11 years of surgery (1964–1974) without the routine use of the microscope (15% mortality in 95 operated aneurysms in 95 patients) with the results of his subsequent 7 years of surgery (1975–1981) during which time microtechnique was used routinely. The overall aneurysm-associated mortality during these latter 7 years was 4% among 191 aneurysms; the overall patient mortality was 5% among 146 patients. All deaths were in single-aneurysm cases. During the last 3 years (1979–1981) there were no deaths in 68 patients harboring 95 aneurysms.

The number of patients recognized to have multiple aneurysms has increased with greater utilization of four-vessel angiography using subtraction techniques, magnification, and special views. A few additional aneurysms are seen at surgery now that the author explores much of the circle of Willis with the operating microscope. Twenty-eight patients harbored more than one operated aneurysm; a total of 73 operated aneurysms were associated with another operated aneurysm (i.e., multiple aneurysms). There were no deaths in these cases. Table 34.3 lists these cases.

Our patients were operated on an average (mean and mode) of 10–14 days after the SAH. Patients in a strict grade 1 or 2 (Botterell's 1973 classification as outlined by Lougheed and Marshall; see classification 25 in Appendix 1, p. 1109) often were operated sooner. Patients not in a grade 1 or 2 classification or a Hunt's grade 1a classification (classification 28 in Appendix 1, p. 1109) at 2 weeks post-SAH were delayed until their status improved. Preoperative medical therapy included bedrest in a quiet and

Table 34.1. Abbreviations Symbolizing Specific Aneurysms

Abbreviation	*Specific artery and aneurysm*
ICA	Internal carotid artery
ICAA	Internal carotid artery aneurysm
ppICAA	Aneurysm on segment of ICA within petrous pyramid
csICAA	Aneurysm on segment of ICA within cavernous sinus
ic/csICAA	Aneurysm on infraclinoid segment of ICA, presumably within cavernous sinus
oaICAA	ICAA at ophthalmic artery take-off
vICAA	Ventral or paraclinoid position of ICAA
pcaICAA	ICAA at posterior communicating artery take-off
achaICAA	ICAA at anterior choroidal artery take-off
bICAA	ICAA at terminal bifurcation of ICA
amcaICAA	ICAA at the accessory middle cerebral artery take-off
OA	Ophthalmic artery
OAA	Ophthalmic artery aneurysm
PCoA	Posterior communicating artery
PCoAA	Posterior communicating artery aneurysm
AChA	Anterior choroidal artery
AChAA	Anterior choroidal artery aneurysm
MCA	Middle cerebral artery
MCAA	Middle cerebral artery aneurysm
ACoA	Anterior communicating artery
ACoAA	Anterior communicating artery aneurysm
ACeA	Anterior cerebral artery
A_1AA	Aneurysm of the A-1 or horizontal segment of the ACeA
ACeAA	Anterior cerebral artery aneurysm (distal to ACoA)
anACeAA	Aneurysm of an anomalous ACeA
azACeAA	Aneurysm of an azygous ACeA
BA	Basilar artery
BAA	Basilar artery aneurysm
bBAA	BAA at terminal bifurcation of BA

continued

darkened room, use of a bedside commode if the patient is alert, moderate elevation of the head, phenobarbital for sedation, diazepam as needed for restlessness, meperidine for headache, stool softeners or mild laxatives, antihypertensive medication (methyldopa most commonly) if patient was not in vasospasm, and epsilon-aminocaproic acid (EACA) for antifibrinolysis. See Chapter 22 for details.

During surgery the patient is started on methylprednisolone or dexamethasone, and this is continued for about 3 days after surgery. Approximately 250 ml of 15% mannitol solution is given intravenously as the skin incision is made. Antibiotics are not used. Diphenylhydantoin usually is given for at least 2 years after surgery.

Moderate hyperventilation is maintained to keep the monitored arterial P_{CO_2} at 25–30 mm Hg. A lumbar puncture needle for CSF drainage is left in place (using the special mattress shown in Fig. 26.1). Often lumbar CSF drainage is not needed, but it is available in case the patient has a communicating hydrocephalus that prevents easy access to the basal cisterns.

Close communication with the anesthesiologist is mandatory. In a normotensive patient the systolic blood pressure is maintained at 100–110 mm Hg (measured at the heart level in a supine patient with the head end of the table elevated about 10 degrees). Upon opening the dura, the ICP becomes essentially atmospheric; at this point the systolic BP is reduced to about 90 mm Hg. As the aneurysm is approached, the BP is reduced further to a systolic level of about 70–75. This degree of arterial hypotension is not used if excess brain retraction is needed, vasospasm is obvious, the carotid

Table 34.1 Abbreviations Symbolizing Specific Aneurysms (continued)

Abbreviation	*Specific artery and aneurysm*
scaBAA	BAA at superior cerebellar artery take-off
aicaBAA	BAA at anterior inferior cerebellar artery take-off
vaBAA	BAA at site where vertebral arteries join (i.e., aneurysm at union of vertebral arteries)
trBAA	BAA involving trunk of BA but exact site not specified
uoBAA	BAA of unknown origin (site not specified)
PCeA	Posterior cerebral artery
P_1AA	Aneurysm of the P-1 or horizontal segment of the PCeA
pcaPCeAA	PCeAA at junction of PCoA and PCeA
PCeAA	Posterior cerebral artery aneurysm (distal to PCoA)
PChA	Posterior choroidal artery
PChAA	Posterior choroidal artery aneurysm
thvChAA	Aneurysm of choroidal arteries in roof of third ventricle
SCA	Superior cerebellar artery
SCAA	Superior cerebellar artery aneurysm
AICA	Anterior inferior cerebellar artery
AICAA	Anterior inferior cerebellar artery aneurysm
VA	Vertebral artery
VAA	Vertebral artery aneurysm
picaVAA	VAA at posterior inferior cerebellar artery take-off
uoVAA	VAA of unknown origin (site not specified)
PICA	Posterior inferior cerebellar artery
PICAA	Posterior inferior cerebellar artery aneurysm
PrTA	Primitive trigeminal artery
PrTAA	Primitive trigeminal artery aneurysm
PrOA	Primitive otic artery
PrOAA	Primitive otic artery aneurysm
PrHA	Primitive hypoglossal artery
PrHAA	Primitive hypoglossal artery aneurysm
perfAA	Aneurysm of perforating arteries of circle of Willis

artery is retracted (for BAA cases), or a major artery is temporarily occluded. If the latter situation exists, we often raise the BP to hypertensive levels in order to maintain good collateral circulation to the brain.

There are certain periods during the operation when the aneurysm is most prone to premature rupture; these are detailed in Chapter 32. In addition, another remote aneurysm may be at risk to bleed at any time. The surgeon must keep the anesthesiologist closely informed of his activities to avoid untoward BP elevations, especially in the presence of ICP reduction.

The reader is referred to Chapter 26 for details of positioning, equipment, and instrumentation used by this author.

The Flap

The right-sided approach is used for all right ICAA, right MCAA, ACoAA, and terminal BAA unless a midline aneurysm is associated with an operated left-sided aneurysm. The left-sided approach is used for all left ICAA, left MCAA, and any ACoAA or terminal BAA associated with an operated left ICAA or MCAA. Rarely, the ACoAA or terminal BAA is approached from the left side if the aneurysm neck cannot be safely clipped from the right side owing to orientation of the aneurysm. We believe the right-sided approach usually is safer because the dominant hemisphere of the brain is not subjected to any risk of retraction pressure or vessel occlusion. Also, such an approach is more comfortable for the right-handed surgeon. We

Table 34.2. Aneurysms Treated by Intracranial Surgery: Results

	Without microscope, 1964–1974		*With microscope, 1975–1981*	
Arterial site	*No. of aneurysms*	*Deaths*	*No. of aneurysms*	*Deaths*
Internal carotid, cavernous sinus	0	0	2	0
Internal carotid, ophthalmic	2	0	8	0
Internal carotid, ventral	0	0	5	0
Internal carotid, posterior communicating	28	4	37	0
Internal carotid, anterior choroidal	2	0	13	0
Internal carotid, bifurcation	3	1	7	1
Middle cerebral	18	2	35	0
Anterior communicating	33	5	42	3
Anterior cerebral, A-1	0	0	1	0
Anterior cerebral, distal	2	1	4	0
Basilar, bifurcation	4	0	21	4
Basilar, superior cerebellar	0	0	7	0
Basilar, AICA	0	0	1	0
Basilar, trunk	1	1	0	0
Superior cerebellar artery	0	0	1	0
Vertebral, PICA	2	0	6	0
Posterior inferior cerebellar	0	0	1	0
Total	95	14	191	8
Percent mortality		15%		4%
1979–1981 Mortality (95 aneurysms)				0%

Table 35.3. Operated Multiple Aneurysms

Doubles in 15 patients				
L-pcaICAA	+ L-achaICAA			
L-pcaICAA	+ L-oaICAA			
R-pcaICAA	+ R-oaICAA			
R-pcaICAA	+ R-achaICAA			
R-pcaICAA	+ L-pcaICAA			
L-pcaICAA	+ L-achaICAA			
L-pcaICAA	+ R-pcaICAA			
R-pcaICAA	+ R-MCAA			
R-vICAA	+ bBAA			
R-vICAA	+ R-achaICAA			
R-MCAA	+ R-MCAA			
L-MCAA	+ ACoAA			
L-bICAA	+ R-bICAA			
ACoAA	+ ACoAA			
bBAA	+ R-oaICAA			
Triples in 10 patients				
L-pcaICAA	+ L-MCAA	+ bBAA		
R-pcaICAA	+ R-MCAA	+ bBAA		
R-pcaICAA	+ ACoAA	+ bBAA		
L-pcaICAA	+ R-achaICAA	+ L-achaICAA		
R-pcaICAA	+ L-achaICAA	+ L-MCAA		
L-pcaICAA	+ L-achaICAA	+ R-MCAA		
L-MCAA	+ ACoAA	+ bBAA		
L-ACeAA	+ L-scaBAA	+ bBAA		
R-achaICAA	+ ACoAA	+ L-scaBAA		
R-MCAA	+ L-MCAA	+ bICAA		
Quadruples in 2 patients				
L-oaICAA	+ R-oaICAA	+ R-MCAA	+ L-vICAA	
L-oaICAA	+ R-oaICAA	+ L-achaICAA	+ L-achaICAA	
Quintuples in 1 patient				
R-MCAA	+ L-MCAA	+ ACoAA	+ L-ACeAA	+ R-aicaBAA

have adopted this practice in most cases even if the midline aneurysm points to the right or arises toward the side of a dominant, left A-1 or P-1 parent artery.

All surgical photographs shown in this and subsequent chapters illustrate the right-sided approach. For teaching purposes, cases done from the left side have had their color photographs reversed to maintain anatomic orientation. To maintain radiographic consistency in this book, most lateral skull x-ray films and most right or left angiograms in the lateral projection have been photographed as if being observed from the left side.

For a right frontolateral craniotomy, the head is held in a three-point skull-fixation apparatus (Fig. 26.3) and turned approximately 45° to the left, tilted 15° to the left, and dropped back about 15° (Fig. 34.1). This brings the "psychopathic point"[1] into the center and to the highest point of the operative field (see Chapter 29, p. 758). For MCAA and bICAA the head is dropped back as far as possible so that the surgeon's line of vision is as perpendicular as possible to the M-1 portion of the middle cerebral artery. However, this makes sphenoid wing

[1] The point where three landmarks meet: the zygomatic process of the frontal bone, the orbital ridge, and the temporal line.

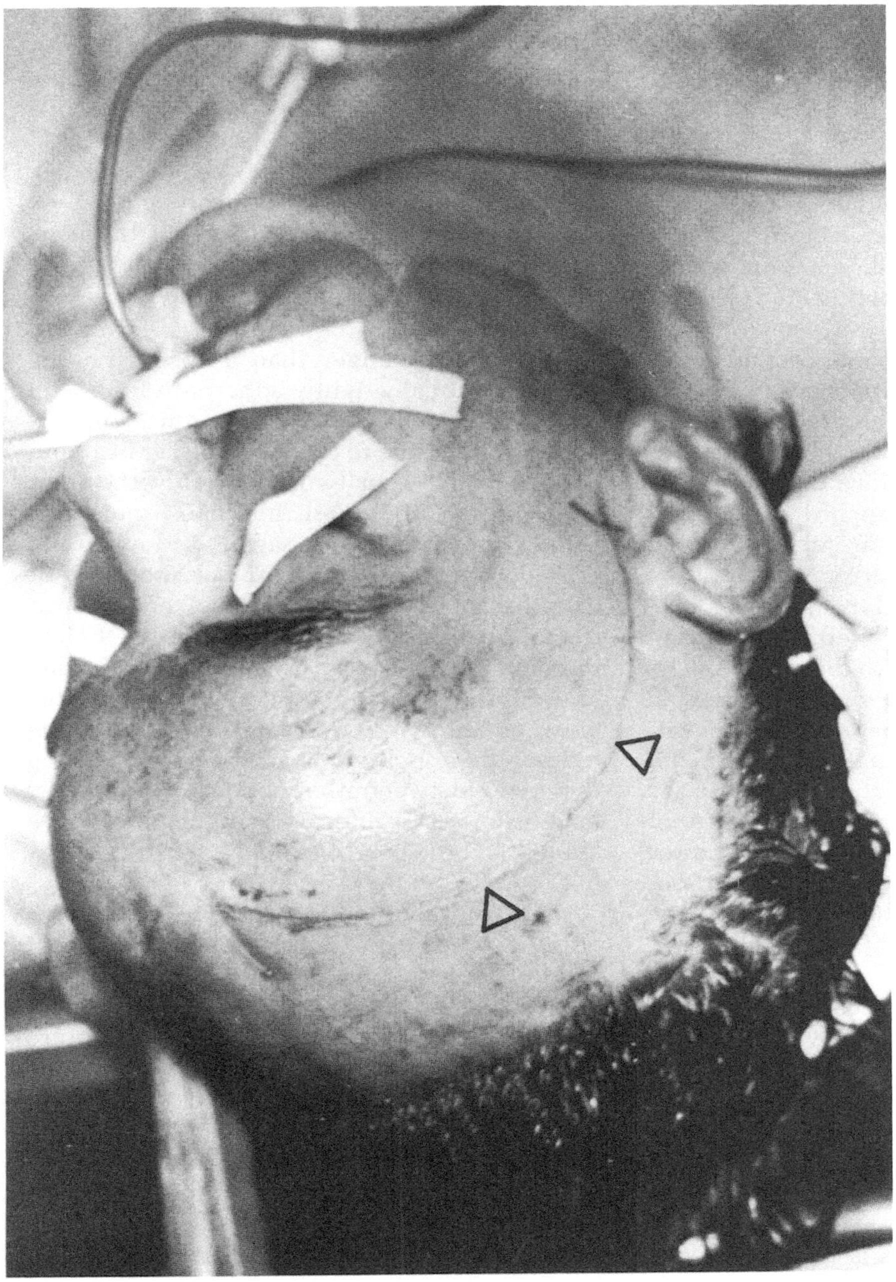

Fig. 34.1. Patient's head in a skull clamp. The incision (*triangles*) is outlined to stay behind the hairline yet allow the bone flap to remain attached to the temporalis muscle. See Fig. 29.19 for alternative incision. From Fox JL, ref. 5.

removal more difficult because the surgeon is working through the inclined binocular tubes of the microscope. With the patient's head dropped back far, the sphenoid wing is thrown relatively upward, requiring the surgeon to extend his own neck as he works on the sphenoid wing with the O.R. table elevated. Nevertheless, such positioning makes the more delicate and hazardous part of the surgery, the dissection of the aneurysm itself, easier and more comfortable for the surgeon.

The skin incision is kept behind the hairline rather than curving forward into the exposed forehead. This requires a longer incision, but the cosmetic result is better after the hair grows back. The incision (Fig. 34.1) begins at the midline, curves laterally behind the hairline, and terminates one fingerbreadth in front of the ear at the level of (or slightly below) the zygomatic arch. The skin flap and galea are stripped from the temporalis fascia and periosteum, covered with oxycellulose gauze (cotton may get caught in the high-speed drills), and pulled forward with fishhook retractors (Fig. 34.2; see also Figs. 26.9 and 26.11).

An incision is made in the anterior and posterior limit of the exposed temporalis muscle. The anterior portion of the temporalis muscle is stripped posteriorly from the zygomatic process of the frontal bone. Here one may have to electrocoagulate two branches of the anterior deep temporal artery (from the internal maxillary artery). Also, tiny arteries perforating the frontal bone just behind its zygomatic process may have to be coagulated (with cutting current) and/or sealed with bone wax. The periosteum is stripped along the line of incision from the exposed frontal, parietal, and temporal bones. However, a triangle of periosteum is preserved anteriorly for later suturing to the temporalis fascia, thereby covering the anterior frontal burr hole at the end of the operation. This piece of periosteum, with its base anteriorly, is laid on the galea of the skin flap, covered with oxycellulose, and held by a fishhook retractor.

The frontotemporal bone flap (Fig. 29.3) itself is similar to that illustrated by Kempe (Fig. 29.19). Figure 34.2 shows the usual four-burr-hole flap used by the author.

1. The first burr hole is just behind the "psychopathic point," and its anterior edge touches on that point.
2. The second burr hole is also in the frontal bone. This hole lies more medial than that illustrated by Kempe (Fig. 29.19). There are three advantages to this: (a) It allows more room for frontal lobe retraction without the retractor striking the frontal bone. (b) It permits plenty of room for maintenance of temporalis muscle attachment to the fronto-tempero-spheno-parietal bone flap, thereby reducing the incidence of later temporalis muscle atrophy. (c) There is enough exposed bone flap for placement of flap-edge holes for suture/rubber band retraction of the bone flap.
3. The third burr hole is placed in the parietal bone just inferior to the temporal line.
4. The fourth burr hole is drilled in the temporal bone just in front of the ear and above the zygomatic arch. If placed too far back, temporal bone air cells may be encountered. The bone dust is saved as it can be put back in the burr holes after closure of the bone flap, thereby helping to prevent any future indentations of the scalp into the burr holes.

In patients younger than 50–55 years, the dura is not usually tightly adherent to the skull bone. In these cases, we often utilize the air-driven craniotome to cut the skull flap in a similar design between two holes: only the most anterior and the most inferoposterior burr holes. Otherwise, a Gigli saw is used to cut the skull bone between the four burr holes. Prior to either of these techniques of craniotomy, rongeurs are used (we usually use the Echlin rongeur) to bite away as much of a channel in the fronto-spheno-temporal bone as possible between the two basal burr holes under the temporalis muscle. Doing this before sawing the bone between the upper calvarial burr holes allows this inferior bony channel to be cut without the bone flap inadvertently fracturing too high above the base.

After the bone flap is cut free, its inferior edge is rongeured (Leksell rongeur) until it presents a smooth, nonprojecting surface. Heavy silk sutures are passed through two of the small edge holes (already drilled for future reattachment of the bone flap to the calvarium). The sutures are each connected to a rubber band which has been wrapped around the rubber tubing shown in Fig. 26.9. In this manner, the bone flap, still attached to the temporalis muscle, is retracted over the zygomatic arch, thereby exposing the dura. The bone flap is waxed at its edges and then covered with wet oxycellulose. The calvarial edges are waxed. The dura then is tacked up with sutures passed through the calvarial edge holes (also to be used for reattachment of the bone flap). The sphenoid wing is rongeured inferiorly as far as possible and then waxed.

The superficial temporal artery (STA) runs in front of the ear and just superficial to the galea. Preservation of this artery is useful, especially if the surgeon plans an STA to middle cerebral artery (STA-MCA) anastomosis. This may be necessary if one plans on a trapping

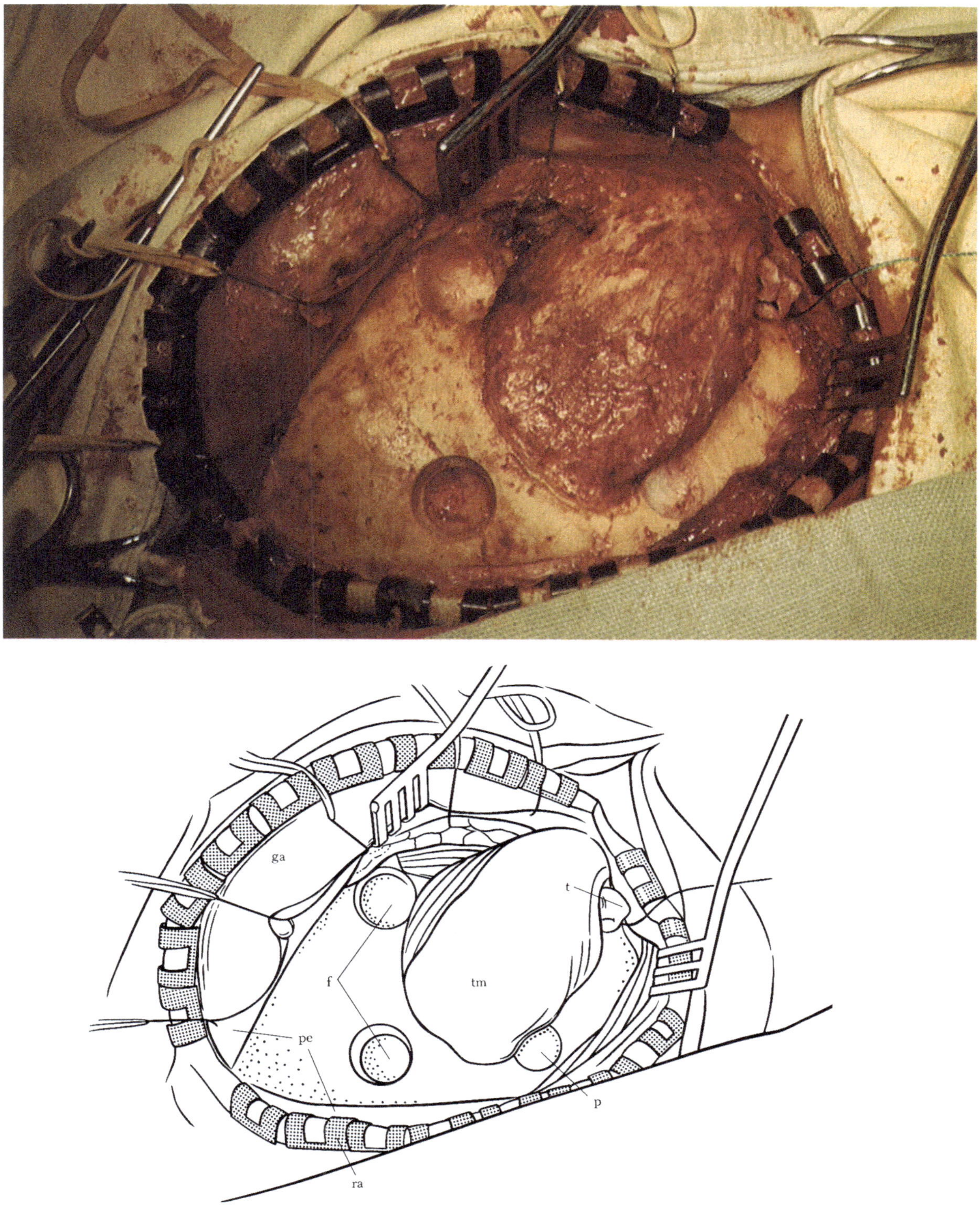

Fig. 34.2. Initial exposure of right frontotemporal craniotomy for approach to aneurysm. There are four burr holes surrounding the temporalis muscle, which covers the bony pterion. The two frontal burr holes (*f*) are obvious. The parietal bone burr hole (*p*) lies behind the superior aspect of the temporalis muscle and contains bone wax. The temporal bone burr hole (*t*) in front of the right ear contains a small cottonoid. *tm,* Temporalis muscle. *ga,* Galea. *pe,* Periosteum retracted. *ra,* Raney scalp clip.

procedure or an ICA or MCA occlusion. In such a circumstance, meticulous technique is needed to prevent STA injury.

The frontalis branches of the facial nerve pass forward between the galea and temporalis fascia, and are usually seen passing anteroinferior to the first burr hole. They can sometimes be preserved by turning a superficial layer of the temporalis fascia forward over the zygomatic process of the frontal bone before incising the temporalis muscle anteriorly. Electrocoagulation in the area must be kept at a minimum. From a practical standpoint, the nerves are often injured and the patient will have an immobile forehead on the ipsilateral side following surgery. In most cases, frontalis muscle function returns within 6 months.

Exposure of Basal Cisterns

The operating microscope is now brought into the surgical field and used until dural closure. See Chapter 26 for information about the instrumentation used as part of this author's microtechnique. The Leyla self-retaining retractors are attached to the O.R. table (Fig. 26.15). The dura of the frontal and temporal lobes are retracted gently from the sphenoid bone and the lateral roof of the orbit. If necessary, some CSF can be drained by the LP needle to relieve pressure on the brain. Ordinarily, this needs to be done only if the patient has hydrocephalus. Release only sufficient CSF to permit a relaxed brain, as excess removal risks premature rupture of the aneurysm or tearing of veins bridging the dura and the brain. The dura of the temporal lobe is often quite vascular and will require bipolar electrocoagulation, oxycellulose application, and occasionally the use of tantalum clips.

With a suction–irrigation apparatus in the left hand and a high-speed air drill (we use the Codman drill) in the right hand (of a right-handed surgeon), the surgeon removes projections of the sphenoid wing and lateral orbital roof. Keep all cottonoids out of the immediate field to avoid injury by their being caught in the drill. The steel drill bit is used initially because of its more rapid bone removal. As the base of the anterior clinoid process is approached, the drill bit is changed to the diamond type, which tends less to tear the nearby dura. The Lempert rongeur is very helpful in removing sliver-like projections of the sphenoid wing. A tiny bit of bone wax on a small cottonoid is applied against the bone with the bipolar forceps to stop bone bleeding. One must be careful to avoid drilling into the orbital cavity. If this occurs, the patient will have greater swelling and ecchymosis of orbital tissues during the postoperative period. In some patients there is a partial, congenital absence of the greater wing of the sphenoid bone behind the orbit.

The sphenoid wing is rongeured and burred down to the base of the anterior clinoid process, a medial depth of about 5 cm (Fig. 34.3). As one approaches this point, the meningoorbital artery is a landmark seen in the dura passing from the middle meningeal artery through its own foramen in the sphenoid wing (or through the superior orbital fissure) to communicate with the lacrimal artery in the orbit (20a). (This artery is one of the remnants of the embryologic stapedial arterial system; see Chapter 15.) The meningoorbital artery usually is electrocoagulated and severed, allowing further drilling of the sphenoid wing. At this point, the faster steel drill bit is switched to a diamond bit. The base of the anterior clinoid process appears as a glistening white bone often containing a single small vascular channel (Fig. 34.3).

Figure 34.4 illustrates the value of removing much of the sphenoid wing. Before the sphenoid wing is removed, the surgeon's view of the suprasellar region is blocked by the lateral projection of the wing unless greater and hazardous brain retraction is applied. Partial removal of the sphenoid wing, practiced for years by Dandy's disciples, permits a lower, basal, tangential approach to the circle of Willis. Once the surgeon uses this technique routinely and then omits it from an operative case, he will appreciate its significant value of permitting easier visualization of basal cisterns. This technique, coupled with the skilled use of self-retaining retractors and the operating microscope on a relaxed brain allows the surgeon to manipulate microinstruments in small but satisfactorily visualized spaces that contain a potentially lethal aneurysm.

The dural opening is considerably smaller than the craniotomy defect. The bony opening is larger for the reasons stated earlier in this chapter. The dura is permitted to cover the brain as much as possible to protect the brain from the drying effects of air and light. The

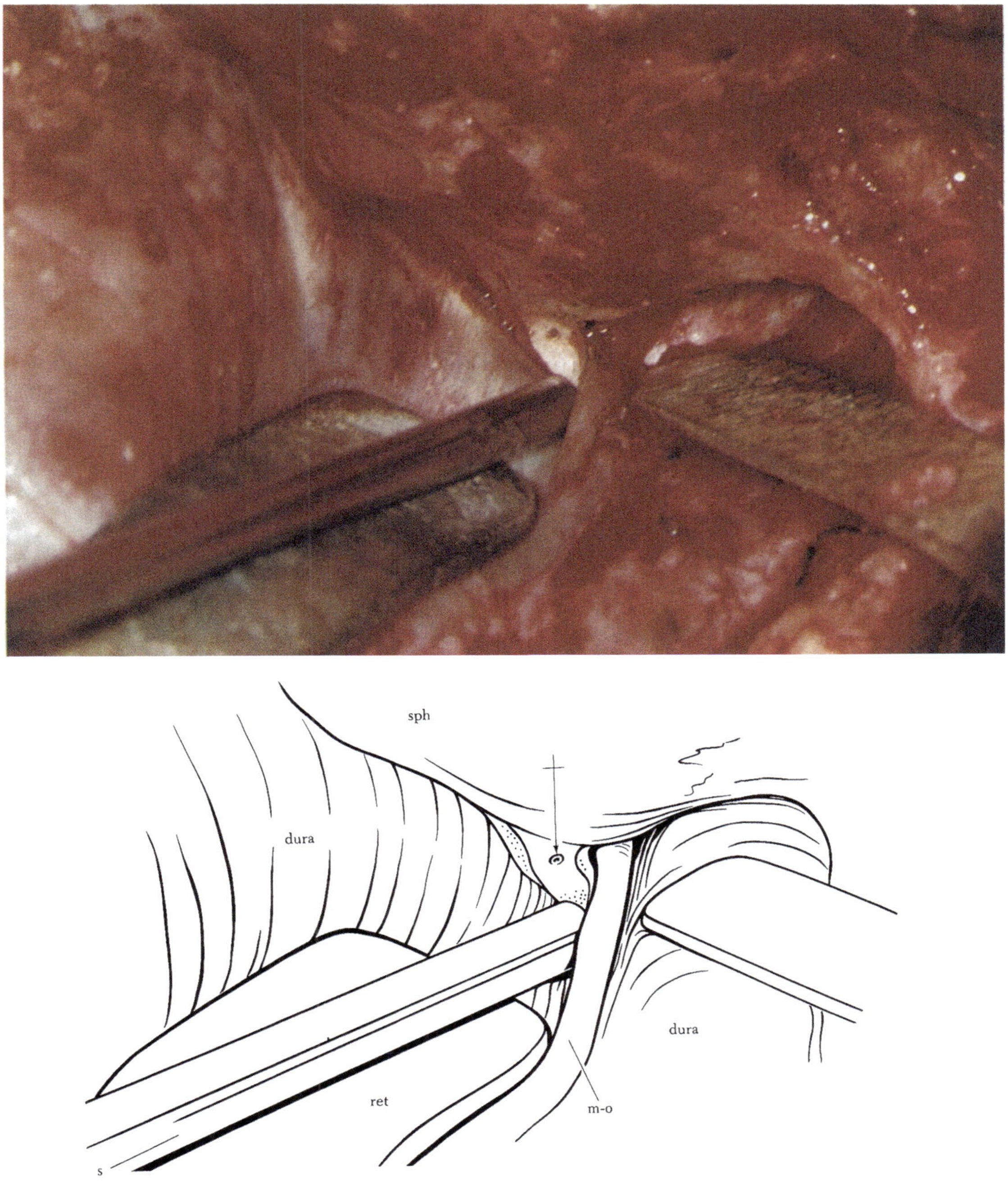

Fig. 34.3. Right sphenoid wing (*sph*) already burred away. *Crossed arrow:* Vascular channel in the base of the white anterior clinoid process. *m-o,* Meningoorbital artery. On right is a retractor on the dura of the temporal lobe. On left is a suction tube (*s*) and retractor (*ret*) on the dura of the right frontal lobe. Zeiss dial set at 10. From Fox JL, ref. 5.

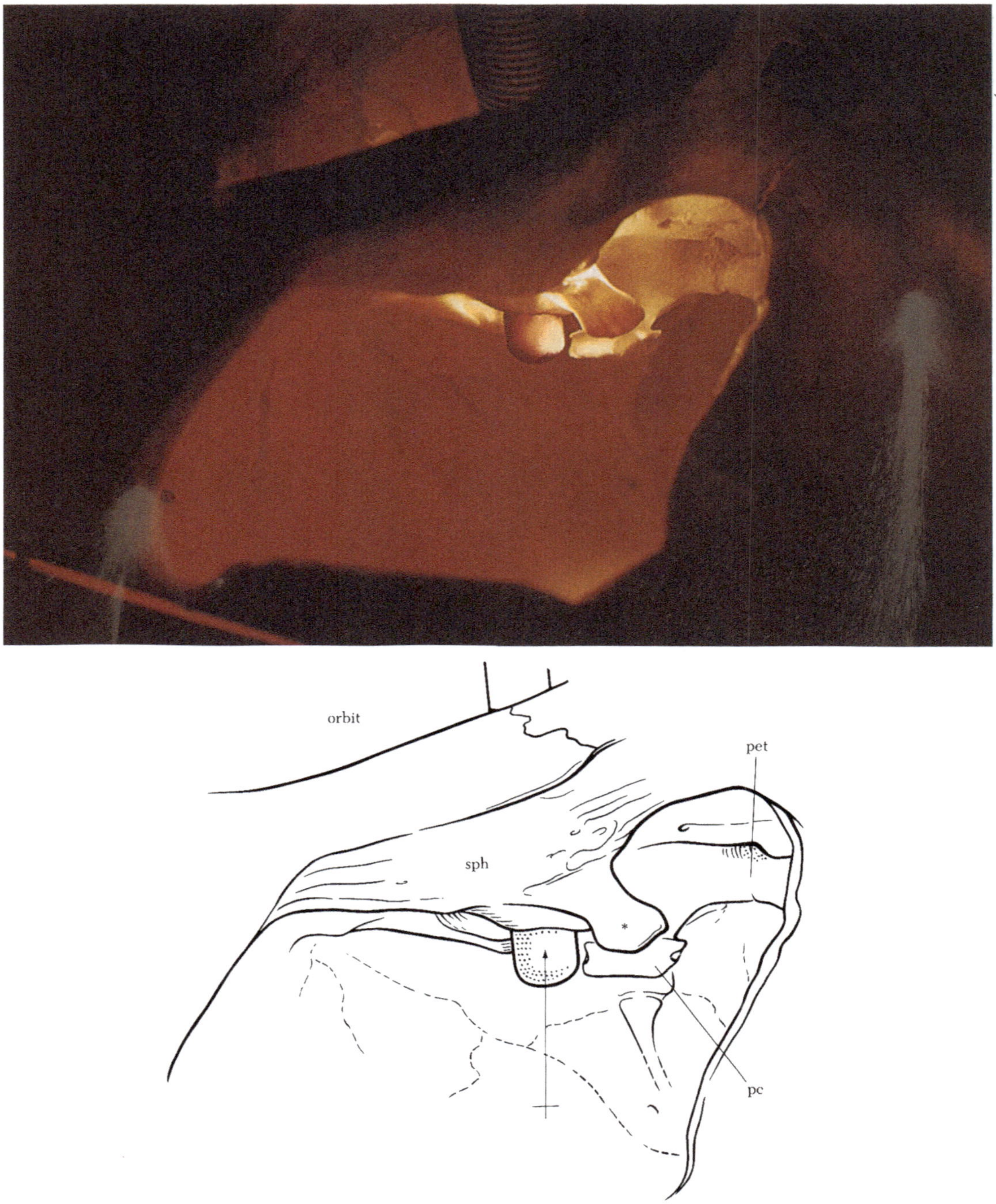

Fig. 34.4. View of a dry skull in the same position as in Figs. 34.1, 34.2, and 34.3. The right orbit is at the upper left corner. The sphenoid wing (*sph*) has been drilled away. *Crossed arrow:* Red rubber eraser ("anterior communicating artery aneurysm") sitting on the tuberculum sellae flanked by both anterior clinoid processes. *, Right anterior clinoid process. *pet,* Right petrous pyramid. *pc,* Right posterior clinoid process. From Fox JL, ref 5.

dura is opened in a modified, shallow horseshoe-shaped manner (Fig. 34.5). The dural flap is retracted over the smoothed-out sphenoid bone by suturing it to the galea. Often a secondary dural incision over the sylvian fissure is needed if the fissure is to be opened widely. At this point, some CSF can be removed by lumbar drainage or by aspiration from the chiasmatic and adjacent cisterns under a minimally elevated frontal lobe (Figs. 34.5 and 34.6). Figure 34.7 shows recent blood under the arachnoid covering the soft, edematous brain of a patient operated 2 days after her SAH. This is the typical appearance of an acute, severe SAH (from a pcaICAA in this case). The difficulties in approaching the basal cisterns in this situation contrast with the greater ease of dissection apparent in the other figures.

Attention must be paid to the one or more veins bridging the temporal lobe and the sphenoparietal sinus. Although it is good practice to preserve venous drainage where possible, we have never seen any complications from electrocoagulating and severing these veins. In cases where minimal temporal lobe retraction is necessary (as in ACoAA cases), these veins may be preserved. However, there is the risk of tearing these veins in the middle of the aneurysm dissection. Therefore we more often than not coagulate and section them.

Attention is next directed to the sylvian fissure. The microscope dial (Zeiss) is set at 16 (third setting). This gives a true 6× magnification as described in Chapter 26, pp. 683–688. As we have gained more experience, we have opened the sylvian fissure more and more. This has several benefits (6): (a) small vessels are not compressed by arachnoidal bands during retraction of the brain; (b) there is less resistance (and hence less brain-retractor pressure) to retraction of the frontal lobe; (c) traction on one lobe does not pull and injure the other lobe; (d) fewer bridging veins need be sacrificed; (e) the olfactory nerve usually can be preserved; and (f) there is minimal traction on perforating arteries and on the aneurysm.

The sylvian fissure is opened usually on the frontal lobe side of the sylvian veins. Initially we use a jeweler's forceps to pick up the arachnoid (Fig. 34.8), which is incised with microscissors. The self-retaining retractor blades are employed to separate the frontal and temporal lobes, thus gently stretching the arachnoid in the fissure. This facilitates exposure of the next, deeper layer of arachnoid and adhesions. We no longer hesitate to coagulate and incise veins and superficial arteries passing between the two lobes. In this manner the surgeon, with the suction tube in his left hand and the bipolar forceps or microscissors in his right hand, works his way down toward the base of the sylvian fissure (Fig. 34.9). If meticulous care is taken with small arachnoidal adhesions adjacent to MCA branches deeper in the fissure, when released they will not compress and compromise vessels as the lobes are separated, and the surgeon will find the fissure suddenly opening up to significant advantage. A small dental cotton ball (counted) is helpful for compressing bleeding vessels with the suction tube prior to their electrocoagulation.

The sylvian fissure is difficult to open in patients in whom frontal and temporal brain tissue has impacted together during growth and development. Even in such cases the fissure eventually can be opened to a significant degree. Of course, a soft, edematous, and boggy brain soon after the SAH makes this procedure considerable more difficult. In such circumstances, pial vessels are very friable and often bleed if touched. In contrast, atrophied brains or the presence of clot in the sylvian fissure permits relatively easy opening of the fissure.

One finally reaches the much tougher arachnoid fibers at the base of the sylvian fissure. When these are cut (Fig. 34.10), the surgeon gains immediate entrance into the carotid cistern (Fig. 34.11) and release of more CSF. In the absence of fibrin and dense adhesions, one should be able to visualize clearly the structures in and near the carotid and chiasmatic cisterns anterior to the arachnoidal membrane of Liliequist. At this stage such structures include the olfactory tract, ipsilateral optic nerve, internal carotid artery and its posterior communicating branch, and oculomotor nerve. Often one can see the white dura of the posterior clinoid process projecting medial to the oculomotor nerve. This structure is illustrated in Figs. 5.2, 7.4, 34.4, 34.11, 34.14, 34.16, 35.10, 36.20, 38.8, 38.13, 38.14, 38.15, and 38.39.

For most aneurysms this amount of sylvian fissure opening is sufficient. However, if one is to approach a BAA by this route, then the fissure must be opened maximally, exposing the M-1 artery and its branches. Figure 34.12 illustrates such an exposure with an exquisite view of the basal cisterns in front of the Liliequist

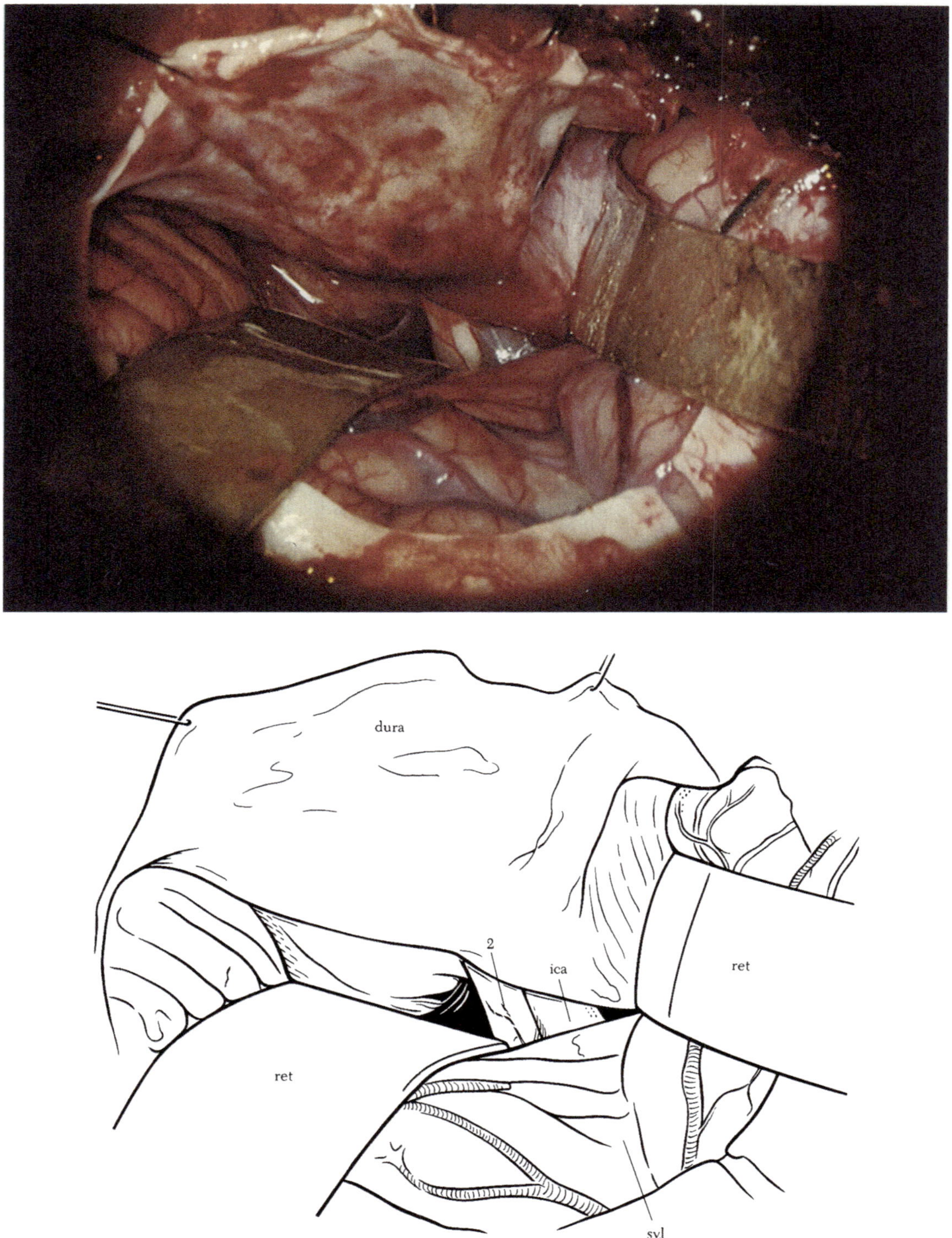

Fig. 34.5. Magnification reduced. Retractors (*ret*) elevating the right temporal lobe (*above*) and the frontal lobe (*below*) 1 cm from the right sphenoid wing. *dura,* Dura reflected over the sphenoid wing. The veins to the sphenoparietal sinus have been electrocoagulated and severed to permit retraction of the temporal lobe. The sylvian fissure (*syl*) is not yet opened. *2,* Optic nerve. *ica,* Internal carotid artery. Zeiss dial set at 6 (First setting). From Fox JL, ref. 5.

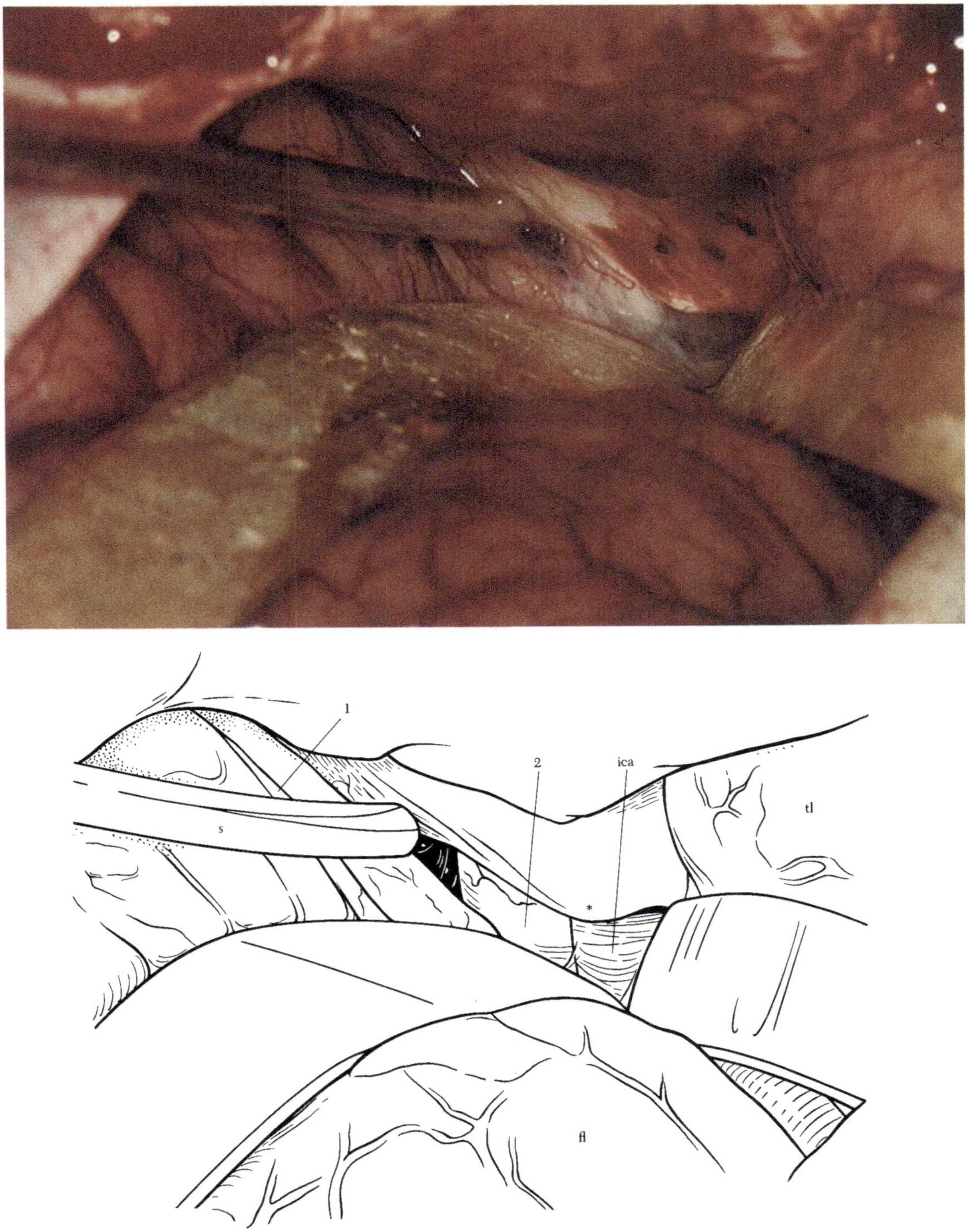

Fig. 34.6. View along the sphenoid wing to the right anterior clinoid process (*). *tl*, Temporal lobe. *fl*, Frontal lobe. The internal carotid artery (*ica*) and optic nerve (*2*) are covered by arachnoid. *1*, Right olfactory tract. *s*, Suction tube. Zeiss dial set at 10 (2nd setting). From Fox JL, ref. 5.

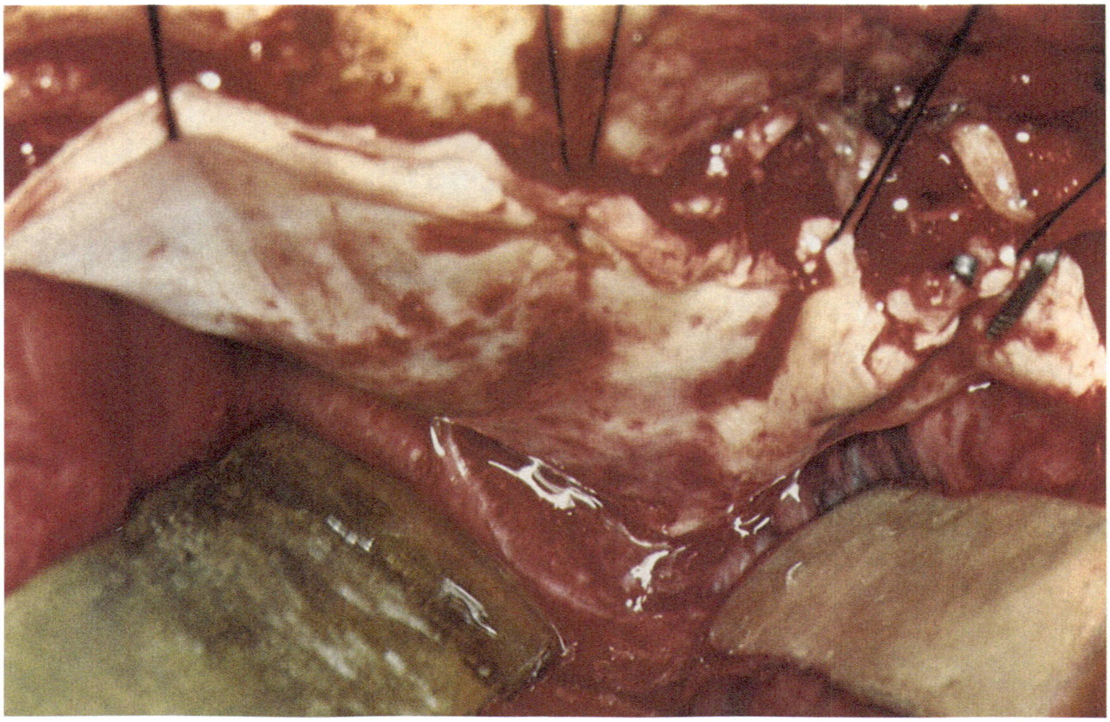

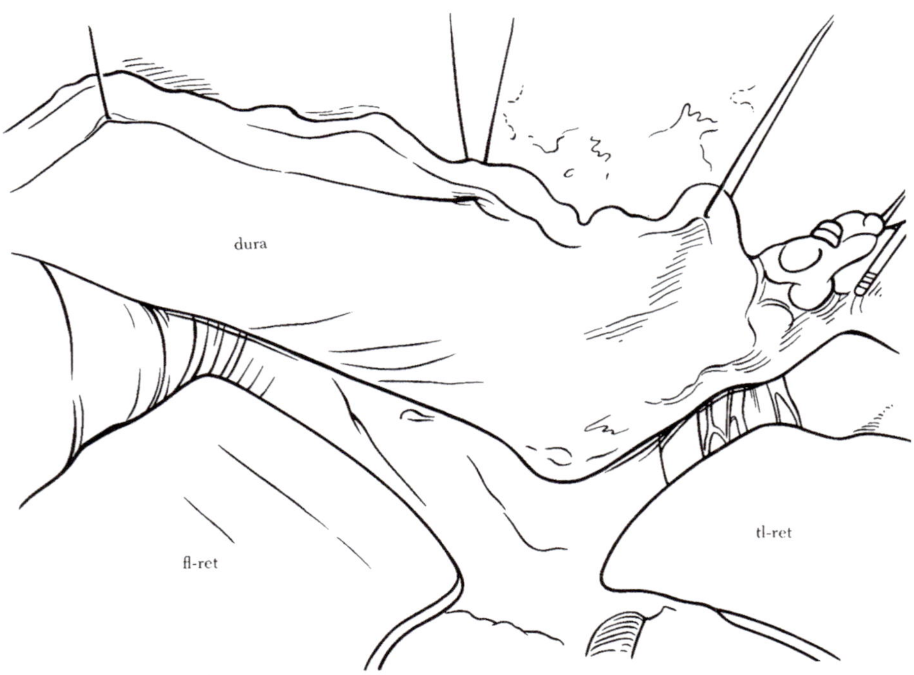

Fig. 34.7. Brain of patient operated 2 days after SAH. *dura,* Dural flap retracted over sphenoid wing. *fl-ret,* Frontal lobe retractor. *tl-ret,* Temporal lobe retractor. The brain is red from red blood cells enmeshed under arachnoid. Zeiss dial set at 10 (2nd setting).

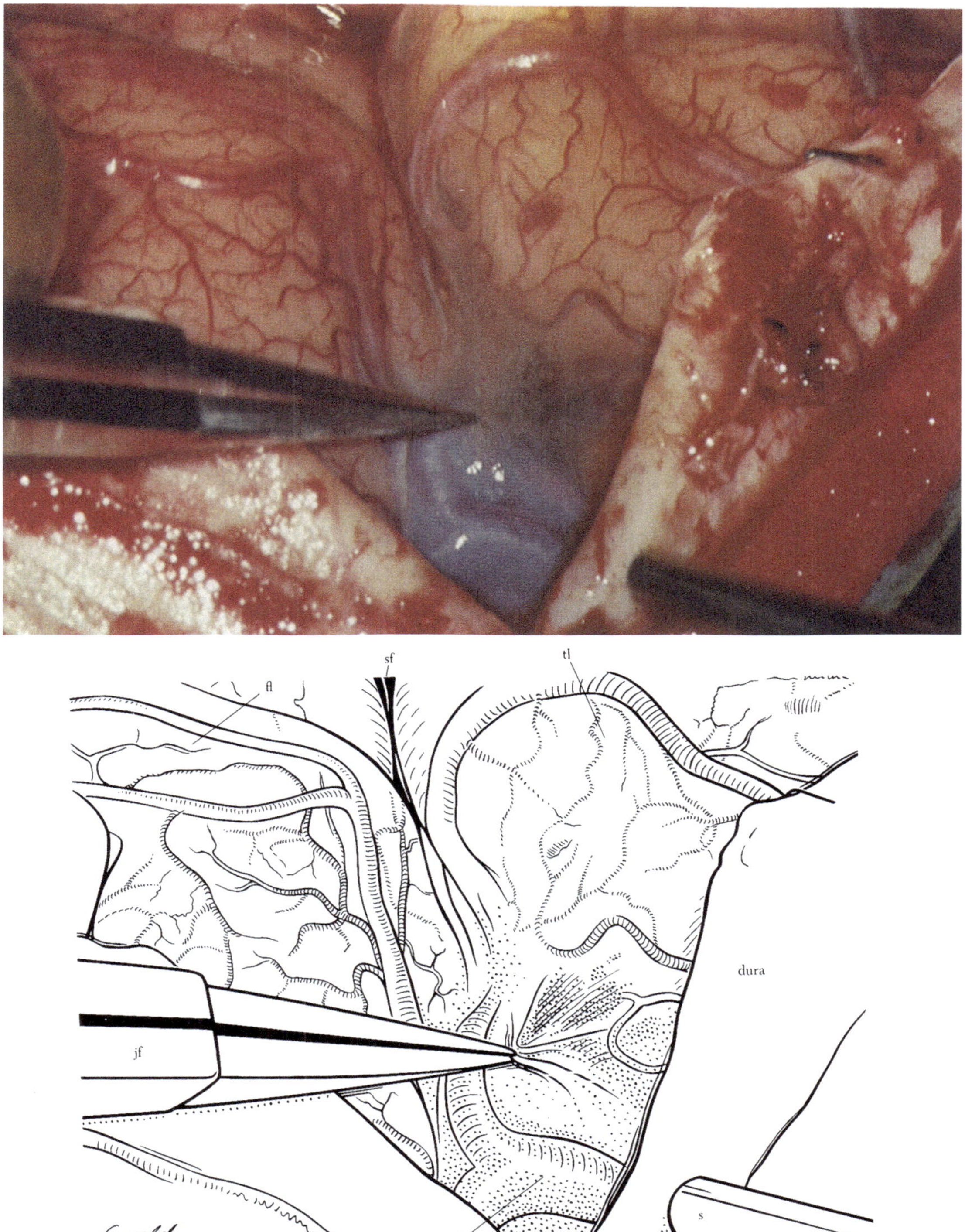

Fig. 34.8. Initial opening of arachnoid over right sylvian fissure (*sf*). *jf,* Jeweler's forceps. *fl,* Frontal lobe. *tl,* Temporal lobe. *dura,* Dural margin. *s,* Suction tube. *v,* Vein. Zeiss dial set at 16. Unless otherwise stated, all subsequent color photographs were taken with the original Zeiss dial set at 16 (3rd setting), giving a true 6× magnification.

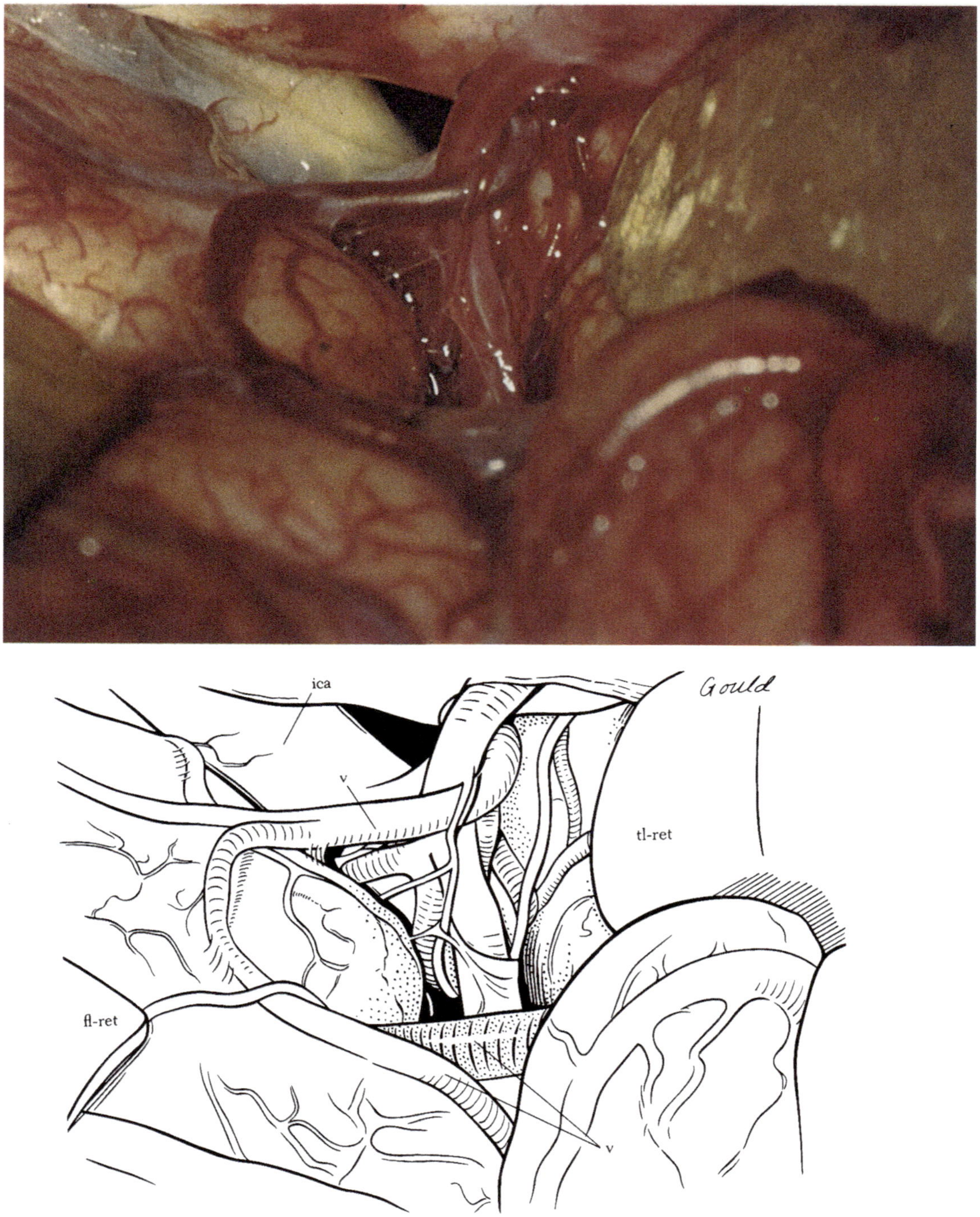

Fig. 34.9. Further opening of sylvian fissure containing entwining vessels. As a next step, the bridging veins (*v*) are electrocoagulated and severed. *tl-ret,* Temporal lobe retractor. *fl-ret,* Frontal lobe retractor. *ica* Internal carotid artery.

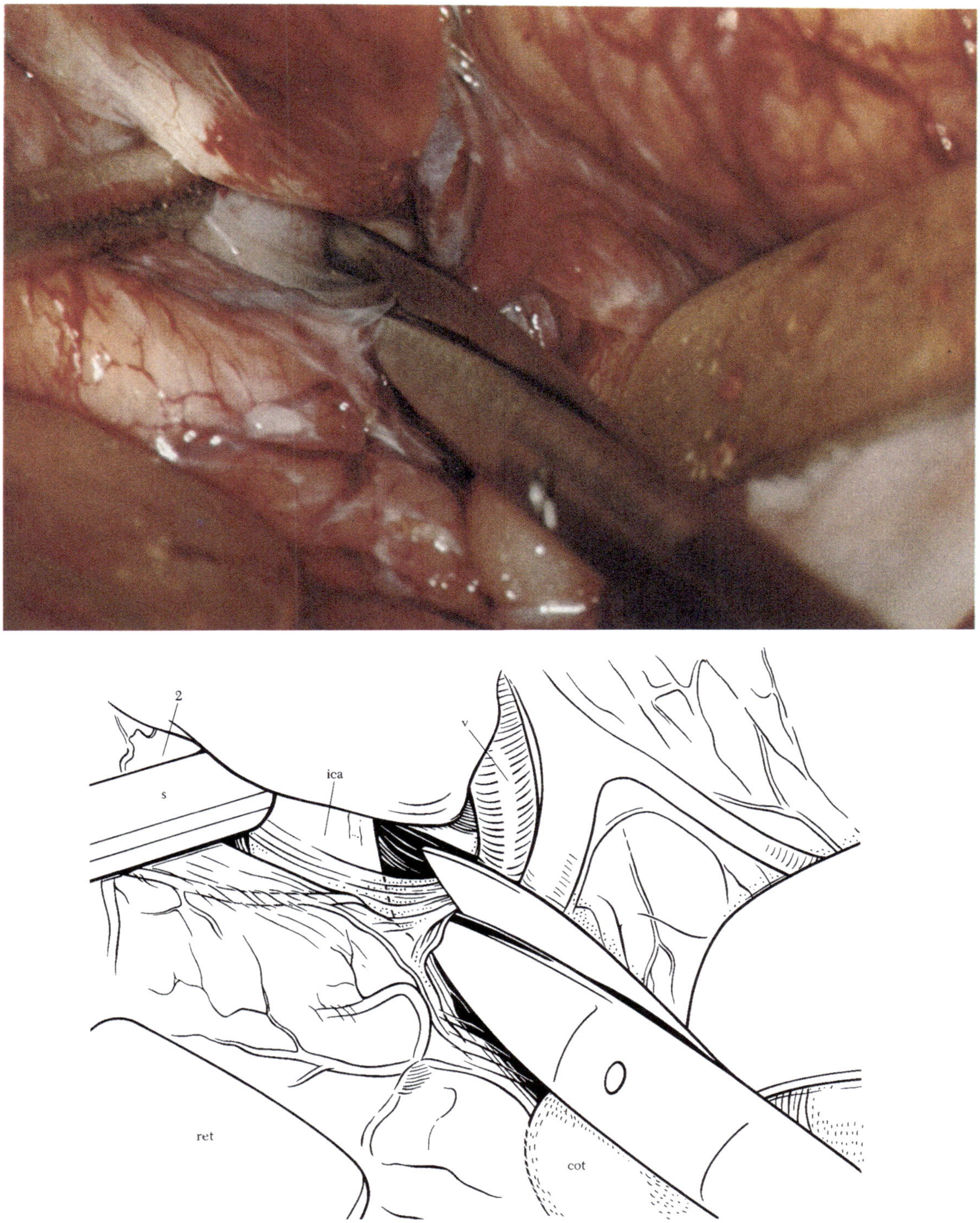

Fig. 34.10. Cutting the arachnoid at the base of the sylvian fissure. A suction tube (*s*) is in the surgeon's left hand, and microscissors are in his right. The optic nerve (*2*) and the internal carotid artery (*ica*) are still covered by arachnoid. *cot,* Small cotton ball. *ret,* Retractor on frontal lobe. *v,* Vein from the temporal lobe to the sphenoparietal sinus. From Fox JL, ref. 5.

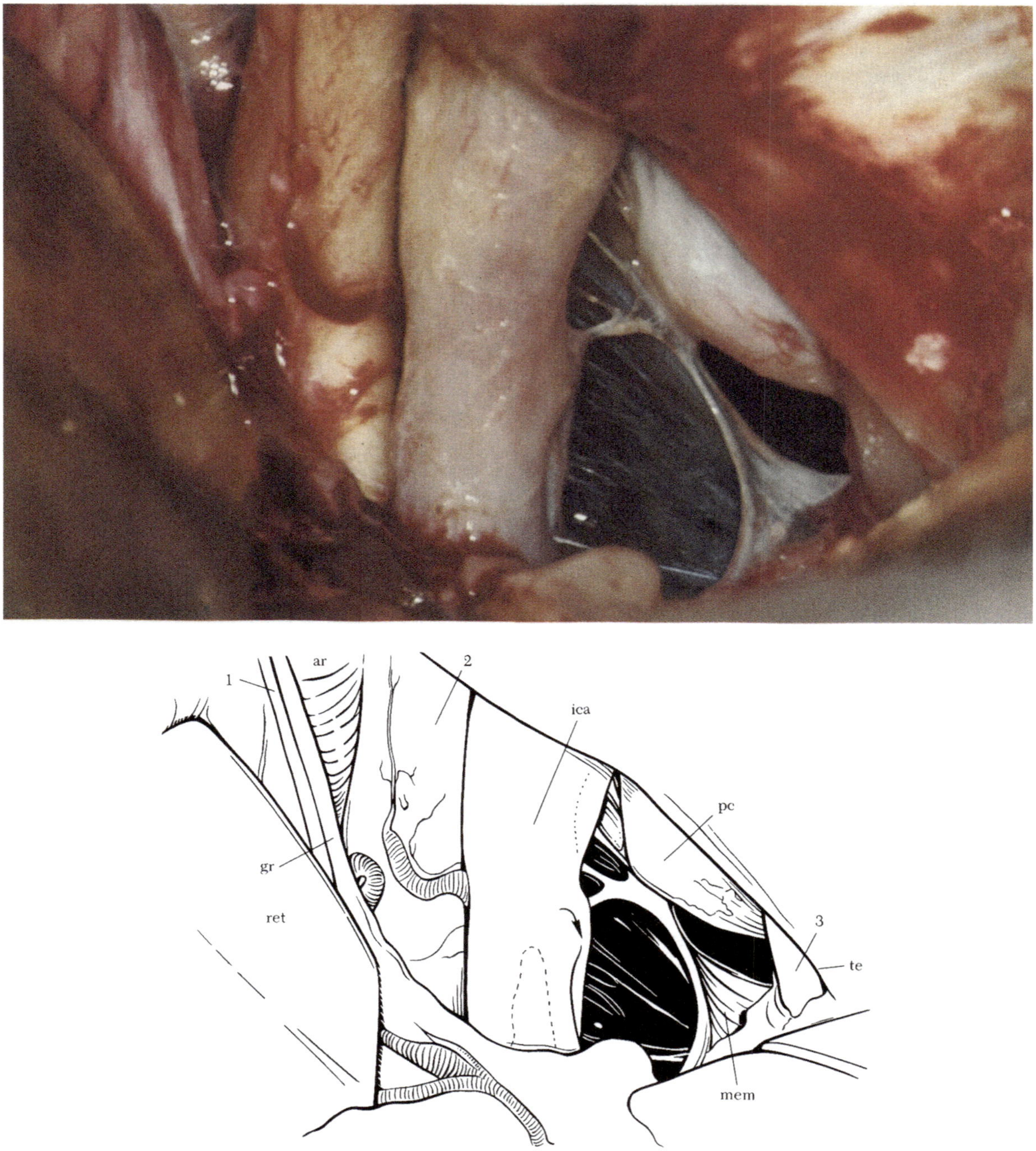

Fig. 34.11. View of carotid cistern and environs. *ar,* Arachnoid membrane between the optic nerves. *1,* Olfactory tract. *gr,* Gyrus rectus. *2,* Right optic nerve. *ret,* Retractor on frontal lobe. *Curved arrow,* Origin of the posterior communicating artery. *ica,* Internal carotid artery. *3,* Oculomotor nerve passing forward under the more lateral tentorial edge (*te*), by the more medial posterior clinoid process (*pc*), and thence into the cavernous sinus. *mem,* A reflection of Liliequist's membrane. Between the oculomotor nerve and Liliequist's membrane is a black, clear CSF passageway into the interpeduncular cistern. Note the attachment of Liliequist's arachnoidal membrane to the posterior clinoid and adjacent dorsum sellae. Opening this membrane between the oculomotor nerve and the ICA is the usual frontolateral route to a terminal basilar artery aneurysm. From Fox JL, ref. 5.

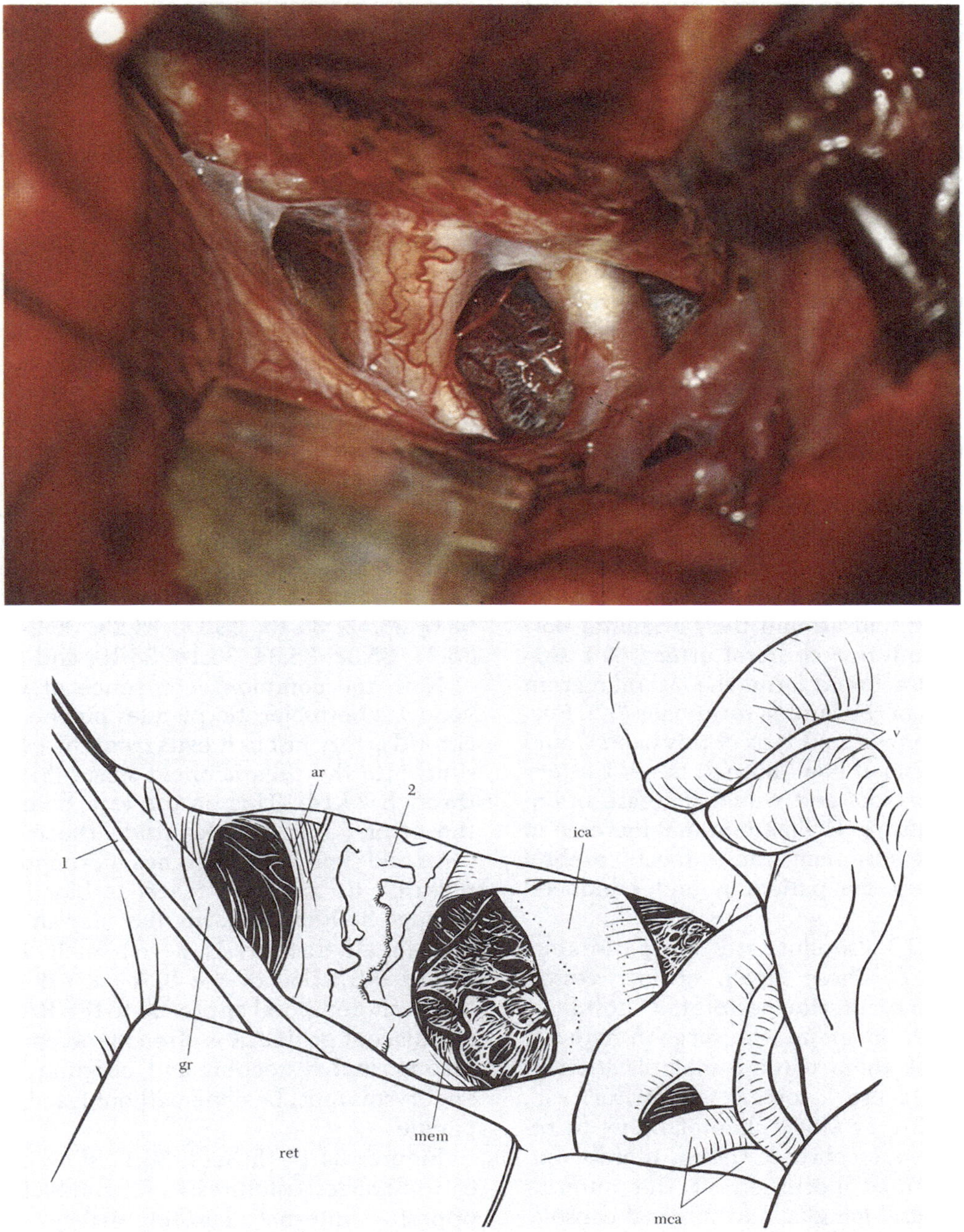

Fig. 34.12. View of the right optic nerve, internal carotid artery, and environs. Retractors (*ret*) are holding up the frontal lobe. Note the complex of middle cerebral branches (*mca*) in the opened sylvian fissure and the small vessels on the optic nerve (*2*). *gr*, Gyrus rectus. *1*, Olfactory tract. The typical atherosclerotic plaque is seen on the internal carotid artery (*ica*). *ar*, Arachnoid between the optic nerves. *mem*, Arachnoidal membrane of Liliequist deep to either side of the carotid artery. In this example the membrane is multiperforated. *v*, Two large veins from the temporal lobe to the sphenoparietal sinus. From Fox JL, ref. 5.

membrane. The line of exposure and attack now depends on the location of the aneurysm(s).

Figures 34.11 and 34.12 as well as the subsequent color photographs in this chapter are best visualized when CSF drainage by lumbar puncture is not done—or at least not continued—as the CSF nicely distends the arachnoid lining of the cisterns, giving the surgeon a better view of the anatomy. This CSF also keeps cerebral tissues and vessels wet and allows diffusion of blood (thus preventing clotting in basilar cisterns).

Some of the major benefits of using the operating microscope in this type of surgery are improved binocular vision, increased illumination, sharper focus, magnification, and fewer parallax problems, allowing the surgeon to visualize anatomy that was never before seen so clearly. An example is shown in Fig. 34.13. The frontal lobe is retracted only 1.5 cm. Note the band of arachnoid around the horizontal portion of the anterior cerebral artery (A-1 segment). This arachnoid forms the lateral margin of the cistern of the lamina terminalis (32). Further retraction without lysis of this band would compromise blood flow through the A-1 artery and its perforators and would increase brain-retractor pressure. Even a minimal increase in retractor pressure can cause focal cerebral ischemia when the patient is under induced hypotension.

Figure 34.13 also illustrates the perforators from the A-1. These small, critical vessels ascend into the anterior perforated substance; when they are in spasm, the surgeon may not be able to see them without magnification. It is advisable to use a topical vasodilator, e.g., 3% papaverine or 0.5% phentolamine, to reduce any acute or chronic spasm, thereby ensuring continued perfusion of the anterior brainstem, basal ganglia, and internal capsule. Note in Fig. 34.13 that Liliequist's membrane has been opened except inferiorly (at the top of Fig. 34.13 between the carotid artery and the optic nerve) with visualization of the basilar artery (in the background). Normally, this membrane is left intact (unless a thickened membrane is causing hydrocephalus) so that blood in the anterior cisterns will not escape into the interpeduncular cistern containing the basilar artery. In this case, the membrane has been divided; part passes behind the pituitary stalk and part passes in front of the stalk while covering the diaphragm sellae behind the right optic nerve. The vascular tuft commonly seen in the arachnoid between the optic nerves is present.

Accurate and gentle placement of the self-retaining retractor blades is critical. Most often we still use cottonoid strips cut to the width of the retractor blade and placed between the retractor blade and brain tissue. They seldom stick to the brain if kept wet with CSF and saline. One must be careful to avoid excess brain retraction pressure, especially when arterial hypotension is used. With the sphenoid wing burred down smoothly and the sylvian fissure opened widely in the presence of good anesthetic technique, excess brain retraction is uncommon. Often the retractor just supports the relaxed brain. Care must be taken to avoid letting the tip of the frontal lobe retractor compress Heubner's artery, which often lies just in front of the A-1 artery (Figs. 5.2, 34.15, 35.3, 35.6, 35.12, 35.13, 35.15, 35.23, 35.24, 35.26, 35.27, 35.33, 35.34, 36.18, 36.19, and 36.30.

Note the common occurrence of white or yellow atherosclerotic plaques on the internal carotid artery just as it exits from the cavernous sinus into the subarachnoid space (Figs. 34.11 through 34.14). This occurs at a point where the artery, rigidly held inside the cavernous sinus and skull base, becomes more mobile and pulsatile in the CSF space as blood courses through it. (Flow patterns may play an etiologic role in atherosclerosis here.) Such a plaque makes retraction of the ICA hazardous (as in the frontotemporal approach to the BAA). Also, an adjacent pcaICAA is often involved with the plaque, and dissection and clipping of these aneurysms must be done without fracturing the plaque.

Figures 34.14 through 34.17 show how one can visualize structures as far medially as the opposite internal carotid artery and its branches. These figures illustrate additional variations in the surgical anatomy of the area. In Fig. 34.14 we see a wide lateral deviation of the posterior communicating artery. Also a very small A-1 artery starts medially at the ICA bifurcation. The typically reddish vascular appearance of the pituitary stalk entering through the diaphragm sellae is seen here and in subsequent figures. The white dura of the dorsum sellae is seen between the ICA and the pituitary stalk. In Fig. 34.15 the frontal lobe is elevated, and we see the opposite, whitish-appearing ICA

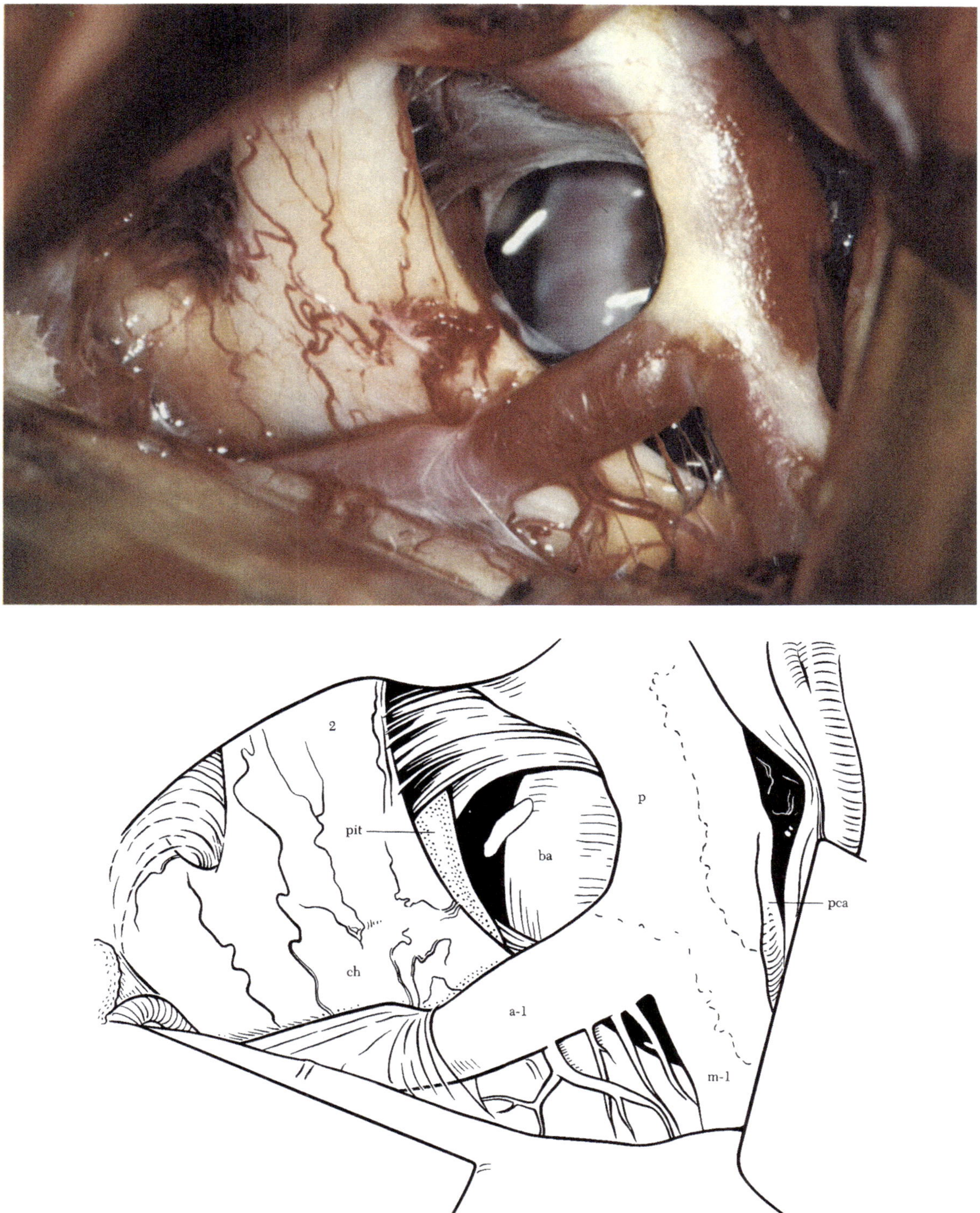

Fig. 34.13. Views of the carotid, chiasmatic, and interpeduncular cisterns. *p*, Atherosclerotic plaque on the internal carotid artery. *pca*, Posterior communicating artery. *a-1*, First portion of the anterior cerebral artery. *m-1*, First portion of the middle cerebral artery. Overlying the basilar artery (*ba*) and seen between the optic nerve (*2*) and the carotid artery are reflections from clear CSF in the interpeduncular cistern. *pit*, Pituitary stalk. *ch*, Optic chiasm. See text for further details. From Fox JL, ref. 5.

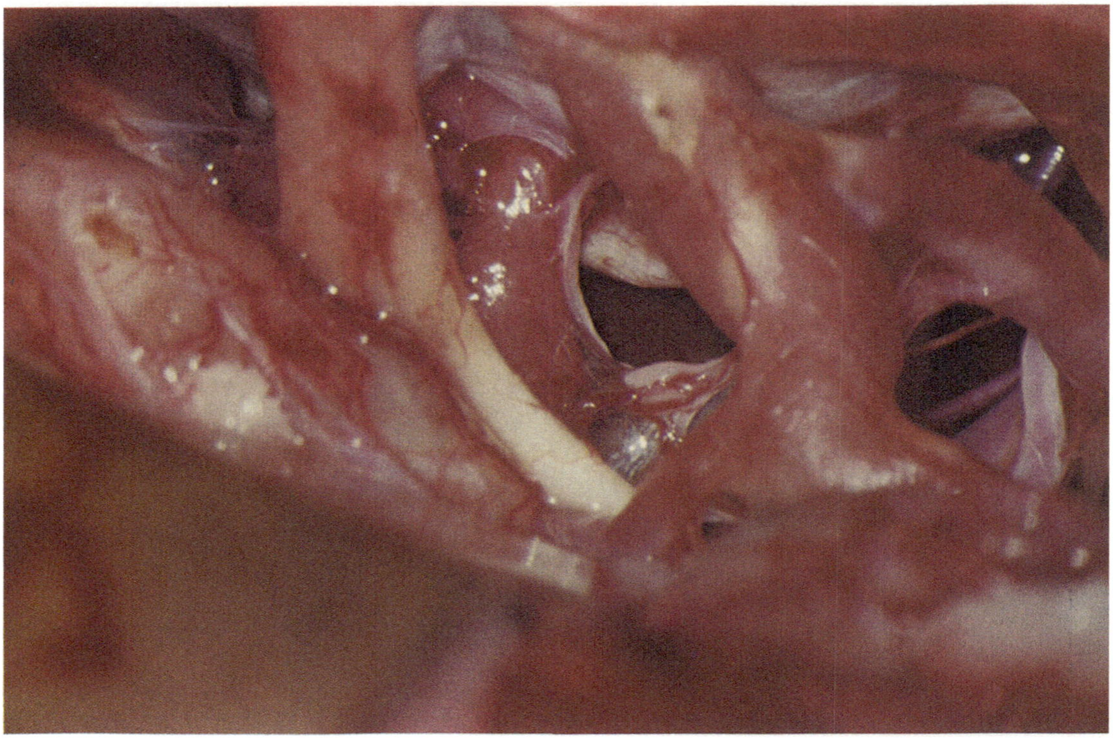

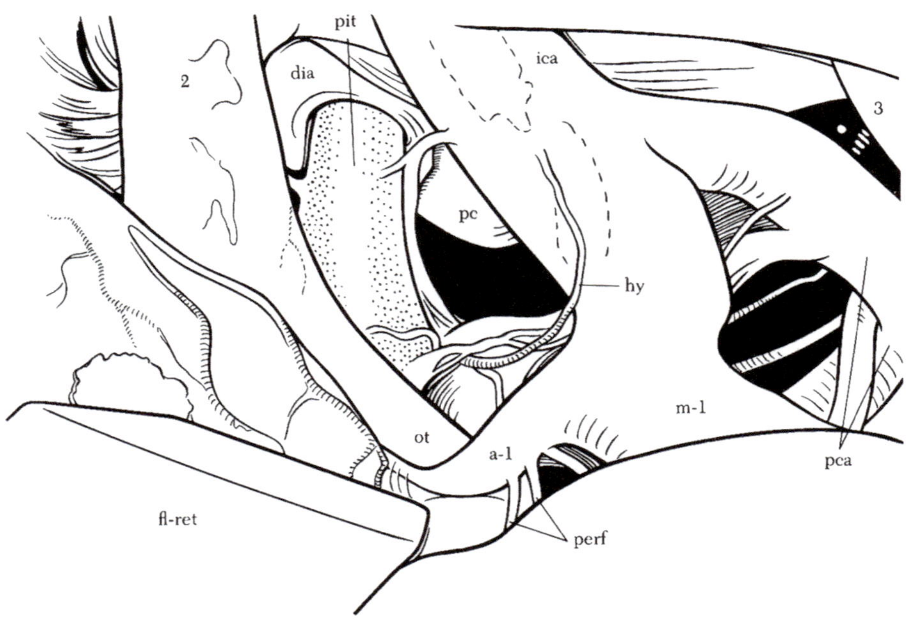

Fig. 34.14. View of carotid and chiasmatic cisterns. *2,* Optic nerve. *dia,* Diaphragm sellae. *pit,* Pituitary stalk. *pc,* Posterior clinoid process. *ica,* Internal carotid artery. *3,* Oculomotor nerve. *pca,* Posterior communicating artery. *m-1,* M-1 part of middle cerebral artery. *perf,* A-1 perforators. *a-1,* A-1 part of anterior cerebral artery. *ot,* Optic tract. *fl-ret,* Frontal lobe retractor. Note hypothalamic perforators (*hy*) from ICA to pituitary stalk and hypothalamus.

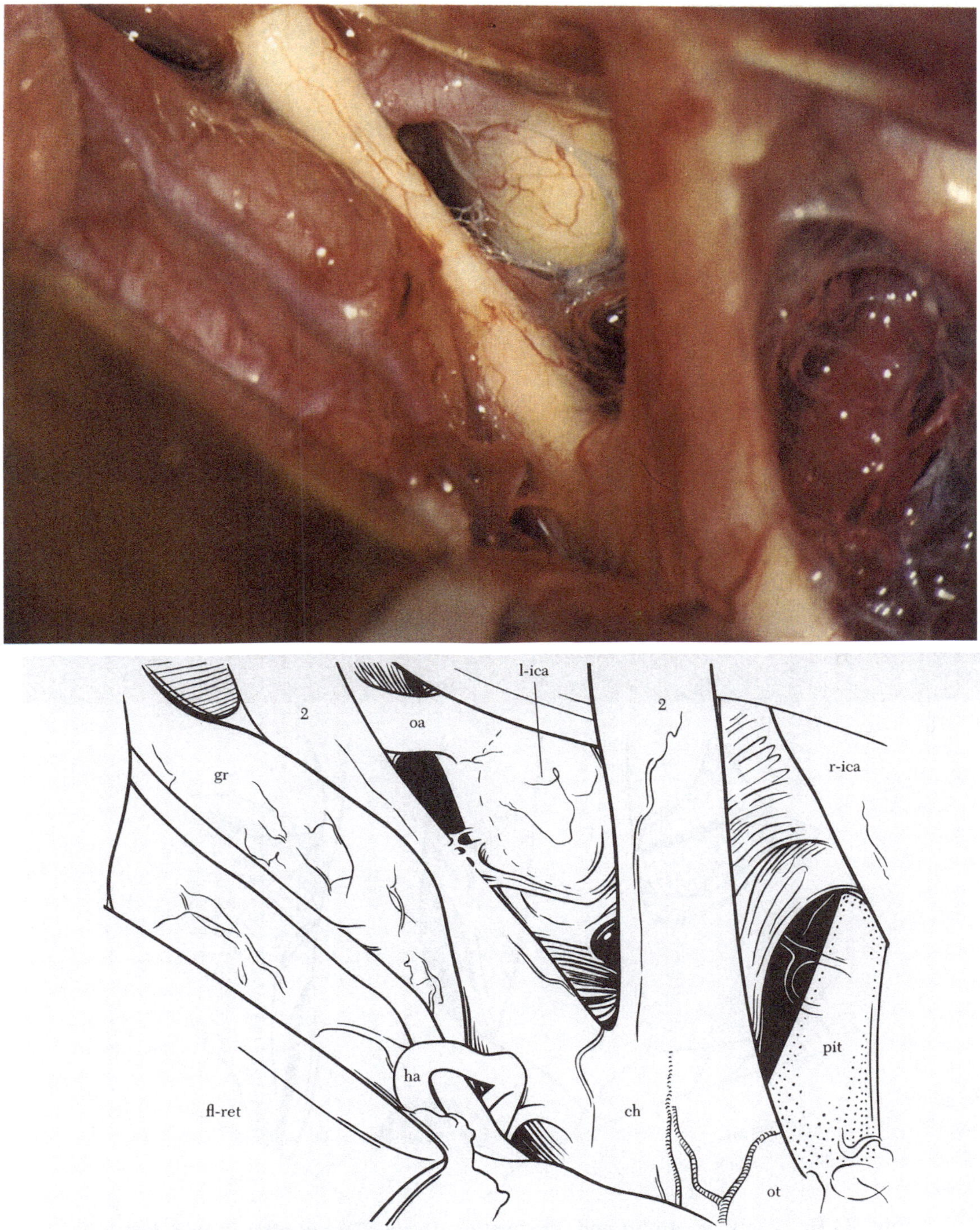

Fig. 34.15. Looking medially across the chiasmatic cistern. *fl-ret,* Frontal lobe retractor. *gr,* Right gyrus rectus. *2,* Right and left optic nerves. *oa,* Left ophthalmic artery. *l-ica,* Left internal carotid artery. *r-ica,* Right internal carotid artery. *pit,* Pituitary stalk. *ch,* Optic chiasm. *ha,* Branch of Heubner's artery. *ot,* Right optic tract.

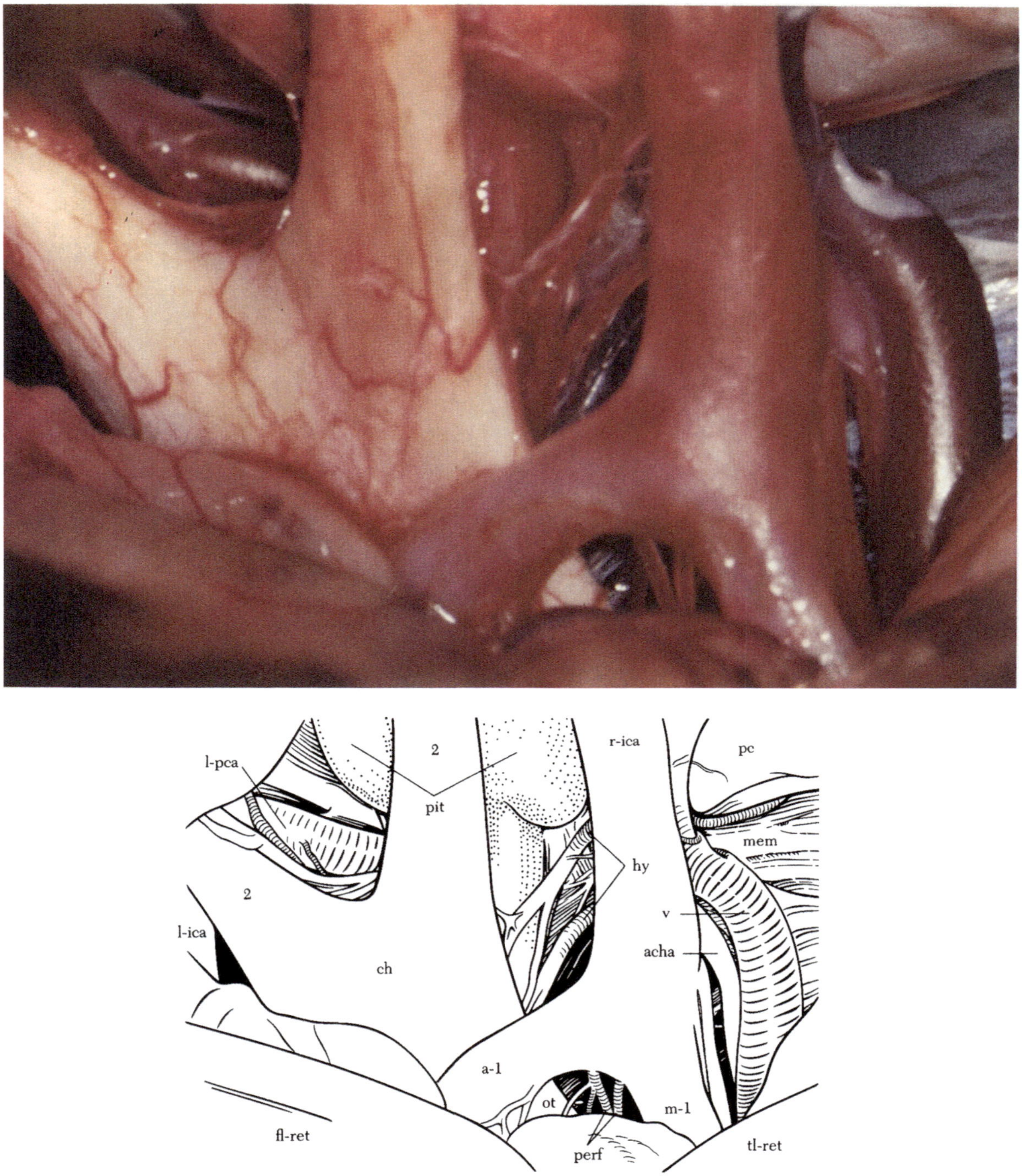

Fig. 34.16. View of carotid and chiasmatic cisterns. The pituitary gland (*pit*) projects superior to the level of the diaphragm sellae. *2,* Optic nerves. *ch,* Optic chiasm. *r-ica,* Right internal carotid artery. *hy,* Hypothalamic perforators from ICA and posterior communicating artery (not seen). *pc,* Dura of posterior clinoid process. *mem:* Membrane of Liliequist. *v,* Unusual vein arising from cavernous sinus. *acha,* Anterior choroidal artery. *tl-ret,* Temporal lobe retractor. *m-1:* M-1 portion of middle cerebral artery. *perf,* Perforators from bifurcation of ICA to anterior perforated substance. *ot,* Right optic tract. *a-1,* A-1 portion of anterior cerebral artery. *fl-ret,* Frontal lobe retractor. *l-ica,* Left internal carotid artery. *l-pca,* Left posterior communicating artery.

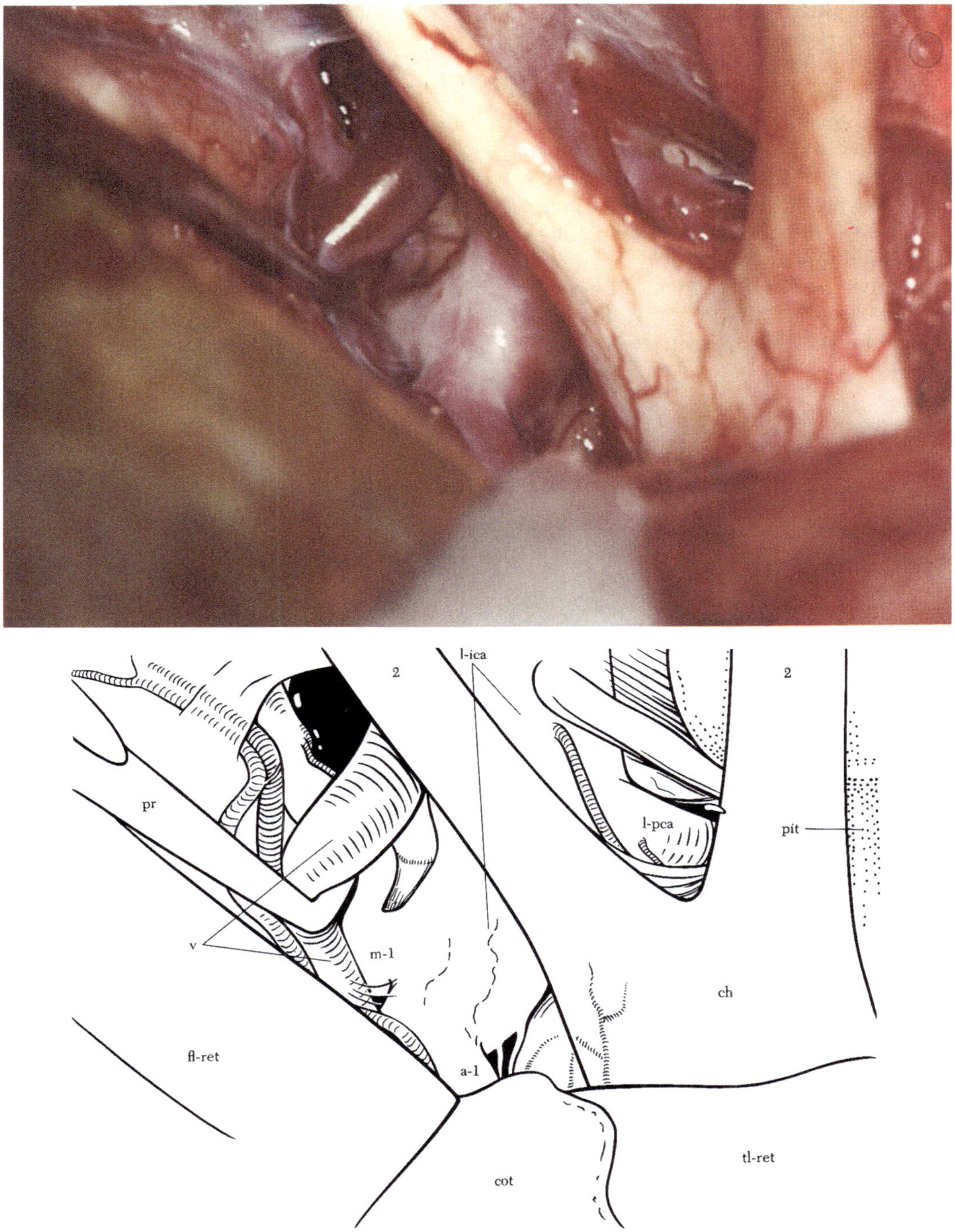

Fig. 34.17. Same case as in Fig. 34.16. View is looking medially toward the left internal carotid artery (*l-ica*). *2,* Optic nerves. *pit,* Pituitary stalk. *l-pca,* Left posterior communicating artery. *ch,* Optic chiasm. *tl-ret,* Temporal lobe retractor. *a-1,* A-1 portion of left anterior cerebral artery. *cot,* Cotton strip. *m-1,* M-1 portion of left middle cerebral artery. *fl-ret,* Frontal lobe retractor. *v,* Unusual vein on left arising from cavernous sinus. *pr,* Probe retracting the vein.

and its pinker ophthalmic artery lying beyond the diverging optic nerves.

Figure 34.16 is remarkable in that we see half of the pituitary gland lying superior to the level of the diaphragm sellae (a biopsy revealed normal pituitary gland). Also there is an unnamed vein (present bilaterally) passing superiorly and backward from the cavernous sinus. This prominent vein coursed behind and lateral to the ICA and disappeared behind the anterior perforated substance. Lying beyond the diverging optic nerves we see the PCoA. In Fig. 34.17 the surgeon can see the opposite (left) ICA, its PCoA, and its bifurcation. A similar large vein is seen lateral to the left ICA.

The membrane of Liliequist, known originally as the membrane of Key and Retzius, is an important arachnoid landmark (18,19,32). During pneumoencephalography, air often is seen outlining this membrane, which separates the interpeduncular and chiasmatic cisterns (Fig. 34.18). The membrane runs from the dorsum sellae and posterior clinoid processes upward toward the mammillary bodies of the hypothalamus (Figs. 34.19 and 34.20). It passes from side to side between both oculomotor

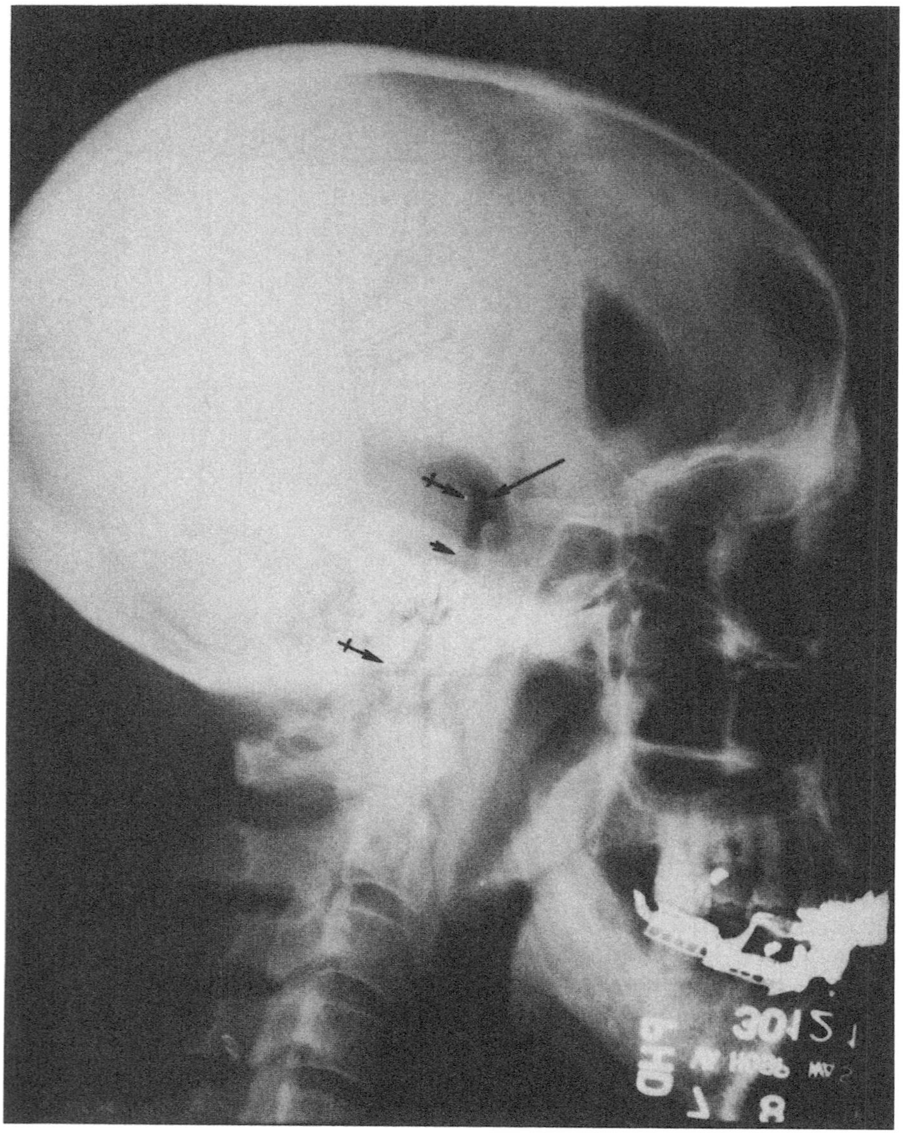

Fig. 34.18. Pneumoencephalogram performed several weeks after an SAH from a bBAA. *Highest uncrossed arrow:* Liliequist membrane (or membrane of Key and Retzius) blocking passage of air from the interpeduncular cistern. From Fox JL, Luessenhop AJ, ref. 8.

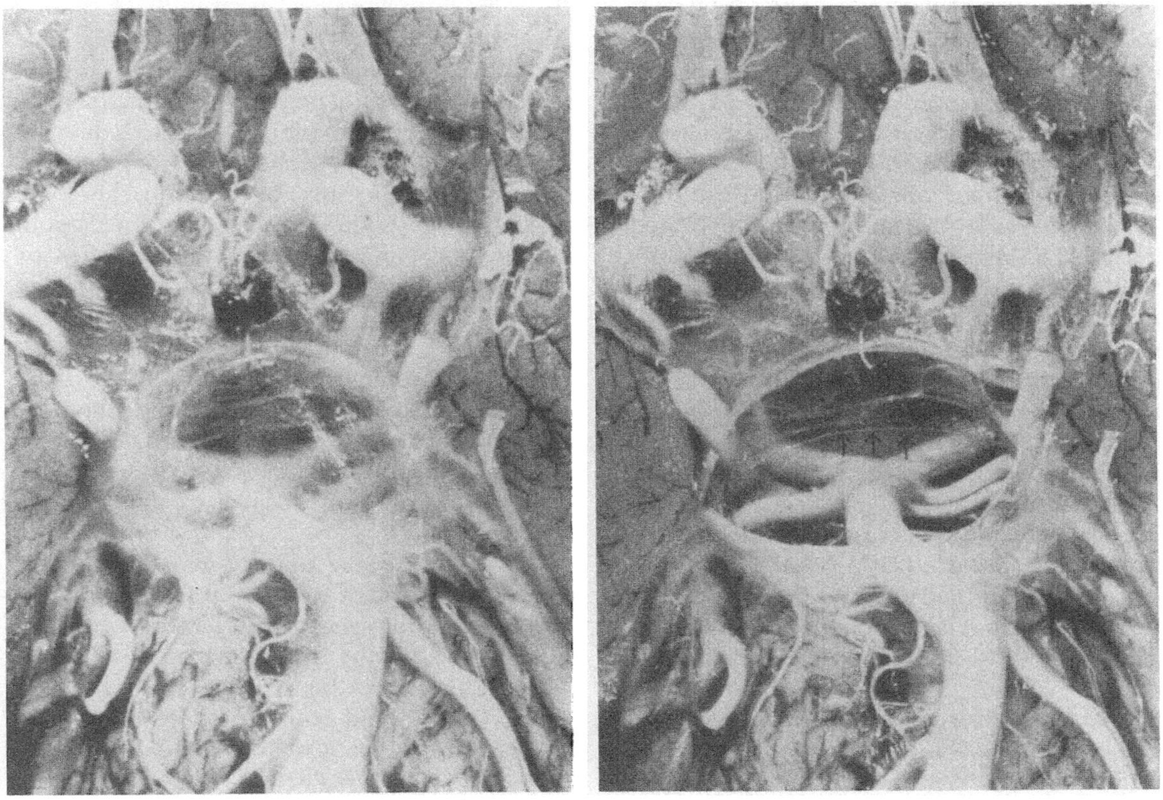

Fig. 34.19. Anatomic dissection of human brain, basal view. Above are olfactory tracts, optic nerves, and internal carotid arteries. ***Left*** In the midzone is the intact arachnoid membrane of the interpeduncular cistern. ***Right*** The membrane has been opened to show the arachnoid membrane of Key and Retzius, or Liliequist, (*arrows*) stretching between the two oculomotor nerves. Below is the basilar artery and its branches in front of the brainstem. From Liliequist B, ref. 19.

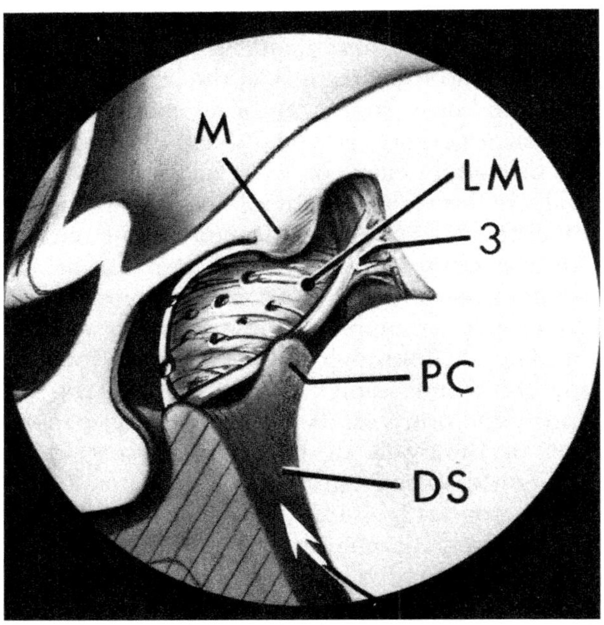

Fig. 34.20. Sagittal section of a normal brain and the sellar region, looking to the right. *M,* Mammillary body. *LM,* Liliequist's membrane. *3,* Right oculomotor nerve. *PC,* Right posterior clinoid process. *DS,* Dorsum sellae. *Arrows,* Normal flow of cerebrospinal fluid through the prepontine and interpeduncular cisterns. From Fox JL, Al-Mefty O, ref. 7.

nerves. Figures 34.11 through 34.13 and 34.16 show the membrane as seen by the surgeon. Normally it is either a solid, translucent sheet with openings on either side (Fig. 34.11) or a multiperforated membrane (Fig. 34.12) allowing passage of CSF from the posterior fossa into the anterior cisterns, from whence CSF circulation continues over the surface of the brain. After an SAH, adhesions along this membrane may seal off CSF passageways and cause a communicating hydrocephalus. Opening either this membrane or the lamina terminalis at surgery releases much CSF and may be a permanent cure for aneurysm patients with hydrocephalus. (See Figs. 35.3, 35.11, 35.12, 35.13, 35.26, 35.33, and 35.34 for examples of the lamina terminalis as seen at surgery.)

Unless one is approaching a terminal BAA or attempting to release CSF from the posterior cisterns, it is better to leave the Liliequist membrane intact. It acts as an effective barrier to surgical blood entering the posterior basal cisterns.

Of anatomic interest is the pituitary stalk, which lies between the membrane of the Liliequist posteriorly and the optic chiasm anteriorly. The stalk appears as a reddish, vascularized projection usually seen passing inferiorly beyond the space between the ICA and optic nerve. Examples are in Figs. 5.2, 34.13 through 34.17, 35.11, 35.13, 35.33, and 36.21. Anterior thalamic and hypothalamic perforators can be seen feeding the hypophyseal stalk from the ICA and PCoA.

Regardless of the aneurysm location, not only do we open the sylvian fissure substantially but we lyse adhesions and arachnoid between the ipsilateral optic nerve and the base of the frontal lobe. This allows: (a) gentle retraction of the frontal lobe without adhesions pulling on the optic nerve; (b) less brain retraction pressure; (c) occasional inspection of the ACoA region for another aneurysm not seen on angiography (Fig. 35.13 is an example); (d) exposure of the lamina terminalis in cases with hydrocephalus; and (e) assessment of local anatomic variations and enhancement of the surgeon's knowledge of surgical anatomy. In our personal experience the latter is done at no risk to the patient and has been extremely important in honing the surgeon's skills. In non-ACoAA cases actual exposure of the ACoA itself is not done in patients in whom significant frontal lobe retraction would be required.

The Aneurysm

The following chapters describe and illustrate specific types of intracranial aneurysm. The reader is referred there for detailed descriptions of specific approaches and microsurgical anatomy of aneurysms. In addition there are artistic, autopsy, and live surgical illustrations of aneurysm anatomy and aneurysm sites by other authors which can be recommended (5,17,21–23,25a,27,31). Regarding giant aneurysms, there are worthwhile publications by Drake (3), Hosobuchi (12), and Sundt and Piepgras (29) which report specialized techniques for the treatment of giant (25 mm diameter or more) intracranial aneurysms. Some special aneurysm therapy techniques are summarized in Chapter 31.

The typical berry aneurysm is found at a branch or forking of the parent intracranial artery. It does not arise at the lateral (proximal) angle but rather at the apical or distal angle (Figs. 34.21 and 34.22). It is the opinion of this author (J.L.F.) that most of these aneurysms arise as a result of long-term blood flow patterns. There is an association with atherosclerosis, vascular hypertension, congenital weakness of bifurcating angles, and/or pituitary or sex hormonal factors in many but not all instances.

Intracranial aneurysm sites are often closely related anatomically to small perforating arteries (13–16). Such arteries have vital significance for the surgeon and the patient. As noted by Kaplan (15), "The arterial supply to the basal masses of the forebrain is through the perforating branches of four major arteries from the internal carotid of each side: the anterior cerebral, middle cerebral, anterior choroidal and posterior cerebral arteries." Such arteries may be intimately close, or even adherent, to the walls of berry aneurysms; however, as noted by others (24,25) and confirmed by our microsurgical observations, perforators or branches do not *arise* from the wall of the typical berry aneurysm. Examples of these vessels are seen in Figs. 34.23 through 34.26. Confusion regarding this point stems from several factors: (a) In premicrosurgery days, small arteries adherent to the walls of berry aneurysms were thought to arise from the wall. (b) As an aneurysm grows (Fig. 34.27), its neck expands and the adjacent branching artery may be drawn into the expanded neck. (c) Fusiform, atherosclerotic aneurysms (ectasias) often have

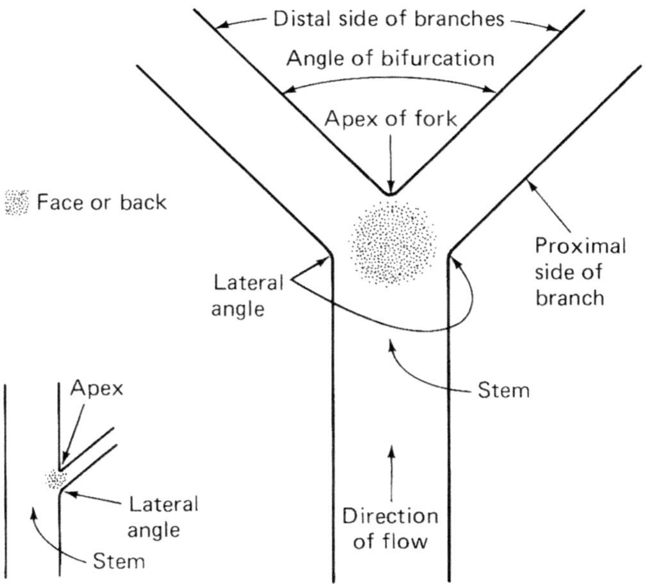

Fig. 34.21. Terminology used for certain anatomic sites about the bifurcation of branching vessels. From Stehbens WE, ref. 26.

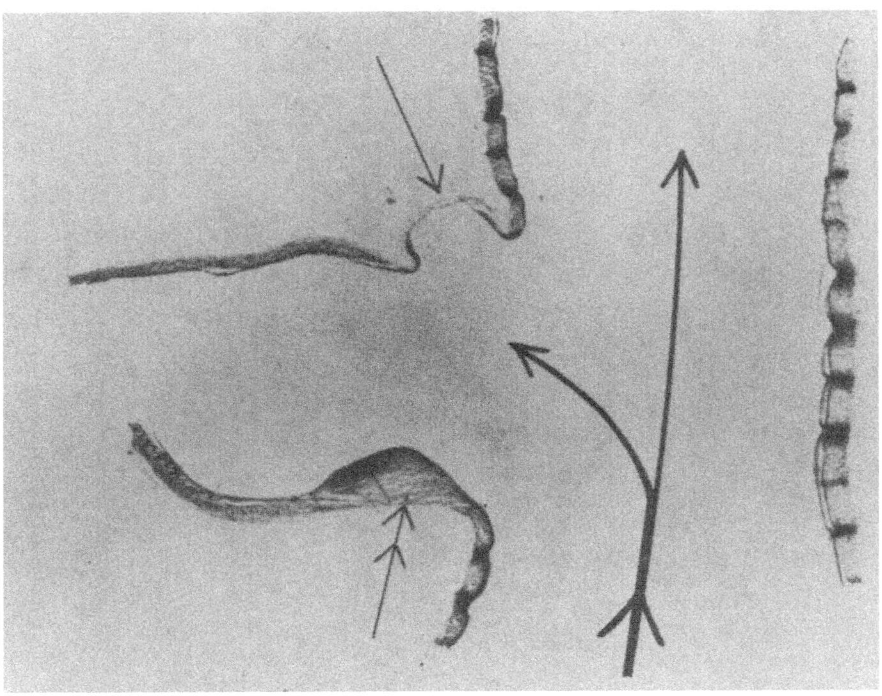

Fig. 34.22. Histologic section of minute aneurysm (*single-headed straight arrow*) at distal angle of bifurcation. *Double-headed arrow:* Intimal cushion. *Internal arrows:* Blood flow pattern. From Hassler O, ref. 11.

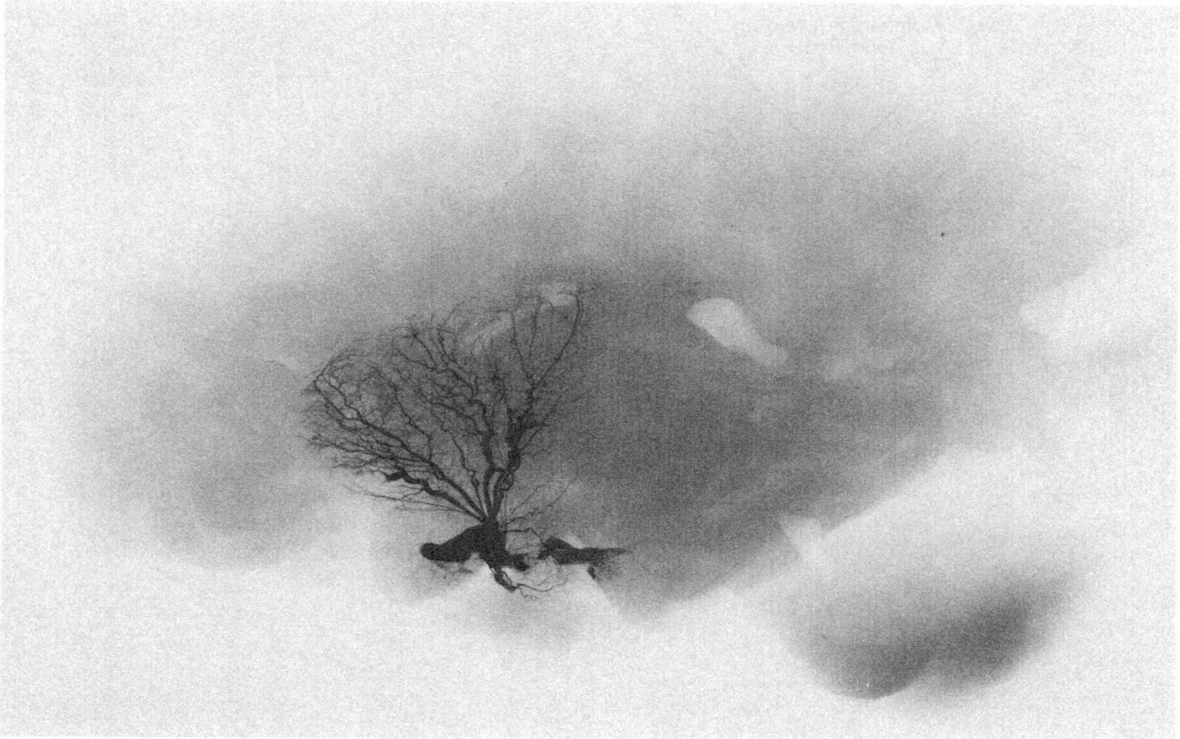

A

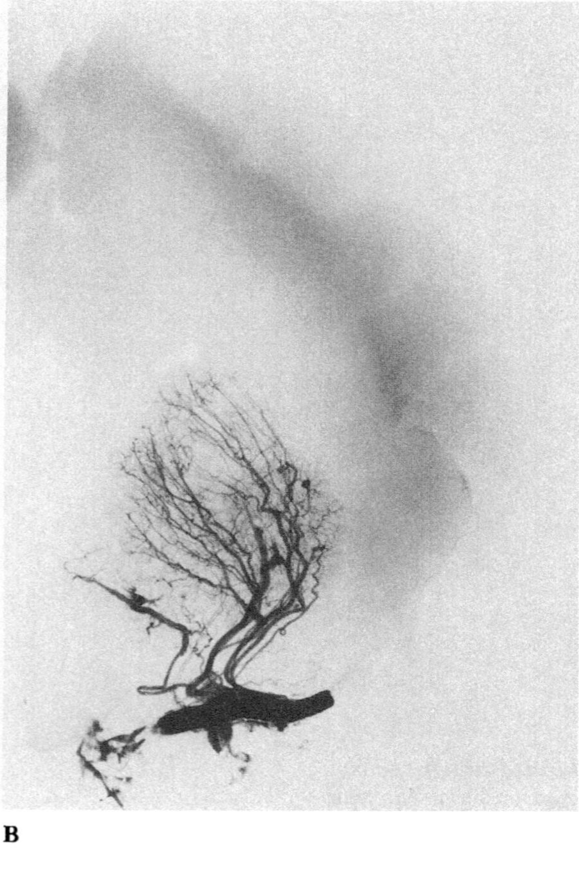

B

Fig. 34.23. Lateral (**A**) and frontal (**B**) views of radiographs showing contrast medium inside perforating arteries of autopsied human brain. These perforators arise from the ICA bifurcation and the A-1 and M-1 arteries. From Kaplan HA, ref. 16.

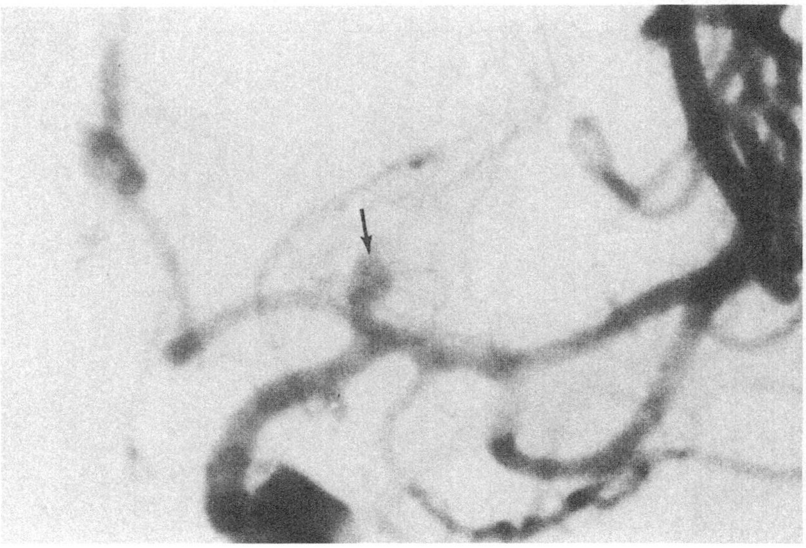

Fig. 34.24. Left carotid angiogram, AP view, subtraction technique. Note aneurysm (*arrow*) arising at junction of ICA and A-1. The aneurysm is surrounded by a leash of vital perforating arteries arising from M-1, ICA bifurcation, and A-1. From Fox JL, Nugent GR, ref. 9.

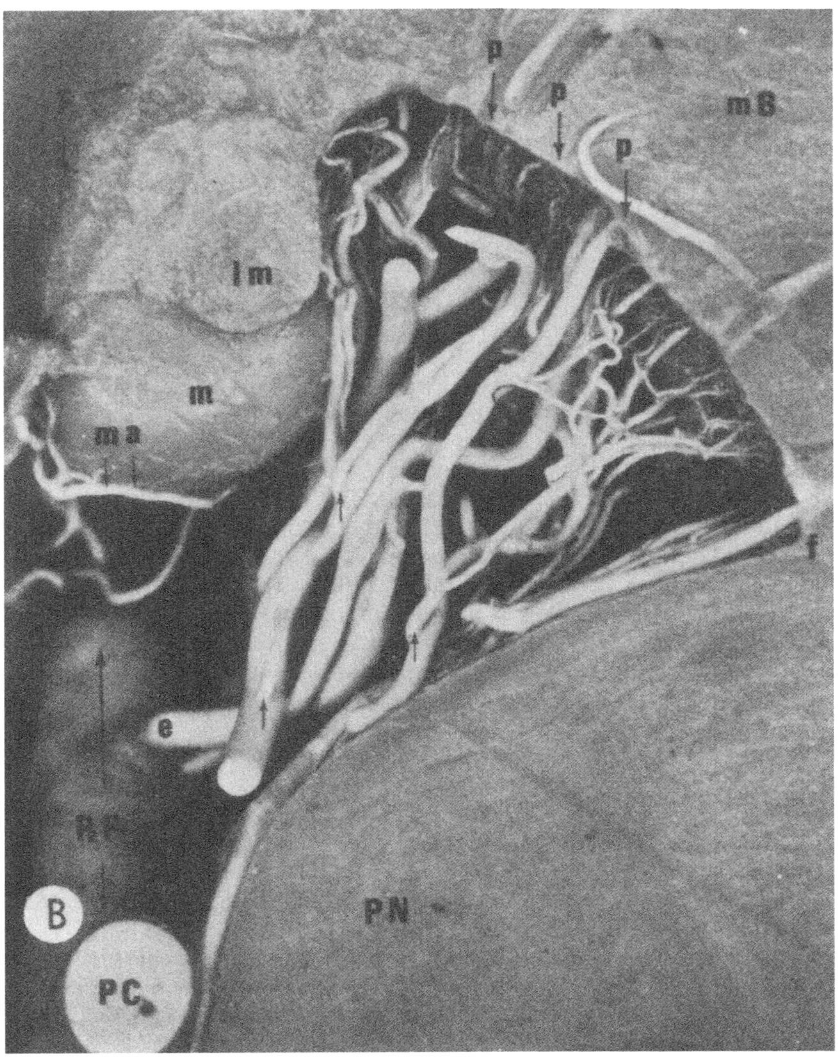

Fig. 34.25. Autopsy dissection of the interpeduncular fossa. *F,* Floor of third ventricle. *m,* Right mammillary body. *lm,* Left mammillary body. *ma,* Mammillary artery. *ppp,* Posterior perforated substance. *f,* Foramen cecum. *PN,* Pons. *mB,* Midbrain. *PC,* Left posterior cerebral artery (P-1 segment). *RP,* Right posterior communicating artery (P-1 segment). *e,* Origin of a posterior thalamoperforating artery. *Unlabeled arrows,* Angiographically nonvisible (usually) perforating arteries within the interpeduncular fossa. From George AE, Raybaud C, Salamon G, et al., ref. 10.

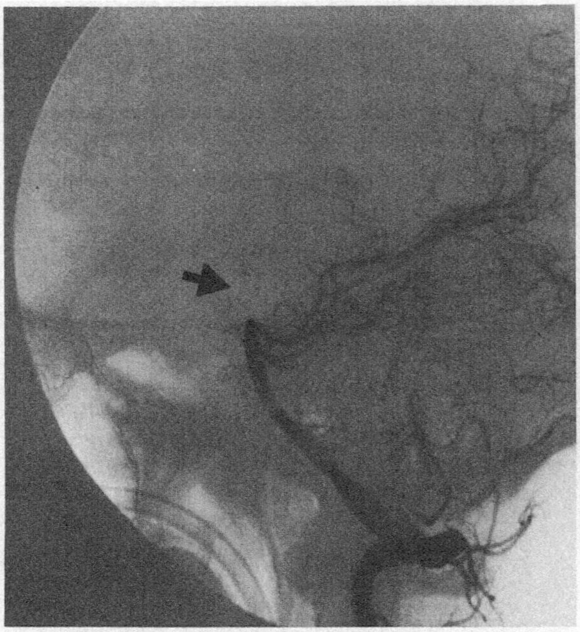

Fig. 34.26. Lateral view of vertebrobasilar arteriogram (subtraction technique) to show example of posterior thalamoperforators (*arrow*) arising from P-1 and the BA bifurcation.

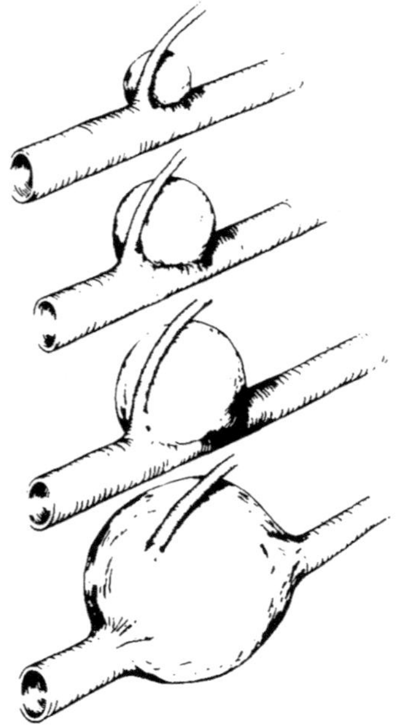

Fig. 34.27. The complexity of an intracranial aneurysm neck as a function of its size. From Drake CG, ref. 4.

branches arising from their walls, but these are not the berry aneurysms discussed here.

Regarding aneurysm size, McCormick (20) studied 177 autopsied aneurysms. Of these, he found that 11 (6%) were 21–50 mm in diameter (91% had evidence of bleeding); 5 (3%) were 16–20 mm (100% had evidence of bleeding); 15 (8%) were 11–15 mm (87% had evidence of bleeding); 49 (28%) were 6–10 mm (41% had evidence of bleeding); 74 (42%) were 3.2–5.0 mm (2.5% had evidence of bleeding); and 23 (13%) were 2–3 mm (none had evidence of bleeding).

Details of the anatomy and related surgical considerations of intracranial aneurysms are given in the following chapters.

Bibliography

1. Dandy WE: Intracranial Arterial Aneurysms. New York, Hafner, 1944, reprinted 1969
2. Drake CG: Advances in the neurosurgical treatment of aneurysms, arteriovenous malformations, and hematomas of the vertebral circulation. Adv Neurol 16:211–225, 1977
3. Drake CG: Giant intracranial aneurysms: experience in 174 patients. Clin Neurosurg 26:12–95, 1979
4. Drake CG: The treatment of aneurysms of the posterior circulation. Clin Neurosurg 26:96–144, 1979
5. Fox JL: Microsurgical exposure of intracranial aneurysms. J Microsurg 1:2–31, 1979
6. Fox JL, Albin MS, Bader DCH, et al.: Microsurgical treatment of neurovascular disease. Neurosurgery 3:285–337, 1978
7. Fox JL, Al-Mefty O: Suprasellar arachnoid cysts: an extension of the membrane of Liliequist. Neurosurgery 7:615–618, 1980
8. Fox JL, Luessenhop AJ: Hydrocephalus secondary to hemorrhage from a basilar artery aneurysm. With a note on embolization technique. Acta Neurochir (Wien) 17:228–235, 1967
9. Fox JL, Nugent GR: Recent advances in intracranial aneurysm surgery. W Va Med J 72:104–105, 1976
10. George AE, Raybaud C, Salamon G, et al.: Anatomy of the thalamoperforating arteries with special emphasis on arteriography of the third ventricle. Part I. Am J Roentgenol 124:220–230, 1975
11. Hassler O: Morphological studies on the large cerebral arteries with reference to the aetiology of subarachnoid haemorrhage. Acta Psy-

chiatr Neurol Scand [Suppl 154]36:1–145, 1961
12. Hosobuchi Y: Direct surgical treatment of giant intracranial aneurysms. J Neurosurg 51:743–756, 1979
13. Kaplan HA: Anatomy and embryology of the arterial system of the forebrain. In Vinken PJ, Bruyn GW (eds.): Handbook of Clinical Neurology, Volume 11: Vascular Diseases of the Nervous System. Part I. Amsterdam, North-Holland, 1972, pp. 1–23
14. Kaplan HA: Embryology and anatomy of the blood vessels of the brain. In Fields WS (ed.): Pathogenesis and Treatment of Cerebrovascular Disease. Springfield, Ill., Thomas, 1961, pp. 5–31
15. Kaplan HA: The anatomy of the perforating arteries of the basal ganglia. In Salamon G (ed.): Advances in Cerebral Angiography. Berlin, Springer-Verlag, 1975, pp. 33–36
16. Kaplan HA: The lateral perforating branches of the anterior and middle cerebral arteries. J Neurosurg 23:305–310, 1965
17. Kempe LG: Operative Neurosurgery, Vol 1: Cranial, Cerebral, and Intracranial Vascular Disease. Berlin, Springer-Verlag, 1968, pp. 1–75, 203–214
18. Key A, Retzius G: Studien in der Anatomie des Nervensystems und des Bindegewebes, Vol 1. Stockholm, Norsted & Söner, 1875, plate III
19. Liliequist B: The subarachnoid cisterns. An anatomic and roentgenologic study. Acta Radiol [Suppl] 185:1–108, 1959
20. McCormick WF: Problems and pathogenesis of intracranial arterial aneurysms. In Toole JF, Moossy J, Janeway R (eds.): Cerebral Vascular Diseases. New York, Grune & Stratton, 1971, pp. 219–231
20a. Pernkopf E: Atlas of Topical and Applied Human Anatomy, Vol 1: Head and Neck. Philadelphia, Saunders, 1963, pp. 20, 30, 31, 63, 185, 186
21. Pia HW: Classification of aneurysms of the internal carotid system. Acta Neurochir (Wien) 40:5–31, 1978
22. Rhoton AL Jr: Anatomy of saccular aneurysms. Surg Neurol 14:59–66, 1980
23. Rhoton AL, Saeki N, Pearlmutter D, et al.: Microsurgical anatomy of common aneurysm sites. Clin Neurosurg 26:248–306, 1979
24. Rodda R: The necropsy demonstration of cerebral aneurysms by intra-arterial injection. Proc Aust Assoc Neurol 7:115–121, 1970
25. Sachs M, Cabezas CC, Posada JT, et al.: Anatomical research on the intracranial arterial aneurysms. Prog Brain Res 30:275–281, 1968
25a. Seeger W: Microsurgery of the Brain. Anatomical and Technical Principles. New York, Springer-Verlag, 1980
26. Stehbens WE: Medial defects of the cerebral arteries of man. J Pathol Bacteriol 78:179–185, 1959
27. Stehbens WE: Pathology of the Cerebral Blood Vessels. St Louis, Mosby, 1972
28. Stehbens WE: The renal artery in normal and cholesterol-fed rabbits. Am J Pathol 43:969–985, 1963
29. Sundt TM Jr, Piepgras DG: Surgical approach to giant intracranial aneurysms. Operative experience with 80 cases. J Neurosurg 51:731–742, 1979
30. Yaşargil MG, Fox JL: The microsurgical approach to intracranial aneurysms. Surg Neurol 3:7–14, 1975
31. Yaşargil MG, Fox JL, Ray MW: The operative approach to aneurysms of the anterior communicating artery. In Krayenbühl H (ed.): Advances and Technical Standards in Neurosurgery, Vol. 2. New York, Springer-Verlag, 1975, pp. 113–170
32. Yaşargil MG, Kasdaglis K, Jain KK, et al.: Anatomical observations of the subarachnoid cisterns of the brain during surgery. J Neurosurg 44:298–302, 1976

35

Technique of Aneurysm Surgery

II. Anterior Communicating and Anterior Cerebral Artery Aneurysms

Anterior Communicating Artery Aneurysms

As noted in Chapter 29, the frontotemporal (frontolateral, or pterional) approach to the ACoAA is one of four standard approaches and is the shortest route to the anterior communicating artery (ACoA). This route also has been a standard approach to all aneurysms of the circle of Willis and nearby branches since the time of Walter Dandy. Hence, when one is dealing with a patient harboring multiple aneurysms, the same craniotomy orientation can be used for all upper BAA, ipsilateral ICAA and MCAA, and ACoAA in the same patient.

As already mentioned in the previous chapter, the arteries entering the anterior perforated substance from ICA, A-1, and M-1 are critical and must not be injured. In the past such injuries have not uncommonly occurred during an attack on an ACoAA. Of importance is the largest of these perforators, the recurrent artery of Heubner. The detailed anatomy and irrigation zones of these arteries can be found elsewhere in the literature (11,16,17,19,28, 29,33,35,37,39,42,45,50,52,55). Heubner's artery is diagramed in Figs. 35.1 and 35.2. In the previous chapter, Figs. 34.13, 34.14, and 34.16 give a surgeon's view of some of the A-1 perforators which must be protected from stretching, injury, and spasm. Examples of Heubner's artery as seen by the surgeon are found in Figs. 5.2, 34.15, 35.3, 35.6, 35.12, 35.13, 35.15, 35.23, 35.24, 35.26, 35.27, 35.33, 35.34, 36.18, 36.19, and 36.30.

As noted in some of the aforementioned figures, the artery of Heubner may be seen before the A-1 artery is identified as the surgeon dissects medially under the frontal lobe. This recurrent artery commonly is found lying just superior and anterior to the A-1 artery as the recurrent artery courses laterally (Fig. 35.3). At times, branches of Heubner's artery may wander anteriorly under the frontal lobe and should not be confused with the frontoorbital artery, which often may be sacrificed as it is followed to the aneurysm.

The surgeon must be cognizant of the various anatomic variations of the circle of Willis. Such variations are the rule rather than the exception (22,44). As illustrated in Fig. 35.4A, one of the A-1 arteries (for example) may be small or absent, often with contralateral A-1 enlargement to feed both ascending anterior cerebral arteries (see Fig. 35.33 for a surgical example). This discrepancy between the diameters (and hence blood flow pattern) of the right and left A-1 arteries is seen in about 80% of patients with an ACoAA (55). This A-1 asymmetry seems to be associated with a higher incidence of ACoAA (7,8,24–27,31,32,43), and it probably is related etiologically to ACoAA formation by flow phenomena rather than congenital maldevelopment per se. Although some authors have described a correlation between many vascular "anomalies" of the circle of Willis and intracranial aneurysm formation (36,38), most workers now do not find any greater incidence of variations in the circle of Willis pattern in aneurysm cases compared to control cases

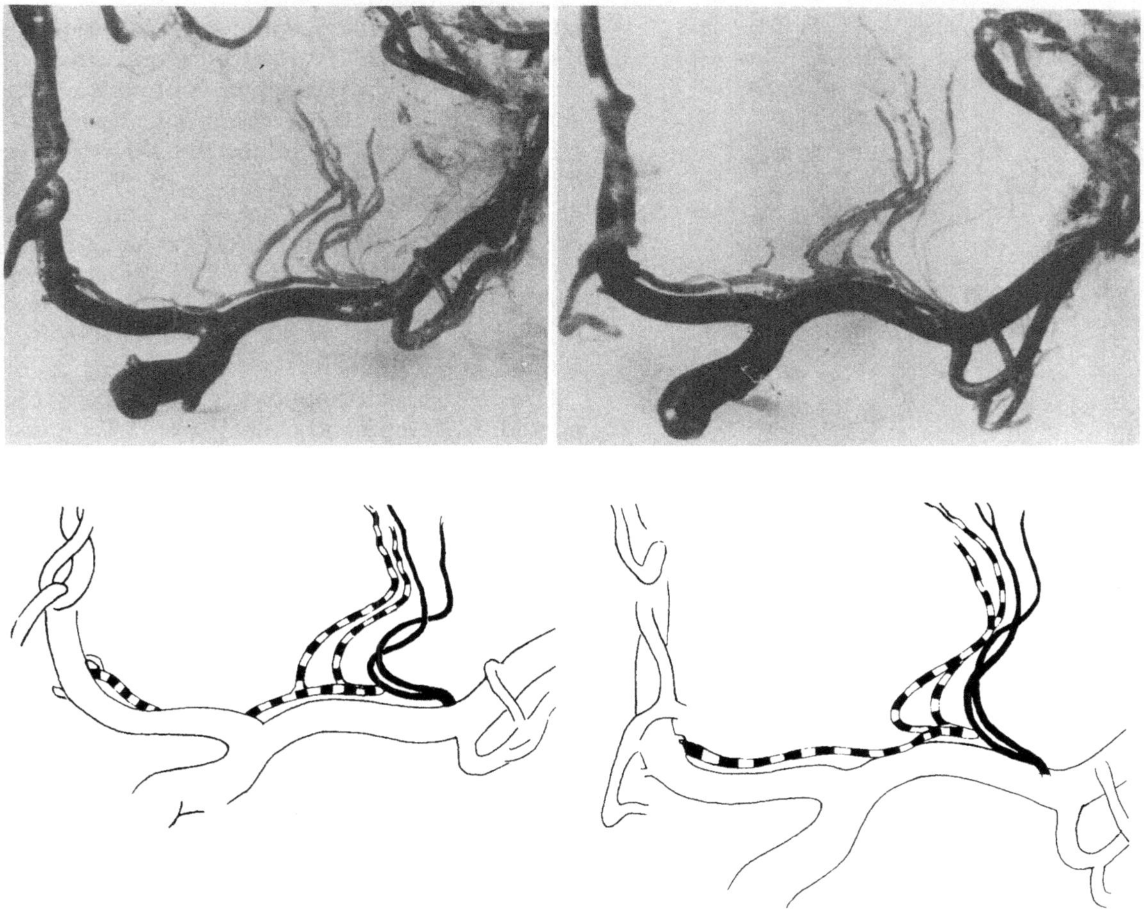

Fig. 35.1. Photograph of a plastic cast (*above*) and diagram (*below*) of the recurrent artery of Heubner as seen from in front with two somewhat different projections. In the diagram, Heubner's artery is shown in interrupted lines. From Westberg G: ref. 50.

except (a) where there is a noticeable difference in the size of the two A-1 arteries as just described (7,8,24–27,31,32,43) and (b) where there is an azygous anterior cerebral artery (18,20). The latter condition is associated with a high incidence of aneurysm of the azygous ACeA. There is no correlation between the ACoA duplication and bridging anomalies (Fig. 35.4B) and the presence of an aneurysm in the same region (24).

Of particular significance for the surgeon is the fact that in cases where one A-1 is larger than the other, the ACoA aneurysm (ACoAA) arises from the ACoA (usually at the ACoA/A-2 junction) on the side of the *larger* A-1 artery. This was illustrated by Voris in 1951 (48) (Fig. 35.5), and confirmed in autopsied brains of 37 ACoAA cases by Stehbens in 1963 (43). More recently, surgeons have noted the same relationships (25,26,47,53–55). Yaşargil and Smith (55) concluded that A-1 was larger on the left side in 49% of their ACoAA cases and larger on the right side in 27% of these cases. They found the ACoAA arising from the side of the smaller A-1 in only 2% of these patients.

Anomalies of the ACoA itself are occasionally seen at surgery. Figure 35.6 presents such an example seen in a patient operated for a bBAA. Duplications, triplications, and/or bridgings of the ACoA are well known (Fig. 35.7). An anomaly of the anterior cerebral artery (ACeA) that may be confused with an ACoAA is a proximal loop in a midline, *accessory* anterior cerebral artery, which arises from the ACoA between

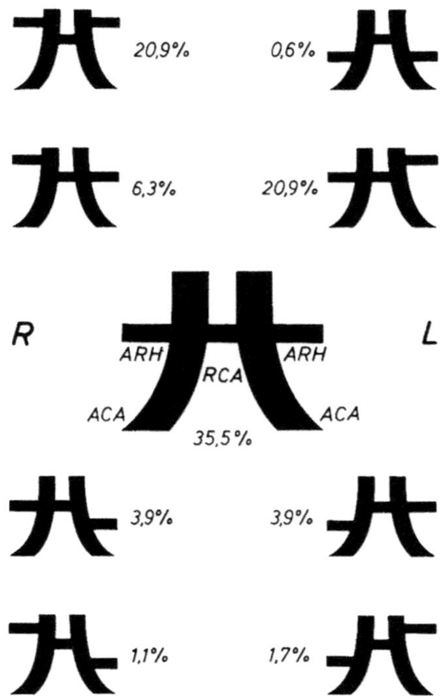

Fig. 35.2. Diagram of variations in origin of right (*R*) and left (*L*) arteries of Heubner (*ARH*). *RCA*, anterior communicating artery; *ACA*, A-1 artery. Note that in most cases the artery originates at or just above the A-1/A-2 junction. From Kribs M, Kleihues P: ref. 23.

the right and left A-2 arteries (Fig. 35.8). As the surgeon exposes the ACoA region, this forward loop initially and erroneously may appear to be an ACoAA arising between the right and left A-2 arteries. Another anomaly is the *azygous* (or *azygos*) anterior cerebral artery (18,30), which is reminiscent of the unpaired ACeA in the chimpanzee and some other lower forms of animals (30,49). The azygous ACeA is the single, midline A-2/A-3 ascending portion of the ACeA. As it turns around the corpus callosum, it divides into its right and left divisions. Unlike the accessory ACeA, which complements a right and left ascending ACeA arising from the ACoA, the azygous ACeA is the only ascending ACeA feeding both cerebral hemispheres before it divides. These anomalies will be discussed again later in this chapter.

The Surgical Exposure

The following is a continuation of the frontotemporal exposure described and illustrated in the previous chapter. Figure 35.9 is an anatomic frontotemporal cut-away illustration of the ACoA region, its aneurysm, and surgical orientation. As the dissection continues medially toward the anterior communicating complex, the surgeon may follow the A-1 segment if it is easily seen (Figs. 34.13, 34.16, 35.3, 35.6, 35.12, and 35.21 are examples). In cases where the ICA is elongated and the A-1 is hidden posteriorly (Figs. 35.28 and 35.29), the surgeon should avoid retraction to expose the A-1 and instead go directly to the gyrus rectus as described below.

The gyrus rectus approach as originally reported by Kempe and colleagues (21,47) is detailed also in Chapter 30; it is an important contribution to the ACoAA approach. We have adopted this technique in most cases. There are a few patients who have both a relatively short ICA with a straight A-1 artery and a directly posteriorly or inferoposteriorly projecting ACoAA, in whom simple and gentle retraction of the frontal lobe will reveal the ACoA complex and not risk traction on and premature rupture of the aneurysm. An example is seen in Figs. 35.10–35.12.

Figure 35.13 is another example where the gyrus rectus incision was not used. However, in this case the aneurysm was not seen on angiography (even in retrospective examination of the films); it was discovered incidentally during exploration of the circle of Willis for treatment of other known, multiple aneurysms. Upon elevation of the frontal lobe, the anteriorly pointing ACoAA was seen and subsequently clipped. Notice the use of a dental cotton ball between the retracting suction tube and the brain. This technique is commonly employed to pull the brain tissue away from an aneurysm in order to gain better exposure of the aneurysm and parent arteries. Alternatively, the aneurysm itself can be retracted from the brain in a like manner under differing circumstances.

Figures 35.14 and 35.15 illustrate two separate aneurysms arising from the ACoA. Only the anteroinferiorly projecting aneurysm is seen in the exposure in Fig. 35.15. In this situation the surgeon must be extremely careful in elevating the frontal lobe from the optic nerves to avoid traction on the aneurysm and rupture. It is clear that the aneurysm is adherent to the left optic nerve near the chiasm. After exposure through the gyrus rectus, the aneurysm was gently freed from the optic nerve, narrowed by electrocoagulation, and then clipped. The

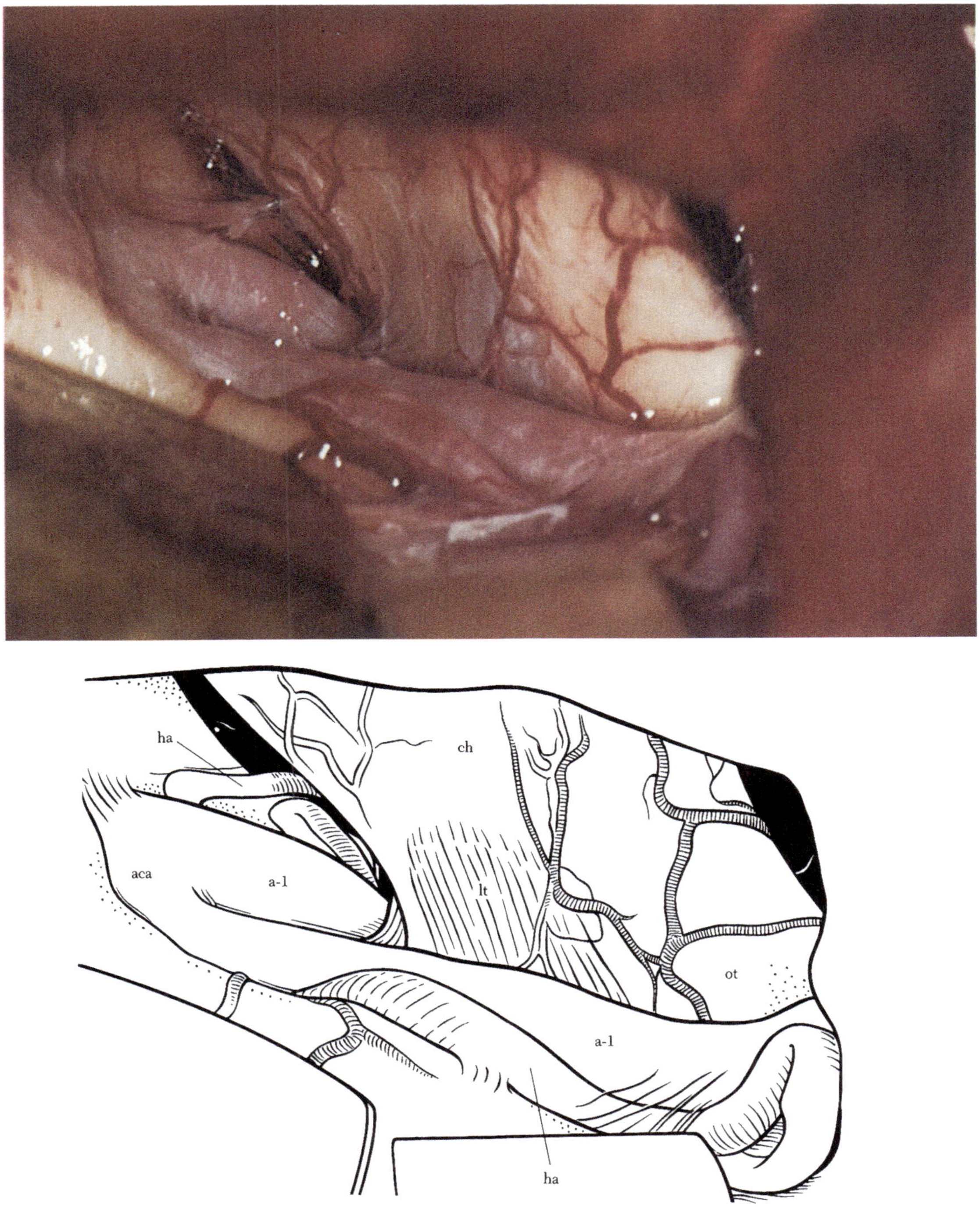

Fig. 35.3. Right frontotemporal view of prefixed chiasm (*ch*) at anterior communicating artery (*aca*) region during approach to an anterior communicating artery aneurysm (same case as in Figs. 35.25–35.27). *a-1*, right and left A-1 arteries; *ha*, right and left Heubner's arteries; *ot;* right optic tract; *lt*, lamina terminalis. Adjacent to left Heubner's artery (*above*) is prominent left A-1 perforator. On close examination the observer sees tiny arteries passing from the A-1 and anterior communicating arteries to the lamina terminalis and optic chiasm. From Fox JL: ref. 12.

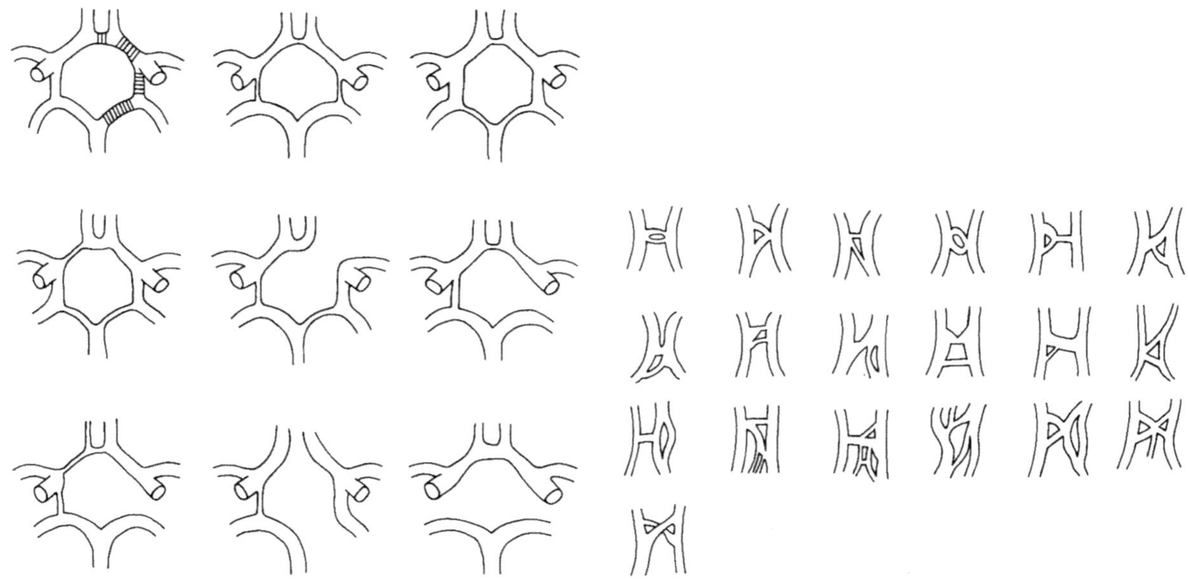

A B

Fig. 35.4. **A** Diagrams of common variations in the circle of Willis. The upper left diagram is the "normal" circle; the arterial portions that often become attenuated are emphasized by a series of parallel lines: tracing clockwise these arteries are ACoA, A-1, PCoA, and P-1. From Greitz T, Lindgren E: ref. 15. **B** Diagrams of common variations in the anterior communicating artery (ACoA) complex. From Crudeli R: ref. 9.

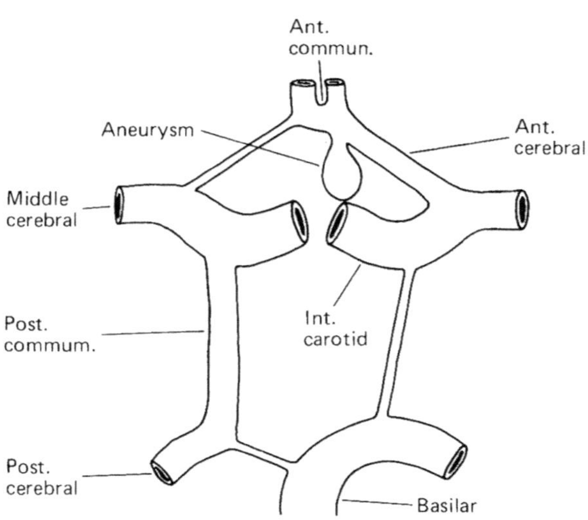

Fig. 35.5. Diagram of circle of Willis with an aneurysm of the anterior communicating artery on the side of the larger A-1 (*ant. cerebral*). From Voris HC: ref. 48.

other (hidden) ACoAA in the same patient was subsequently visualized and clipped by elevating the right A-2 artery. The dome of the aneurysm was stuck to prominent hypothalamic perforators from which it was separated before clipping.

Figures 35.16 and 35.17 are two more angiographic examples of ACoAA cases in which retraction of the frontal lobe must be carried out with delicacy. In such circumstances, it cannot be emphasized strongly enough that the surgeon should avoid any exposure of the aneurysm until the ACoA complex is visualized via a partial gyrus rectus excision. In this way, the neck of the aneurysm can be seen and controlled before the dome, adherent to the optic nerves or tuberculum sellae, is mobilized (and possibly torn by premature or excess frontal lobe retraction).

Whether the surgeon follows A-1 medially from the ICA bifurcation or goes directly

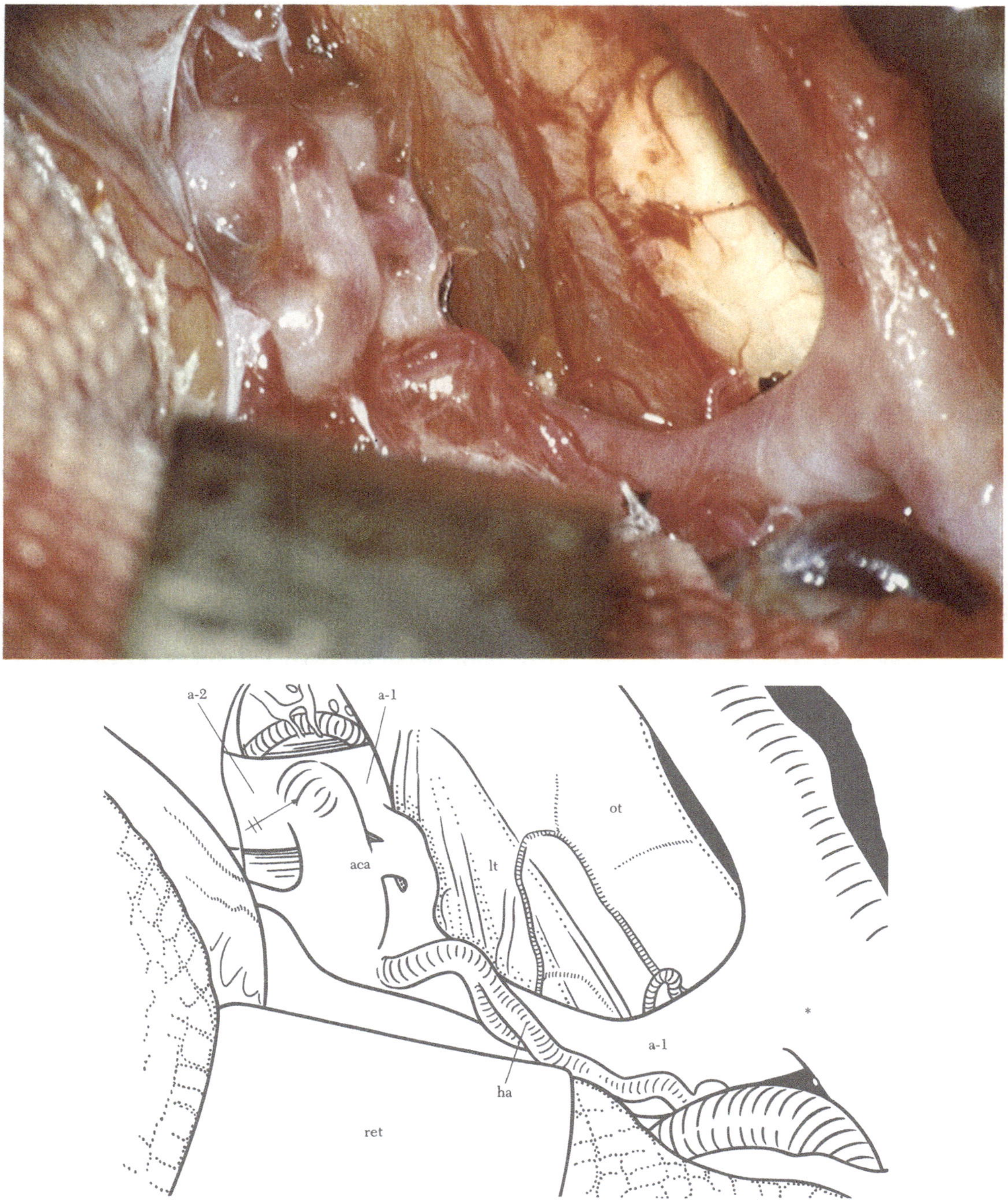

Fig. 35.6. Photograph of ACoA anomaly. On the right (*) is the right ICA and its bifurcation into A-1 and M-1. A retractor blade (*ret*) pulls the frontal lobe from the right A-1 (*a-1*) coursing medially (*leftward*) over the right optic tract (*ot*) and lamina terminalis (*lt*). At the medial limit of A-1 is part of Heubner's artery (*ha*) arising and running laterally over it. At that same point the ACoA (*aca*) is seen to arise as a duplicated artery with a vertical bridge like a "lazy," or horizontal, H. (Actually it is a triplicated ACoA, but the third portion is hidden.) Beyond the ACoA anomaly (upper left corner) is the left A-1 (*a-1*) and A-2 (*a-2*) union. At the left A-1, A-2, and ACoA union there is a red microaneurysm (*double-crossed arrow*) of the ACoA.

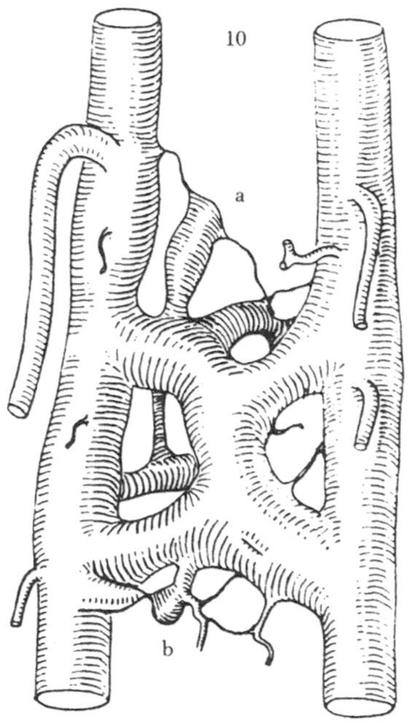

Fig. 35.7. A historic, diagrammatic example of an ACoA anomaly forming duplications and bridges. On either side are the left and right A-1/A-2 junctions. From Bremer JL: ref. 4.

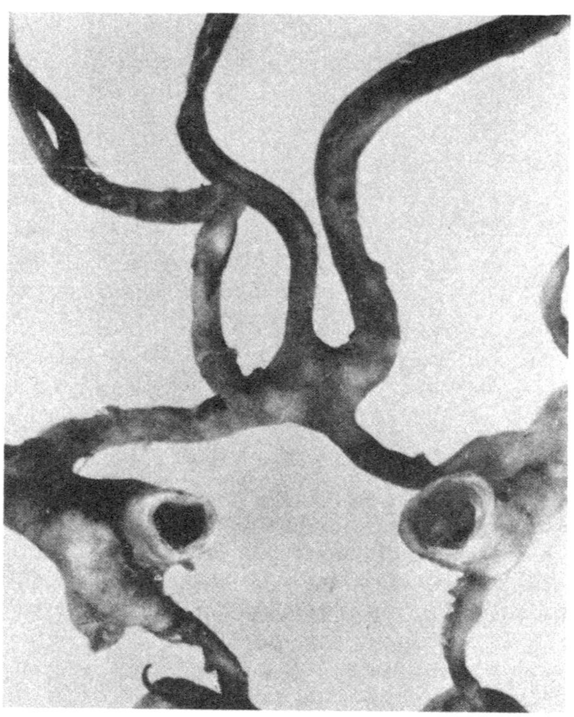

Fig. 35.8. Postmortem example of an accessory anterior cerebral artery passing upward between the right and left anterior cerebral arteries. From Castillo R, et al.: ref. 6.

through the gyrus rectus without visualizing A-1 initially, care must be taken not to injure Heubner's artery or confuse it with the orbitofrontal (frontoorbital) artery. There may be one or two additional Heubner's arteries arising from A-1 or A-2. It may divide into one or more prominent branches. We have seen a common trunk arise from A-1 and bifurcate into Heubner's artery going laterally along A-1 and the orbitofrontal artery coursing anterosuperiorly around the frontal pole.

In the majority of ACoAA cases we go through the gyrus rectus regardless of the direction the aneurysm points. Kempe (21) has a diagram of the incision which need only be 1 cm in length (Fig. 35.18). The initial exposure of the gyrus rectus and the site of its incision are nicely demonstrated in Figs. 35.19–35.21. There is often a triangular or quadrangular zone formed by (a) the optic nerve/frontal lobe junction (or A-1/frontal lobe junction), (b) the olfactory tract and retractor blade, and (c) the orbitofrontal artery as the self-retaining retractor blade first exposes the gyrus rectus medial to the olfactory tract. The initial incision is made in the gyrus rectus within this zone. The pia is cauterized and incised with a knife blade. Then with suction, bipolar forceps, and microscissors, a zone of brain tissue 1 cm in length is removed down to the medial pia-arachnoid layer.

We have found that if the orbitofrontal (fronto-orbital) artery is followed, it will lead the surgeon directly to the ACoA complex. However, extreme care must be taken since this artery often is adherent to the dome of the aneurysm. As the aneurysm is approached, this artery can be electrocoagulated and severed. In this way, any retraction on the frontal lobe with a consequent pulling on the orbitofrontal artery will not result in traction on the ACoAA wall (a not uncommon cause of intraoperative rupture). Once the medial pia-arachnoid layer of the gyrus rectus is reached, fibrin and clot obscuring the aneurysm may be encountered. The pia-arachnoid layer is carefully opened and any fibrin and clot around the ACoA, its A-1/A-2 branches, and the neck of the aneurysm are removed by suction and forceps. Adhesions are lysed. The dome of the aneurysm initially is avoided and the self-retaining retractors maintained in proper position to permit exposure of the neck without movement of the dome of the aneurysm.

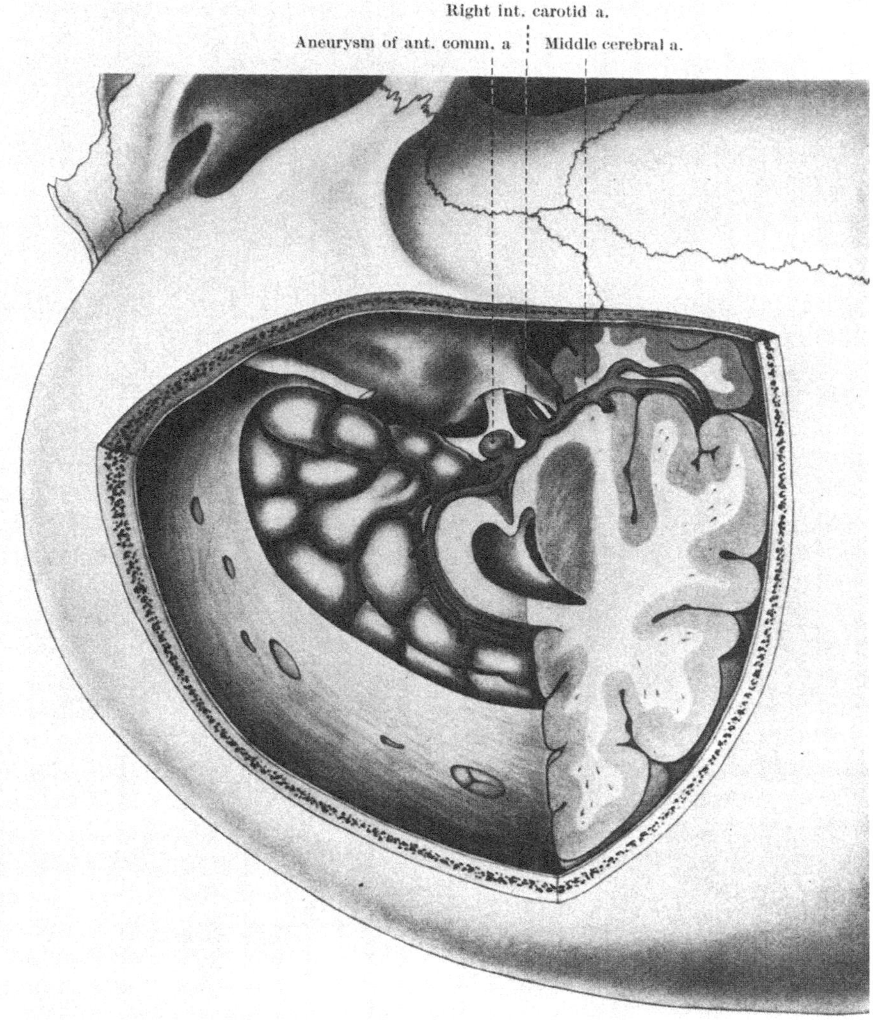

Fig. 35.9. Drawing of ACoAA and environs in a frontotemporal orientation. The right frontal and temporal lobes are cut away anteriorly to expose the ICA, MCA, and ACeA. From Kempe LG: ref. 21.

The ACoAA being approached in Fig. 35.21 is demonstrated angiographically in Fig. 35.22. In our experience, this superior projection of the aneurysm into the interhemispheric fissure between the frontal lobes is the commonest one. It arises from the ACoA/A-2 junction on the side of the larger A-1 artery in most instances. Its dome is flanked or surrounded by the right and left A-2 arteries (Fig. 35.23). Perforating arteries from A-1 and ACoA may be in spasm. At this point, lay a small cottonoid soaked with vasodilators (such as 0.5% phentolamine or 3% papaverine solution) on the arteries for a minute. This will help maintain good perfusion to vital structures. This should be repeated as needed and after clipping.

With the blood pressure reduced, the neck (and dome in most of our cases) of the ACoAA (Fig. 35.23) must be dissected free of its adjacent A-2 arteries and any hypothalamic perforators on the posterior and inferior (hidden) surface of the aneurysm. The delicate dissection with microvascular instruments may take considerable time (see Figs. 26.13, 26.16, and 26.17 for those instruments used by this author [J.L.F.]). The back wall of the aneurysm may be seen best by gentle separation of the right A-2 from the aneurysm and brain tissue and

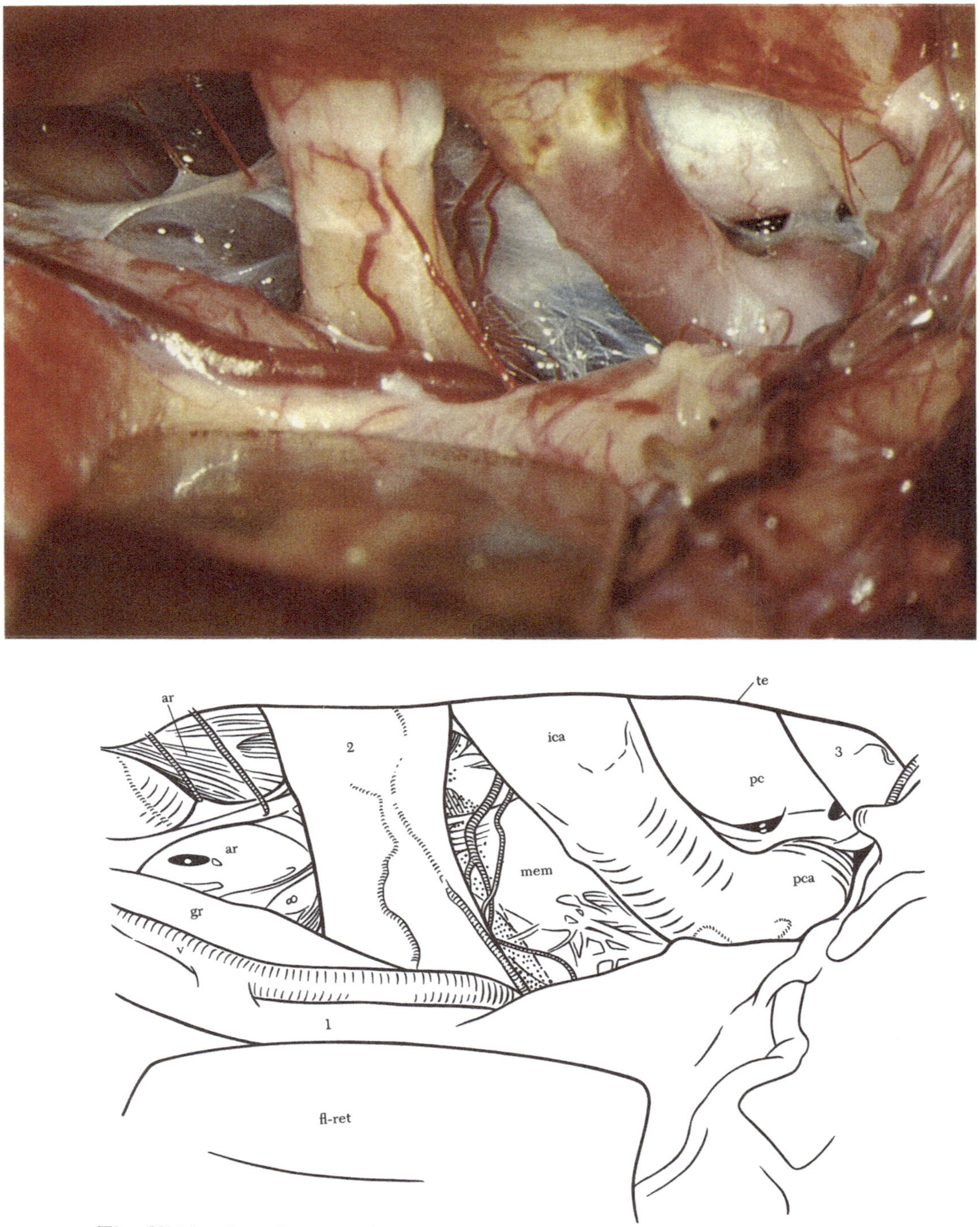

Fig. 35.10. Initial approach to ACoAA. The gyrus rectus (*gr*) approach is not used in this case. *ar,* arachnoid between optic nerves; *2,* right optic nerve; *ica,* internal carotid artery; *te,* anterior reflection of tentorial edge; *3,* oculomotor nerve passing lateral to dura on posterior clinoid process (*pc*); *pca,* posterior communicating artery; *mem,* membrane of Liliequist; *fl-ret,* frontal lobe retractor; *1,* olfactory tract; *v,* vein on gyrus rectus (*gr*).

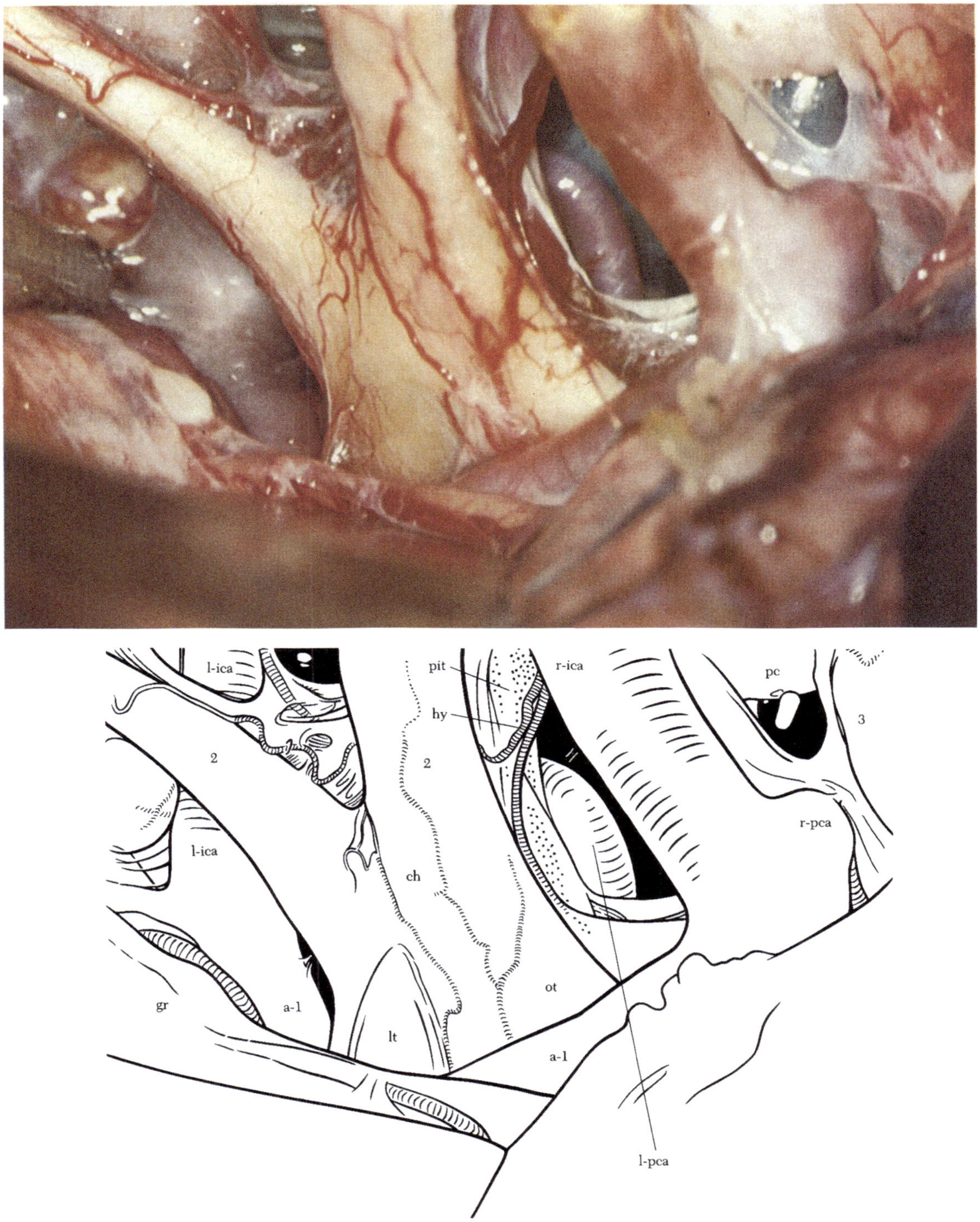

Fig. 35.11. Medial exposure of same case as in Fig. 35.10 by retraction of right frontal lobe. Both left and right A-1 arteries (*a-1*) are coming into view. *2*, left and right optic nerves; *ch*, optic chiasm; *ot*, right optic tract; *lt*, lamina terminalis; *pit*, pituitary stalk; *hy*, hypothalamic perforators from right internal carotid artery (*r-ica*); *pc*, posterior clinoid process; *3*, oculomotor nerve; *r-pca*, right posterior communicating artery; *l-pca*, left posterior communicating artery; *gr*, right gyrus rectus; *l-ica*, left internal carotid artery.

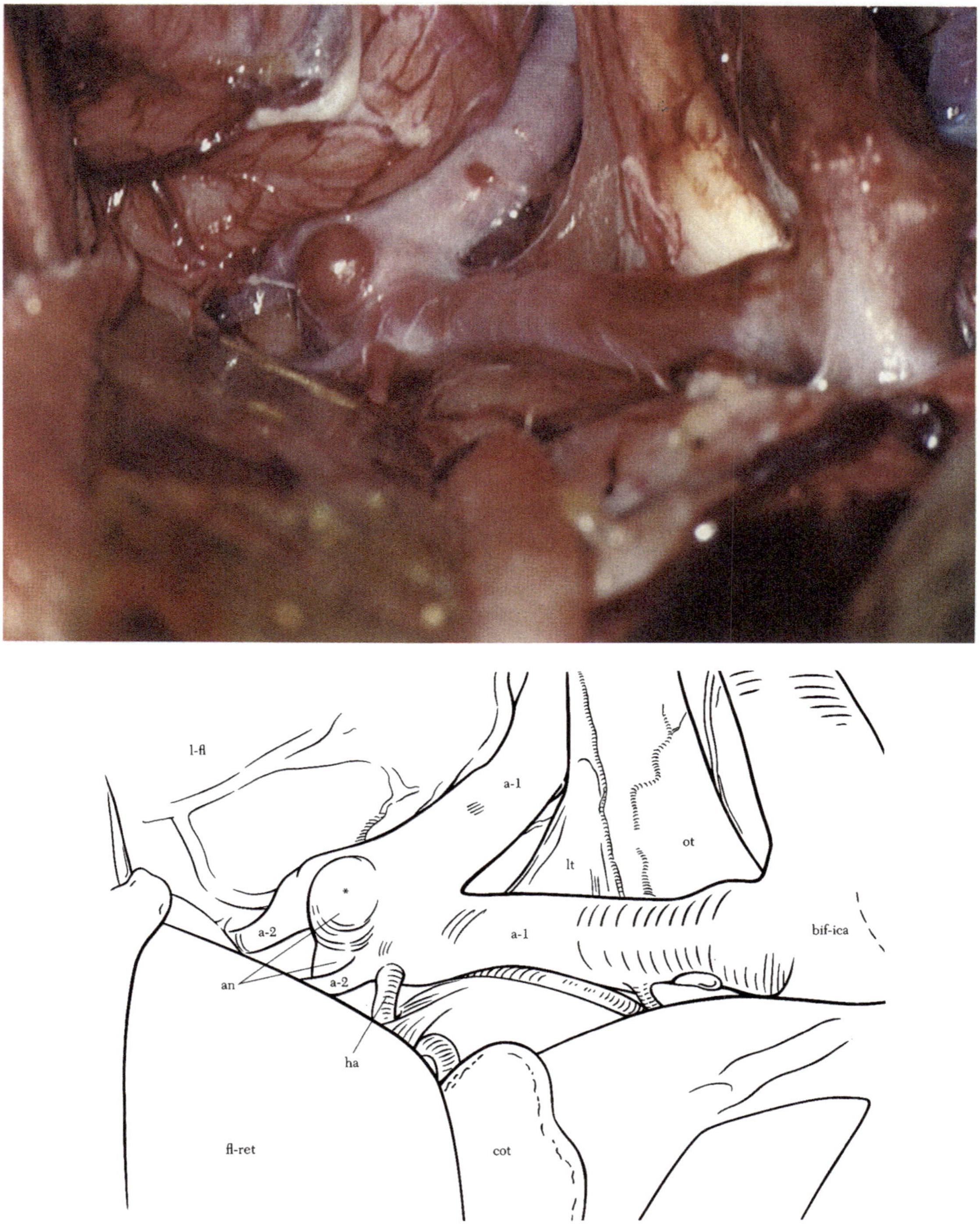

Fig. 35.12. Exposure of two aneurysms (*an*) on the ACoA (same case as in Figs. 35.10 and 35.11). The small red blister (*) pointing anterosuperiorly is obvious. The large aneurysm pointing inferoposteriorly is hidden and passes down between the left (*above*) and right (*below*) A-2 arteries (*a-2*). *l-fl*, left frontal lobe; *a-1*, left (*above*) and right (*below*) A-1 arteries; *lt*, lamina terminalis; *ot*, right optic tract; *bif-ica*, bifurcation of right ICA; *cot*, cotton strip under right frontal lobe retractor (*fl-ret*); *ha*, right Heubner's artery.

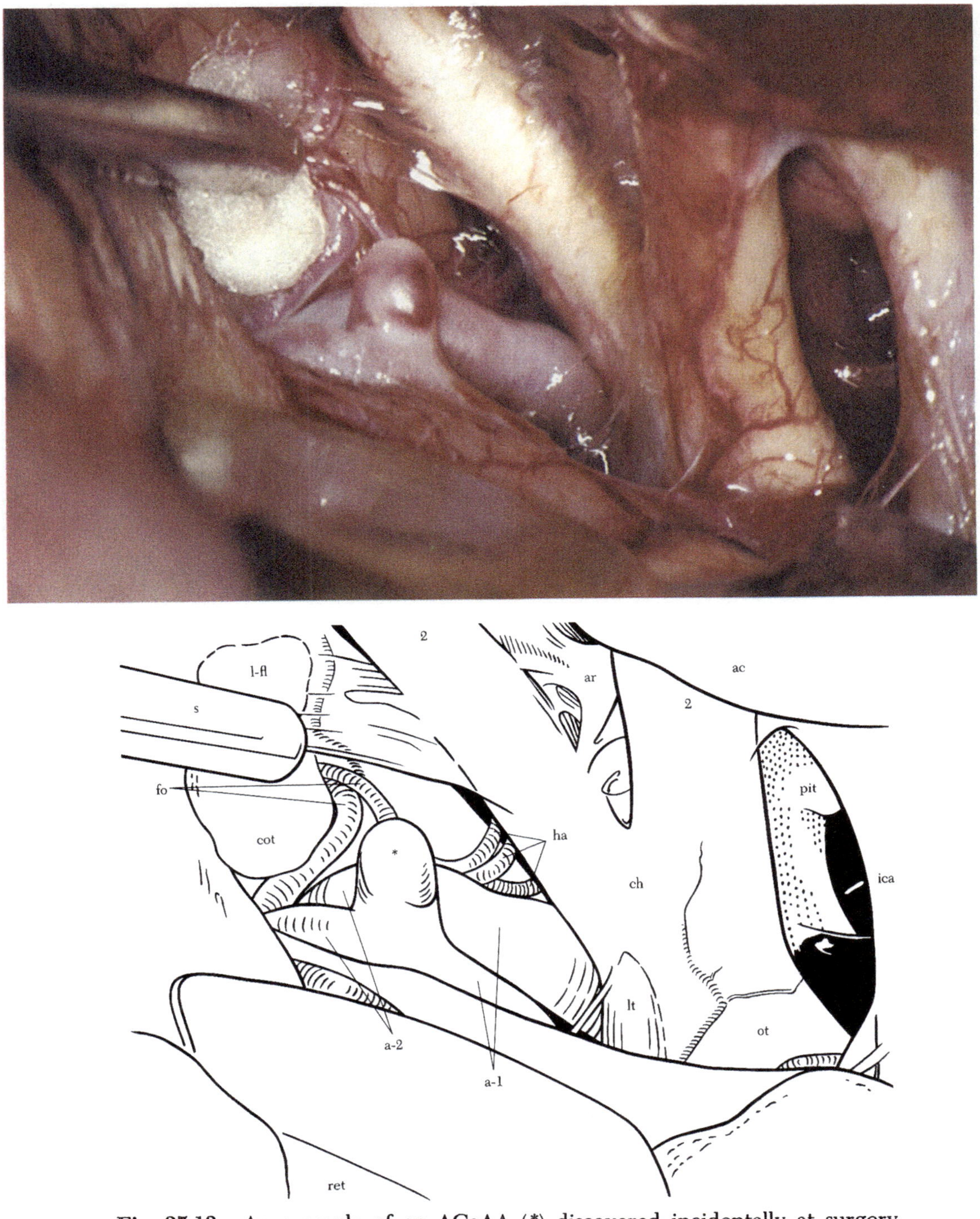

Fig. 35.13. An example of an ACoAA (*) discovered incidentally at surgery upon elevation of the right frontal lobe by the retractor (*ret*). The aneurysm projects forward but has not adhered to the optic nerves (*2*) or chiasm (*ch*). *ar,* arachnoid between optic nerves; *ac,* right anterior clinoid process; *pit,* superior aspect of pituitary gland; *ot,* right optic tract; *lt,* lamina terminalis; *a-1,* left (*above*) and right (*below*) A-1 arteries; *a-2,* left (*above*) and right (*below*) A-2 arteries; *cot,* cotton ball (*dental*) used to assist in retraction of the left frontal lobe (*l-fl*) by the suction tube (*s*); *fo,* left (*above*) and right (*below*) frontoorbital arteries; *ha,* left Heubner's artery with two accessory Heubner's arteries (or perforators).

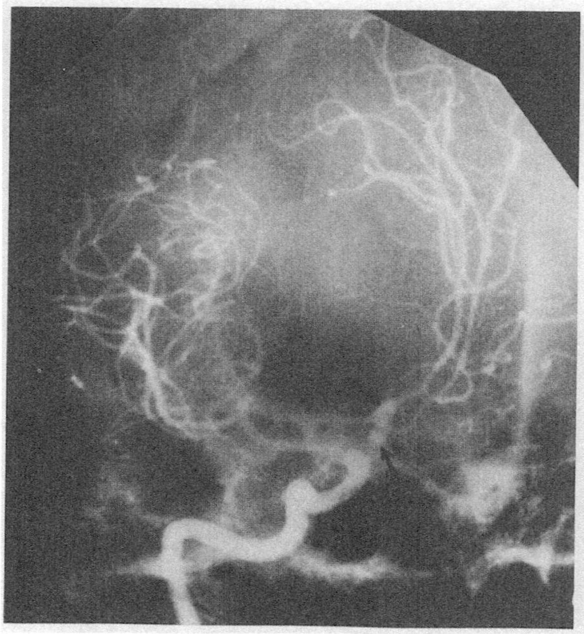

A

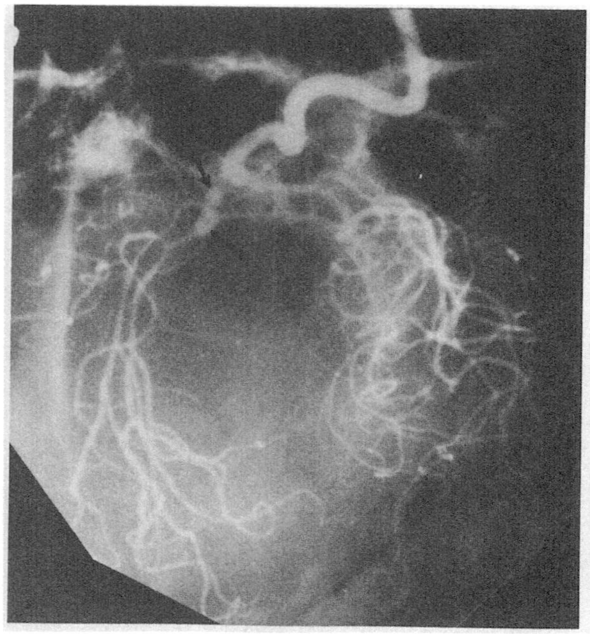

B

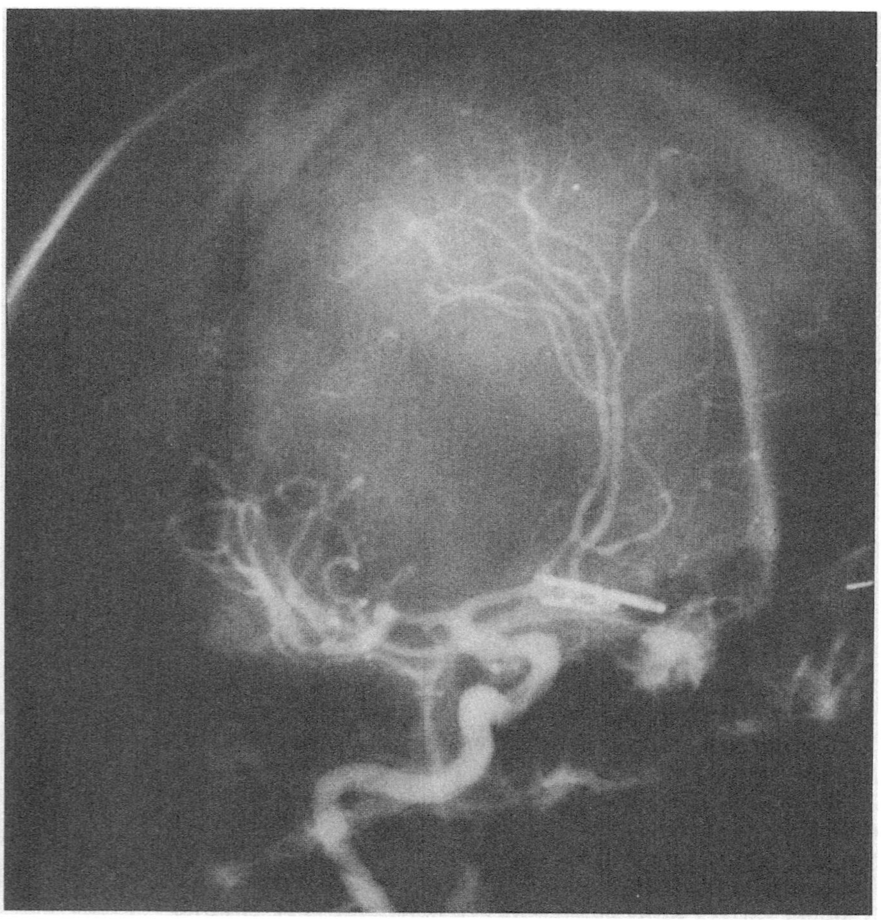

C

Fig. 35.14. A Oblique Towne view of right carotid angiogram demonstrating two separate aneurysms (*arrows*) on the ACoA. One projects downward and forward toward the optic nerves or tuberculum sellae, and the other projects upward and backward into the interhemispheric fissure. B Same as A except the film is upside down as the surgeon sees the vessels and aneurysms in the operating room. C Postoperative angiogram. Both aneurysms clipped separately.

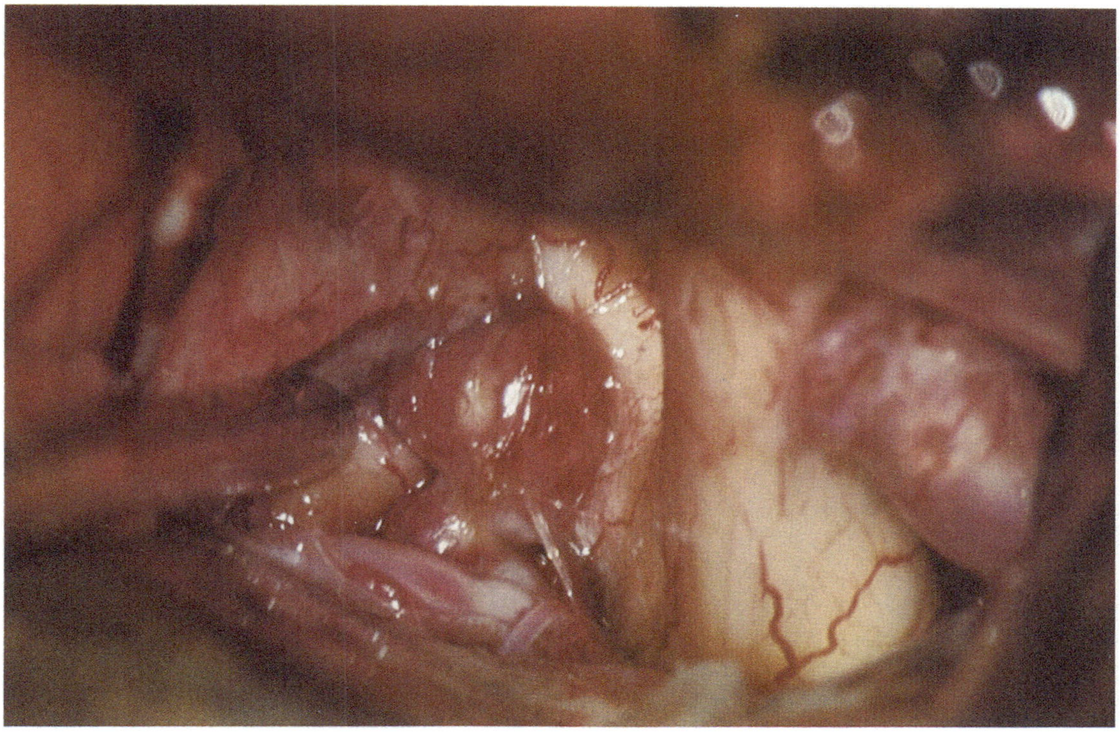

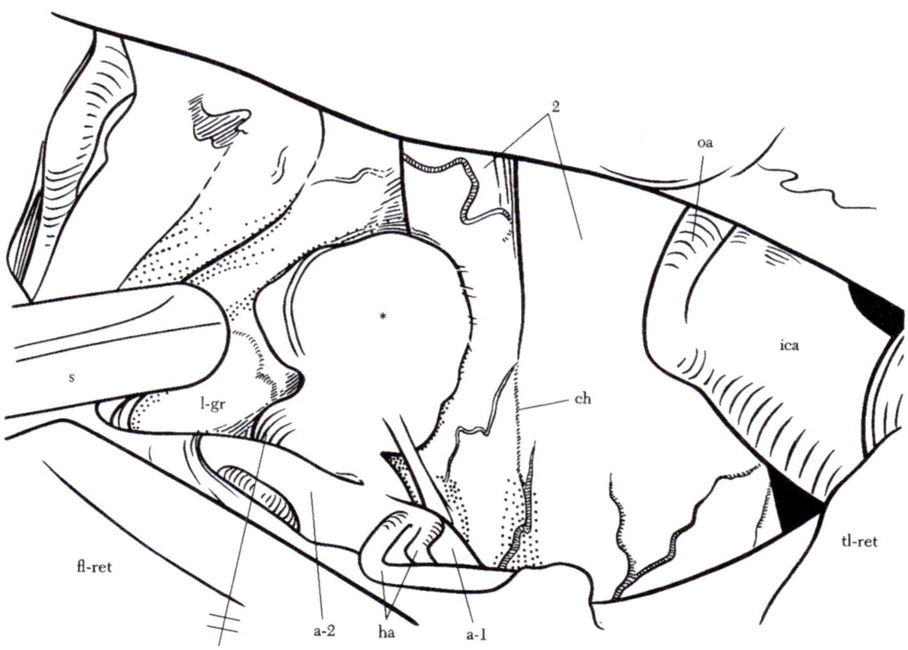

Fig. 35.15. Right frontolateral exposure of the inferoanteriorly projecting ACoAA (*) seen in the angiogram of Fig. 35.14. Only the beginning of the posterosuperiorly projecting ACoAA is seen arising from the ACoA (*double-crossed arrow*). The aneurysm was exposed by removal of part of the right gyrus rectus. Notice the aneurysm (*) is adherent to the left optic nerve just in front of the chiasm (*ch*). *2*, left and right optic nerves; *oa*, ophthalmic artery; *ica*, right internal carotid artery; *tl-ret*, temporal lobe retractor; *a-1*, right A-1 artery; *ha*, two right Heubner's arteries; *a-2*, right A-2 artery; *fl-ret*, frontal lobe retractor; *l-gr*, left (medial surface) gyrus rectus; *s*, suction tube.

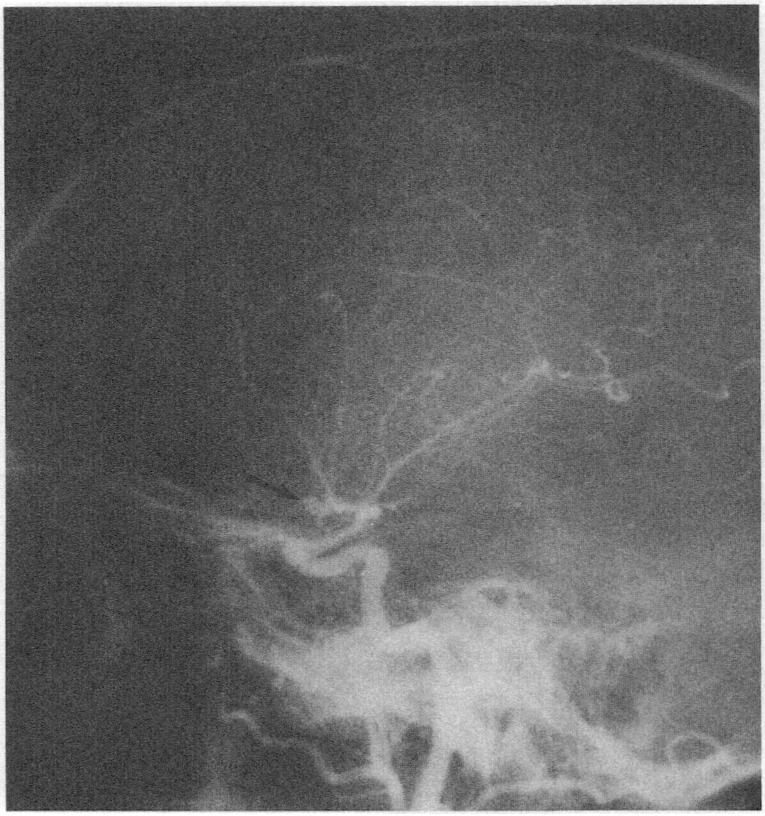

Fig. 35.16. Lateral view of angiogram illustrating an anteriorly projecting ACoAA (*arrow*).

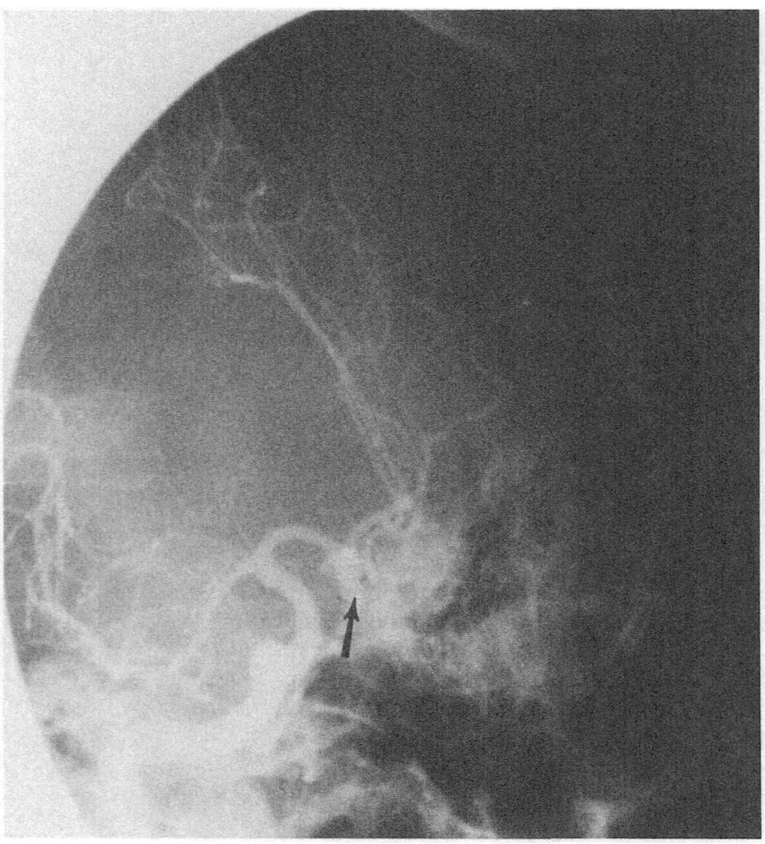

Fig. 35.17. A right oblique Towne view of another anteroinferiorly projecting ACoAA (*arrow*).

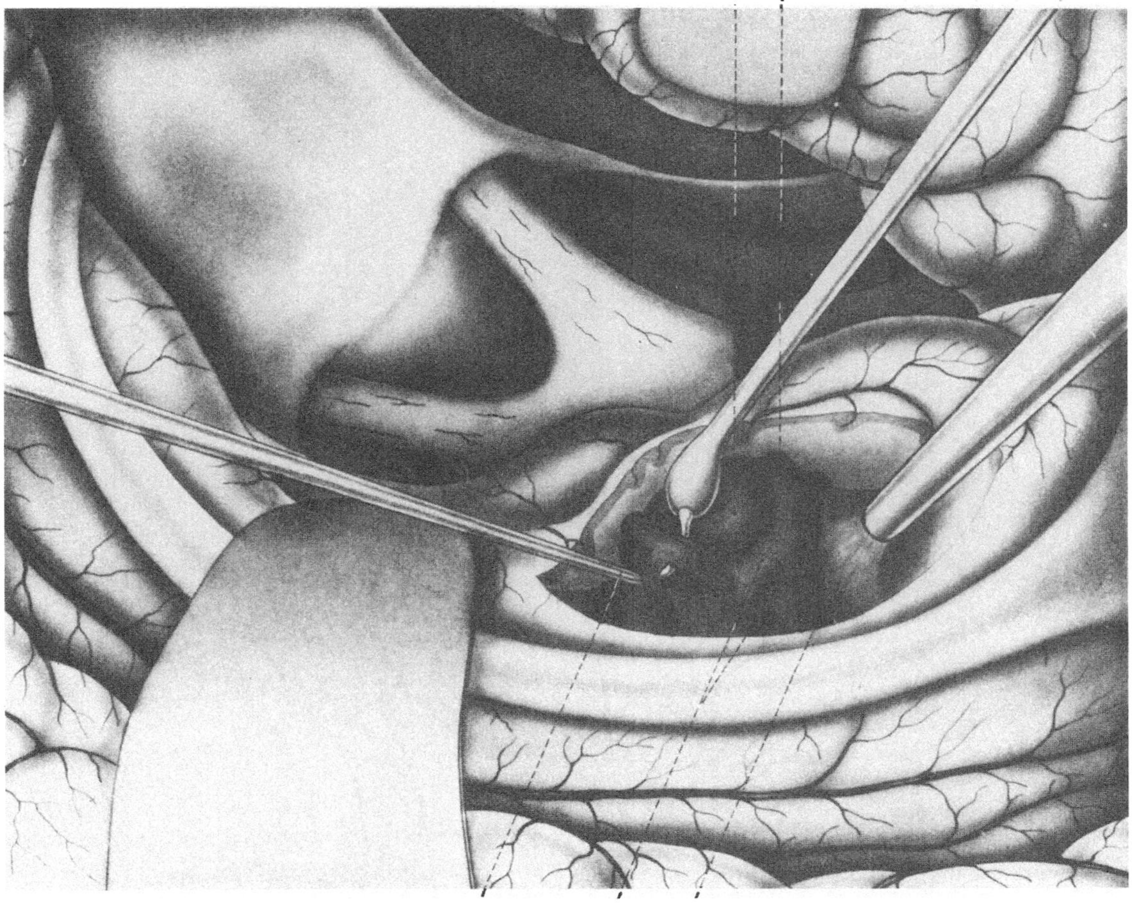

Fig. 35.18. Diagram of exposure of ACoAA via right gyrus rectus approach. At a later stage the superficial pial layer and brain tissue between the aneurysm and optic chiasm usually are removed. From Kempe LG: ref. 21.

then elevation of A-2. This maneuver can be important because the aneurysm dome may be considerably larger and project backward, perhaps as a secondary lobule—in which case the surgeon may choose an inadequate clip were he not to realize this. As the aneurysm is separated from both A-2 arteries, the surgeon must be careful not to confuse aneurysm/A-2 adhesions near the ACoA with an aneurysm/A-2 common wall. This junctional zone is a not uncommon site of aneurysm rupture during the dissection. A bleed here is extremely difficult to control compared to a rupture at the dome.

Clipping the Aneurysm

The old adage of exposing only the neck, applying the clip, and getting out fast is history. With the aid of microtechnique and hypotensive anesthesia, the surgeon usually can safely dissect out the fundus (or most of it). This allows one to apply the clip without tearing the junction of the neck with its parent artery—for if the dome is not free, the neck of the aneurysm may, in some cases (especially in the presence of atherosclerosis), be stretched between the fixed dome and the parent artery as the clip

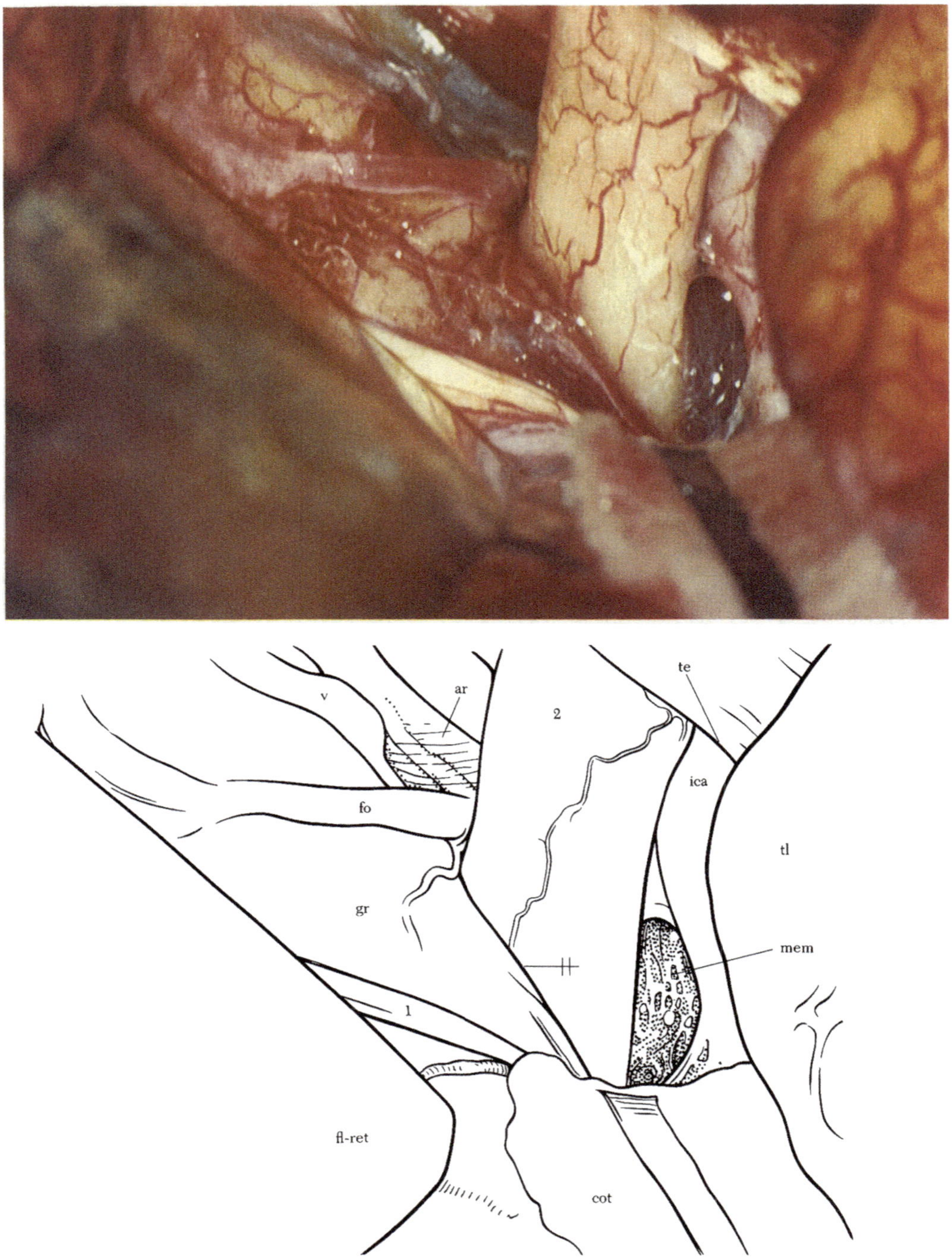

Fig. 35.19. Initial exposure of gyrus rectus (*gr*) during an approach to an ACoAA where the A-1 artery is not followed medially. Note the quadrangular zone bounded by the edge of the frontal lobe retractor blade (*fl-ret*), the frontoorbital artery (*fo*), the frontal lobe/optic nerve junction (*double-crossed arrow*), and the olfactory tract (*1*). The incision in the gyrus rectus is made here and the frontoorbital artery is followed to the aneurysm. *v,* vein; *ar,* arachnoid between optic nerves; *2,* right optic nerve; *ica,* internal carotid artery; *te,* anterior reflection of tentorial edge; *tl,* temporal lobe; *mem* membrane of Liliequist; *cot,* cotton strip lying on sylvian fissure.

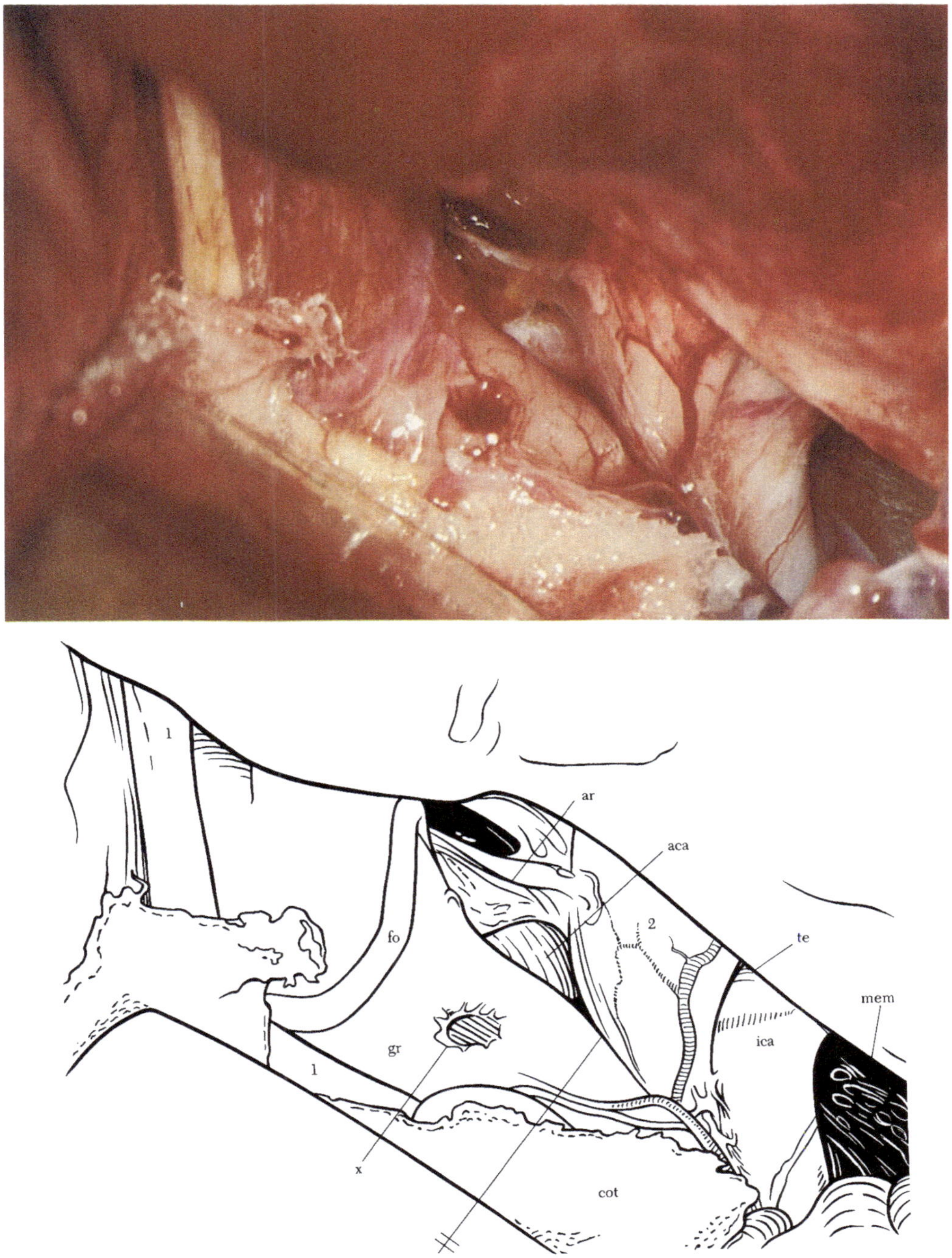

Fig. 35.20. Initial exposure of gyrus rectus (*gr*) during an approach to an ACoAA (same case as in Figs. 35.28–35.30) where the A-1 artery is not followed medially. Note quadrangular zone bounded by medial edge of gyrus rectus and its junction (*double-crossed arrow*) with the optic nerve, a cotton strip (*cot*) under frontal lobe retractor, the olfactory tract (*1*), and the frontoorbital artery (*fo*). An initial incision (*x*) has been made within this zone. *ar*, arachnoid between optic nerves; *aca*, anterior communicating artery; *2*, right optic nerve; *te*, anterior reflection of tentorial edge; *ica*, internal carotid artery; *mem*, membrane of Liliequist.

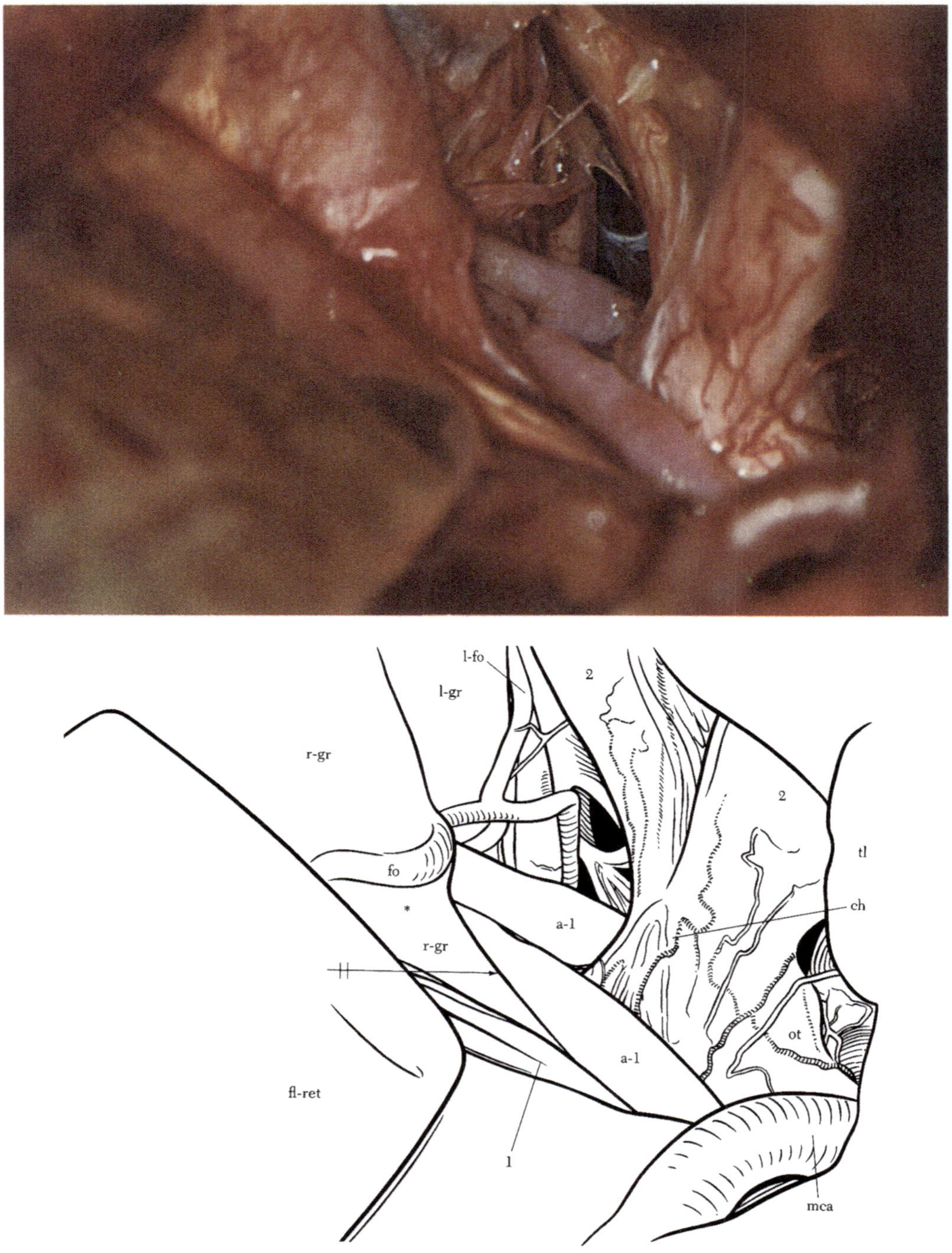

Fig. 35.21. Initial exposure of gyrus rectus on the right (*r-gr*) during an approach to an ACoAA (same case as in Figs. 35.22–35.24) where the right A-1 artery (*a-1*, below) is followed medially but not as far as the ACoAA. Note quadrangular zone bounded by the frontal lobe and right A-1 junction (*double-crossed arrow*), the olfactory tract (*1*), the frontal lobe retractor blade (*fl-ret*), and the frontoorbital artery (*fo*). The initial incision is made within this zone (*). *r-gr,* right gyrus rectus; *l-gr,* medial surface of left gyrus rectus; *l-fo,* left frontoorbital artery; *2,* left and right optic nerves; *tl,* temporal lobe; *ch,* optic chiasm; *ot,* right optic tract; *mca,* branch of middle cerebral artery in sylvian fissure; *a-1,* left (*above*) and right (*below*) A-1 arteries converging toward the hidden ACoA.

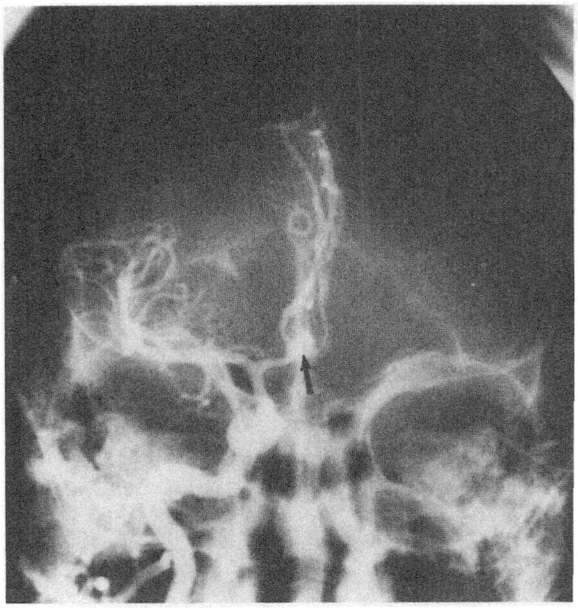

A

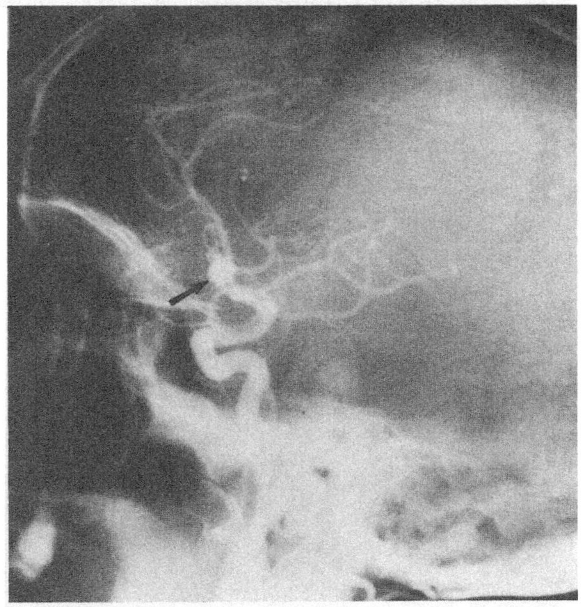

B

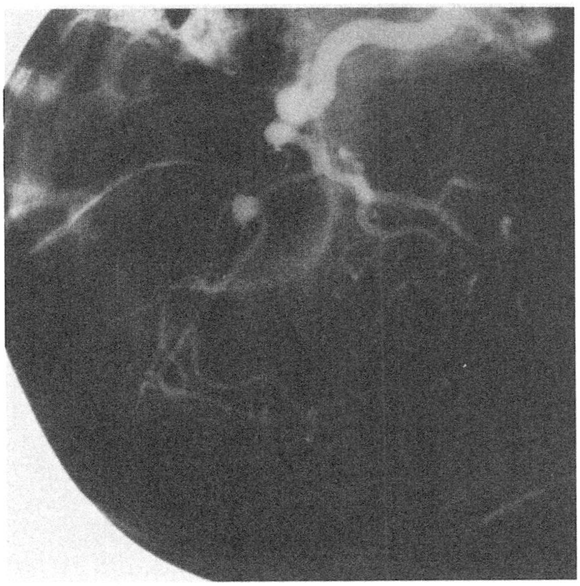

C

Fig. 35.22. Angiogram of case shown in Figs. 35.21, 35.23, and 35.24. A Frontal view revealing typical ACoAA (*arrow*). B Lateral view indicating ACoAA (*arrow*) projects upward between frontal lobes. C Upside-down oblique view illustrating aneurysm as surgeon sees it projecting between both A-2 arteries. From Fox JL: ref. 12.

squeezes down on it. It is easier to deal with a dome ruptured by dissection than with a tear in the neck caused by clipping. Figures 35.23 and 35.27 reveal an aneurysm with a very broad neck. The fundus is dissected free anterosuperiorly. The next step is to dissect it free posteroinferiorly, a step that requires meticulous microtechnique.

Before application of the clip, the surgeon and anesthesiologist must confer regarding blood pressure and any other pertinent assessments. The surgeon should already have selected any clips most likely to be used (in case of a sudden, premature rupture). We have Heifetz clips available for temporary A-1 clipping (uncommonly needed) since they are weaker than many aneurysm clips and tend to be less injurious to the arterial wall. At this time, the surgeon selects the specific clip to be applied and tests it near the aneurysm without actually applying the clip. Adjustments may have to be made in the length and angle of the clip blade. The surgeon may determine the clip must be applied with his left hand instead of his dominant right hand. We never use an "encircling" type of clip around the ACoA, for it may occlude vital perforators. A Yaşargil, Drake, or McFadden clip (see Chapter 27) has been used most commonly by us. The Yaşargil clip-holder has the advantage of being bayonet in shape. Final dissections are completed. The surgeon takes the clip-holder and unlocks it *before* the clip is applied (otherwise the tremor of the un-

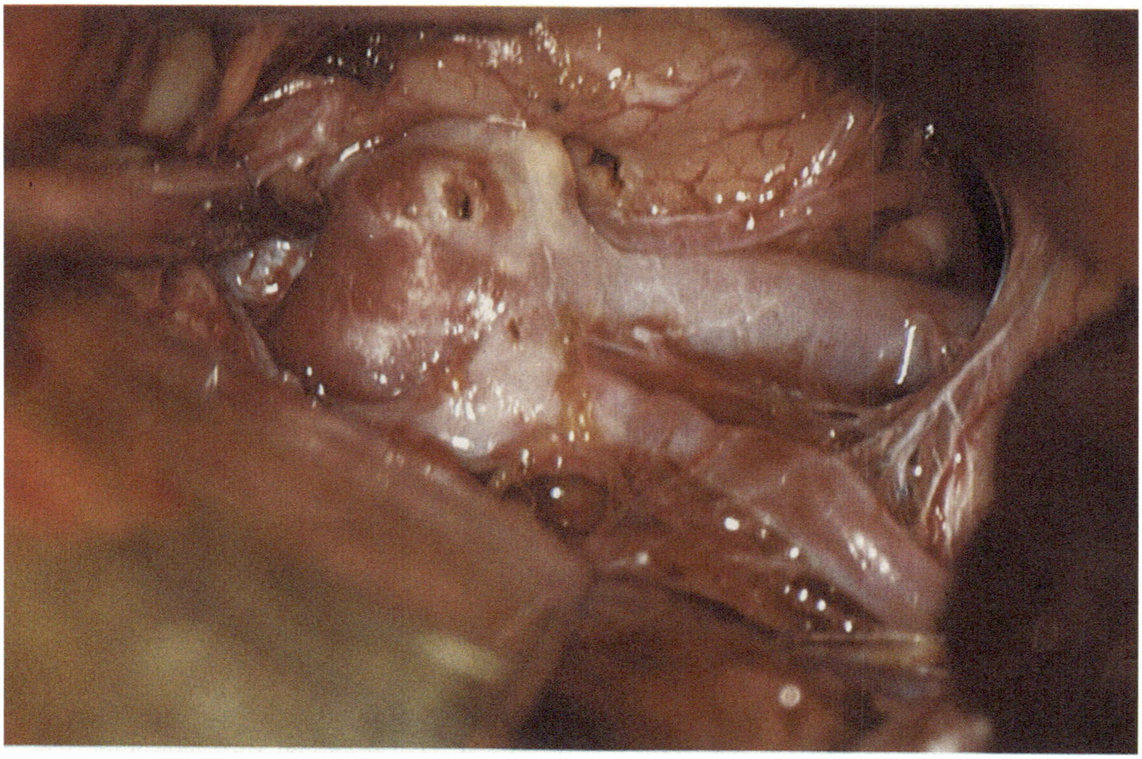

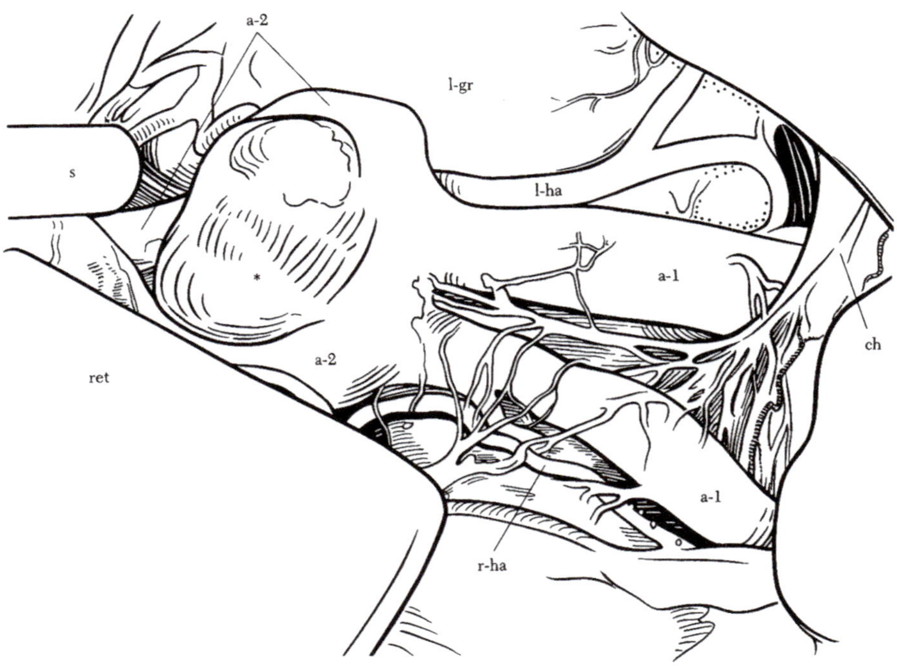

Fig. 35.23. ACoAA (*) exposed after a 1-cm length of right gyrus rectus has been removed. Same case as in Figs. 35.21, 35.22, and 35.24. On angiography (Fig. 35.22B) the aneurysm projects upward, but the surgeon sees it projecting to his left at operation. The suction tube (*s*) is retracting the right gyrus rectus to expose part of the left A-2 artery (*a-2, above*). Between the retractor blade (*ret*) and the aneurysm (*) is the right A-2 artery (*a-2,* below). *l-gr,* medial surface of left gyrus rectus; *l-ha,* left Heubner's artery; *ch,* optic chiasm; *a-1,* left (*above*) and right (*below*) A-1 arteries; *r-ha,* tiny right Heubner's artery.

locking motion may tear and rupture the aneurysm).

The wings of the clip are spread to encircle the aneurysm. They are used to dissect between the neck and adjacent tissues before closure around the aneurysm. Slow, deliberate movements are required. Do not apply the clip as close as possible to the ACoA —especially if one is not applying the clip with its wings parallel to the ACoA. Otherwise, there is a high risk of tearing the A-2/ACoAA junction. The clip should be about 1 mm from the ACoA to allow the aneurysm wall at that junctional point to bend as it is pulled inward by the clip blade. We often apply a larger clip on the center of the dome first to collapse the aneurysm and then follow with a second, smaller clip about the neck. The wings of the clip must strangle the neck gradually, followed by slow and cautious disengagement and removal of the clip-applier.

Figure 35.24 shows two clips applied to the ACoAA in the previous figure. In this case the first (anterior) clip had been applied too close to the atherosclerotic left A-2/ACoA junction. This caused the brittle wall to crack with resulting hemorrhage, which was controlled by slight advancement of the clip against the wall of the left A-2 artery. A second (posterior) clip was applied on the fundus and parallel to the first clip. (We often have applied an extra clip to buttress the first clip rather than use any tissue adhesive.) If any unsecured aneurysm remains and cannot be clipped safely, we cover that part of the aneurysm with cotton fibers followed by Gelfoam (the latter to separate the future cotton foreign body reaction from the optic chiasm and nerves).

After the first clip has been applied, one must make a diligent search to confirm that the aneurysm is entirely barred from the arterial circulation without entrapment of any perforator or parent arteries in the clip. If such is the case or if the clip is not exactly placed correctly to secure the patient from any future bleed, the surgeon will have to readjust the clip or remove it and apply another clip in its place. Such maneuvers are done in about 80% of our cases. Any encroachment on a parent artery or perforator may lead to a serious postoperative ischemic complication.

For methods of handling premature (i.e., unplanned) rupture of an intracranial aneurysm, the reader is referred to Chapter 32. There are several techniques for preclipping decompression of an aneurysm or narrowing of its neck; these are summarized in Chapter 31. In our experience, clipping is the principal method of treating accessible aneurysms. Other methods are detailed in Chapter 31.

Figure 35.3 and Figs. 35.25–35.27 are photographs of the same ACoAA case where the anatomy is nicely demonstrated. In this patient the ICA is short, and thus only minimal frontal lobe retraction is required before the A-1 artery and Heubner's artery are well seen. Hence A-1 easily can be followed medially toward the ACoA complex. However, even here the frontal pole is not retracted so as to prevent pulling on the aneurysm. Instead the gyrus rectus incision again is employed. Notice the prefixed optic chiasm in this case (Fig. 35.26) permitting early exposure of the optic tract and adjacent lamina terminalis. The latter can be punctured in cases with hydrocephalus.

In Fig. 35.27 notice the saccule with the eponym, "Murphey's tit," a weak protrusion from which the bleed most likely occurs (41,46). In this same figure, one can imagine the red blood swirling about within the thin walls of the pulsating aneurysm. Such is clearly seen by the surgeon during operation. Of interest is Botterell's comment in 1951 about an observation made by Sir Geoffrey Jefferson (3):

> I am reminded of the occasion last fall when I took Professor Jefferson to see Niagara Falls for the first time and as we were standing up on the lookout tower gazing down upon the rapids and the whirlpool with its narrow neck and circular circulation of water, I thought he was impressed with the scenery and suddenly he said, "I say, Botterell, what a magnificent example of the circulation in an aneurysm!"

There are a number of occasions when the A-1 artery cannot easily be followed from the ICA bifurcation. Figures 35.28–35.31 demonstrate just such an example. A small excision of part of the gyrus rectus permitted adequate exposure of the ACoA complex and aneurysm (Fig. 35.29), bipolar electrocoagulation of the aneurysm (Fig. 35.30), and clipping (Fig. 35.31). A-1 was never seen except at its junction with the ACoA. In these cases, the surgeon must rely on skills provided by experience to know where to find the aneurysm and where to open through the gyrus rectus. The anatomic de-

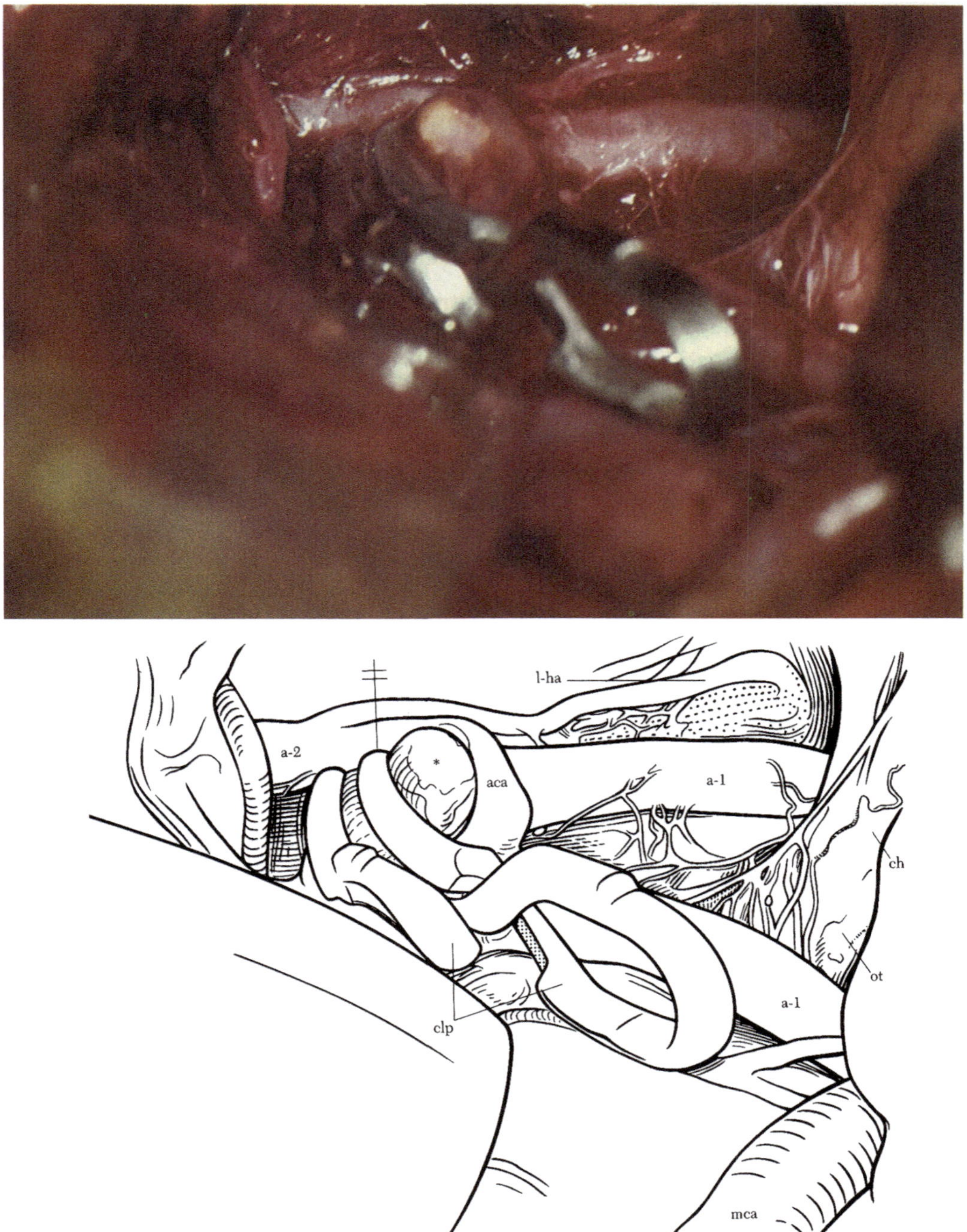

Fig. 35.24. View after clipping of the ACoAA seen in Figs. 35.21–35.23. See text for details. *clp,* shank of two Yaşargil clips; *a-2,* left A-2 artery; *aca,* anterior communicating artery (not aneurysm); *l-ha,* left Heubner's artery; *a-1,* left (*above*) and right (*below*) A-1 arteries; *ch,* optic chiasm; *ot,* right optic tract; *mca,* branch of middle cerebral artery (out of focus) in sylvian fissure. The more anterior clip (on viewer's right) was advanced to minimally compromise the left A-2 artery in order to occlude a junctional A-2/ACoAA rent (*double-crossed arrow*) that occurred during placement of the clip. Note atherosclerosis (*) at base of aneurysm on the left.

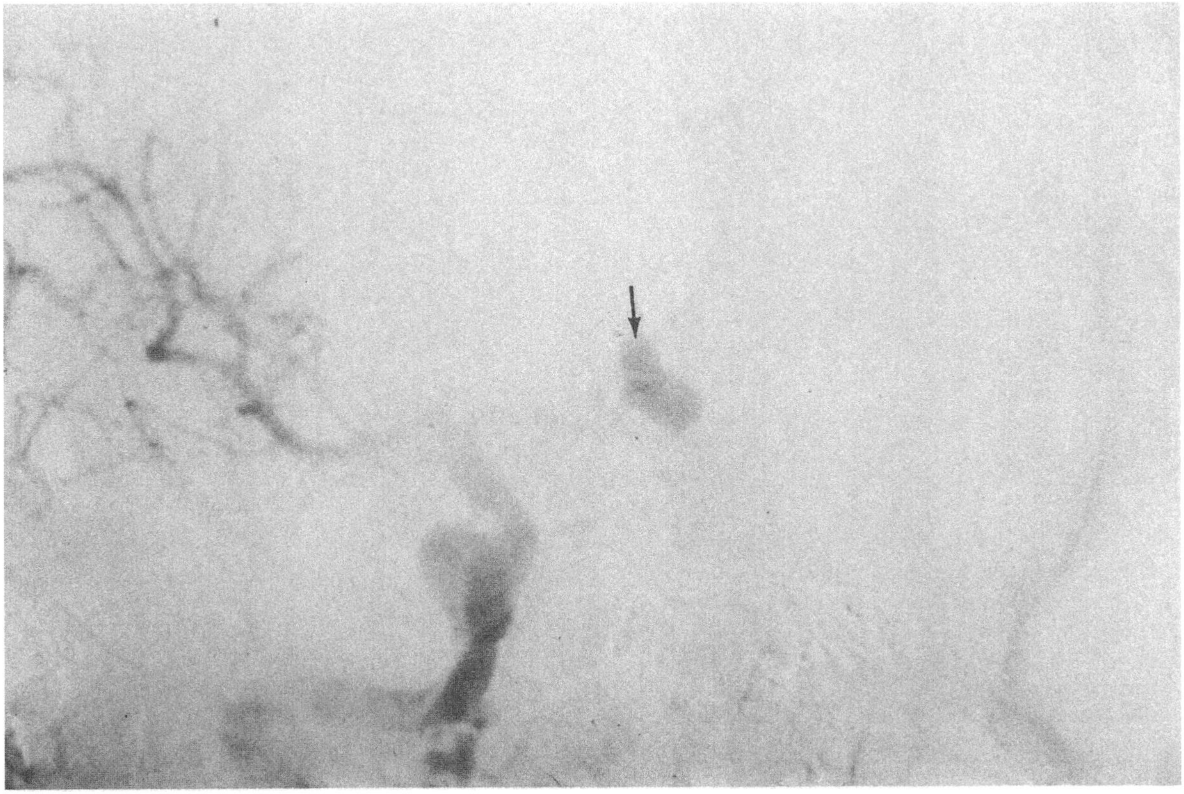

Fig. 35.25. Oblique view of right carotid angiogram (subtraction technique) illustrating very broad-based ACoAA flanked by both A-2 arteries. The surgeon must beware of the secondary dome (*arrow*) projecting posteriorly and hidden from the surgeon's view by the primary dome. Same case as in Figs. 35.3, 35.26, and 35.27.

tails are not easily seen but accurate identification of structures and vessels is mandatory.

Occasionally the surgeon is confronted with an ACoAA which projects directly posteriorly or inferoposteriorly against the hypothalamus. Figures 35.32–35.34 provide an example. In this case the right A-1 artery was hypoplastic, and the aneurysm filled via a left carotid injection during angiography. The somewhat confusing and anomalous vasculature of the anterior circle of Willis in this case is seen in Fig. 35.33. As predicted the ACoAA arose on the side (left) of the larger A-1 artery. Figure 35.34 is an excellent example of the required preservation of vital hypothalamic perforators. Considerable time was taken by the surgeon to free these adherent arteries from the wall of the aneurysm prior to clipping.

Closure

Once the aneurysm(s) is satisfactorily clipped, the patient's blood pressure is returned to normal, topical vasodilators are applied, and the retractors are readjusted for good cerebral perfusion. Any remaining cottonoids and cotton balls used intracranially are removed and recounted. Any bleeding points are controlled. The dura is closed with a 4–0 running nylon or silk suture. The dura is tacked up securely with sutures and the bone flap is replaced. Temporalis muscle, galea, and skin are approximated in a standard fashion. We use a Jackson-Pratt subgaleal drain for about 18 h after surgery.

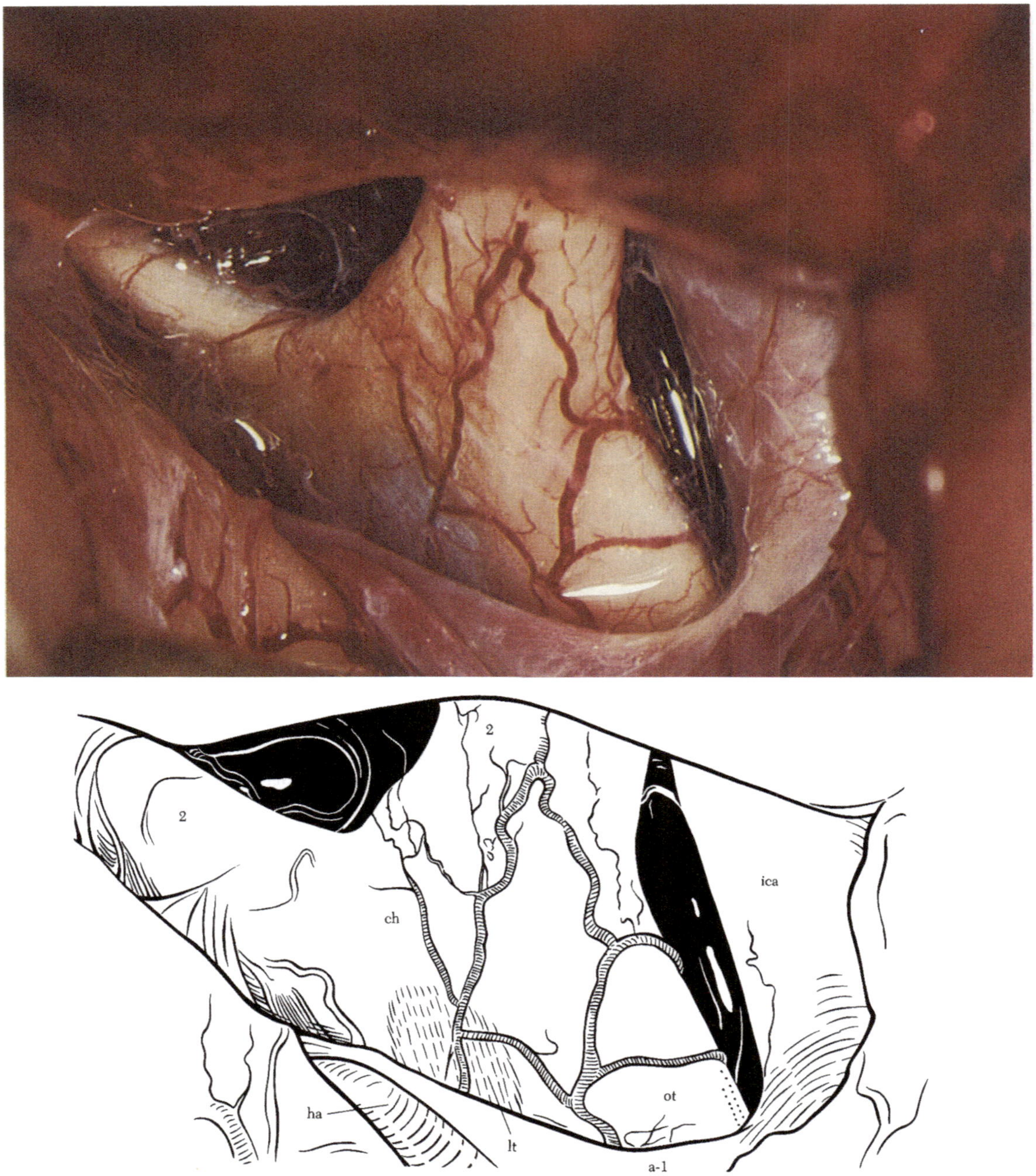

Fig. 35.26. Same case as in Figs. 35.3, 35.25, and 35.27. Exposure of the chiasmatic and lamina terminalis cisterns. The chiasm is prefixed. *lt,* lamina terminalis; *ch,* optic chiasm; *2,* both optic nerves; *ot,* right optic tract; *a-1,* horizontal anterior cerebral artery; *ica,* internal carotid artery; *ha,* recurrent artery of Heubner running laterally anterior to and above (*below* in photograph) the A-1 segment. From Fox JL: ref. 12.

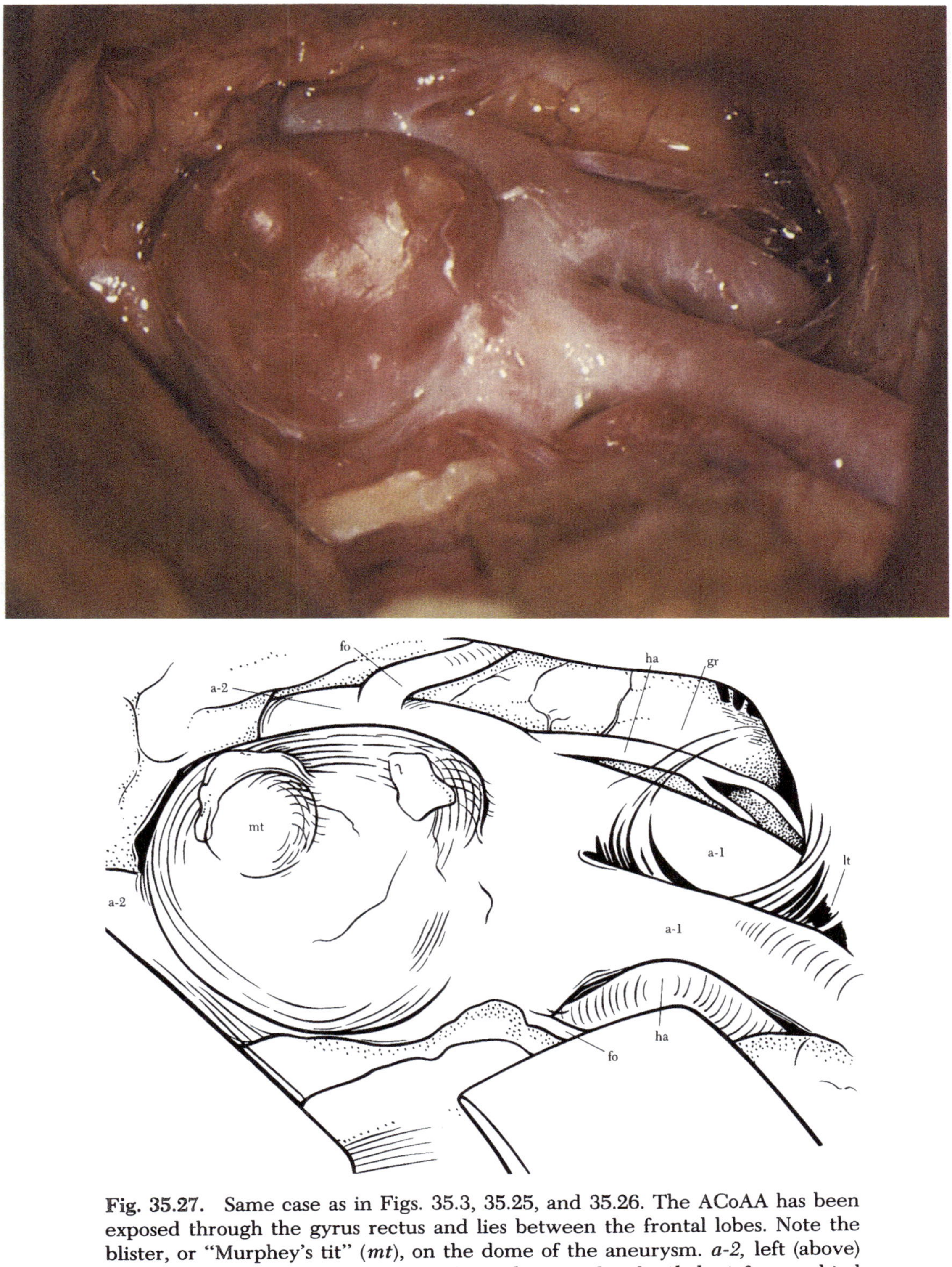

Fig. 35.27. Same case as in Figs. 35.3, 35.25, and 35.26. The ACoAA has been exposed through the gyrus rectus and lies between the frontal lobes. Note the blister, or "Murphey's tit" (*mt*), on the dome of the aneurysm. *a-2,* left (above) and right (*below*) A-2 segments; *fo,* left (*above*) and right (*below*) frontoorbital arteries; *ha,* left (*above*) and right (*below*) Heubner's arteries; *a-1,* left (*above*) and right (*below*) A-1 segments; *gr,* left gyrus rectus; *lt,* lamina terminalis. From Fox JL: ref. 12.

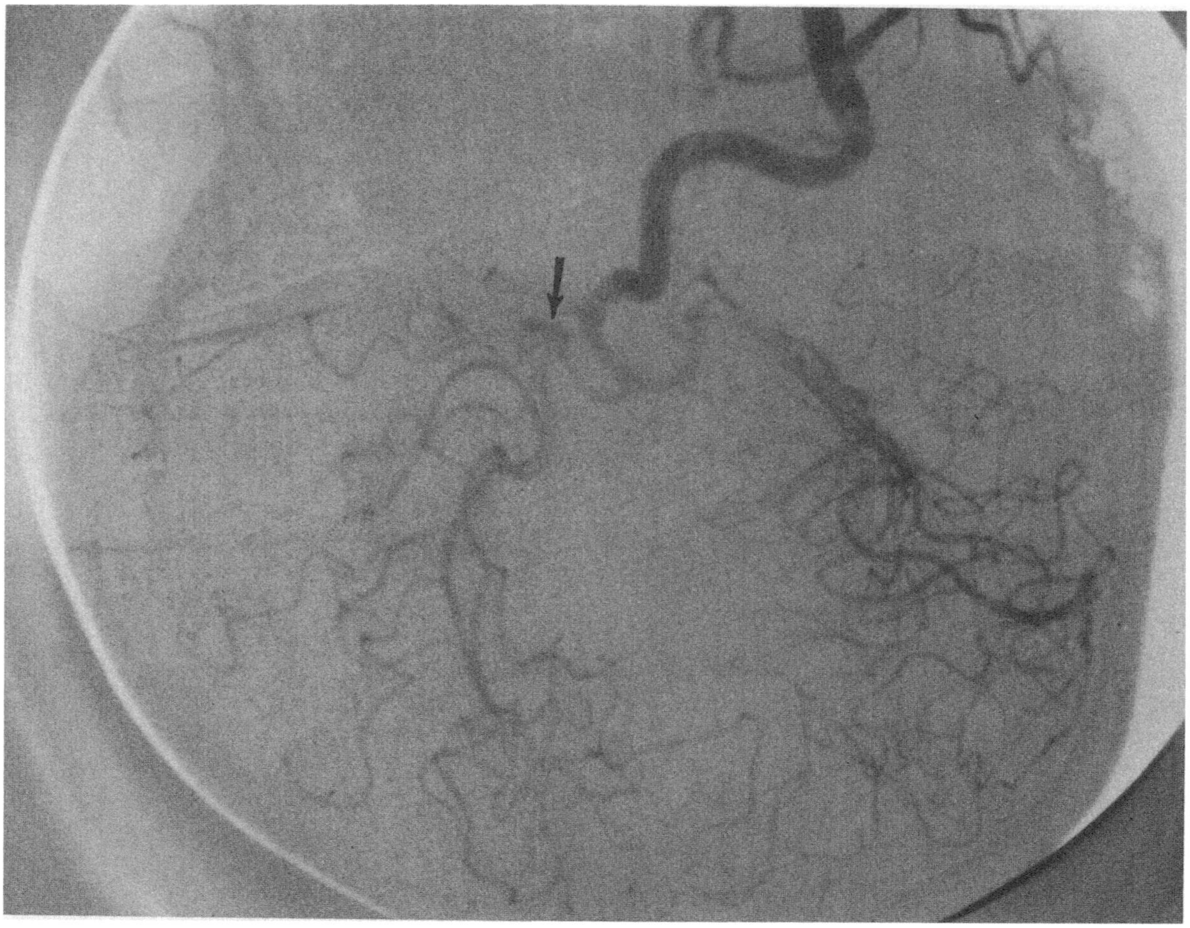

Fig. 35.28. Right carotid angiogram of patient with ACoAA (*arrow*). The view is oblique and upside down as seen at surgery. Note elongated internal carotid artery (*arrowhead*) with forward curvature to its A-1 branch. This places the ICA bifurcation more posteriorly under the anterior perforated substance. Compare this angiogram with Fig. 35.22C where the ICA is shorter and its A-1 branch makes a direct route medially.

Anterior Cerebral Artery Aneurysms

Aneurysms of the A-1 Artery

The horizontal portion, or A-1 portion, of the anterior cerebral artery (ACeA) rarely contains an aneurysm (an A_1AA). We have only one on which we have operated (Fig. 35.35). Many aneurysms so diagnosed in the past were, in fact, bICAA or ACoAA. When a true A_1AA occurs, it usually is at the take-off of a perforator or an A-1 take-off of Heubner's artery (1).

The surgical approach is identical to that for an ACoAA if the A_1AA is medially located. If it is laterally located, then one uses an approach similar to that for a bICAA. The difference may not be great except that if one is approaching an aneurysm on A-1 near the bifurcation of the ICA, then the head should be dropped back more than usual and the sylvian fissure opened as widely as possible. The difficulties are greater if the ICA is elongated since more frontal lobe retraction is required.

Distal ACeA Aneurysms

We have designated aneurysms of the parasagittal, or distal (beyond the anterior communicating artery), anterior cerebral artery as ACeAA. These ACeAA make up about 5% of intracranial aneurysms (compared with

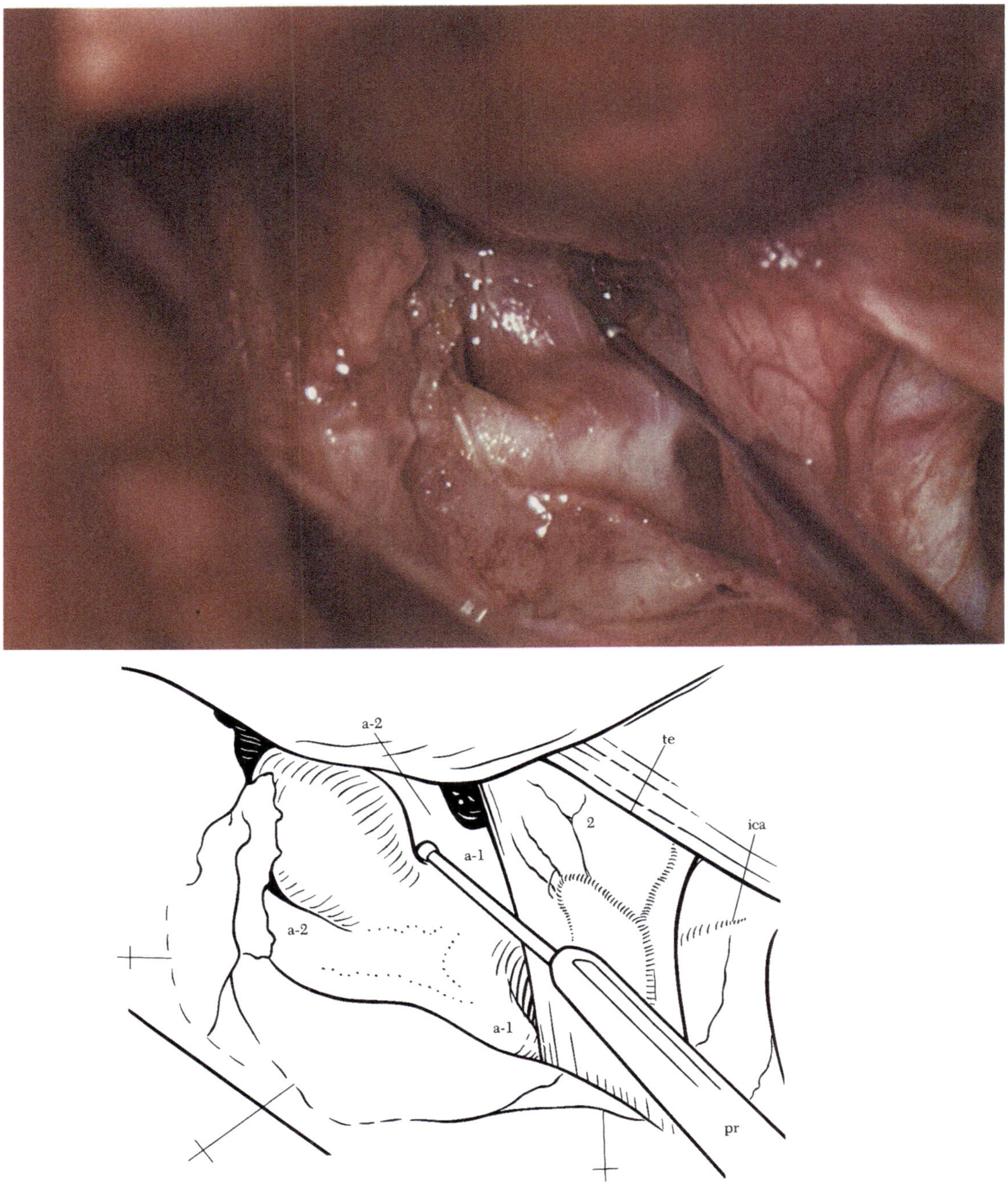

Fig. 35.29. A small ACoAA exposed through a right frontotemporal craniotomy and a 1-cm gyrus rectus incision (*crossed arrows*). Probe (*pr*) tip lies between the neck of the aneurysm and the origin of the left A-2 artery. *a-2,* left (*above*) and right (*below*) A-2 segments; *a-1,* left (*above*) and right (*below*) A-1 segments; *2,* right optic nerve; *te,* reflection of the tentorium toward the anterior clinoid process; *ica,* internal carotid artery. From Fox JL: ref. 12.

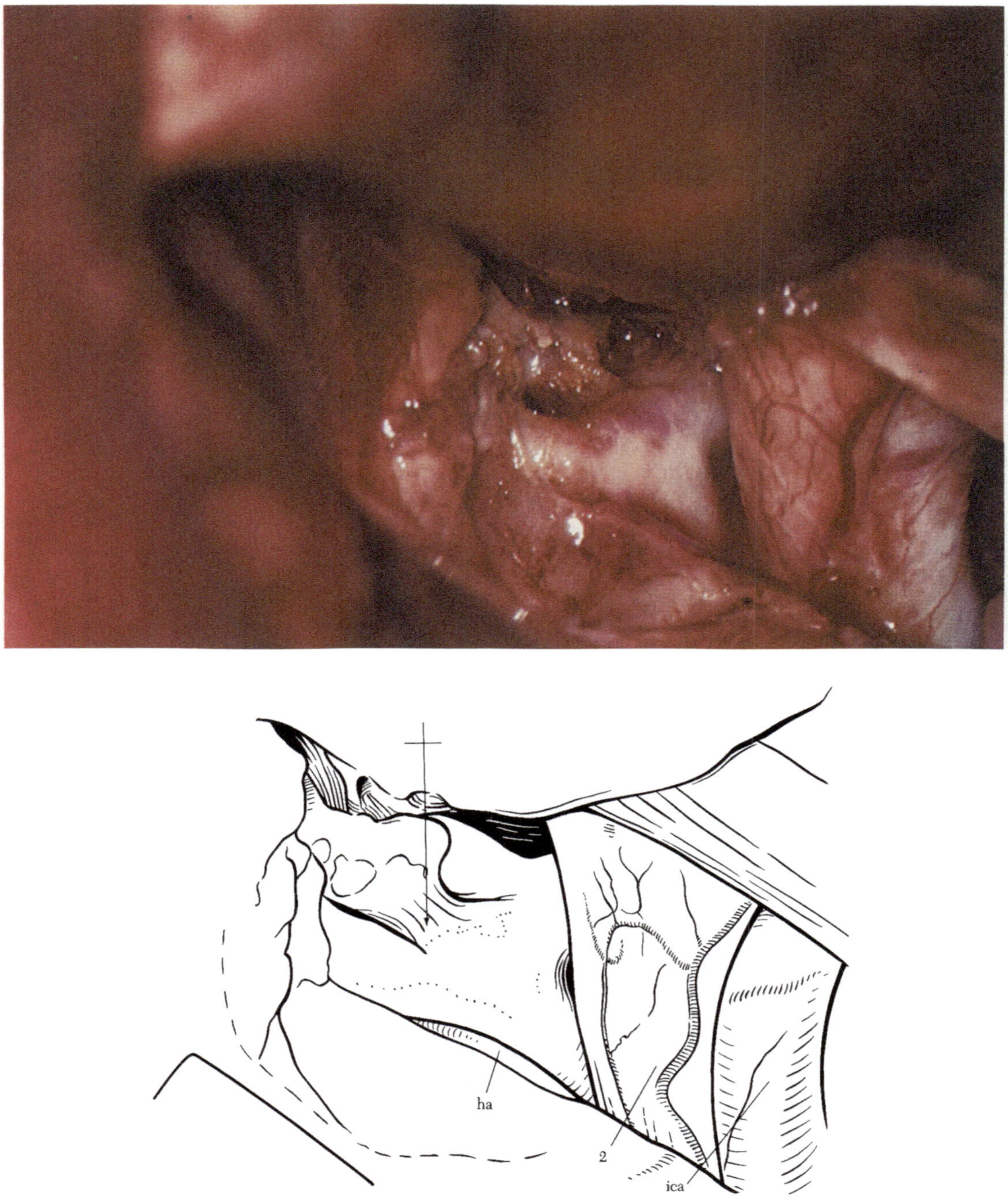

Fig. 35.30. Aneurysm in Fig. 35.29 after bipolar electrocoagulation of the neck (*crossed arrow*). *ha,* right Heubner's artery partially covered by gyrus rectus; *2,* right optic nerve; *ica,* internal carotid artery. From Fox JL: ref. 12.

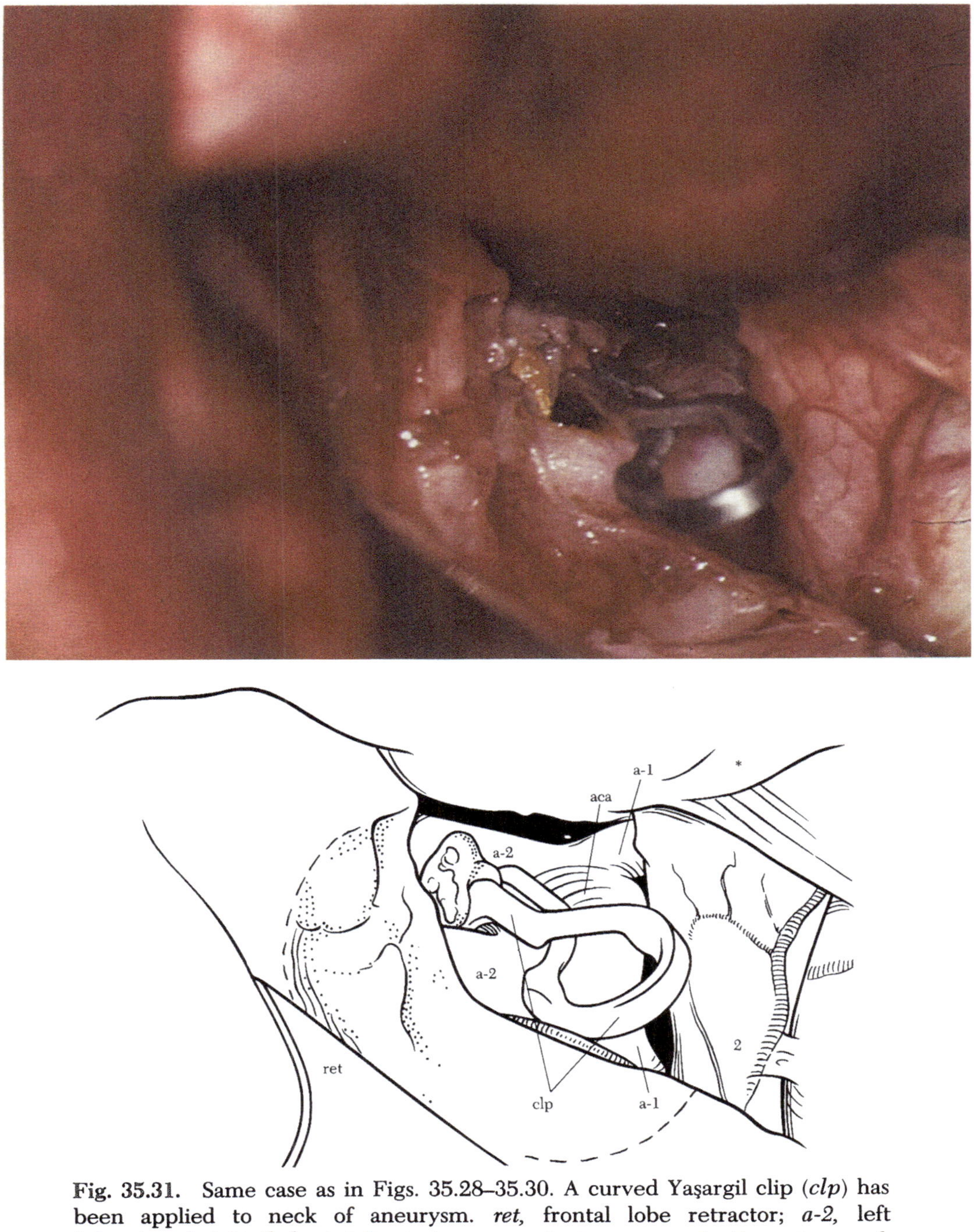

Fig. 35.31. Same case as in Figs. 35.28–35.30. A curved Yaşargil clip (*clp*) has been applied to neck of aneurysm. *ret,* frontal lobe retractor; *a-2,* left (*above*) and right (*below*) A-2 arteries; *aca,* anterior communicating artery; *a-1,* left (*above*) and right (*below*) A-1 arteries; *, anterior clinoid process; *2,* right optic nerve.

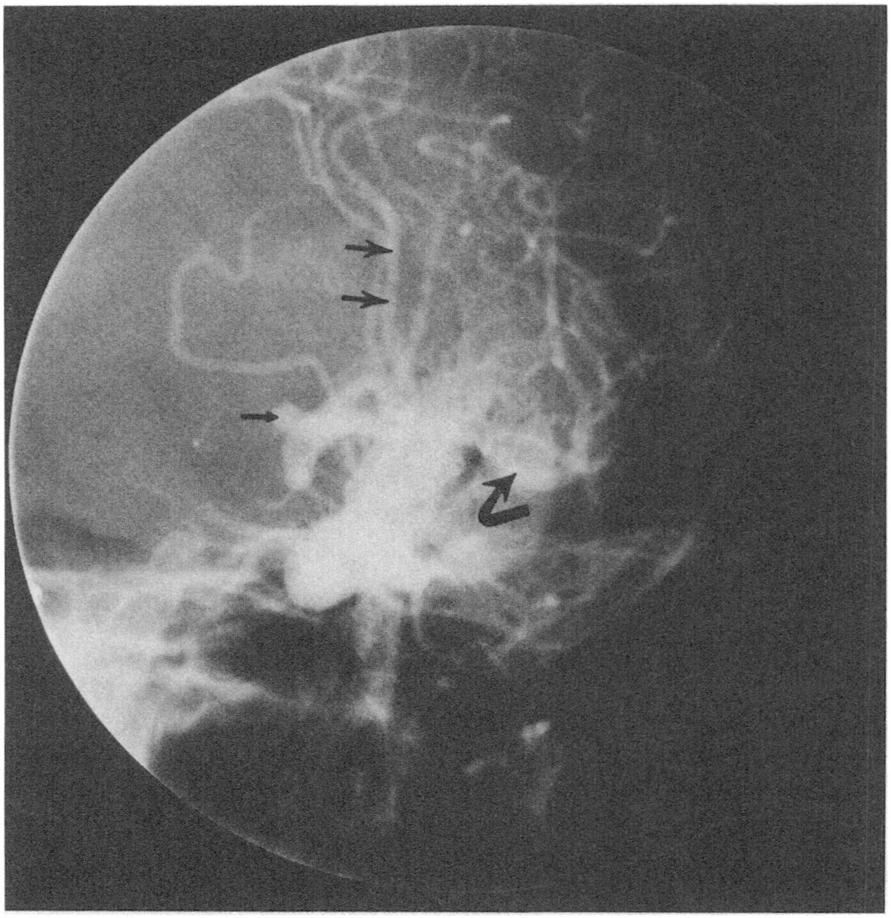

Fig. 35.32. Left carotid angiogram as viewed through a right orbital (oblique) Towne projection (not turned upside down). ACoAA (*single arrow*) projects posteriorly. Other views poorly demonstrated the aneurysm. Same case as in Figs. 35.33 and 35.34. One can predict that this aneurysm will project toward the hypothalamus. *Double arrows,* anterior cerebral artery; *curved arrow,* middle cerebral artery.

ACoAA, which make up about 25%). The majority of these ACeAA occur at the fork between the pericallosal and callosomarginal branches (Fig. 35.36) (1,2,10,51). Pertuiset et al. (40) described five sites: (a) immediately distal to the ACoA (probably at the orbitofrontal branch); (b) at the frontopolar branch (Fig. 35.37); (c) at the callosomarginal branch (Fig. 35.36); (d) on the pericallosal artery distal to the callosomarginal branch; and (4) on the callosomarginal artery distal to its origin.

The azygous anterior cerebral artery is the condition in which there is only one ACeA (i.e., one midline trunk instead of a right and left artery) in its ascending A-2 and A-3 portions. At that point (near the genu of the corpus callosum) the single azygous artery (from the united right and left A-1 arteries) bifurcates into right and left pericallosal arteries. It is at this bifurcation that azygous anterior cerebral artery aneurysms (azACeAA), although rare, may occur (Fig. 35.38) (14,18,20,30,34,41).

The principal techniques of approach to the ACeA are summarized in Chapter 29. Basically, we use a frontal or a frontoparietal craniotomy flap (free bone flap), which is on the side of the aneurysm and parasagittal in location (see Fig. 29.24B). The bone flap extends 2 cm across the midline, and the dura is opened with its base at the superior sagittal sinus. A wide retractor blade holds the falx to the contralateral side. Standard microtechnique is used to approach the pericallosal cistern. Caution must be used to avoid rupture of the aneurysm dur-

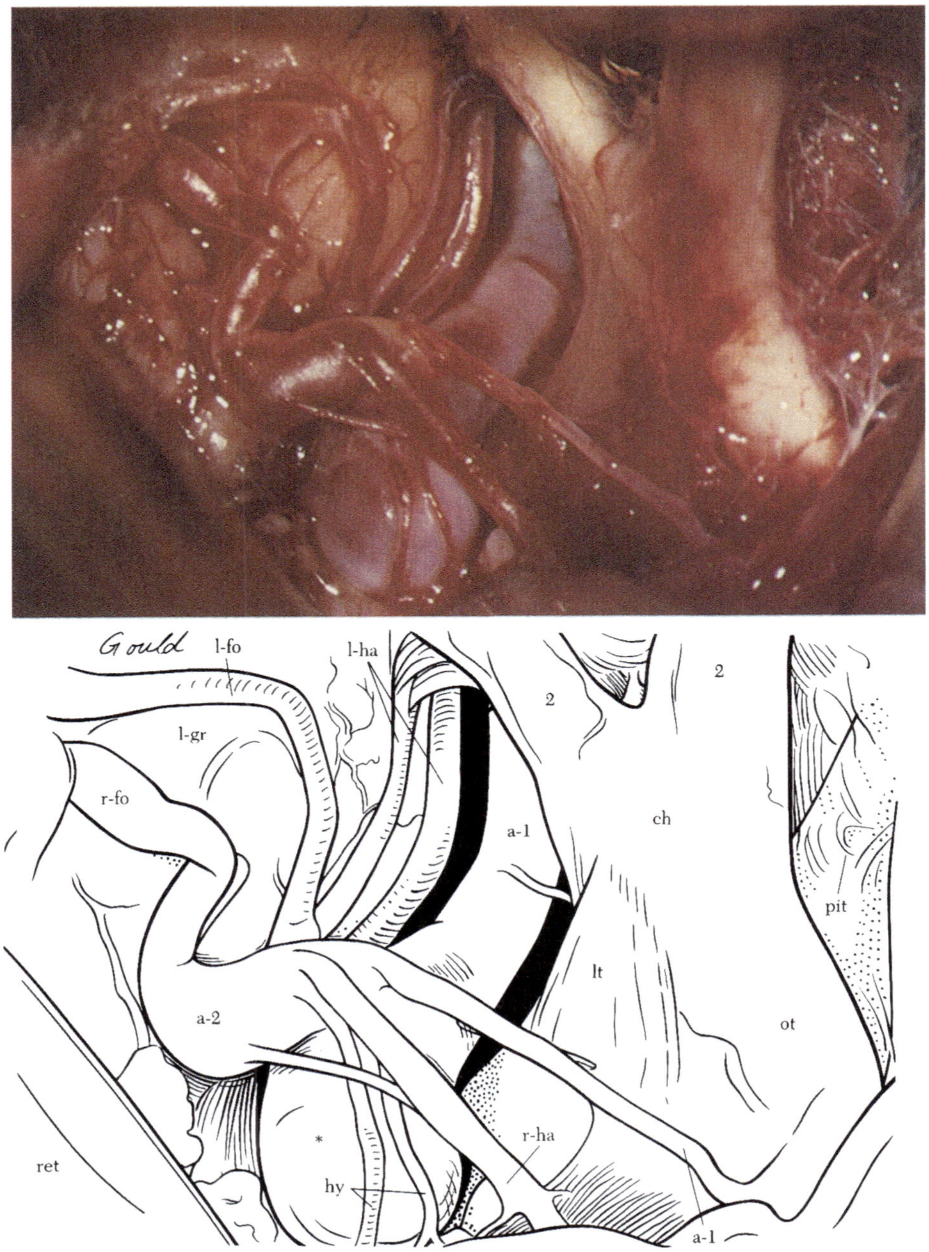

Fig. 35.33. Same case as in Figs. 35.32 and 35.34. The ACoAA (*) projects posteriorly against hypothalamus and superior part of lamina terminalis (*lt*). With the obliqued and extended position of the patient's head, the aneurysm appears to the surgeon to project downward. Note vital hypothalamic perforators (*hy*) stuck to dome of aneurysm. The right A-1 artery (lower *a-1*) is hypoplastic and even thinner than its adjacent Heubner's artery (*r-ha*). The left A-1 artery (upper *a-1*) is large and supplies the large right A-2 artery (*a-2*) and the left A-2 artery (hidden by the right A-2). A pair of left Heubner's arteries (*l-ha*) course leftward above the left A-1. The right and left frontoorbital arteries (*r-fo* and *l-fo*) course superiorly on the gyrus rectus (they may actually be frontopolar arteries with a low-lying take-off). *l-gr*, medial surface of left gyrus rectus; *2*, optic nerves; *ch*, optic chiasm; *pit*, pituitary stalk; *ot*, right optic tract; *ret*, right frontal lobe retractor.

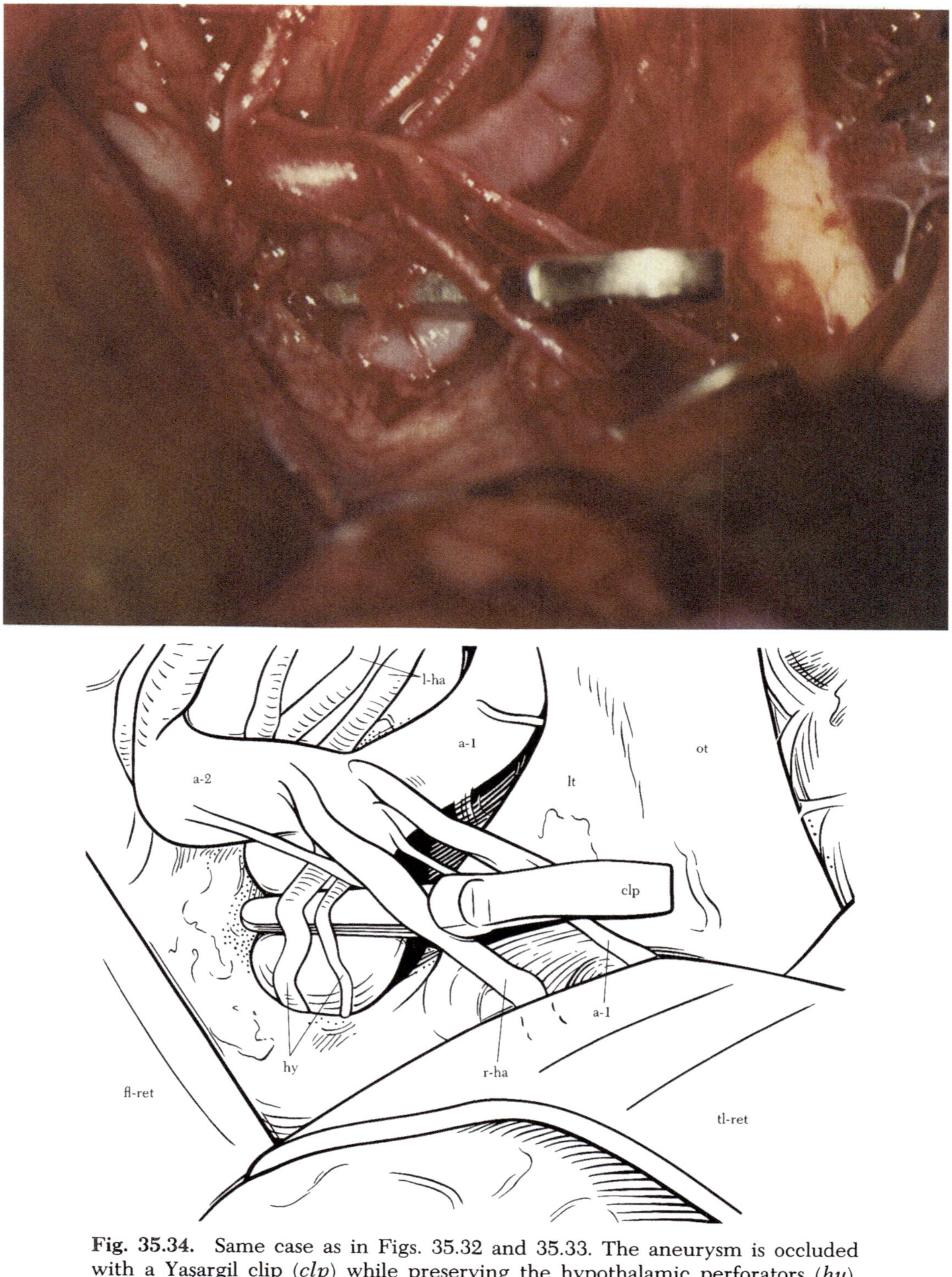

Fig. 35.34. Same case as in Figs. 35.32 and 35.33. The aneurysm is occluded with a Yaşargil clip (*clp*) while preserving the hypothalamic perforators (*hy*). The clip passes between the right A-1 artery (lower *a-1*) and Heubner's artery (*r-ha*). *tl-ret,* temporal lobe retractor; *fl-ret,* frontal lobe retractor; *a-2,* right A-2 artery; *l-ha,* two left Heubner's arteries; *a-1,* left (above) and right (below) A-1 arteries; *lt,* lamina terminalis; *ot,* right optic tract.

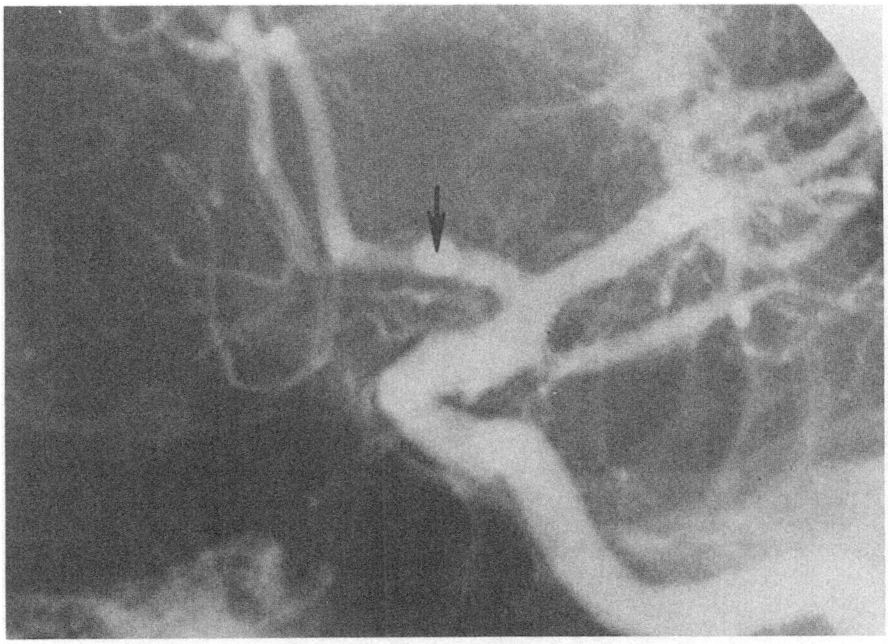

A

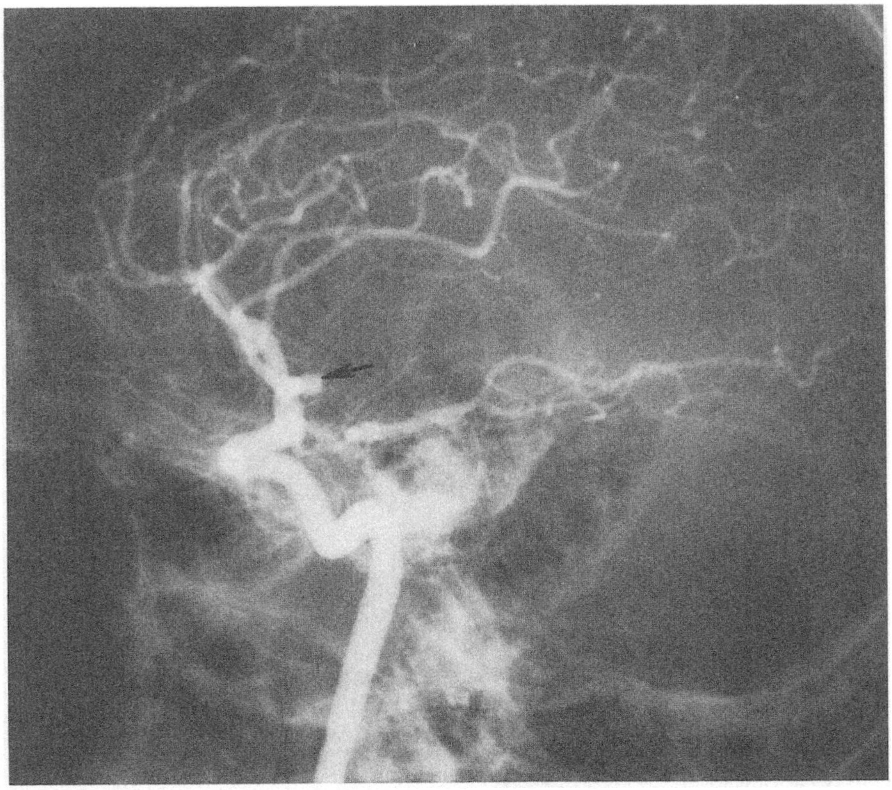

B

Fig. 35.35. A Left carotid angiogram, oblique view through left orbit. A-1 artery round density (*arrow*) is a backward projecting A-1 aneurysm (A_1AA). **B** Same case, lateral Haughton view. Aneurysm (*arrow*) projects back into anterior perforated substance of frontal lobe. The patient was a 50-year-old woman with SAH and a left frontal hematoma seen on CT scan. Aneurysm successfully clipped in October 1980.

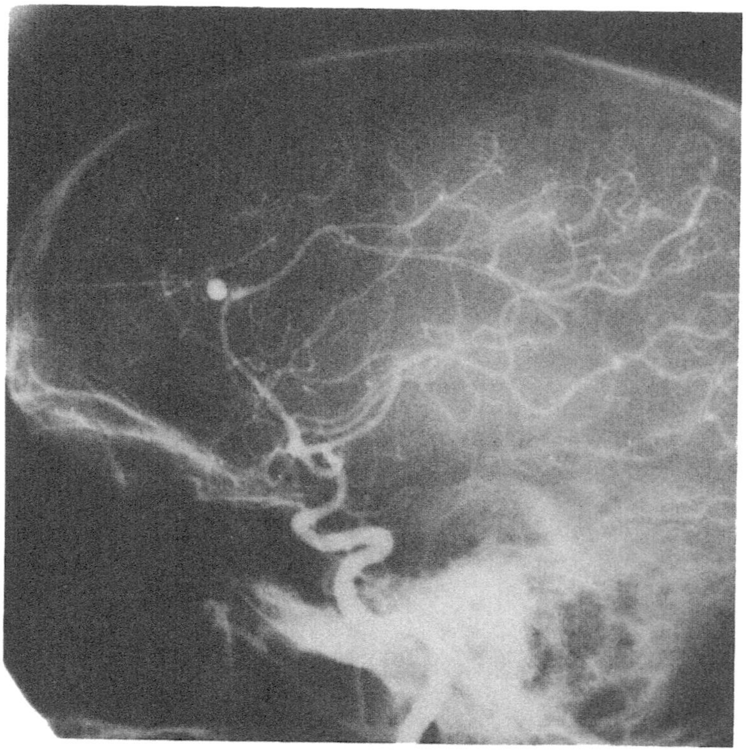

A

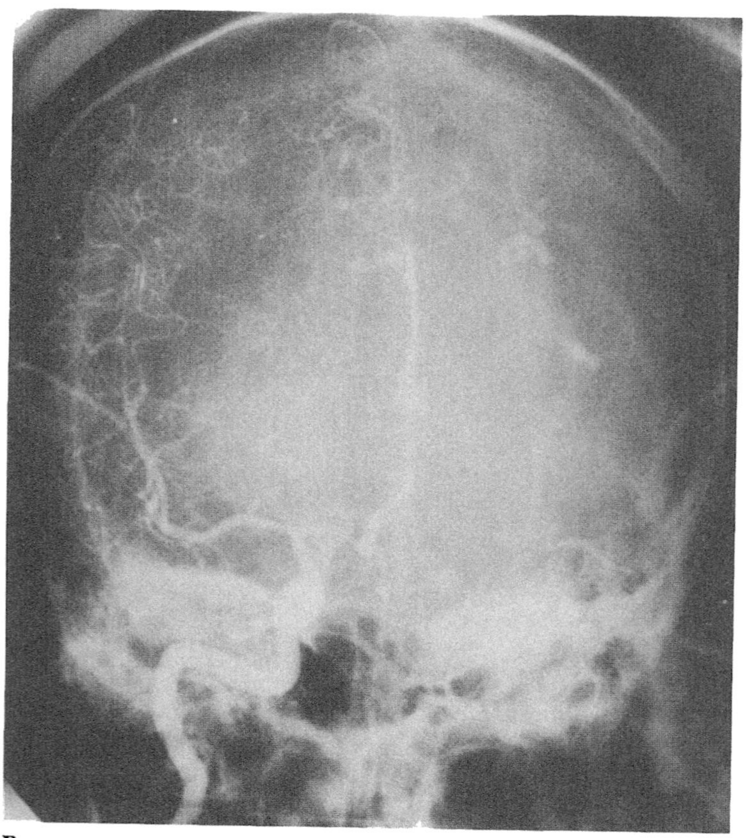

B

Fig. 35.36. Right carotid angiogram demonstrating the usual location of an anterior cerebral artery aneurysm (ACeAA): at the fork between the pericallosal and callosomarginal arteries. A Lateral view. B Frontal (Towne) view.

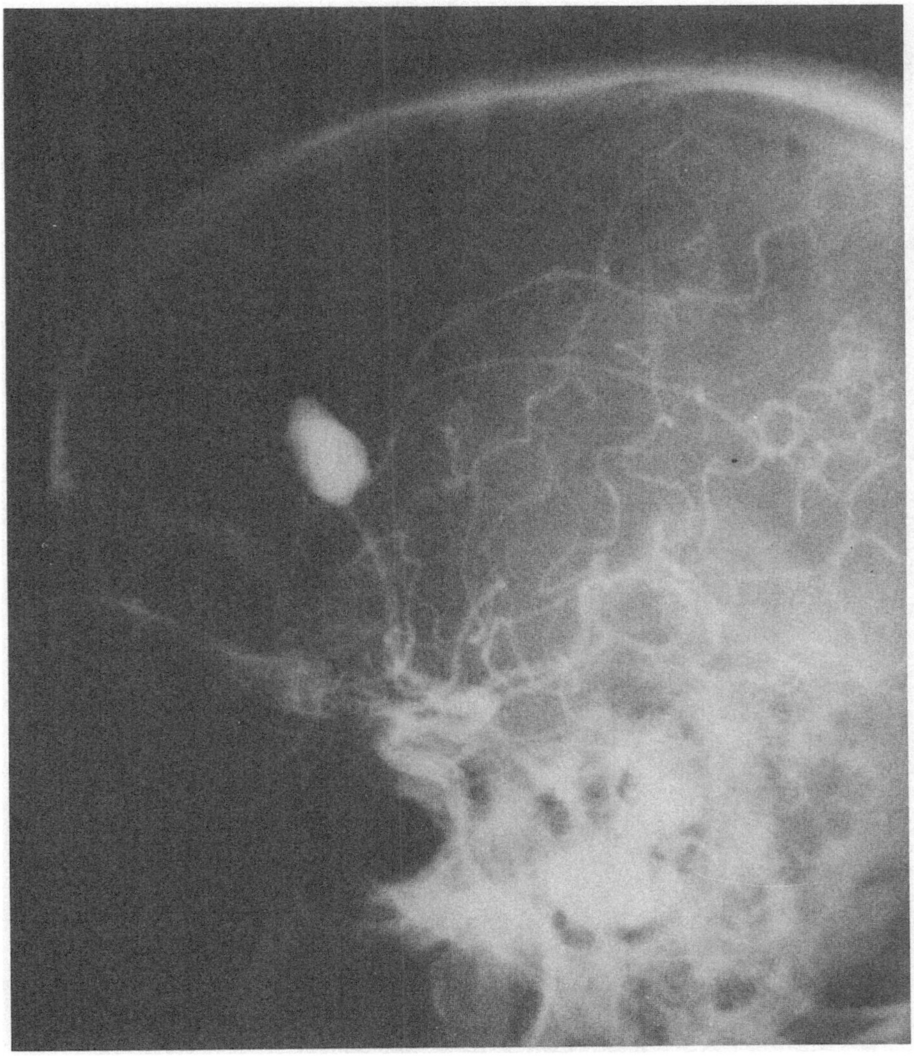

Fig. 35.37. Left carotid angiogram, lateral view, illustrating a prominent ACeAA at the take-off of the frontopolar artery. There is associated hematoma in the left frontal lobe.

ing retraction; the ACeAA may be stuck to the medial surfaces of both cerebral hemispheres. If the aneurysm is not obvious, do not hesitate to obtain a lateral skull Xray during the approach to the pericallosal cistern. This simple maneuver may save time exploring for the aneurysm in the long run. It is easy to continue mistakenly dissecting further and further away from the target along the interhemispheric fissure.

Care must be taken to avoid retractor injury to the contralateral hemisphere and ACeA. If this occurs in the presence of an ipsilateral ACeA compromise during aneurysm dissection or clipping, serious ischemic sequelae will occur. Rarely one may have to permanently trap

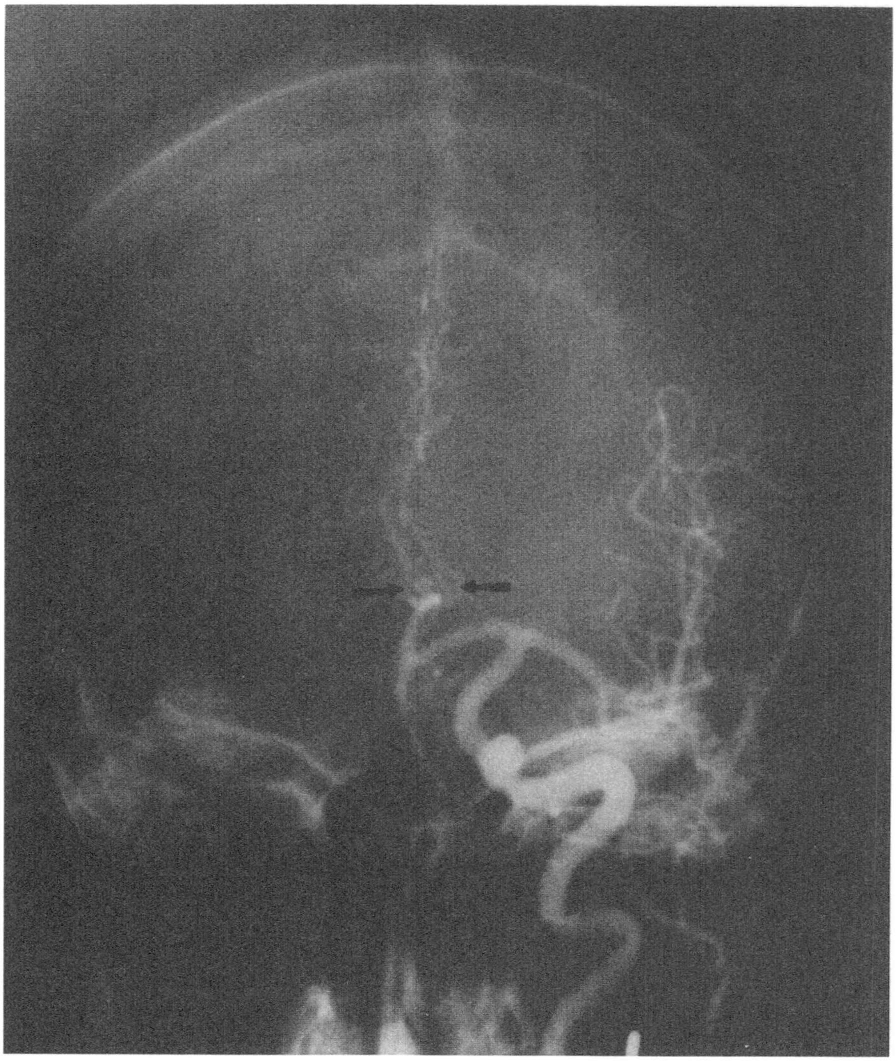

Fig. 35.38. Frontal (Towne) view of left carotid angiogram revealing an azygous anterior cerebral artery aneurysm (azACeAA). The common ACeA trunk, or azygous ACeA, ascends from A-1 and divides into a right and left pericallosal artery (*arrows*). The aneurysm arises from the azygous ACeA at its bifurcation. This was an incidental finding in a 49-year-old man hospitalized in 1975 for basal cell carcinoma of the neck. No surgery was performed on the aneurysm.

the ACeAA. Operative and postoperative BP elevation, fluid maintenance, and delay in sitting the patient up in a chair should be carried out in that circumstance. With modern surgical techniques, the often reported complications of the ACeAA clipping procedure have become considerably less.

Bibliography

1. Allcock JM: Aneurysms. In Newton TH, Potts DG (eds.): Radiology of the Skull and Brain, Vol. 2, Book 4. St. Louis, Mosby, 1974, pp. 2435–2489
2. Becker DH, Newton TH: Distal anterior cere-

bral artery aneurysm. Neurosurgery 4:495–503, 1979
3. Botterell EH: Discussion. Trans Am Neurol Assoc 76:154, 1951
4. Bremer JL: Congenital aneurysms of the cerebral arteries. An embryologic study. Arch Pathol 35:819–831, 1943
5. Busse O: Aneurysmen und Bildungsfehler der Arteria communicans anterior. Virchow's Arch Pathol Anat 229:178–200, 1921
6. Castillo R, Dominiguez A, Serpa A: Study of the structure of aneurysms of the circle of Willis. Excerpta Med ICS No. 110:647–650, 1966
7. Cohen MM, Kristiansen K: Association of aneurysm with anomalies of arteries at base of the brain. Zbl Ges Neurol Psychiat 143:11, 1957
8. Crompton MR: The pathogenesis of cerebral aneurysms. Brain 89:797–814, 1966
9. Crudeli R: Observations sur les aspects anatomiques de l'artère communicante artérieure. Neuro-chirurgie (Paris) 6:29–37, 1960
10. Dechaume JP, Aimard G, Michel D, et al.: Les anévrysmes de l'artère péri-calleuse. A propos d'une série de 12 observations. Neuro-chirurgie (Paris) 19:135–150, 1973
11. Dunker RO, Harris AB: Surgical anatomy of the proximal anterior cerebral artery. J Neurosurg 44:359–367, 1976
12. Fox JL: Microsurgical exposure of intracranial aneurysms. J Microsurg 1:2–31, 1979
13. Fox JL, Albin MS, Bader DCH, et al.: Microsurgical treatment of neurovascular disease. Neurosurgery 3:285–337, 1978
14. Gastaldo JA: Microsurgical anatomy. Letter-to-the-editor. J Neurosurg 46:266–267, 1977
15. Greitz T, Lindgren E: Cerebral vascular anatomy. In Abrams HL (ed.): Angiography, Vol 1. Boston, Little, Brown, 1961, pp. 51–80
16. Heubner O: Die leutische Erkrankungen der Hirnarterien. Leipzig, FCW Vogel, 1874, p. 183
17. Heubner O: Zur Topographie der Ernährungsgebiete der einzelnen Hirnarterien. Zentralbl Med Wissenschaft 10:817–821, 1872
18. Huber P, Braun J, Hirschmann D, Agyeman JF: Incidence of berry aneurysms of the unpaired pericallosal artery: angiographic study. Neuroradiology 19:143–147, 1980
19. Kaplan HA: The lateral perforating branches of the anterior and middle cerebral arteries. J Neurosurg 23:305–310, 1965
20. Katz RS, Horoupian DS, Zingesser L: Aneurysm of azygous anterior cerebral artery. Case report. J Neurosurg 48:804–808, 1978
21. Kempe LG: Operative Neurosurgery, Vol. 1. Cranial, Cerebral, and Intracranial Vascular Disease. New York, Springer-Verlag, 1968, pp. 1–75, 203–214
22. Kleiss E: Die verschiedenen Formen des Circulus arteriosus cerebralis Willisi. Anat Anz 92:216–230, 1942
23. Kribs M, Kleihues P: The recurrent artery of Heubner. A morphological study of the blood supply of the rostral basal ganglia in normal and pathological conditions. In Zülch KJ (ed.): Cerebral Circulation and Stroke. New York, Springer-Verlag, 1971, pp. 40–56
24. Kwak R, Niizuma H, Hatanaka M, et al.: Anterior communicating artery aneurysms with associated anomalies. J Neurosurg 52:162–164, 1980
25. Kwak R, Ohi T, Niizuma H, et al.: Afferent artery and the site of neck of anterior communicating aneurysms. Surg Neurol 13:221–223, 1980
26. Kwak R, Ohi T, Niizuma H, et al.: Hemodynamics in the anterior part of the circle of Willis in patients with anterior communicating artery aneurysm. Neurol Surg (Tokyo) 6:1065–1069, 1978
27. Kwak R, Takahashi M, Suzuki J: Anterior communicating artery aneurysm and the blood circulation at the anterior part of the circle of Willis and its vascular anomalies. Brain Nerve (Tokyo) 22:439–443, 1970
28. Lazorthes G, Gaubert J, Poulhes J: La distribution centrale et corticale de l'artère cérébrale antérieure. Étude anatomique et incidences neurochirurgicales. Neuro-chirurgie (Paris) 2:237–253, 1956
29. Leeds NE: The striate (lenticulostriate) arteries and the artery of Heubner. In Newton TH, Potts DG (eds.): Radiology of the Skull and Brain. Angiography, Vol. 2, Book 2. St. Louis, Mosby, 1974, pp. 1527–1539
30. LeMay M, Gooding CA: The clinical significance of the azygous anterior cerebral artery (A. C. A.). Am J Roentgenol 98:602–610, 1966
31. McCormick WF: Intracranial arterial aneurysm: a pathologist's view. Stroke 8:15–19, 1973
32. McCormick WF: Problems and pathogenesis of intracranial arterial aneurysms. In Toole JF, Moossy J, Janeway R (eds.): Cerebral Vascular Diseases. New York, Grune & Stratton, 1971, pp. 219–231
33. Newton TH, Potts DG (eds.): Radiology of the Skull and Brain. Angiography, Vol. 2, Book 2. St. Louis, Mosby, 1974, pp. 1145–1848
34. Niizuma H, Kwak R, Uchida K, et al.: Aneurysms of the azygos anterior cerebral artery. Surg Neurol 15:225–228, 1981
35. Ostrowski AZ, Webster JE, Gurdjian ES: The proximal anterior cerebral artery: an anatomic study. Arch Neurol 3:661–664, 1960
36. Padget DH: The circle of Willis. Its embryology and anatomy. In Dandy WE (ed.): Intracranial Arterial Aneurysms. New York, Hafner, 1944, pp. 67–90 [reprinted 1969]
37. Padget DH: The development of the cranial ar-

teries in the human embryo. Contr Embryol Carneg Inst No. 212 32:205–261, 1948
38. Peisker R: Über das gemeinsame Vorkommen von angeborenen (Forbusschen) Aneurysmen und Anomalien im Bereich des basalen Gefässringes. Acta Neurochir 12:69–79, 1964
39. Perlmutter D, Rhoton AL Jr: Microsurgical anatomy of the anterior cerebral-anterior communicating-recurrent artery complex. J Neurosurg 45:259–272, 1976
40. Pertuiset B, Lepoire J, Boudin G, et al.: Les anévrysmes de l'artère pericalleuse. (Étude anatomoclinique et thérapeutique à propos de 5 observations). Neuro-chirurgie (Paris) 7:321–338, 1961
41. Pool JL, Potts DG: Aneurysms and Arteriovenous Anomalies of the Brain. Diagnosis and Treatment. New York, Harper & Row, 1965
42. Rubinstein HS: The anterior communicating artery in man. J Neuropathol Exp Neurol 3:196–198, 1944
43. Stehbens WE: Aneurysms and anatomical variation of cerebral arteries. Arch Pathol 75:45–64, 1963
44. Stehbens WE: Pathology of the Cerebral Blood Vessels. St. Louis, Mosby 1972
45. Stephens RB, Stilwell DL: Arteries and Veins of the Human Brain. Springfield, Ill., Thomas, 1969
46. Sundt TM Jr: Francis Murphey, M.D. Surg Neurol 8:141–142, 1977
47. VanderArk GD, Kempe LC: Classification of anterior communicating aneurysms as a basis for surgical approach. J Neurosurg 32:300–303, 1970
48. Voris HC: Complications of ligation of the internal carotid artery. J Neurosurg 8:119–131, 1951
49. Watts JW: A comparative study of the anterior cerebral artery and the circle of Willis in primates. J Anat (London) 68:534–550, 1934
50. Westberg G: The recurrent artery of Heubner and the arteries of the central ganglia. Acta Radiol [Diagn] 1:949–954, 1963
51. Wilson CB, Christensen FK, Subrahmanian MV: Intracranial aneurysms at the pericallosol artery bifurcation. Am Surg 31:386–393, 1965
52. Wollschlaeger G, Wollschlaeger PB: The circle of Willis. In Newton TH, Potts DG (eds.): Radiology of the Skull and Brain. Angiography, Vol. 2, Book 2. St. Louis, Mosby, 1974, pp. 1171–1201
53. Yaşargil MG, Fox JL: The microsurgical approach to intracranial aneurysms. Surg Neurol 3:7–14, 1975
54. Yaşargil MG, Fox JL, Ray MW: The operative approach to aneurysms of the anterior communicating artery. In Krayenbühl H (ed.): Advances and Technical Standards in Neurosurgery, Vol. 2. New York, Springer-Verlag, 1975, pp. 113–170
55. Yaşargil MG, Smith RD: Surgery on the carotid system in the treatment of hemorrhagic stroke. In Thompson RH, Green JR (eds.): Advances in Neurology, Vol. 16. Stroke. New York, Raven Press, 1977, pp. 181–209

36

Technique of Aneurysm Surgery

III. Internal Carotid Artery Aneurysms

Approximately one-third of all intracranial berry aneurysms occur on the internal carotid artery. This chapter will address the surgical approach to these lesions in the following order of site: (a) pcaICAA; (b) achaICAA; (c) bICAA; (d) oaICAA and vICAA; and (e) csICAA. We are beginning with pcaICAA since these are the most common type of ICAA; the approach to the others, while differing significantly, still begins in the carotid cistern at the PCoA take-off region.

This chapter is a continuation of the frontotemporal approach described in Chapters 34 and 35. Therefore some technical aspects already covered will not be repeated here.

Posterior Communicating Artery–Internal Carotid Artery Aneurysms

On the usual lateral angiogram (Fig. 36.1) the pcaICAA *appears* to arise at the proximal angle between the internal carotid artery (ICA) and the posterior communicating artery (PCoA). In fact it arises at the *distal* angle (Fig. 36.2). The common illusion seen in Fig. 36.1 is due to the PCoA passing medial to the neck of the aneurysm as it courses posteriorly. Figure 36.3 demonstrates the typical medial position of PCoA in relation to the aneurysm. The PCoA may wander laterally in an occasional case. It may be a large "fetal" type of artery (in about one-third of cases [57]), small, a fibrous band, or absent (5,39).

Occasionally, the base of the aneurysm may be broad and involve the origin of the anterior choroidal artery (AChA) also (65). Although the pcaICAA may come in a multitude of shapes and projections, Selverstone (48) described four principal types: (a) flask-shaped, with a neck long enough to be clipped; (b) globular, ellipsoidal, or irregular, with an extremely short neck; (c) sessile, with a sac at least as wide as the base; and (d) dome-shaped, with the base of the sac at its widest point.

Most of these aneurysms project laterally, posterolaterally, posteriorly, or posteroinferiorly (3). VanderArk and colleagues (57) analyzed 78 cases and concluded that 24% project laterally above the tentorium (Fig. 36.4); 24%, laterally and inferiorly below the tentorium (Fig. 36.3); 36%, directly backward or posteroinferiorly (Fig. 36.5); 13%, upward and medially; and 3%, downward and medially. The importance of assessing the projection, or direction, of the aneurysm is exemplified in Fig. 36.6. A lateral or posterolateral projection often is associated with adhesions between the dome of the aneurysm and the temporal lobe. In this circumstance even slight traction on the temporal lobe may distort or pull on the aneurysm and cause its rupture at surgery.

True posterior communicating artery aneurysms (PCoAA), although rare, do occur (10, 41,65). Most likely, they arise at a take-off of an anterior thalamic perforator. Their exposure naturally requires this same frontolateral approach, and the PCoA is followed back to the aneurysm. However, as Dandy once remarked (10), "Most of these aneurysms arise at or very

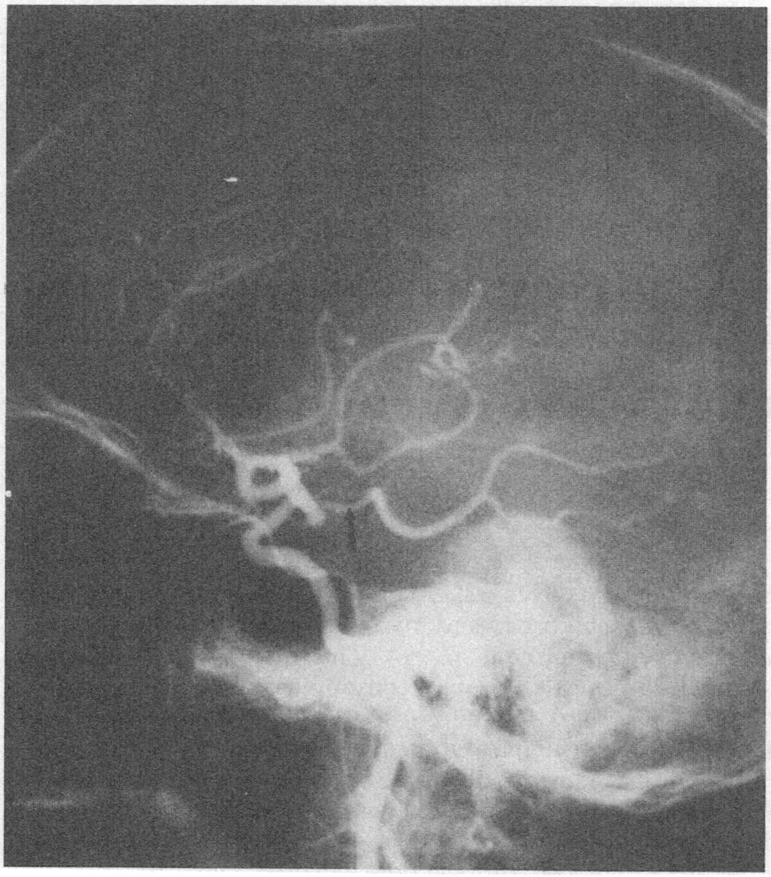

Fig. 36.1. Lateral view of pcaICAA on angiogram. The prominent posterior communicating artery (*arrow*) appears to arise from the internal carotid artery distal to the neck of the aneurysm. It actually arises proximal to the neck of the aneurysm (following the rule that aneurysms originate at the distal angle of the bifurcation) and passes medial to the aneurysm.

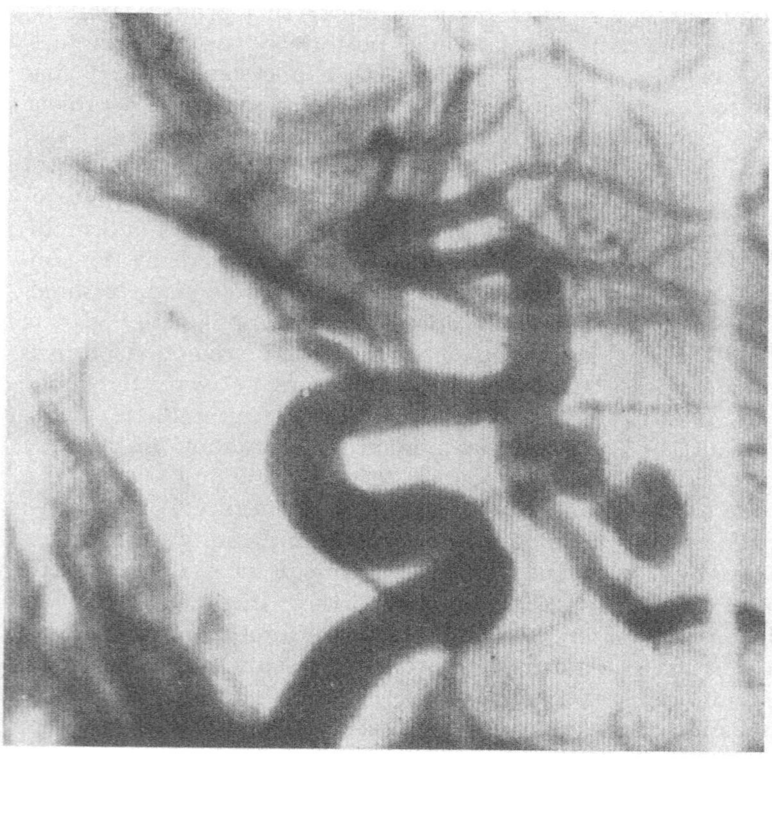

Fig. 36.2. Lateral angiogram illustrating more clearly the origin of the posterior communicating artery in relation to the pcaICAA. In this case the PCoA courses downward before going posteriorly. From af Björkesten G, Troupp H: ref. 2.

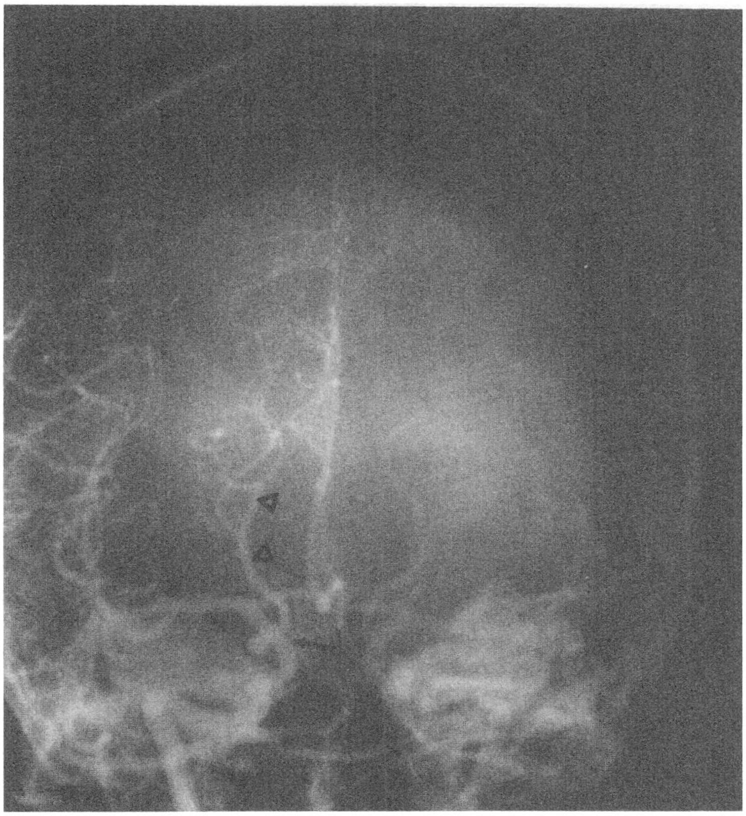

Fig. 36.3. Right carotid angiogram, AP view. *Arrow* points toward origin of the PCoA on the posterolateral wall of the ICA. The PCoA actually arises at the proximal angle between the ICA and the aneurysm. *Triangles,* posterior cerebral artery coursing around brain stem.

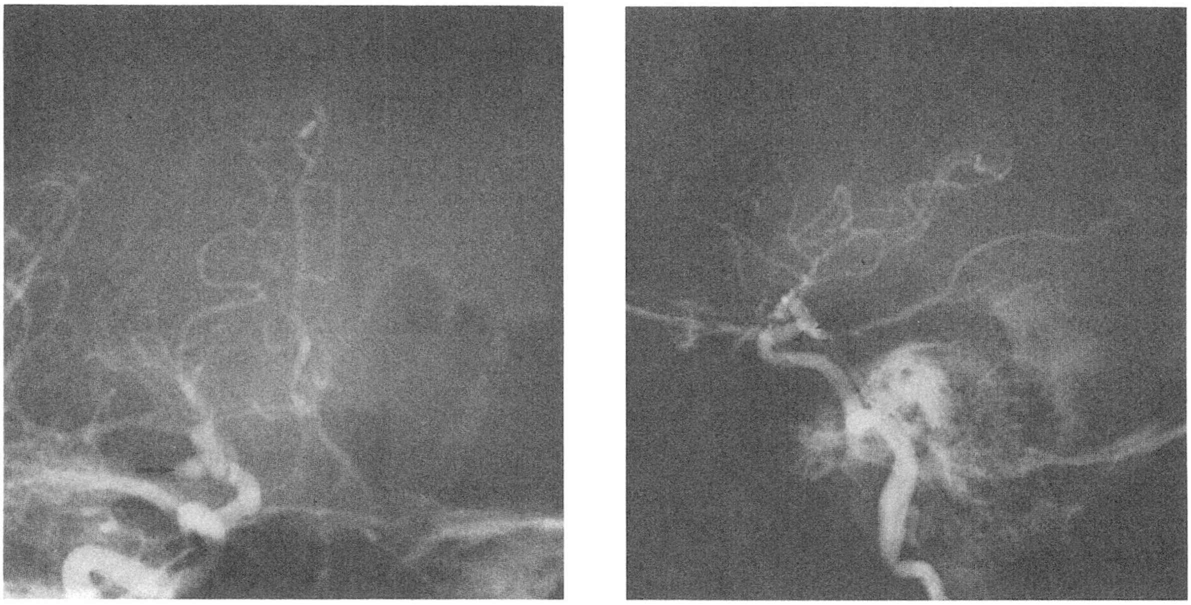

A B

Fig. 36.4. A Frontal view of right carotid angiogram. The aneurysm (*arrow*) projects laterally against the temporal lobe and tentorium. B Lateral view. *Arrow,* aneurysm; *arrowhead,* origin of the PCoA.

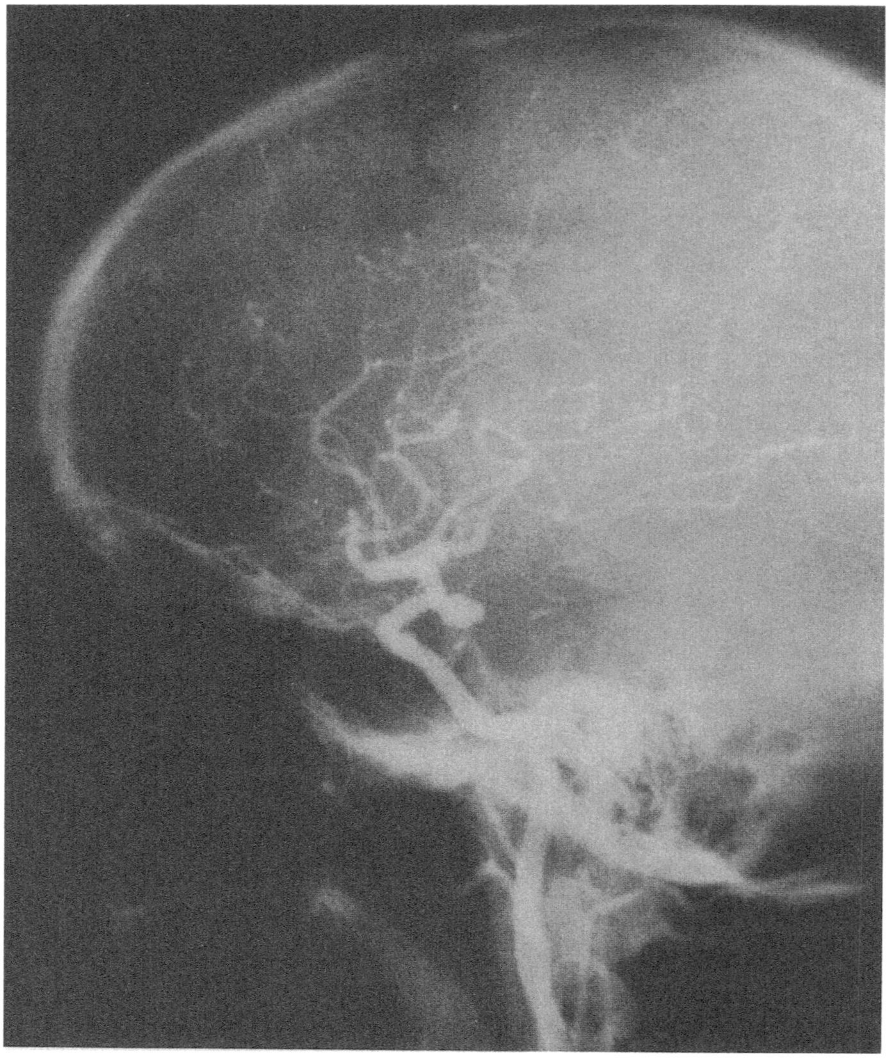

A

Fig. 36.5. Angiogram demonstrating common type of pcaICAA projecting straight backward. (A small csICAA also is present.) **A** Lateral view. **B** Frontal view showing aneurysm (*arrow*) superimposed on ICA.

near the junction of these two trunks and they usually lie on the posterior communicating artery, frequently concealing it and giving the superficial impression that the sac arises from it, but if the orifice is carefully examined it will usually be found to enter the carotid."

Surgical Exposure

The carotid cistern is exposed as illustrated in Chapter 34. The approach is between the sphenoid wing and sylvian fissure as shown in Fig. 36.7 and 36.8. In this example, note how the PCoA takes its typical course, arising at the proximal ICA/aneurysm junction on the posterolateral side of the ICA and then passing behind the ICA to reappear deep to the space between the ICA and optic chiasm. Figure 36.9 is the same case seen at high magnification. Here are illustrated the vital brain stem perforators which must be protected by careful microtechnique, application of topical 3% papaverine or 0.5% phentolamine, and avoidance of their entrapment in the aneurysm clip. They may be enclosed in a layer of arachnoid.

Figures 36.10–36.13 show the gradual exposure and cauterization of a pcaICAA, which projects down and laterally under the anterior

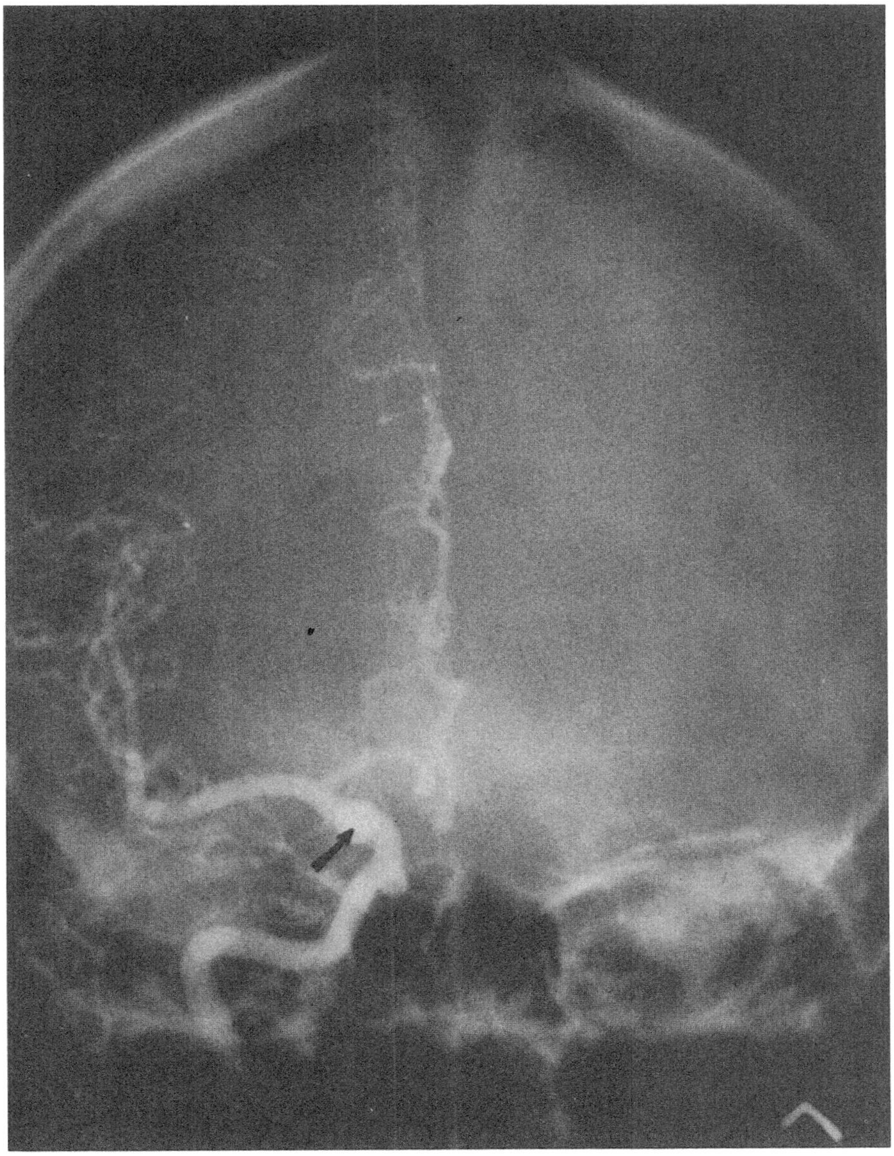

B

reflection of the tentorium. The dome is hidden by and adherent to the tentorial edge. Figures 36.11 and 36.12 demonstrate removal of sympathetic fibers from the wall of the ICA, a step which some (62) have considered possibly beneficial in reducing vasospasm. The membrane of Liliequist is left intact to keep blood out of the posterior cisterns. The temporal lobe has been retracted just enough to expose the aneurysm. After removal of all adhesions around the aneurysm, bipolar coagulation was carried out to shrink the size of the aneurysm. In this patient such a step was helpful by allowing the surgeon to see clearly the PCoA (Fig. 36.13), which arose on the posterior wall of the ICA. This PCoA origin was hidden by the aneurysm but should be identified before application of the clip to avoid its entrapment in the clip.

The technique of narrowing the waist of an aneurysm with bipolar electrocautery is already detailed in Chapter 31. When used on the pcaICAA, the forceps tip must be entirely around the aneurysm and directed away from any anterior thalamoperforators on the other side of the artery. Prior to electrocoagulation and clipping, we gently free the dome from the tentorium to which it is often adherent. This allows the surgeon to narrow the neck by

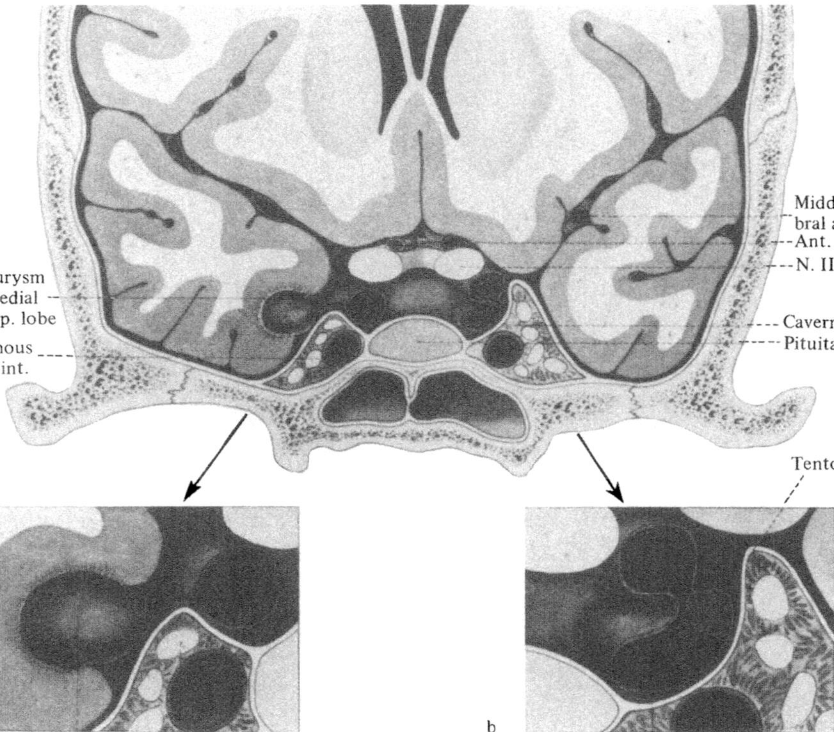
Middle cerebral a.
Ant. comm. a.
N. II
Dome of aneurysm covered by medial aspect of temp. lobe
Cavernous sinus
Pituitary
Intracavernous portion of int. carotid a.
Tentorial edge
a
b
Aneurysm above and lateral to tentorial edge
N. III
Int. carotid a.
Aneurysm medial to tentorial edge

A

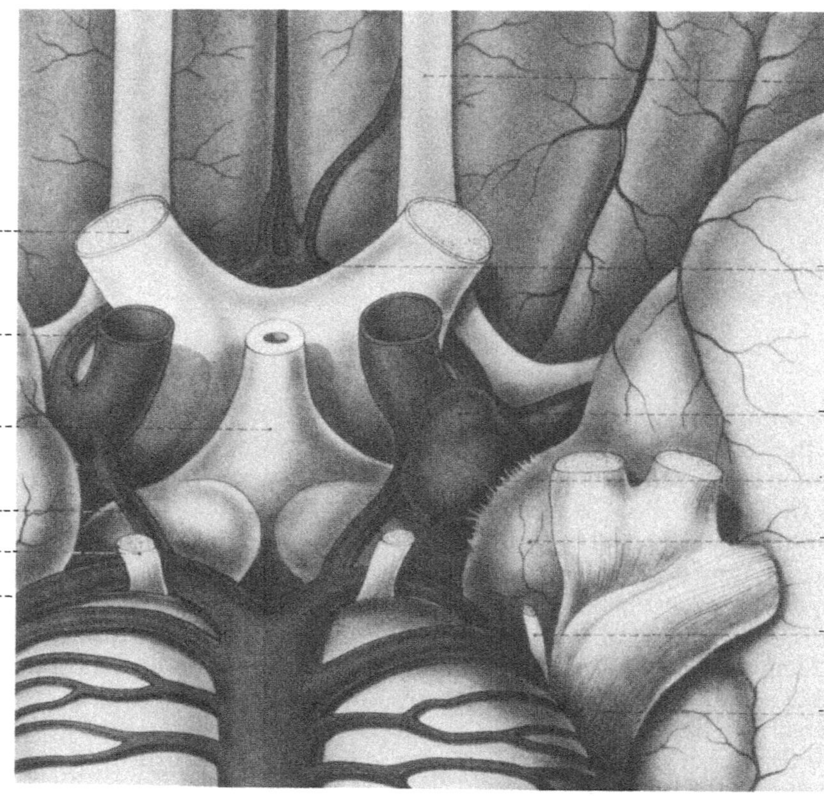
Olfactory tract
N. II
Ant. comm. a.
Rt. int. carotid a.
Aneurysm
Infundibulum
Adhesions between aneurysm and temp. lobe
Post. comm. a.
N. III
Uncus
Post. cerebral a.
N. IV
N. V

B

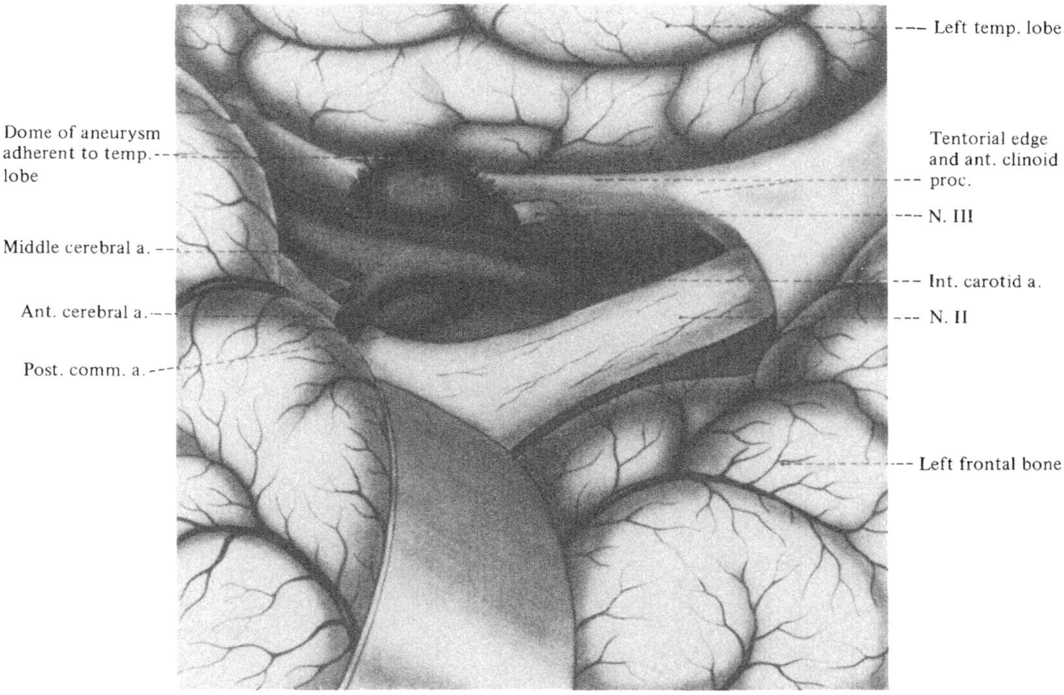

C

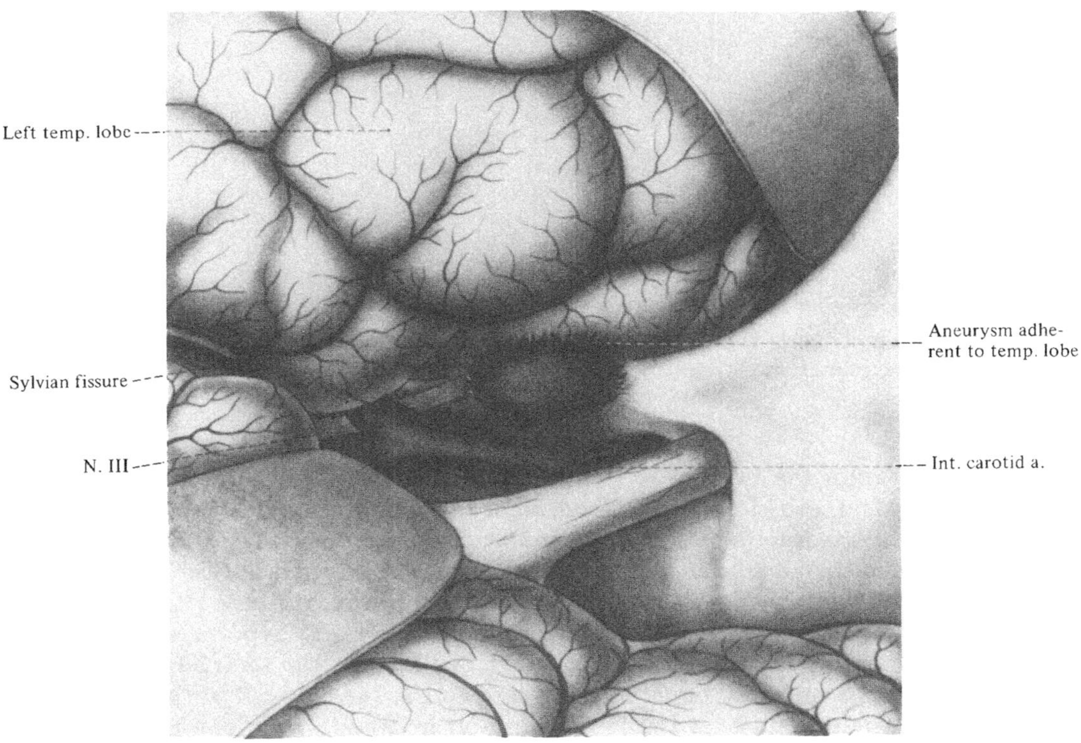

D

Fig. 36.6. Diagrams of a pcaICAA projecting laterally. Adhesions to the aneurysm dome are illustrated. From Kempe LG: ref. 31. **A** Coronal section. **B** Basal view. Note adhesions between uncus of left temporal lobe and aneurysm. **C** and **D** Variations on site of left pcaICAA adhesions to temporal lobe and tentorial edge.

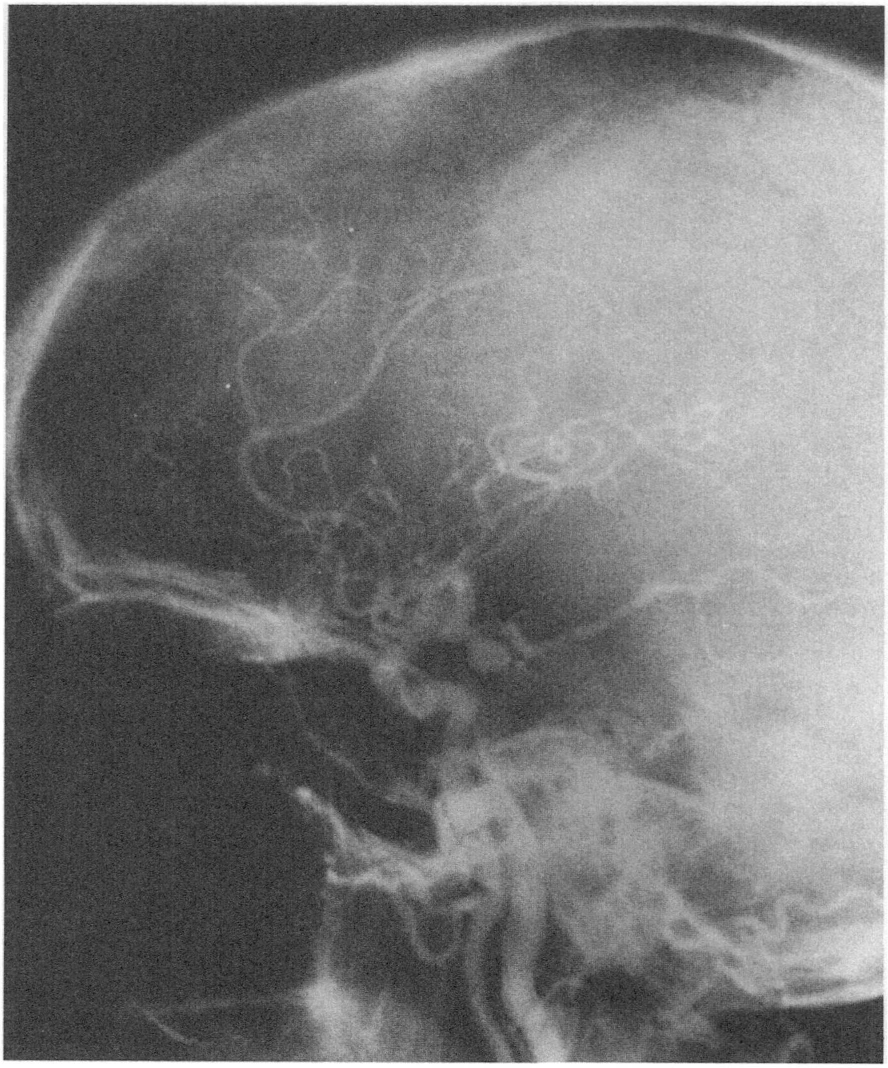

Fig. 36.7. Lateral angiogram showing the pcaICAA and environs exposed in Figs. 36.8 and 36.9. The *triangles* mark the origin and termination of the posterior communicating artery.

forceps or clip without tearing the neck as it is stretched between a rigid, atherosclerotic artery and the tentorial edge. A tear in the dome is much more easily handled than a tear at the neck. Notice in Fig. 36.13 how the electrocoagulation has narrowed the waist of the aneurysm, making it firmer, more cylindrical, and more elongated. This permits not only easier clip application but also a better view of the surrounding anatomy requiring protection. Such electrocoagulation of an aneurysm, of course, is not necessary in most cases but is helpful in many.

Figures 36.14–36.16 portray a prominent pcaICAA fixed between a short, rigid, atherosclerotic ICA and the tentorium. Exposure with minimal retraction was facilitated by removal of much of the sphenoid wing and opening the sylvian fissure. The origin of the PCoA lies behind the aneurysm and the ICA. Anterior thalamoperforators and hypothalamic perforators (Fig. 36.9) are not yet seen but are partially adherent to the medial wall of the aneurysm. These must be freed from the aneurysm prior to clipping. The clip is applied slowly by inserting its posteromedial wing between the anterior thalamoperforators and the aneurysm and its anterolateral wing about 1 mm beyond the PCoA take-off zone.

A straight clip is used if the PCoA can be

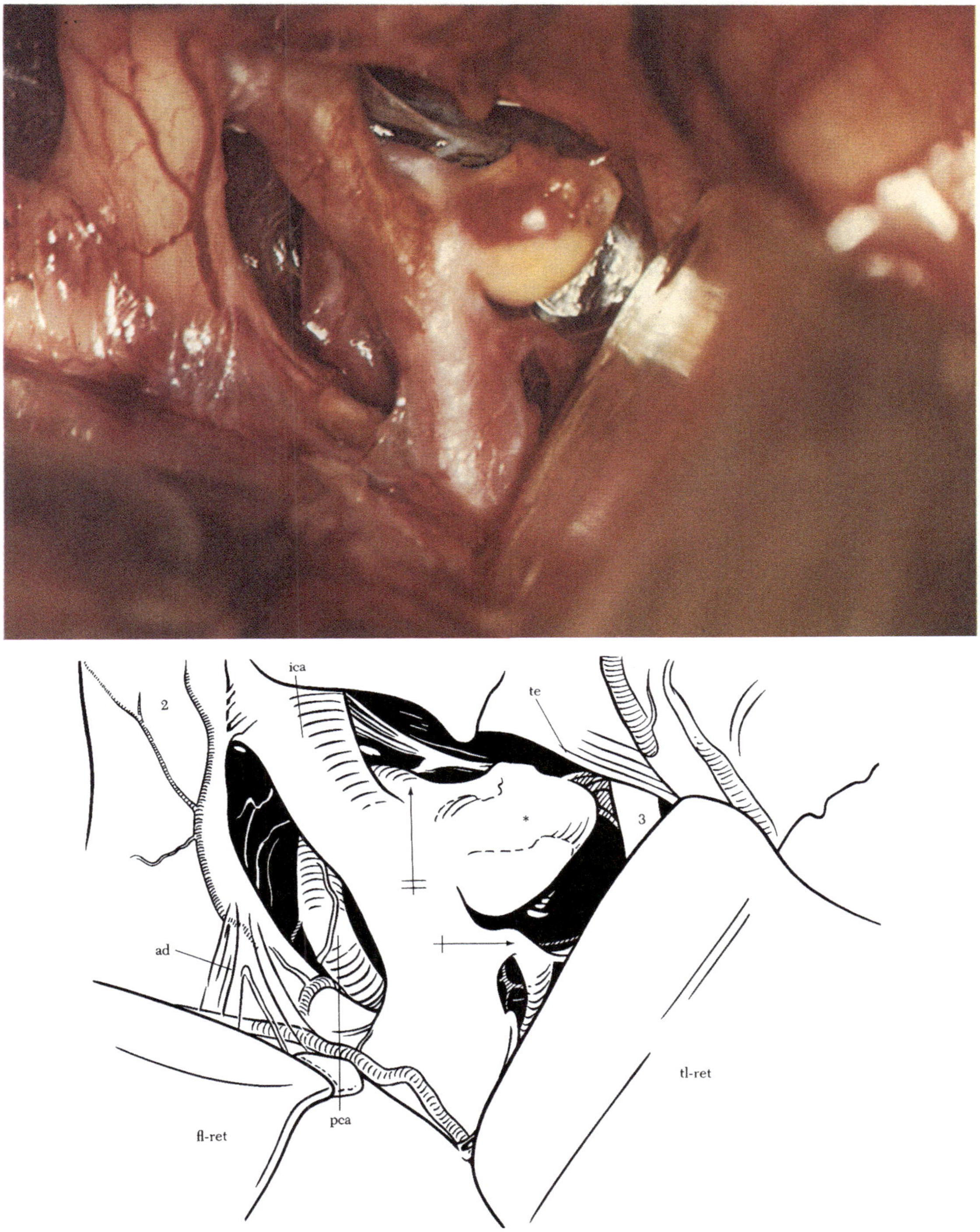

Fig. 36.8. An example of a typical pcaICAA (*) projecting laterally and inferiorly under the tentorial edge (*te*). The aneurysm has already been shrunken by bipolar electrocoagulation. This gave a clear view of its relationship to the origin (*double-crossed arrow*) of the posterior communicating artery (*pca*) and the origin of the anterior choroidal artery (*single-crossed arrow*) entering the crural cistern. A few adhesions remain between the dome of the aneurysm and the oculomotor nerve (*3*). *tl-ret,* temporal lobe retractor; *fl-ret,* frontal lobe retractor; *ad,* adhesions between optic tract and frontal lobe; *2,* right optic nerve; *ica,* internal carotid artery.

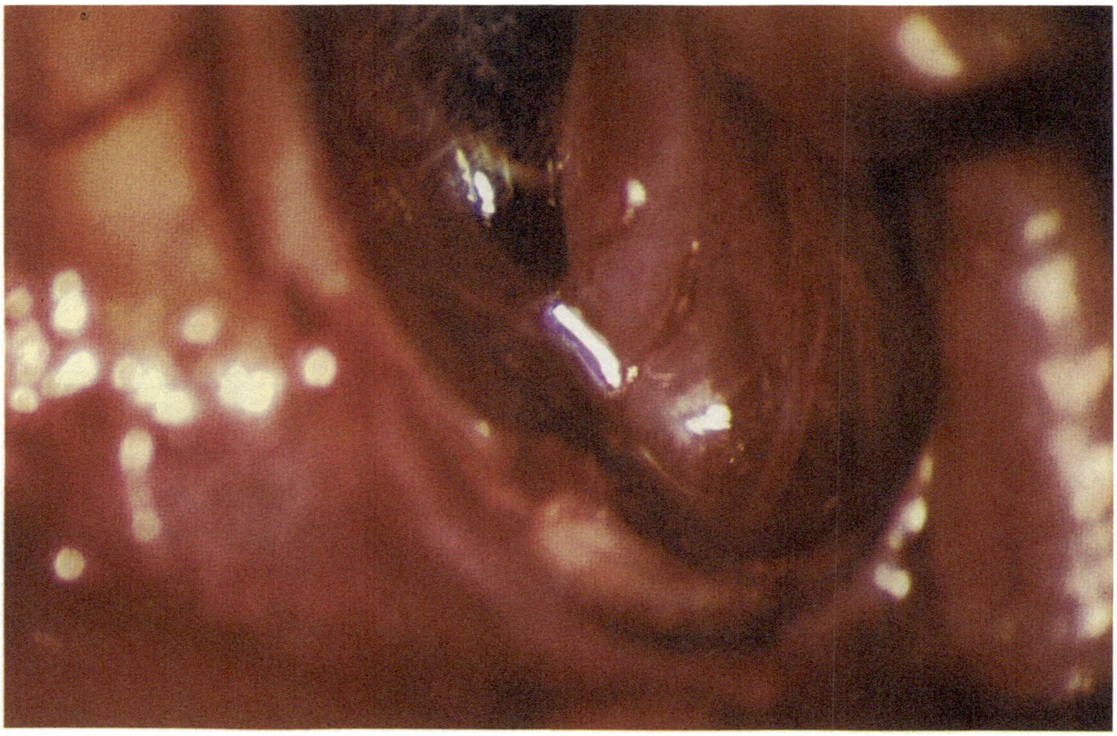

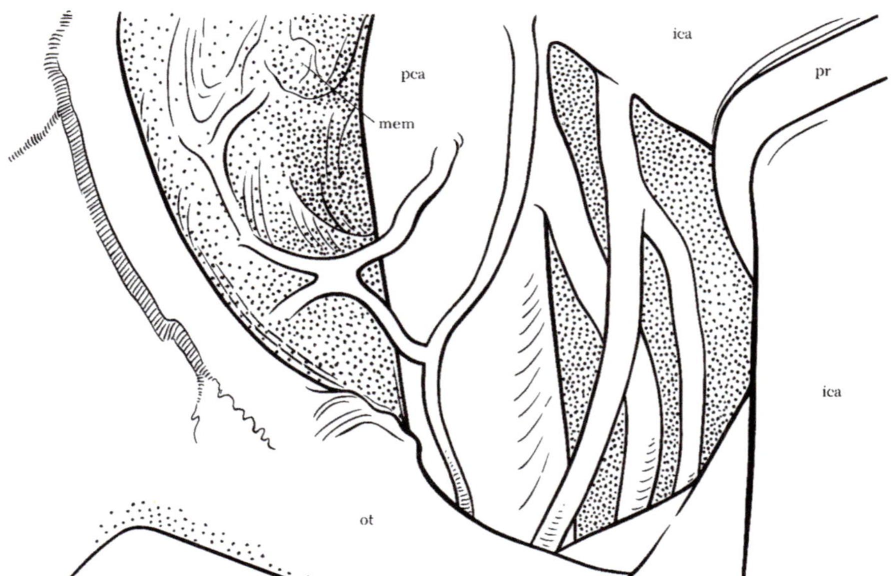

Fig. 36.9. Magnified view between the optic tract (*ot*) and the internal carotid artery (*ica*) of Fig. 36.8. Zeiss dial set at 40 (highest magnification). Note important anterior thalamic and hypothalamic perforators arising from the internal carotid artery (*ica*) being retracted by a probe (*pr*) and arising from the posterior communicating artery (*pca*). *mem*, membrane of Liliequist. From Fox JL: ref. 20.

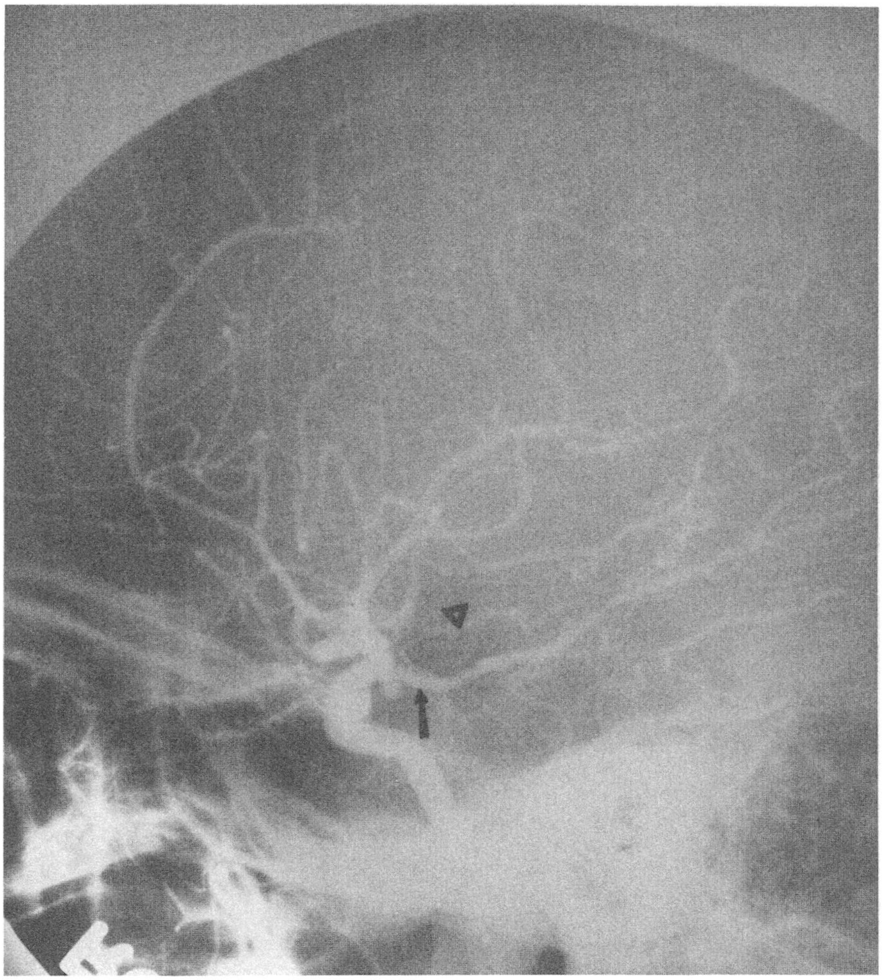

Fig. 36.10. Lateral angiogram of pcaICAA illustrated in Figs. 36.11–36.13. (There also is a small csICAA.) *Arrow,* "fetal" type of posterior communicating artery; *triangle,* anterior choroidal artery.

seen (as in Fig. 36.15) coursing medial to the back wall of the ICA. A gently curving clip (its *convexity* toward the ICA) is applied if the origin of the PCoA is not clear or if the PCoA courses lateral to the back wall of the ICA. This prevents the clip from compromising any perforators of PCoA origin since its tips curve away from these arteries. It is injury to the perforators or the AChA which causes ischemic damage. Occlusion of the PCoA itself will not result in ischemia if the P-1 artery is normal and intact. We have not hesitated to apply a second clip (Fig. 36.16) to buttress the first clip (rather than use tissue adhesives or acrylate). Clip readjustment often is necessary. We usually aspirate or open the dome of the aneurysm to collapse it, confirm that it is secured, take any pressure off nearby neural structures (such as the oculomotor nerve), and remove any distending pressure tending to hold the clip blades open (especially in large aneurysms). This step is not always necessary.

One of the times when aneurysm rupture may occur is during clip application and during clip-applicator withdrawal. If the tear occurs at the ICA/aneurysm-neck junction, control of the hemorrhage is most difficult—especially if the ICA is rigid with atherosclerosis. It is for this reason that the clip must be applied a defined distance from the ICA so that 1 or 2 mm of aneurysm neck is permitted to roll in with the approximation and closure of the clip blades. Thus, this part of the aneurysm neck forms the "wall" enclosing the parent artery

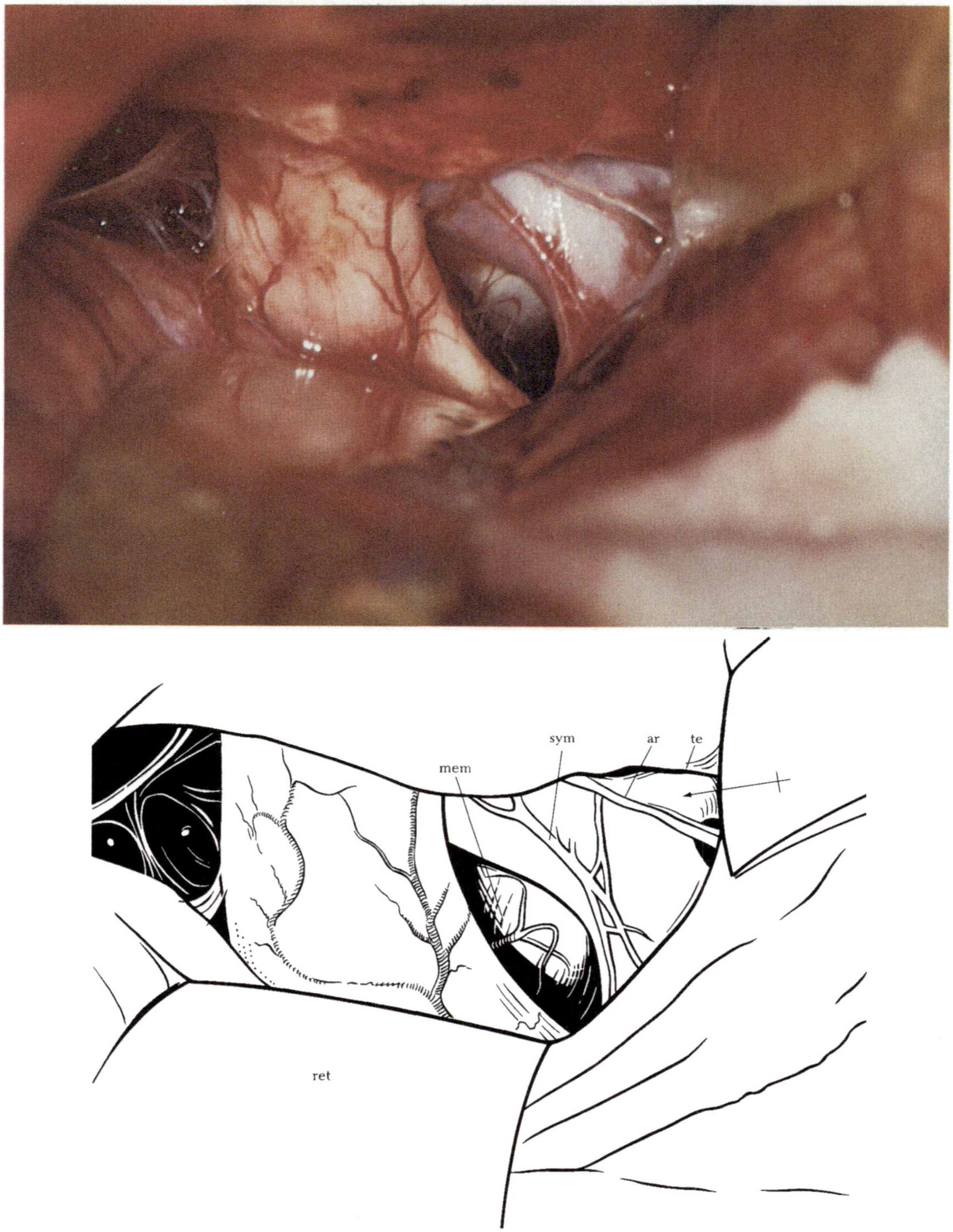

Fig. 36.11. Right internal carotid artery aneurysm at the posterior communicating artery. This aneurysm (*crossed arrow*) lies under the anterior reflection of the tentorium (*te*). An arachnoid strand (*ar*) crosses its neck. *sym,* probable sympathetic fibers on the internal carotid artery; *mem,* membrane of Liliequist in the background; *ret,* retractor on the frontal lobe. From Fox JL: ref. 20.

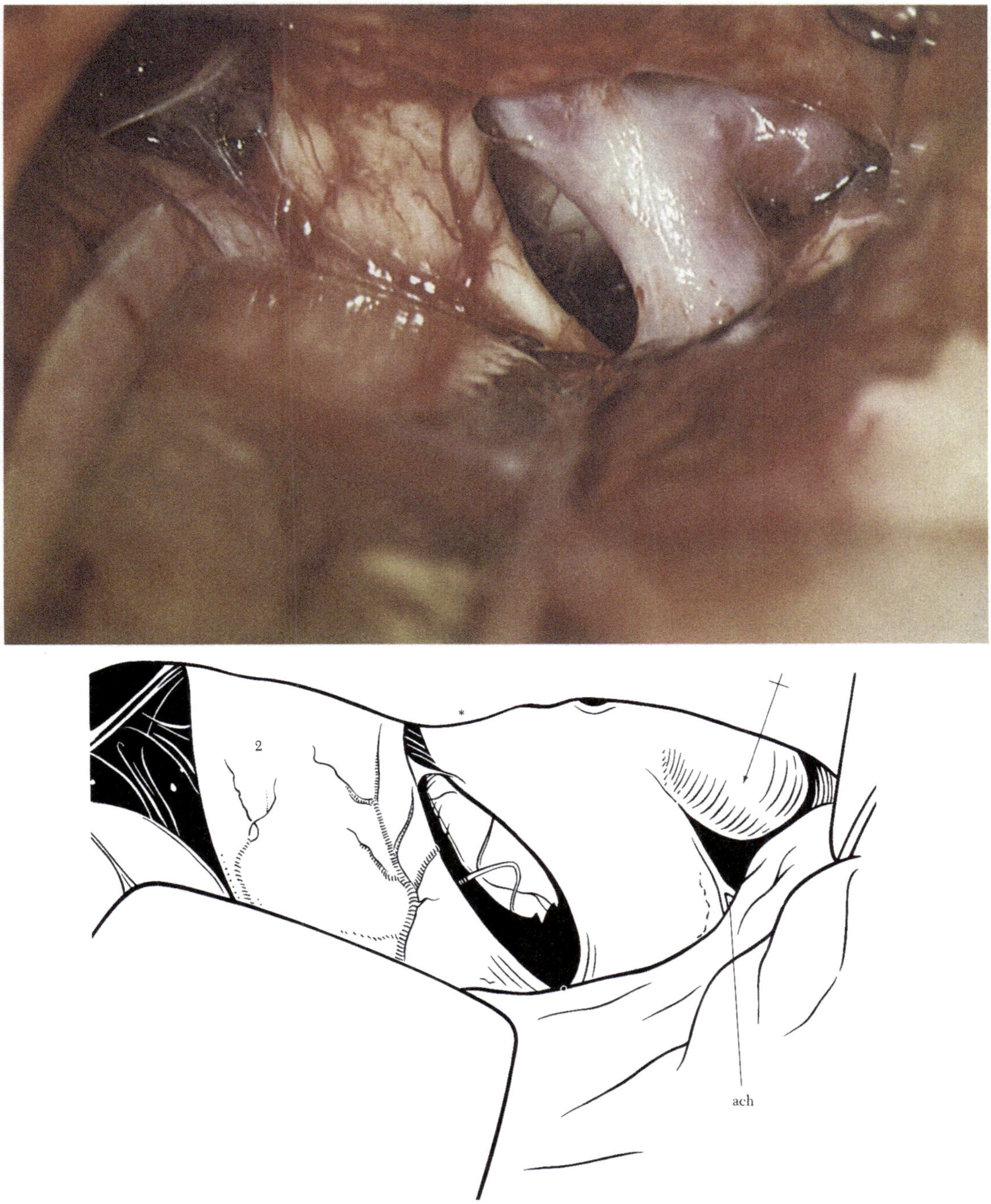

Fig. 36.12. Further exposure of the aneurysm in figs. 36.10 and 36.11. The arachnoid and sympathetic fibers over the carotid artery have been excised. *ach*, anterior choroidal artery origin; *2*, right optic nerve; *, anterior clinoid process; *crossed arrow*, aneurysm under the tentorial edge. From Fox JL: ref. 20.

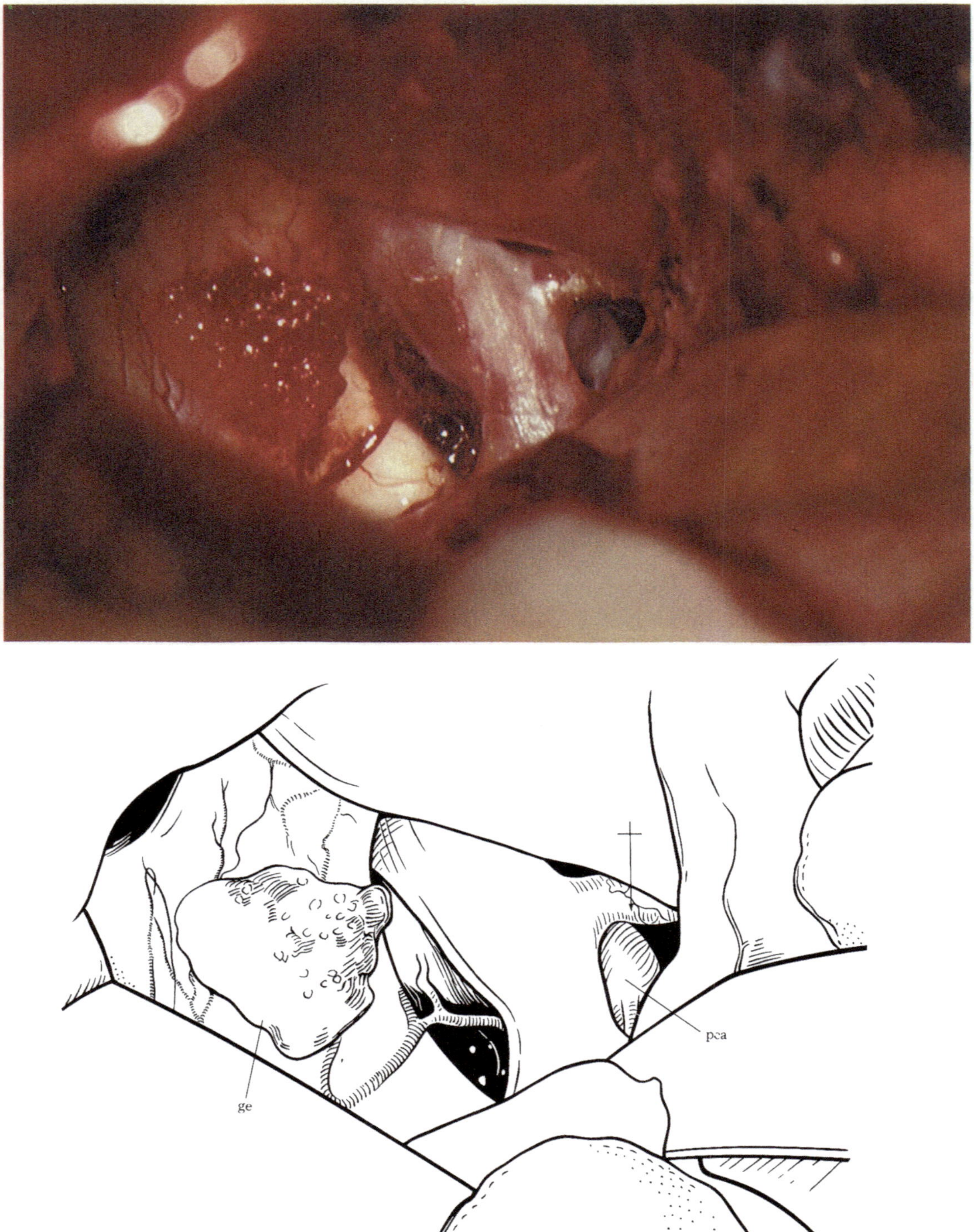

Fig. 36.13. Aneurysm (*crossed arrow*) of the internal carotid artery shrunken by bipolar electrocoagulation. The origin of the posterior communicating artery (*pca*) is hidden by the neck of the aneurysm. *ge,* Gelfoam on the optic chiasm. From Fox JL: ref. 20.

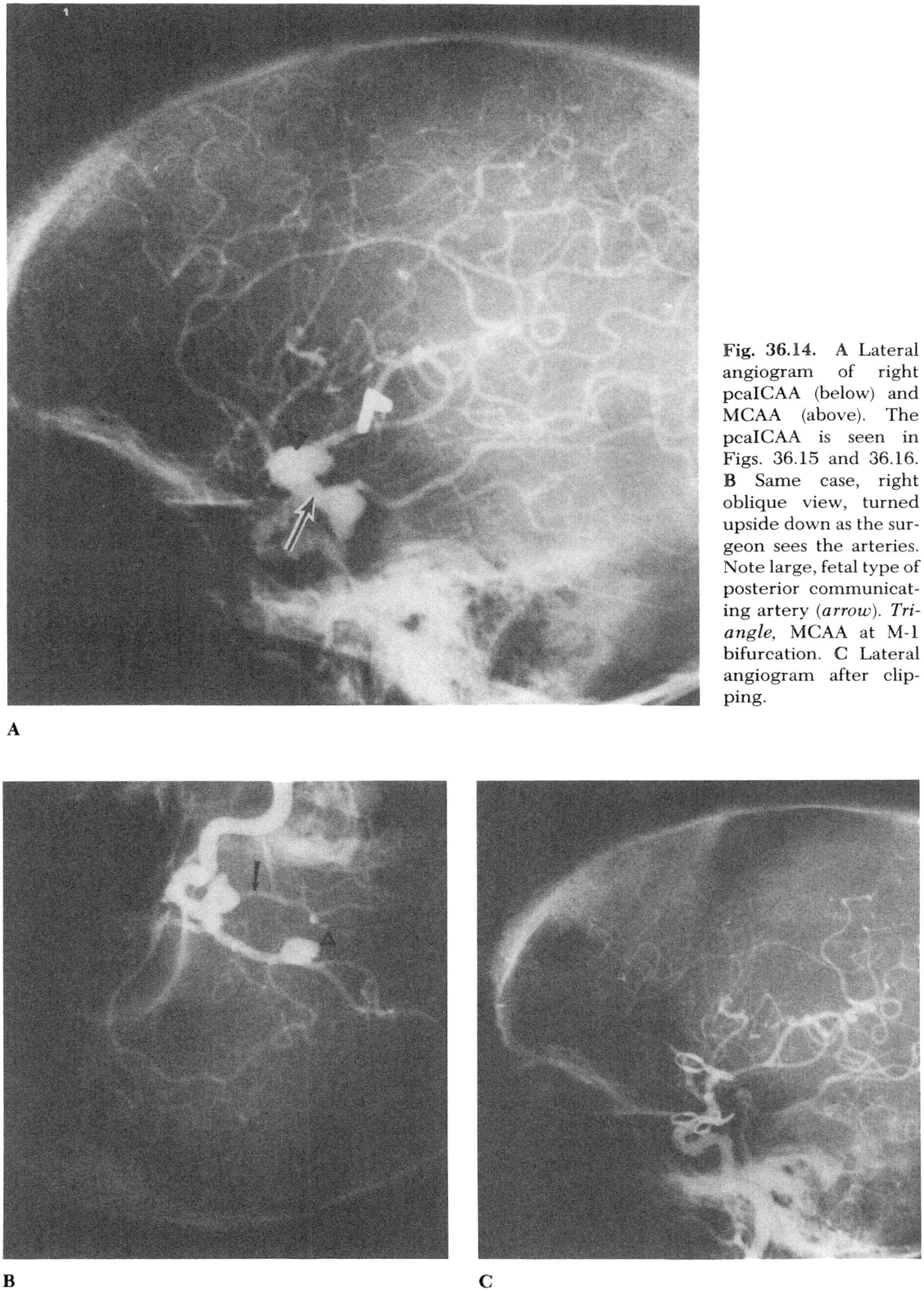

Fig. 36.14. **A** Lateral angiogram of right pcaICAA (below) and MCAA (above). The pcaICAA is seen in Figs. 36.15 and 36.16. **B** Same case, right oblique view, turned upside down as the surgeon sees the arteries. Note large, fetal type of posterior communicating artery (*arrow*). *Triangle,* MCAA at M-1 bifurcation. **C** Lateral angiogram after clipping.

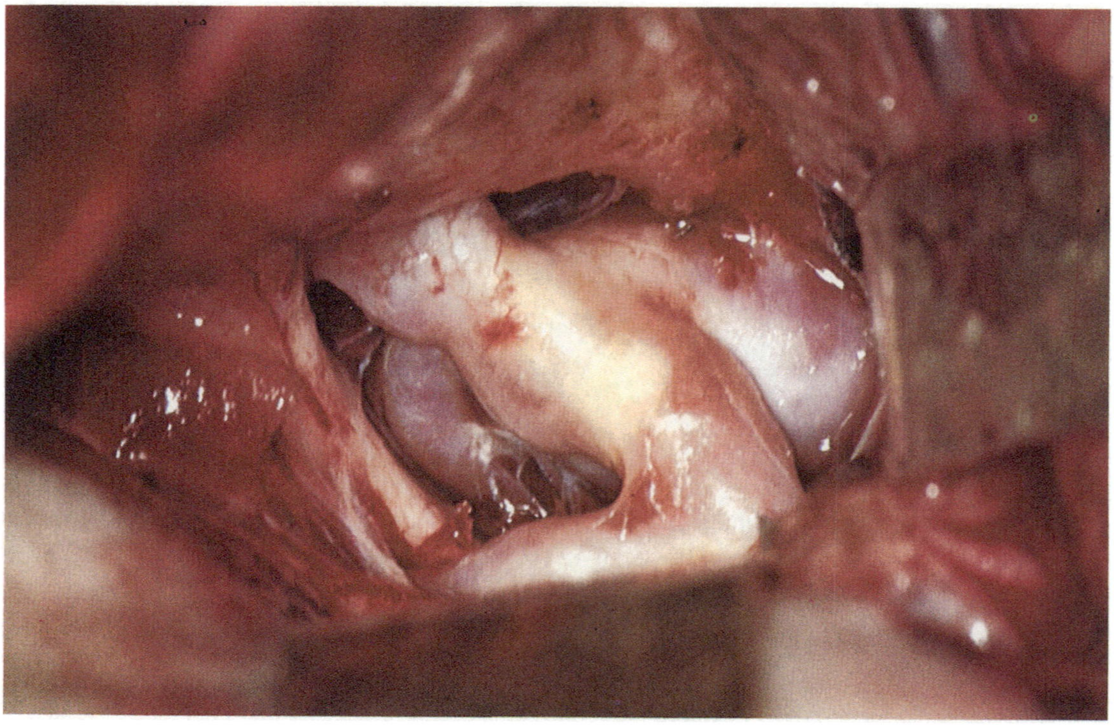

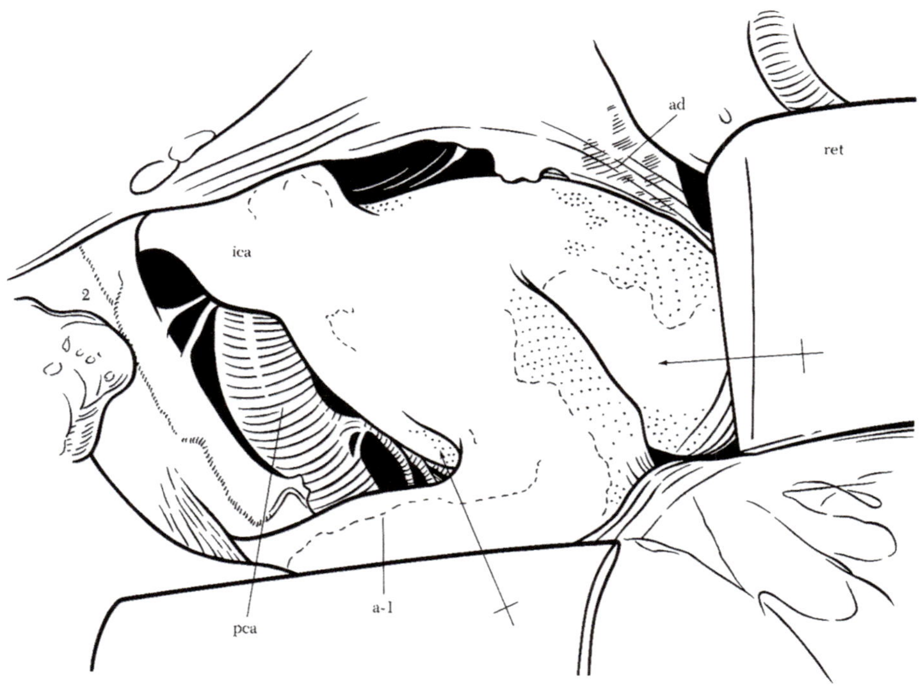

Fig. 36.15. Internal carotid artery aneurysm (*crossed arrows*) seen in Fig. 36.14. This is a large "posterior communicating artery" aneurysm arising at the distal angle between the carotid (*ica*) and posterior communicating (*pca*) arteries. *2*, right optic nerve; *a-1*, A-1 artery; *ret*, retractor on the temporal lobe; *ad*, adhesions between the dome of the aneurysm and the tentorial edge. From Fox JL: ref. 20.

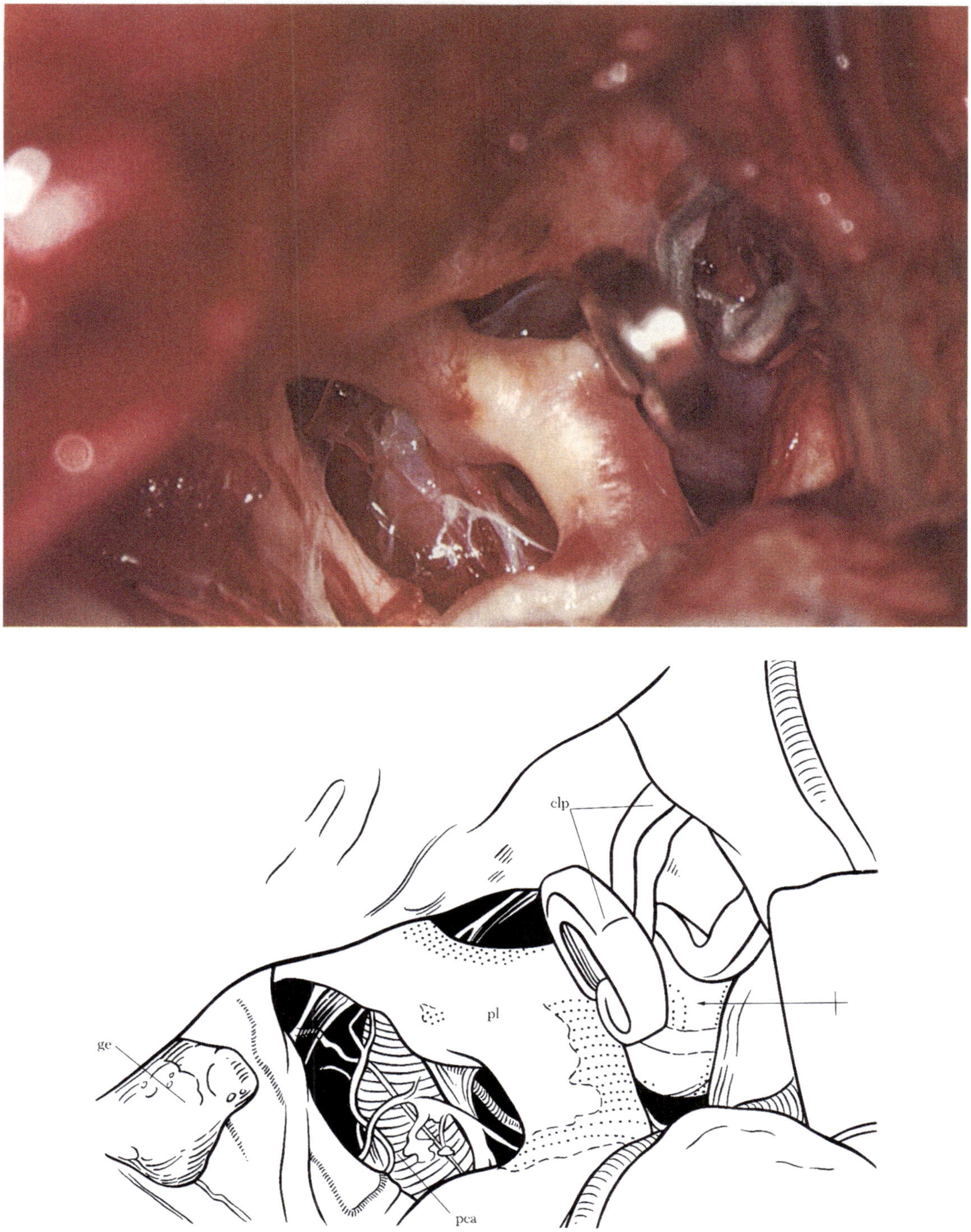

Fig. 36.16. Same case as in Figs. 36.14 and 36.15 after two Yaşargil clips (*clp*) have been placed on neck of aneurysm (*single-crossed arrow*). *pca,* posterior communicating artery (arising on posteroinferior side of the internal carotid artery); *ge,* Gelfoam on optic nerve; *pl,* atherosclerotic plaque in wall of the internal carotid artery; *clp,* shanks of two clips.

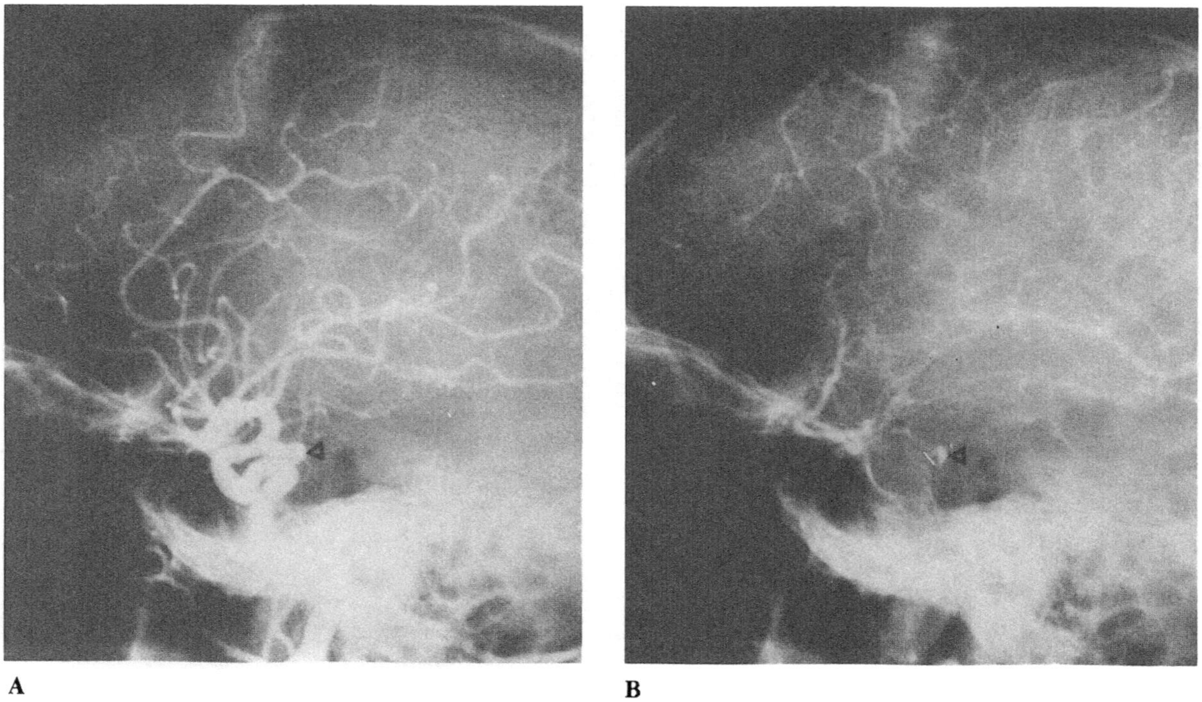

Fig. 36.17. Lateral carotid angiogram of pcaICAA shown in Figs. 36.18 and 36.19. **A** Arterial phase showing aneurysm (*triangle*). **B** Venous phase demonstrating contrast media still in aneurysm (*triangle*) due to slow run-off.

where the opening into the aneurysm once existed. If the clip is set too close to the parent artery, there will be too much stress at the ICA/aneurysm-neck junction. If the clip is set too far from the parent artery, the surgeon can always readjust the clip or apply a second clip as indicated.

The oculomotor nerve (CN-3) is an important nearby structure frequently hidden by the aneurysm. The aneurysm often compresses or is adherent to this nerve between its appearance from under the uncus of the temporal lobe and its exit into the cavernous sinus. These patients often have signs relating to compromise of this nerve (see Chapter 7). The surgeon must employ care so as to avoid injury to CN-3 during temporal lobe retraction, dissection, and clipping. Examples of the surgeon's view of CN-3 are found in Figs. 5.2, 7.4, 34.11, 35.10, 36.8, 36.20, 36.23, 36.40, 36.50, 36.56, 36.57, 36.59, and most of the color photographs in Chapter 38.

Figures 36.17–36.19 exemplify the advantages of shrinking the neck of an ICAA. In this case the relationship of the aneurysm neck to the AChA in Fig. 36.18 was not clear until the neck was narrowed, revealing that the pcaICAA did not involve the origin of the AChA. A slightly curved clip was then applied with its convex side toward the ICA and the PCoA. Additional observations here include Heubner's artery (protected from retractor injury), adhesions between the aneurysm and the temporal lobe as well as the tentorium, the blue-gray Liliequist membrane in the background (Fig. 36.19), and the origin of the PCoA seen only after shrinking of the aneurysm neck (Fig. 36.19).

The Infundibulum

There are occasions where the small aneurysm, usually an incidental aneurysm discovered during surgery (Fig. 36.20), cannot be clipped. We treat these by covering with cotton fibers (Fig. 36.21). The aneurysmal dilatation in Fig. 36.20 may represent (a) the beginning of a pcaICAA (note the dilatation is at a distal angle between the ICA and the PCoA) or (b) a PCoA "infundibulum." There is considerable discussion in the literature regarding whether a PCoA infundibulum is a preaneurysmal phenomenon (6, 8, 13, 14, 17, 18, 23, 24, 28–30, 43–47, 51–55, 58–60, 67).

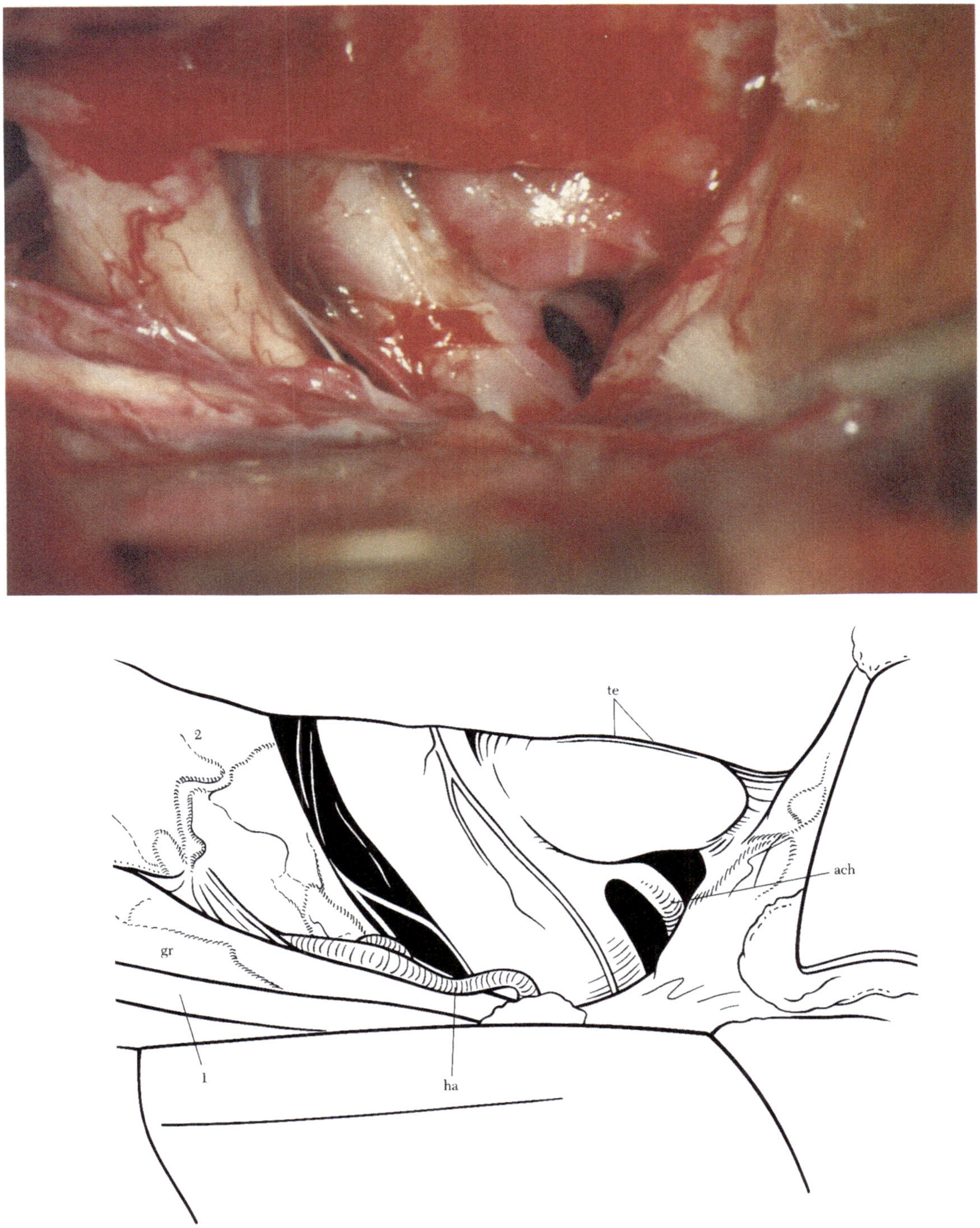

Fig. 36.18. Another right internal carotid artery aneurysm lying under the anterior reflection of the tentorium (*te*). *ach,* anterior choroidal artery touching the aneurysm; *ha,* recurrent artery of Heubner (avoid retractor injury!); *1,* right olfactory tract; *gr,* gyrus rectus; *2,* optic nerve. From Fox JL: ref. 20.

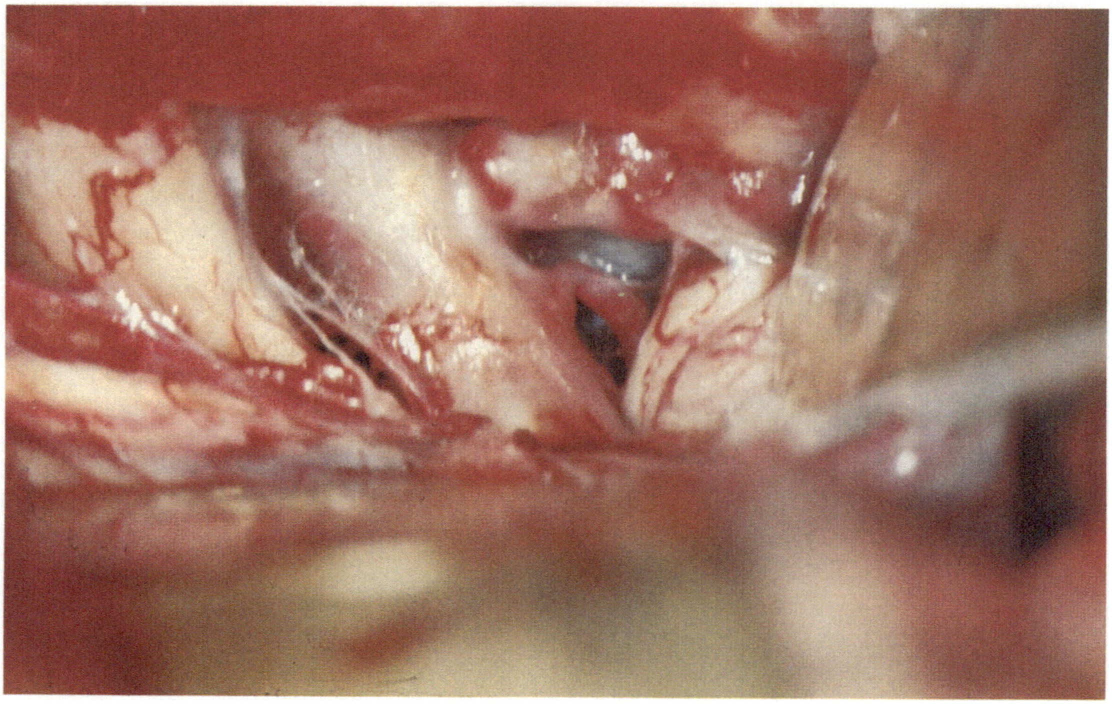

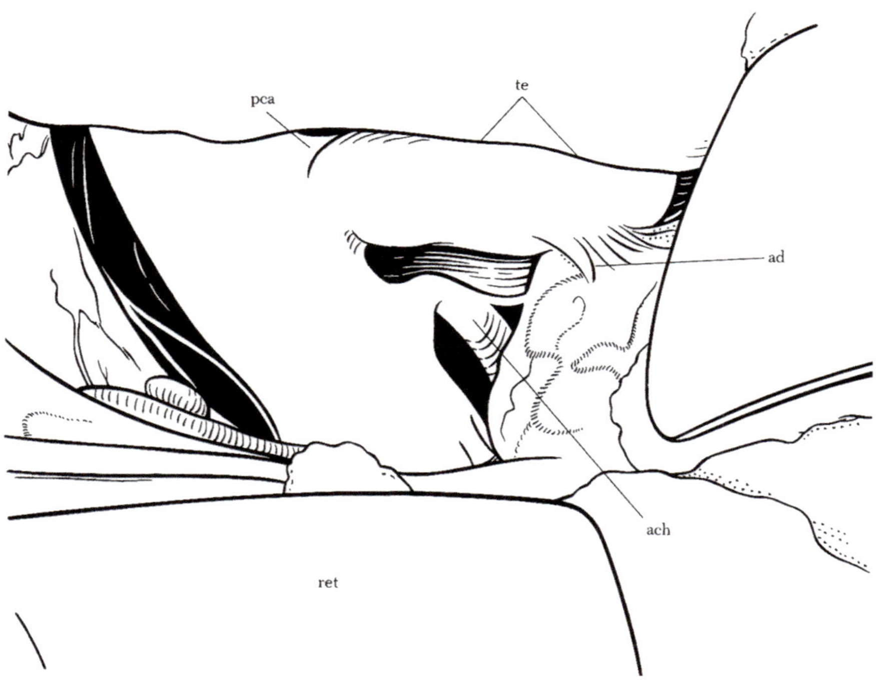

Fig. 36.19. Same aneurysm as in Figs. 36.17 and 36.18 following bipolar electrocoagulation. The anterior choroidal artery (*ach*) is clearly seen entering the crural cistern (64). *ad,* adhesions between the temporal lobe and the aneurysm; *te,* tentorial edge; *pca,* origin of the hidden posterior communicating artery; *ret,* retractor on the frontal lobe. This aneurysm originated at the take-off of the posterior communicating artery. From Fox JL: ref. 20.

The angiographic and autopsy incidence of the PCoA infundibulum (Fig. 36.22) appears to be between 6 and 16% (8,29,45,59,60), and the incidence increases with age. There are case reports of growth of an infundibulum into an aneurysm (13,58,67) and one report of actual subarachnoid hemorrhage from a PCoA infundibulum itself (6). Certainly the thin wall of the infundibulum, or preaneurysmal dilatation, portrayed in Fig. 36.20 strongly suggests that in some cases these can grow into a typical pcaICAA. See Chapter 12 (pp. 379–383) for further discussion.

Anterior Choroidal Artery–Internal Carotid Artery Aneurysms

The surgical approach to an achaICAA is similar to that for a pcaICAA. However, it is even more important here to open the sylvian fissure since the aneurysm will be a bit higher on the ICA.

On the angiogram the aneurysm may appear as a pcaICAA (3). The aneurysm may project laterally into the temporal lobe (Fig. 36.23) or against the tentorial edge or project medially against the optic tract (Fig. 36.24) (15,38,66). Most commonly they point laterally or posterolaterally and arise at the distal angle between the ICA and the AChA. At surgery the aneurysm may obscure the origin of the AChA and its branches. There may be one or two such arteries coursing posteriorly toward the choroid fissure (Figs. 36.8, 36.19, 36.20, and 38.29). An incidental, small achaICAA is seen in Fig. 38.38.

Preservation of the AChA is mandatory. An accessory AChA and/or adjacent anterior thalamoperforators should be looked for and protected. The AChA may project laterally before starting its medial and posterior course, or it may arise on the posterior wall of the ICA. It follows the optic tract and enters the choroid fissure of the temporal lobe (Fig. 36.25).

If the aneurysm points laterally, extreme caution must be taken during any temporal lobe retraction. The achaICAA may be embedded in the brain here. If the aneurysm projects medially it may be adherent to the optic tract, in which case any movement or retraction of the ICA may effect rupture. Occasionally, the surgeon will have to dissect over the top of the ICA bifurcation to get at the posterior wall. The technique of isolation and clipping of the aneurysm is similar to methods already described for other aneurysms.

Aneurysms at the Bifurcation of the Internal Carotid Artery

Aneurysms at the terminal bifurcation of the ICA (Fig. 36.26) are particularly hazardous to treat surgically because of the vital perforating arteries often surrounding and adherent to the aneurysm (11,27,32,50,66). The surgeon must look for and protect (a) Heubner's artery; (b) the medial lenticulostriate arteries from A-1 (see Fig. 34.13); (c) the lateral lenticulostriate arteries from M-1; (d) perforators from the ICA bifurcation passing along the back (hidden) wall of the aneurysm (see Fig. 34.16); (e) anterior thalamoperforators from the ICA and PCoA; and (f) branches of the AChA as well as the AChA itself. They may have to be gently stripped from the wall or neck of the aneurysm before clipping.

In most cases the bICAA projects superiorly or posterosuperiorly (Figs. 36.27 and 36.28) into the anterior perforated substance, which makes exposure particularly difficult. The aneurysm may angle laterally or medially. Rarely they project forward. They tend more often to arise at the ICA/A-1 junction (Fig. 36.29) than at the ICA/M-1 junction.

Surgical Exposure

In these cases of bICAA, the patient's head should be dropped back more than in most aneurysm cases so that, after a wide opening of the sylvian fissure, the axis of the neck of the aneurysm is as perpendicular as possible to the surgeon's line of site (via the angled binocular microscope). An example is illustrated in Figs. 36.30 and 36.31. If the carotid artery is elongated, greater brain retraction is necessary to gain access to the termination of the ICA. Once the neck of the aneurysm is seen (Fig. 36.30), one can either drop the BP during dissection *or* apply a temporary Heifetz clip on the ICA (don't occlude the PCoA, the AChA, or any back-wall perforators!) and *raise* the BP during the occlusion time. In Fig. 36.30 Heubner's artery can be seen crossing the neck of the aneurysm. The next steps involve dissecting the neck and proximal part of the fundus out

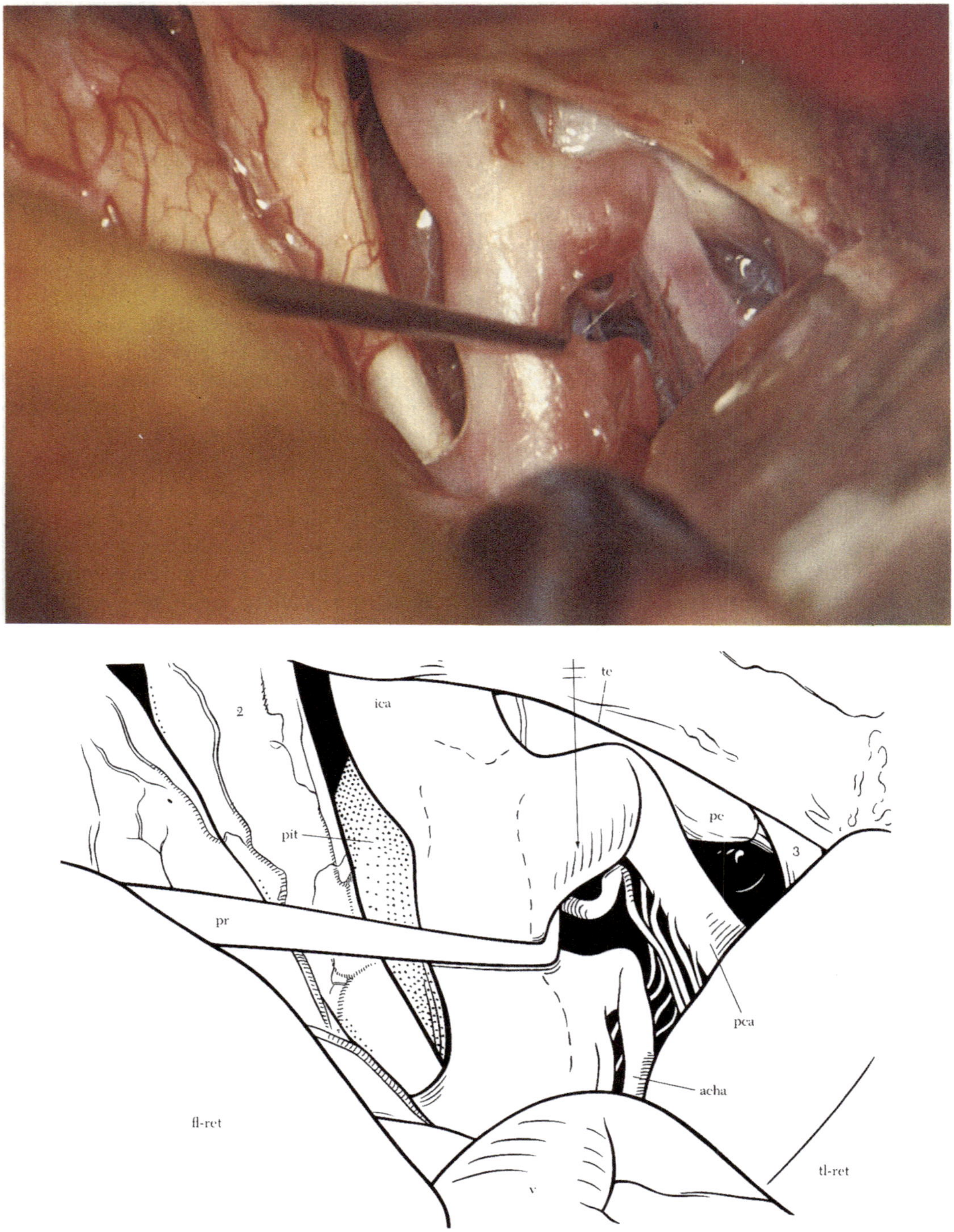

Fig. 36.20. Example of preaneurysmal type of infundibulum (*double-crossed arrow*) of the posterior communicating artery (*pca*). *acha,* anterior choroidal artery; *tl-ret,* temporal lobe retractor; *v,* sylvian vein; *fl-ret,* frontal lobe retractor; *pr,* probe retracting internal carotid artery; *pit,* pituitary stalk; *2,* optic nerve; *ica,* internal carotid artery; *te,* anterior reflection of tentorial edge; *pc,* posterior clinoid; *3,* oculomotor nerve.

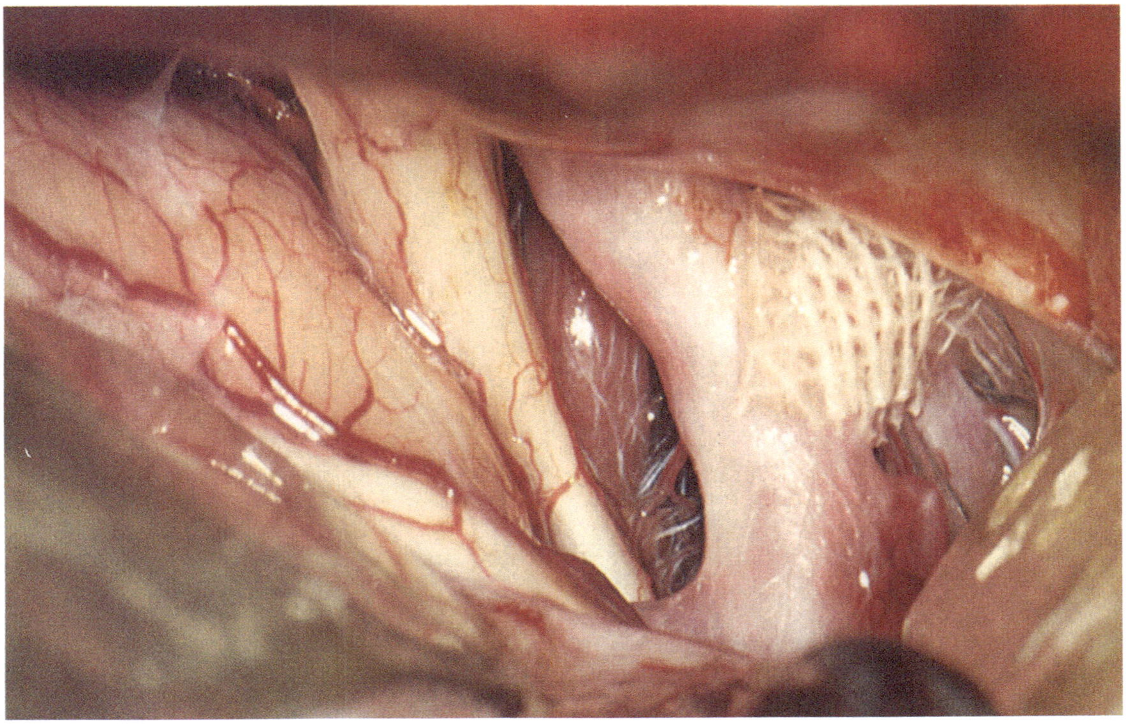

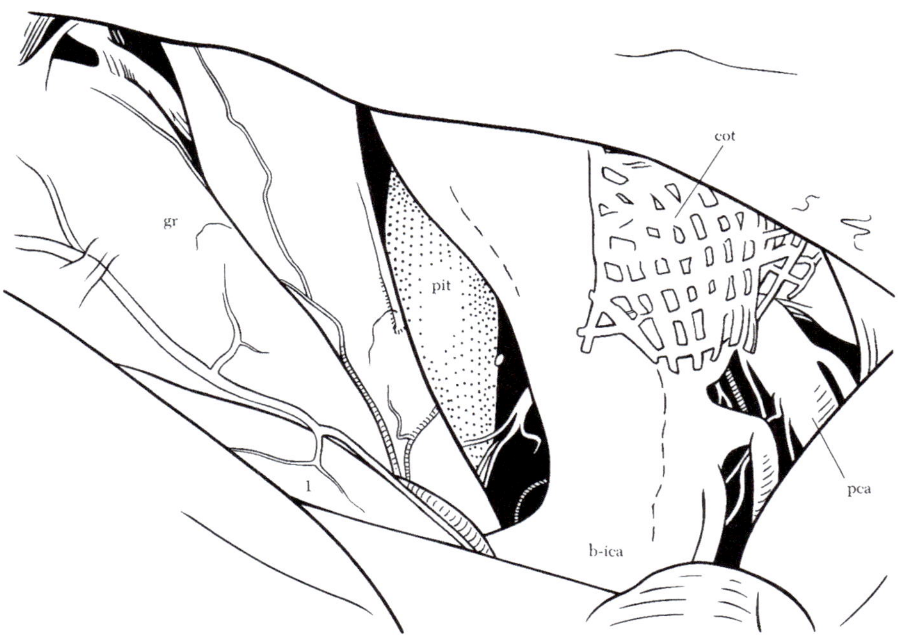

Fig. 36.21. After coating of infundibular region seen in Fig. 36.20. Cotton (*cot*) was used to coat the area. *pca,* posterior communicating artery; *b-ica,* bifurcation of internal carotid artery; *1,* olfactory tract; *gr,* gyrus rectus; *pit,* pituitary stalk.

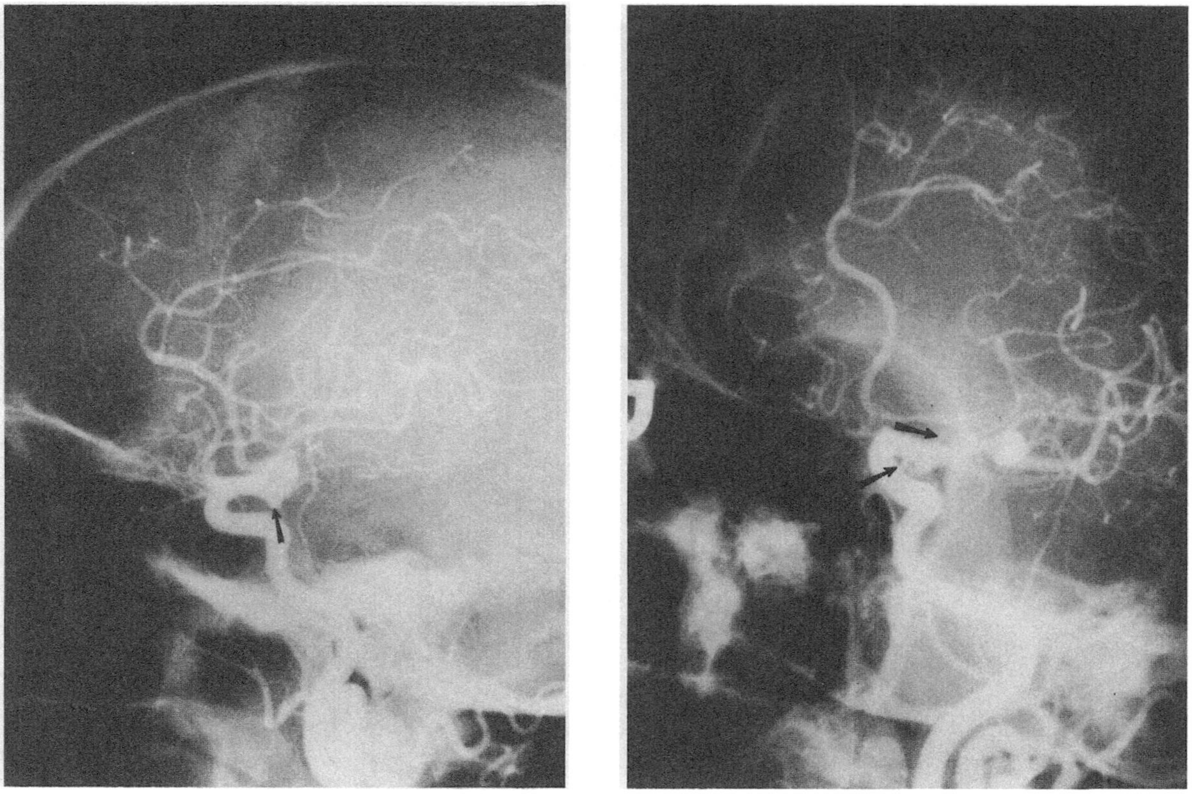

A B

Fig. 36.22. Carotid angiogram illustrating another posterior communicating artery infundibulum. A Lateral view. *Arrow,* infundibulum. B Special oblique view. *Arrows,* posterior communicating artery arising from infundibulum.

of the anterior perforated substance, identifying and clearing away all surrounding perforators, and then applying the clip(s) in such a way as to avoid stress at the aneurysm-neck/parent-artery junction zones. In this case it was necessary to apply the clip with its wings parallel to the A-1 and M-1 arteries (Fig. 36.31).

Figures 36.32 and 36.33 illustrate a giant bICAA compressing the anterior perforated substance of the frontal lobe. This case was particularly difficult due to the fact that, as the aneurysm expanded (see Fig. 34.27), it incorporated M-1 in its expanding neck. In addition, the anterior choroidal artery had its origin at the ICA/aneurysm junction. After isolating the entire aneurysm, a long Drake clip was used to collapse the center of the dome of the aneurysm. Then two McFadden clips and three Yaşargil clips were applied in order to approximate the aneurysm walls of variable thickness while permitting circulation into M-1, A-1, perforators, and the AChA. As is often true of large aneurysms, the greater thickness of the opposing walls at one end of the clip-blades holds the clip-blades open enough so that blood can continue to enter the aneurysm at the other end of the clip-blades where the opposing walls are thinner. Hence the frequent necessity to use multiple, accurately placed clips for effective obliteration of the aneurysm sac. The angiogram on the eighth postoperative day (Fig. 36.32D) confirmed satisfactory clip placement and demonstrated a small intravascular clot (?) near the bifurcation of the ICA. This was treated prophylactically using temporary heparin/Coumadin therapy with an excellent result.

Another technical problem with large aneurysms is the common presence of a prominent atherosclerotic plaque and/or thrombus formation within the aneurysm itself (Fig. 36.34). Temporary trapping of the parent vessels with the systolic blood pressure *elevated* to about 160–180 mmHg, opening the wall of the aneurysm, removal of the clot or plaque, and final

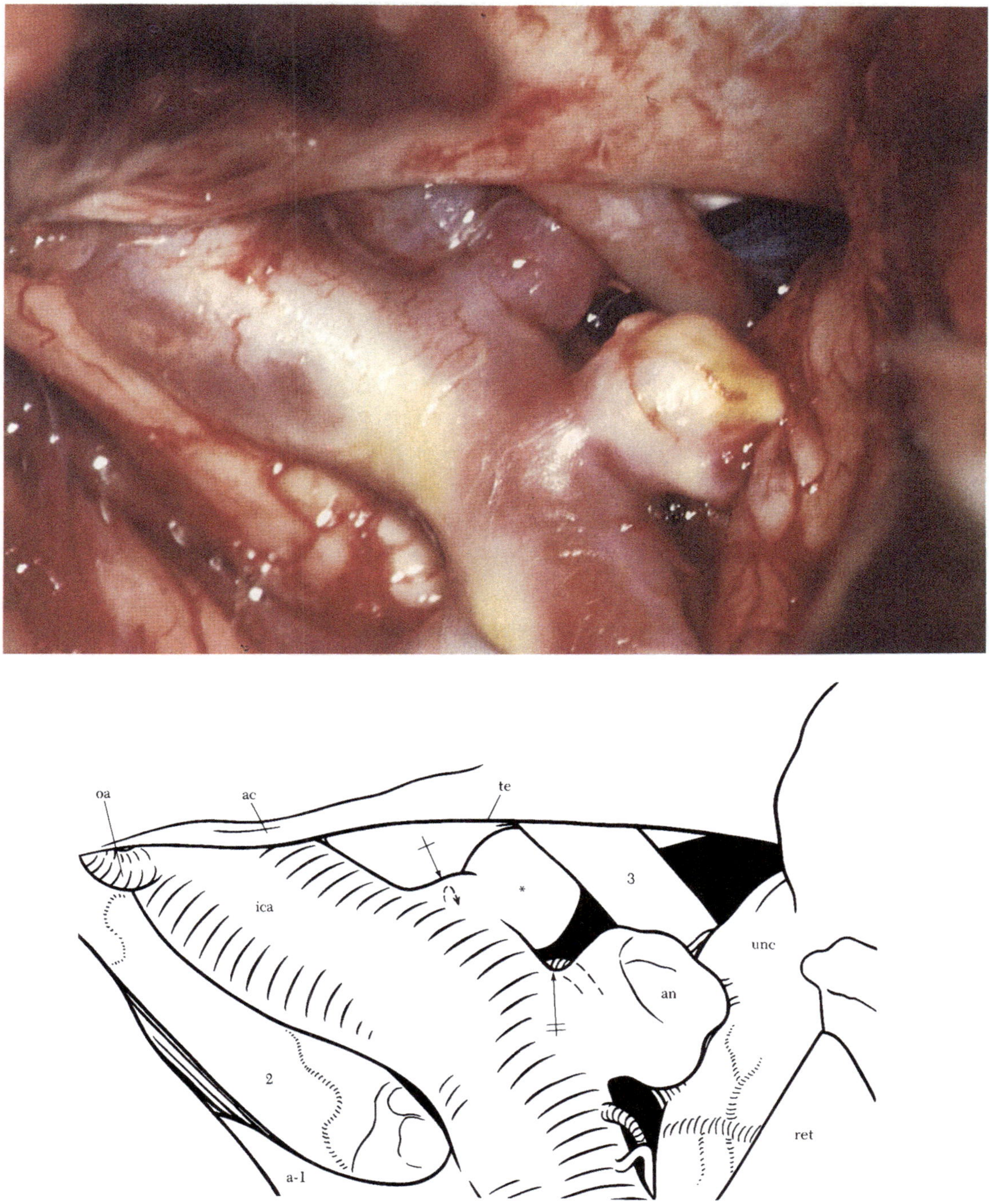

Fig. 36.23. Example of aneurysm (*an*) of the ICA (*ica*) at the take-off (*double-crossed arrow*) of the anterior choroidal artery (i.e., an achaICAA). The dome of this atherosclerotic aneurysm is adherent to the uncus (*unc*) of the temporal lobe. There is a second aneurysm (*) at the take-off (*single-crossed arrow*) of the hidden posterior communicating artery. *oa,* ophthalmic artery origin; *ac,* anterior clinoid process; *te,* edge of tentorium; *3,* oculomotor nerve; *ret,* temporal lobe retractor; *a-1,* A-1 artery; *2,* optic nerve.

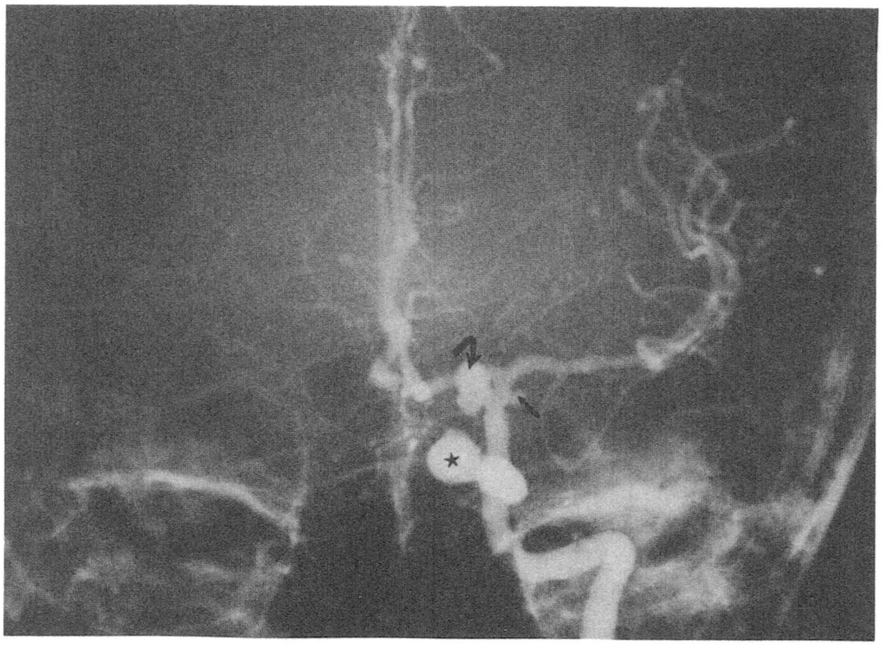

A

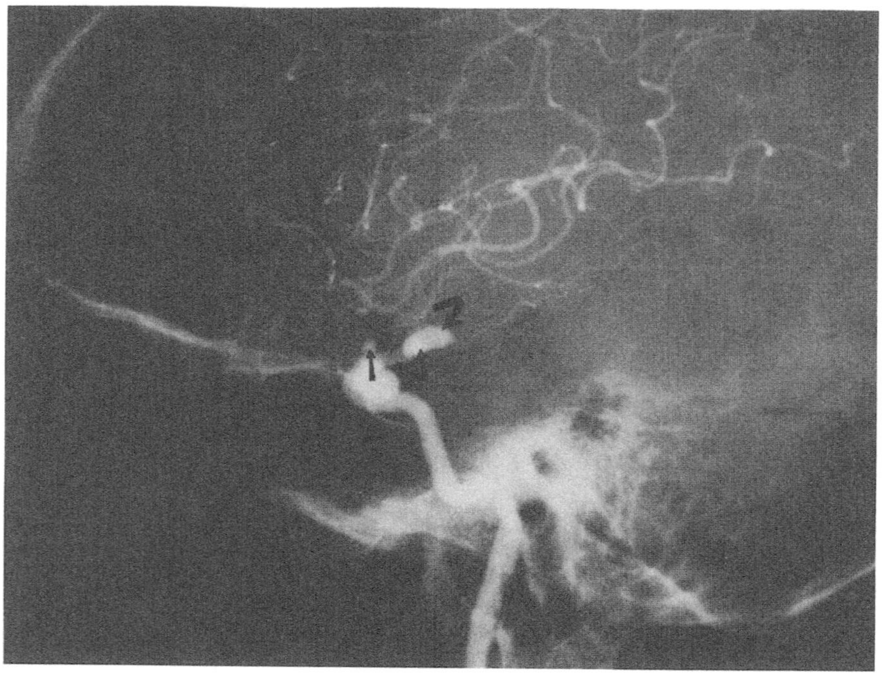

B

Fig. 36.24. A Frontal view of a left carotid angiogram demonstrating multiple aneurysms. *Curved arrow,* medially projecting achaICAA (ruptured); *straight arrow,* laterally projecting achaICAA; *star,* csICAA. **B** Lateral angiographic view of same case. *Curved arrow,* large (medial) achaICAA; *posterior straight arrow,* superimposed smaller (lateral) achaICAA; *anterior straight arrow,* small oaICAA (arrow crosses the csICAA). This 52-year-old woman also had a right oaICAA (see Figs. 36.39 and 36.40). All aneurysms except the left csICAA and left oaICAA were successfully clipped. The latter incidental aneurysm was hidden by the anterior clinoid process.

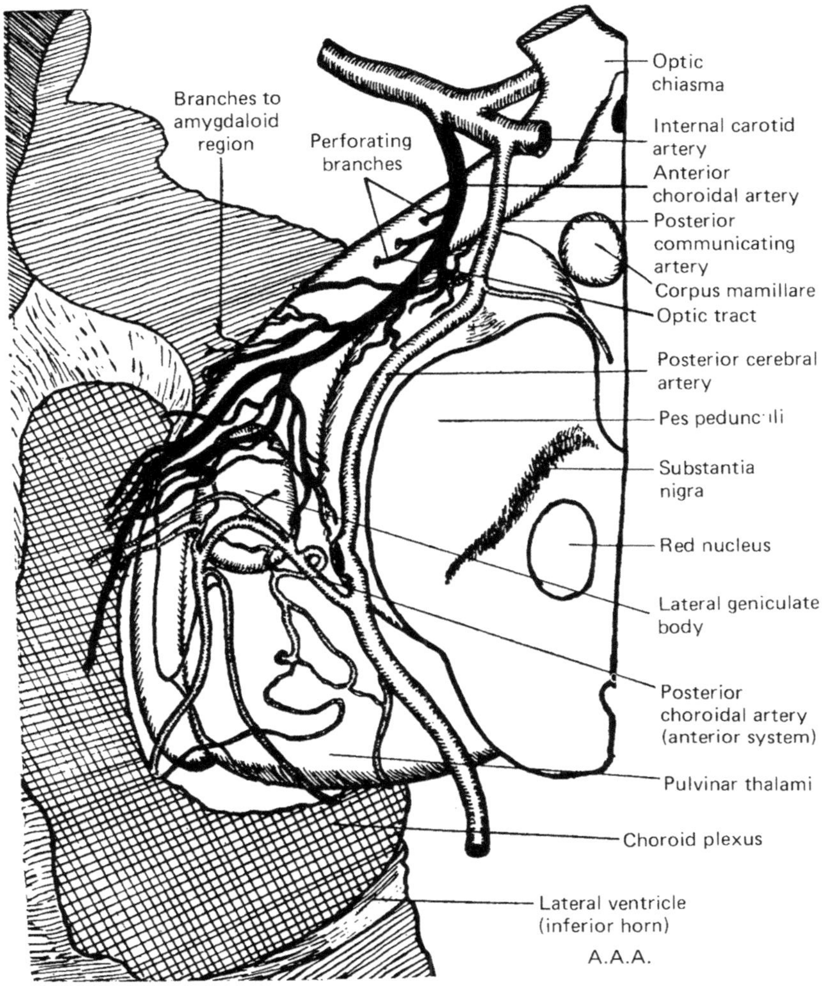

Fig. 36.25. Diagram of the anterior choroidal artery (in black) and environs. From Abbie AA: ref. 1.

clipping or excision and oversewing of the wall (see Chapter 31) may resolve the problem. Additional methods of handling these aneurysms are discussed in Chapter 31.

Ophthalmic Artery–Internal Carotid Artery Aneurysms

These aneurysms (oaICAA) arise at the distal angle between the ophthalmic artery and the internal carotid artery as the latter exits from the cavernous sinus. They are in close relation to the anterior clinoid process, which may partially or completely obstruct the surgeon's view of the aneurysm. The types of projection of the oaICAA can be classified into four basic patterns (3,4,16,25,26,33,37,42,49,56,63): (a) supraoptic type projecting superomedially above optic nerve (most common; see Figs. 36.35A and 36.36 [*2*]); (b) suboptic type projecting medially under optic nerve (Fig. 36.35B and 36.36 [*1*]); (c) supraclinoid type projecting forward over anterior clinoid process (Figs. 36.35C and 36.36 [*3*]); and (d) ventral, or paraclinoid, type projecting inferiorly from the underside of the optic nerve opposite the ophthalmic artery take-off (Fig. 36.37).

In the vast majority of cases the aneurysm arises from the medial or superomedial wall of the ICA. Nutik (37) and Yaşargil (62) have separated those arising from the inferior wall (pattern d above) and called them "paraclinoid," or "ventral," internal carotid artery aneurysms (vICAA). Whether these should be excluded from the oaICAA group can be debated. They do originate away from the common "distal angle" site, project downward (sometimes into the cavernous sinus), have a broad neck, and require a somewhat different surgical approach. Some of the "infraclinoid"

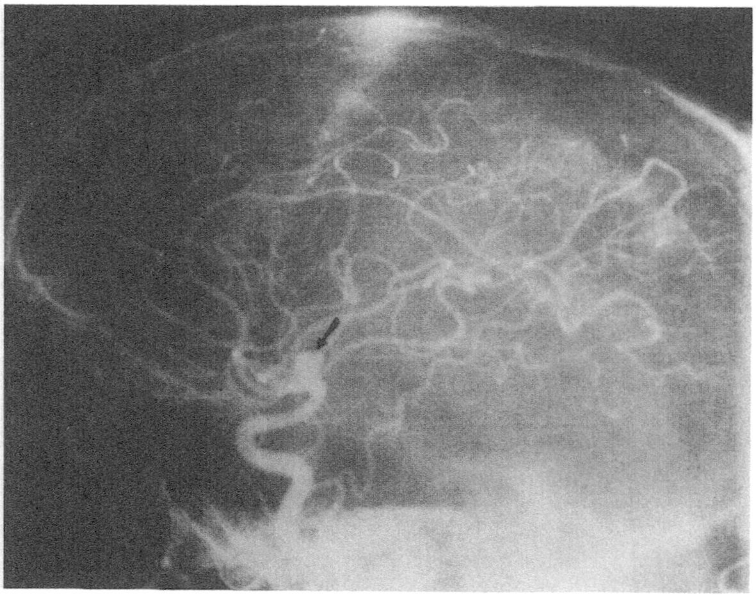

A

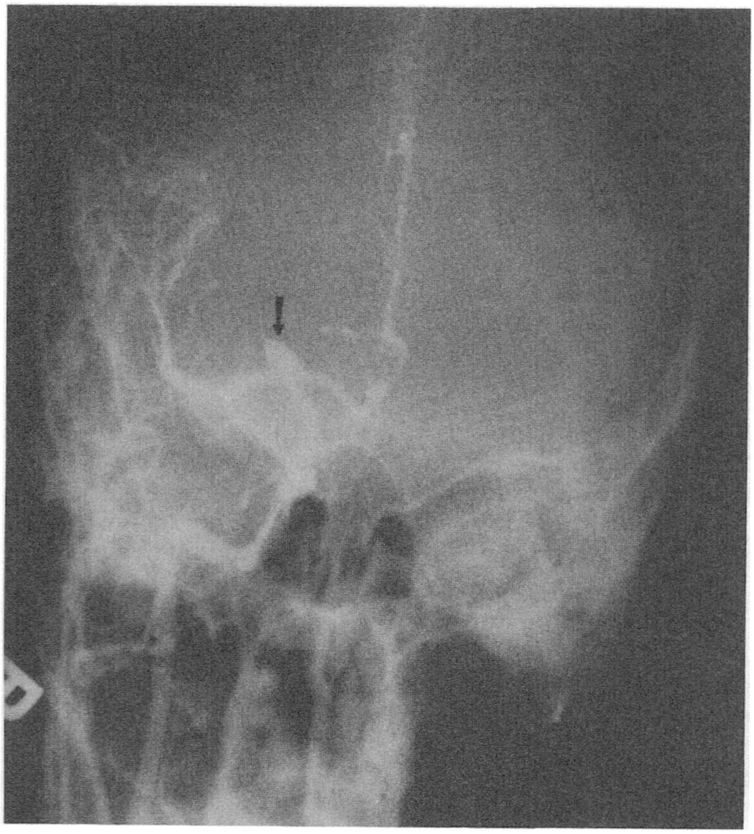

B

Fig. 36.26. A Lateral angiogram demonstrating a bICAA (*arrow*) projecting superiorly into the anterior perforated substance. **B** Frontal view, same case. **C** Oblique view, same case. The film is turned upside down to show the aneurysm and environs as the surgeon sees them. In this case, the arrow points to the right A-1/aneurysm junction.

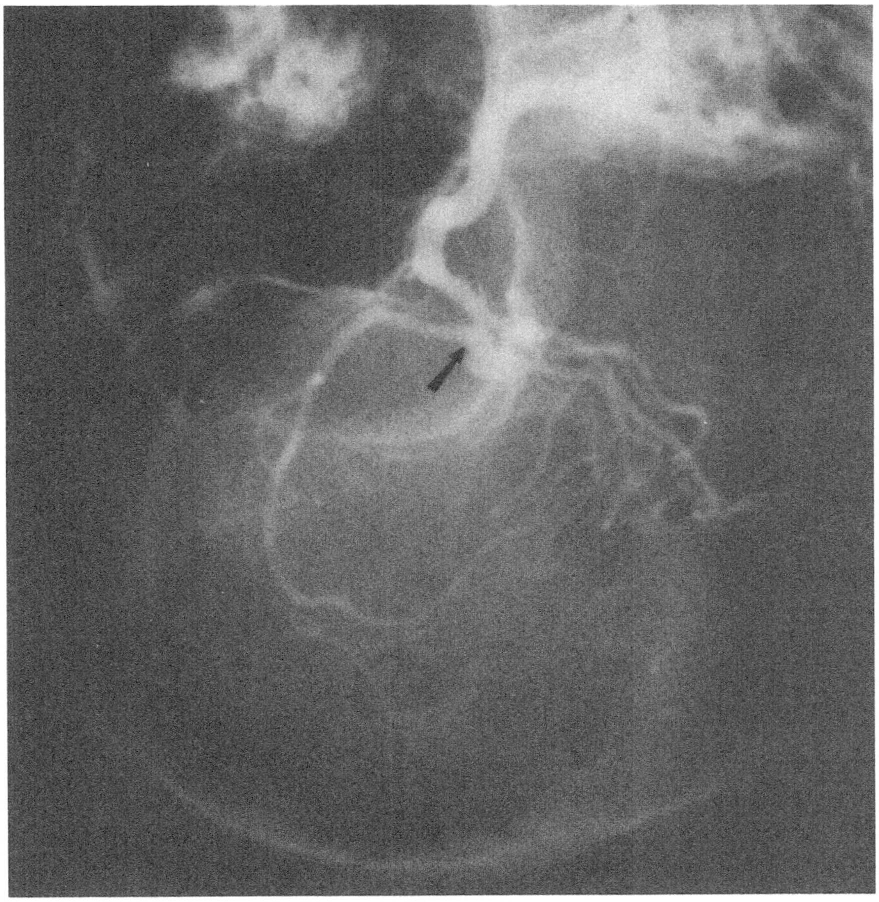

Fig. 36.26C

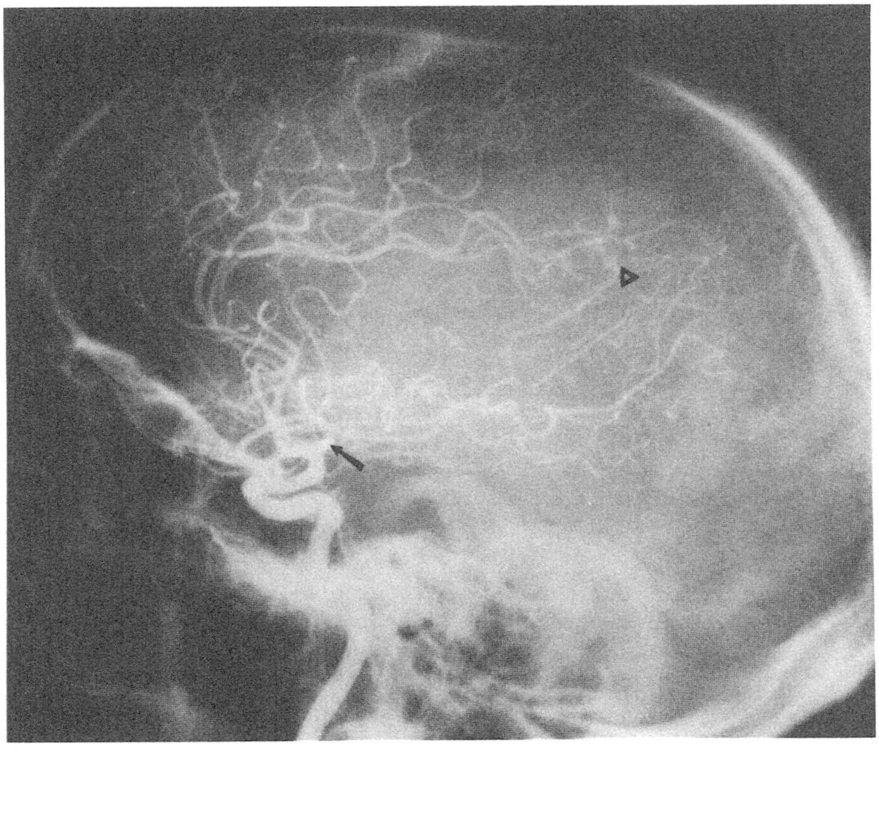

Fig. 36.27. Lateral angiogram revealing incidental bICAA (*arrow*) in patient with metastatic carcinoma to the brain (*triangle*). The aneurysm points posterosuperiorly.

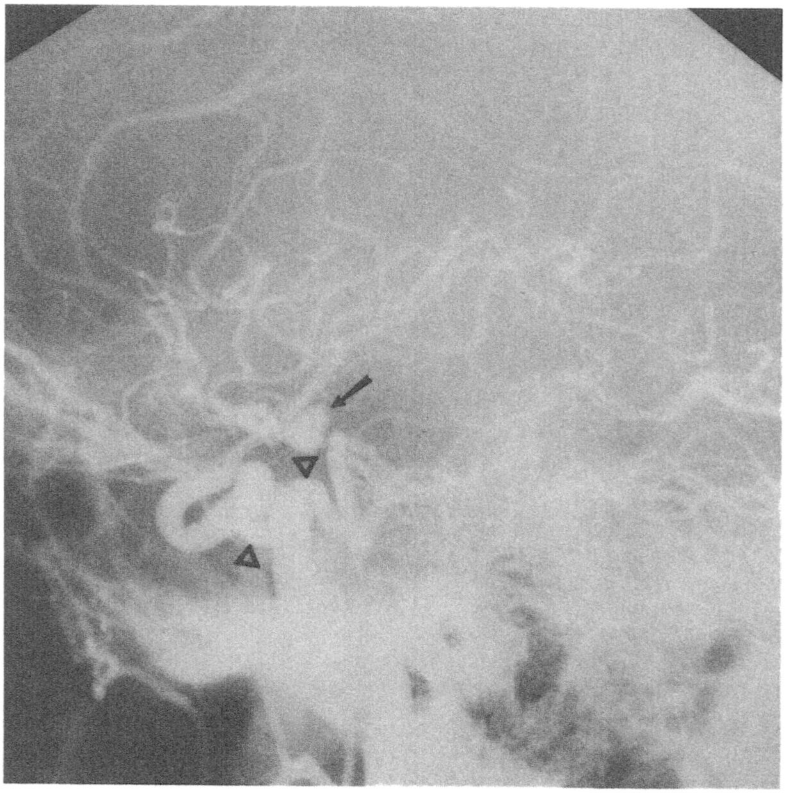

A

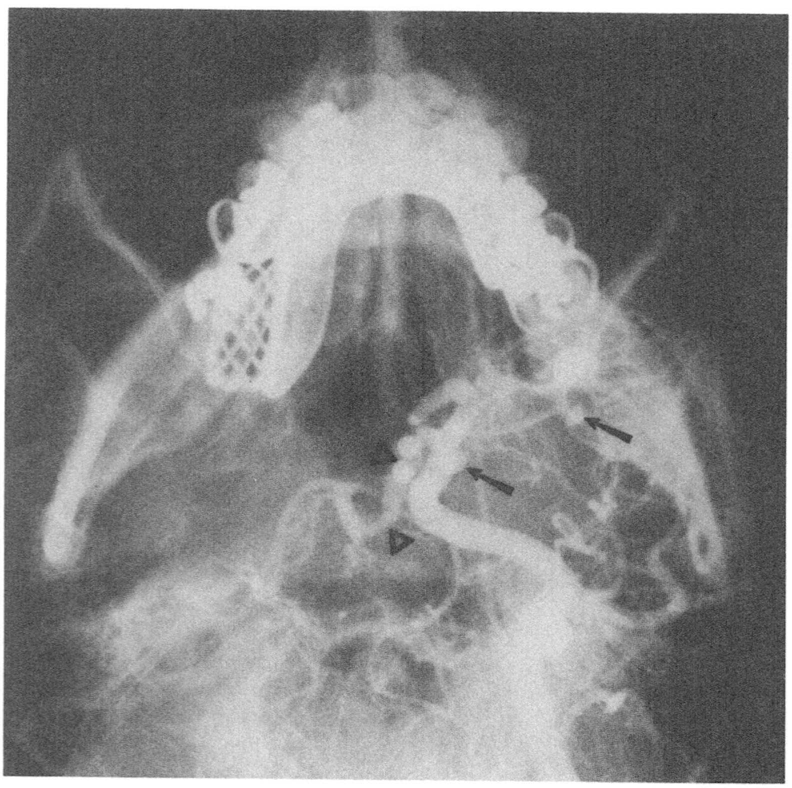

B

Fig. 36.28. **A** Lateral angiogram of a 52-year-old woman with SAH from a left backward-projecting bICAA (*arrow*). She also had bilateral MCAA. All were successfully clipped. Note primitive trigeminal artery (*triangles*). The PCoA was absent but the AChA was present at surgery. **B** Basal view of same case. *Medial arrow*, bICAA; *lateral arrow*, MCAA; *triangles*, primitive trigeminal artery.

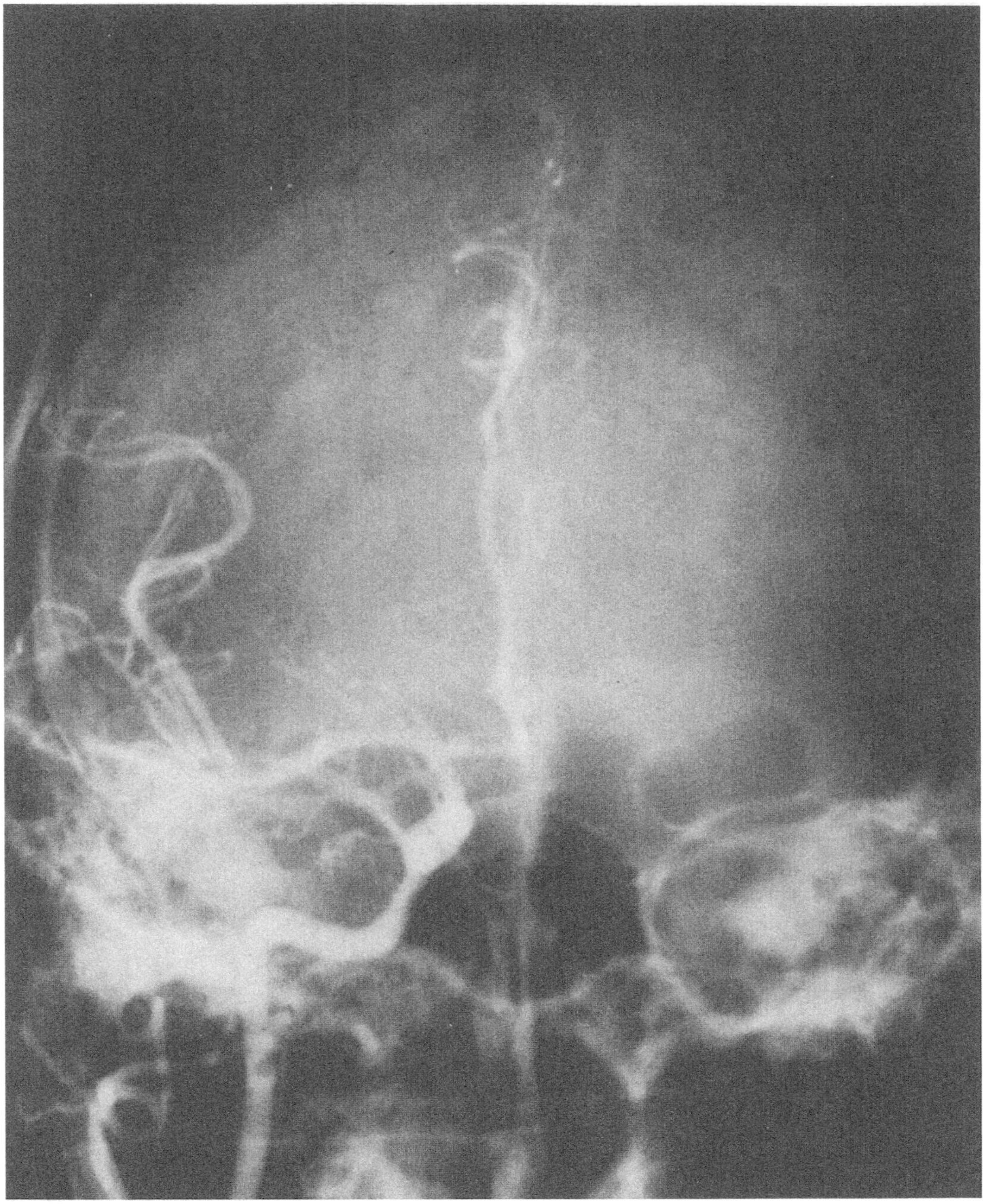

Fig. 36.29. Right carotid angiogram, frontal view, portraying a small aneurysm arising at the ICA/A-1 junction.

or "cavernous sinus" ICAA (ic/csICAA) described in the older literature may have actually been vICAA, or ventrally projecting oaICAA, which usually present with signs of SAH rather than signs of a carotid-cavernous fistula.

On lateral angiograms Punt (44) used a line drawn 1 mm proximal to the take-off of the OA to define the dura of the cavernous sinus (i.e., ICAA below this line were said to lie in the cavernous sinus and so are called csICAA). He concluded that this is a better landmark than the anterior clinoid process since use of the latter landmark would give the false impression that all of the ICA below the anterior clinoid process lies within the cavernous sinus.

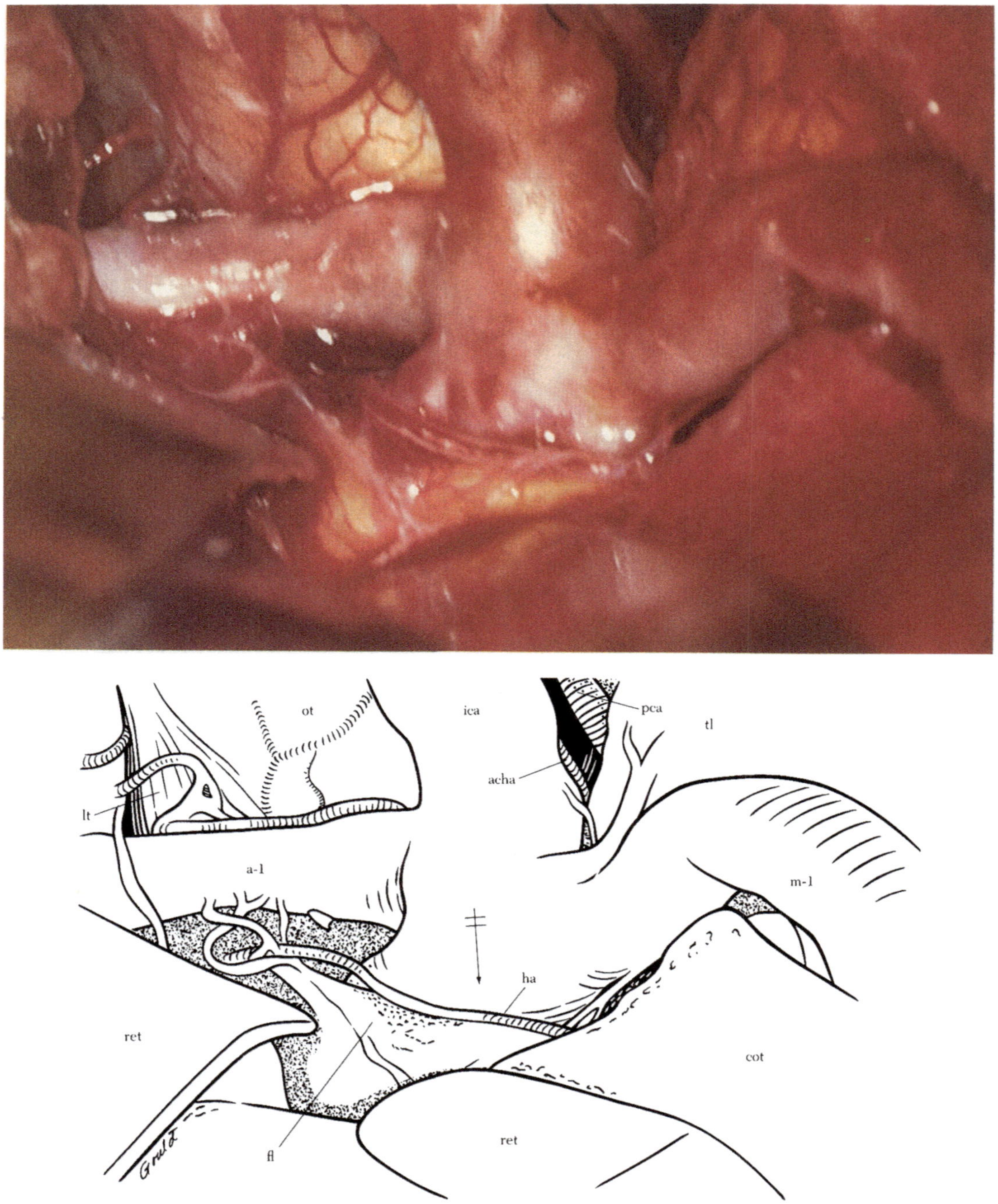

Fig. 36.30. Surgical exposure of an aneurysm at the bifurcation of the internal carotid artery. At this point only the broad neck (*double-crossed arrow*) and an adherent Heubner's artery (*ha*) are exposed. *cot,* cotton strip; *ret,* frontal lobe retractors; *fl,* portion of frontal lobe encasing aneurysm; *a-1,* A-1 artery; *lt,* lamina terminalis; *ot,* optic tract; *ica,* right internal carotid artery; *pca,* posterior communicating artery; *acha,* anterior choroidal artery; *tl,* temporal lobe; *m-1,* M-1 artery.

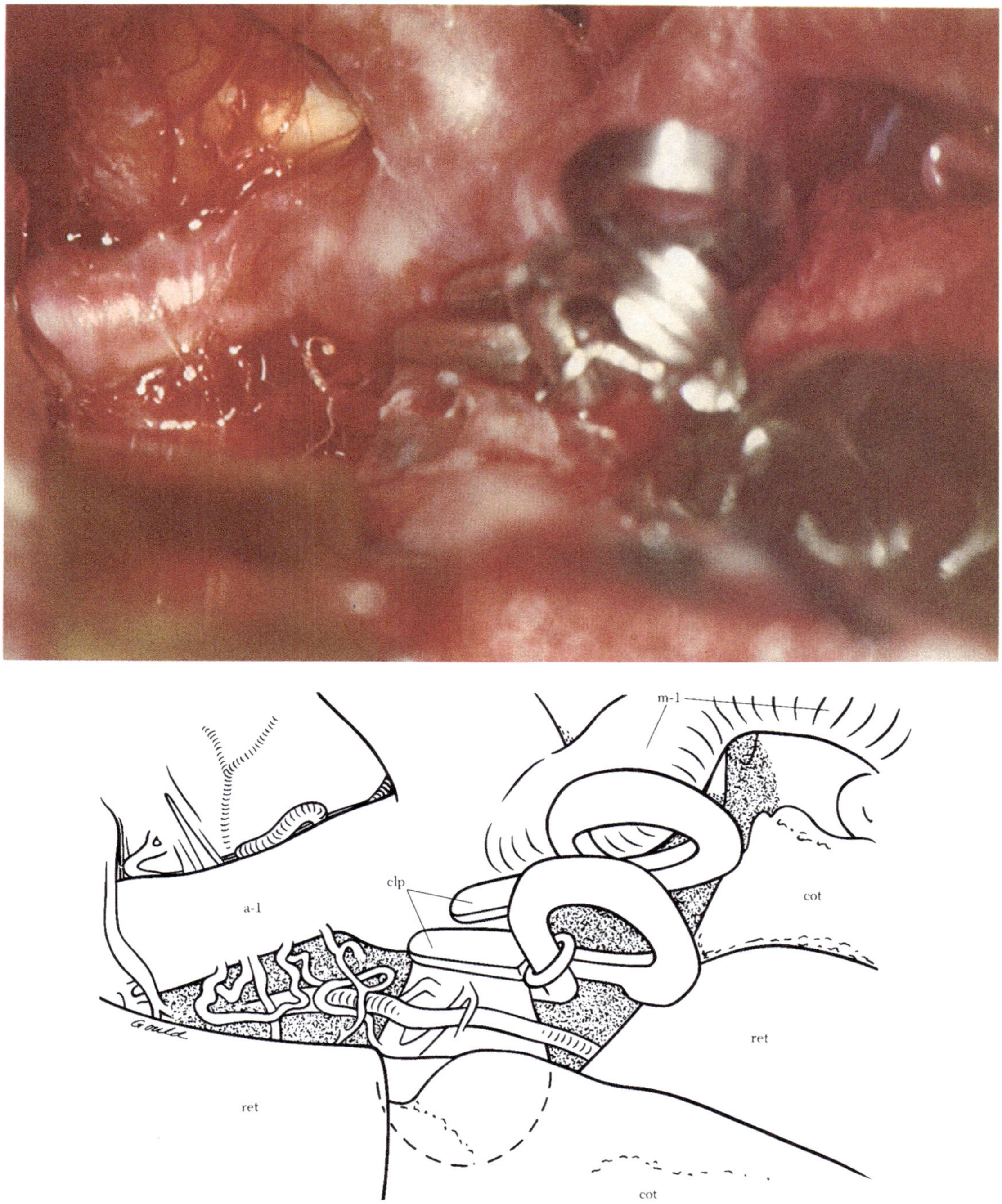

Fig. 36.31. Same case as in Fig. 36.30 after application of two Yaşargil clips on the neck of the aneurysm. Note the wings of the clips (*clp*) are applied parallel to A-1 (*a-1*) and M-1 (*m-1*) in this case (see text). *cot*, cotton strip; *ret*, frontal lobe retractors (the shanks of the clips are reflected from the laterally placed retractor blade); *dotted lines*, hidden portion of aneurysm.

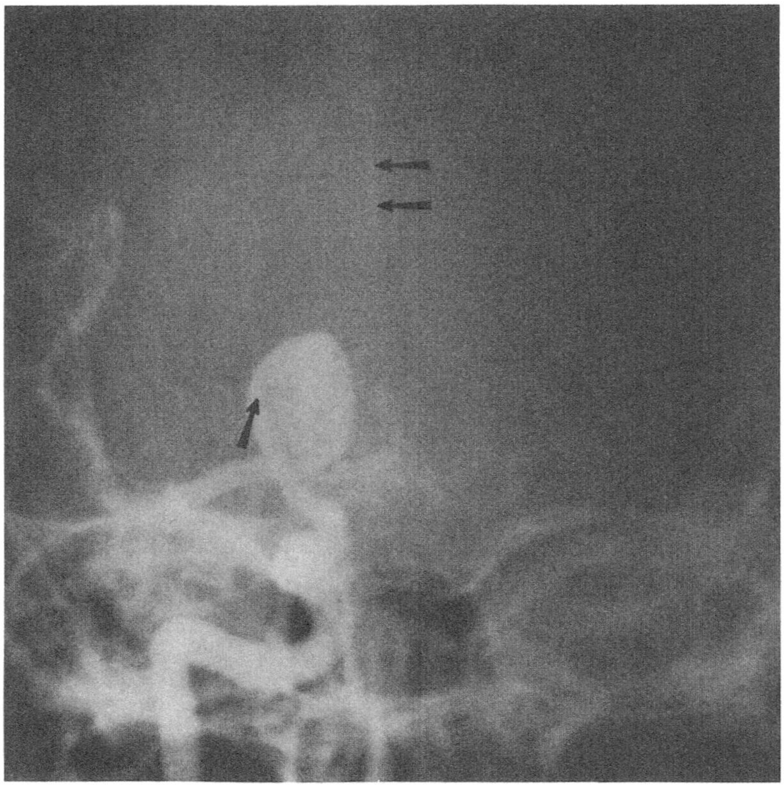

A

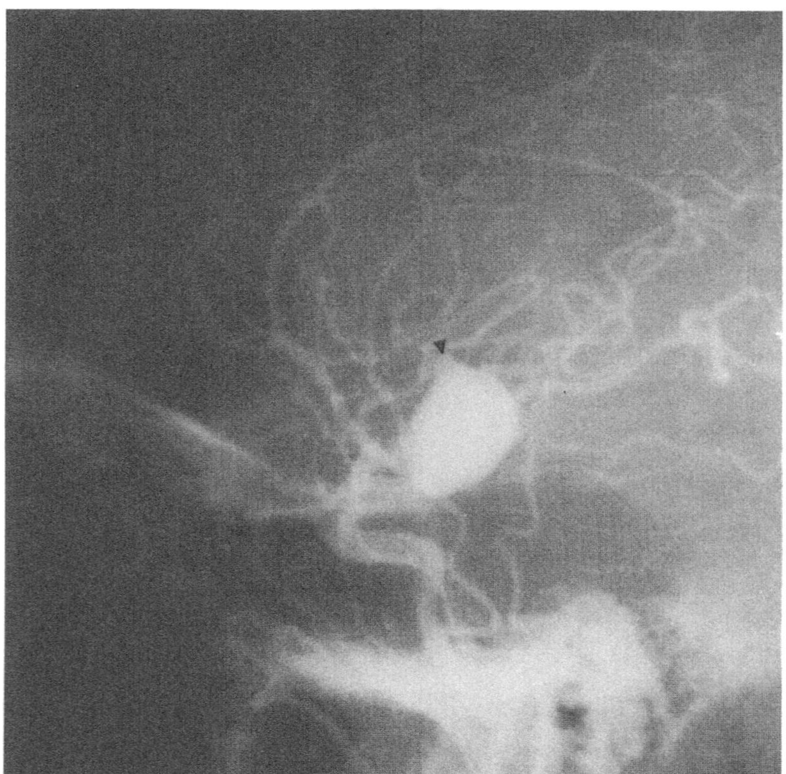

B

Fig. 36.32. Angiogram of giant internal carotid artery aneurysm arising at the ICA bifurcation. The patient was a 33-year-old man who had a subarachnoid bleed from this aneurysm. Although the aneurysm was on the left, the films have been reversed to match the surgical anatomy seen in Fig. 36.33. The patient also had a smaller bICAA on the opposite (right) side. Both were treated successfully by clipping. **A** Frontal view. *Single arrow,* flow of contrast media in aneurysm; *double arrows,* faintly filling anterior cerebral artery. **B** Lateral view. *Arrowhead,* saccule on aneurysm. Note aneurysm projects posterosuperiorly. **C** Upside-down oblique view as the surgeon sees the aneurysm at operation. *Triangle,* saccule on aneurysm. **D** Frontal view. Six aneurysm clips were used to collapse aneurysm effectively without compromising A-1 or M-1 circulation. *Single arrow,* probable focal spasm or intraluminal ICA clot on medial wall; *double arrows,* anterior cerebral artery. The patient returned to his vocation.

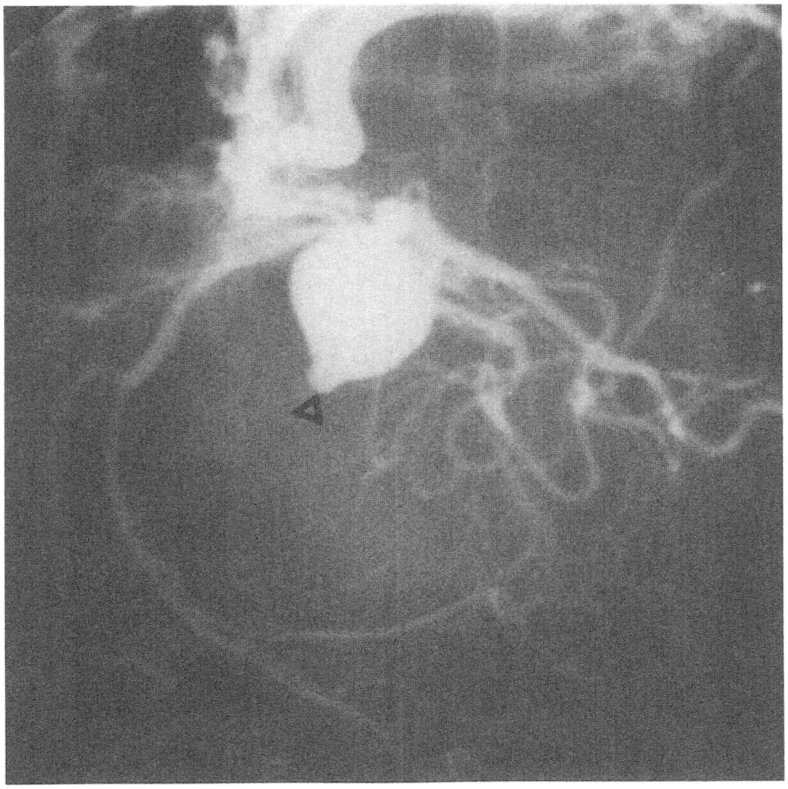

C

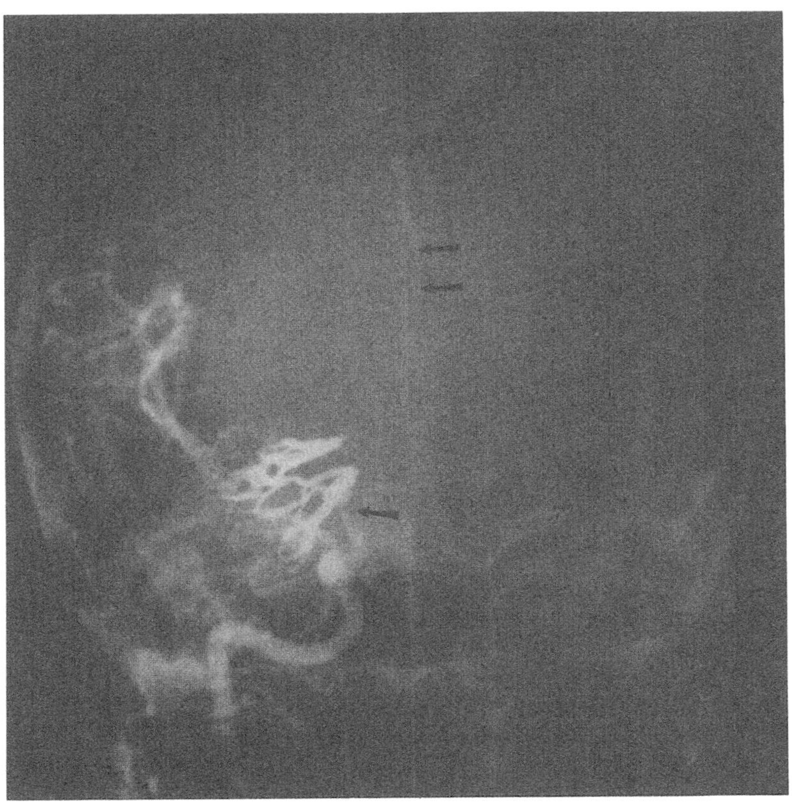

D

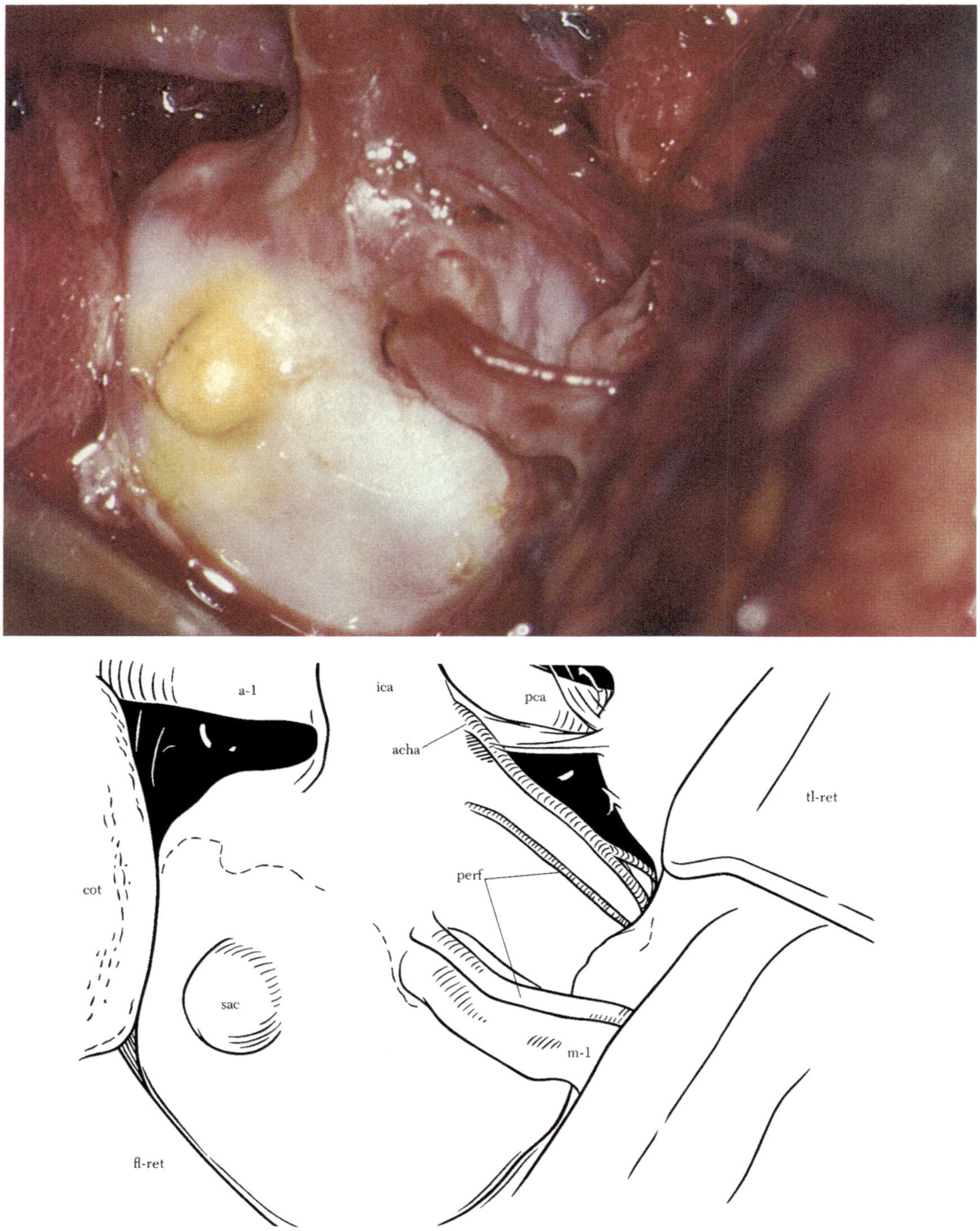

Fig. 36.33. Operative view of bICAA aneurysm shown in Fig. 36.32. Note the aneurysm has expanded to the point where M-1 (*m-1*) and some perforators (*perf*) have been incorporated in the neck of this giant aneurysm. *fl-ret,* frontal lobe retractor; *sac,* atherosclerotic saccule on dome of aneurysm; *cot,* cotton strip; *a-1,* A-1 artery; *ica,* termination of internal carotid artery; *pca,* posterior communicating artery; *acha,* anterior choroidal artery; *tl-ret,* temporal lobe retractor. (Viewed as if operated on right side).

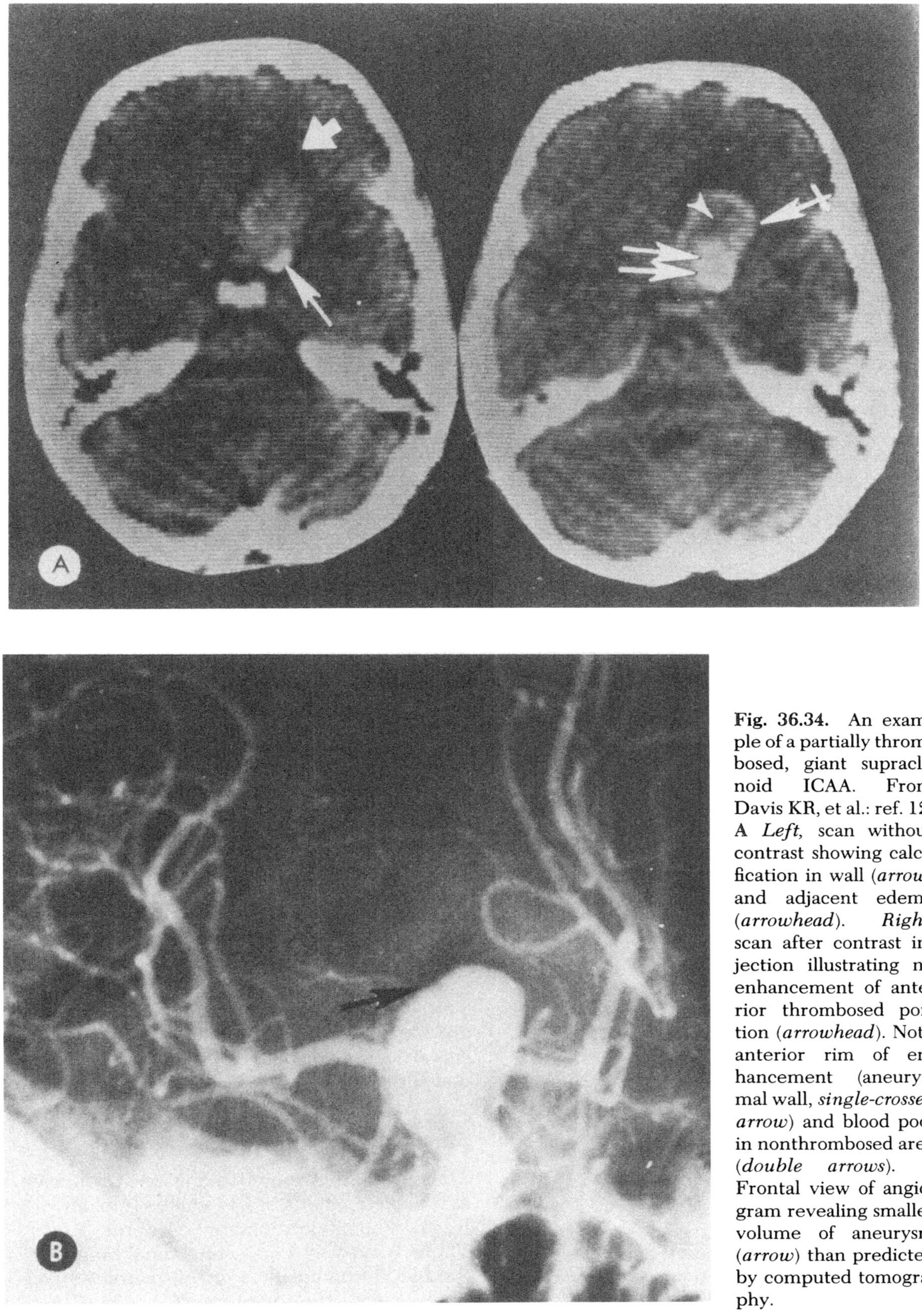

Fig. 36.34. An example of a partially thrombosed, giant supraclinoid ICAA. From Davis KR, et al.: ref. 12. A *Left,* scan without contrast showing calcification in wall (*arrow*) and adjacent edema (*arrowhead*). *Right,* scan after contrast injection illustrating no enhancement of anterior thrombosed portion (*arrowhead*). Note anterior rim of enhancement (aneurysmal wall, *single-crossed arrow*) and blood pool in nonthrombosed area (*double arrows*). **B** Frontal view of angiogram revealing smaller volume of aneurysm (*arrow*) than predicted by computed tomography.

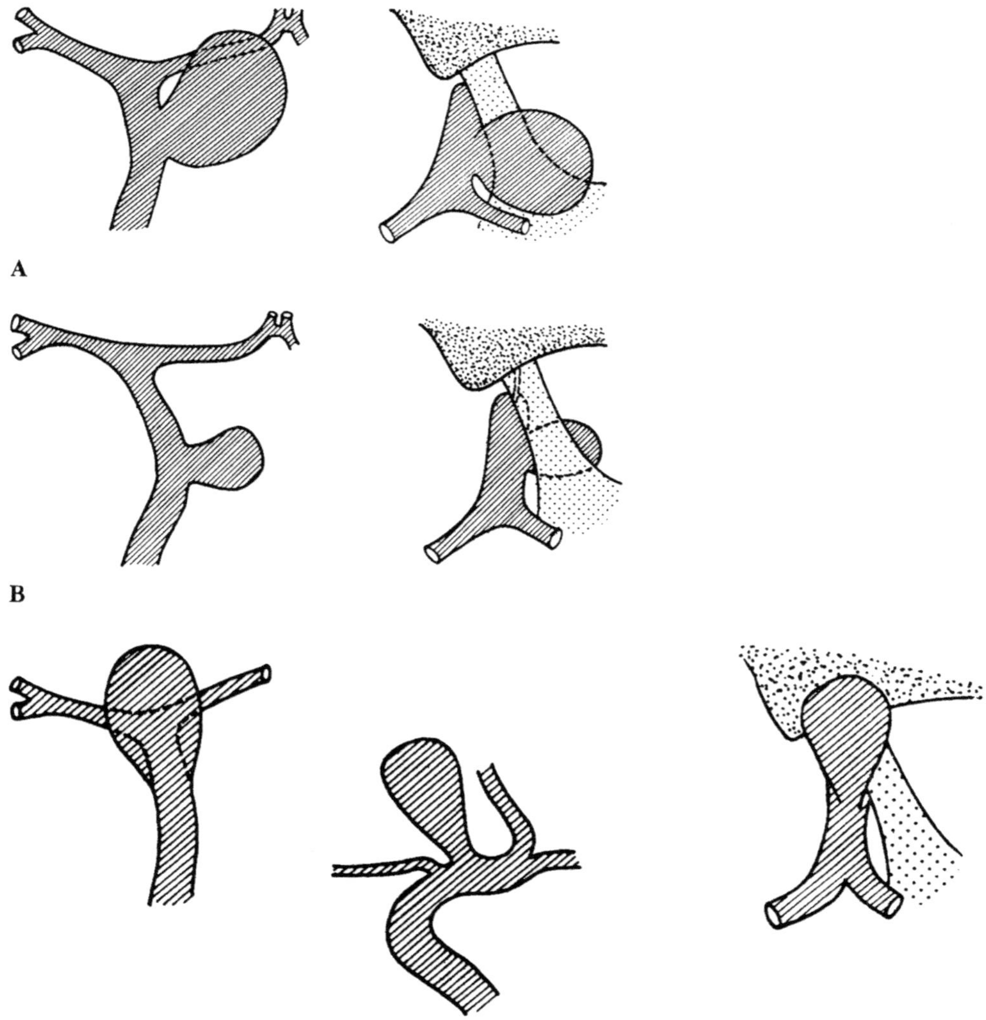

Fig. 36.35. Diagrams of various types of left oaICAA. **A** Supraoptic, projecting superomedially above optic nerve and chiasm. **B** Suboptic, projecting medially below optic nerve and chiasm. **C** Supraclinoid, projecting forward over anterior clinoid process. From Thurel C. et al.: ref. 56.

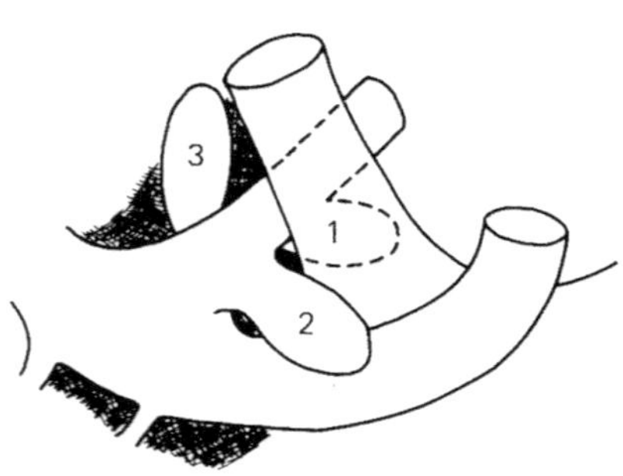

Fig. 36.36. Diagram of various types of left oaICAA. *1*, suboptic; *2*, supraoptic; *3*, supraclinoid. From Kothandaram P, et al.: ref. 33.

This, of course, is not always the case, and there are some oaICAA and so-called vICAA which can arise, in part, between the cavernous sinus and the anterior clinoid region.

Surgical Exposure

The small, "innocuous-looking" oaICAA, such as is depicted in Fig. 36.38, can be fraught with hazard should intraoperative rupture occur. There is no way to gain proximal control of the ICA intracranially. For this reason we routinely expose the ipsilateral ICA and ECA in

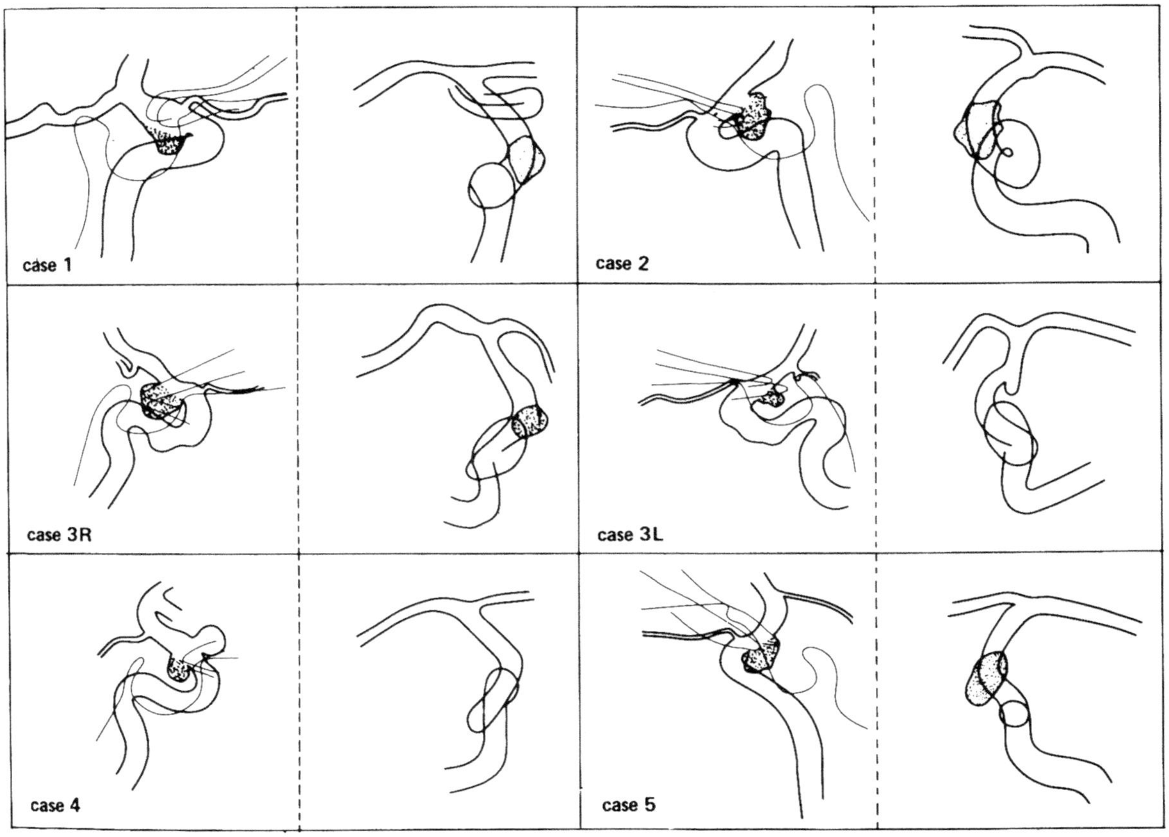

Fig. 36.37. Diagrams of six cases of "paraclinoid," or "ventral," internal carotid artery aneurysms (vICAA). Some consider this a variant of the oaICAA (see text), but they arise on the ICA wall opposite from the OA take-off. From Nutik S: ref. 37.

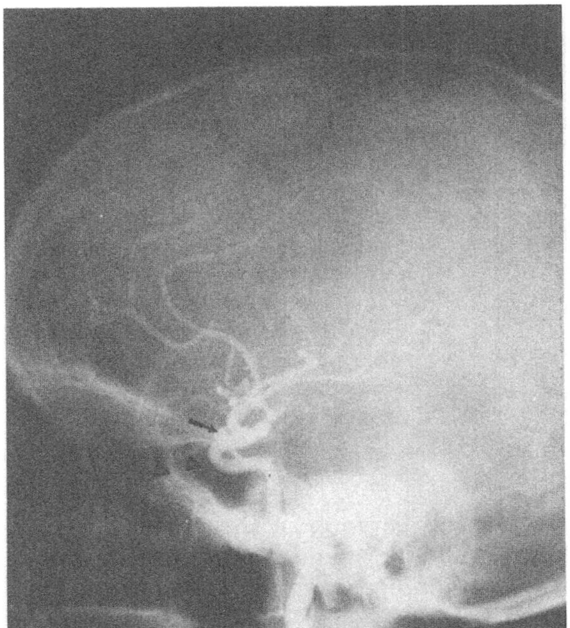

Fig. 36.38. Lateral angiogram revealing a small oaICAA (*arrow*) projecting superiorly just distal to the take-off of the ophthalmic artery (*triangles*).

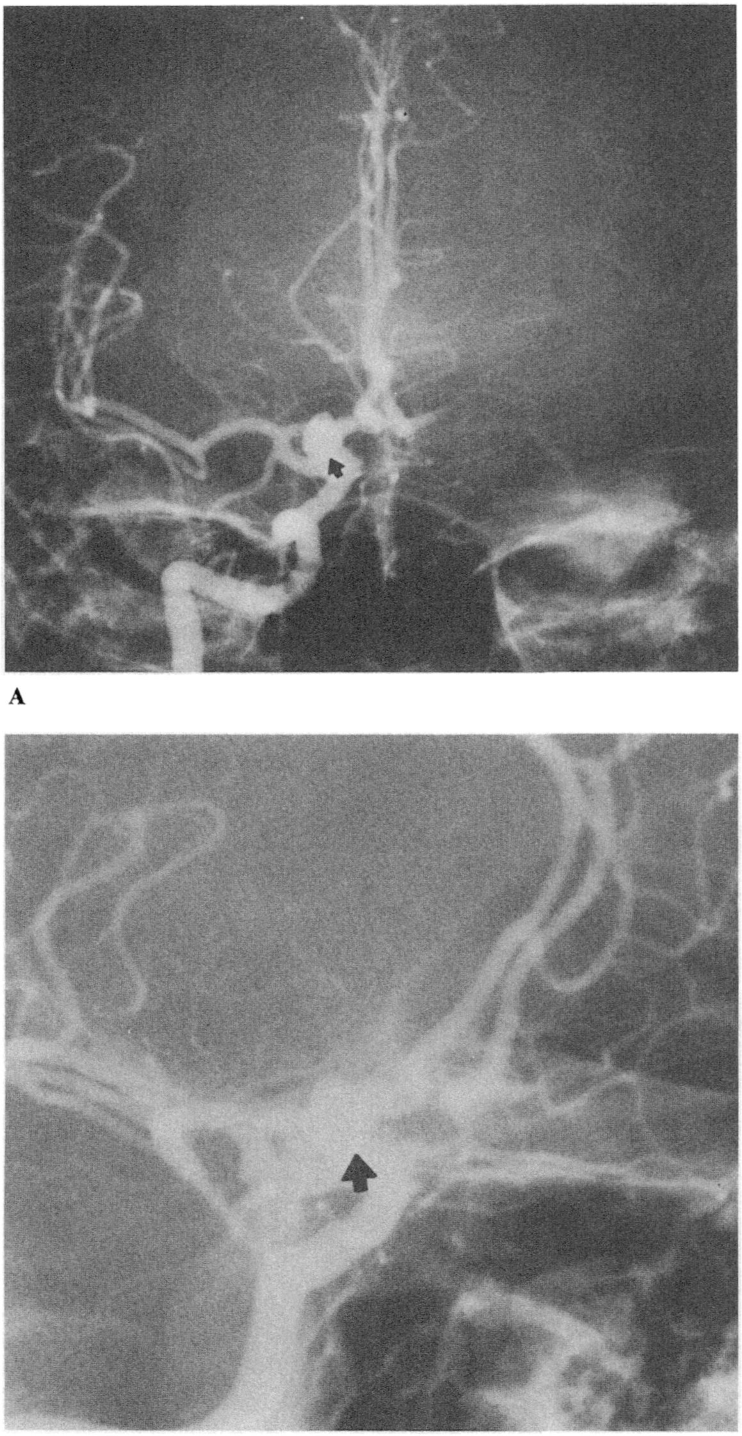

A

B

Fig. 36.39. **A** Frontal view of right carotid angiogram showing an oaICAA. *Arrow,* origin of aneurysm. **B** Oblique view of same. *Arrow,* origin of aneurysm. This is the same patient with multiple aneurysms illustrated in Fig. 36.24. The surgical view is seen in Fig. 36.40.

the neck and place temporary umbilical tapes around these arteries before starting the craniotomy. These ligatures remain loose and within the sterile operative field. Often we will occlude both the ICA *and* the ECA transiently *instead of* dropping the blood pressure during dissection and clipping of the aneurysm (see below). Should the aneurysm rupture, a temporary trapping procedure thus is available to the surgeon.

Figures 36.39–36.41 demonstrate a case in which a superomedially projecting oaICAA was

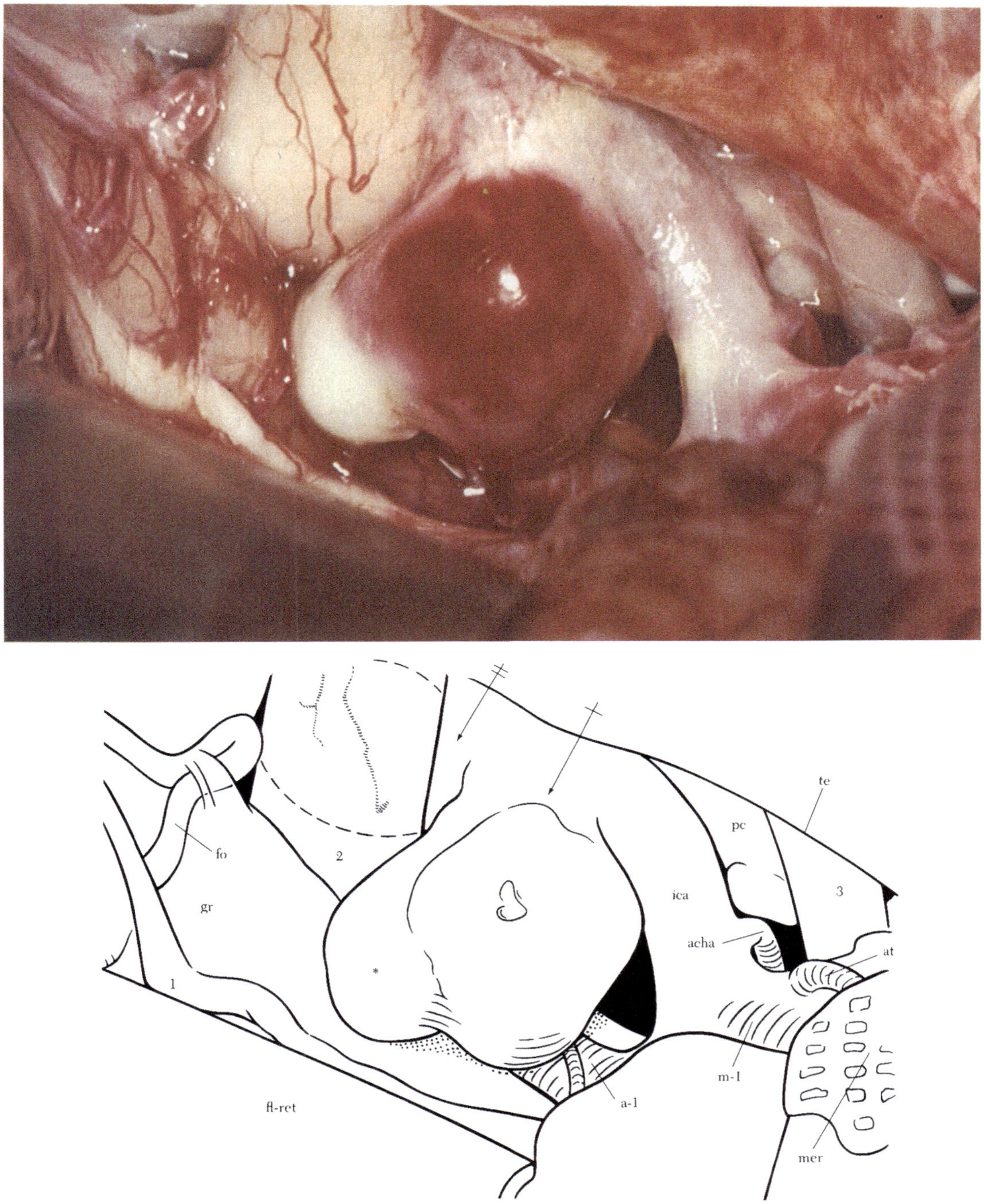

Fig. 36.40. Surgical exposure of the oaICAA shown in Fig. 36.39 projecting superomedially over the optic nerve (*2*). *Single-crossed arrow,* neck (origin) of aneurysm at internal carotid artery (*ica*); *double-crossed arrow,* origin of thrombosed second oaICAA projecting medially (*dotted lines*) under optic nerve (*2*); *pc,* posterior clinoid process in background between the internal carotid artery (*ica*) and the oculomotor nerve (*3*); *te,* anterior reflection of tentorial edge; *acha,* origin of anterior choroidal artery; *at,* anterior temporal artery; *m-1,* origin of M-1 artery; *mer,* Mersilene gauze under temporal lobe retractor; *a-1,* origin of A-1 artery, *fl-ret,* frontal lobe retractor; *1,* olfactory tract; *gr,* gyrus rectus; *2,* optic nerve; *fo,* frontoorbital artery; *, atherosclerotic plaque in wall of aneurysm.

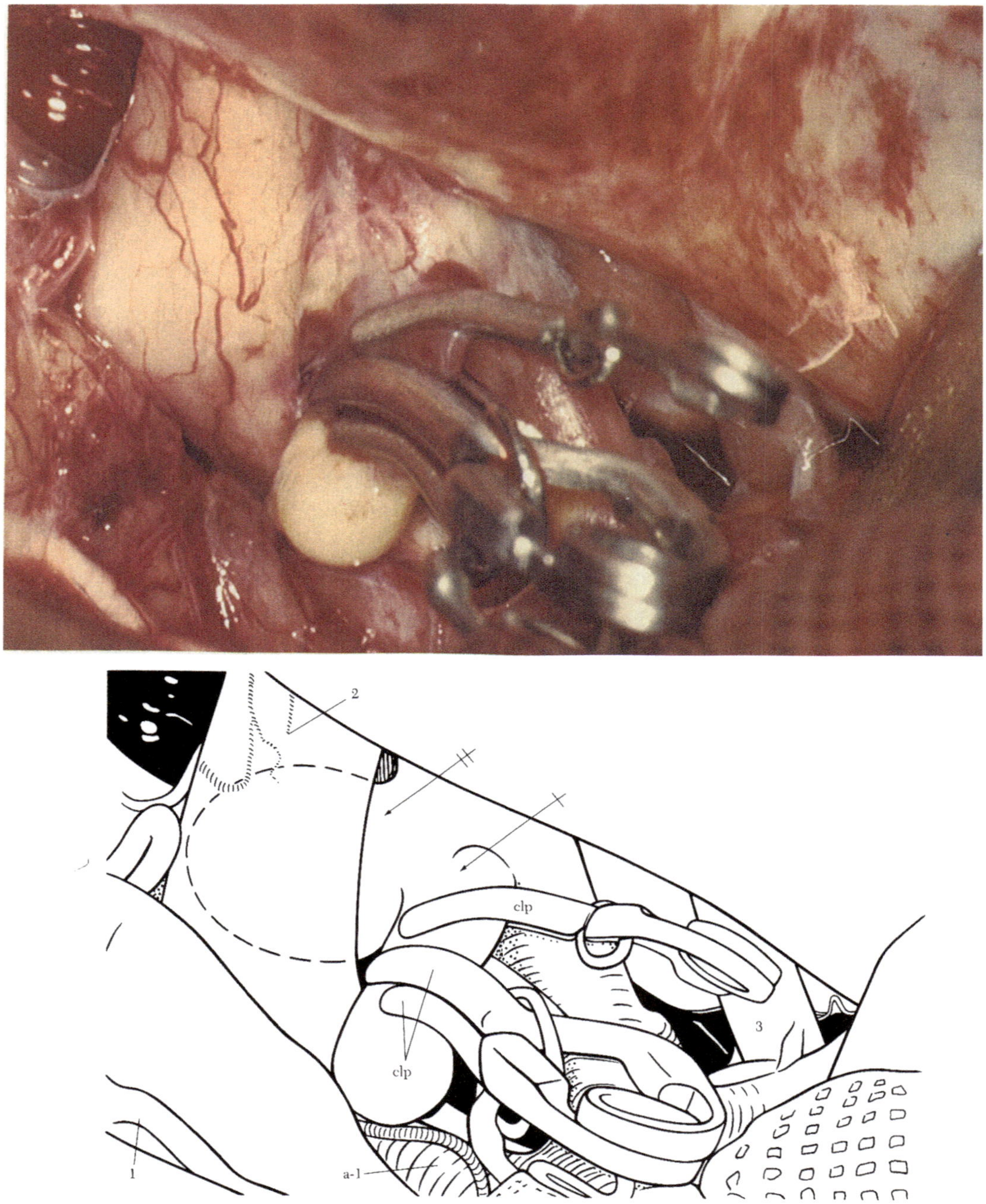

Fig. 36.41. Same case as in Figs. 36.39 and 36.40 after application of three Yaşargil clips (*clp*). *Double-crossed arrow,* thrombosed oaICAA under optic nerve (*2*); *single-crossed arrow,* origin of clipped oaICAA; *3,* oculomotor nerve; *a-1,* A-1 artery; *1,* olfactory tract.

seen on the angiogram; but at surgery a second, thrombosed, medially projecting oaICAA was also found under the optic nerve. Because the neck of the aneurysm was not covered by the anterior clinoid process, it was not necessary to drill down the bony process. Since the medial portion of the aneurysm wall was thickened with atherosclerosis, the primary clip was held open near its shank. This prevented collapse of the aneurysm. Two additional clips placed on either side of the main clip and not including the thicker medial wall resolved that problem.

Occasionally, a small oaICAA may be partially or completely obscured by a prominent anterior clinoid. In this circumstance, it is advisable to raise the blood pressure and temporarily trap the aneurysm between the ligatures in the neck and a temporary Heifetz clip in the head (between the aneurysm and PCoA). Then the dura is removed and a high-speed diamond drill used to remove the bony protrusion as detailed in Chapter 30 (page 800). If the drilling time is prolonged, it may be wise to stop and transiently release the temporary ligatures and clip every 5 to 10 min. One must beware not to confuse an anterior clinoid process with dura covering a small oaICAA under an eroded anterior clinoid. In such a case, one may need only to dissect and cut the dural envelope away from the wall of the aneurysm.

Figures 36.42–36.47 nicely exemplify the surgical exposure and treatment of a large, or giant, oaICAA. Many of these oaICAA grow to a large size, yet their neck may be such as to permit appropriate clipping. Again, exposure with minimal brain retraction is facilitated by partial sphenoid wing removal and a wide opening of the sylvian fissure. This case exhibits another not uncommon problem: how to approach the giant oaICAA when a small (ruptured in this case) MCAA is in the surgeon's path. The problem is that (a) if the MCAA is not clipped, it may rupture again during the prolonged operation on the oaICAA or (b) if it is clipped with standard spring clips, the shank of the clip(s) may project into and interfere with the line of sight and instrumentation pathway. As noted in Fig. 36.43, this problem was solved by using a series of malleable, tantalum clips to obliterate the MCAA.

In Figs. 36.44 and 36.45 it can be seen that although the giant, pulsating aneurysm projects superoposteromedially and disappears under the frontal lobe and optic nerve, the neck is fairly well defined at the distal OA/ICA junction. This neck was not seen until the dura of the anterior clinoid process was removed (we use the cutting current on a probe for this); in this case it was not necessary to drill away the anterior clinoid process. At this point, the systolic blood pressure is *raised* to about 160–170 mmHg and the aneurysm is temporarily trapped. The trapping procedure involves (a) ligatures on both the ICA *and* the ECA in the previously prepared neck and (b) a Heifetz clip on the intracranial ICA between the PCoA take-off and the aneurysm. It is critical to raise the BP (as one does for carotid endarterectomy cases during carotid artery occlusion) to provide a better cerebral perfusion pressure. Observation of the status of the two A-1 arteries and ACoA complex as well as the PCoA will help indicate the extent of collateral circulation during the trapping. Also, if there remain good ipsilateral A-1 and M-1 pulsations during the temporary trapping, adequate cerebral perfusion is likely.

In our experience it is necessary to occlude both the ICA and the ECA in the neck in this circumstance, for if the ICA only is occluded and the aneurysm then opened, a remarkable flow of arterial blood can persist into the aneurysm via the external carotid artery collaterals and hence retrograde into the ophthalmic artery. Even with closure of the ECA and trapping of the ICA, some blood will enter the opened aneurysm retrograde via petrous and cavernous branches of the ICA, via contralateral ECA collaterals to the ipsilateral OA, and via ethmoidal arteries. After the trapping procedure has been initiated, the aneurysm is opened with a Beaver knife or a No. 11 scalpel blade (21) or collapsed with a needle attached to suction (19).

In this case we opened with a knife and scissors while aspirating the minimal blood effluent from the neck of the aneurysm. The dome was left attached to the frontal lobe, olfactory tract, optic nerve and chiasm, and A-1 (Figs. 36.46 and 36.47). The neck was secured with a McFadden clip followed by a Yaşargil clip to occlude the neck remaining between the first clip and the ICA, yet preserving OA blood flow (Fig. 36.47). Although the use of clips of varying metallic mixtures adjacent to each other has been said to create a "battery" effect and unwanted tissue reaction (34–36), we are unaware of any clinical problems from the presence of

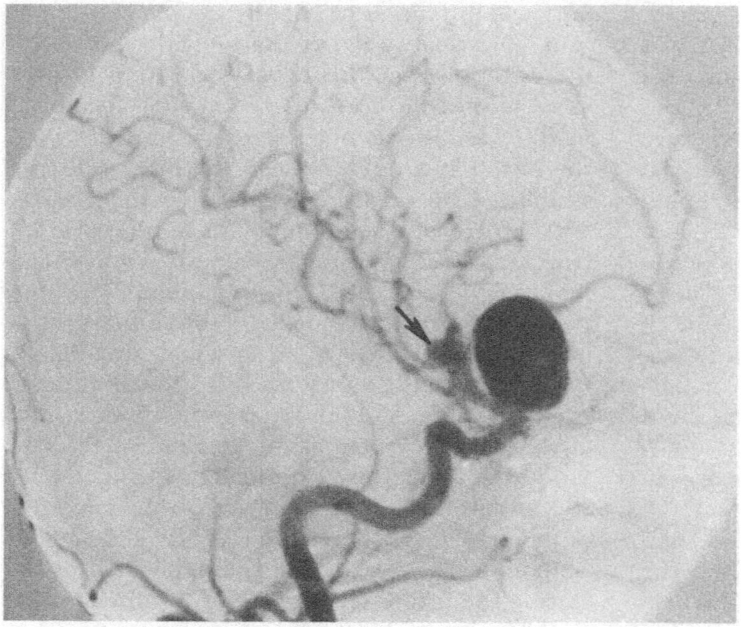

A

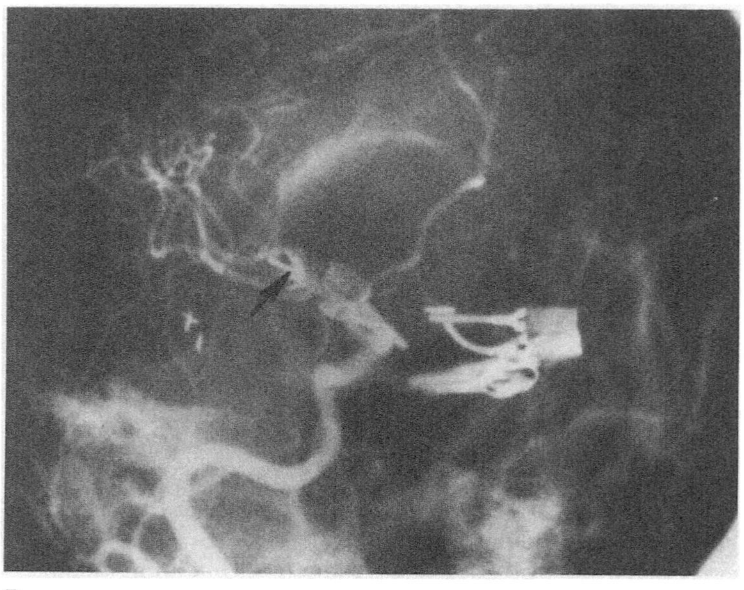

B

Fig. 36.42. Right carotid angiograms, oblique views, of a 49-year-old woman with multiple intracranial aneurysms: giant right oaICAA (Figs. 36.43–36.47); small ruptured right MCAA (Fig. 36.43); giant left oaICAA (Figs. 36.49 and 36.50, reversed); and giant left vICAA (Figs. 36.49 and 36.50, reversed). From Fox JL: ref. 21. **A** Preoperative angiogram revealing giant right oaICAA and ruptured MCAA (*arrow*). **B** Postoperative angiogram demonstrating occlusion of both aneurysms on the right. Multiple tantalum clips (*arrow*) were used on the MCAA. The clips on the patient's left side are on the left vICAA and left oaICAA, which also were occluded successfully with similar preservation of the parent arteries. See original publication for details (21).

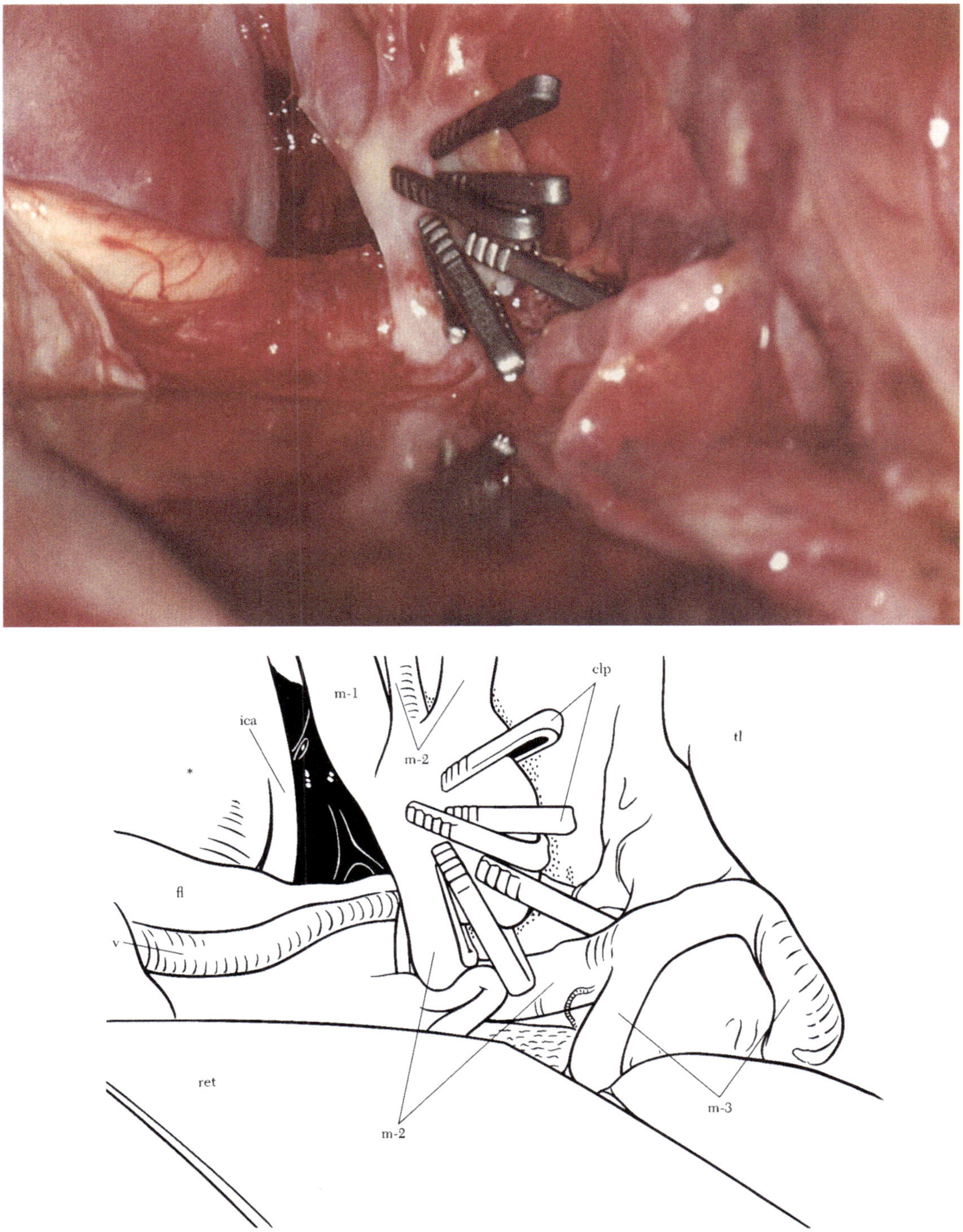

Fig. 36.43. Operative view of clipped MCAA in sylvian fissure and portion of giant oaICAA (*) under frontal lobe (*fl*). Same case as in Figs. 36.42 and 36.44–36.47. *ica*, right internal carotid artery; *m-1*, M-1 artery; *m-2*, three M-2 branches; *m-3*, two M-3 branches of middle cerebral artery; *clp*, tantalum Ligaclips on middle cerebral artery aneurysm; *tl*, temporal lobe; *ret*, frontal lobe retractor, *v*, vein; *fl*, frontal lobe.

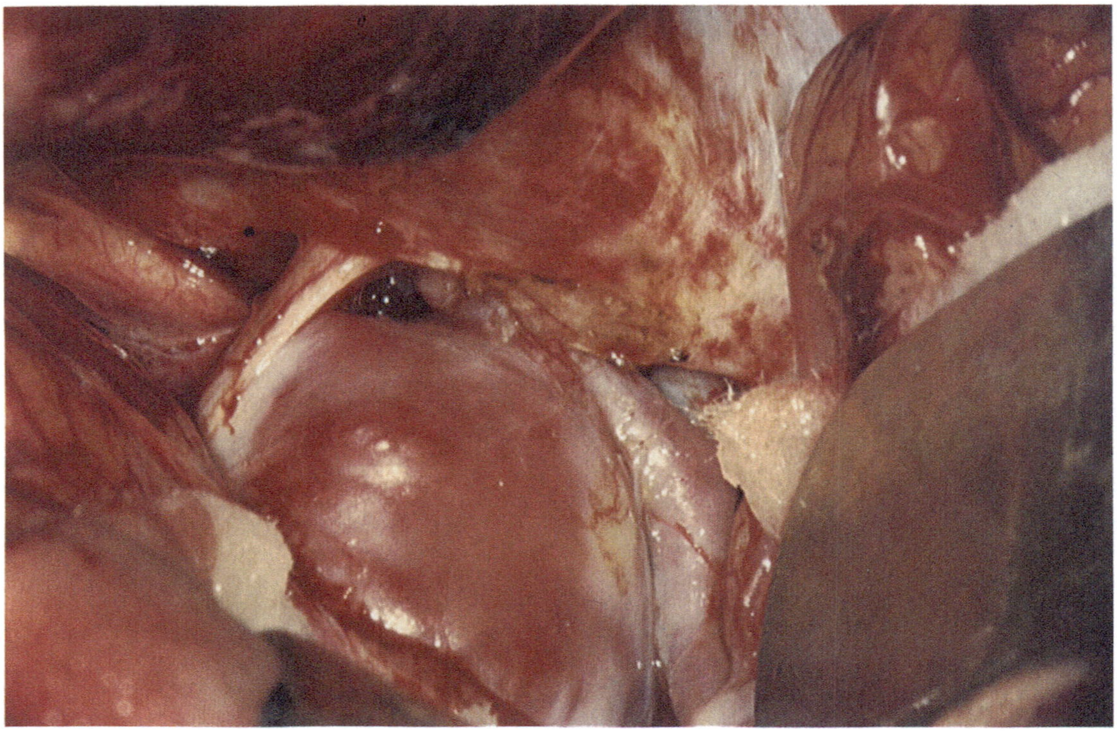

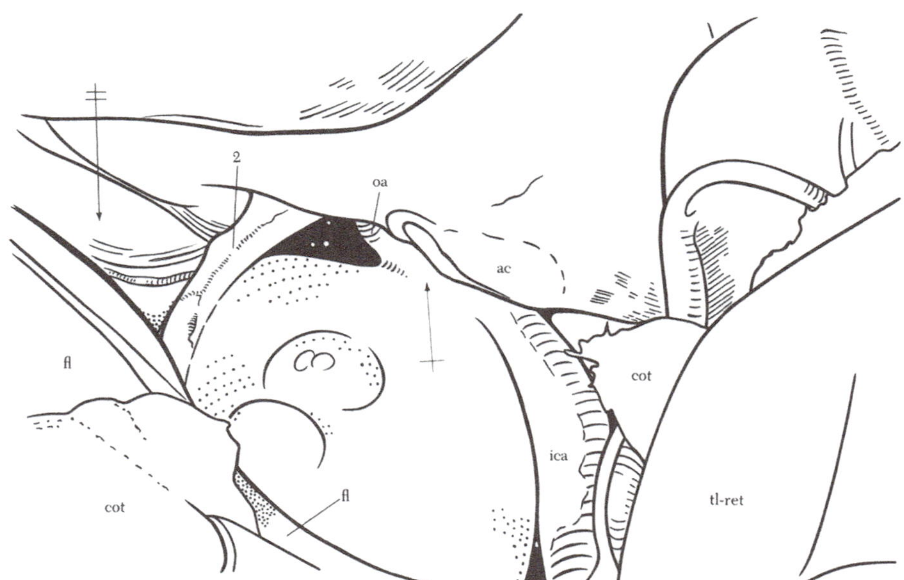

Fig. 36.44. Exposure of giant right oaICAA. Same case as in Figs. 36.42, 36.43, and 36.45–36.47. Magnification reduced with Zeiss dial set at No. 10. *2,* optic nerve stretched over aneurysm; *oa,* ophthalmic artery; *ac,* dura removed from anterior clinoid process; *cot,* edge of cottonoid strip; *tl-ret,* temporal lobe retractor; *ica,* internal carotid artery; *fl,* frontal lobe; *double-crossed arrow,* medial dome of another giant left oaICAA (see Figs. 36.49 and 36.50); *single-crossed arrow,* origin of right oaICAA.

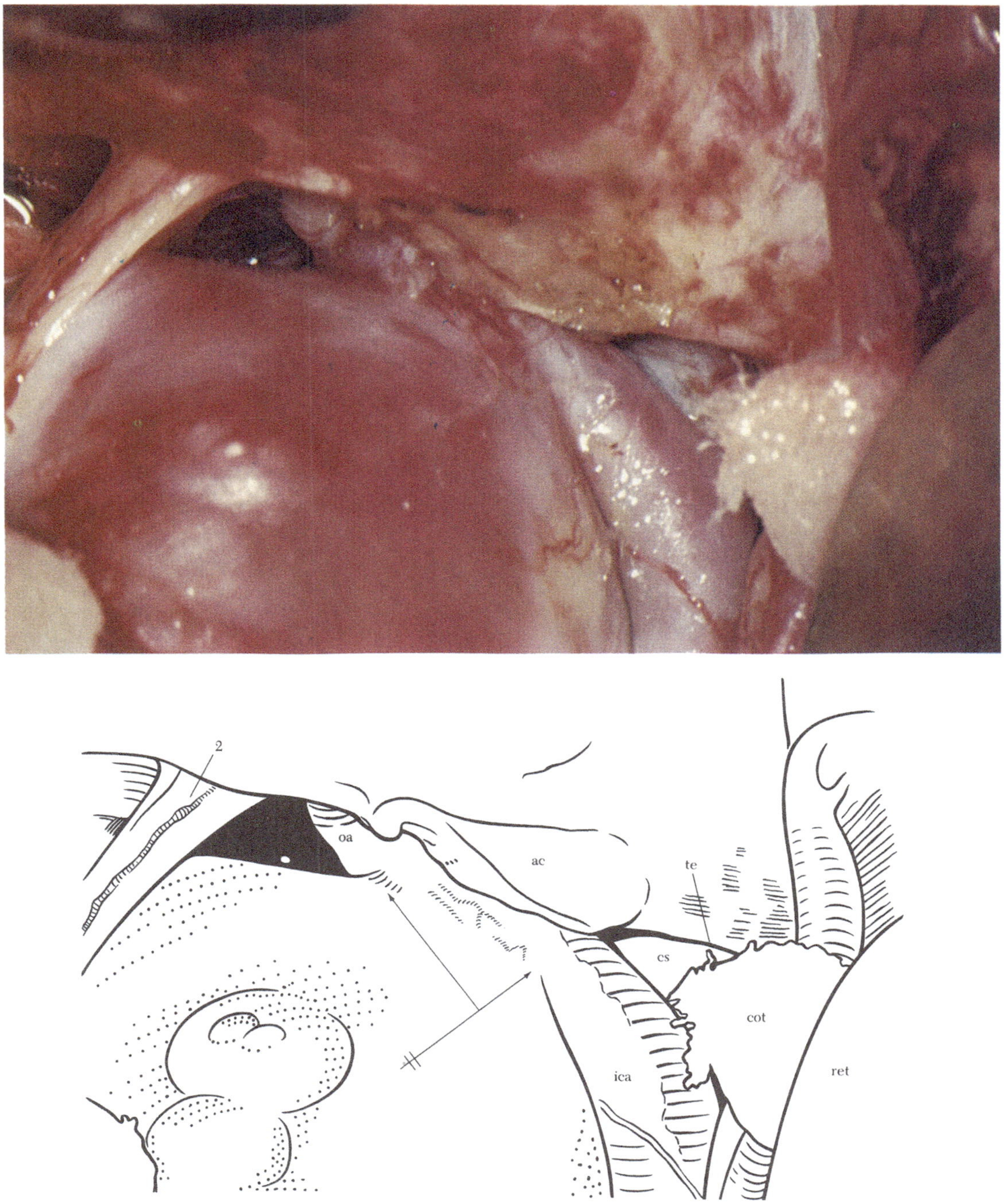

Fig. 36.45. Same view as in Fig. 36.44 except at higher magnification to show more clearly the relationship of neck of aneurysm (*double-crossed arrow*) to ophthalmic artery (*oa*), internal carotid artery (*ica*), and anterior clinoid process with dura removed (*ac*). *cs,* roof of cavernous sinus; *te,* anterior reflection of tentorial edge; *cot,* cottonoid strip; *ret,* retractor; *2,* stretched optic nerve. From Fox JL: ref. 21.

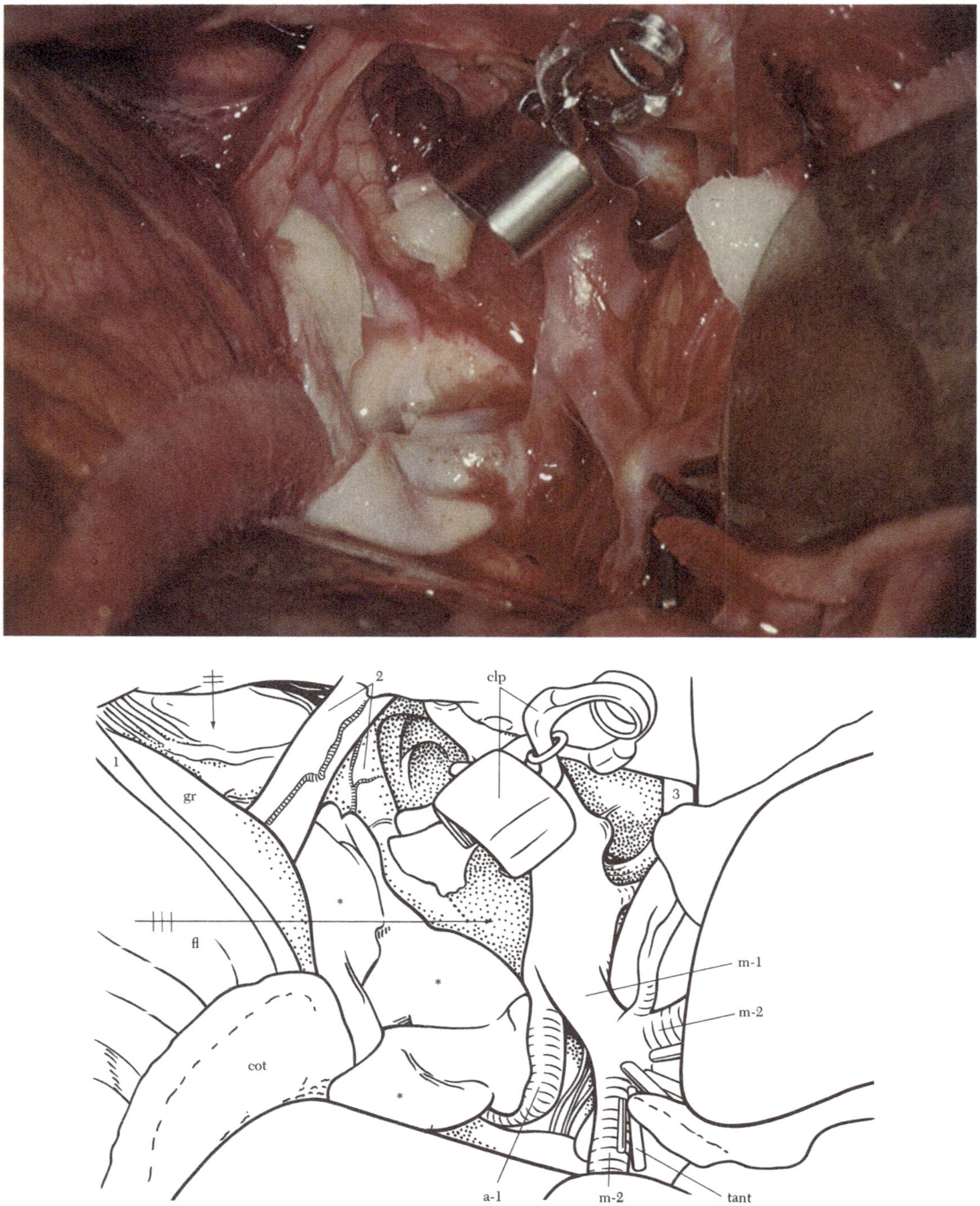

Fig. 36.46. Similar view and magnification as in Fig. 36.44 following opening and clipping of aneurysm. *2,* flattened and splayed right optic nerve; *clp,* shanks of McFadden (below) and Yaşargil (above) clips on neck of oaICAA; *3,* oculomotor nerve; *m-1,* M-1 artery; *m-2,* M-2 branches; *tant,* tantalum clips on middle cerebral artery aneurysm; *a-1,* A-1 artery passing behind remains of dome of aneurysm (*) and then between dome and frontal lobe (*fl*); *cot,* cottonoid strip; *triple-crossed arrow,* medial dome of a giant left vICAA; *gr,* gyrus rectus; *1,* olfactory tract; *double-crossed arrow,* medial dome of another giant left oaICAA.

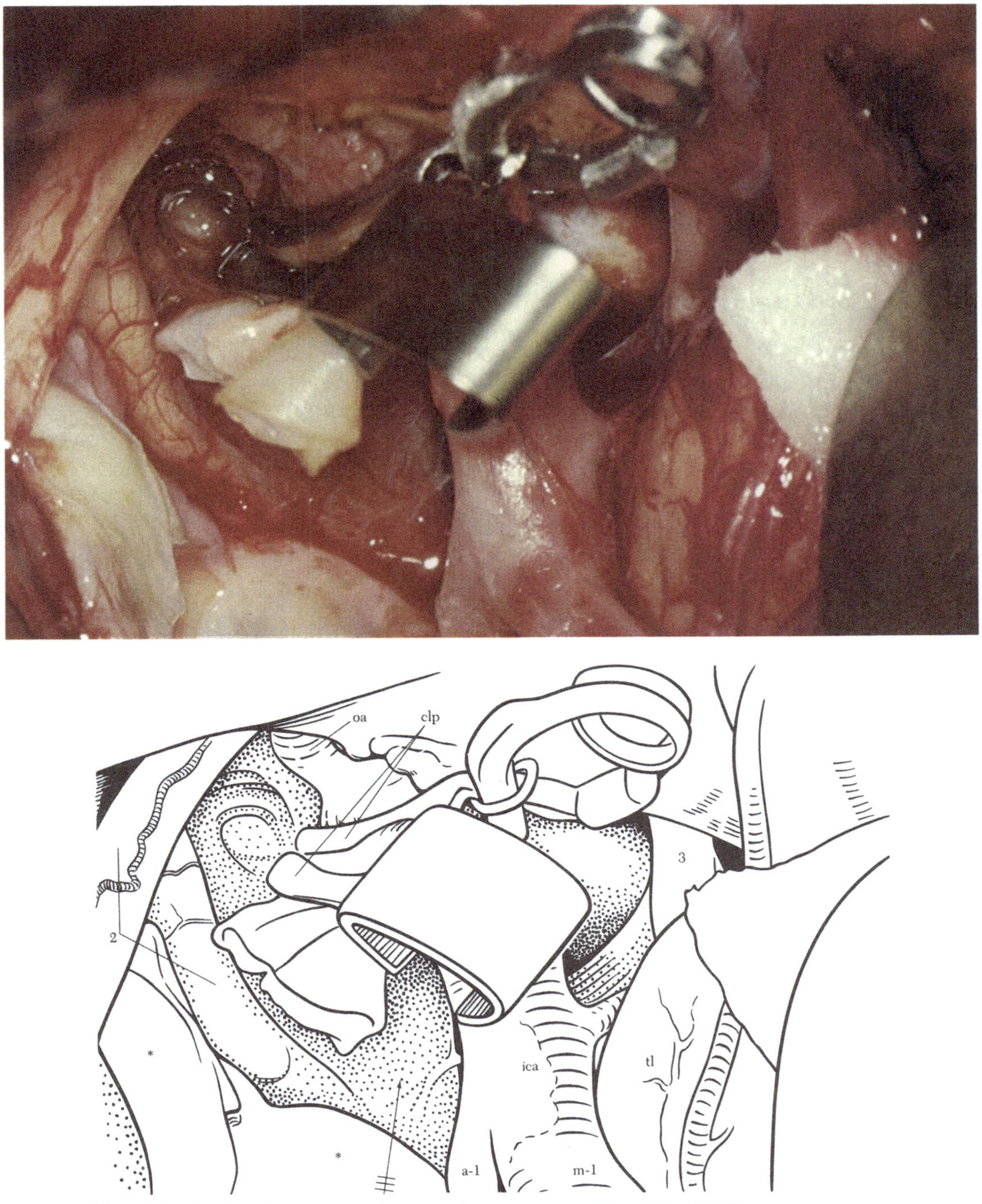

Fig. 36.47. Similar view and magnification as in Fig. 36.45 following opening and clipping of aneurysm. *, inner wall of dome of aneurysm (stuck to frontal lobe and optic nerve); *2*, flattened and splayed portion of right optic nerve; *oa*, ophthalmic artery; *clp*, wings of McFadden clip (below) and Yaşargil clip (above); *3*, oculomotor nerve; *tl*, temporal lobe; *m-1*, origin of M-1 artery; *ica*, termination of internal carotid artery; *a-1*, origin of A-1 artery; *triple-crossed arrow*, medial wall of giant left vICAA.

adjacent, standard, intracranial aneurysm clips made by different manufacturers. After clipping of the aneurysm, the temporary clips are removed, the BP returned to normal, and the arteries topically bathed in 3% papaverine or 0.5% phentolamine soaked in a cottonoid. Postoperative angiography (Fig. 36.42B) confirmed obliteration of the aneurysms and patency of the parent arteries.

Ventral Internal Carotid Artery Aneurysms

The ventral internal carotid artery aneurysm (Fig. 36.48) poses special problems: (a) the neck is on the ventral side of the ICA and hence the artery partially or completely obscures the neck from the surgeon's view unless the aneurysm projects ventrolaterally; (b) the neck is usually very broad; (c) atherosclerosis of the ICA and aneurysm is not uncommon; (d) the portion of the ICA containing the neck of the aneurysm frequently is obscured by the anterior clinoid process; (e) the dome may project into the cavernous sinus; and (f) the dome may be adherent to anterior thalamoperforators and hypothalamic perforators from the ICA and the PCoA, to the PCoA itself, to the oculomotor nerve laterally, and to the pituitary stalk medially. The vICAA pictured in Figs. 36.49 and 36.50 exemplifies most of these characteristics. Both of the aneurysms in Fig. 36.50 were treated successfully in a manner described above for the other giant oaICAA (see original publication for details [21]).

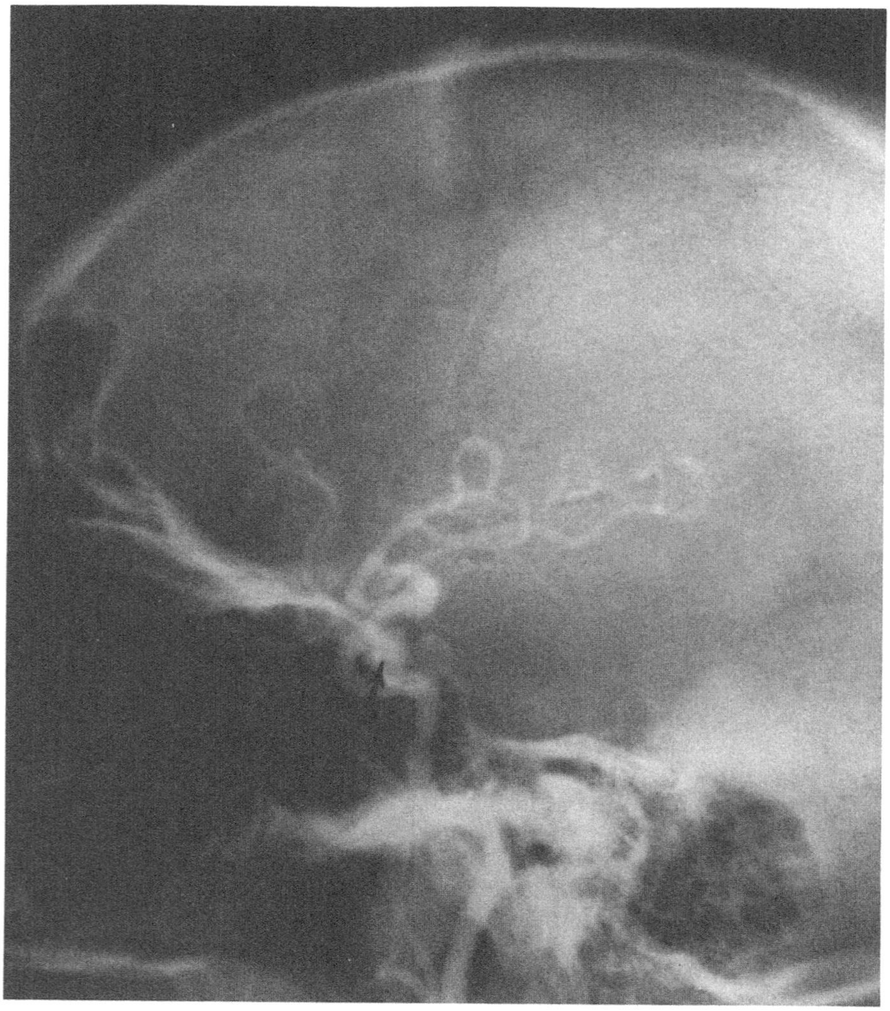

Fig. 36.48. Lateral angiogram revealing a right vICAA (*arrow*) projecting downward into the cavernous sinus.

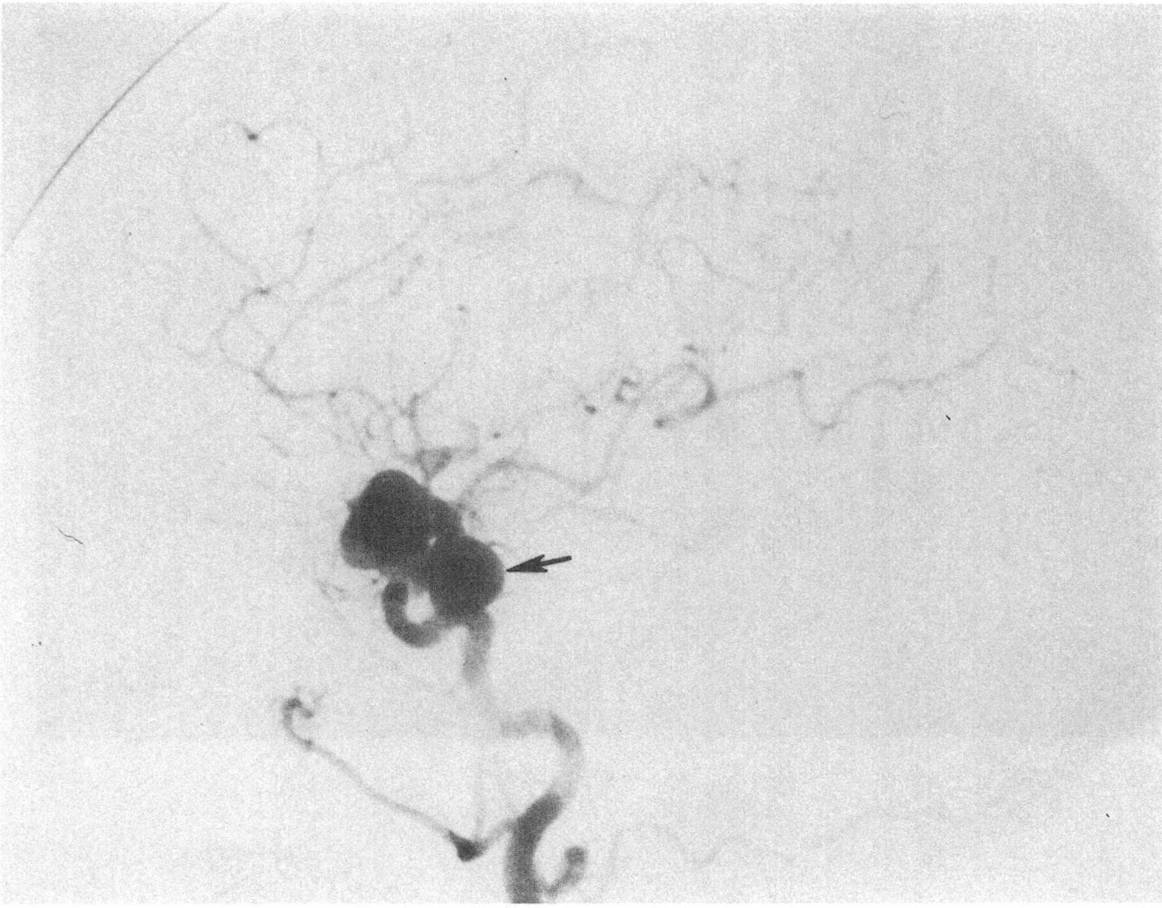

Fig. 36.49. Left lateral angiogram illustrating two large aneurysms on the left side: a superomedially projecting oaICAA and a ventrally projecting vICAA (*arrow*). This is the same patient seen in Figs. 36.42–36.47 and 36.50 (reversed). All aneurysms were successfully clipped. From Fox JL: ref. 21.

Cavernous Sinus–Internal Carotid Artery Aneurysms

Aneurysms in the cavernous sinus normally have not been treated by clipping procedures but rather by carotid artery ligation, trapping procedures, intraluminal thrombosis techniques (e.g., with wire), intravascular balloon occlusion, and other unusual methods. Often no surgical therapy is recommended. Once rupture takes place into the cavernous sinus, the treatment is that for a C-C fistula.

Aneurysms in the cavernous sinus may appear angiographically as small, incidental sacs (Fig. 36.51). They tend to expand laterally and superiorly between CN-3 and CN-4 above *and* CN-5 and CN-6 below (Fig. 7.5) (7). Eventually the csICAA may grow to the point of causing a cavernous sinus syndrome (see Chapter 7) and then erode its nearby bony structures (Fig. 36.52A). Once it achieves giant proportions, intraluminal clot often collects (Fig. 36.52B). Figure 36.53 depicts the complicated anatomy of the cavernous sinus and environs.

Two Case Reports

Although a direct attack upon a csICAA is rare, the following illustrates what has been done by the senior author (JLF) with two cases. Although entrapment with an extracranial-intracranial anastomosis was considered, we elected

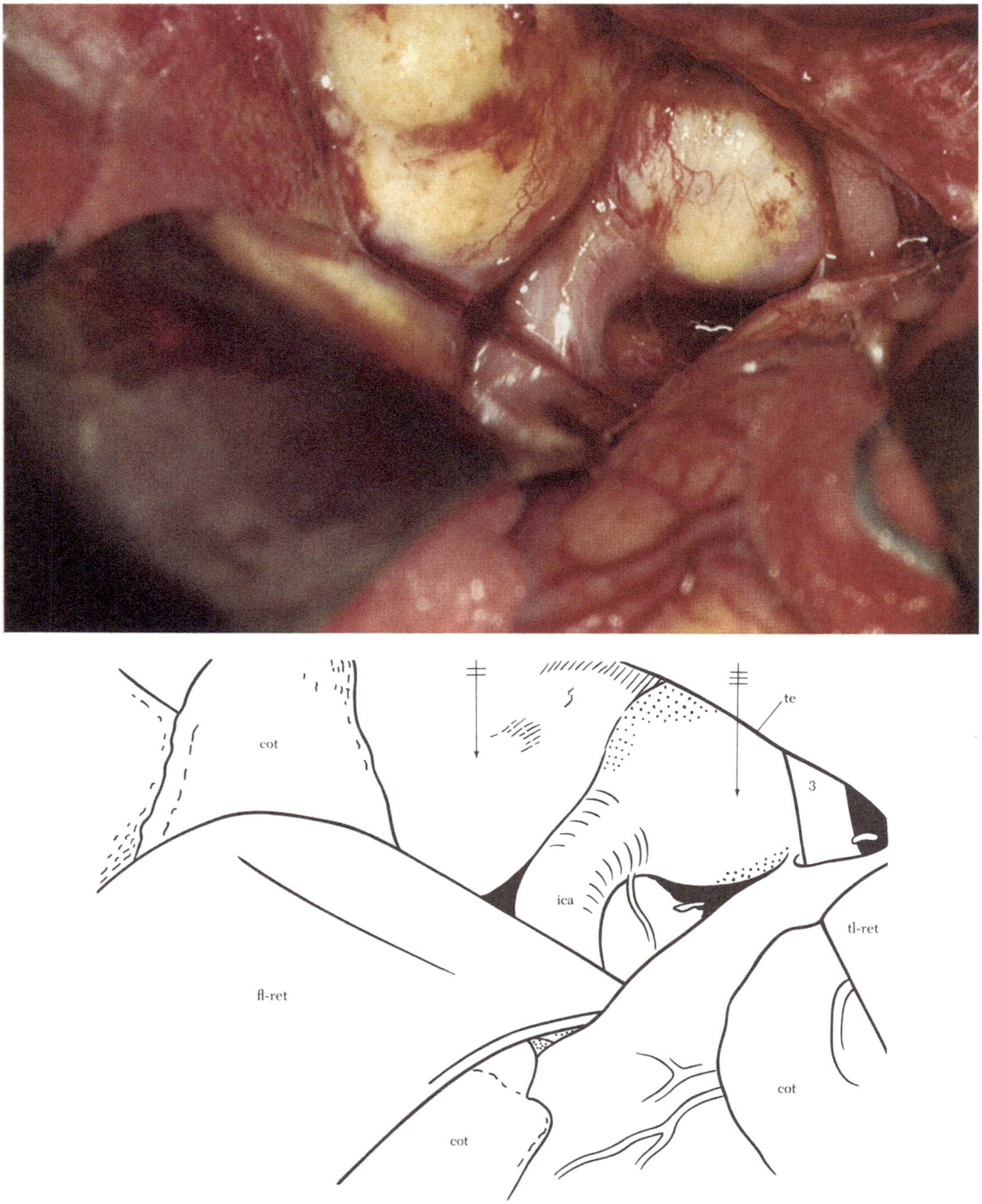

Fig. 36.50. Surgical view of a giant oaICAA (*double-crossed arrow*) and a giant vICAA (*triple-crossed arrow*). The oaICAA extended between the ICA (*ica*) and the ipsilateral optic nerve (hidden). The vICAA extended between the oculomotor nerve (*3*) and the pituitary stalk (hidden). *te,* anterior reflection of tentorial edge; *cot,* cottonoid strips under retractors; *tl-ret,* temporal lobe retractor; *fl-ret,* frontal lobe retractor. Note walls of aneurysms are yellow with atherosclerosis. Viewed as if operated on right side. From Fox JL: ref. 21.

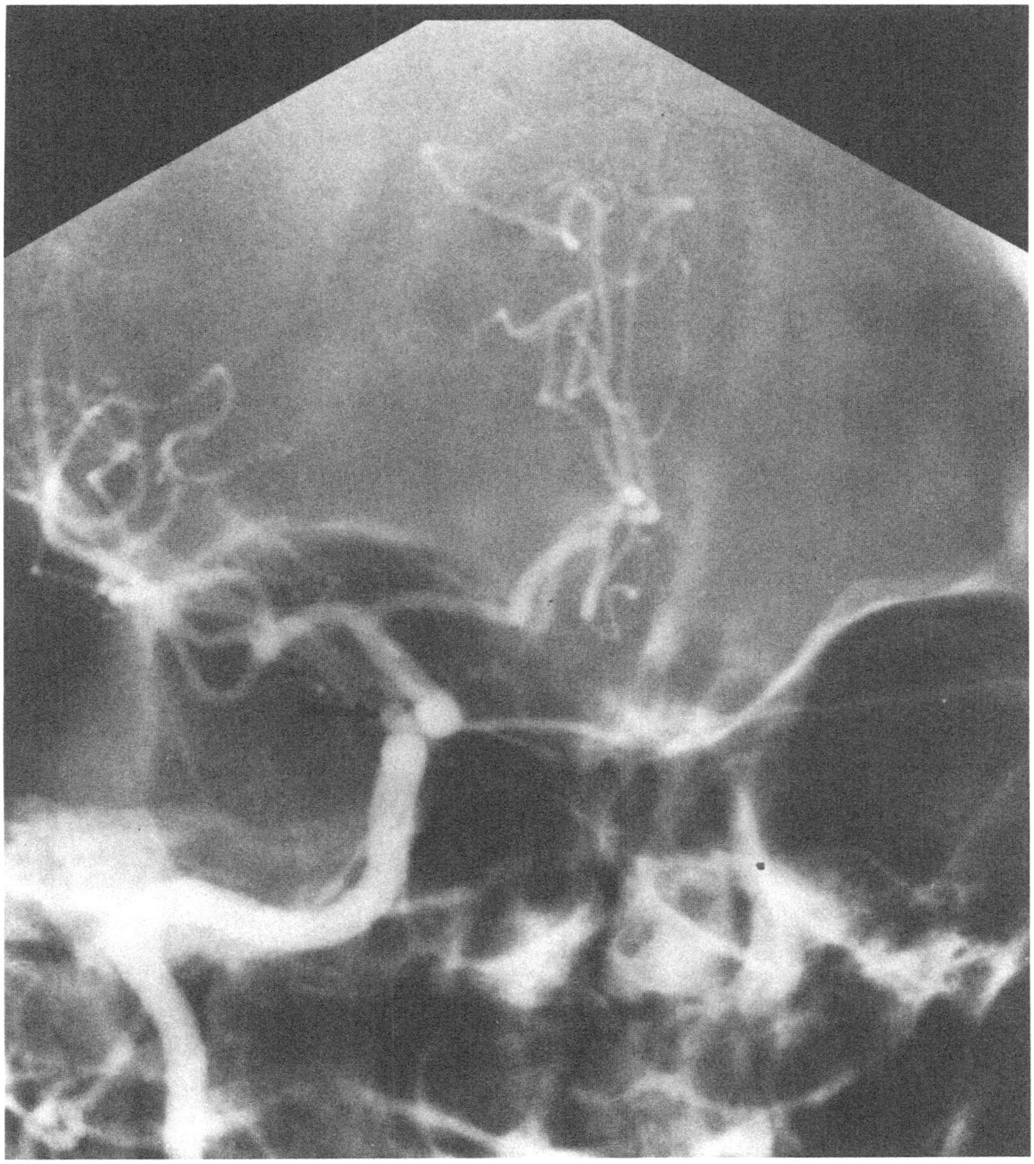

Fig. 36.51. Frontal view of a small csICAA (*arrow*) seen on angiography.

to expose the giant aneurysm (Fig. 36.54) and attempt to reconstitute a neck to the aneurysm for ligation or clipping. Failing that, it was planned to fill the aneurysm with preformed Ivalon sponge in the hope that an ICA channel might be preserved.

Case 1 was a 47-year-old, normotensive woman with a 7-year history of progressively worsening right CN-6 paresis. There were no other deficits. Skull x-rays and CT scan revealed a right temporal fossa mass with erosion of the petrous pyramid. Angiography (Fig. 36.54) confirmed the presence of a giant right csICAA. The patient returned home after a successful operative procedure illustrated below.

Case 2 was a 64-year-old hypertensive woman with a 3-day history of left-sided headache, total left ophthalmoplegia, and sensory loss in the first two divisions (slight in the third division) of the trigeminal nerve. Skull x-rays and CT scan were negative. Angiography revealed a large, partially clotted csICAA on the left. The patient returned home after a successful operative procedure illustrated below. The ophthalmoplegia completely cleared over a year's time except for some mild ptosis.

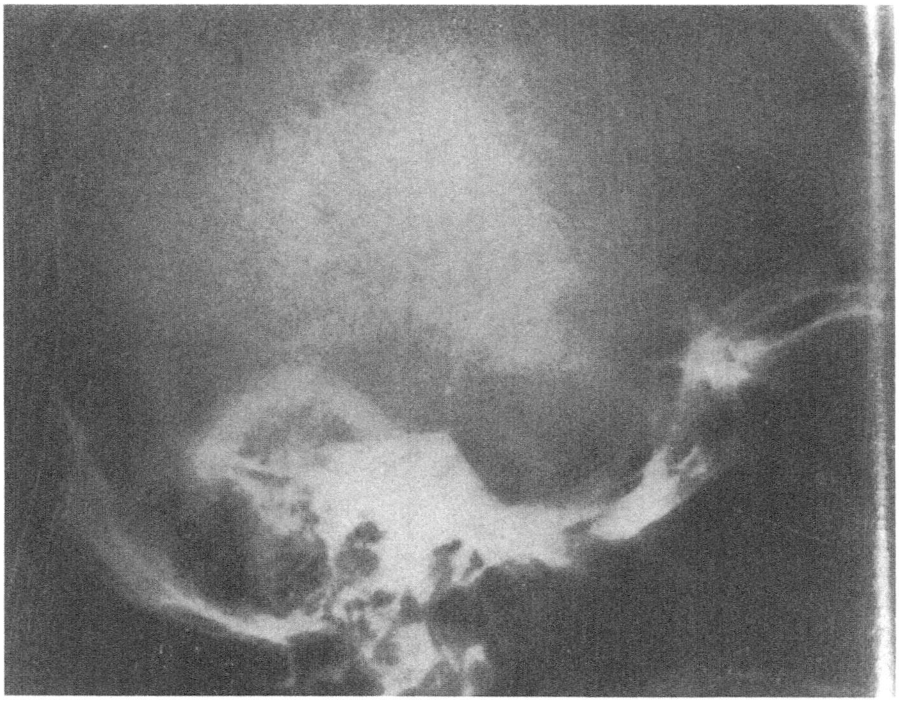

A

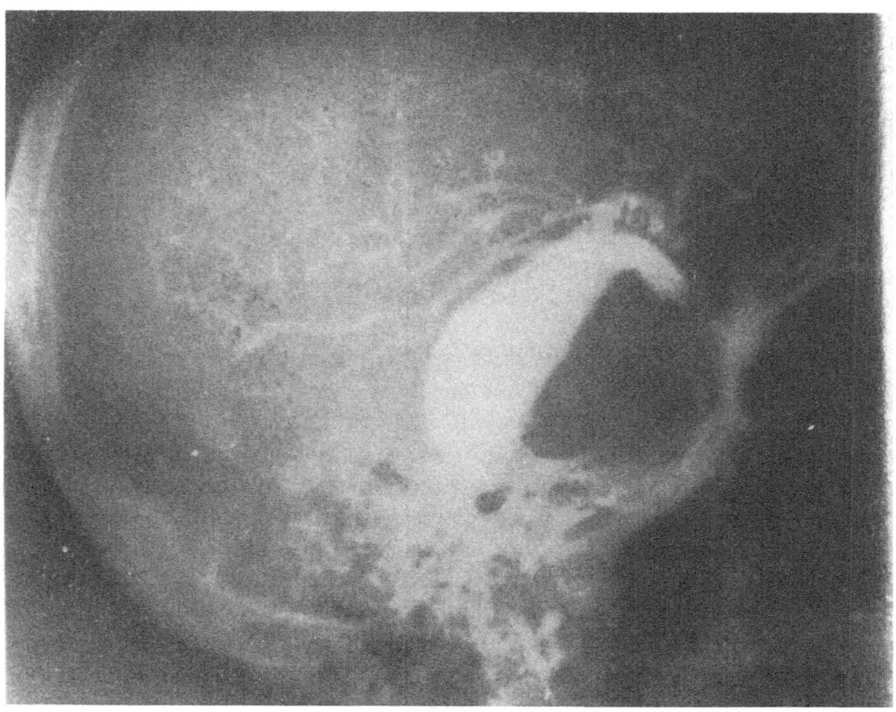

B

Fig. 36.52. Radiograms illustrating a giant csICAA. From Calmettes L, et al.: ref. 9. **A** Lateral skull X ray demonstrating erosion of the skull base. **B** Angiogram revealing a massive csICAA with considerable intraluminal clot formation.

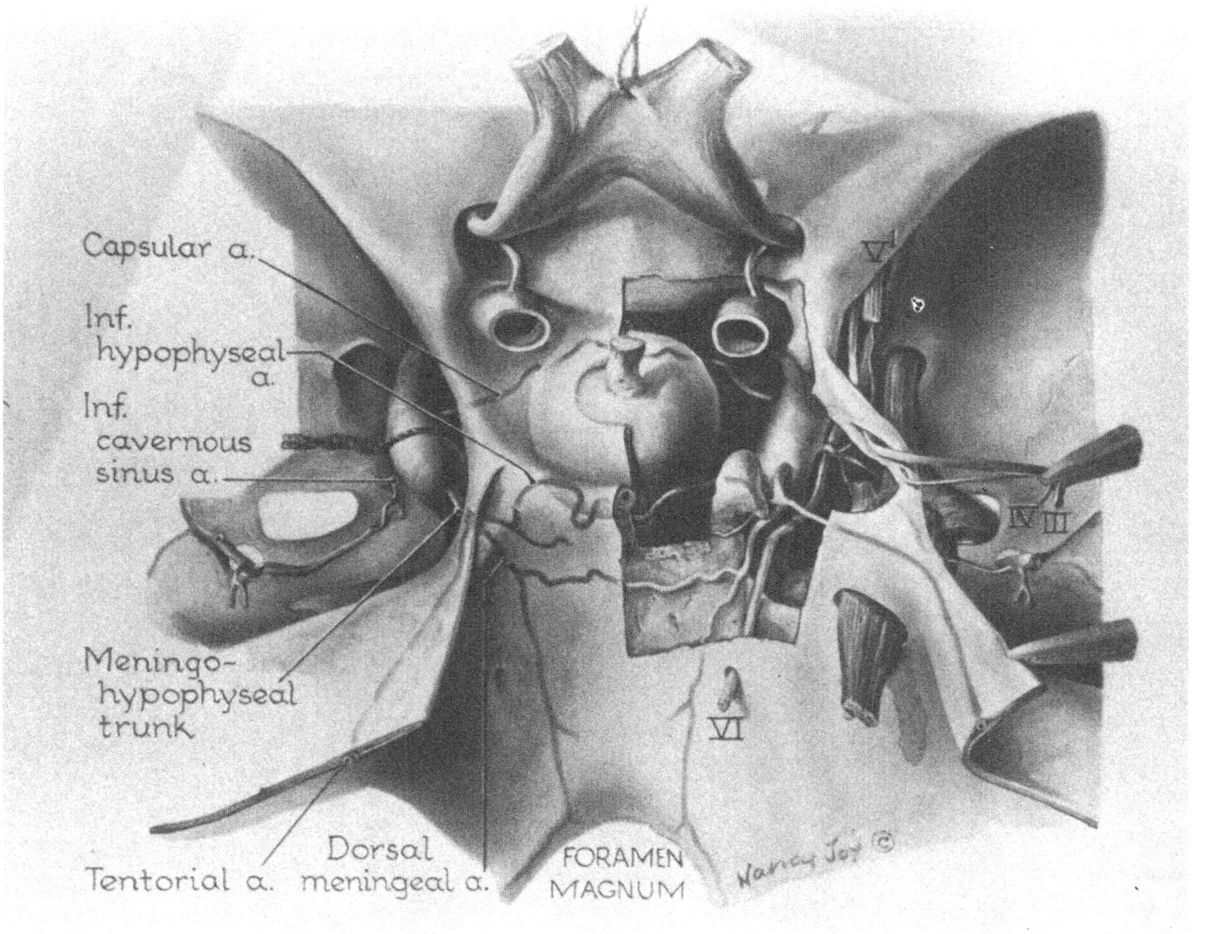

Fig. 36.53. Drawing of structures within and adjacent to the cavernous sinus and pituitary gland. From Parkinson D: ref. 40.

Surgical Exposure

The operative photographs from case number 1 (Figs. 36.55, 36.56, and 36.58) and case number 2 (Figs. 36.57 and 36.59, both reversed) are combined in order to elucidate the step-by-step surgical anatomy. Again, partial sphenoid wing removal and a wide opening of the sylvian fissure permitted an excellent exposure without adverse brain retraction pressure (Fig. 36.55). The temporal lobe had been elevated by the mass pushing the dural roof of the cavernous sinus upward, outward, and backward. Figure 36.56 portrays the relationship of the aneurysmal mass to the oculomotor nerve (CN-3).

Temporary ligatures were placed around the cervical ICA and ECA, and a temporary Heifetz clip was applied around the ICA between the aneurysm and the PCoA (Fig. 36.57) after the BP was elevated as previously described in this chapter. An incision was made in the dura forming the compressed roof of the cavernous sinus and aneurysm (Fig. 36.57). Finally, the wall of the aneurysm was opened and retracted with stay sutures (Fig. 36.58).

We attempted to isolate the aneurysm in each case, but the walls were too atherosclerotic and brittle. A neck could not be formed. Also, inferiorly, venous bleeding from the otherwise compressed cavernous sinus began as dissection continued toward the neck. Ivalon sponge was cut to proper size and shape, inserted into the aneurysm, and the walls approximated (Fig. 36.59). No extracranial-intracranial bypass was done since there were well-devel-

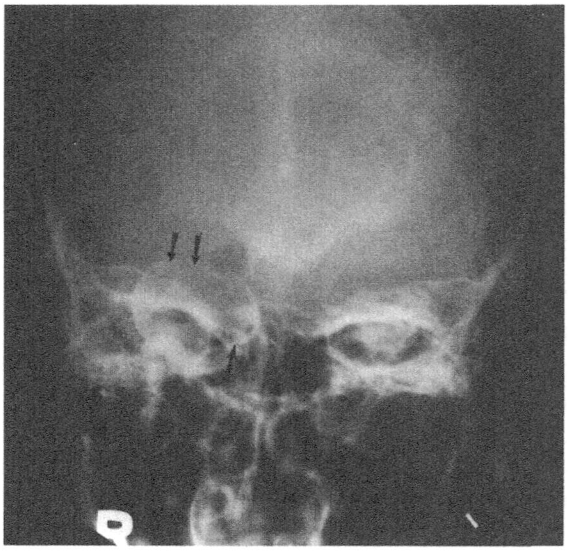

A

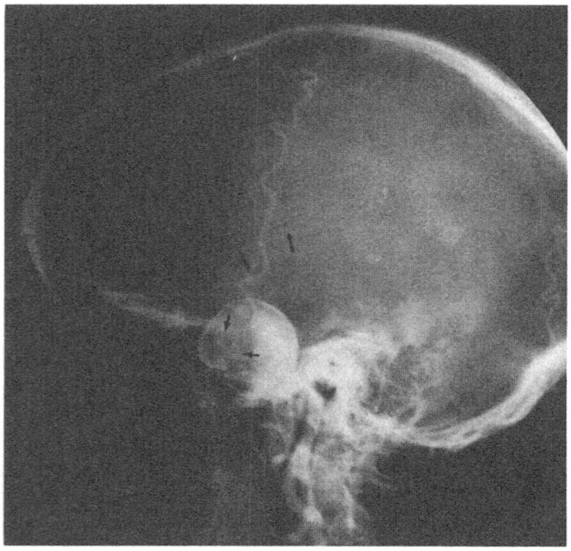

B

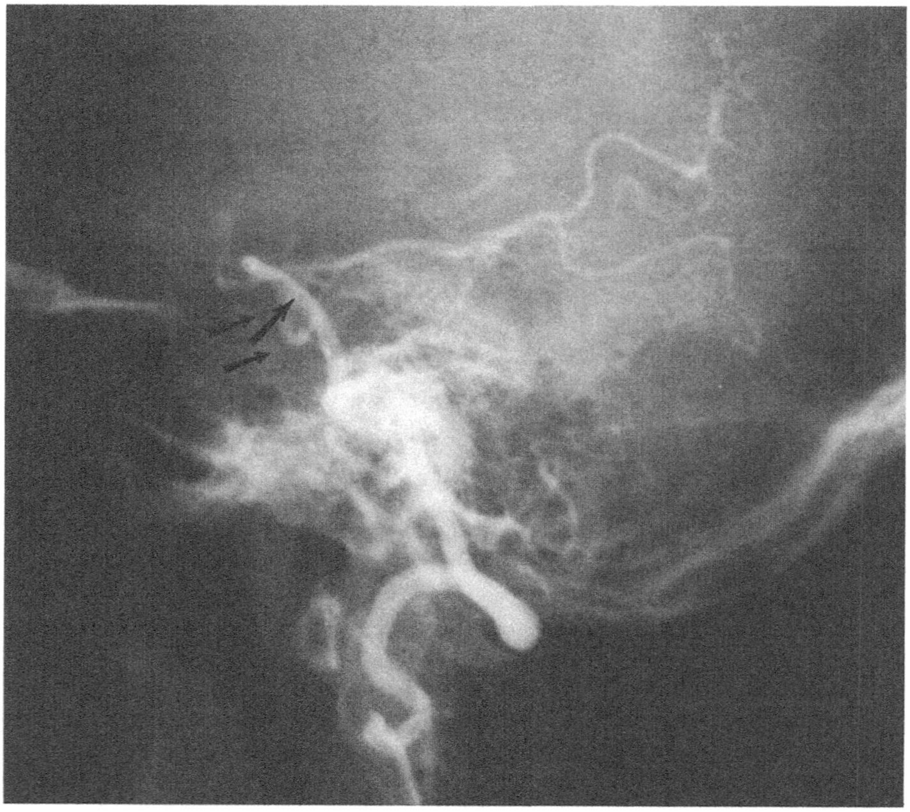

C

Fig. 36.54. Angiogram of same csICAA shown in Figs. 36.55, 36.56, and 36.58. **A** Frontal view of carotid angiogram. *Double arrows,* upper limit of aneurysm; *single arrow,* flow of contrast from ICA into aneurysm. **B** Lateral view of carotid angiogram. *Two lower arrows,* entrance and exit points of contrast media into and out of aneurysm; *two upper arrows,* middle cerebral artery. **C** Vertebrobasilar angiogram showing the basilar artery (*single arrow*) pushed backward by the aneurysm. *Double arrows,* dorsum sellae.

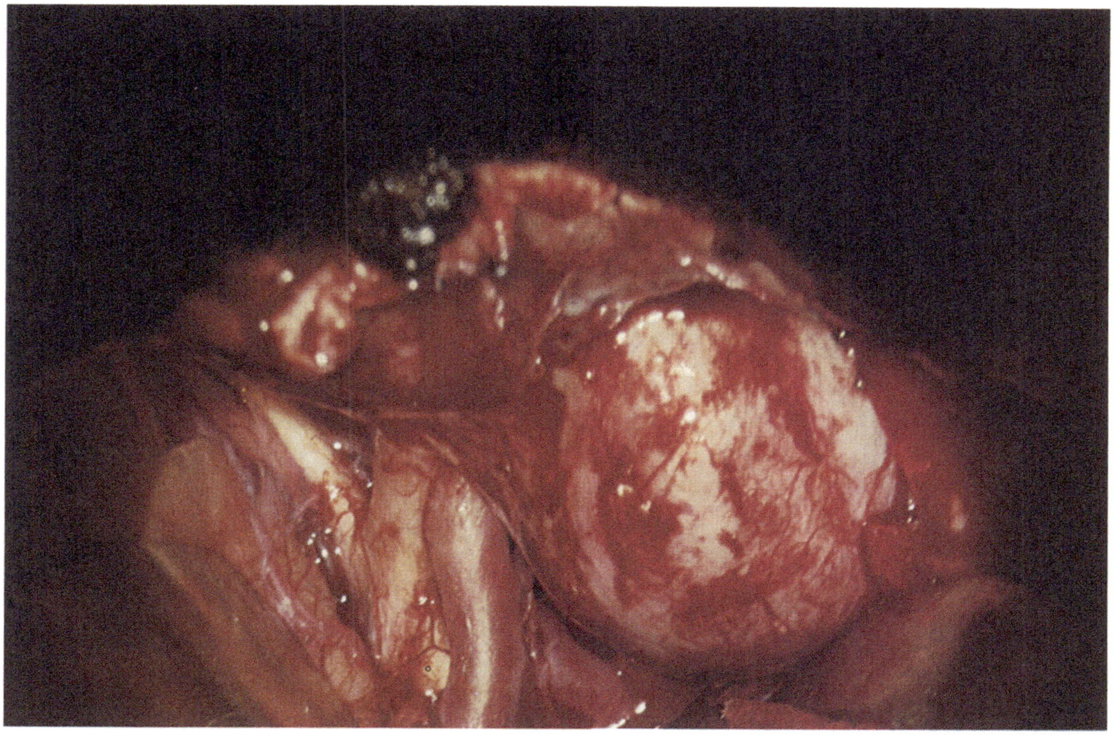

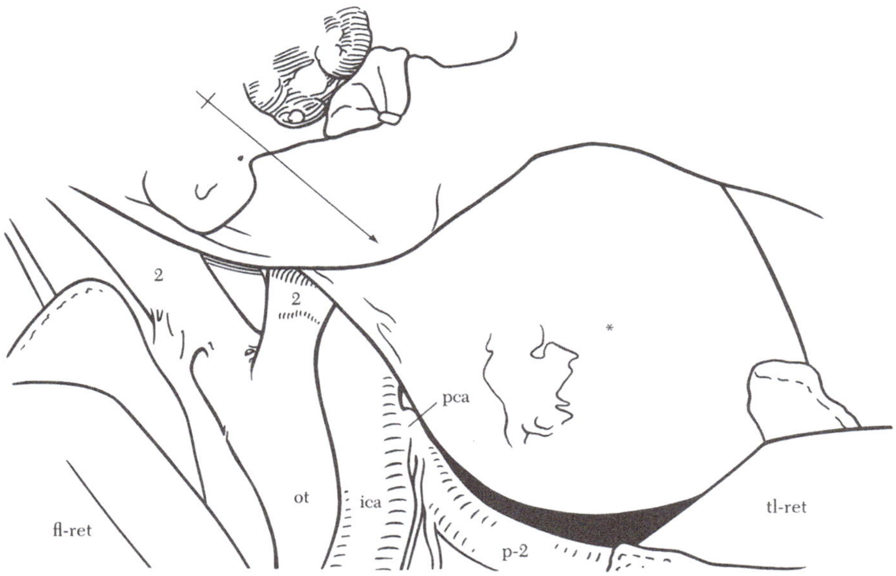

Fig. 36.55. Initial operative exposure of a giant csICAA (case 1) shown under low power (Zeiss magnification dial at No. 6). *, dura of cavernous sinus massively expanded upward, outward, and backward by underlying giant csICAA (Fig. 36.54); *single-crossed arrow*, anterior clinoid process; *tl-ret*, temporal lobe retractor; *p-2*, P-2 portion of posterior cerebral artery; *pca*, part of posterior communicating artery seen on end and hidden by the internal carotid artery (*ica*); *ot*, right optic tract; *fl-ret*, frontal lobe retractor; *2*, both optic nerves.

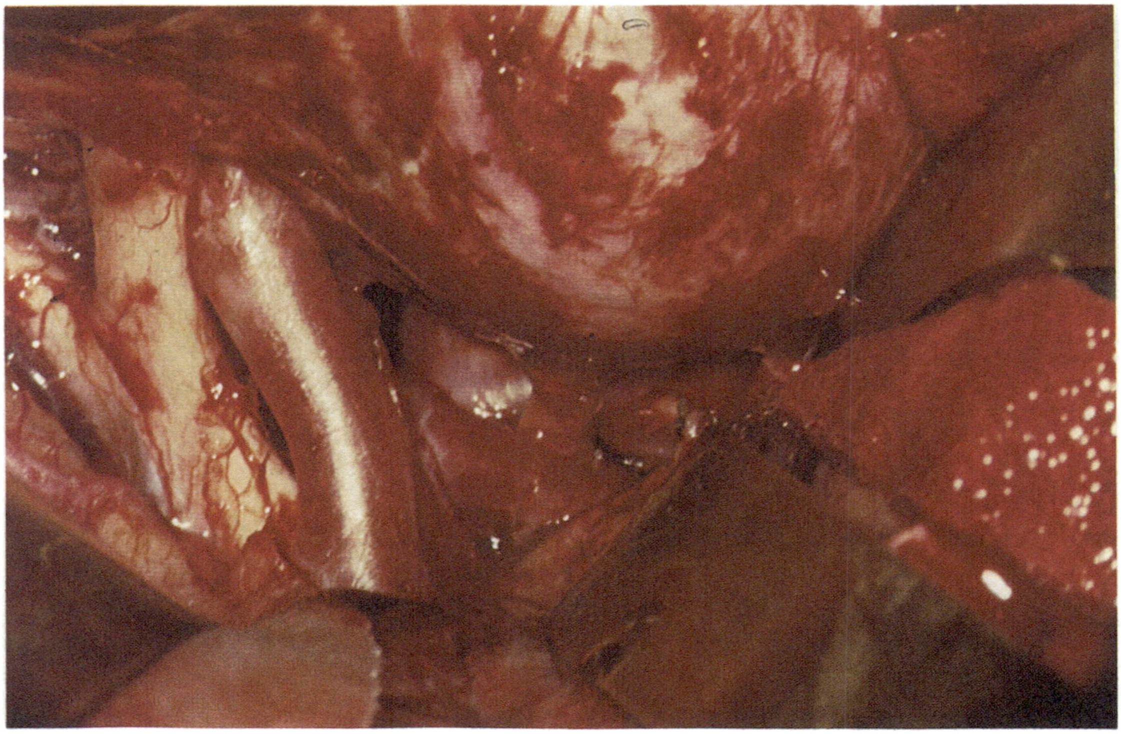

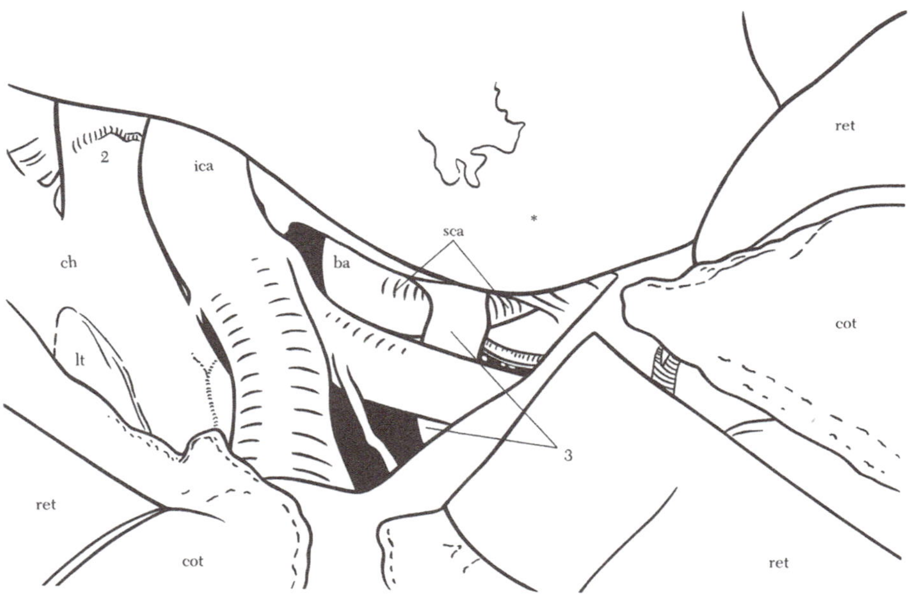

Fig. 36.56. Magnified view of Fig. 36.55. *, dura over mass of aneurysm; *ret*, retractors; *cot*, cottonoid strips; *3*, oculomotor nerve; *lt*, lamina terminalis; *ch*, optic chiasm; *2*, right optic nerve; *ica*, internal carotid artery exiting from cavernous sinus; *ba*, tip of basilar artery in interpeduncular cistern; *sca*, superior cerebellar artery behind oculomotor nerve. Note how oculomotor nerve (*3*) passes behind P-2 and enters cavernous sinus in a much more posterior position due to its displacement by the aneurysm.

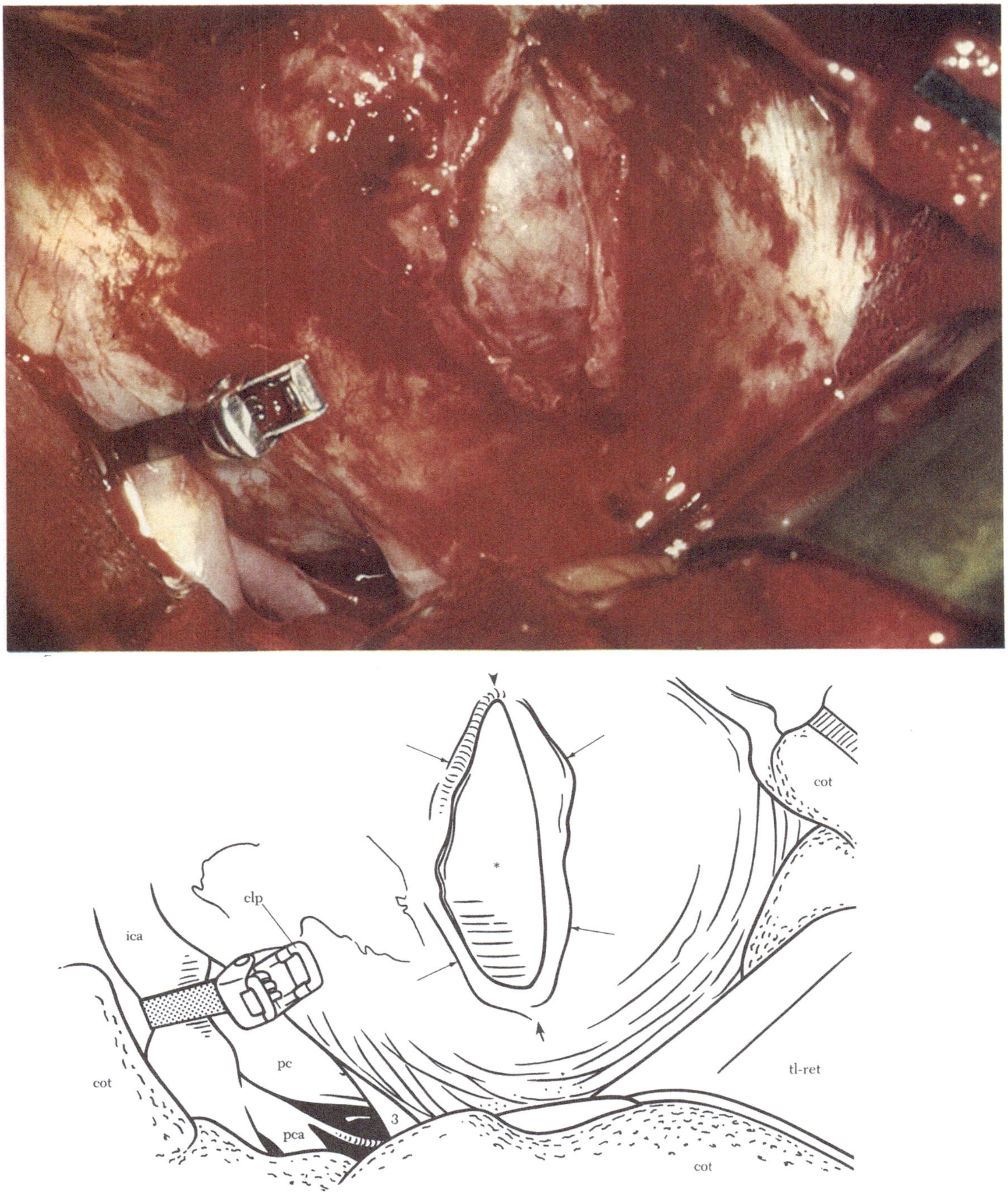

Fig. 36.57. Initial opening of dura forming compressed roof of cavernous sinus and aneurysm (case 2, photograph reversed). *, exposed wall of dome of csICAA; *arrows,* reflected dural edge after initial dural incision; *cot,* cottonoid strips; *tl-ret,* temporal lobe retractor; *3,* oculomotor nerve going under edge of tentorium; *pc,* posterior clinoid process; *pca,* posterior communicating artery; *ica,* internal carotid artery exiting from cavernous sinus; *clp,* Heifetz clip (while aneurysm temporarily trapped).

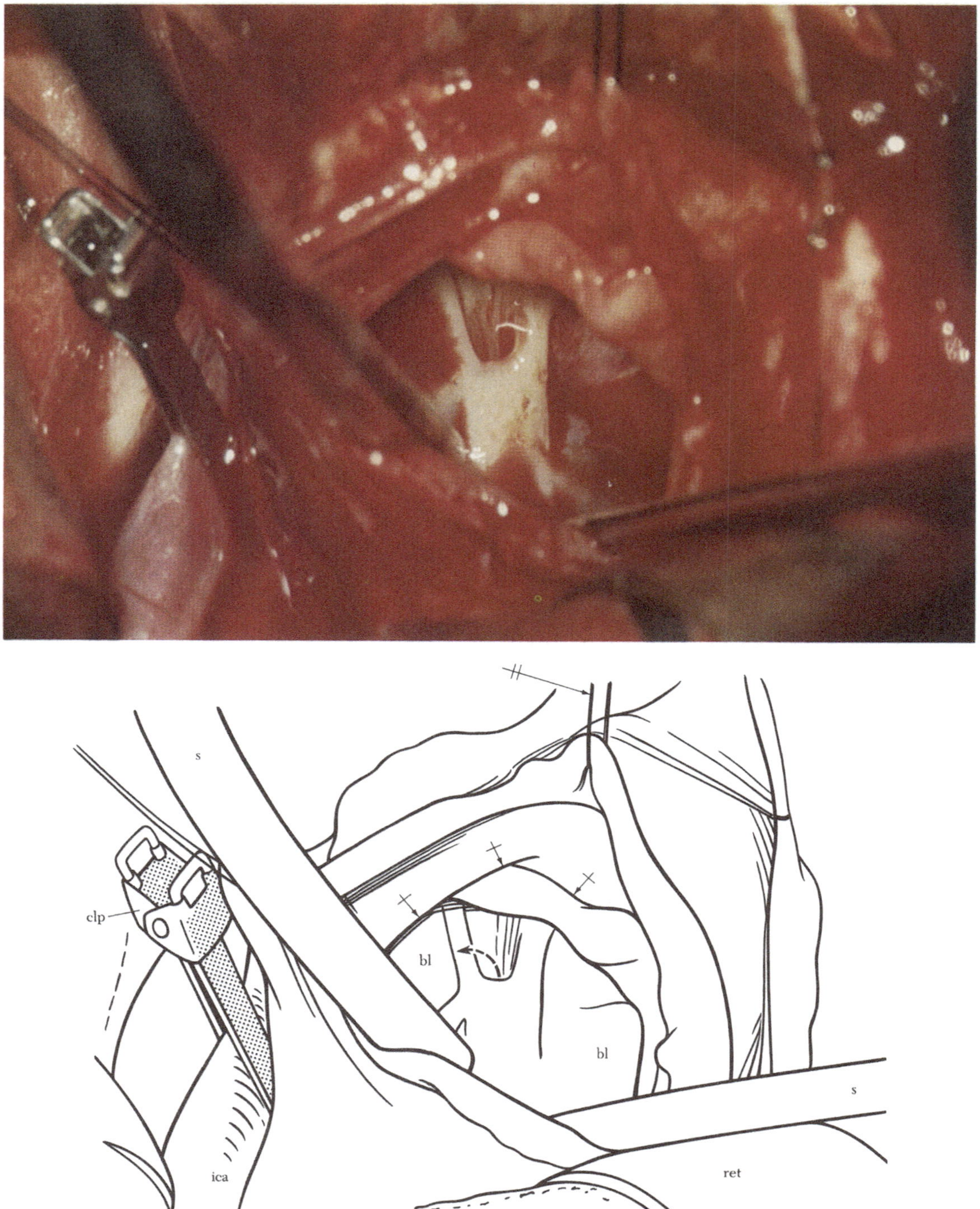

Fig. 36.58. Aneurysm opened. *s,* suction tubes; *single-crossed arrows,* edge of wall of aneurysm opening; *double-crossed arrow,* traction suture on dural roof of cavernous sinus; *ret,* retractor blade; *bl,* blood inside aneurysm; *ica,* internal carotid artery distal to temporary Heifetz clip (*clp*); *curved arrow,* pathway of blood out of proximal opening from internal carotid artery into aneurysm (distal exit higher up and hidden by anterior wall of aneurysm).

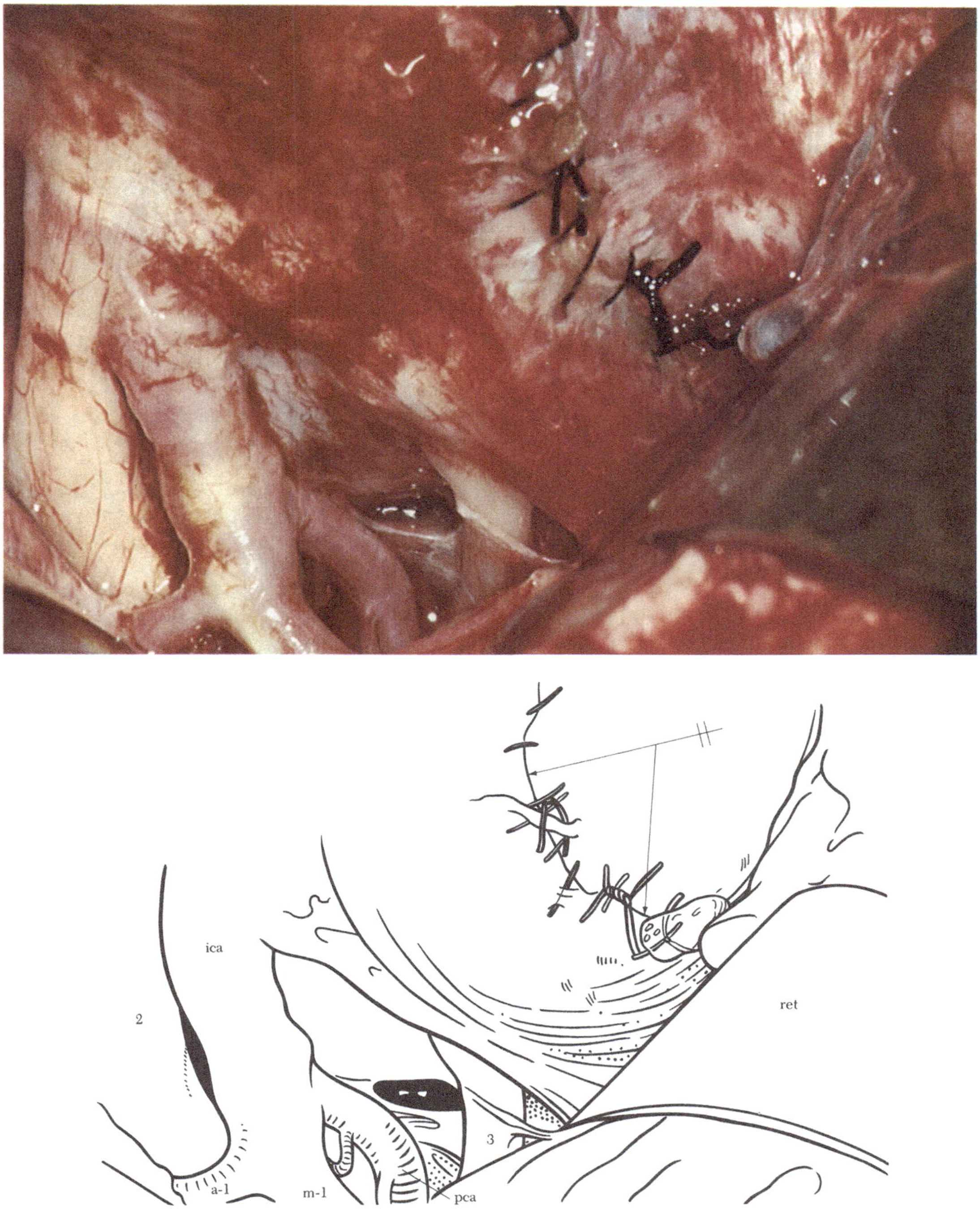

Fig. 36.59. Final closure of incision (*double-crossed arrow*) in cavernous sinus dural roof (and aneurysm wall covered by the dura). *ret,* retractor; *3,* oculomotor nerve; *pca,* posterior communicating artery; *m-1,* origin of M-1 artery; *a-1,* origin of A-1 artery; *2,* optic nerve; *ica,* internal carotid artery exiting from cavernous sinus.

oped PCoA and A-1 arteries, OA flow was preserved (reversed), and there were excellent arterial pulsations seen at surgery. Postoperatively, the blood pressure was maintained at a high level for a few days. Angiography revealed occlusion of the aneurysm and the ICA, but there was good collateral circulation, including circulation via the ophthalmic artery (which a trapping procedure would have obviated). Hopefully, in the future an internal graft-like stent may be utilized to maintain postoperative blood flow between the two separated openings of the ICA into the aneurysm.

Bibliography

1. Abbie AA: The clinical significance of the anterior choroidal artery. Brain 56:233–246, 1933
2. af Björkesten G, Troupp H: Changes in the size of intracranial arterial aneurysms. J Neurosurg 19:583–588, 1962
3. Allcock JM: Aneurysms. In Newton TH, Potts DG (eds.): Radiology of the Skull and Brain, Vol 2, Book 4. St. Louis, Mosby, 1974, pp. 2435–2489
4. Almeida GM, Shibata MK, Bianco E: Carotid-ophthalmic aneurysms. Surg Neurol 5:41–45, 1976
5. Alpers BJ, Berry RG, Paddison, RM: Anatomical studies of the circle of Willis in normal brain. Arch Neurol Psychiat 81:409–418, 1959
6. Archer CR, Silbert S: Infundibula may be clinically significant. Neuroradiology 15:247–251, 1978
7. Barr HWK, Blackwood W, Meadows SP: Intracavernous carotid aneurysms. A clinical-pathological report. Brain 94:607–622, 1971
8. Borghi PL, Romagnoli R, Monaco V: La dilatazione infundibulare dell'arteria communicante posteriore. Rilievi angiografici in 74 casi. Radiol Med (Torino) 55:913–922, 1969
9. Calmettes L, Déodati F, Arbus L, et al.: Volumineux anévrysme carotidien intracranien révélé par des manifestations oculaires. Rev Oto-Neuro-Ophtal 38:157–159, 1966
10. Dandy WE: Intracranial Arterial Aneurysms. New York, Hafner, 1944 [reprinted 1969]
11. Da Pian R, Pasqualin A, Scienza R: Direct microsurgical approach to aneurysms of the internal carotid bifurcation. Surg Neurol 13:27–37, 1980
12. Davis KR, New PFJ, Ojemann RG, et al.: Computed tomographic evaluation of hemorrhage secondary to intracranial aneurysm. Am J Roentgenol 127:143–153, 1976
13. Drake CG: On the surgical treatment of ruptured intracranial aneurysms. Clin Neurosurg 13:122–155, 1965
14. Drake CG, Vanderlinden RG: The late consequences of incomplete surgical treatment of cerebral aneurysms. J Neurosurg 27:226–238, 1967
15. Drake CG, Vanderlinden RG, Amacher AL: Carotid-choroidal aneurysms. J Neurosurg 29:32–36, 1968
16. Drake CG, Vanderlinden RG, Amacher AL: Carotid-ophthalmic aneurysms. J Neurosurg 29:24–31, 1968
17. Edelsohn L, Caplan L, Rosenbaum, AE: Familial aneurysms and infundibular widening. Neurology 22:1056–1060, 1972
18. Epstein F, Ransohoff J, Budzilovich GN: The clinical significance of junctional dilation of the posterior communicating artery. J Neurosurg 33:529–531, 1970
19. Flamm ES: Suction decompression of aneurysms. Technical note. J Neurosurg 54:275–276, 1981
20. Fox JL: Microsurgical exposure of intracranial aneurysms. J Microsurg 1:2–31, 1979
21. Fox JL: Multiple giant aneurysms. Surt Neurol 12:147–151, 1979
22. Fox JL, Albin MS, Bader DCH, et al.: Microsurgical treatment of neurovascular disease. Neurosurgery 3:285–337, 1978
23. Fox JL, Baiz TC, Jakoby RK: Differentiation of aneurism from infundibulum of the posterior communicating artery. J Neurosurg 21:135–138, 1964
24. Gryspeerdt GL: Angiographic studies of the blood flow in the circle of Willis. The value of various arterial compression tests. Acta Radiol [Diagn] 1(Part 1):298–313, 1963
25. Guidetti B, La Torre E: Carotid-ophthalmic aneurysms. A series of 16 cases treated by direct approach. Acta Neurochir 22:289–304, 1970
26. Guidetti B, La Torre E: Management of carotid-ophthalmic aneurysms. J Neurosurg 42:438–442, 1975
27. Hamby WB: Intracranial surgery for aneurysms. Progr Neurol Surg 3:1–65, 1969
28. Harwood-Nash DC, Fitz CR: Aneurysms. In Harwood-Nash DC, Fritz CR (eds.): Neuroradiology in Infants and Children, Vol. 3. St. Louis, Mosby, 1976, pp. 906–913
29. Hassler O, Saltzman G-F: Angiographic and histological changes in infundibular widening of the posterior communicating artery. Acta Radiol 1:321–327, 1963
30. Hassler O, Saltzman G-F: Histological changes in infundibular widening of the posterior communicating artery. A preliminary report. Acta Pathol Microbiol Scand 46:305–312, 1959
31. Kempe LG: Operative Neurosurgery, Vol. 1. Cranial, Cerebral, and Intracranial Vascular Disease. New York, Springer-Verlag, 1968, pp. 1–75, 203–214
32. Kodama N, Koshu K, Ebina T, et al.: Surgical

treatment of internal carotid bifurcation aneurysm. No To Shinkei 30:669–675, 1978
33. Kothandaram P, Dawson BH, Kruyt RC: Carotid-ophthalmic aneurysms. A study of 19 patients. J Neurosurg 34:544–548, 1971
34. McFadden JT: Aneurysm clips, J Neurosurg 46:129, 1977
35. McFadden JT: Metallurgical principles in neurosurgery. J Neurosurg 31:373–385, 1969
36. McFadden JT: Tissue reactions to standard neurosurgical metallic implants. J Neurosurg 36:598–603, 1972
37. Nutik S: Carotid paraclinoid aneurysms with intradural origin and intracavernous location. J Neurosurg 48:526–533, 1978
38. Okawara S: Aneurysm of the anterior choroidal artery. Brain Nerve (Tokyo) 19:1185–1192, 1967
39. Padget DH: The circle of Willis. Its embryology and anatomy. In Dandy WE (ed.): Intracranial Arterial Aneurysms. New York, Hafner, 1944, pp. 67–90 [reprinted 1969]
40. Parkinson D: Collateral circulation of the cavernous carotid artery: anatomy. Canad J Surg 7:251–268, 1964
41. Pertuiset B: Les anévrysmes de l'artère communicante postérieure. Diagnostic et indications thérapeutiques (sans la pathogénie). Presse Med 70:935–937, 1962
42. Pia HW: Classification of aneurysms of the internal carotid system. Acta Neurochir 40:5–31, 1978
43. Pool JL, Potts DG: Aneurysms and Arteriovenous Anomalies of the Brain. Diagnosis and Treatment. New York, Harper & Row, 1965
44. Punt J: Some observations on aneurysms of the proximal internal carotid artery. J Neurosurg 51:151–154, 1979
45. Salan A, Massazza G: La dilatazione infundibulare dell'arteria communicante posteriore. Uno studio di anatomia radiologica su 500 angiografie carotidee. Il Policlinico 71:953–959, 1964
46. Saltzman G-F: Circulation through the posterior communicating artery in different compression tests. A preliminary report. Acta Radiol 51:10–16, 1959
47. Saltzman G-F: Infundibular widening of the posterior communicating artery studied by carotid angiography. Acta Radiol 51:415–421, 1959
48. Selverstone B: Coating of intracranial aneurysms with nontoxic adherent plastics. In Schmidek HH, Sweet WH (eds.): Current Techniques in Operative Neurosurgery. New York, Grune & Stratton, 1977, pp. 31–40
49. Sengupta RP, Gryspeerdt GL, Hankinson J: Carotid-ophthalmic aneurysms. J Neurol Neurosurg Psychiat 39:837–853, 1976
50. Sengupta RP, Lassman LP, de Moraes AA, et al.: Treatment of internal carotid bifurcation aneurysms by direct surgery. J Neurosurg 43:343–351, 1975
51. Stehbens WE: Aneurysms and anatomical variation of cerebral arteries. Arch Pathol 75:45–64, 1963
52. Stehbens WE: Histopathology of cerebral aneurysms. Arch Neurol 8:272–285, 1963
53. Stehbens WE: Ultrastructure of aneurysms. Arch Neurol 32:798–807, 1975
54. Taveras JM, Wood EH: Diagnostic Neuroradiology, Vol. 2, end ed. Baltimore, Williams & Wilkins, 1976, pp. 585, 855–857, 911–952, 1021–1045
55. Thiébaut F, Wackenheim A, Vrousos C: La dilatation infundibulaire de l'artère communicante postérieure. J Radiol Electrol 44:768–770, 1963
56. Thurel C, Rey A, Thiébaut JB, et al.: Anévrysmes carotid-ophtalmiques. Neuro-chirurgie (Paris) 20:25–39, 1974
57. VanderArk GD, Kempe LG, Kobrine A: Classification of internal carotid aneurysms as a basis for surgical approach. Neurochirurgia (Stuttgart) 15:81–85, 1972
58. Waga S, Morikawa A: Aneurysm developing on the infundibular widening of the posterior communicating artery. Surg Neurol 11:125–127, 1979
59. Watanabe M, In S, Kuramoto S: Junctional dilation of the posterior communicating artery. Neurol Surg (Tokoyo) 3:917–924, 1975
60. Wollschlaeger G, Wollschlaeger PB, Lucas FV, et al.: Experience and result with postmortem cerebral angiography performed as routine procedure of the autopsy. Am J Roentgenol 101:68–87, 1967
61. Yaşargil MG, Boehm WB, Ho REM: Microsurgical treatment of cerebral aneurysms at the bifurcation of the internal carotid artery. Acta Neurochir 41:61–72, 1978
62. Yaşargil MG, Fox JL: The microsurgical approach to intracranial aneurysms. Surg. Neurol 3:7–14, 1975
63. Yaşargil MG, Gasser JC, Hodosh RM, et al.: Carotid-ophthalmic aneurysms: direct microsurgical approach. Surg Neurol 8:155–165, 1977
64. Yaşargil MG, Kasdaglis K, Jain KK, et al.: Anatomical observations of the subarachnoid cisterns of the brain during surgery. J Neurosurg 44:298–302, 1976
65. Yaşargil MG, Smith RD: Surgery on the carotid system in the treatment of hemorrhagic stroke. In Thompson RH, Green JR (eds.): Advances in Neurology, Vol. 16. Stroke. New York, Raven Press, 1977, pp. 181–209
66. Yaşargil MG, Yonas H, Gasser JC: Anterior choroidal artery aneurysms: their anatomy and surgical significance. Surg Neurol 9:129–138, 1978
67. Yoshimoto T, Suzuki J: Surgical treatment of an aneurysm on the funnel-shaped bulge of the posterior communicating artery. Case report. J Neurosurg 41:377–379, 1974

37

Technique of Aneurysm Surgery

IV. Middle Cerebral Artery Aneurysms

The early treatment of middle cerebral artery aneurysms (MCAA) was associated with a high incidence of mortality and morbidity (2). This was related in part to (a) the frequent intracerebral hematoma; (b) the necessity for separation of and/or dissection into the frontal and temporal lobes; and (c) the close relationship of the parent arteries and lateral lenticulostriate vessels to basal ganglia, internal capsule, optic radiations, and cortical zones concerned with motor, sensory, and speech activity. The results began to improve in the 1950s (4).

The vast majority of MCAA arise at the M-1 bifurcation. They can project in most directions such as laterally (Fig. 37.1), forward (Fig. 37.2), upward (Fig. 37.3), or downward (Fig. 37.4) (1). Backward projections certainly occur, but medial projections are uncommon. Figure 37.5 is an angiogram of an unusual MCAA arising from M-1 at the anterior temporal artery origin. Uncommon MCAA sites are at M-2 or M-3 bifurcations or on more distal branches. Aneurysms at more distal sites commonly are associated with infection (mycotic), cancer (oncotic), or other associated conditions. In such cases their surgical or nonsurgical therapy must relate also to the treatment of the associated disease or anomaly.

Of vital concern are the MCA perforators, or lateral lenticulostriate arteries. They are not readily seen at surgery, for they arise on the back surface of the M-1 and proximal M-2 arteries, these arteries and the aneurysm obscuring the view of the perforators. There are many variations in the numbers and patterns of lenticulostriate vessel origins, which must be preserved. These M-1 perforators often arise in multiple sets on the undersurface of the M-1 artery. Each set contains two to five small arteries passing into the frontal lobe and a smaller number passing into the temporal lobe. One set, which arises at the M-1 artery bifurcation, is often hidden by the aneurysm. The temporal polar and anterior temporal arteries also arise from the M-1 artery, the latter often at the M-1 bifurcation.

The M-1 artery usually *bifurcates* into the two main trunks (5): (a) the superior (frontal) M-2 trunk sends ascending branches to the frontal lobe and central zones; and (b) the inferior (temporal) M-2 trunk sends out middle and posterior temporal branches before dividing into posterior parietal and angular branches. Not infrequently the M-1 artery terminates in a *trifurcation*. The additional trunk may be the anterior temporal artery which, instead of arising proximally from M-1, occasionally may originate at the M-1 termination. Or one of the more distal MCA branches may originate instead at the M-1 termination.

The Surgical Exposure

As is done for patients with aneurysms arising at the ICA bifurcation, patients with MCAA also should have the head considerably extended during the frontotemporal exposure. This allows the surgeon to view the MCAA somewhat perpendicular to its main axis. Otherwise the dome may obscure the neck of the aneurysm. This attitude of the brain also permits a more comfortable opening of the sylvian fissure in the frontotemporal approach

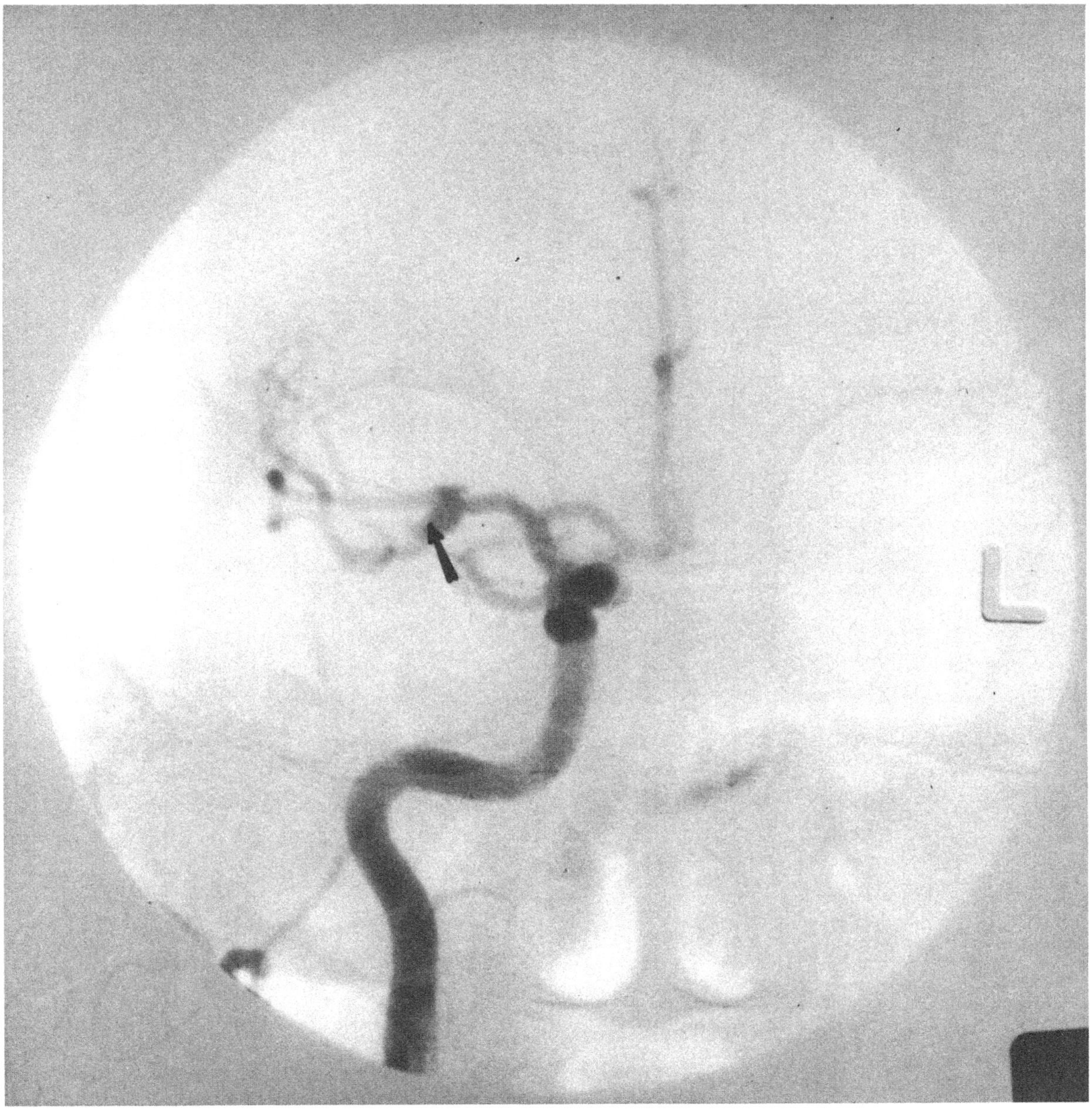

Fig. 37.1. Frontal transorbital view of laterally projecting MCAA (*arrow*). Note short M-1 segment.

(but makes sphenoid wing removal more awkward).

In most instances, we first open the sylvian fissure superficially and then begin the M-1 dissection by following it up from the ICA bifurcation. This permits proximal control of M-1 (with temporary clips if needed) should the aneurysm rupture. We raise the BP in cases where M-1 is deliberately, temporarily occluded. In cases (as in Fig. 37.6) where the ICA is short, M-1 is short, the sylvian fissure is easily opened, adhesions are minimal, and edema is absent, the aneurysm can be isolated with relative ease. In other cases (as in Figs. 37.7 and 37.8) where the ICA is elongated, M-1 is long, the frontal and temporal lobes are tightly adherent, and/or brain edema exists, then exposure of the aneurysm may require a more prolonged, meticulous, and difficult dissection.

If the sylvian fissure is already a prominent

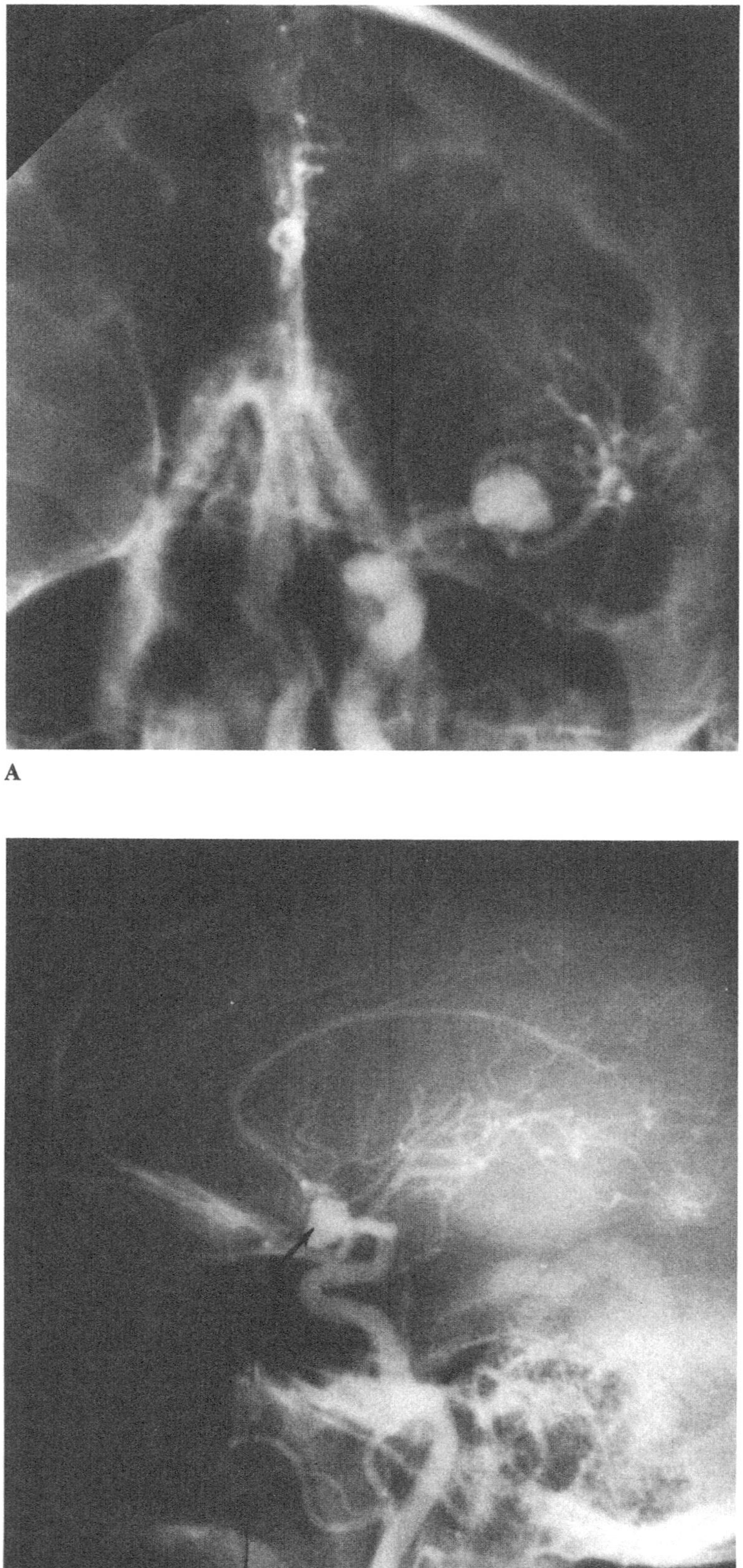

A

B

Fig. 37.2. Frontal transorbital view (A) and lateral view (B) of laterally and anteriorly projecting MCAA. Note short M-1 segment on frontal view.

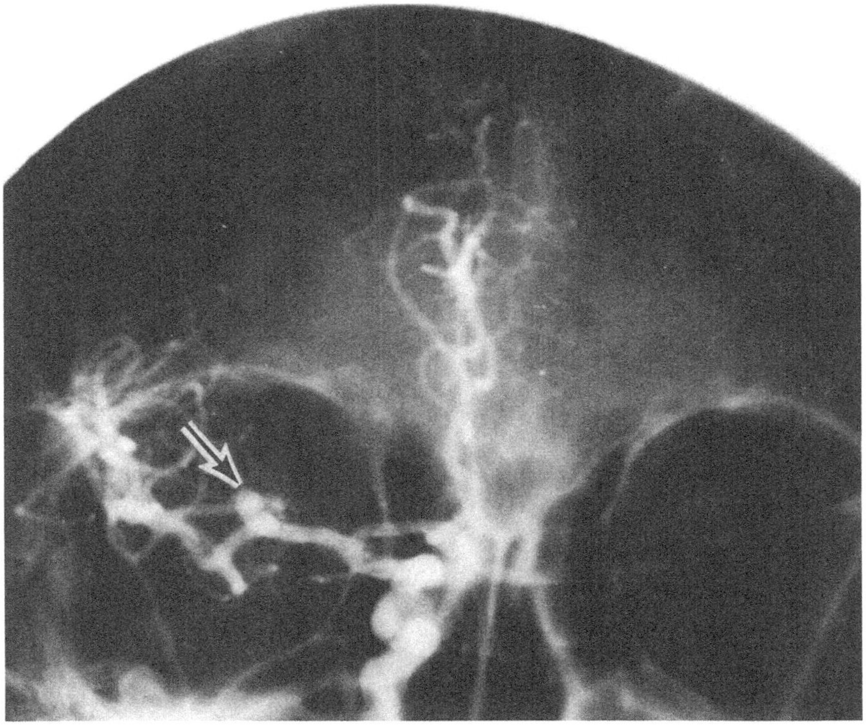

Fig. 37.3. Frontal transorbital view of superiorly projecting MCAA (*arrow*).

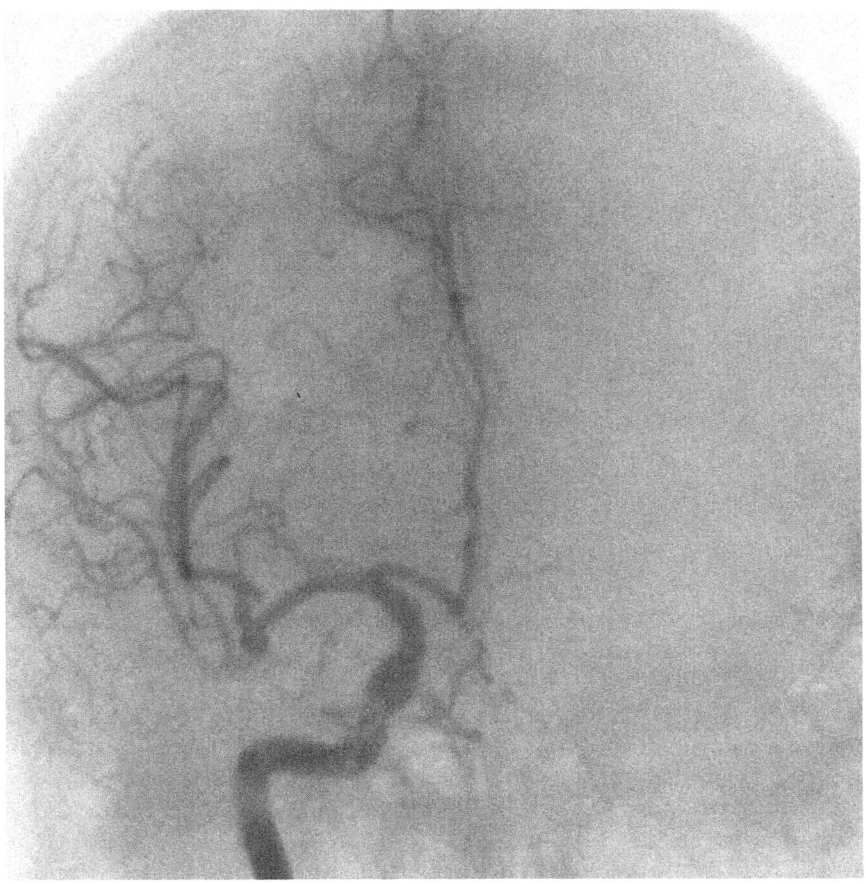

Fig. 37.4. Frontal view of inferiorly projecting MCAA. Note fairly long M-1 segment.

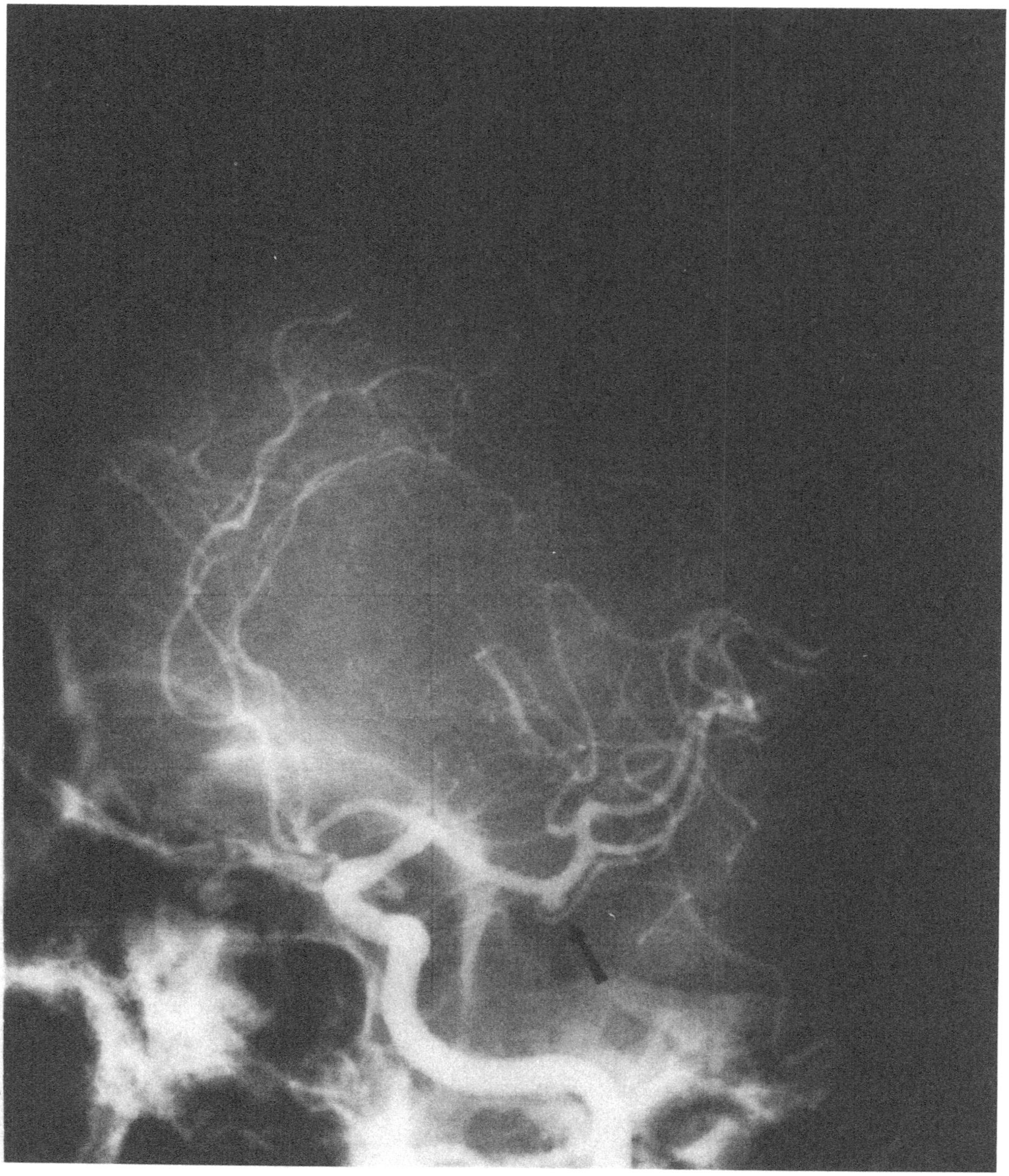

Fig. 37.5. Oblique view of MCAA arising from M-1 at take-off of the anterior temporal branch. The M-1 segment is unusually long.

space due to contained hematoma or due to relative cerebral atrophy, one instead can easily follow the fissure from outside inward to the aneurysm. Removal of the superior temporal gyrus is rarely necessary. A word of caution regarding opening a sylvian fissure distended by clot: cutting the tense arachnoid between the frontal and temporal lobes may suddenly release pressure on the aneurysm, resulting in MCAA rupture. Figures 37.9–37.11 demon-

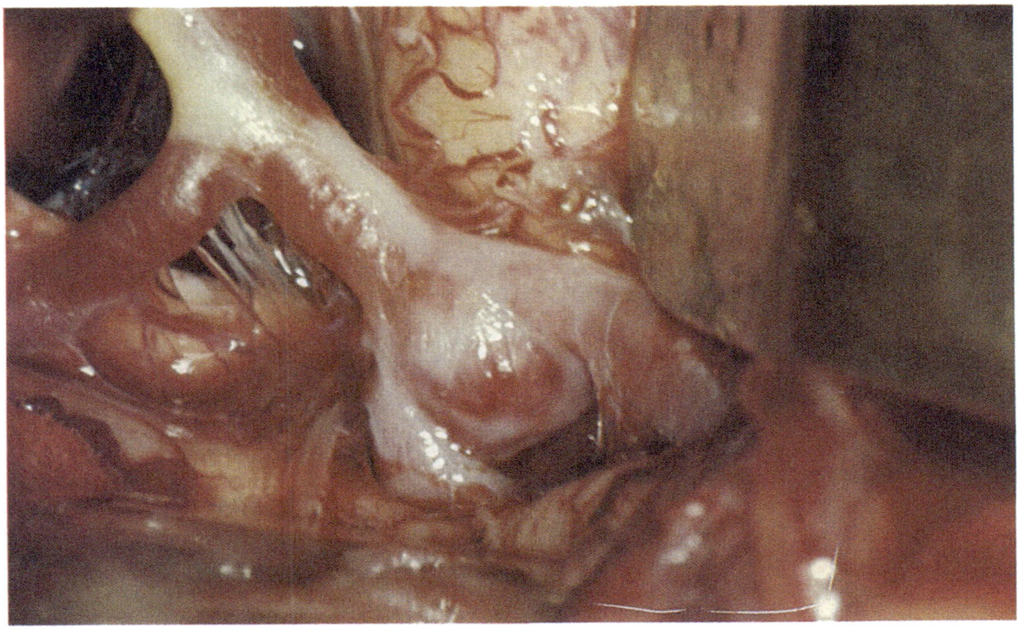

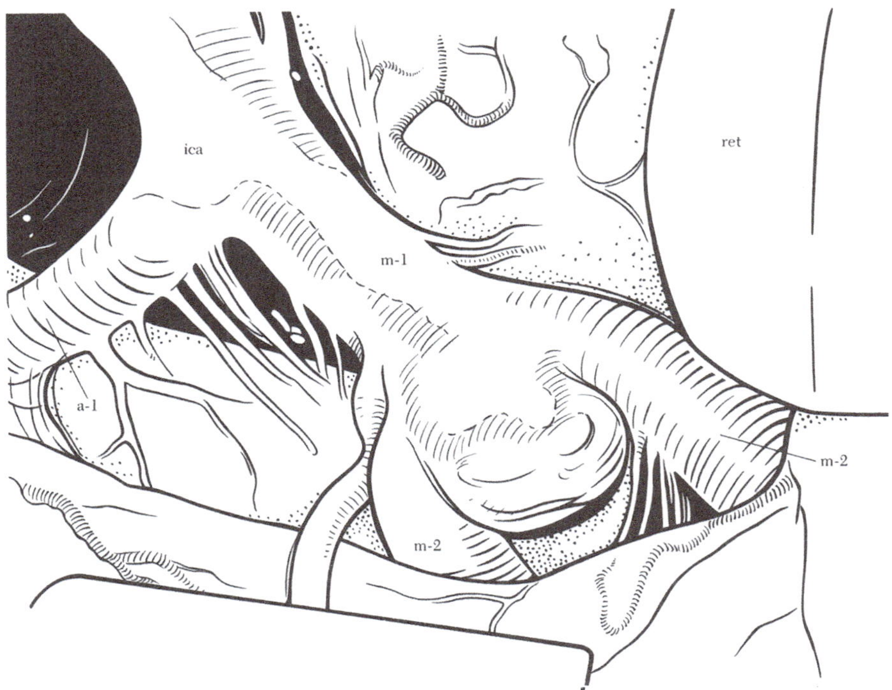

Fig. 37.6. Small right middle cerebral artery aneurysm. *ica,* bifurcation of the short internal carotid artery; *ret,* retractor on the temporal lobe; *a-1,* A-1 segment with leash of perforators going into the anterior perforated substance of the frontal lobe; *m-1,* M-1 segment with perforators (most hidden by parent artery); *m-2,* temporal (above) and frontal (below) M-2 segments of the middle cerebral artery flanking the aneurysm. From Fox JL: ref. 3.

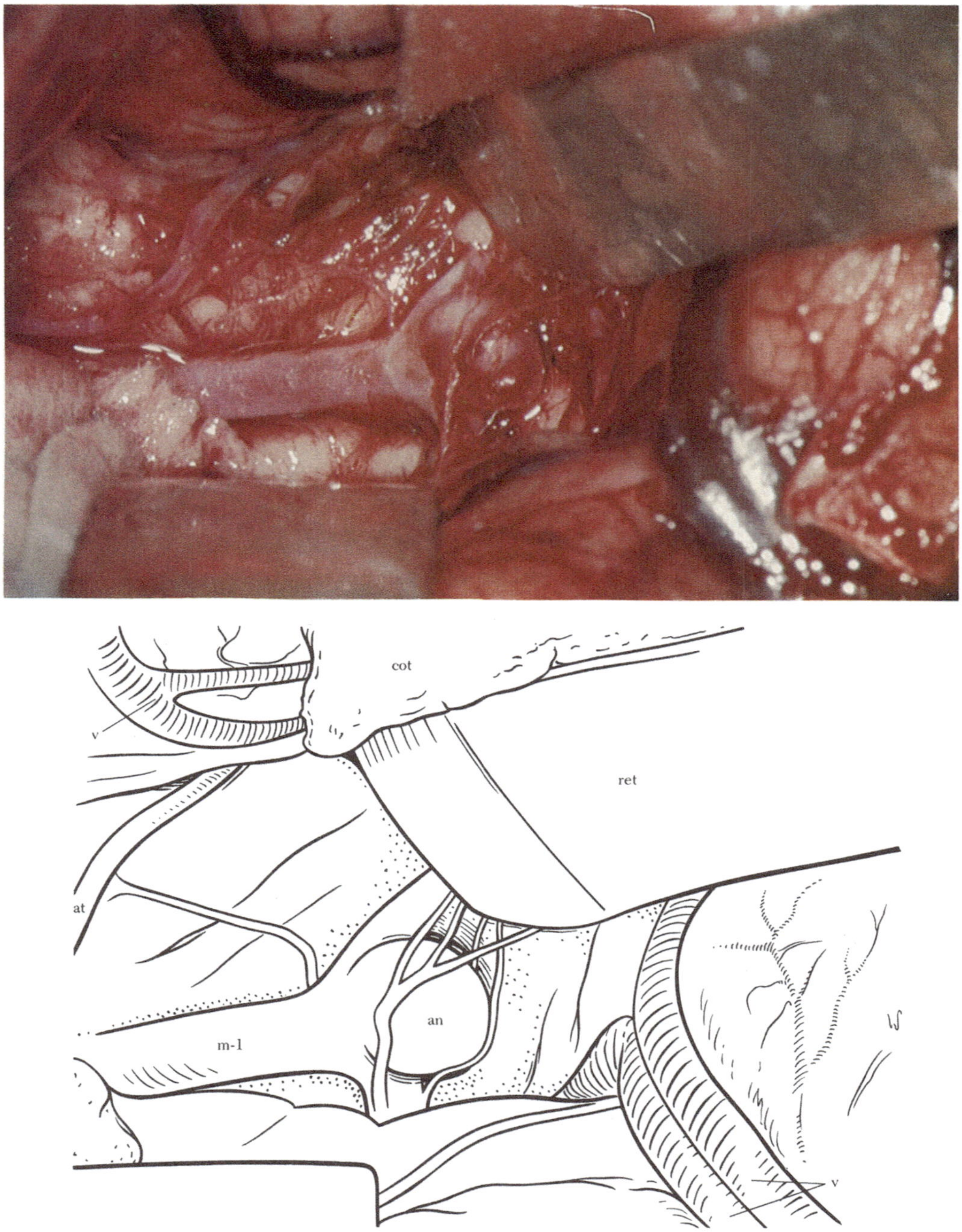

Fig. 37.7. Small middle cerebral artery aneurysm at the end of the long right M-1 artery (*m-1*). *ret,* retractor on the temporal lobe; *cot,* cottonoid sponge; *v,* veins; *an,* aneurysm flanked by M-2 temporal division (above) and M-2 frontal division (below). Note the perforators stuck to the dome of the aneurysm. *at,* anterior temporal artery (arises from the M-1 segment). From Fox JL: ref. 3.

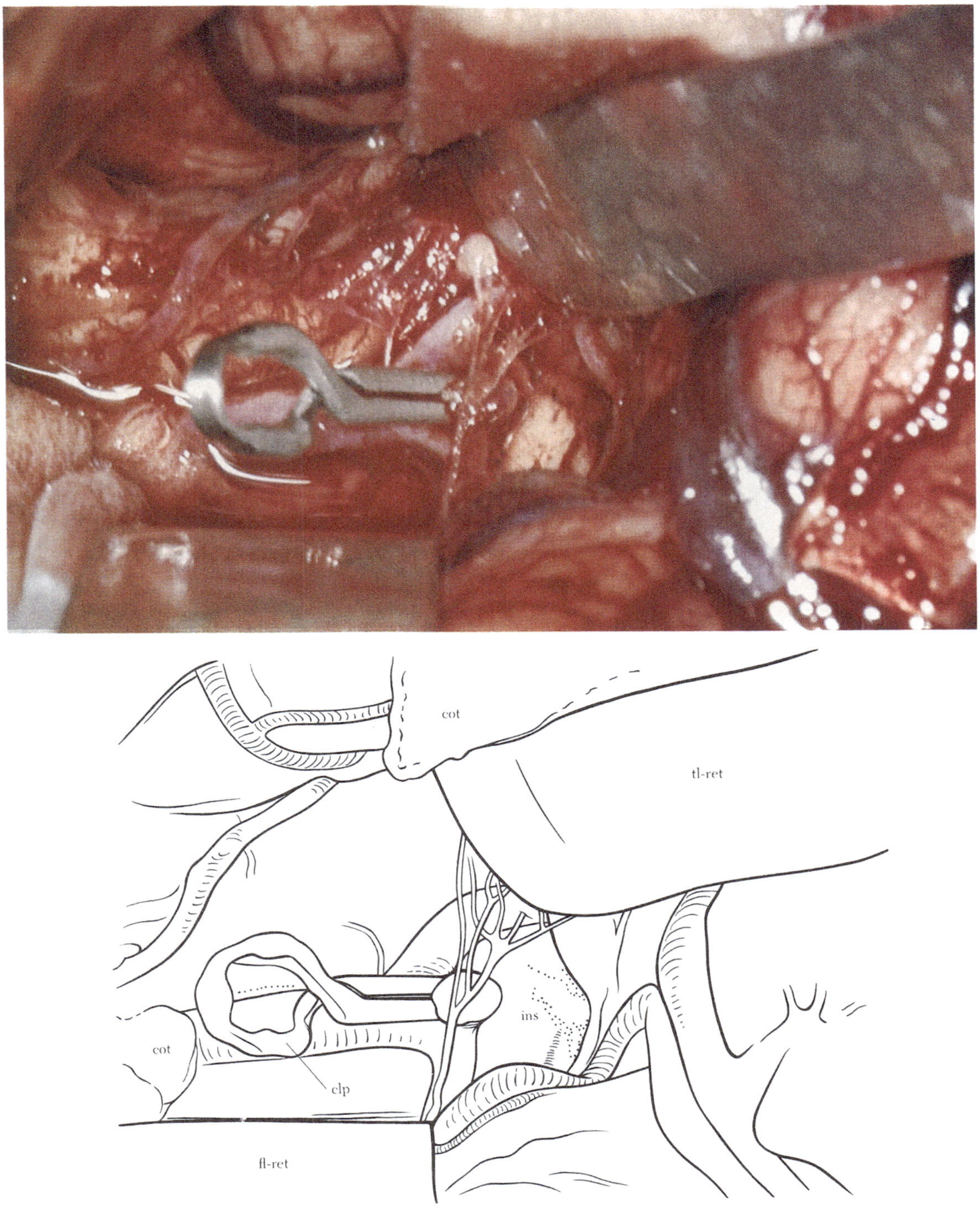

Fig. 37.8. Same case as in Fig. 37.7 after aneurysm was clipped. *cot,* cottonoid strips; *tl-ret,* temporal lobe retractor; *ins,* portion of insula (island of Reil); *clp,* shank of Yaşargil aneurysm clip; *fl-ret,* frontal lobe retractor. In this case the tiny arteries stuck to the dome of the aneurysm were left unmolested and the circumstances did not require their dissection from the dome before application of the clip to the neck.

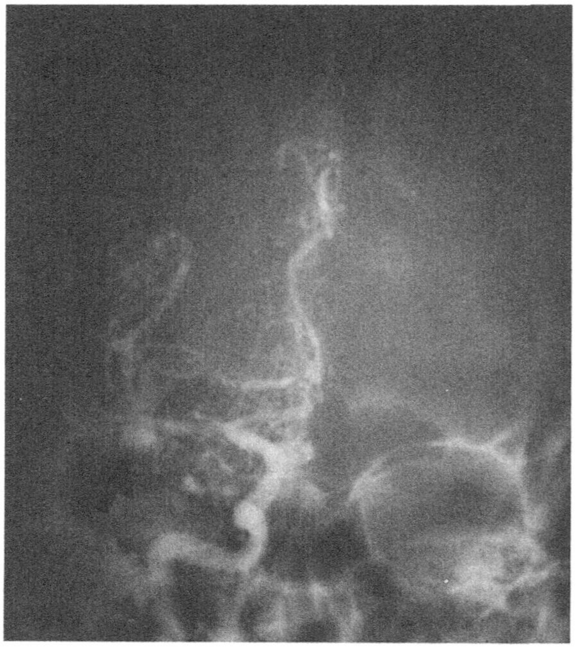

A

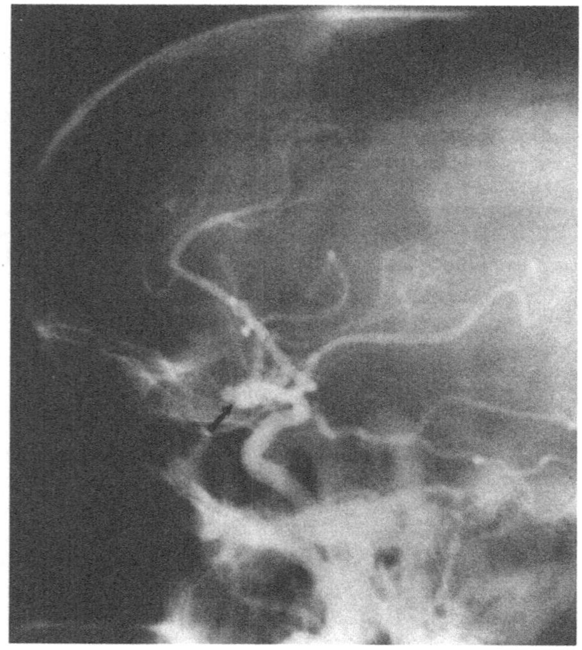

B

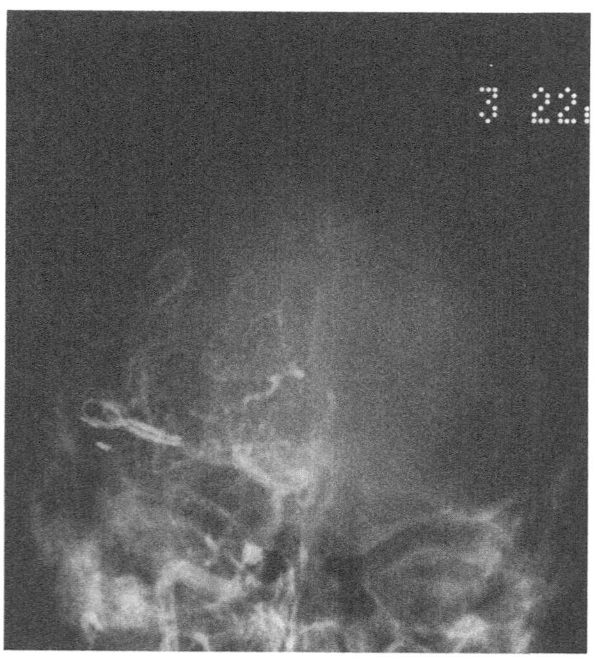

C

Fig. 37.9. A Prominent right MCAA (*arrow*) seen in frontal view of angiogram (same case as in Figs. 37.10 and 37.11). **B** Lateral view of same aneurysm (*arrow*) projecting forward and downward. **C** Postoperative angiogram showing occlusion of the aneurysm and preservation of parent arteries (some vasospasm apparent). The patient recovered nicely.

strate a large, multiloculated middle cerebral aneurysm. This was approached directly through the lateral sylvian fissure because of surrounding hematoma. Each blister or loculus was shrunken by bipolar electrocoagulation before the clips were applied. Although the aneurysm could have been encased in plastic, the above technique effectively isolated the aneurysm from its parent vessel and the perforators (Fig. 37.9C).

Aneurysms which are located on more distal M-2 or M-3 bifurcations and still lie within the sylvian fissure (especially if the fissure is not opened by clot or brain atrophy) can be particularly difficult to approach and isolate. Such MCAA will lie near or upon the island of Reil (insula) and be encased with vital areas of juxtaposed frontal and temporal lobes. An example is shown in the angiogram of Fig. 37.12. This small ruptured aneurysm was missed during the first craniotomy because we did not expose deeply and posteriorly enough into the fissure. An intraoperative angiogram would have helped. Instead we found a 2-mm aneurysm more proximally, covered it with cotton, and mistakenly assumed it was the culprit. Postoperative angiography (Fig. 37.12) demonstrated persistence of the aneurysm, which was reoperated and successfully clipped.

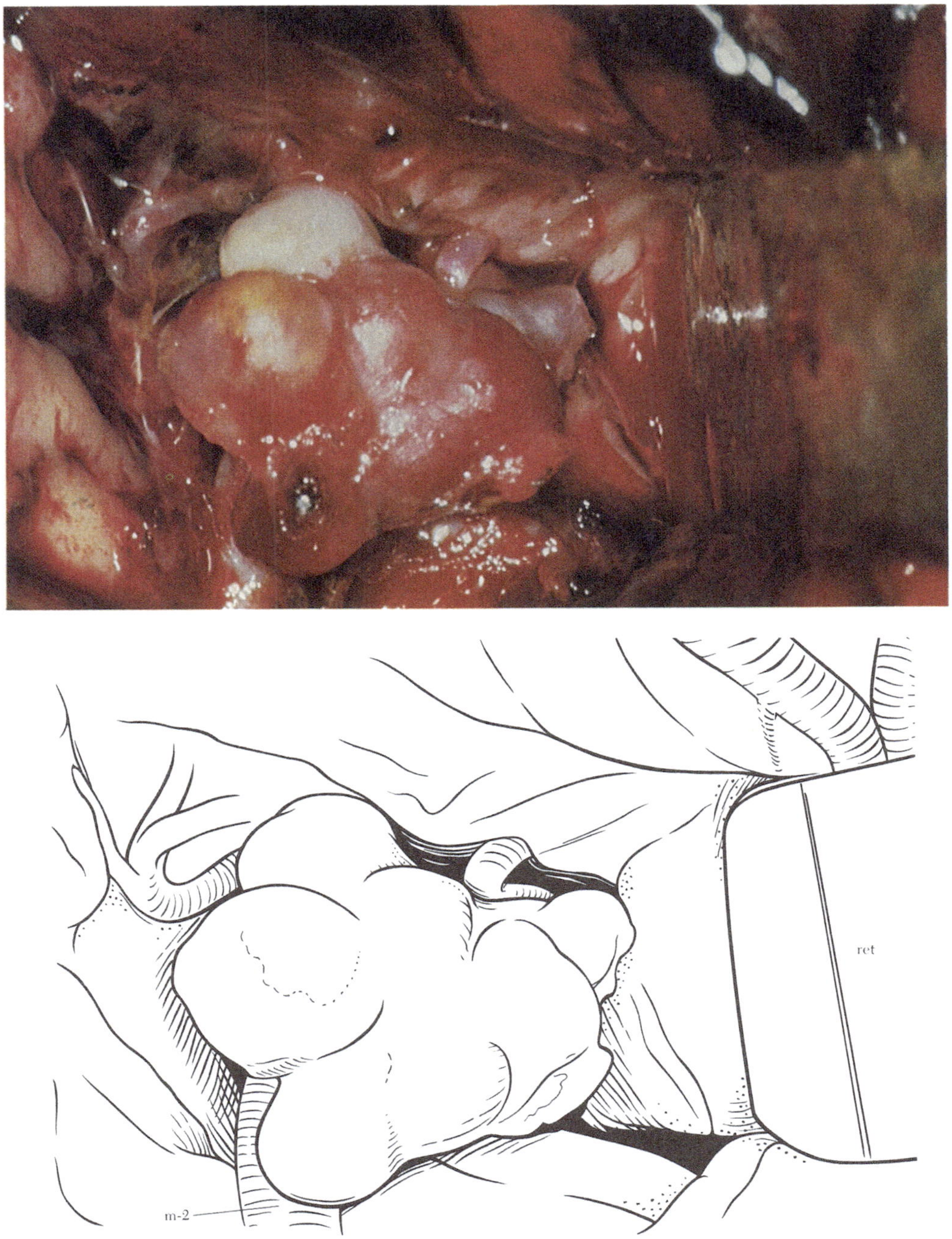

Fig. 37.10. Right middle cerebral artery aneurysm with six or seven locules. M-1 and temporal M-2 arteries are hidden. *m-2,* frontal M-2 artery; *ret,* retractor on the temporal lobe. The area was encased in hematoma. From Fox JL: ref. 3.

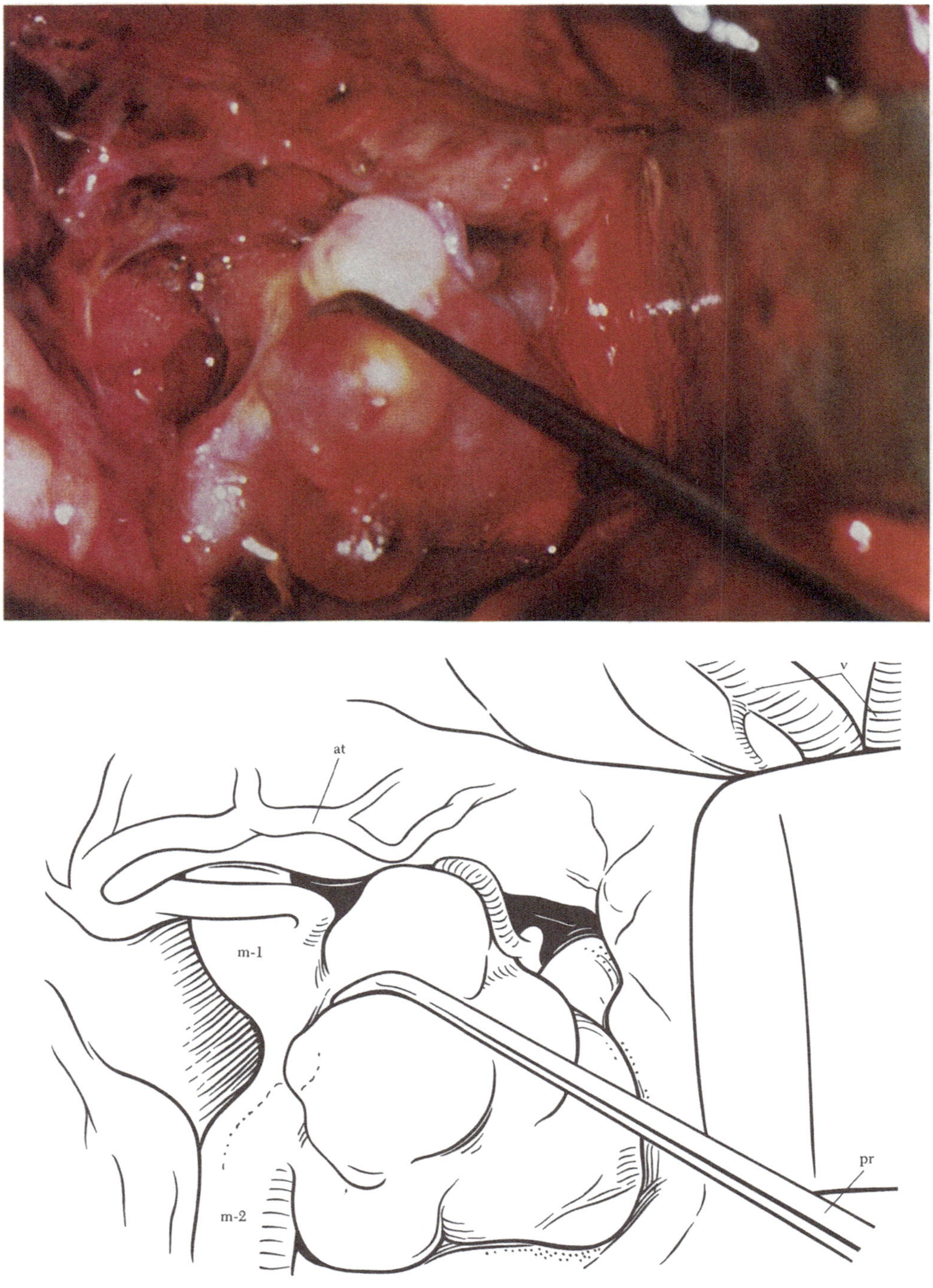

Fig. 37.11. Aneurysm shown in Figs. 37.9 and 37.10 retracted by probe (*pr*) to expose the M-1 segment (*m-1*) and the frontal M-2 origin (*m-2*). *at*, anterior temporal artery; *v*, veins on the temporal lobe. From Fox JL: ref. 3.

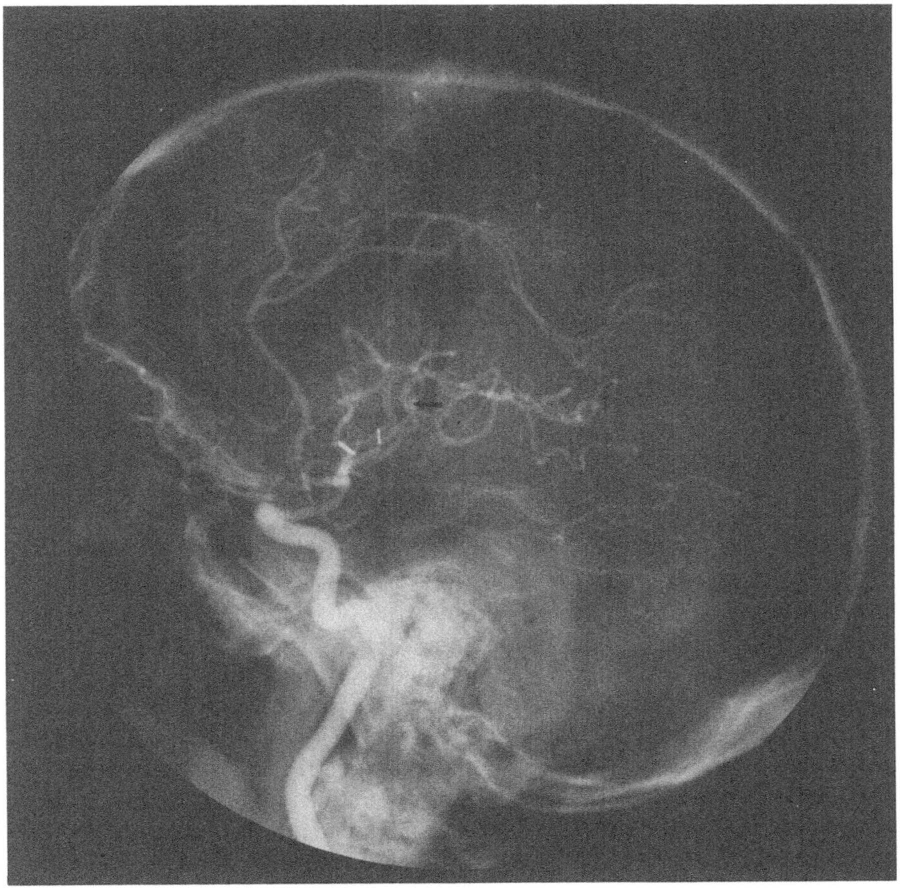

Fig. 37.12. Lateral view of angiogram after first craniotomy to clip the left MCAA (*arrow*). See text for details. The anterior, larger metal clip marked the microaneurysm covered with cotton. The posterior, smaller metal clip marked the posterior limit of the first dissection along the insula. The aneurysm (*arrow*) was later successfully clipped.

Bibliography

1. Allcock JM: Aneurysms. In Newton TH, Potts DG (eds.): Radiology of the Skull and Brain, Vol. 2, Book 4. St. Louis, Mosby, 1974, pp. 2435–2489
2. Dandy WE: Intracranial Arterial Aneurysms. New York, Hafner, 1944 [reprinted 1969]
3. Fox JL: Microsurgical exposure of intracranial aneurysms. J Neurosurg 1:2–31, 1979
4. Höök O, Norlén G: Aneurysms of the middle cerebral artery. A report of 80 cases. Acta Chir Scand(Suppl)235:1–39, 1958
5. Yaşargil MG, Smith RD: Surgery on the carotid system in the treatment of hemorrhagic stroke. In Thompson RH, Green JR (eds.): Advances in Neurology, Vol. 16. Stroke. New York, Raven Press, 1977, pp. 181–209

38

Technique of Aneurysm Surgery

V. Basilar Artery Aneurysms

This chapter is an extension of the preceding Chapters 34–37 on the frontotemporal route to anterior circulation aneurysms. The frontotemporal (transsylvian) approach to basilar artery aneurysms (BAA), especially the bifurcation basilar artery aneurysms (bBAA) and basilar artery aneurysms arising at the superior cerebellar artery take-off (scaBAA), is illustrated in this chapter. The more commonly used subtemporal approach and other approaches used by other surgeons are described in Chapter 29.

This author (JLF) has changed from the subtemporal to the frontotemporal route after carrying out the frontotemporal approach on patients with multiple aneurysms, patients in whom the anterior circulation and basilar artery aneurysms were successfully exposed and clipped via the same craniotomy. Also the ability to see the bBAA *en face* on its rostroventral aspect is impressive (see below). The advantages and disadvantages of the frontotemporal approach, which is being used more widely now than before, are detailed in Chapter 29.

The BA normally tends to enlarge at its bifurcation (14). The preaneurysmal stage may begin as a slight outpouching (Fig. 38.1) and expand into a bBAA as the years progress. A number of authors, most notably Charles Drake, have written on the surgical anatomy and treatment of aneurysms at or near the basilar artery bifurcation (1,3–11,13–15,17–22). The bBAA tends to point (a) rostrally as a direct continuation of the BA (Figs. 38.2 and 38.3); (b) upward toward the midbrain-thalamic junction (Fig. 38.4); (c) backward toward the midbrain and between the cerebral peduncles (Fig. 38.5); (d) anteriorly (rare) over the dorsum sellae (Fig. 38.6); or (e) laterally (rare). The neck of the aneurysm is an extension of the BA and tends to be broad. The aneurysm may be elongated, bulbous and overlapping the P-1 arteries, or enlarged into a spherical or bilobed mass which incorporates the P-2 arteries in its expanding neck. If there is a marked difference in the size of the two P-1 arteries, the aneurysm tends to arise on the side of the larger P-1 (21).

The termination of the BA may lie lower down on the dorsum sellae, in which case one or both P-1 arteries initially will course rostrally around the side of the aneurysm. In this situation P-1 and its posterior thalamoperforators may be adherent to the dome of the aneurysm. A rostrally projecting aneurysm arising at the level of the posterior clinoid processes may have no adherent posterior thalamoperforators; but if the aneurysm is large and bulbous, it may extend laterally to the anterior thalamoperforators coming off the PCoA. A superiorly and posteriorly projecting bBAA may have perforators stuck to its back wall. These tiny arteries arise from P-1 and the termination of the BA. Such perforators are more difficult to see by the frontotemporal route, but they must be cleared away from the aneurysm and clip application area.

Figure 38.7 diagrams various relationships of the basilar artery termination to the dorsum sellae and third ventricle. The bBAA is an extension of the direction of this termination. Notice the height of the basilar artery bifurcation. Typically it is at or just above the dorsum sellae. It may be higher and encroach on the mammil-

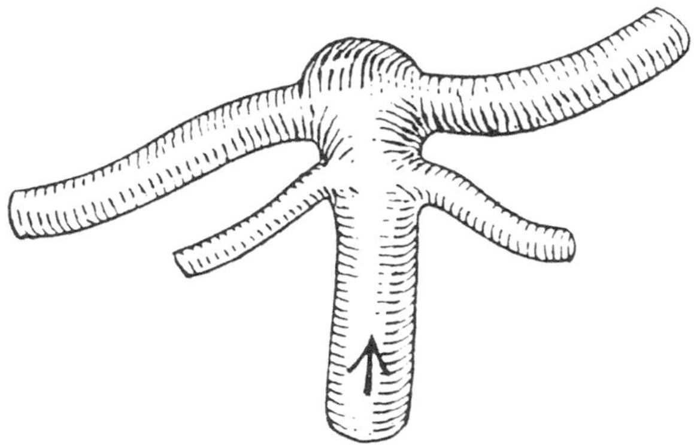

Fig. 38.1. Diagram of basilar artery examined at autopsy. Note outpouching of basilar artery tip between the two horizontal posterior cerebral arteries in this 42-mm human embryo. Sugar (16) described this as "surely the earliest 'berry aneurysm' known!" From Bremer JL: ref. 2.

lary bodies or even push into the floor of the third ventricle. Greater brain retraction is needed to visualize a highly placed BA termination. Occasionally the BA termination is below the top of the dorsum sellae. In such cases, the posterior clinoid process may partially obstruct the view of the neck of the aneurysm.

The Surgical Exposure

Bifurcation Basilar Artery Aneurysms

The reader should reexamine Figs. 34.3–34.11 to review the surgical exposure to this point. The patient's head is in the standard position previously described in Chapter 34. Basically this is a transsylvian approach and requires maximum and meticulous opening of the sylvian fissure opposite a well–drilled-down sphenoid wing. The ICA bifurcation, M-1, and A-1 will be exposed and clearly visualized in most cases. Adequate exposure of the upper basilar

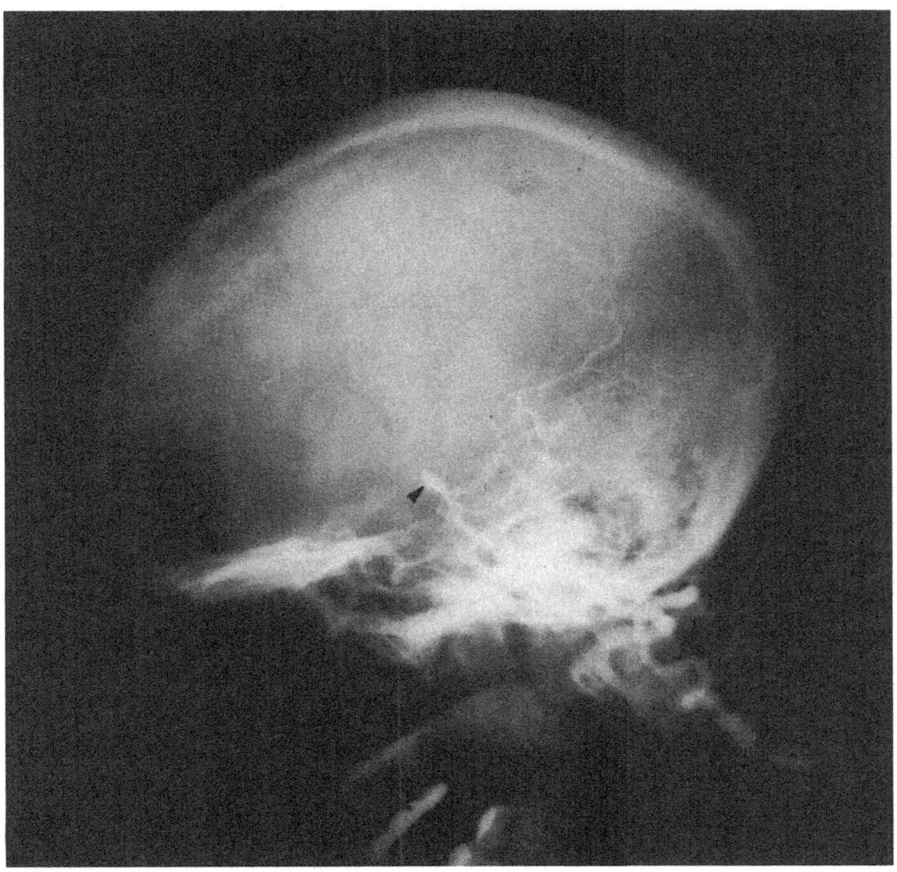

Fig. 38.2. Lateral angiographic view of a rostrally projecting bBAA (*arrowhead*).

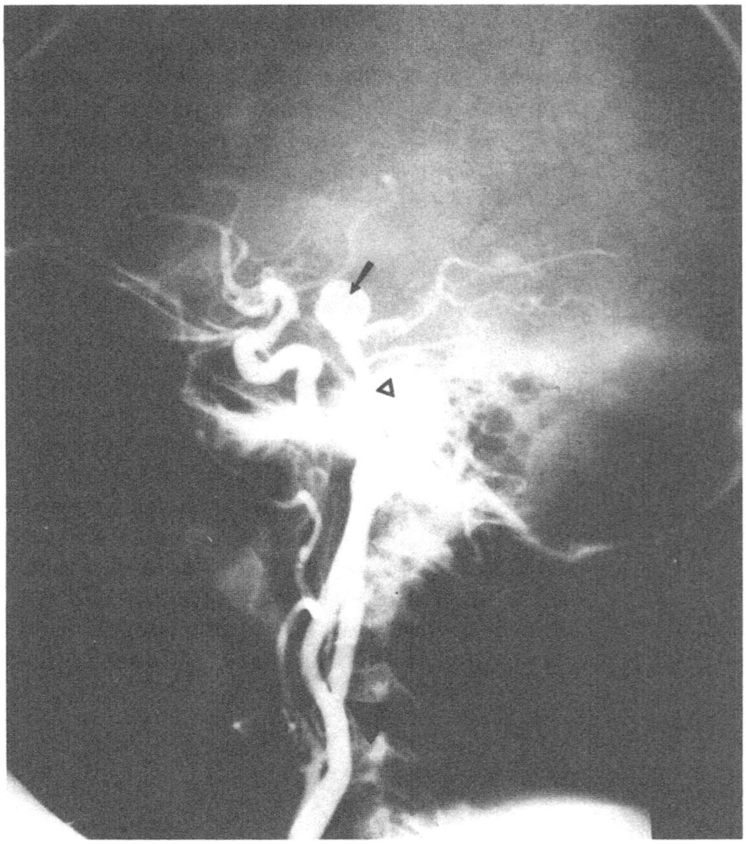

A

Fig. 38.3. A Lateral angiogram of bulbous bBAA (*arrow*) arising from basilar artery supplied via a primitive hypoglossal artery. This unusual carotid-basilar anastomosis arises from the cervical internal carotid artery, passes through the anterior condyloid foramen, and joins the lower basilar artery (*triangle*). **B** Same. A small amount of contrast media remains in aneurysm (*arrow*). **C** Frontal view. Note circulation within aneurysm (*arrow*).

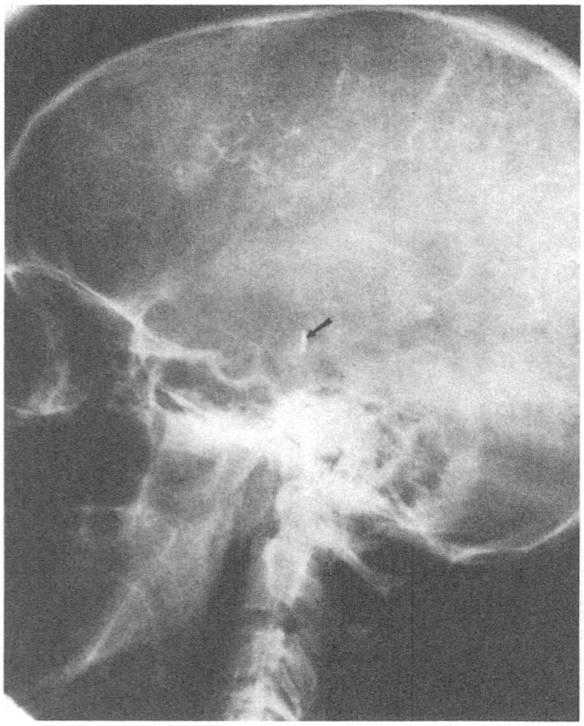

B

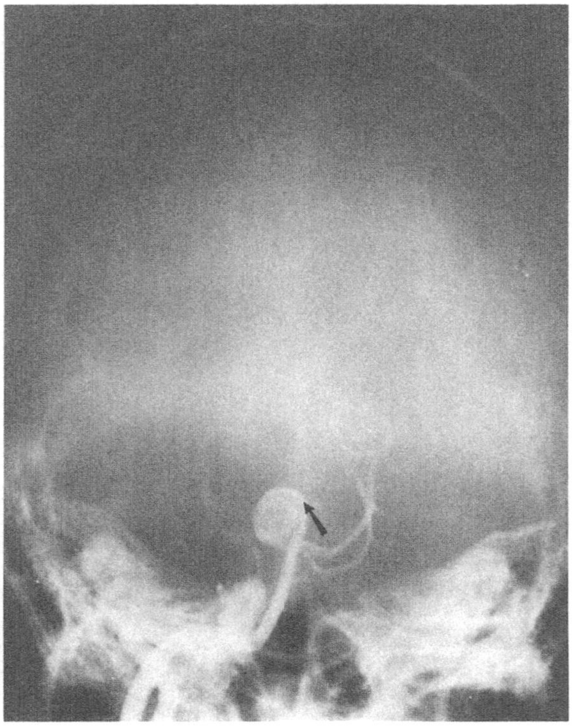

C

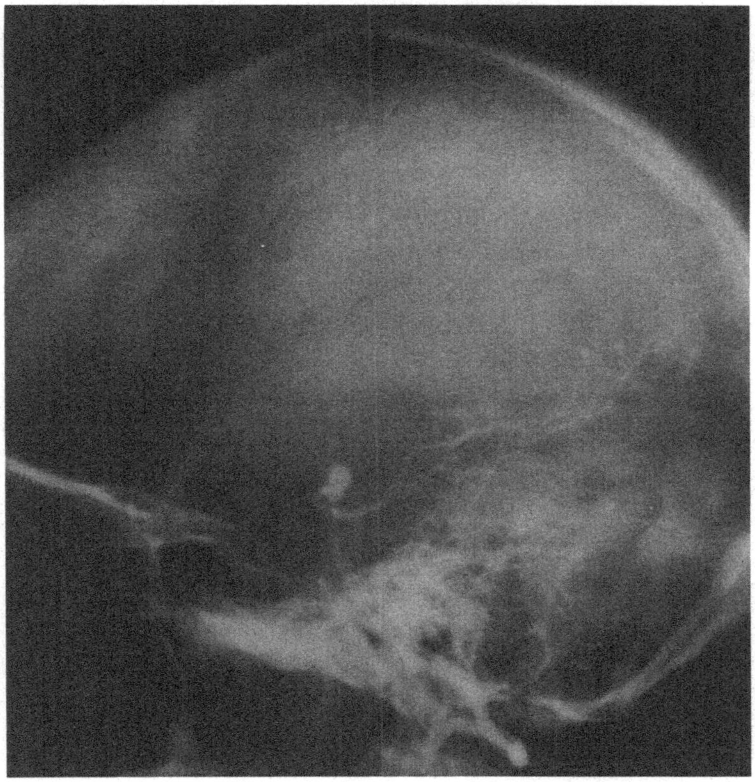

A

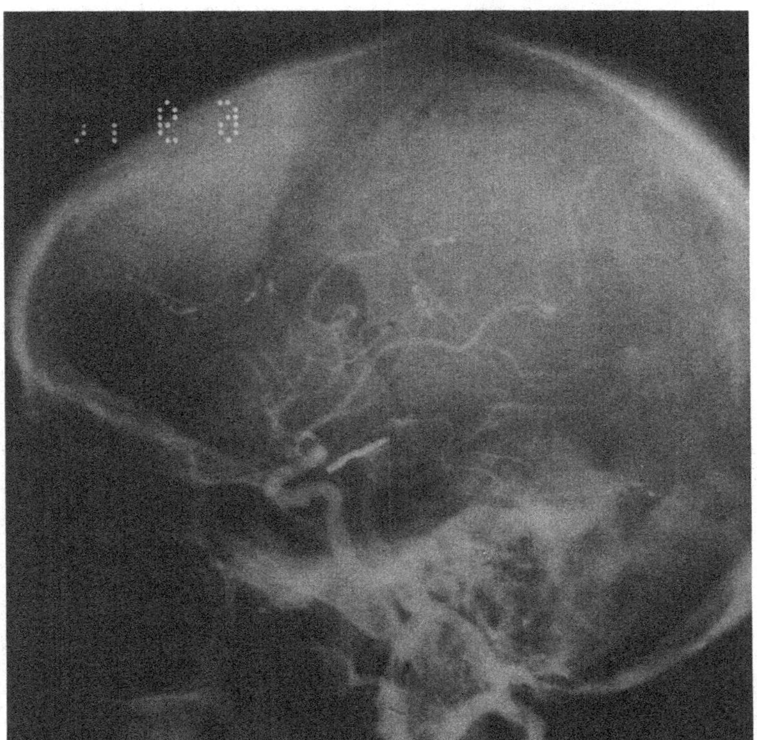

B

Fig. 38.4. **A** Lateral angiogram revealing superiorly projecting bBAA. **B** Same patient after clipping to show frontotemporal craniotomy flap.

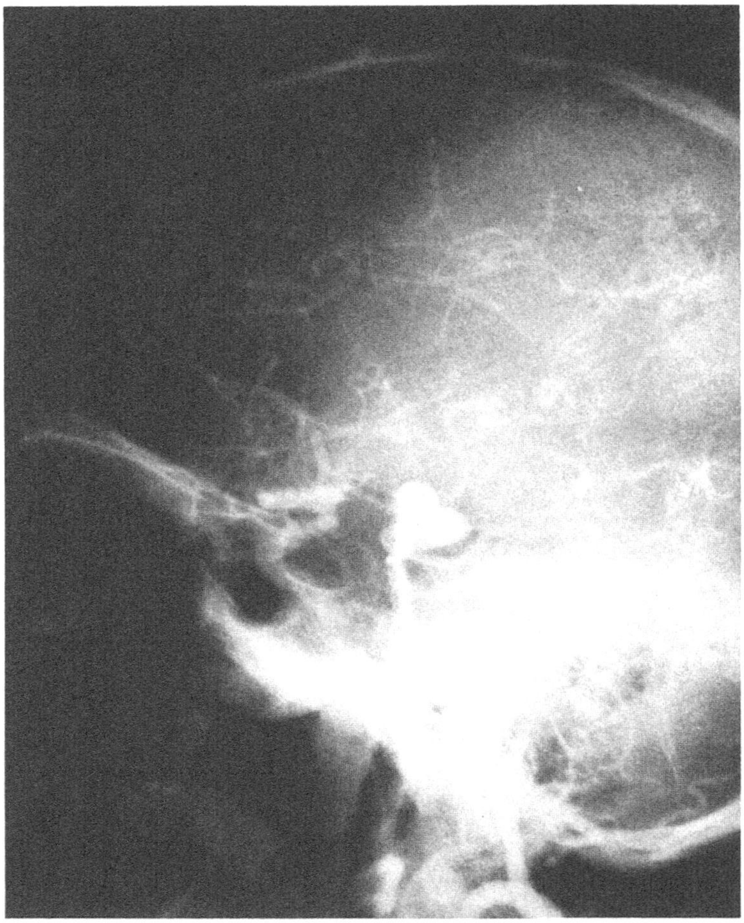

Fig. 38.5. Lateral angiogram illustrating superiorly and posteriorly projecting bilobed bBAA.

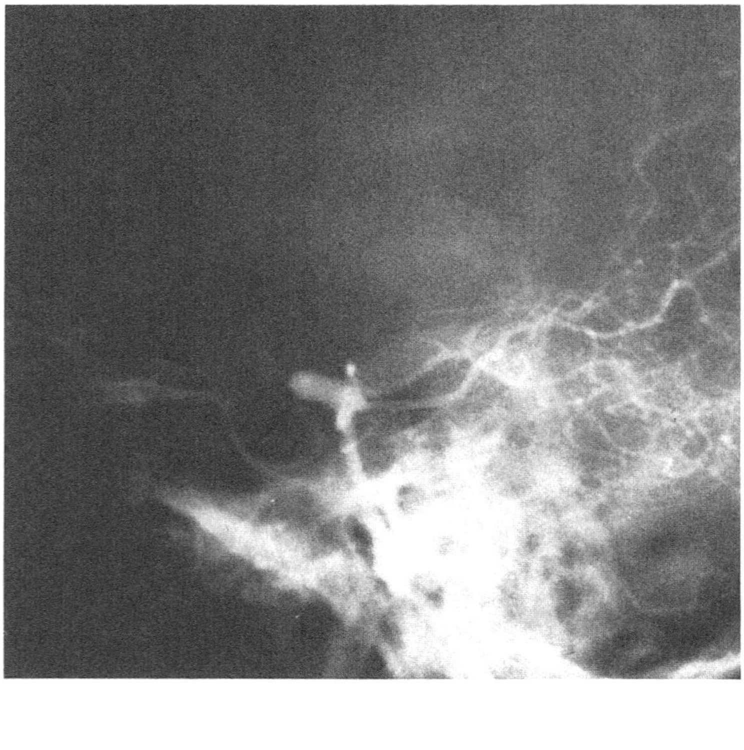

Fig. 38.6. Lateral angiogram portraying anteriorly projecting bBAA. Note how the aneurysm projects forward over the top of the dorsum sellae (*arrow*).

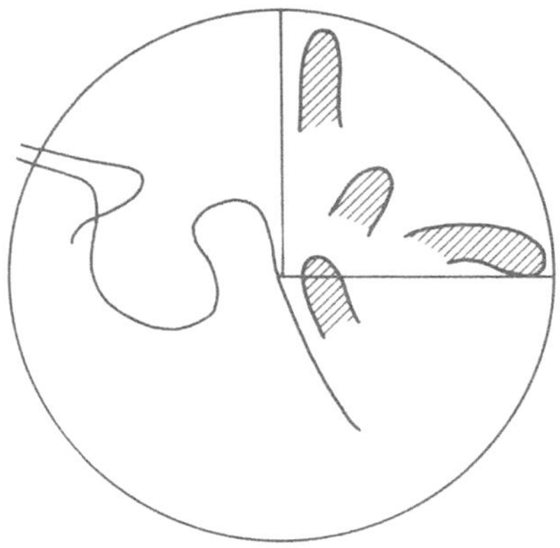

A

Fig. 38.7. Diagrams illustrating various relationships of the basilar artery termination to the dorsum sellae (**A**) and the third ventricle (**B**). From Greitz T, Löfsted S: ref. 12.

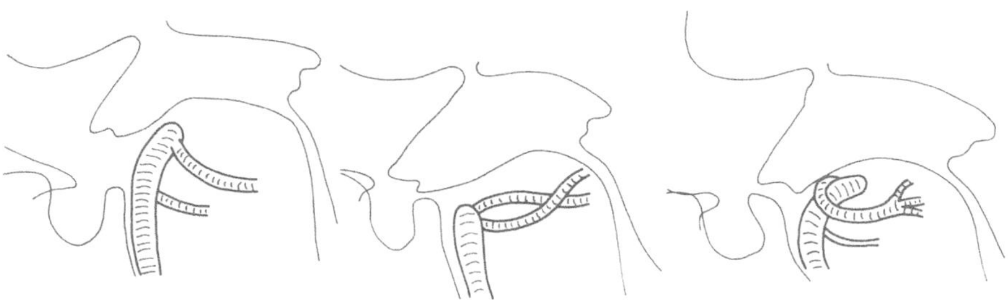

B

artery requires close attention to many small details, the accumulation of which results in a very satisfactory exposure. Omission of any of these points in the end will result in dissatisfaction with the frontotemporal approach to basilar artery aneurysms. Figure 38.8 shows the relationship of the basilar artery to the skull as seen by the surgeon using this approach.

After a wide opening of the sylvian fissure, the frontal lobe is freed of adhesions between itself and the optic nerve/chiasm and A-1. Initially a self-retaining retractor is used on the frontal lobe; but later when the ICA/M-1 area is retracted with a narrow retractor blade, the frontal lobe may fall away by itself and the frontal lobe retractor may not be required.

Veins between the temporal lobe and sphenoparietal sinus are electrocoagulated and severed. The temporal lobe is gently retracted to expose the zone between the oculomotor nerve (CN-3) and the internal carotid artery (Fig. 38.9). Although it may be advantageous not to separate the uncus of the temporal lobe from CN-3 when the subtemporal route (retro–oculomotor nerve route) is used (9), it is mandatory to dissect the uncus off CN-3 when the frontotemporal route in front of CN-3 is followed. The uncus often is adherent to CN-3; gentle dissection will sufficiently disengage this brain tissue to expose the path of the PCoA, the P-1 and P-2 portions of the posterior cerebral artery, the origin of the oculomotor nerve, the superior cerebellar artery (SCA), and the rostral end of the pons (Fig. 38.9).

If the ICA is deviated laterally, a narrow, self-retaining retractor blade should be placed on the ICA, on M-1, or on their juncture (depending on the anatomic orientation and relationships). The ICA is retracted medially (Fig. 38.10) just sufficient to provide exposure without occluding the ICA or MCA. Vascular hypotension should be minimized during such retraction. One must be careful of retracting a very atherosclerotic ICA, which may crack and hemorrhage. If the ICA does not deviate laterally, one can delay the time at which such vascular retraction is initiated. The next step is opening the membrane of Liliequist (Fig. 38.11), which may be thickened with adhesions from a previous SAH. Care must be exercised

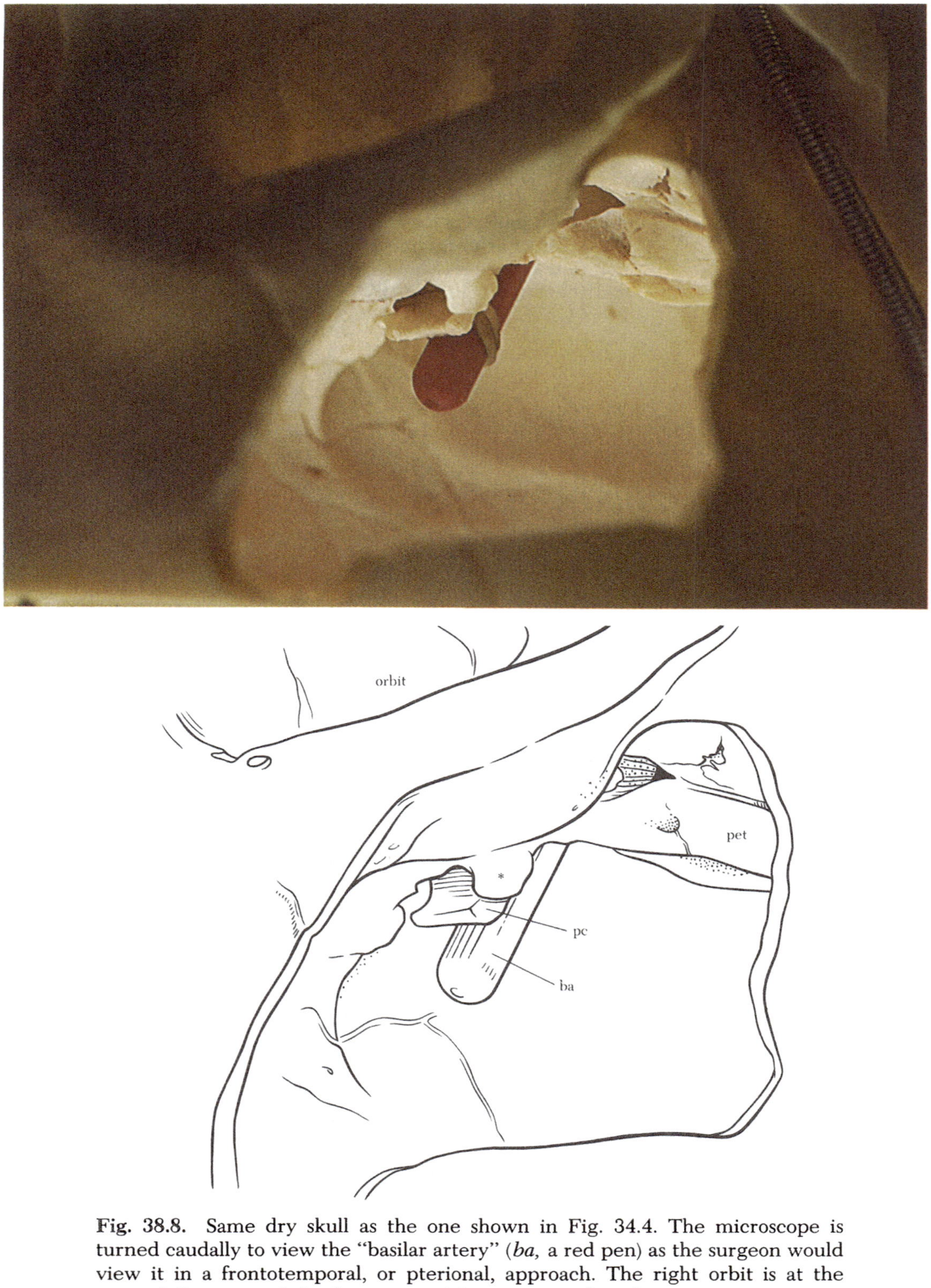

Fig. 38.8. Same dry skull as the one shown in Fig. 34.4. The microscope is turned caudally to view the "basilar artery" (*ba,* a red pen) as the surgeon would view it in a frontotemporal, or pterional, approach. The right orbit is at the upper left corner of the figure. *pc,* right posterior clinoid process; *pet,* petrous pyramid; *, right anterior clinoid process. From Fox JL: ref. 11.

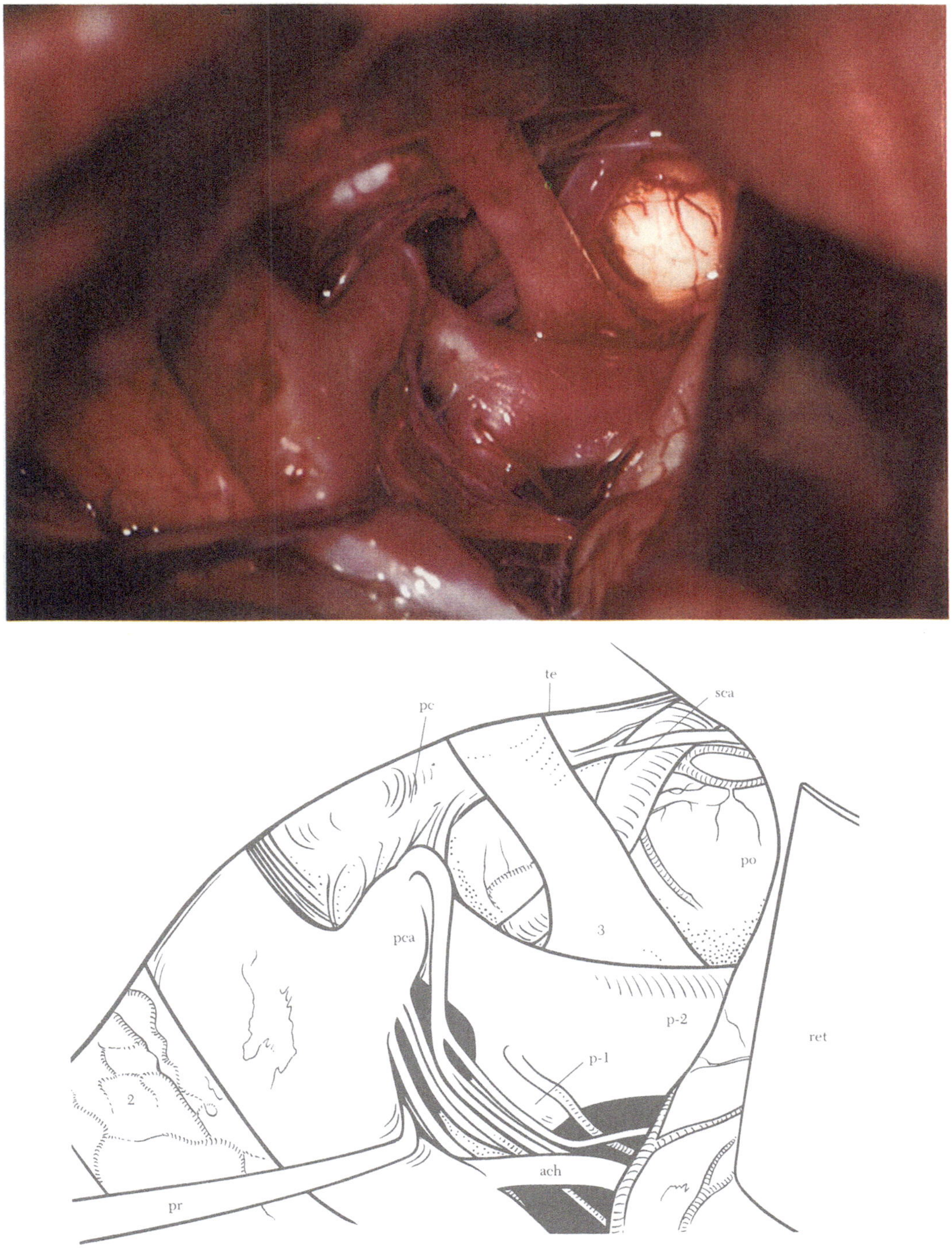

Fig. 38.9. Anatomy at the origin (*3*) of the right oculomotor nerve from the interpeduncular fossa of the midbrain. *po*, pons; *sca*, right superior cerebellar artery; *te*, tentorial edge; *pc*, posterior clinoid process medial to the oculomotor nerve; *pr*, probe retracting internal carotid artery medially; *2*, optic nerve; *pca*, posterior communicating artery with leash of anterior thalamic perforators; *ach*, anterior choroidal artery passing under the temporal lobe; *p-1*, P-1 segment of the posterior cerebral artery (toward hidden basilar artery); *p-2*, P-2 segment passing between the brain stem and the temporal lobe; *ret*, retractor on the right temporal lobe. From Fox JL: ref. 11.

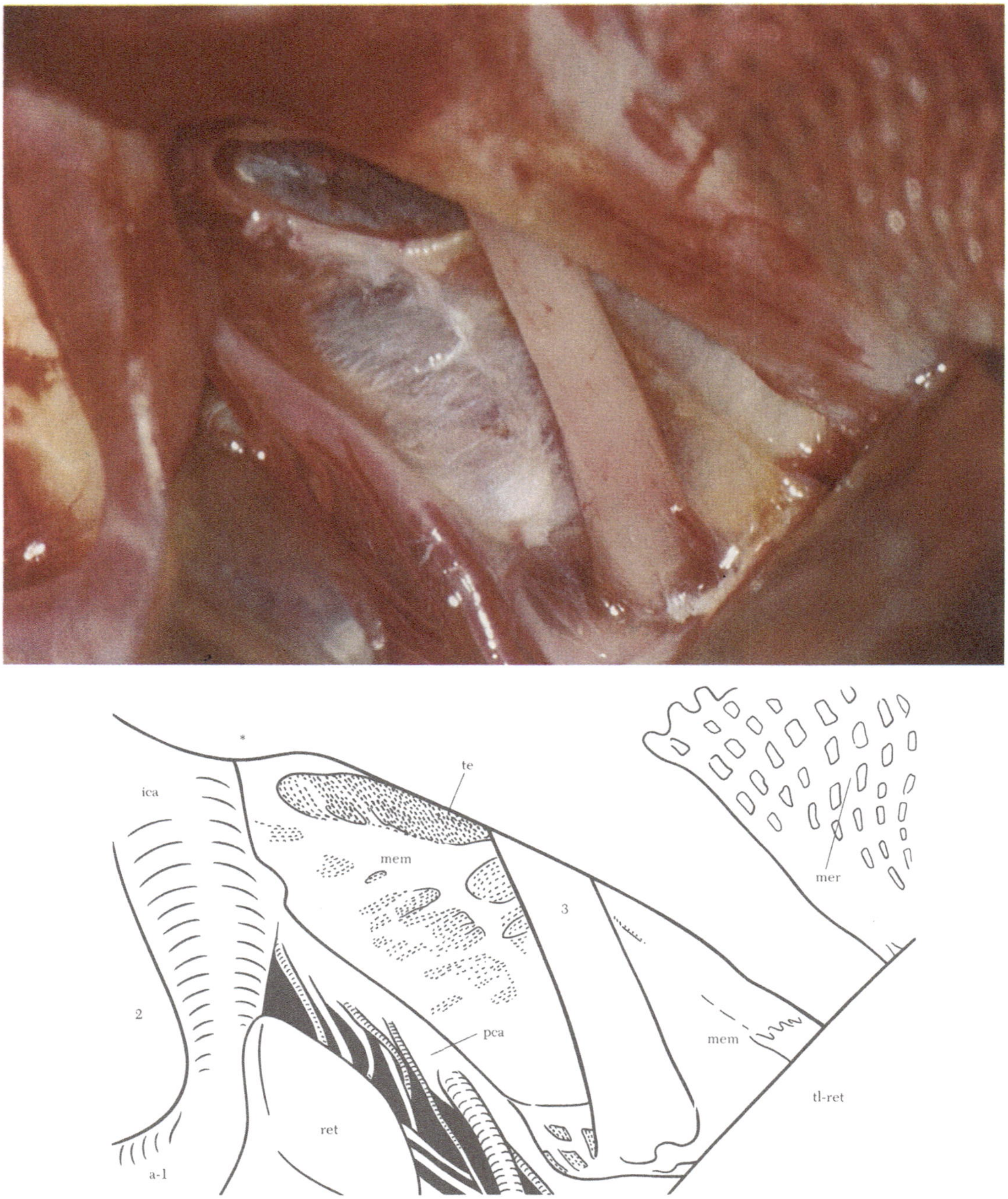

Fig. 38.10. Exposure between the internal carotid artery (*ica*) and oculomotor nerve (*3*). The arachnoid membrane of Liliequist (*mem*) is thickened by adhesions. A narrow retractor (*ret*) is holding the ICA bifurcation and M-1 medially. Note the anterior thalamoperforators coming off the posterior communicating artery (*pca*). The dome of a large, anteriorly or rostrally projecting basilar-tip aneurysm will lie medial to these perforators. *, anterior clinoid process; *te*, anterior reflection of tentorial edge; *mer*, Mersilene mesh over temporal lobe; *tl-ret*, temporal lobe retractor; *a-1*, origin of A-1 artery; *2*, optic nerve.

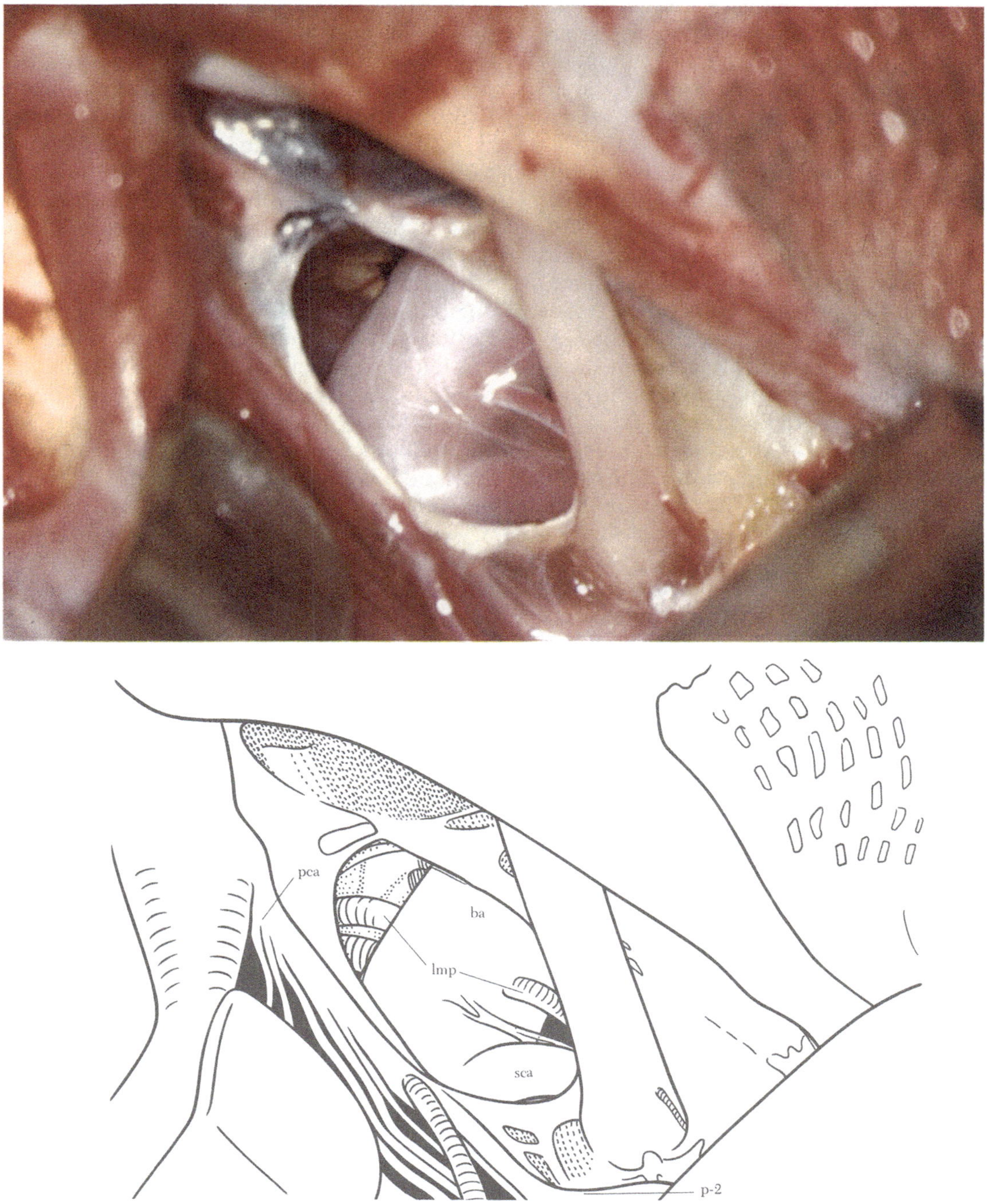

Fig. 38.11. Same view as in Fig. 38.10 after the membrane of Liliequist has been opened to expose the interpeduncular cistern containing the basilar artery (*ba*), the right superior cerebellar artery (*sca*), and left and right lateral medullary perforators (*lmp*). *p-2,* part of P-2 artery; *pca,* posterior communicating artery.

to avoid injury to the fundus of a large, anteriorly or rostrally projecting aneurysm. Such may lie immediately medial to the PCoA and its leash of perforators. These perforators should be dilated with topical 3% papaverine or 0.5% phentolamine.

The posterior clinoid process is an important landmark which should be identified. Examples are shown in Figs. 5.2, 7.4, 34.4, 34.11, 34.14, 34.16, 35.10, 36.20, 38.8, 38.13–38.15, and 38.39. The oculomotor nerve passes immediately lateral to this process before going under the tentorial edge and into the roof of the cavernous sinus. The posterior clinoid process may partially obstruct the surgeon's view of the neck of a low-lying bBAA (15,20), but so far it has not prevented enough exposure in our cases to allow satisfactory clipping. An example of a case of a low-lying bBAA is shown in Figs. 38.12–38.15.

The next step is consideration of clipping and sectioning of the PCoA. This permits greater retraction of the ICA and exposure of the aneurysm (Figs. 38.14 and 38.15). We use small tantalum Ligaclips or Hemoclips placed where there are no perforators and placed so as to allow persisting perfusion of anterior thalamoperforators on either side of the clips via the ICA and the BA systems. The main risk is brain ischemia if the aneurysm clip should compromise the ipsilateral P-1 artery. If P-1 is small compared to the PCoA, P-1, instead, can be clipped and sectioned. In most, but not all, cases we have had to clip and section the PCoA in this manner. *Warning:* keep an eye on the ICA/M-1 retractor blade to be sure there are adequate ICA, PCoA, AChA, and M-1 artery pulsations. Occasionally one should test and, perhaps, release the retractor.

One of the major advantages of the frontotemporal approach to bBAA is the ability to see the ventral and rostral surfaces of *both* P-1 arteries and their perforators. An example is given in Figs. 38.16–38.19. Again, note the exposure of the ICA bifurcation, A-1, and M-1 in Figs. 38.17 and 38.18 and the *en face* view of both P-1 arteries and oculomotor nerves in Fig. 38.19. From this point the left and right sides of the aneurysm neck are freed of adhesions and perforators. More of the dome is isolated from the midbrain and peduncles, retracted with microinstruments to see the back wall, and cleared of any hidden perforators before the clip is applied.

Figures 38.20–38.24 exemplify a large bBAA projecting posteriorly from an erected basilar artery. After the origin of the aneurysm is exposed between the oculomotor nerve and the ICA (Fig. 38.21), the contralateral P-1 and aneurysm neck are examined (Fig. 38.22). In this case the right P-1 originated within the expanded, atherosclerotic neck of the aneurysm (Fig. 38.23) in a more-rostral-than-usual fashion. A Drake clip was applied to the neck of the aneurysm with the right P-1 protected by the encircling portion of the clip (Fig. 38.24). Postoperative angiography demonstrated obliteration of the aneurysm, but the clip had compromised the right P-1 orifice. This was our one complication (infarction and death) that could be attributed to loss of the PCoA (deliberately sectioned between clips) and the P-1 artery blood flow.

Another disadvantage of the frontotemporal route is the frequent inability to clip the bBAA neck with the clip blades parallel to the P-1 arteries. This is compensated for by the excellent bilateral exposure of the aneurysm neck, but one must use care as the clip blades encircle the neck in a direction oblique to the P-1 artery direction. Similar to the problem with clipping an ACoAA where stress is placed at the ACoAA/A-2 junction, in this case stress is placed at the bBAA/P-1 junction. Hence the blades of the clip, as they pass between P-1 and the aneurysm on either side, often must remain a good millimeter from the tip of the basilar artery as the clip is closed. This maneuver will avoid a tear at the origin of the atherosclerotic neck. Figures 38.25–38.27 show such an aneurysm. In addition note that the left P-1 (Fig. 38.25) arises higher up on the neck of the aneurysm and, unlike the right P-1, courses upward a few millimeters beside the aneurysm. One must take this into account during clip application. In this patient, we placed one clip diagonally from right to left but not all the way across the neck. A second clip just distal to the first clip reached across the aneurysm and collapsed the dome just above the left P-1 take-off.

The Multiple Aneurysm Case

Patients may present with a BAA plus another aneurysm on the anterior circulation. If it is an ACoAA, the right-sided approach is used, and the exposure is as previously described. If

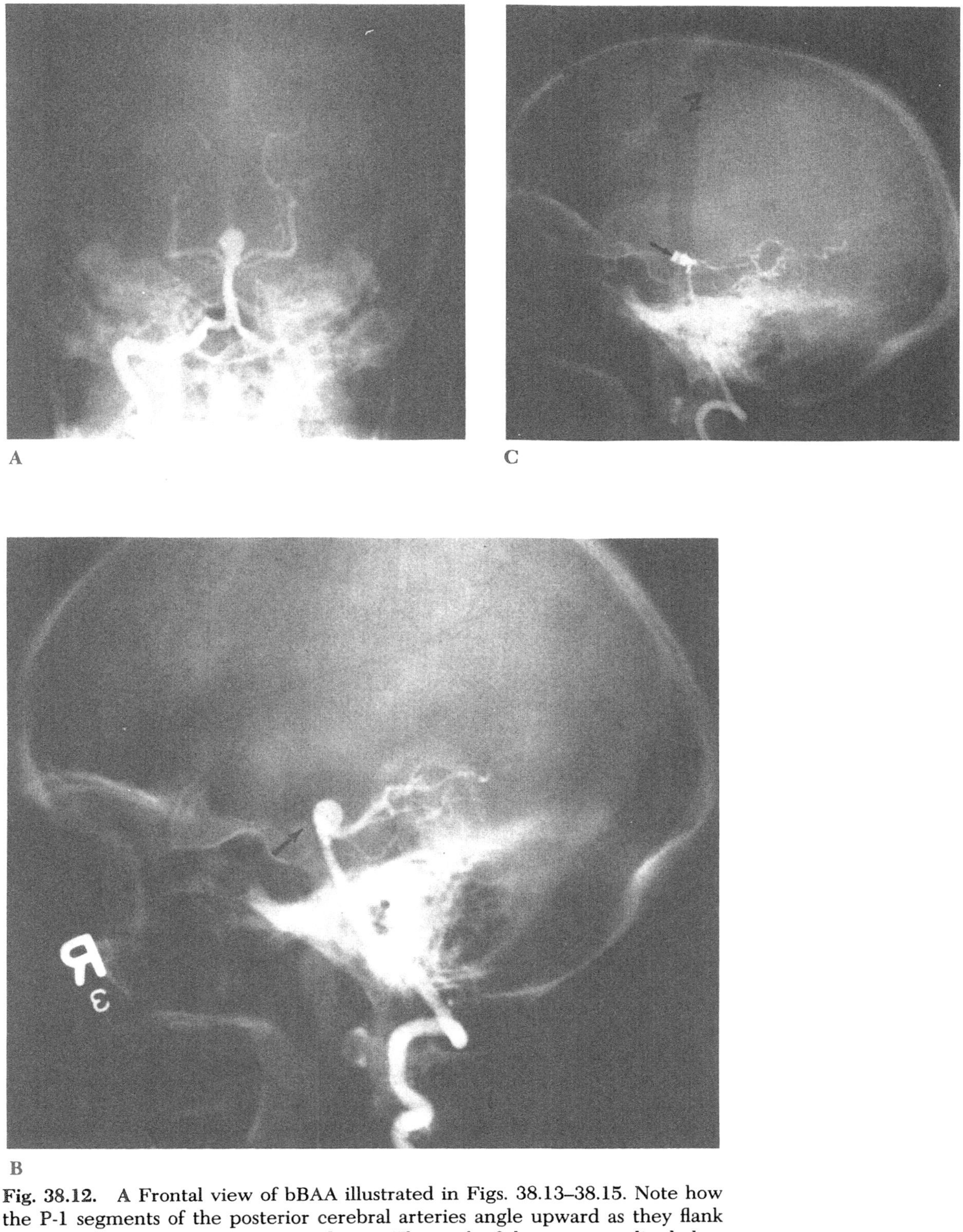

A C B

Fig. 38.12. A Frontal view of bBAA illustrated in Figs. 38.13–38.15. Note how the P-1 segments of the posterior cerebral arteries angle upward as they flank the dome of the aneurysm. B Lateral view. The neck of the aneurysm lies below the level of the posterior clinoid processes (*arrow*). C Lateral postoperative angiogram confirming occlusion of the aneurysm with a Drake clip (*straight arrow*). *Curved arrows*, two of the burr holes of the frontotemporal craniotomy flap. The clinical result was excellent.

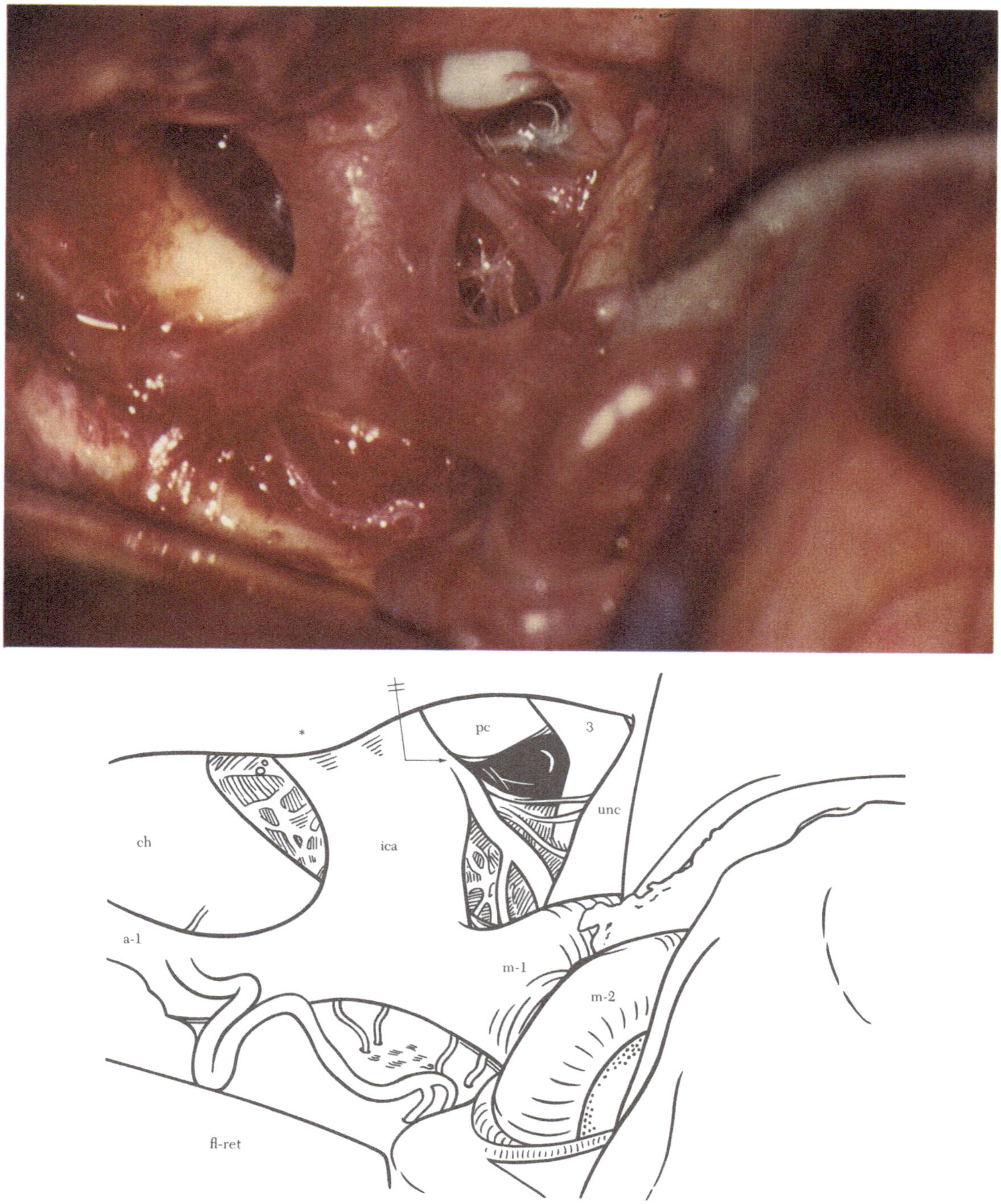

Fig. 38.13. Same case as in Figs. 38.12, 38.14, and 38.15. the sylvian fissure has been widely opened, revealing M-1 arteries (*m-1*), M-2 arteries (*m-2*), and perforators at the bifurcation of the internal carotid artery. Slight retraction on the uncus (*unc*) of the temporal lobe causes traction on and angulation of the oculomotor nerve (*3*). *fl-ret,* frontal lobe retractor; *a-1,* A-1 artery; *ch,* optic chiasm; *, anterior clinoid process; *ica,* internal carotid artery; *double-crossed arrow,* origin of posterior communicating artery; *pc,* posterior clinoid process.

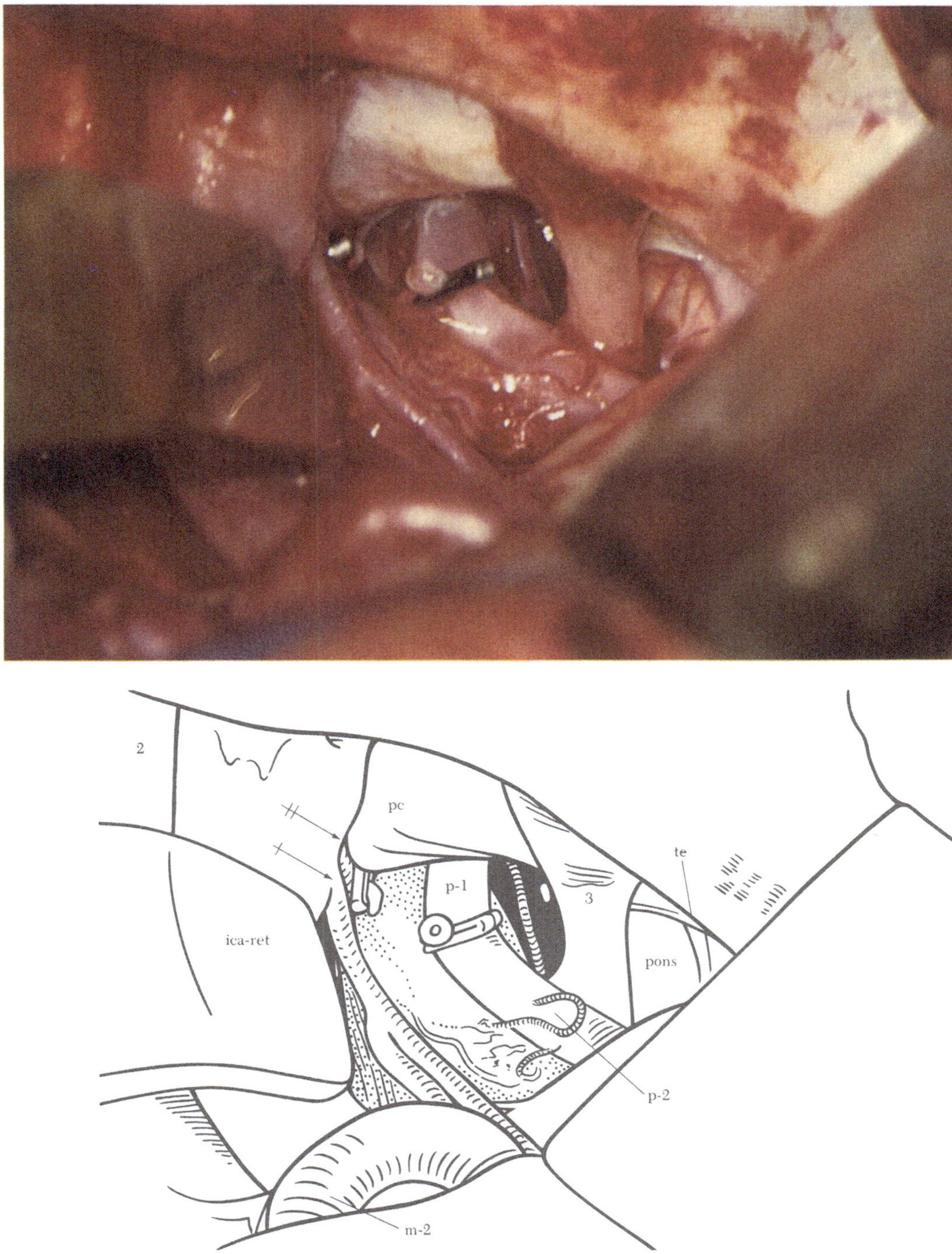

Fig. 38.14. Same case as in Figs. 38.12, 38.13, and 38.15. Tantalum clips are on the ends of the severed posterior communicating artery. The temporal lobe uncus has been disengaged from the oculomotor nerve (*3*), which now is straightened. *te,* edge of tentorium; *pons,* rostral end of pons; *p-2,* P-2 artery distal to tantalum clip; *m-2,* M-2 branch; *ica-ret,* retractor on internal carotid artery; *2,* optic nerve; *single-crossed arrow,* origin of anterior choroidal artery; *double-crossed arrow,* origin of proximal end of posterior communicating artery; *pc,* posterior clinoid process; *p-1,* P-1 artery proximal to tantalum clip; *3,* oculomotor nerve.

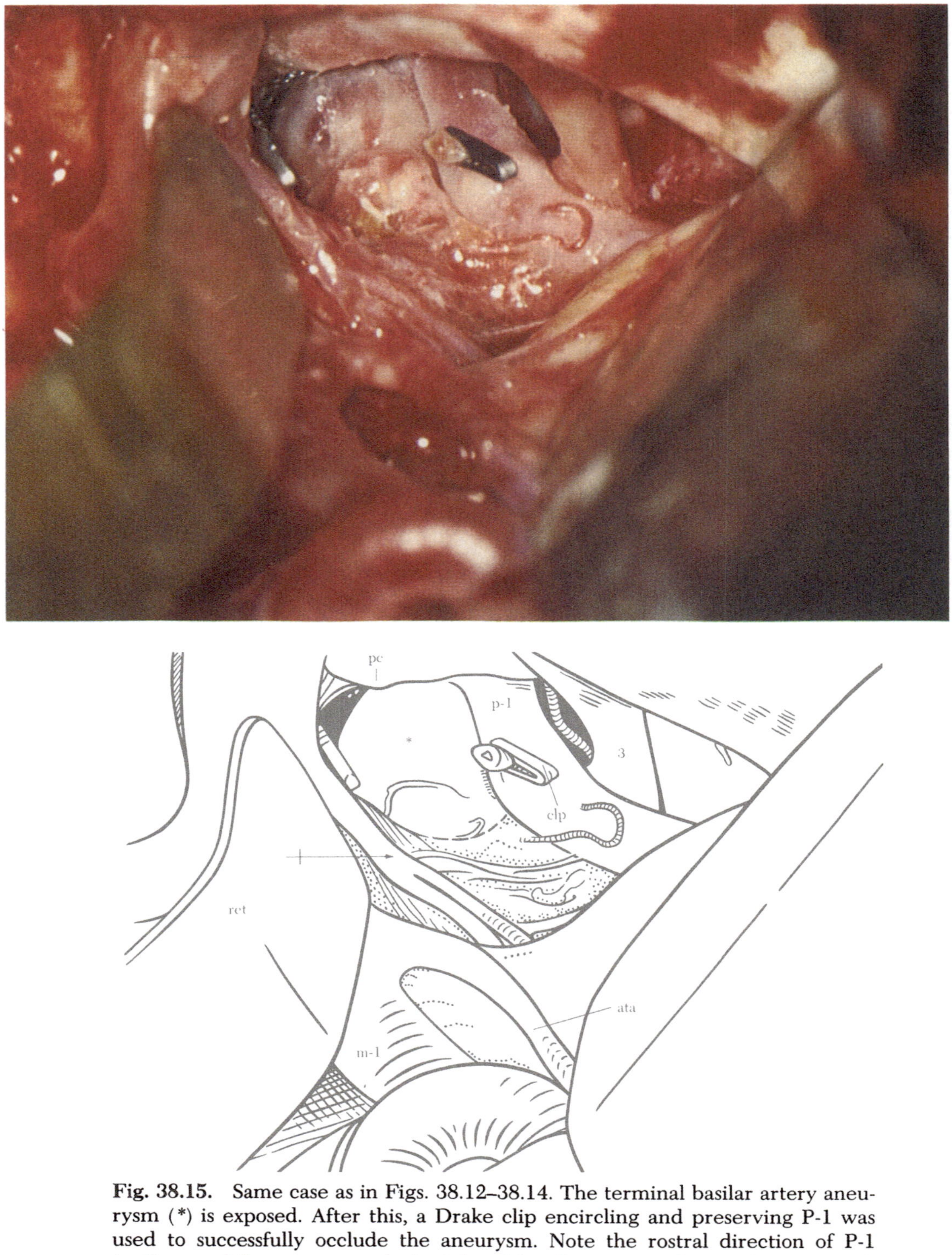

Fig. 38.15. Same case as in Figs. 38.12–38.14. The terminal basilar artery aneurysm (*) is exposed. After this, a Drake clip encircling and preserving P-1 was used to successfully occlude the aneurysm. Note the rostral direction of P-1 (*p-1*) around the aneurysm. *clp,* tantalum Ligaclip on severed posterior communicating artery; *3,* oculomotor nerve; *ata,* anterior temporal artery; *m-1,* M-1 artery; *ret,* retractor on bifurcation of internal carotid artery; *pc,* posterior clinoid process.

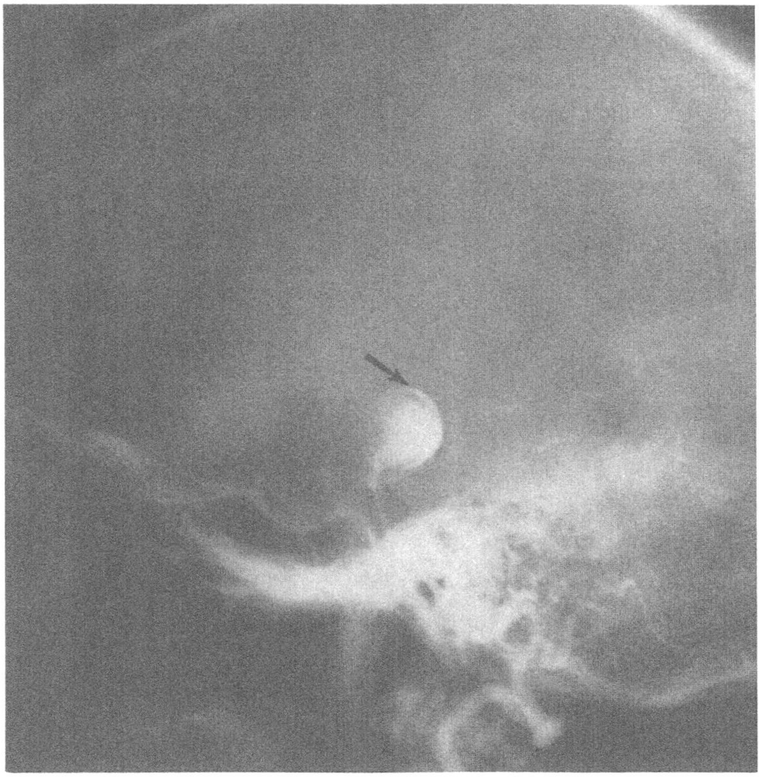

A

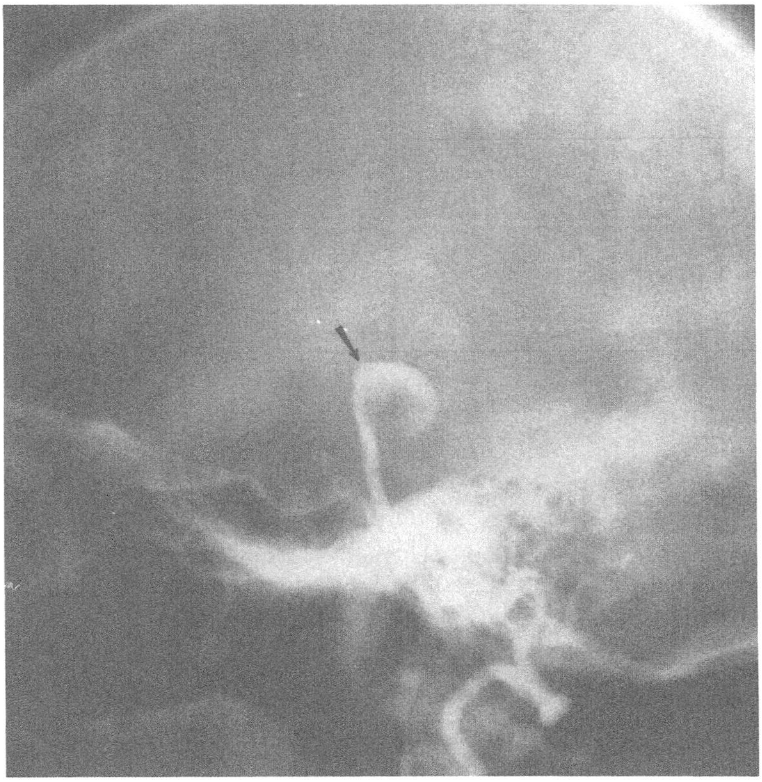

B

Fig. 38.16. **A** Lateral angiogram of large bBAA. Same case as in Figs. 38.17–38.19. Note circular streaming along front and top of the sac (*arrow*). **B** Same case, earlier phase demonstrating saccule (*arrow*) where rupture is likely. This saccule receives the brunt of the pressure from the stream out of the basilar artery. This streaming effect and its continual impingement on the same area of the aneurysm where the stream is deflected may be responsible for the saccule formation.

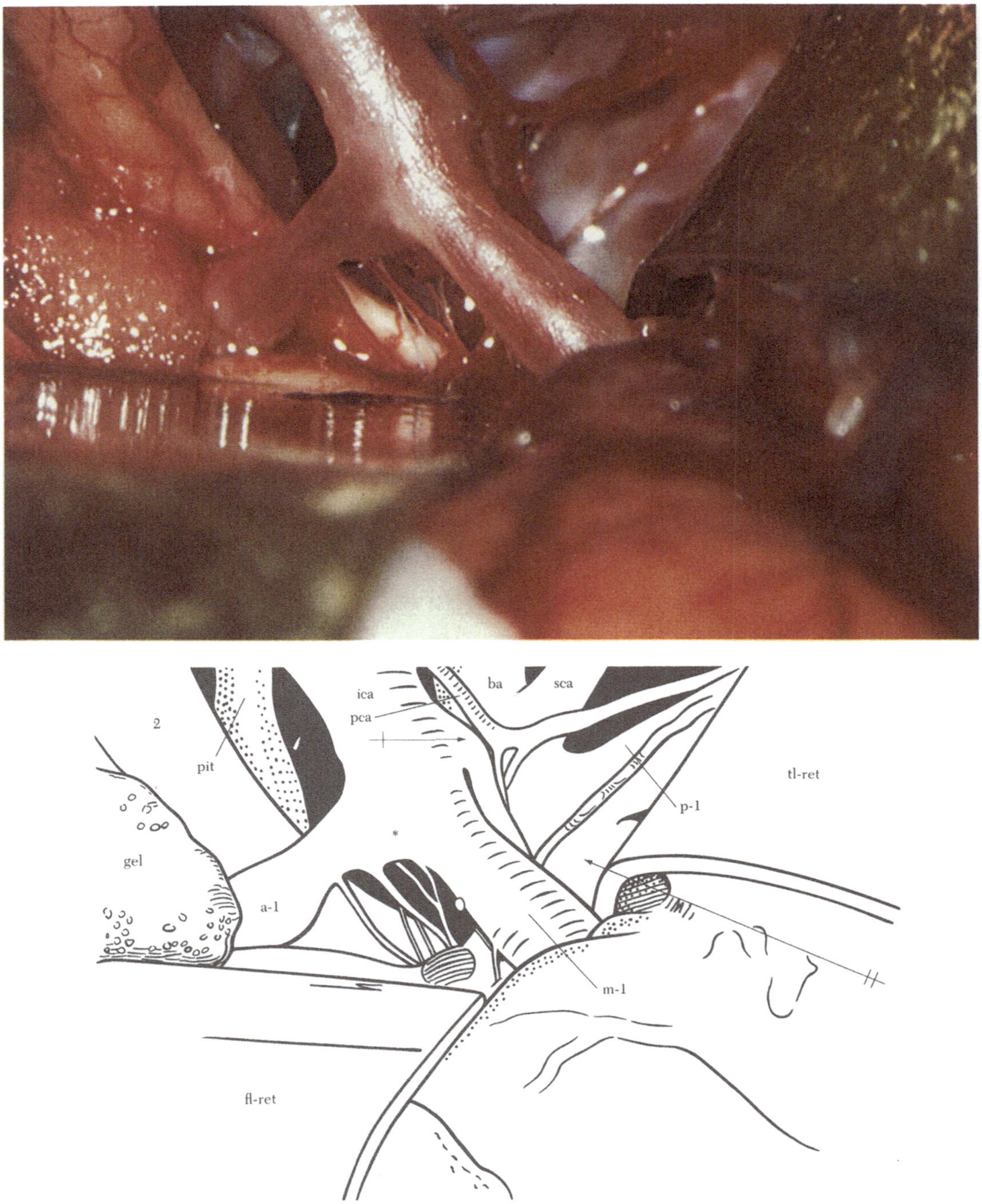

Fig. 38.17. Transylvian view of carotid and interpeduncular cisterns. Same case as in Figs. 38.16, 38.18, and 38.19. *ica,* internal carotid artery; *pca,* miniscule posterior communicating artery (with a couple of important perforators of same size); *single-crossed arrow,* origin of anterior choroidal artery; *ba,* portion of basilar artery; *sca,* right superior cerebellar artery; *tl-ret,* temporal lobe retractor; *p-1,* right P-1 artery; *double-crossed arrow,* portion of aneurysm; *m-1,* M-1 artery; *, bifurcation of internal carotid artery and its perforators; *fl-ret,* frontal lobe retractor; *a-1,* A-1 artery crossing optic tract; *gel,* Gelfoam; *2,* right optic nerve; *pit,* pituitary stalk.

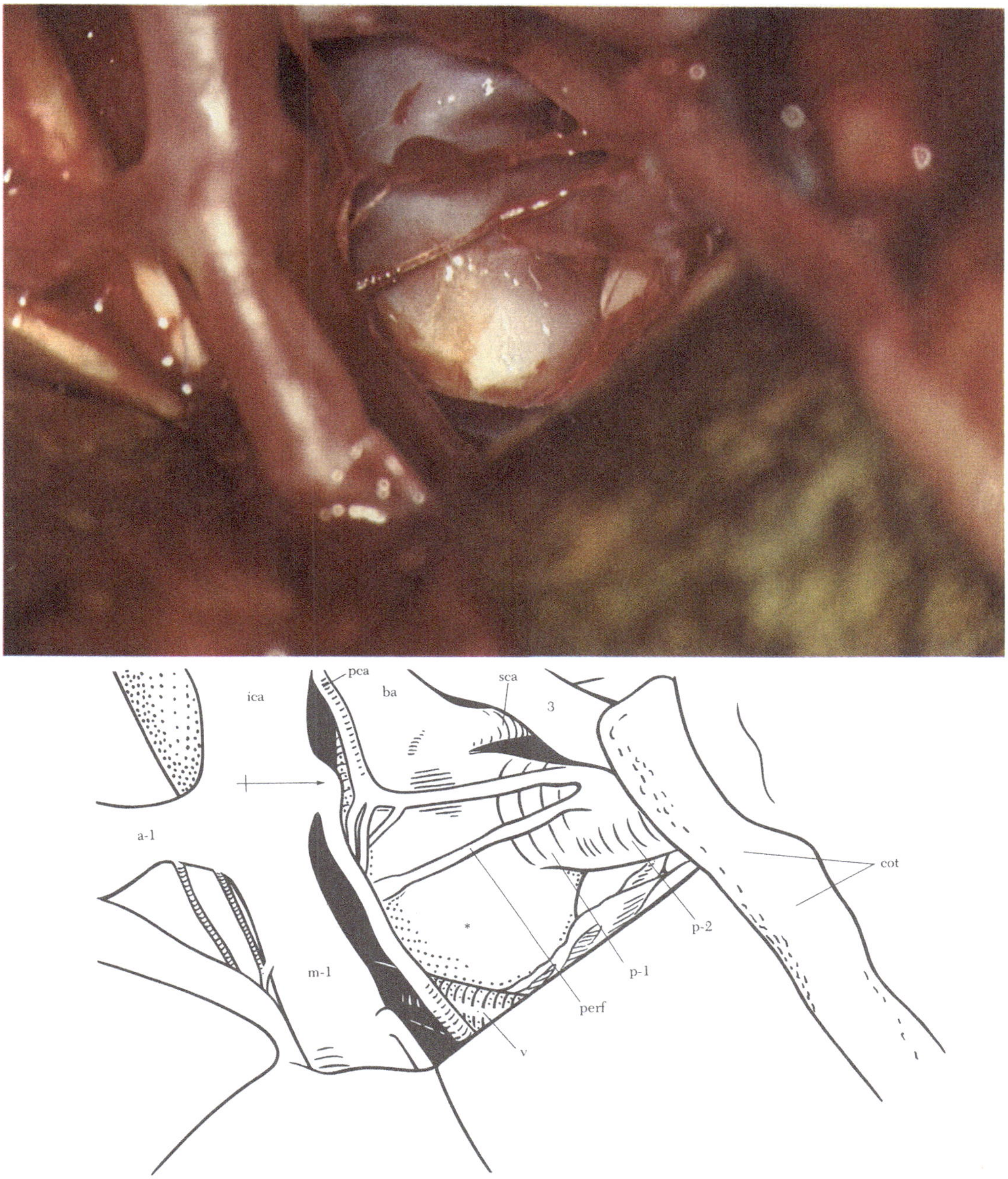

Fig. 38.18. Same case as in Figs. 38.16, 38.17, and 38.19. The direction of the microscope has been altered to reveal more of the dome of the aneruysm (*). Note tiny posterior communicating artery (*pca*), its perforators, and its junction with the posterior cerebral artery (*p-1* and *p-2*) where another perforator (*perf*) takes off. *ica*, internal carotid artery; *single-crossed arrow*, origin of anterior choroidal artery; *ba*, tip of basilar artery; *sca*, right superior cerebellar artery going behind the oculomotor nerve (*3*); *cot*, cottonoid strip under temporal lobe retractor; *v*, vein; *m-1*, M-1 artery; *a-1*, A-1 artery.

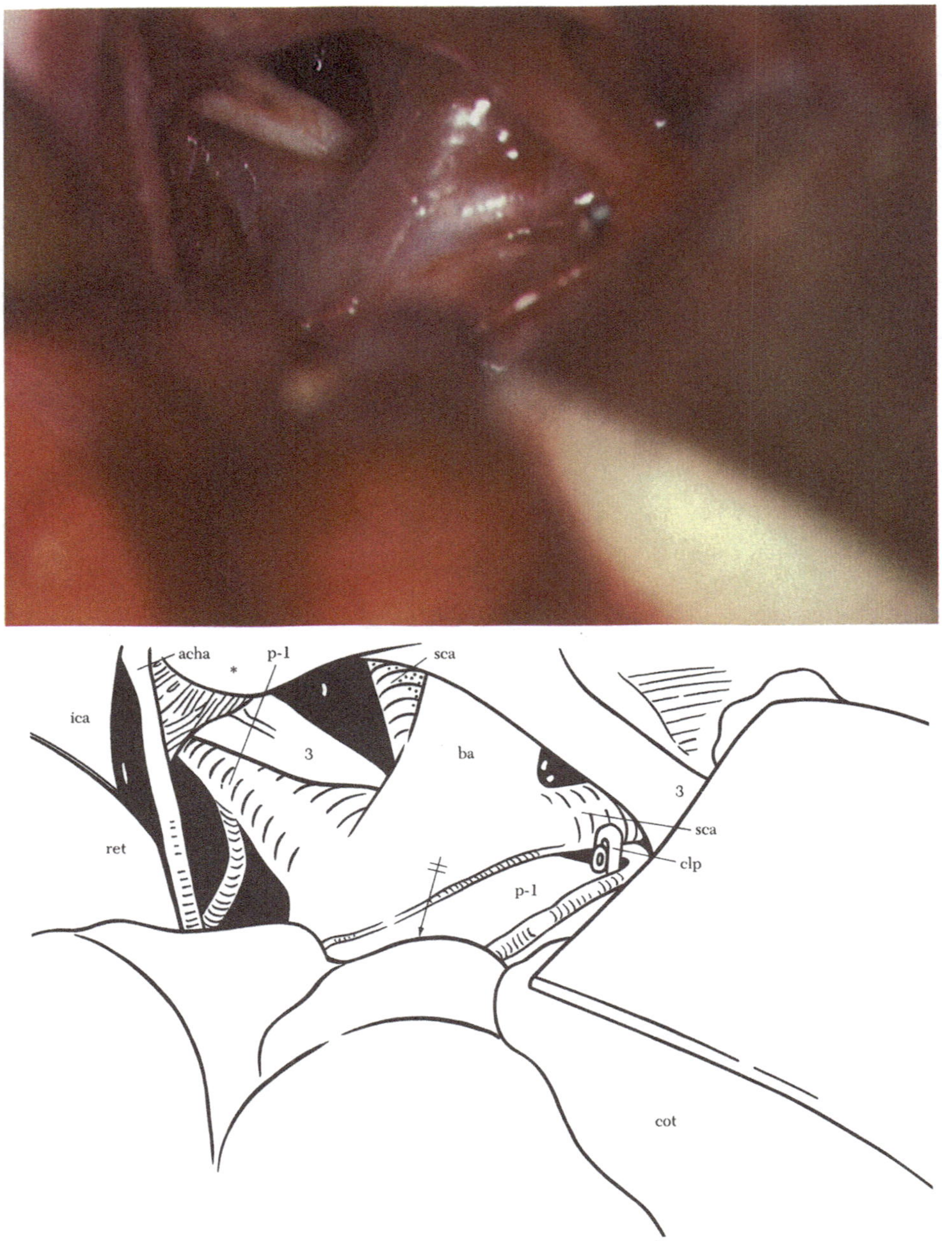

Fig. 38.19. Same case as in Figs. 38.16–38.18. The microscope has been tilted to look leftward between dorsum sellae (*) and basilar artery (*ba*). The origin of the aneurysm (*double-crossed arrow*) is seen *en face.* The surgeon now can define the relationship of any left posterior thalamoperforators to the aneurysm as they arise from the left P-1 (*p-1,* above). Above are seen the left P-1 (*p-1*), the left oculomotor nerve (*3*), and the left superior cerebellar artery (*sca*). On the right are seen the right oculomotor nerve (*3*), the right superior cerebellar artery (*sca*), and the right P-1 (*p-1*). *cot,* cottonoid strip under temporal lobe retractor; *ret,* retractor on right internal carotid artery (*ica*); *acha,* anterior choroidal artery; *, right posterior clinoid process; *clp,* tantalum clip on distal end of severed posterior communicating artery.

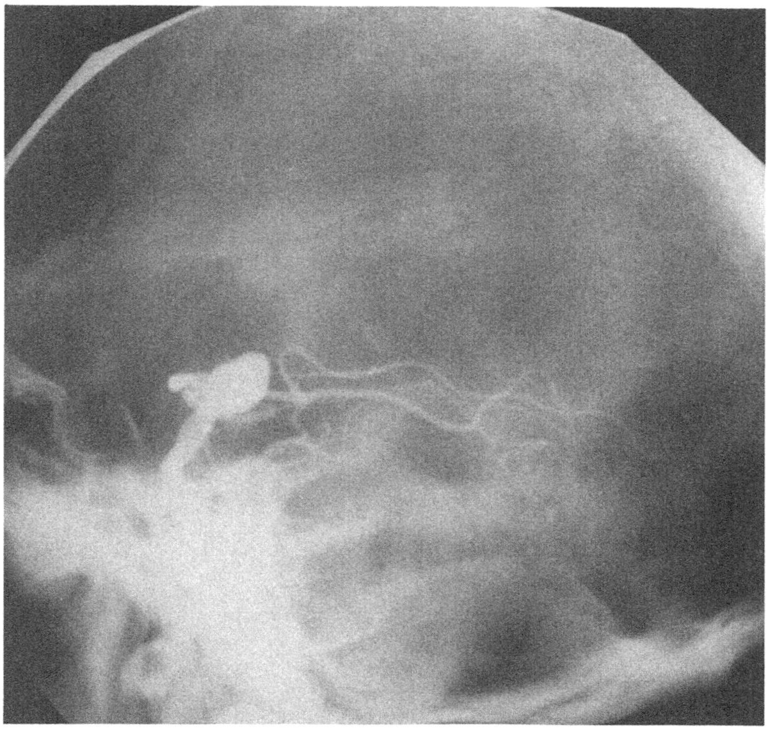

A

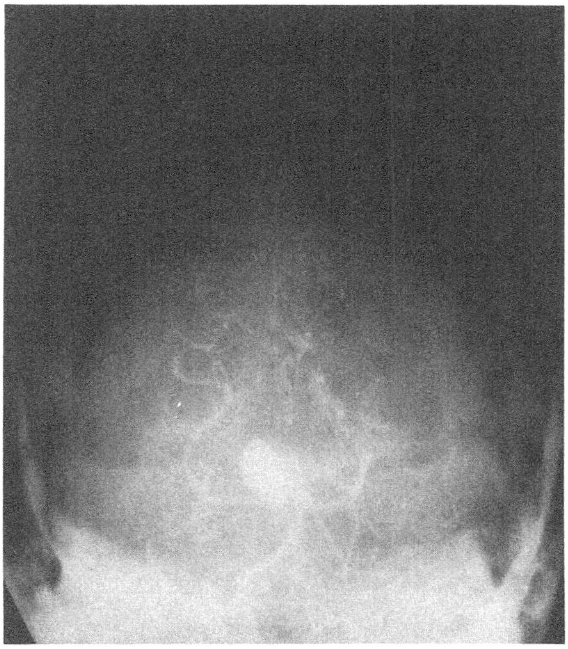

B

Fig. 38.20. **A** Lateral angiogram of large bBAA on a posteriorly erected basilar artery. Same case as in Figs. 38.21–38.24. **B** Frontal view. Aneurysm tilts to right and the right P-1 appears to originate in the neck of the aneurysm (compare with Fig. 38.23).

there is a left MCAA or left ICAA, a left-sided exposure is used for access to the tip of the basilar artery. Retraction injury of the dominant cerebral hemisphere, ischemia of the speech area, and relative inexperience with the left-sided route to a BAA are the main risks. If the MCAA and/or the ICAA are on the right side, the right-handed surgeon is more comfortable with the exposure.

The BAA patient with a MCAA and/or an ICAA presents a special problem: What to do with the MCAA and ICAA which are in the pathway toward the BAA? If these more proximal aneurysms are not clipped, they may rupture during retraction and exposure of the BAA. If they are clipped, the clips themselves may interfere with the exposure of the BAA. Where possible, we have used malleable, tantalum clips on these more proximal aneurysms so that there is not the shank of a spring clip projecting into the field. In other cases, the MCAA aneurysm is covered with Gelfoam and cottonoids and later clipped after obliteration of the BAA. Also, on occasion, we have retracted the ICA and its aneurysm together with the internal carotid retractor blade and later clipped the ICAA after dealing with the BAA.

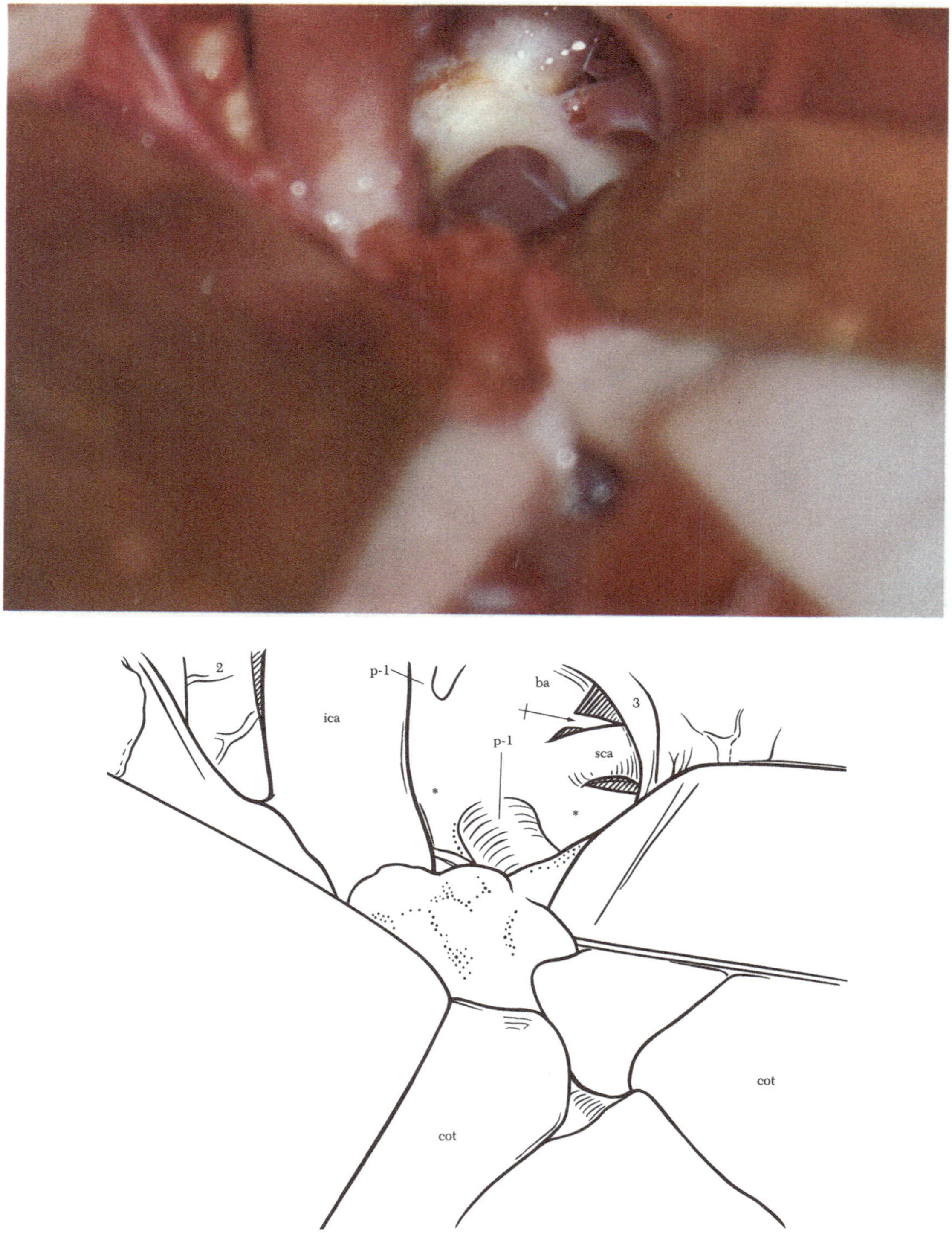

Fig. 38.21. Initial exposure of origin of aneurysm (*) beyond the space between the internal carotid artery (*ica*) and oculomotor nerve (*3*). *ba,* tip of basilar artery; *single-crossed arrow,* lateral medullary perforator; *sca,* right superior cerebellar artery; *cot;* cottonoid strips under retractors; *2,* optic nerve; *p-1,* left (above) and right (below) origins of P-1 arteries. This is the same case as in Figs. 38.20 and 38.22–38.24.

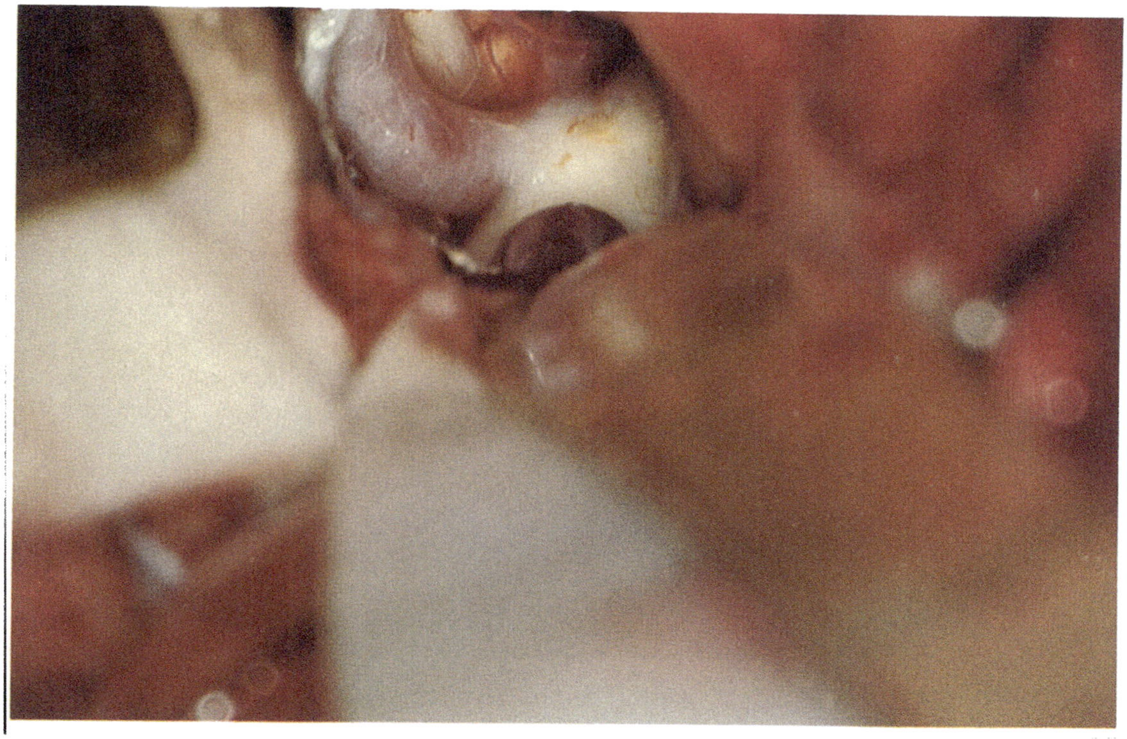

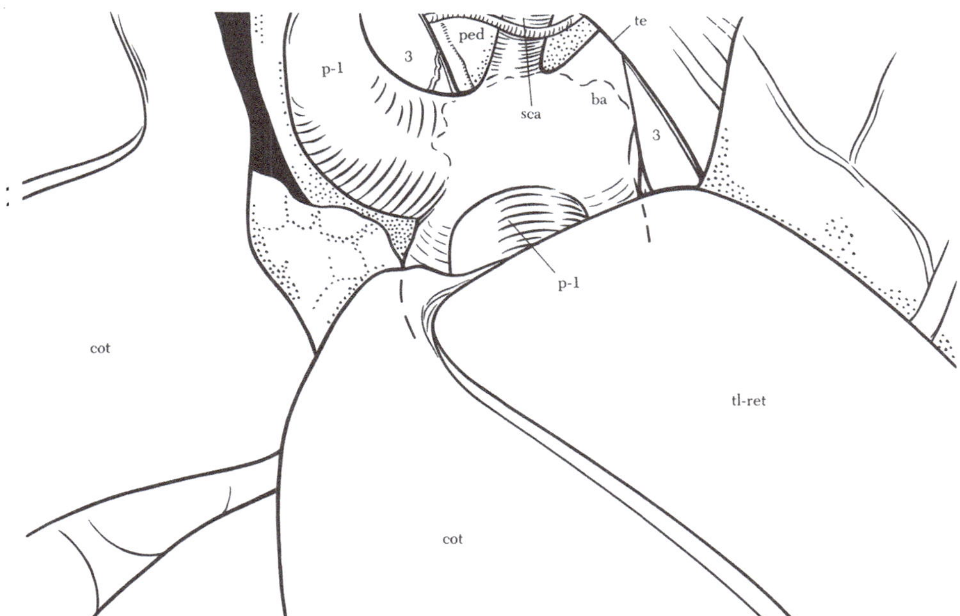

Fig. 38.22. Same case as in Figs. 38.20, 38.21, 38.23, and 38.24. View under dorsum sellae to see environs of tip of basilar artery (*ba*). Above are the left P-1 (*p-1*), left oculomotor nerve (*3*), left peduncle (*ped*), and left superior cerebellar artery (*sca*). Below and to the right are the right oculomotor nerve (*3*) and right P-1 (*p-1*). *te*, tentorial edge; *tl-ret*, temporal lobe retractor; *cot*, cottonoid strips.

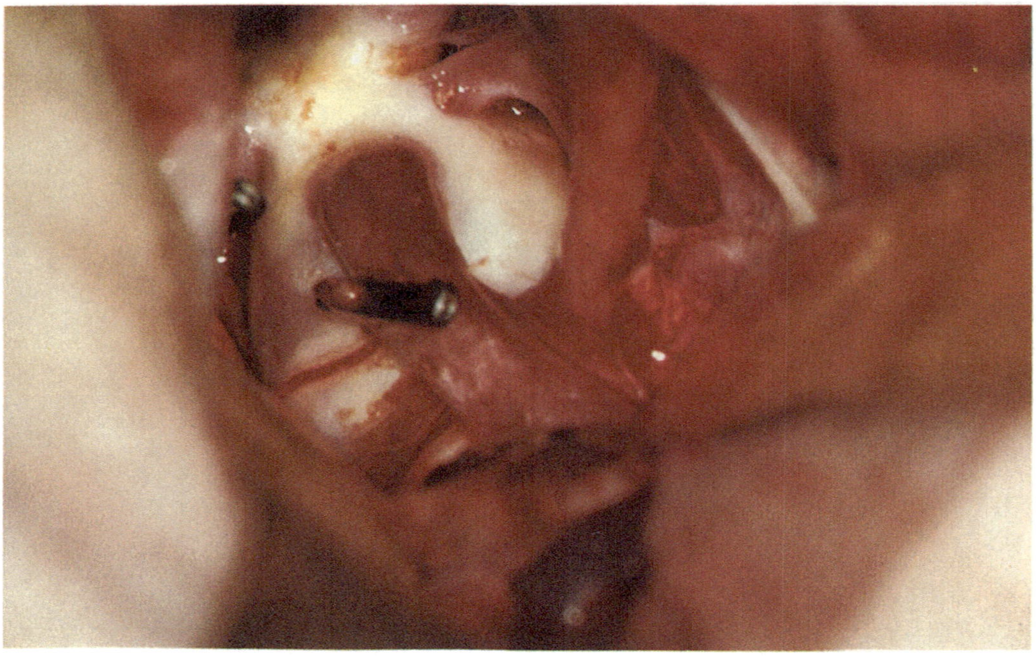

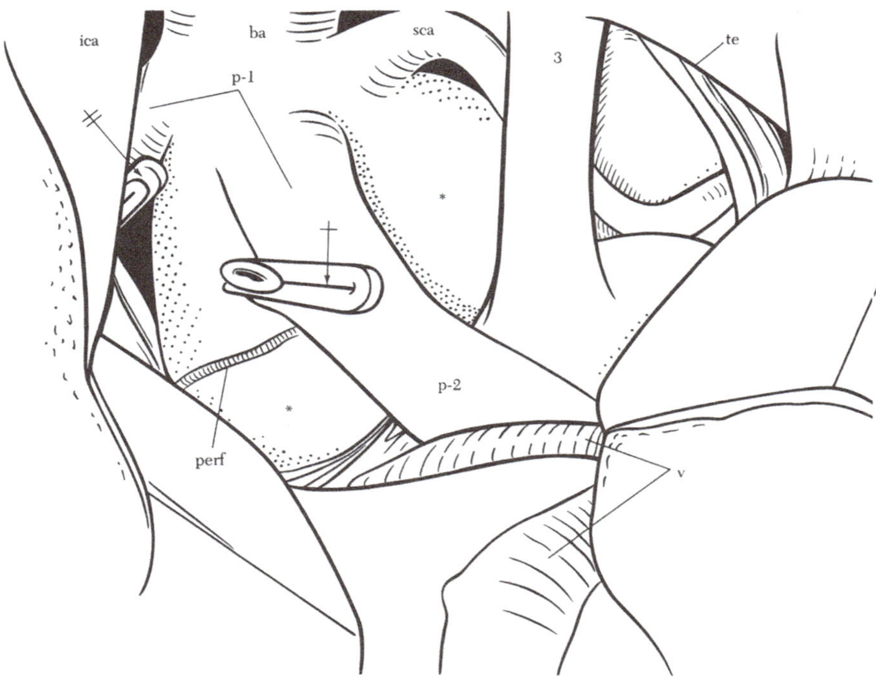

Fig. 38.23. Same case as in Figs. 38.20–38.22 and 38.24. About half of the fundus of the aneurysm (*) has been exposed. Note how the right P-1 (*p-1,* below) has been incorporated in the expanded neck of the aneurysm. *ica,* internal carotid artery (out of focus); *double-crossed arrow,* tantalum clip on proximal end of severed posterior communicating artery; *single-crossed arrow,* tantalum clip on distal end of severed posterior communicating artery; *p-1,* origins of left (above) and right (below) P-1 arteries; *ba,* tip of basilar artery; *sca,* right superior cerebellar artery; *3,* right oculomotor nerve; *te,* tentorial edge; *v,* veins; *p-2,* right P-2 artery; *perf,* perforator from P-1 coursing around dome of aneurysm. From Fox JL: ref. 11.

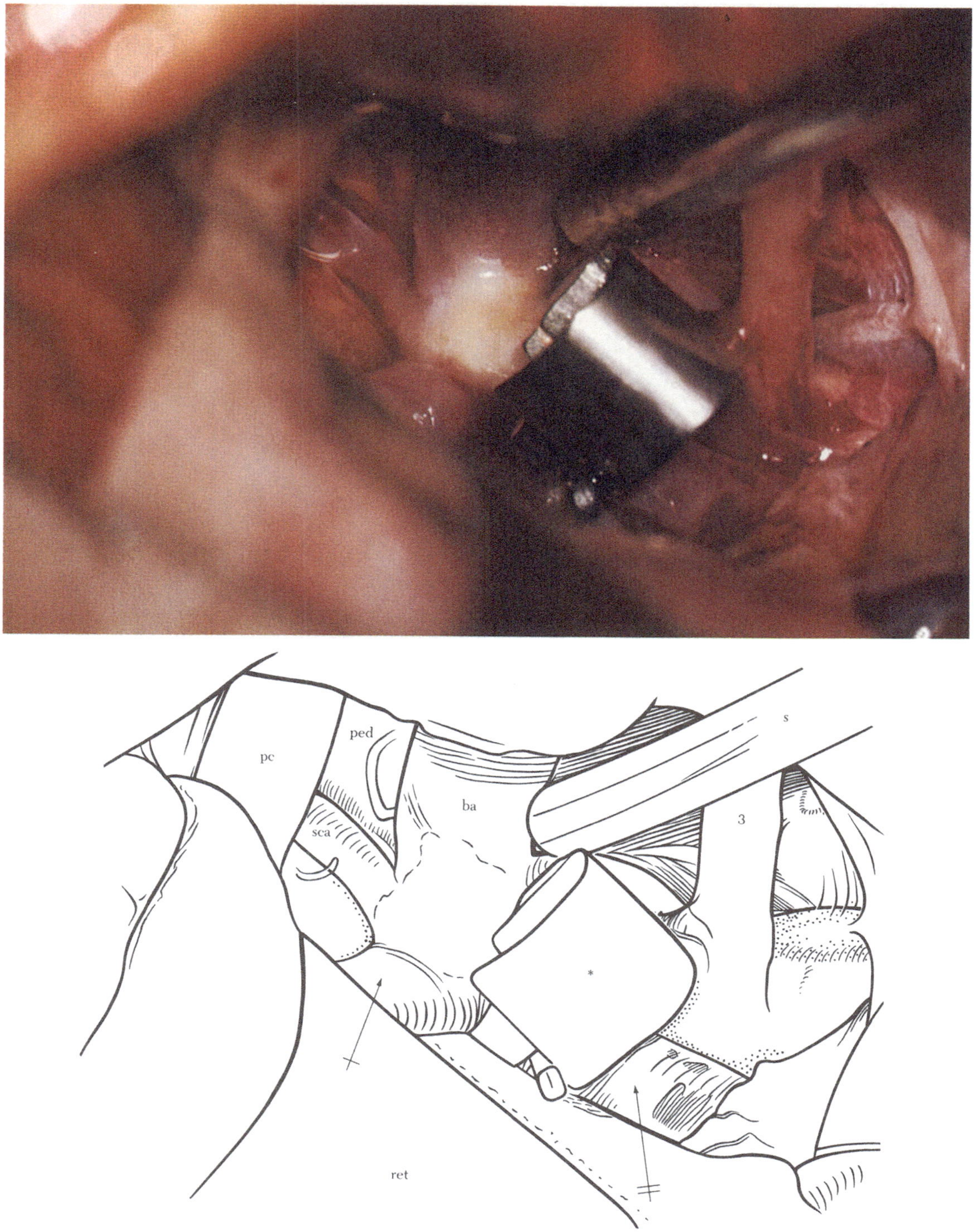

Fig. 38.24. Same case as in Figs. 38.20–38.23 after application of Drake clip (*) so as to encircle the right posterior cerebral artery (*double-crossed arrow*) and collapse the aneurysm. *pc,* posterior clinoid process; *ped,* left peduncle; *sca,* left superior cerebellar artery; *ba,* basilar artery; *s,* suction tube (tip at origin of right superior cerebellar artery); *3,* right oculomotor nerve arising from midbrain; *ret,* retractor blades; *single-crossed arrow,* left P-1; *, shank of Drake clip.

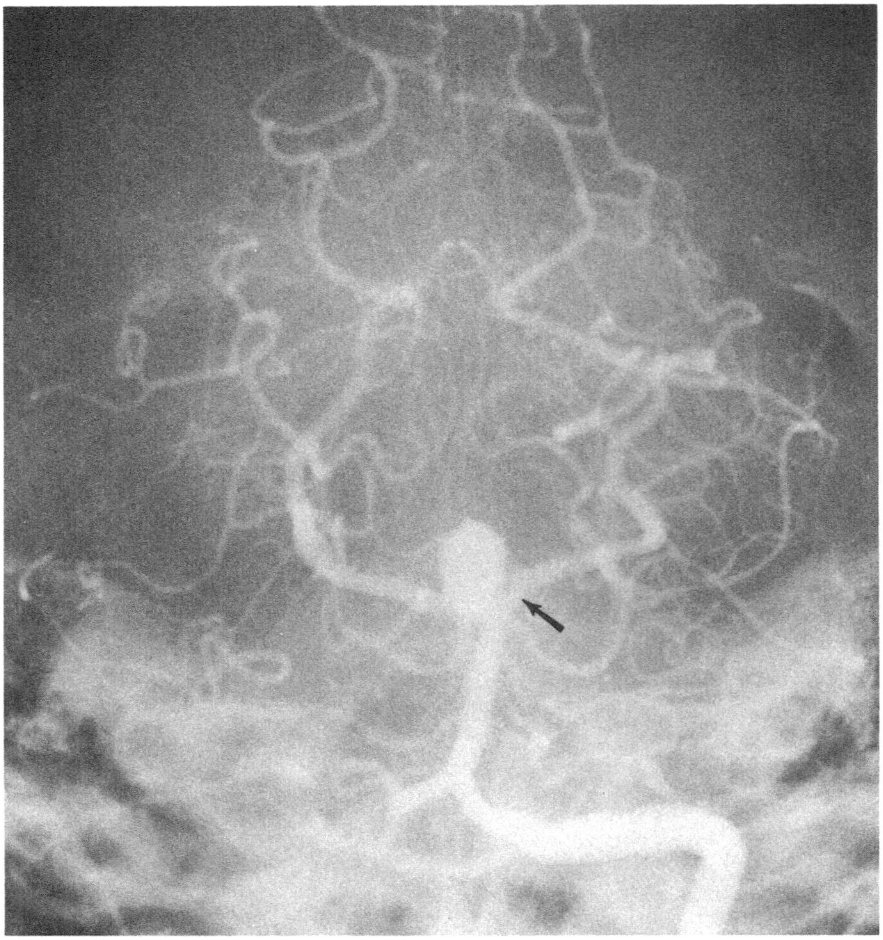

Fig. 38.25. Frontal angiogram of prominent bBAA. Note relationship of aneurysm neck to the P-1 arteries, where the left P-1 (*arrow*) originates higher up on the neck of the aneurysm and goes rostrally before turning laterally. Same case as in Figs. 38.26 and 38.27.

Figures 38.28–38.36 are an example of a patient with three aneurysms: bBAA, MCAA, and pcaICAA. Although the aneurysms were attacked from the left side in this 60-year-old woman, the color photographs here have been reversed for the sake of anatomic orientation and consistency. Initially the sylvian fissure is widely opened (Fig. 38.29). The multilobulated MCAA was covered with gelfoam and cottonoids and clipped with three Yaşargil clips after the BAA was treated.

Figure 38.30 looks like an impassable avenue between the ICAA and the oculomotor nerve. After shrinking of the aneurysm with bipolar electrocautery (Fig. 38.31), tantalum clips can be applied (Fig. 38.32) and the pcaICAA dome excised. Spring clips are not used because their shank will interfere with the approach to the bBAA. The ICA and its remaining aneurysm neck are retracted gently, exposing the membrane of Liliequist (Fig. 38.33). This arachnoid membrane is opened into the interpenduncular cistern (Fig. 38.34). The PCoA is followed to the P-1/P-2 junction; clipped with small, malleable, tantalum clips; and severed between clips in a manner preserving blood flow from P-1 and from the ICA to the PCoA perforators (Fig. 38.35). The bBAA is thus exposed. All posterior thalamic perforators are cleared from around the aneurysm. Figure 38.36 differs from the previous figure by the critical demonstration of a perforator from the left P-1 artery.

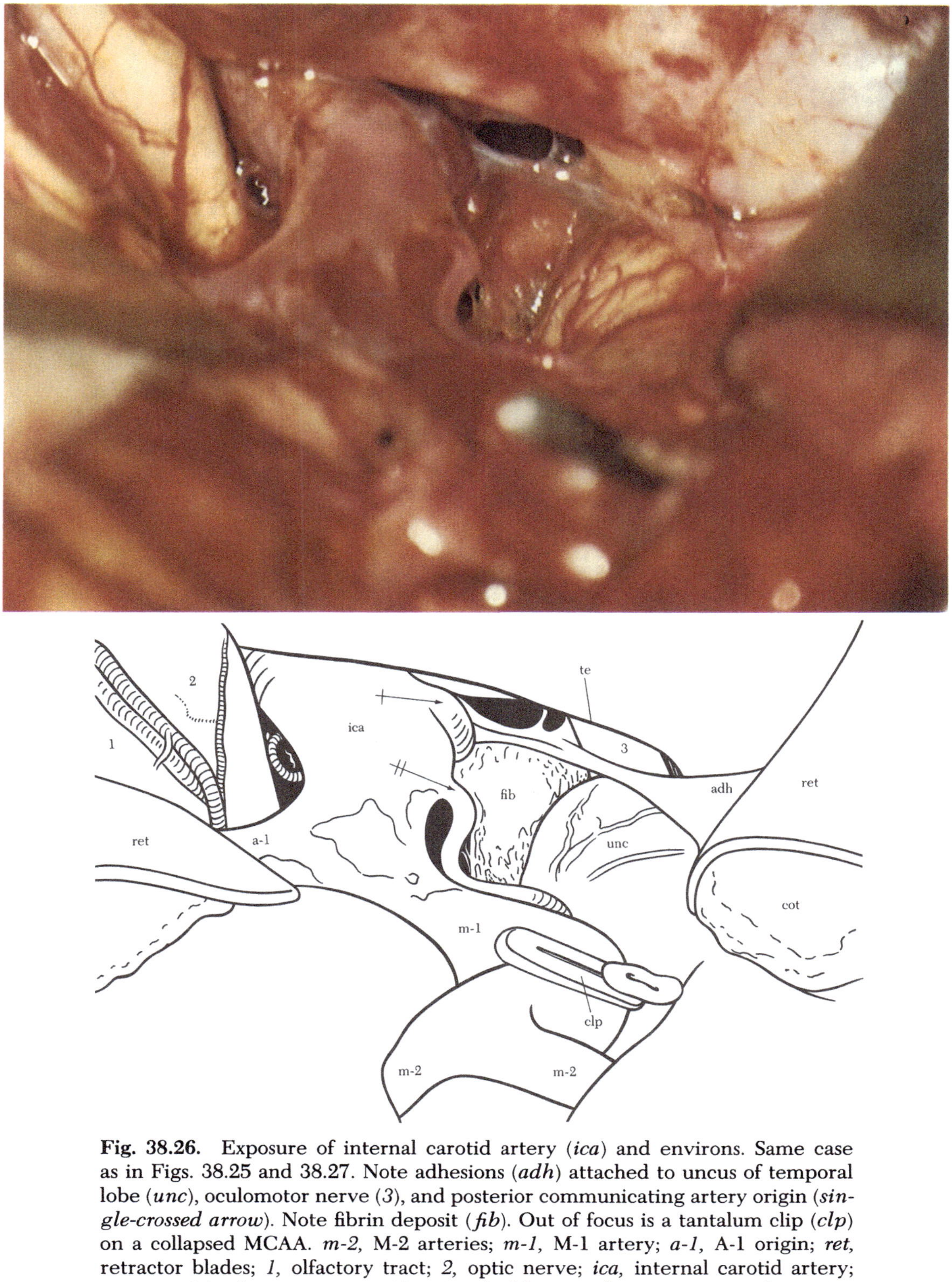

Fig. 38.26. Exposure of internal carotid artery (*ica*) and environs. Same case as in Figs. 38.25 and 38.27. Note adhesions (*adh*) attached to uncus of temporal lobe (*unc*), oculomotor nerve (*3*), and posterior communicating artery origin (*single-crossed arrow*). Note fibrin deposit (*fib*). Out of focus is a tantalum clip (*clp*) on a collapsed MCAA. *m-2,* M-2 arteries; *m-1,* M-1 artery; *a-1,* A-1 origin; *ret,* retractor blades; *1,* olfactory tract; *2,* optic nerve; *ica,* internal carotid artery; *te,* tentorial edge; *cot,* cottonoid strip; *double-crossed arrow,* origin of anterior choroidal artery.

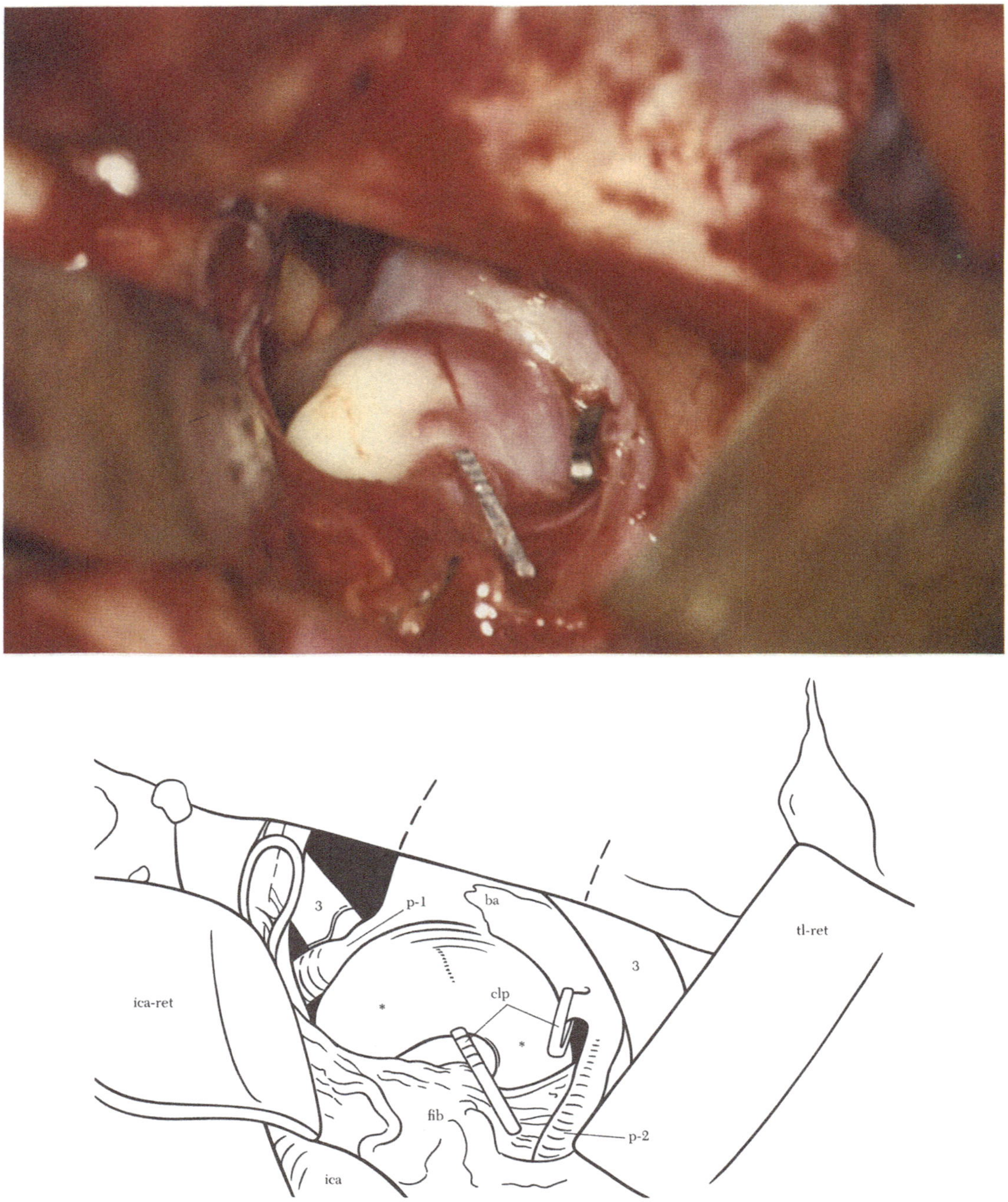

Fig. 38.27. Same case as in Figs. 38.25 and 38.26. The rostroventral face of the aneurysm (*) is exposed. Above and to the left are the left P-1 artery (*p-1*) and left oculomotor nerve (*3*). To the right are the right P-1 artery and right oculomotor nerve (*3*). *ba,* tip of basilar artery; *tl-ret,* temporal lobe retractor; *p-2,* right P-2 artery; *fib,* fibrin deposit; *ica,* internal carotid artery; *ica-ret,* internal carotid artery retractor. *Dotted lines,* path of BA.

In this case, one McFadden clip first was used across the dome of the aneurysm to collapse it. This was followed by a Yaşargil clip on the neck of the aneurysm. The clip often fails to close completely and the pulsating aneurysm causes the clip either to slip down onto the parent artery or its branches or to slip off the aneurysm entirely. A clip applied to the equator of the aneurysm usually will force distending blood out of the dome and help partially collapse the neck. It will not tend to slip onto the parent artery since, by straddling the equator, the clip will not be on the curvature toward the neck of the aneurysm. This technique worked well in this case. Angiography demonstrated occlusion of all aneurysms (Fig. 38.28C and D), and the patient returned home 10 days after the operation.

Superior Cerebellar Artery–Basilar Artery Aneurysms

These scaBAA are uncommon. They lie so close to the termination of the basilar artery that the approach is nearly identical to that for the previously described bBAA. However, the question of on which side should the frontotemporal craniotomy be performed arises. Should it be on the side ipsilateral to the side of the aneurysm, on the right (nondominant) side of the brain, or on the side contralateral to the side of the aneurysm? An ipsilateral approach may be difficult in some cases where the dome of the aneurysm obscures its neck and where the oculomotor nerve lies between the surgeon and the aneurysm. Although in such situations a meticulous dissection will still usually allow adequate aneurysm clipping from the ipsilateral side, serious consideration should be given to the contralateral approach—especially if the aneurysm lies on the left side of the basilar artery or if there is a second aneurysm on the contralateral anterior circulation.

Figures 38.37–38.40 illustrate a case with two aneurysms on the ACoA, a tiny achaICAA on the right, and a left-sided scaBAA. An approach from the right side was utilized with successful clipping of the aneurysms. After the usual frontotemporal exposure of the carotid cistern (Fig. 38.38), the ICA and its aneurysm is retracted; the temporal lobe uncus is moved off the oculomotor nerve; the PCoA is clipped and severed; and the basilar artery is exposed (Fig. 38.39). In Fig. 38.39 one can see the nice exposure of the scaICAA projecting leftward. The neck was quite accessible with the dome pointing away from the surgeon and with no oculomotor nerve interference. The neck was dissected away from fibrin and clot (this aneurysm had bled originally), from the left P-1 artery, and from the left superior cerebellar artery. After bipolar electrocoagulation to shrink the aneurysm, a gently curved spring clip was applied about the aneurysm neck. Following this, the ACoAA and the achaICAA were clipped (Fig. 38.40). This 56-year-old woman returned home 7 days after surgery.

Lower Basilar Artery Aneurysms

In most instances, one may have to use the subtemporal approach to the aicaBAA and vaBAA. Details are presented in Chapter 29. However, in some cases it is still possible to clip a basilar artery aneurysm at the AICA take-off by the frontotemporal approach.

Figures 38.41–38.43 illustrate just such a case. This 52-year-old woman had a ruptured right MCAA plus four more incidental aneurysms: a left MCAA, a left ACeAA at the genu of the corpus callosum, an ACoAA (not seen on the angiogram; see Fig. 35.13), and a right aicaBAA. At her first surgery, a right frontotemporal craniotomy was performed. Upon dissecting the frontal lobe off A-1 and the optic nerve, a previously unrecognized ACoAA was found (Fig. 35.13) and clipped. The MCAA was protected, and the aicaBAA was exposed lying deep to the oculomotor nerve (Fig. 38.42).

The problem here is to clip the aneurysm with the wings of the clip parallel to the basilar artery in order to lessen the risk of tearing the neck of the aneurysm. This required a very delicate insertion of a Yaşargil clip with its wings angled to the surgeon's right but in the same plane as the shank of the clip. The clip had to be inserted deep between the ICA and CN-3 without injury to either (Fig. 38.43). Thereafter the MCAA was dissected free of its adhesions and clipped. Later the left-sided aneurysms were successfully treated, and the patient has done well.

Summary

Chapters 34–38 have shown examples of anterior circulation aneurysms and upper basilar artery aneurysms that can be approached effec-

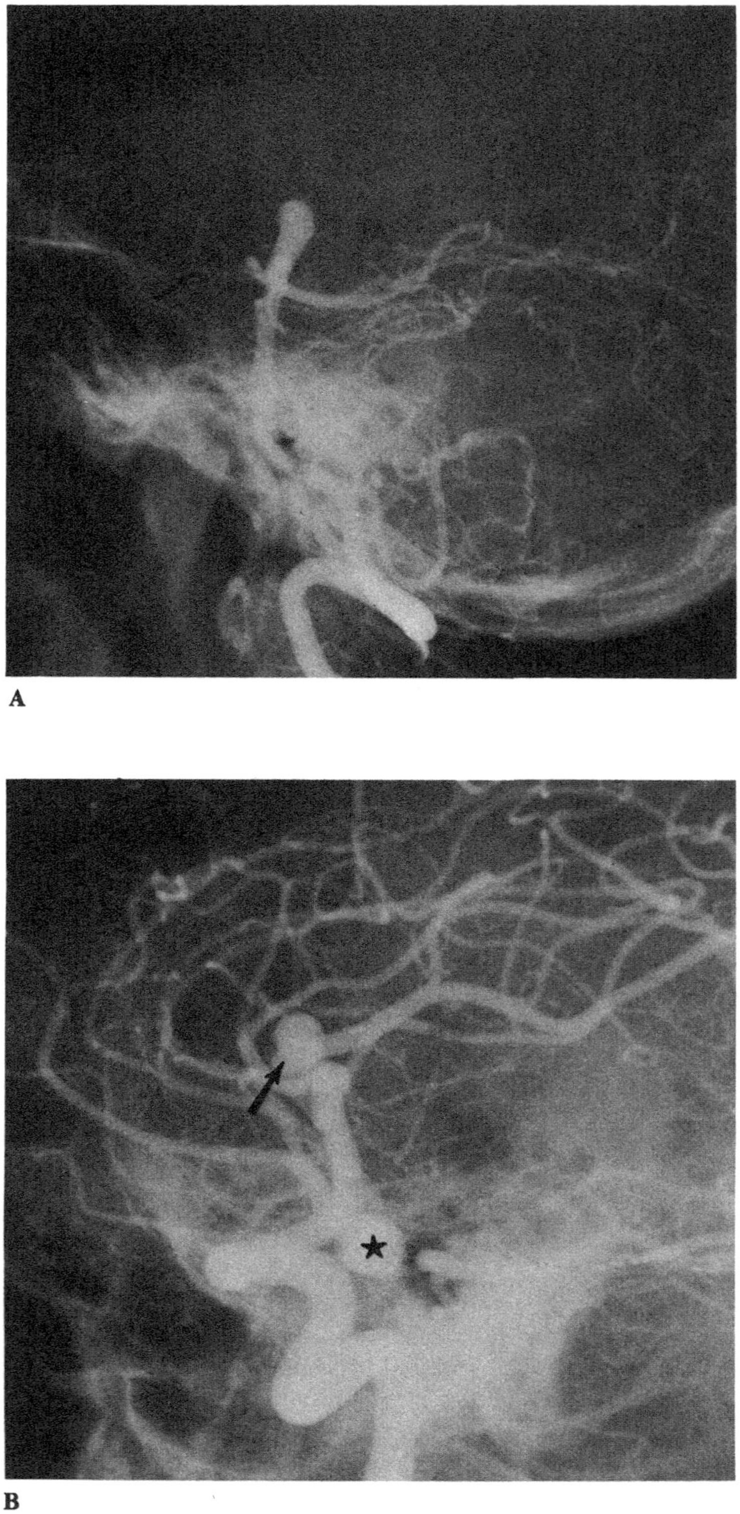

Fig. 38.28. **A** Lateral vertebrobasilar angiogram of an elongated bBAA. Note relation of its ectatic neck to the posterior clinoid processes (*arrow*). Same case as in Figs. 38.29–38.36. **B** Lateral carotid angiogram, Haughton view, of same patient. *Arrow,* MCAA at M-1 bifurcation; *star,* pcaICAA.

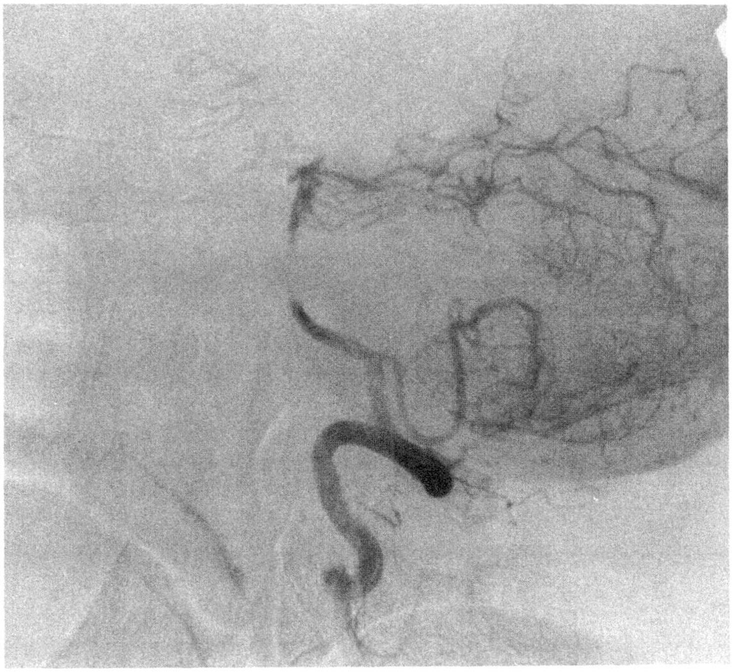

C

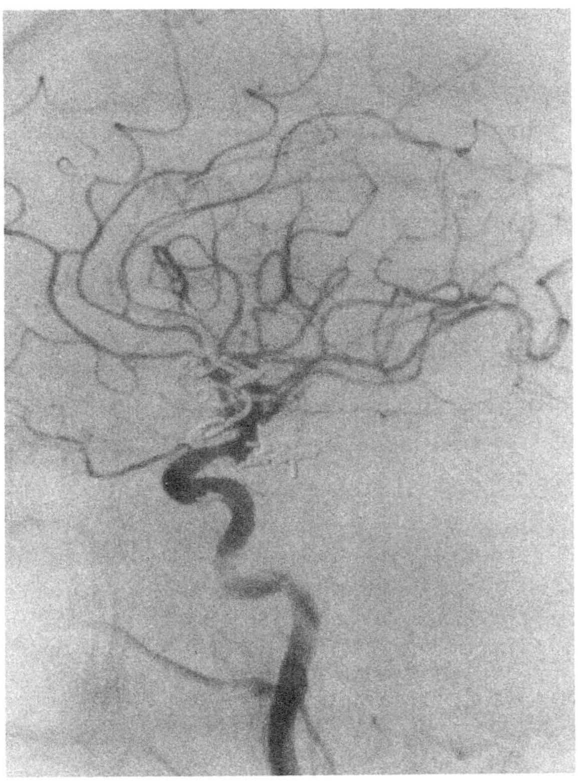

D

C and **D** Postoperative angiograms, subtraction technique. The patient had an excellent clinical result.

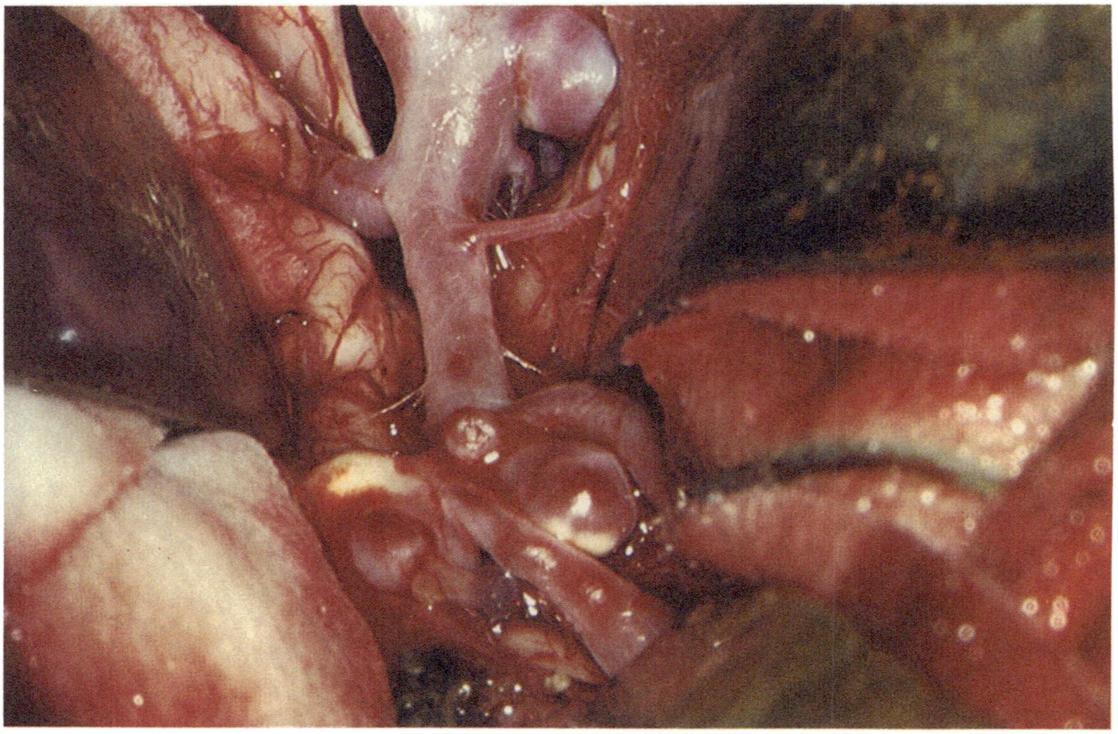

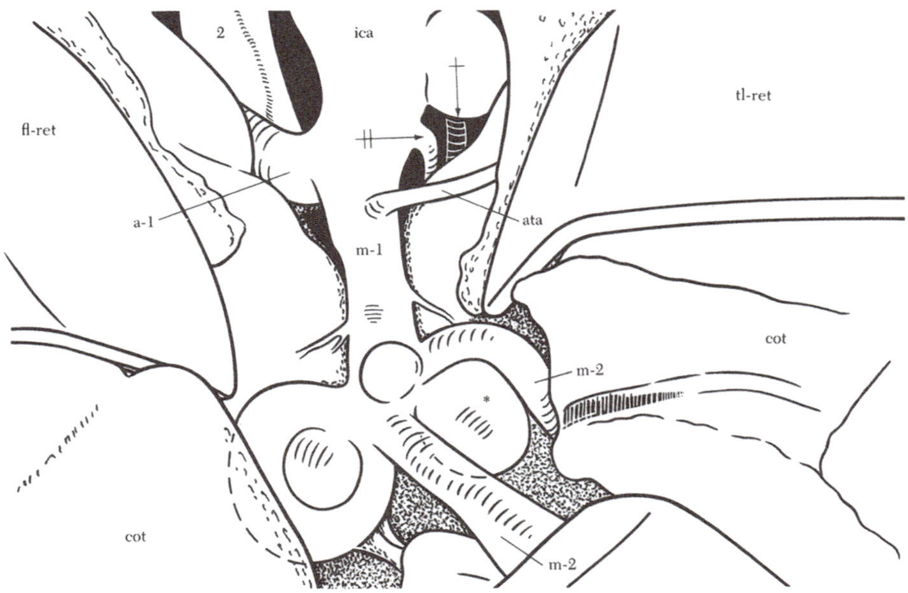

Fig. 38.29. View along sylvian fissure of same case as in Fig. 38.28 and 38.30–38.36. Zeiss magnification dial set at No. 10. *ica,* internal carotid artery; *single-crossed arrow* crosses internal carotid artery aneurysm and points to deep-lying posterior communicating artery; *double-crossed arrow,* origin of anterior choroidal artery; *ata,* anterior temporal artery; *tl-ret,* temporal lobe retractor; *cot,* cottonoid strips; *m-2,* M-2 branches surrounding one of several lobules (*) of a multilobulated middle cerebral artery aneurysm; *m-1,* M-1 artery; *a-1,* A-1 artery; *fl-ret,* frontal lobe retractor; *2,* optic nerve.

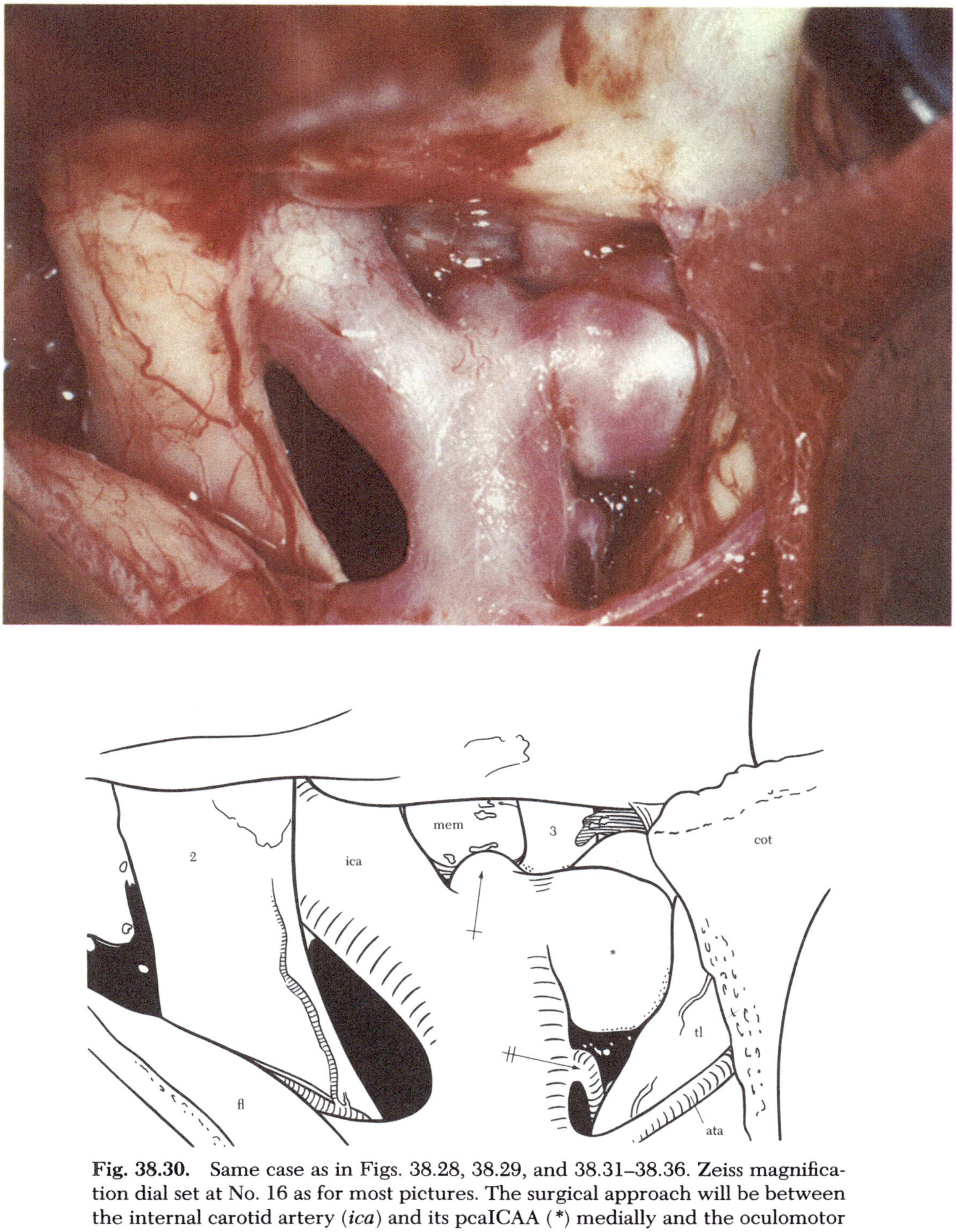

Fig. 38.30. Same case as in Figs. 38.28, 38.29, and 38.31–38.36. Zeiss magnification dial set at No. 16 as for most pictures. The surgical approach will be between the internal carotid artery (*ica*) and its pcaICAA (*) medially and the oculomotor nerve (*3*) laterally. *mem*, membrane of Liliequist; *cot*, cottonoid strip; *tl*, temporal lobe; *ata*, anterior temporal artery; *fl*, frontal lobe; *2*, optic nerve; *single-crossed arrow*, origin of posterior communicating artery; *double-crossed arrow*, origin of anterior choroidal artery.

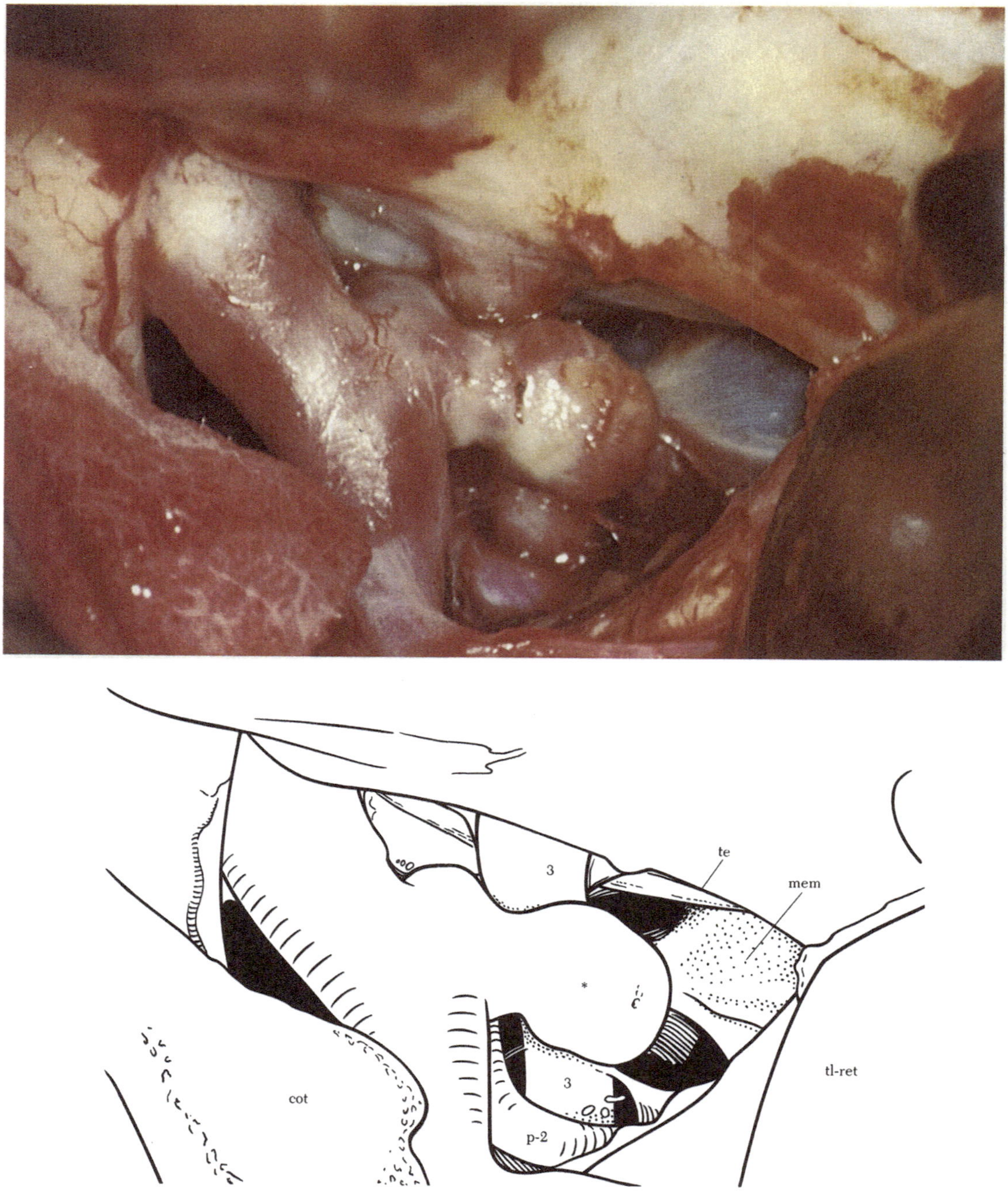

Fig. 38.31. Same case as in Figs. 38.28–38.30 and 38.32–38.36. The internal carotid artery aneurysm (*) has been shrunken by bipolar electrocoagulation, revealing adjacent surgical anatomy. *p-2,* P-2 segment of posterior cerebral artery in front of oculomotor nerve (*3,* seen above and below aneurysm); *cot,* cottonoid strip on frontal lobe; *te,* tentorial edge; *mem,* membrane of Liliequist (or Key and Retzius); *tl-ret,* temporal lobe retractor; *3,* oculomotor nerve.

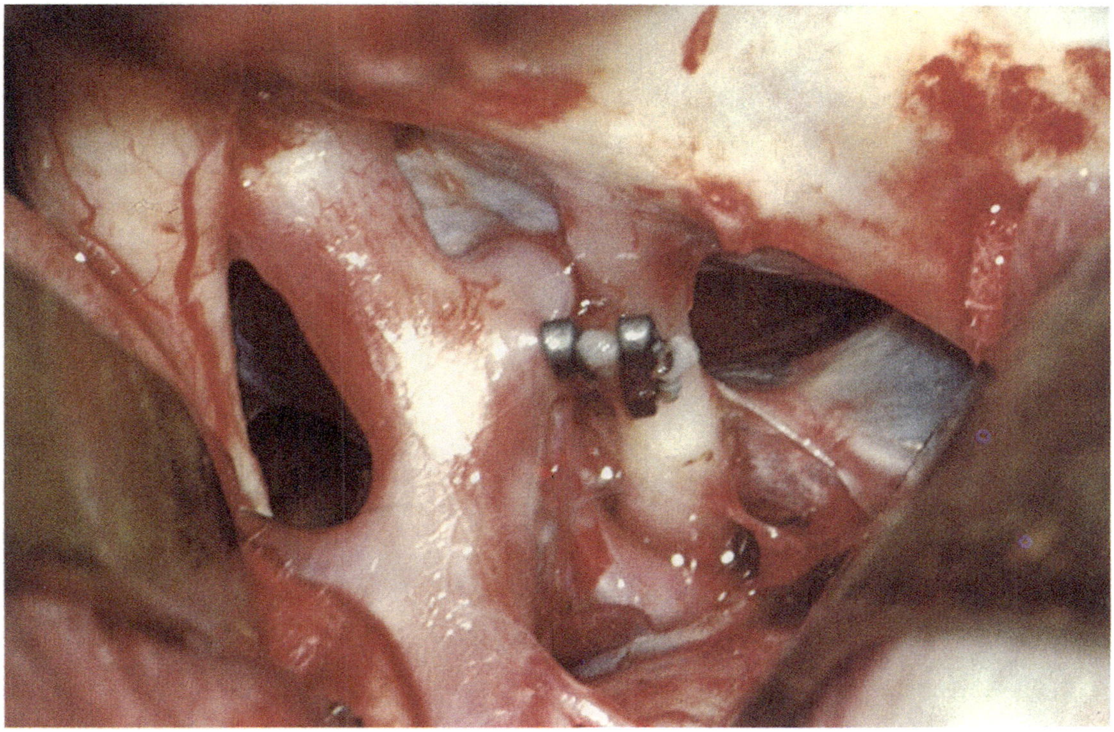

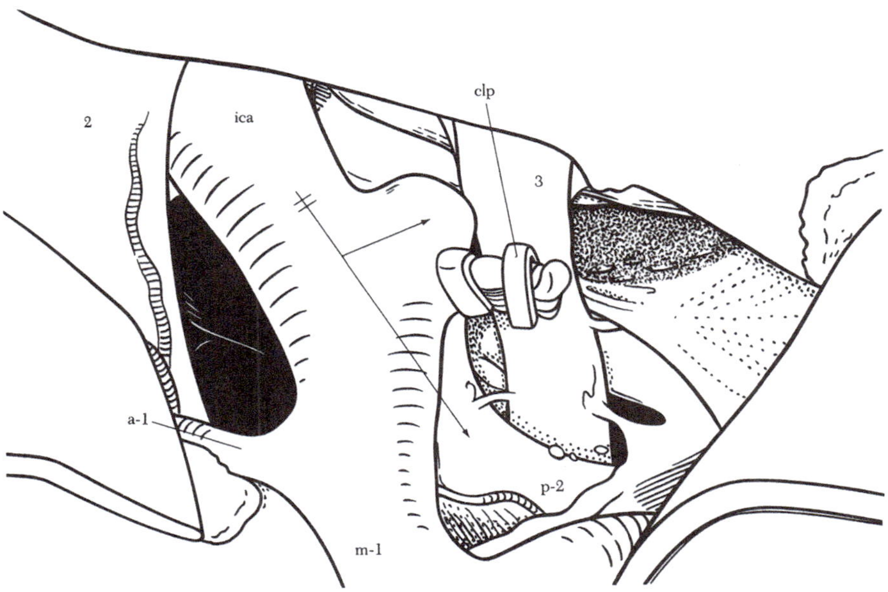

Fig. 38.32. Same case as in Figs. 38.28–38.31 and 38.33–38.36. Shrunken aneurysm has been clipped with two malleable, tantalum Ligaclips (*clp*) and then the dome excised. *3,* oculomotor nerve; *p-2,* P-2 artery; *m-1,* origin of M-1 artery; *a-1,* origin of A-1 artery; *2,* optic nerve; *ica,* internal carotid artery; *double-crossed arrows,* posterior communicating artery; *clp,* one of two tantalum clips on neck of excised aneurysm.

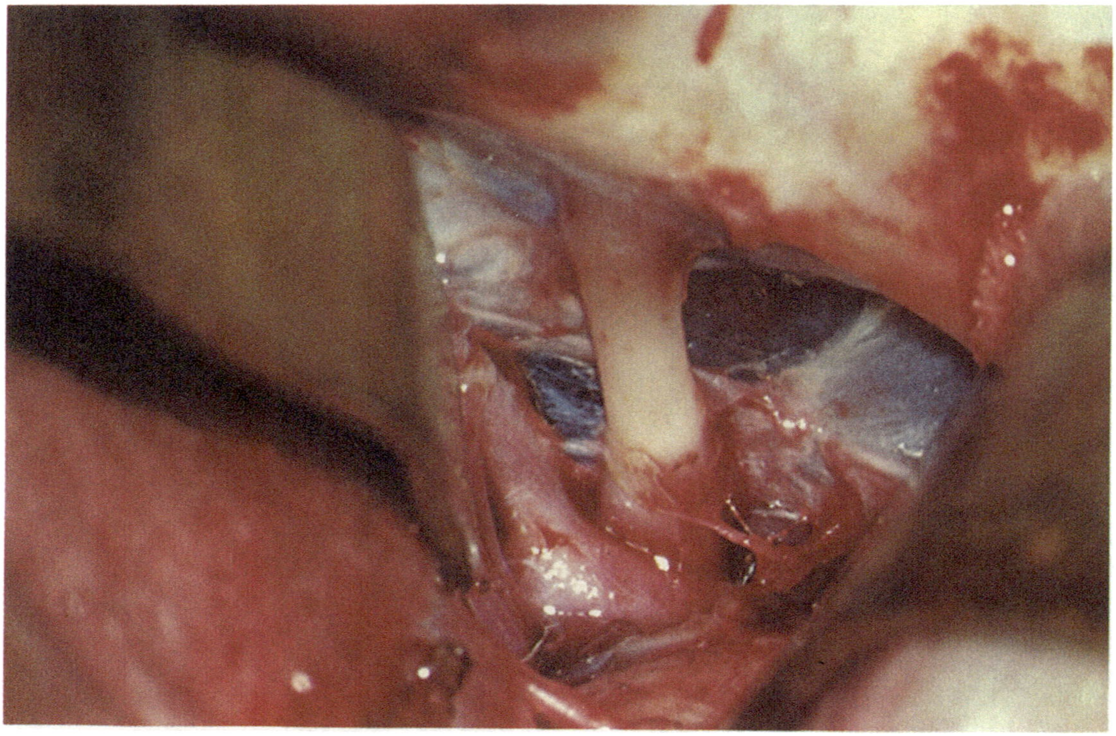

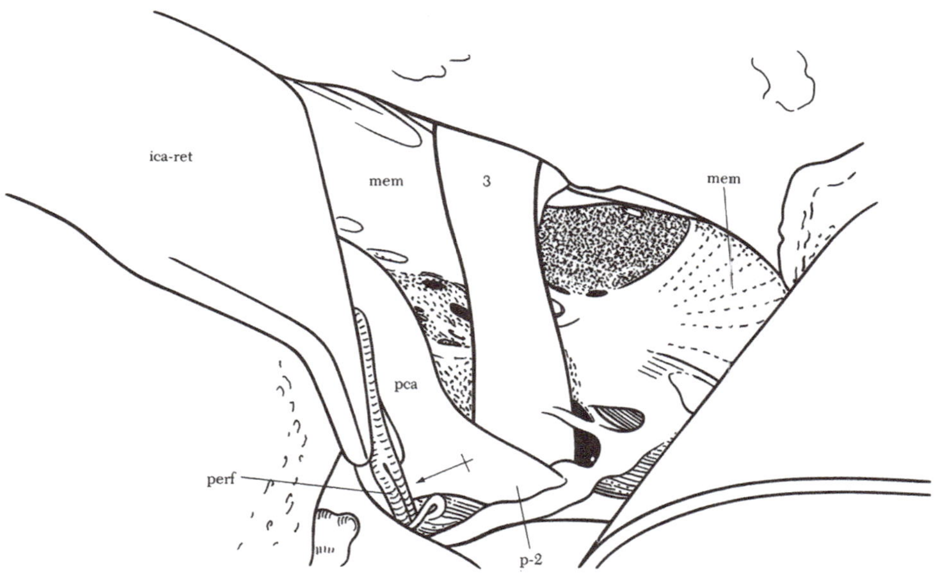

Fig. 38.33. Same case as in Figs. 38.28–38.32 and 38.34–38.36, following posterior communicating artery (*pca*) back to its junction with the P-2 artery (*p-2*) and P-1 artery (*single-crossed arrow*). The retractor (*ica-ret*) is pulling the internal carotid artery, proximal part of posterior communicating artery, and clipped remains of the carotid aneurysm medially. *3,* oculomotor nerve; *mem,* membrane of Liliequist; *perf,* arterial perforator.

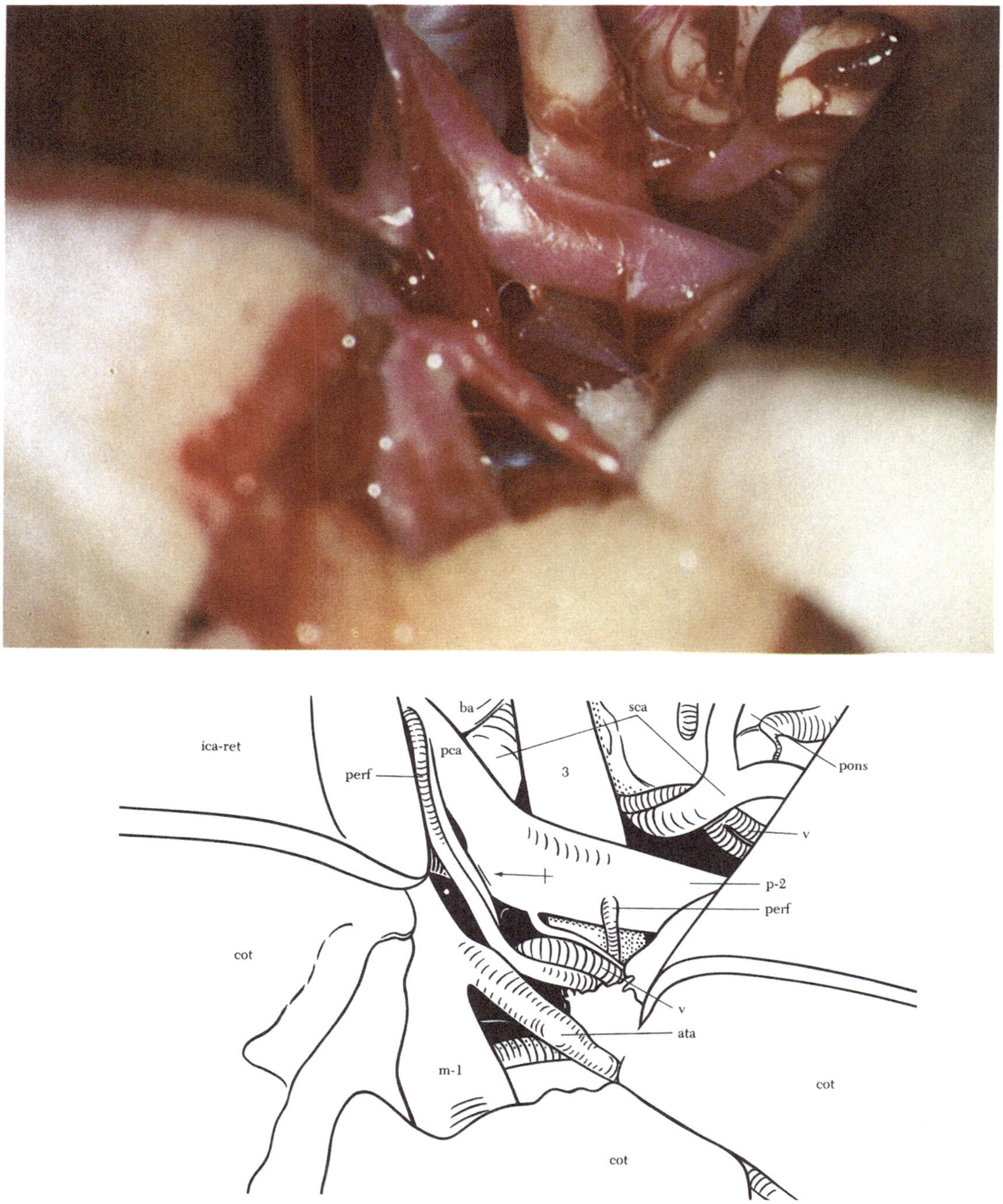

Fig. 38.34. Same case as in Figs. 38.28–38.33, 38.35, and 38.36. Liliequist membrane has been removed, exposing the interpeduncular cistern. *pca,* posterior communicating artery; *ba,* part of basilar artery; *sca,* superior cerebellar artery; *3,* oculomotor nerve; *pons,* rostral part of pons; *v,* vein; *p-2,* P-2 artery; ***single-crossed arrow*** points toward hidden P-1 artery; *perf,* arterial perforator; *ata,* anterior temporal artery; *cot,* cottonoid strips; *m-1,* M-1 artery; *ica-ret,* internal carotid artery retractor.

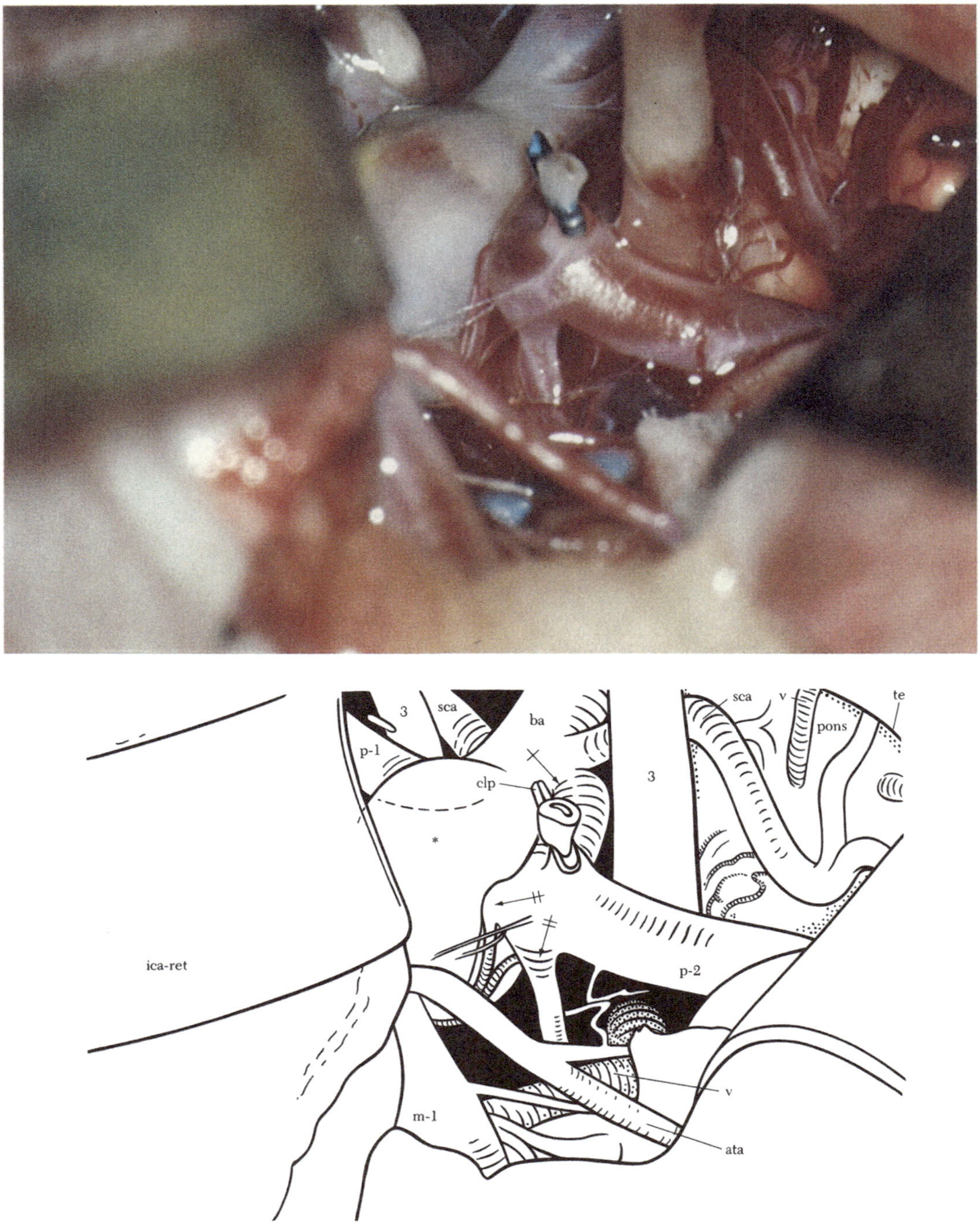

Fig. 38.35. Same case as in Figs. 38.28–38.34 and 38.36. Exposure of basilar tip aneurysm (*) after clipping (*clp*) and section of the posterior communicating artery. *Single-crossed arrow*, origin of P-1 artery looping rostrally around aneurysm; *double-crossed arrows*, perforators from PCoA/P-1/P-2 junctional zone. Above are seen the left P-1 artery (*p-1*), the left oculomotor nerve (*3*), and the left superior cerebellar artery (*sca*). To the observer's right are seen the right oculomotor nerve (*3*), the right superior cerebellar artery (*sca*), and the right P-1 artery (*single-crossed arrow*). *ba*, basilar artery; *v*, vein; *pons*, rostral part of pons; *te*, tentorial edge; *p-2*, right P-2 artery; *ata*, anterior temporal artery; *m-1*, M-1 artery; *ica-ret*, internal carotid artery retractor; *clp*, malleable, tantalum Ligaclip on distal end of transected posterior communicating artery.

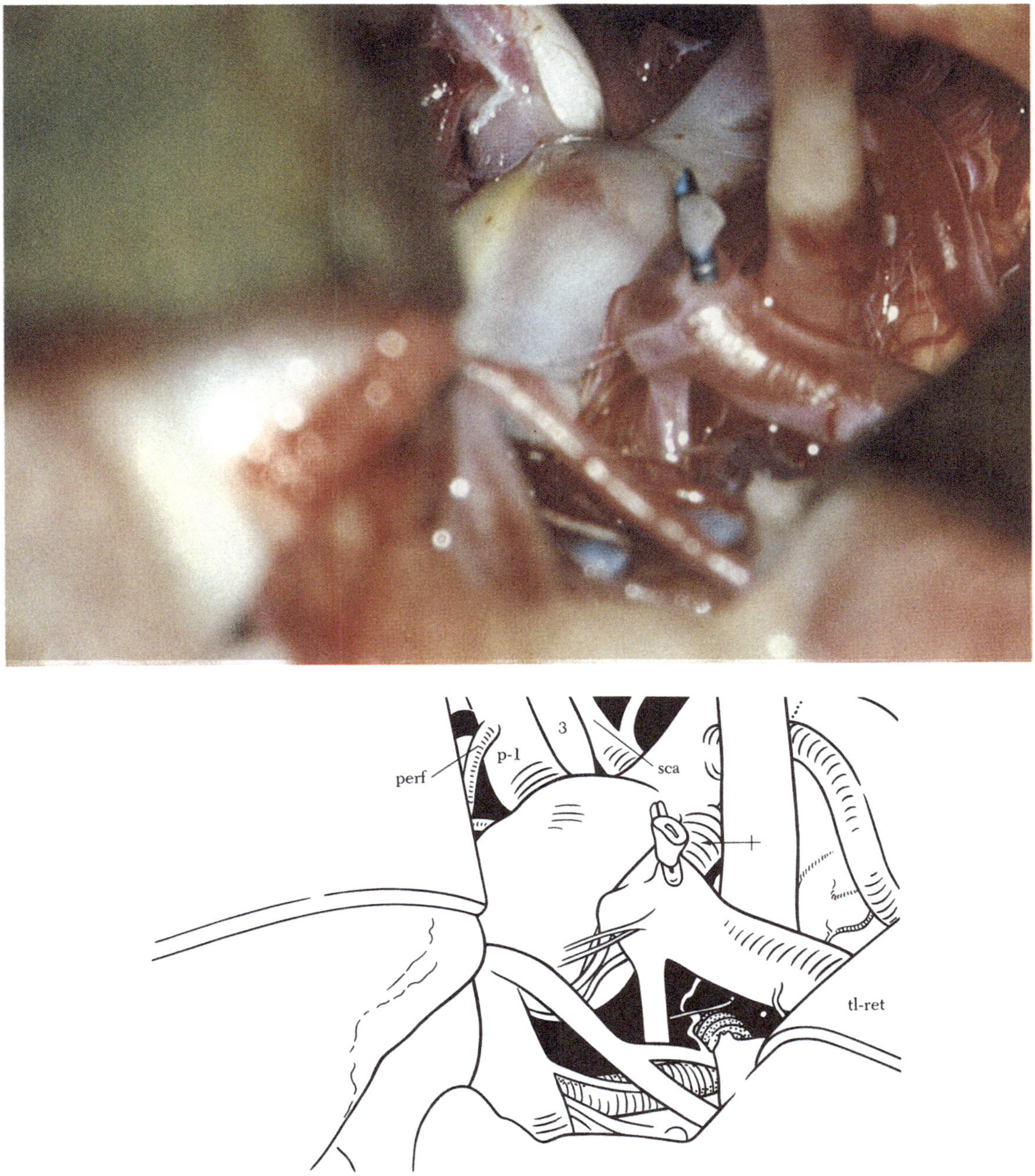

Fig. 38.36. Same case as in Figs. 38.26–38.35. Nearly the same view as in Fig. 38.35 except we now visualize an important perforator (*perf*) coming from the left P-1 artery (*p-1*). *3,* left oculomotor nerve; *sca,* left superior cerebellar artery; *single-crossed arrow,* right P-1 artery; *tl-ret,* temporal lobe retractor. After further dissection of the aneurysm, the aneurysm was clipped with an excellent result (see angiogram, Fig. 38.28C and D).

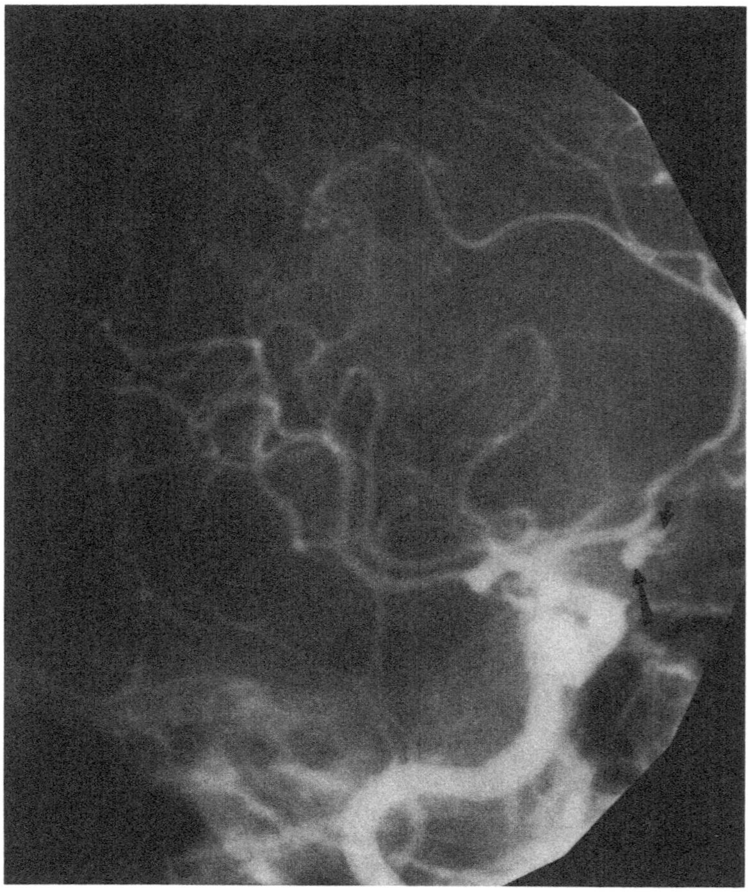

A

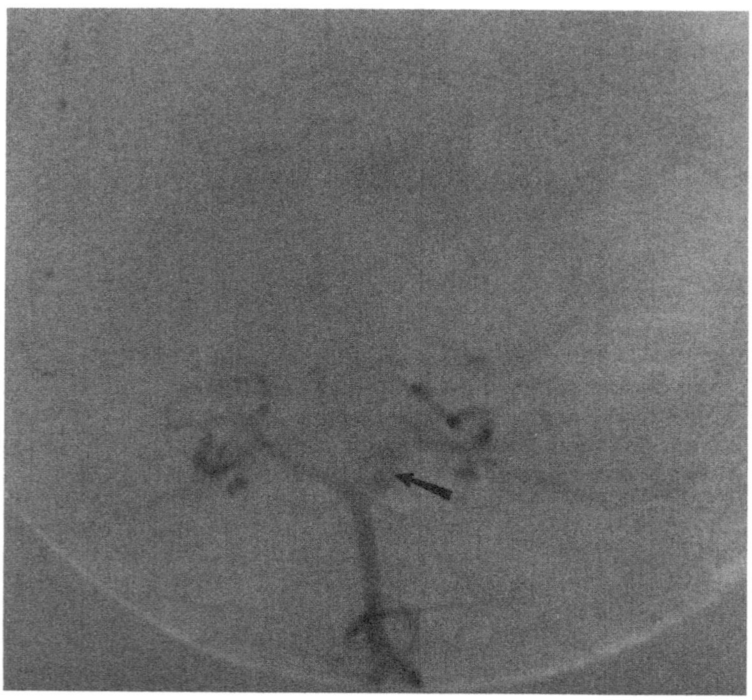

B

Fig. 38.37. A Carotid angiogram, oblique view, demonstrating two aneurysms of the ACoA (*arrows*) and a tiny pouch of contrast media between the PCoA take-off and the ICA bifurcation. At surgery, this latter pouch was an achaICAA. This is the same case as pictured in Figs. 38.38–38.40. **B** Vertebrobasilar angiogram, frontal view, showing a basilar artery aneurysm (*arrow*) lying between the left superior cerebellar artery below and the left P-1 artery above. Although this scaBAA was on the left, the actual surgical exposure was from the patient's right.

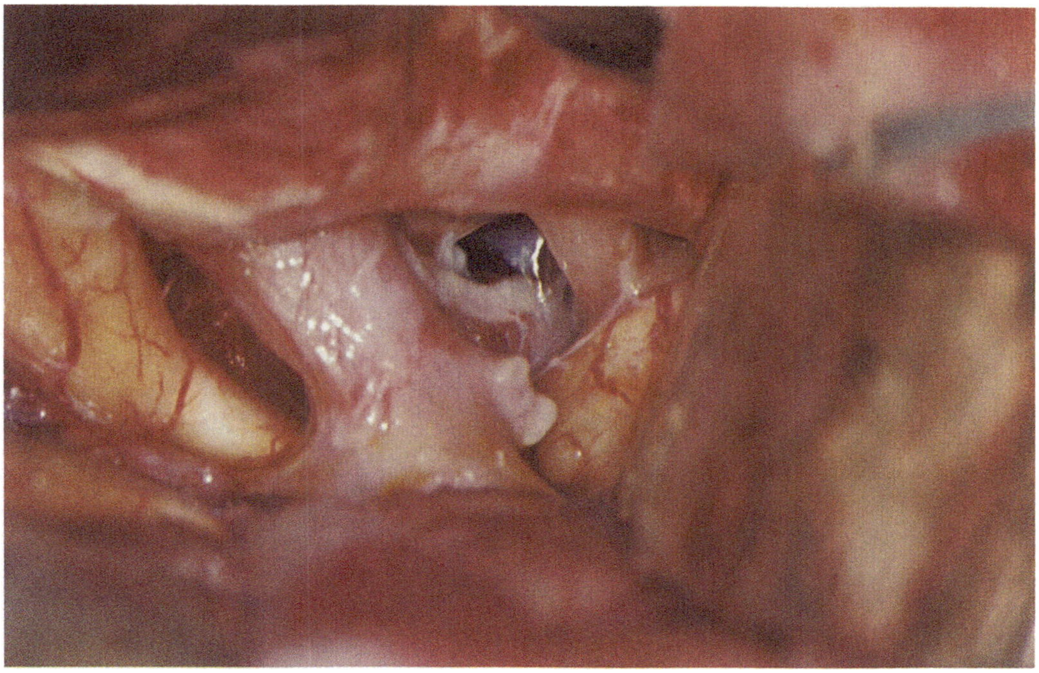

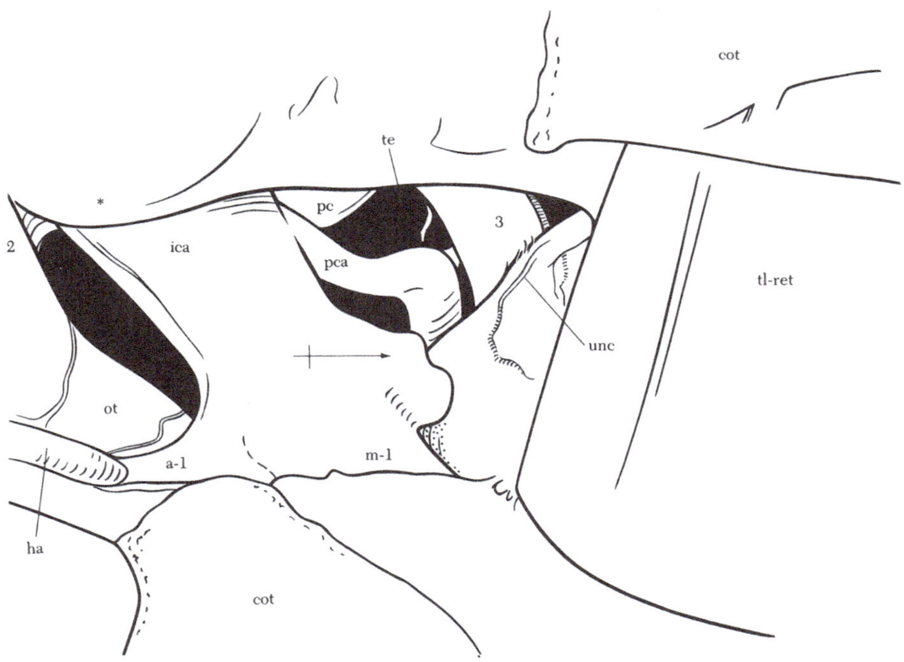

Fig. 38.38. Initial exposure toward the scaBAA. Same case as in Figs. 38.37, 38.39, and 38.40. This patient has a short right internal carotid artery (*ica*) from which a rather small posterior communicating artery arises (*pca*). *Single-crossed arrow,* tiny bilobed aneurysm at the take-off of the hidden anterior choroidal artery; *pc,* posterior clinoid process; *te,* tentorial edge; *3,* oculomotor nerve; *cot,* cottonoid strips; *tl-ret,* temporal lobe retractor; *unc,* uncus adherent to the oculomotor nerve; *m-1,* origin of M-1 artery; *a-1,* origin of A-1 artery; *ha,* Heubner's artery; *ot,* optic tract; *2,* optic nerve; *, anterior clinoid process.

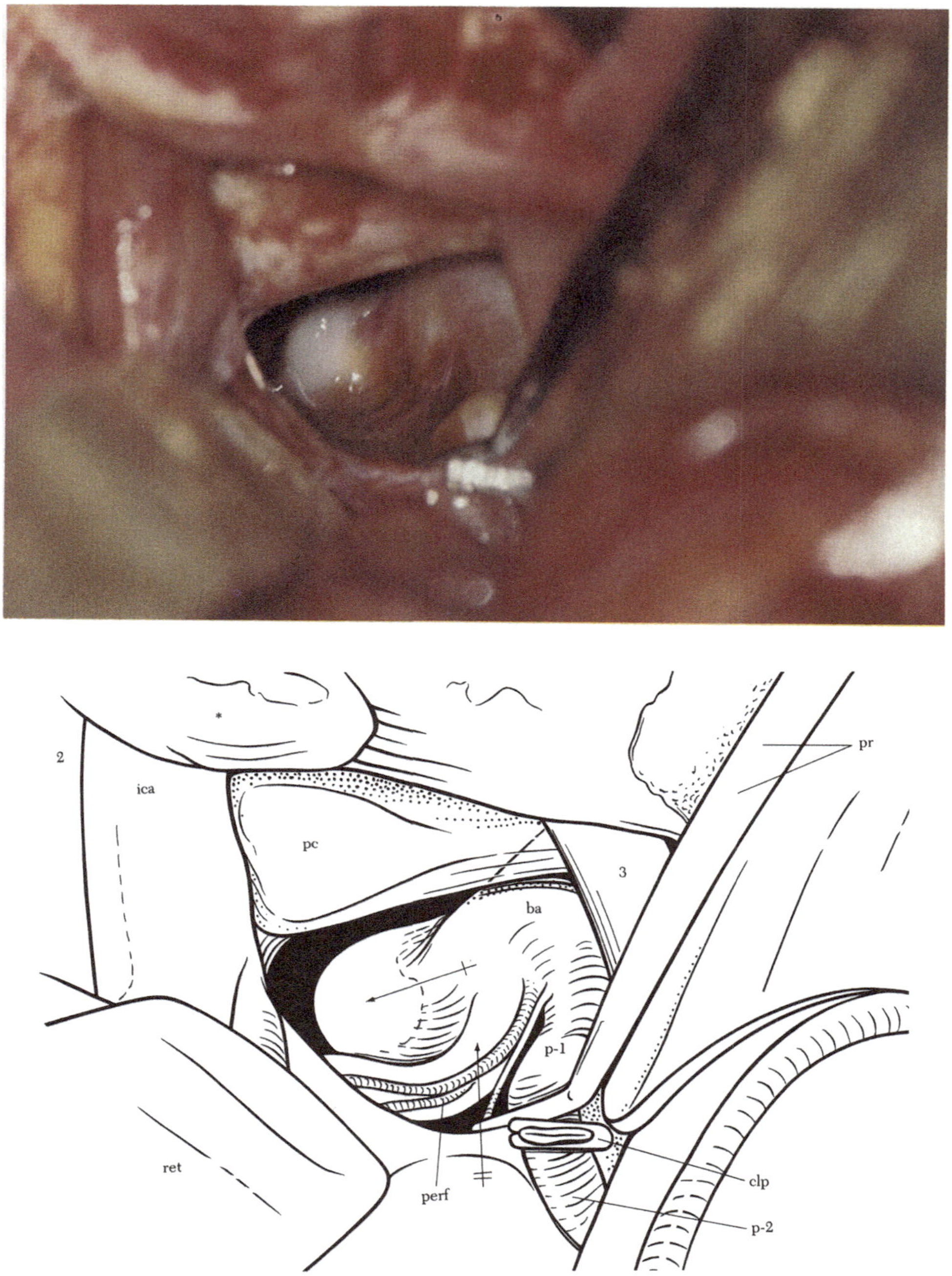

Fig. 38.39. Same case as in Figs. 38.37, 38.38, and 38.40. The left scaBAA (*single-crossed arrow*) is identified within the interpreduncular cistern. This arrow crosses the neck of the aneurysm and points to the fundus. The left superior cerebellar artery on the other side of the aneurysm is hidden by shadows in this picture. The aneurysm is clearly seen beyond the projecting right posterior clinoid process (*pc*). *ba,* terminus of basilar artery; *pr,* probe retracting the right P-1 artery (*p-1*); *3,* oculomotor nerve; *clp,* tantalum clip on distal end of severed posterior communicating artery; *p-2,* right P-2 artery; *double-crossed arrow,* left P-1 artery; *perf,* perforators; *ret,* retractor on the internal carotid artery (*ica*); *2,* optic nerve; *, anterior clinoid process.

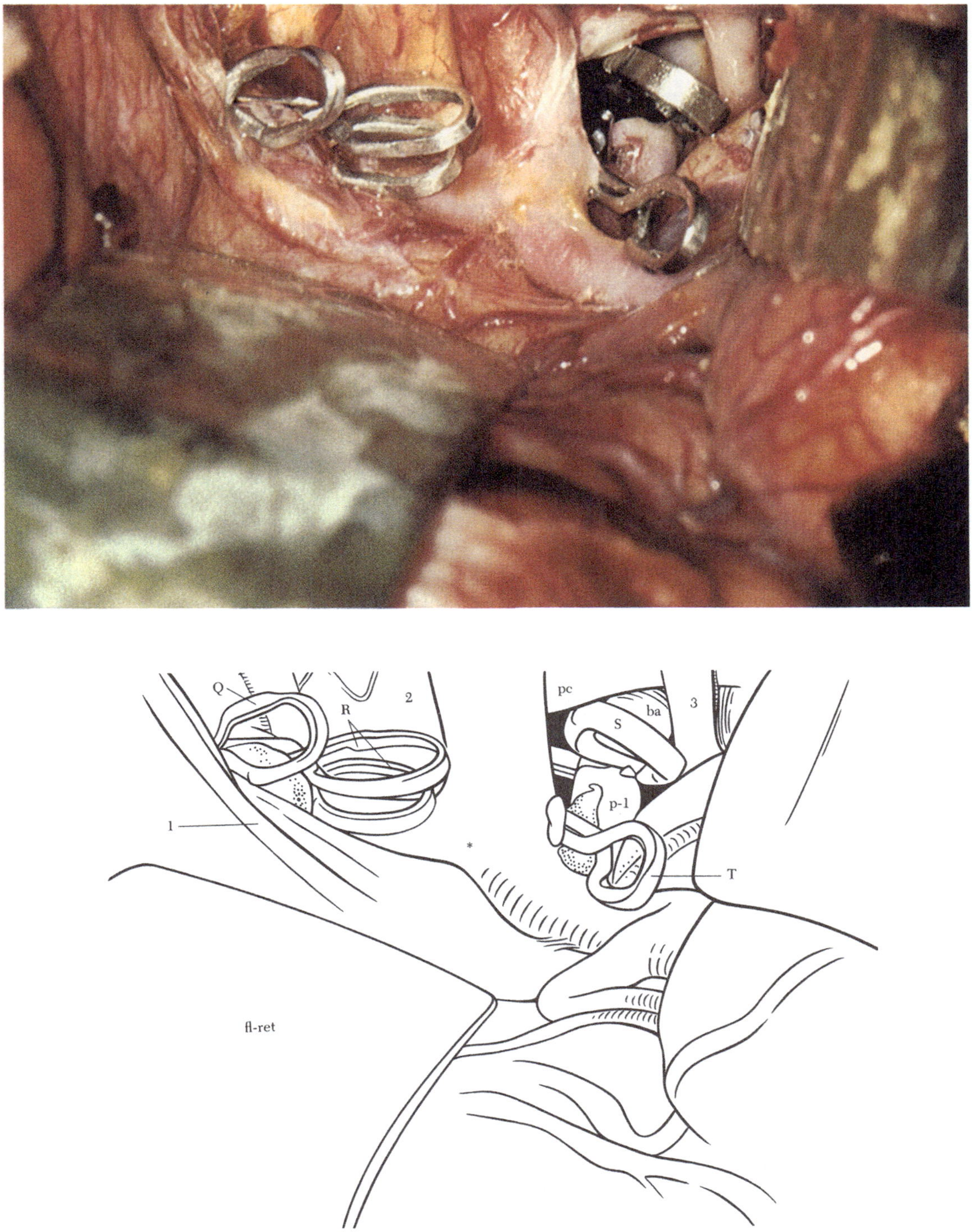

Fig. 38.40. Same case as in Figs. 38.37–38.39. All aneurysms have been clipped. *Q,* clip on upward projecting ACoAA; *R,* two clips on downward projecting ACoAA; *S,* clip on left scaBAA; *T,* clip on right achaICAA; *fl-ret,* frontal lobe retractor; *1,* olfactory tract; *2,* optic nerve; *pc,* posterior clinoid process; *ba,* basilar artery; *3,* oculomotor nerve; *p-1,* P-1 artery; **,* bifurcation of the internal carotid artery.

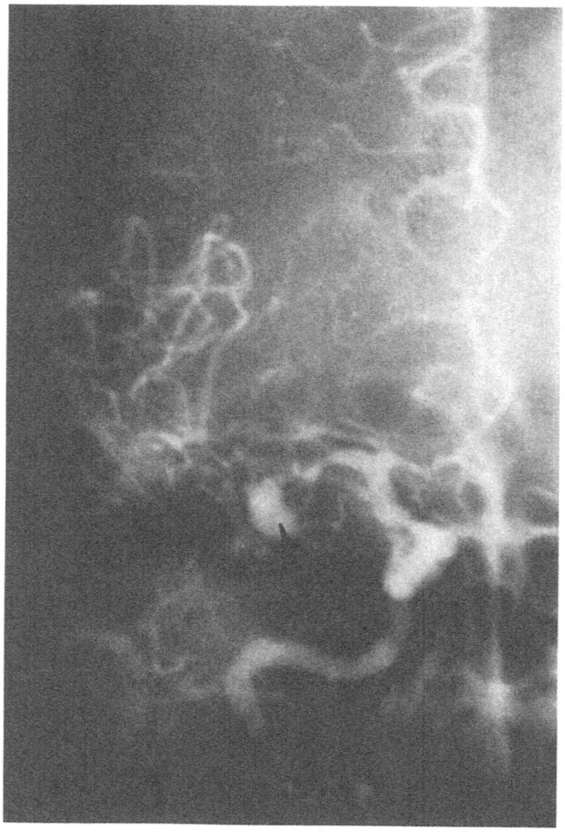

A

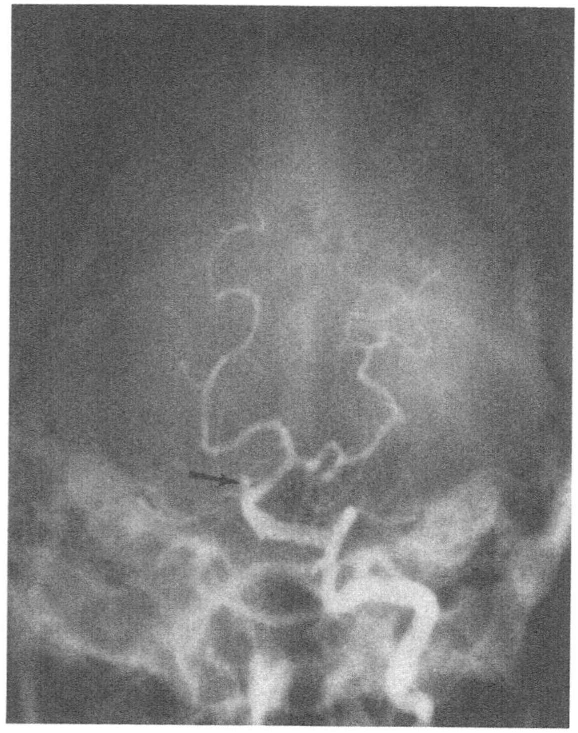

C

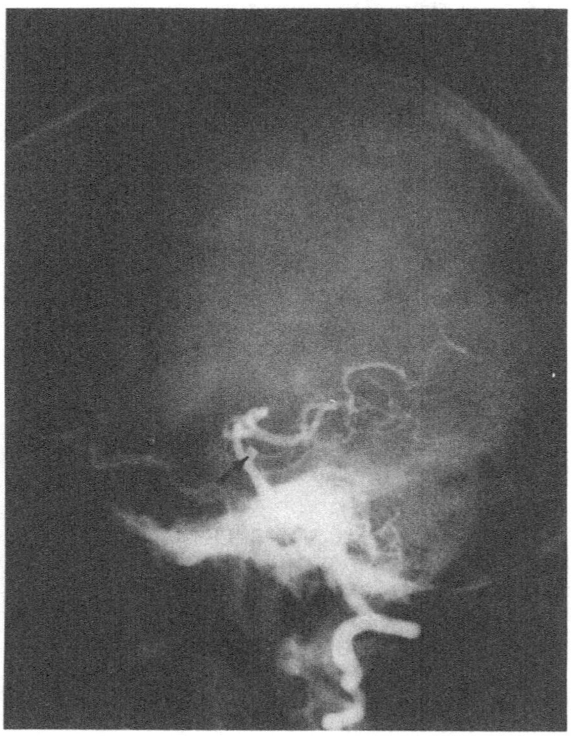

B

Fig. 38.41. A Right carotid angiogram, frontal view, illustrating ruptured MCAA (*arrow*). This is the same case as in Figs. 35.13, 38.42, and 38.43. B Vertebrobasilar angiogram, lateral view, revealing the aicaBAA (*arrow*). Its position was rather high up in relation to the dorsum sellae. C Same, frontal view, showing aneurysm (*arrow*) at the take-off of the anterior inferior cerebellar artery.

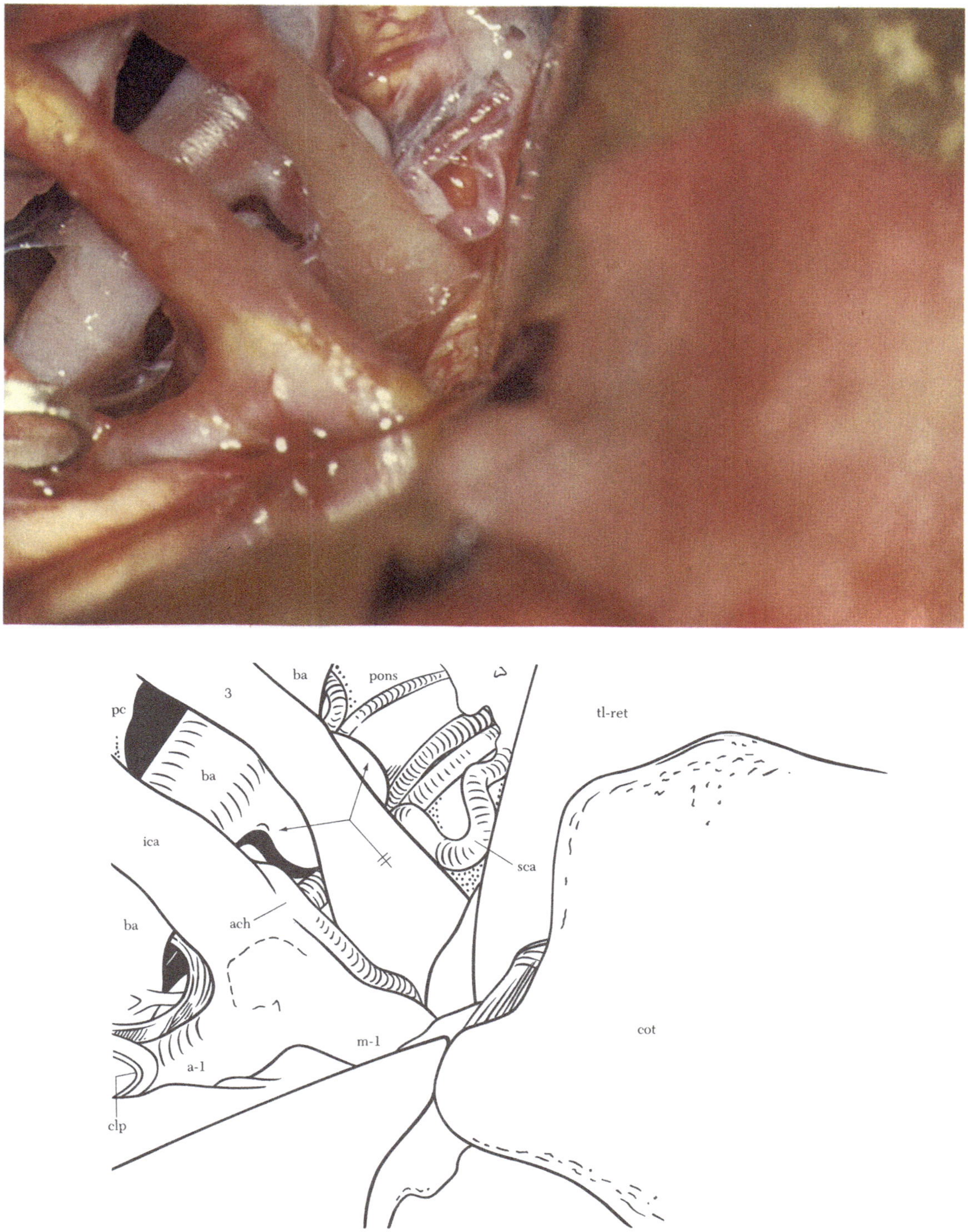

Fig. 38.42. Exposure of aicaBAA (*double-crossed arrows*) behind the oculomotor nerve (*3*). *ba,* basilar artery; *pons,* rostral part of the pons; *tl-ret,* temporal lobe retractor; *sca,* branches of superior cerebellar artery; *cot,* cottonoid strips; *m-1,* M-1 artery; *a-1,* A-1 artery; *clp,* shank of clip on the anterior communicating artery aneurysm (Fig. 35.13); *ica,* internal carotid artery; *pc,* posterior clinoid process; *ach,* anterior choroidal artery. Same case as in Figs. 38.41 and 38.43.

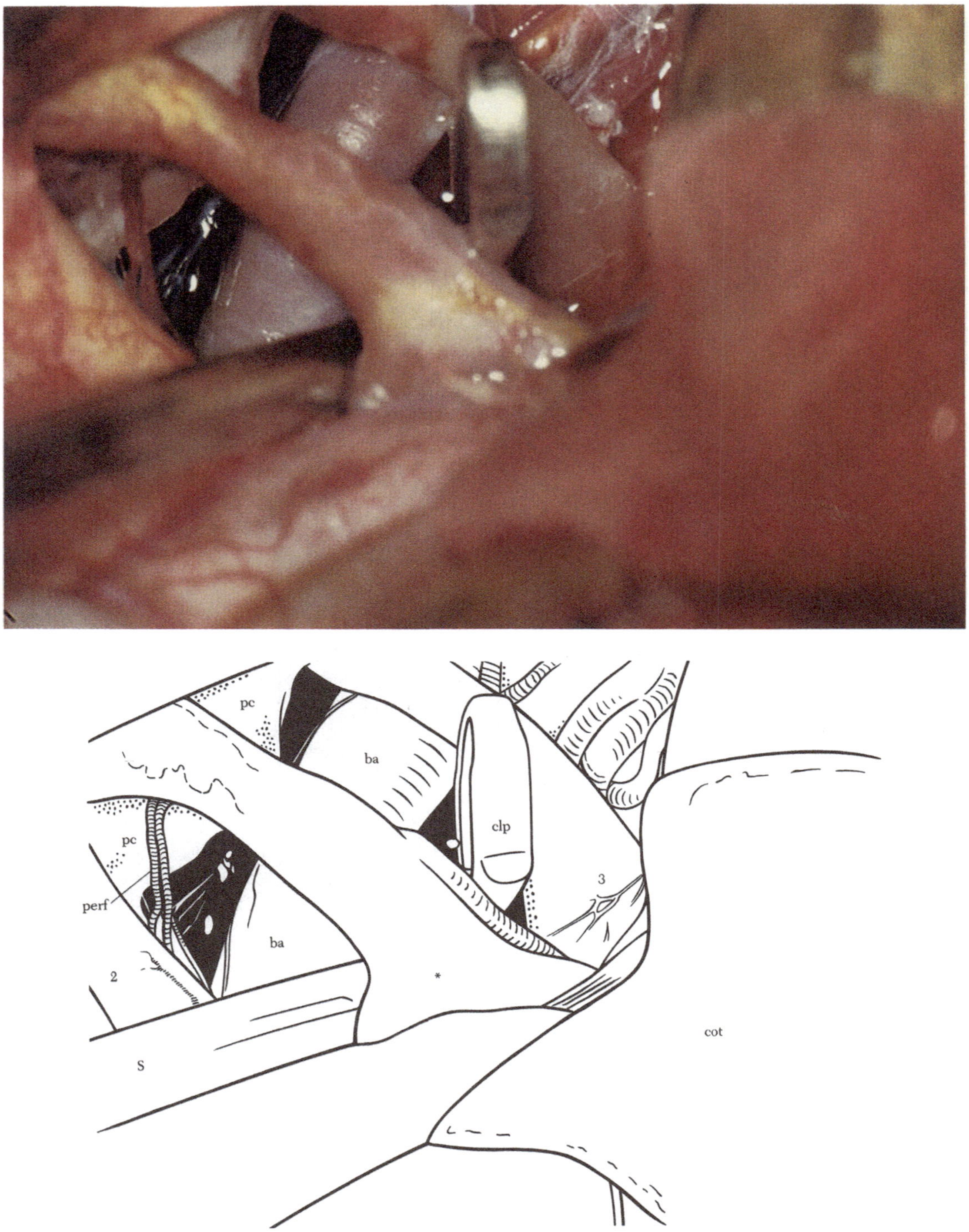

Fig. 38.43. Same case as in Figs. 38.41 and 38.42. The aicaBAA has been clipped. *clp,* shank of clip (see text); *3,* origin of oculomotor nerve from the midbrain; *cot,* cottonoid strip protecting the middle cerebral artery aneurysm in the sylvian fissure; *, bifurcation of the internal carotid artery; *s,* suction tube; *2,* optic nerve; *perf,* hypothalamic perforator from the internal carotid artery; *pc,* posterior clinoid process; *ba,* basilar artery.

tively via the same frontotemporal route. This is a modification of the basic frontolateral approach described originally by Walter Dandy (see Chapter 29) and continued in evolution by a number of surgeons. Yaşargil was the first to illustrate a similar approach for the basilar artery aneurysms. It is apparent that, overall, the advantages of this route outweigh the disadvantages, the approach gaining more and more proponents as the years pass. The next chapter on vertebral artery aneurysms will give examples utilizing the unilateral, suboccipital approach to the posterior fossa.

Bibliography

1. Allcock JM: Aneurysms: In Newton TH, Potts DG (eds.): Radiology of the Skull and Brain, Vol. 2, Book 4. St. Louis, Mosby, 1974, pp. 2435–2489
2. Bremer JL: Congenital aneurysms of the cerebral arteries. An embryologic study. Arch Pathol 35:819–831, 1943
3. Drake CG: Advances in the neurosurgical treatment of aneurysms, arteriovenous malformations, and hematomas of the vertebral circulation. In Thompson RA, Green JR (eds.): Advances in Neurology, Vol. 16. Stroke. New York, Raven Press, 1977, pp. 211–225
4. Drake CG: Cerebral aneurysm surgery—an update. In Scheinberg P (ed.): Cerebrovascular Diseases. Tenth Princeton Conference. New York, Raven Press, 1976, pp. 289–310
5. Drake CG: Management of aneurysms of posterior circulation. In Youmans JR (ed.): Neurological Surgery, Vol. 2. Philadelphia, Saunders, 1973, pp. 787–806
6. Drake CG: Surgical treatment of vertebrobasilar aneurysms. In Koos WT, Böck FW, Spetzler RF (eds.): Clinical Microneurosurgery. Stuttgart, Georg Thieme Verlag, 1976, pp. 213–219
7. Drake CG: The surgical treatment of vertebral-basilar aneurysms. Excerpta Med ICS No. 320:183–190, 1974
8. Drake CG: The surgical treatment of vertebral-basilar aneurysms. Clin Neurosurg 16:114–169, 1969
9. Drake CG: The treatment of aneurysms of the posterior circulation. Clin Neurosurg 26:96–144, 1979
10. Drake CG, Amacher AL: Aneurysms of the posterior cerebral artery. J Neurosurg 30:468–474, 1969
11. Fox JL: Microsurgical exposure of intracranial aneurysms. J Microsurg 1:2–31, 1979
12. Greitz T, Löfsted S: The relationship between the third ventricle and the basilar artery. Acta Radiol 42:85–100, 1954
13. Kempe LG: Operative Neurosurgery, Vol. 1, Cranial, Cerebral, and Intracranial Vascular Disease. New York, Springer-Verlag, 1968, pp. 1–75, 203–214
14. Laine E: Arterial vertebro-basilar aneurysms. Progr Brain Res 30:323–346, 1968
15. Samson DS, Hodosh RM, Clark WK: Microsurgical evaluation of the pterional approach to aneurysms of the distal basilar circulation. Neurosurgery 3:135–141, 1978
16. Sugar O: Pathological anatomy and angiography of intracranial vascular anomalies. J Neurosurg 8:3–22, 1951
17. Sugita K, Kobayashi S, Shintani A, et al.: Microneurosurgery for aneurysms of the basilar artery. J Neurosurg 51:615–620, 1979
18. Sugita K, Kobayashi S, Takemae T, et al.: Direct retraction method in aneurysm surgery. Technical note. J Neurosurg 53:417–419, 1980
19. Wilson CB, U HS: Surgical treatment for aneurysms of the upper basilar artery. J Neurosurg 44:537–543, 1976
20. Wright DC, Wilson CB: Surgical treatment of basilar aneurysms. Neurosurgery 5:325–333, 1979
21. Yaşargil MG, Antic J, Laciga R, et al.: Microsurgical pterional approach to aneurysms of the basilar bifurcation. Surg Neurol 6:83–91, 1976
22. Yaşargil MG, Fox JL: The microsurgical approach to intracranial aneurysms. Surg Neurol 3:7–14, 1975

39

Technique of Aneurysm Surgery

VI. Vertebral Artery Aneurysms

As noted by others (1–4), vertebral artery aneurysms most often arise at the distal (superior) angle between the vertebral artery and the posterior inferior cerebellar artery. An example is seen in Fig. 39.1. As the forthcoming examples will illustrate, picaVAA may arise low down near the foramen magnum or high up near the pontomedullary junction. They may originate at the midline or out laterally depending on the direction and tortuosity of the vertebral arteries. The aneurysm itself may point superomedially into the brain stem, superiorly into the cerebellum, or superolaterally toward the petrous pyramid. Although most are berry-shaped and of varying configuration, there is a high incidence of locally fusiform VAA and picaVAA, many of which will cause a subarachnoid hemorrhage (3–6).

About 15% of intracranial aneurysms are on the V-B circulation: 10% on the basilar artery and 5% on the vertebral arteries. Thus in a negative angiographic study if the radiologist fails to see one of the vertebral arteries, there is a 2 to 3% chance of missing a VAA. We have one case of a patient with SAH in which three-vessel angiography demonstrated a left pcaICAA. A few days after it was clipped, the patient rebled and died. Autopsy revealed a right picaVAA, the original culprit. The right VA had not been seen on the angiogram. If there is not adequate reflux of contrast media down the contralateral VA when the ipsilateral VA is injected (Fig. 39.2), then a direct injection of the fourth vessel, the other VA, is advisable. On the other hand, if a VAA is found, the other VA should be examined for competency in case a planned or emergency intraoperative VAA trapping procedure is done later.

The Surgical Exposure

Whether one places the patient in the sitting position or the lateral "park bench" position (see Chapter 29), the basic exposure to the VAA is via a unilateral suboccipital craniotomy or craniectomy. We have been using the sitting position with blood pressure measurements referred to the head level.

The position of the patient is very important and is identical to that used for cerebellopontine angle tumors. We place the patient in the sitting position (see Fig. 26.2), the feet elevated and wrapped in elastic wrappings. With the surgeon's elbows resting on the padded, turned-down head rest of the operating table, the patient's suboccipital region is at the height of the surgeon's hands. In some instances the patient will need to be elevated on firm cushions to achieve this height. The head is rotated about 20° with the nose pointed toward the side of the aneurysm. This brings the brain stem structures in better alignment with the surgeon's vision. The neck is flexed with care taken to avoid compression of the jugular veins and trachea. The skull is maintained in this position with the 3-pinned skull clamp.

During the draping of the patient the Aesculap retractor support bar is connected to the table with the bar extending over the head of the patient. Later the connector piece is at-

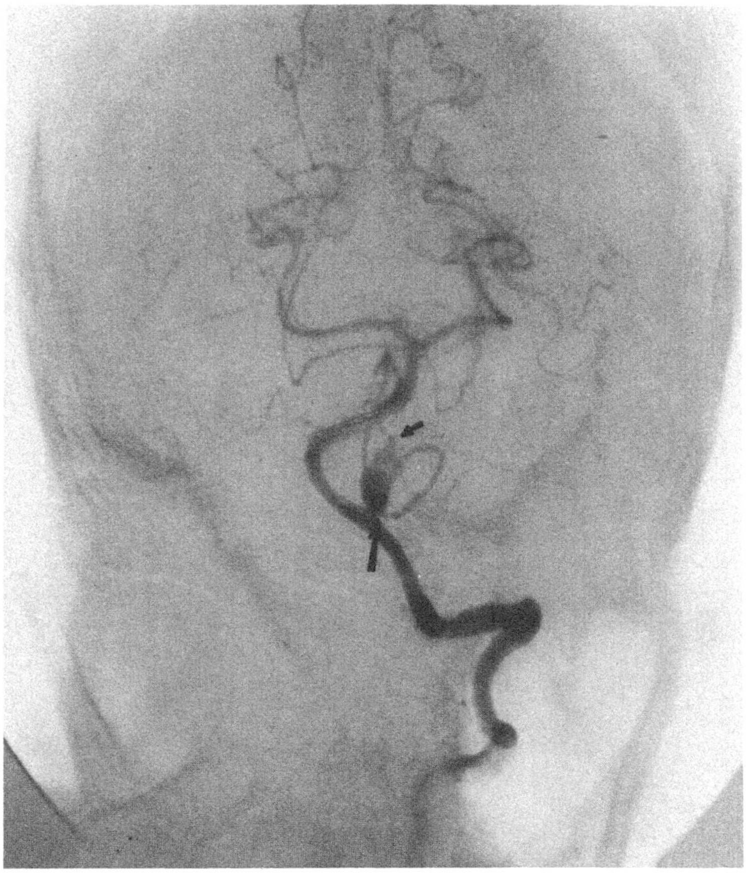

A

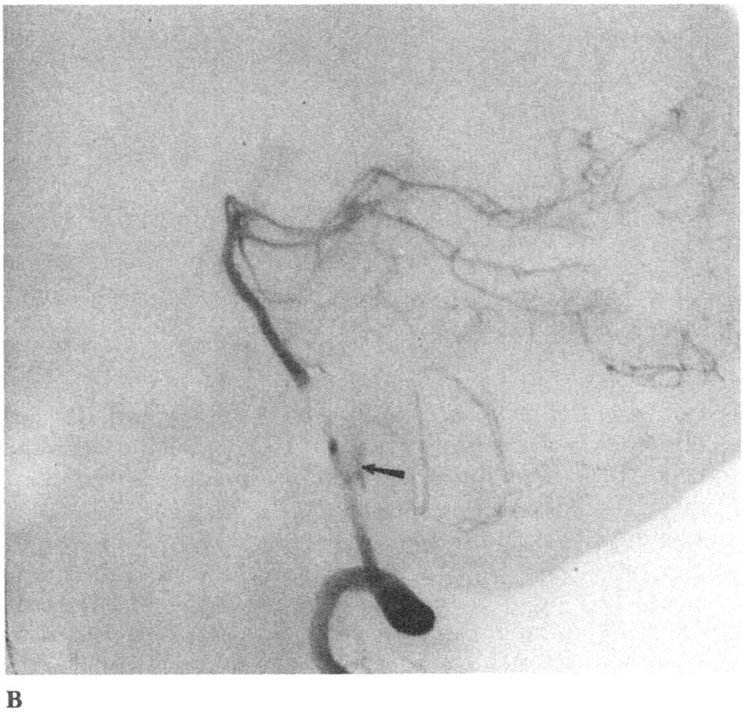

B

Fig. 39.1. **A** Frontal view of picaVAA. PICA originates proximal to the neck of the aneurysm (*long arrow*). This 74-year-old woman died from an intraangiographic rebleed. *Short arrow*, contrast media exiting from aneurysm. **B** Lateral view of same case. *Arrow*, picaVAA.

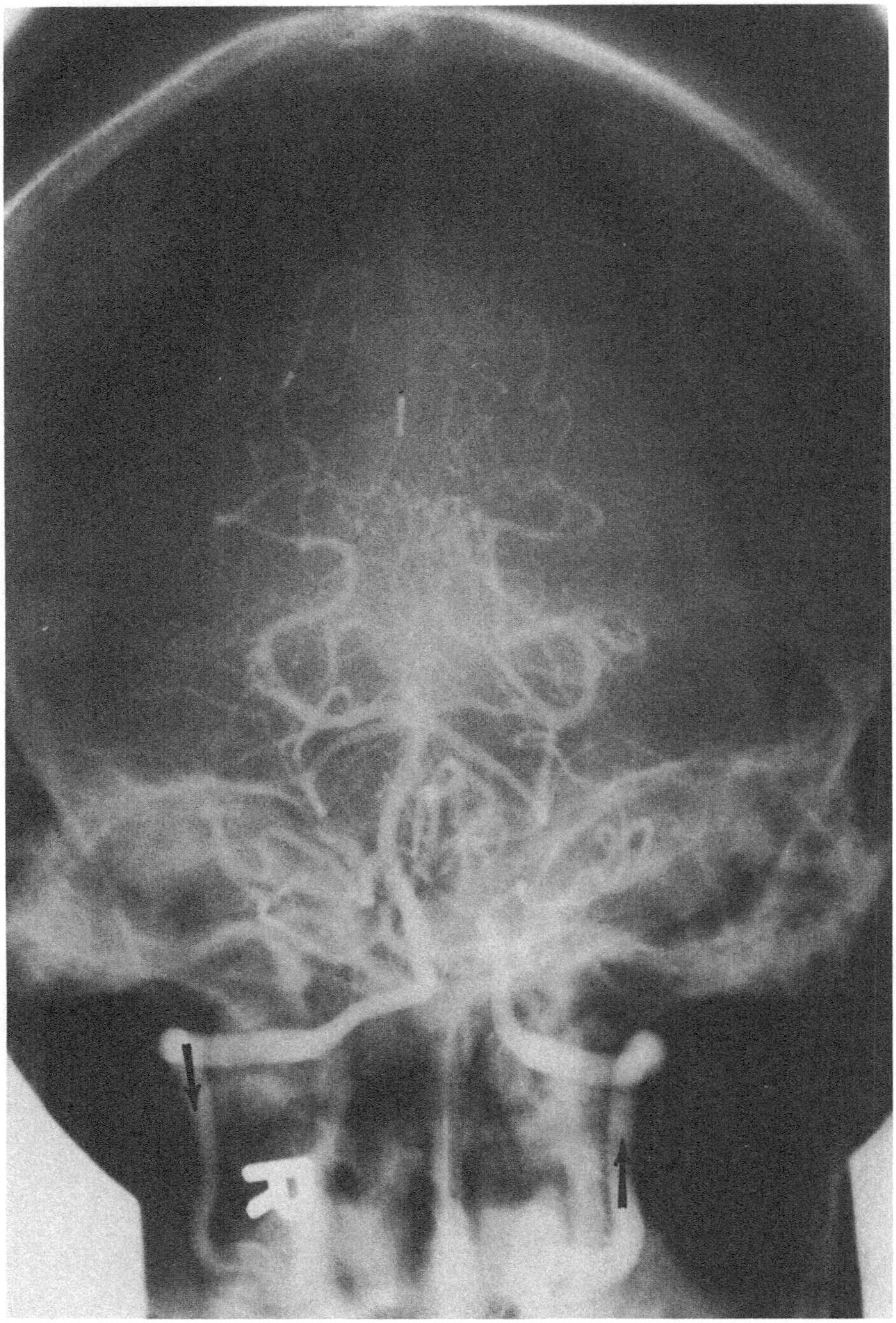

Fig. 39.2. Normal VA angiogram, frontal view. The left VA was injected, and there was good reflux down the right VA beyond the PICA take-off.

tached to this bar allowing attachment of one (usually) or more flexible Aesculap retractor arms. With the retractor in position and elevating the cerebellar hemisphere, no surgical assistants are needed and there is no movement of brain tissues. Drift is minimal if part of the flexible arm is resting on the top of the head. Many surgeons may prefer other types of self-retaining retractors.

As the following surgical photographs illustrate, the surgeon's line of sight will be straight ahead and parallel to the floor and the base of the posterior fossa. Hence, for the sitting patient the straight binocular tube for the microscope eyepieces is used.

The retroauricular-retromastoidal incision is 6–8 cm long and lies 2 cm medial to the medial edge of the mastoid process (7). It begins just above the transverse sinus and extends down to the lowest level of the mastoid tip. The skin is under-cut and retracted. Then the muscle (splenium) and its fascia are incised down to the bone and carefully peeled away from the skull with the aid of electrocautery. The fascia is retracted but preserved for resuturing at the end of the operation. Three burr holes are drilled: (a) at the upper corner of the incision above the transverse sinus (in case the lateral ventricle needs to be drained); (b) against the mastoid process; and (c) at the inferior medial corner of the wound. The upper burr hole is connected to the other two burr holes by use of the Gigli saw. From the lower two burr holes a rongeur is used to remove bone down toward the base of the skull. The teardrop-shaped craniotomy flap of bone is removed and preserved for replacement later. The arch of the first cervical vertebra and its muscular attachments are not disturbed. Laterally bone is removed until the sigmoid sinus is seen. The opened air cells in the mastoid process are sealed with bone wax.

This relatively small opening still allows excellent surgical exposure, for the microscope brings the surgeon's eyes close to the opening (reducing problems of parallax), allows stereoscopic focusing on objects inside a deep wound, and provides direct lighting not achieved by conventional methods. A modified stellate dural incision is made with the main flap turned medially. The remaining dura mater is incised and pulled over the lateral and sigmoid sinuses and the lateral and inferior bony edges. The Aesculap self-retaining brain retractor is inserted under the cerebellum and slowly retracted so as to expose the lateral cerebellomedullary angle and adjacent medulla oblongata (Fig. 39.3). Excessive retraction or excision of parts of the cerebellum are not necessary when this retractor and the microscope are used along with the adjuncts to reduce intracranial pressure. After the surgeon exposes the cerebellomedullary angle, the arachnoid is opened and cerebrospinal fluid is released from the lateral cistern below the 9th, 10th, and 11th cranial nerve bundles.

If the aneurysm lies inferior to most of the CN-9 and CN-10 rootlets, it will be immediately recognized (Figs. 39.4–39.6). Although the aneurysm may be enmeshed in clot and fibrin, most of the cranial nerve rootlets will not be in the way. In Figure 39.5, the aneurysm is freed from the medulla, PICA, and the vertebral artery. The only rootlets in jeopardy here are a CN-11 rootlet overlying the origin of PICA and a CN-10 rootlet caught between the anterior surface of the aneurysm and the posterior surface of the VA. As is often the case, the VA beyond the origin of the aneurysm is hidden by the aneurysm as the VA courses to join its opposite under the brain stem. Hence one must be careful not to trap the VA above the PICA origin in a long clip. Two spring clips secured the aneurysm in this case (Fig. 39.6).

One must be extremely careful during elevation of the cerebellum. The dome of even a small picaVAA may be adherent to the cerebellum and must be dissected off prior to further retraction. Figure 39.7 demonstrates a case in which a small superiorly projecting picaVAA ruptured during cerebellar retraction.

If the aneurysm is located high up on the VA and projects superolaterally, there will be difficulties dissecting the aneurysm from the many rootlets of CN-9, CN-10, and at times CN-12. Figures 39.8–39.12 are from just such a case. Upon opening into the cerebellomedullary angle and elevation of the cerebellum, fibrin (indicating the presence of a previous SAH) is seen (Fig. 39.9), but the picaVAA is too high up to be identified as yet. Further gentle retraction of the cerebellum reveals the aneurysm obscured by fibrin, blood, and branches of CN-9 and CN-10 (Figs. 39.10 and 39.11). Four hypoglossal rootlets emerge from between the pyramid and inferior olive, gather together, and loop over PICA in such a way as to cross the neck of the aneurysm (Fig. 39.11). Isolation of the broad neck while preserving the nerves and not disturbing the dome requires considerable time in such cases.

One can apply a temporary clip on the vertebral artery proximal to PICA. But the multitude of nerves makes placement difficult, the shank of the clip interferes with dissection, and the hazards are increased if the patient is in a sitting position where the intracranial blood pressure already is hydraulically lowered. The status of the contralateral VA should be known prior to surgery in case proximal ligation of the VA or trapping of the VAA is done. Finally, the clip is placed to secure the aneurysm (Fig. 39.12) without compromising the ascending VA hidden beyond the aneurysm, the PICA, or any of the cranial nerves.

If the aneurysm is located high up on the VA and projects superomedially, there will be difficulties dissecting the aneurysm from the ventrolateral surface of the medulla oblongata and the root-entry zones of the cranial nerves.

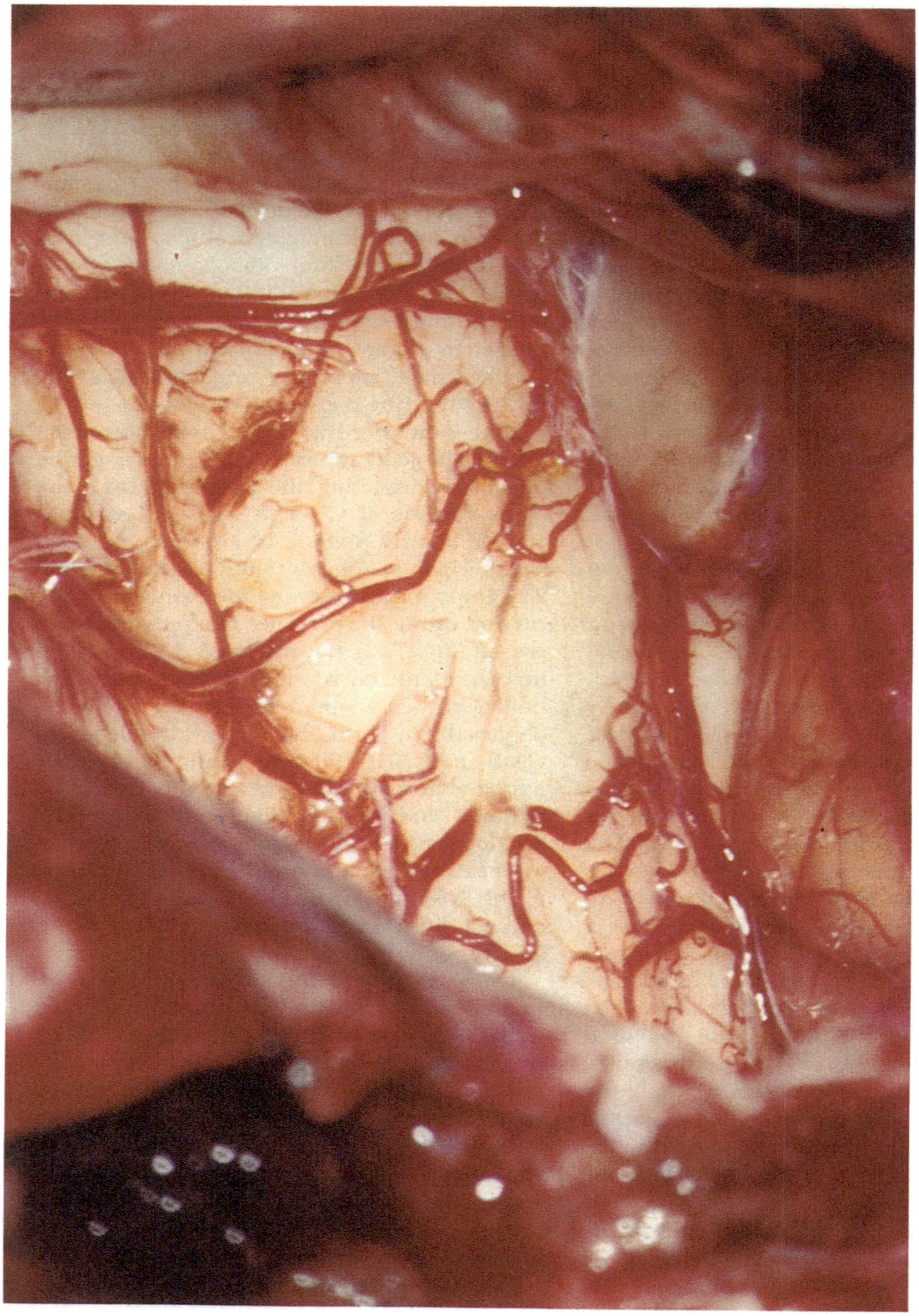

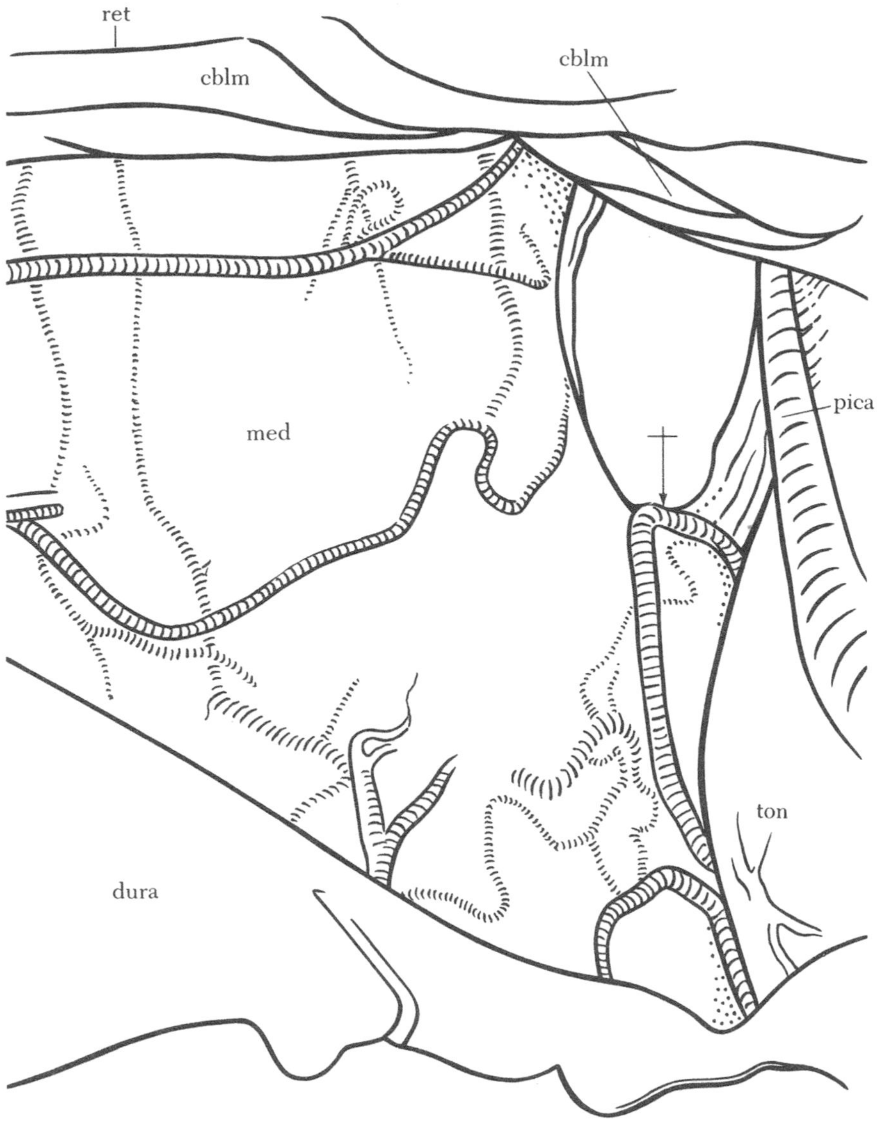

Fig. 39.3. Surgeon's view of left side of medulla oblongata after cerebellum is elevated. Same case as in Figs. 39.4–39.6. *ret,* retractor blade; *cblm,* left cerebellum retracted upward; *single-crossed arrow* lies in 4th ventricle and points to the obex; *pica,* tonsillar branch of the contralateral posterior inferior cerebellar artery; *ton,* contralateral cerebellar tonsil; *dura,* dura folded over lower edge of cranial opening; *med,* medulla oblongata. All color photographs will be from the left side to maintain anatomic consistency and orientation.

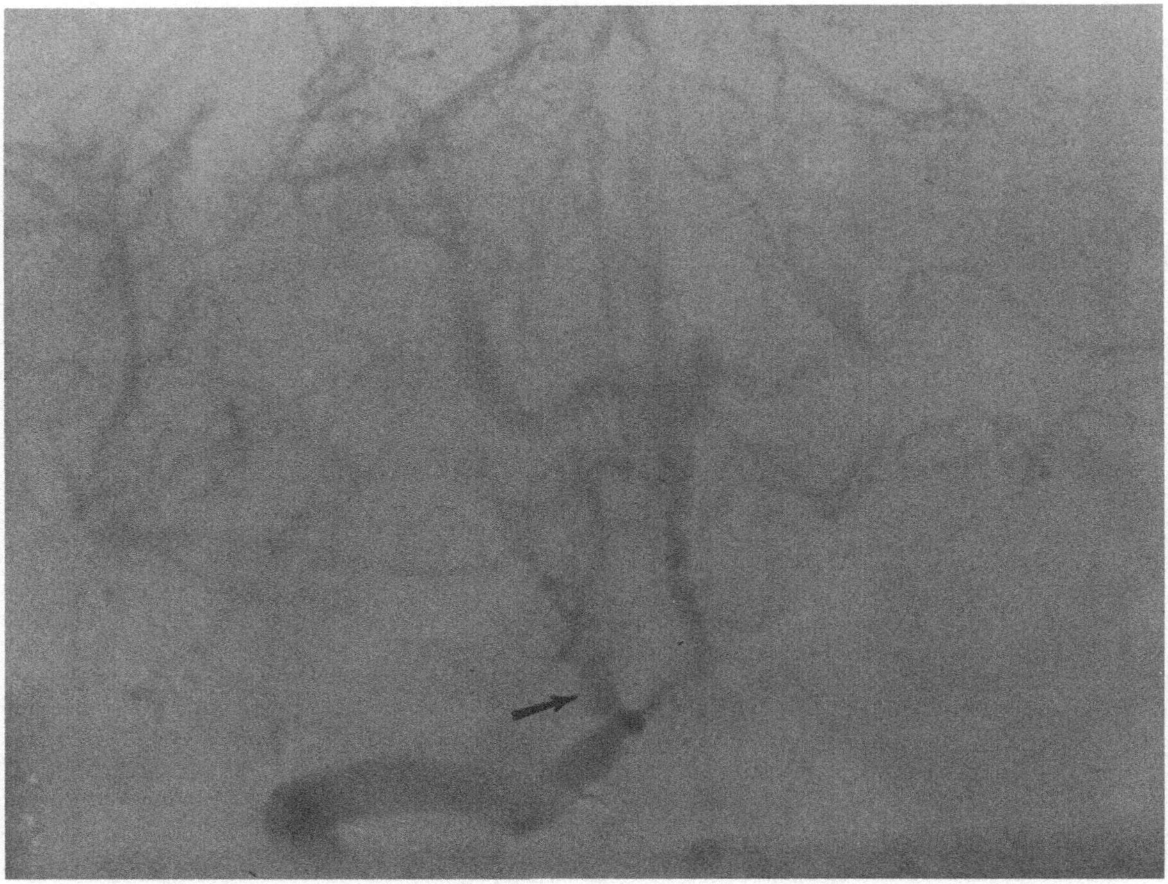

A

Fig. 39.4. **A** Frontal view of picaVAA (*arrow*). **B** Lateral view of aneurysm (*arrow*). Same case as in Figs. 39.3, 39.5, and 39.6.

Figures 39.13–39.18 represent a case of this type. Upon opening into the cerebellomedullary angle (Fig. 39.14), the aneurysm is not immediately obvious. The rootlets of CN-9–CN-12 are seen. As usual, rootlets of CN-12 course over the vertebral artery near PICA, but PICA actually originates higher up than is apparent in the figure. Further elevation of the retractor demonstrates a mass of fibrin (Fig. 39.15) hiding the aneurysm above the rootlets of CN-9 and CN-10. The fibrin is dissected away, exposing a large atherosclerotic aneurysm buried in the left lateral wall of the medulla oblongata (Fig. 39.16). A long, flat microdissector is used to separate the aneurysm from the brain stem. Then the fragile blister, or saccule, projecting superolaterally is freed from adhesions and fibrin (Fig. 39.17). Finally, bipolar electrocoagulation is extremely helpful in this situation to shrink the mass of the aneurysm and permit inspection of the environs prior to clipping (Fig. 39.18). In this way, the vertebral artery, hidden by the aneurysm, can be identified and not caught in the clip. Postoperatively this patient had transient dysphagia and a left vocal cord paralysis, which improved before discharge home.

As already mentioned there are a number of VAA that present with SAH, but the aneurysm is a localized fusiform dilation without any neck that can be clipped. An example is illustrated in Figs. 39.19 and 39.20. Inspection of all sites of the aneurysm at operation (Fig. 39.20) confirmed this. Treatment in this case consisted of clipping the vertebral artery proximal to the PICA take-off. A higher-than-normal

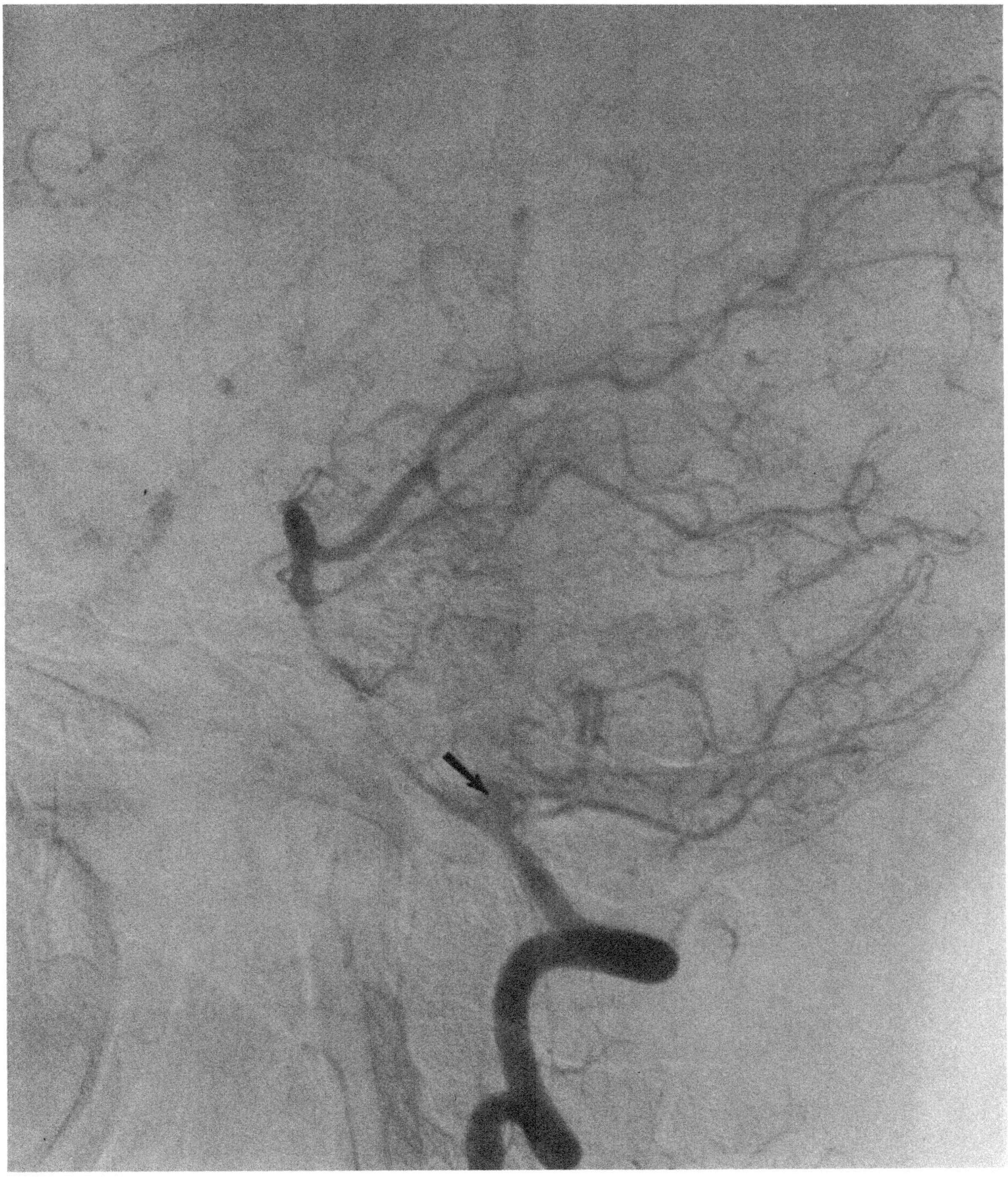

B

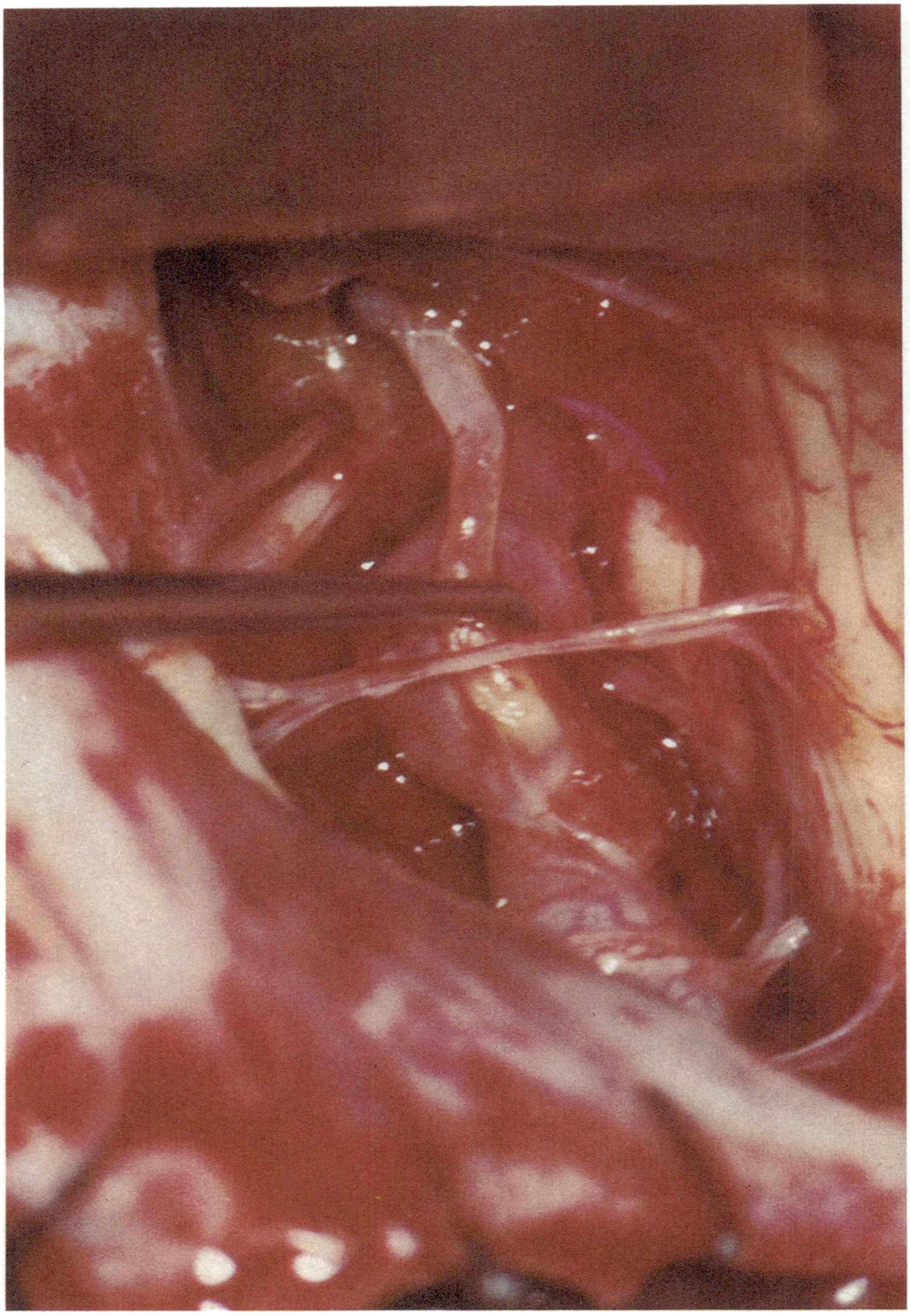

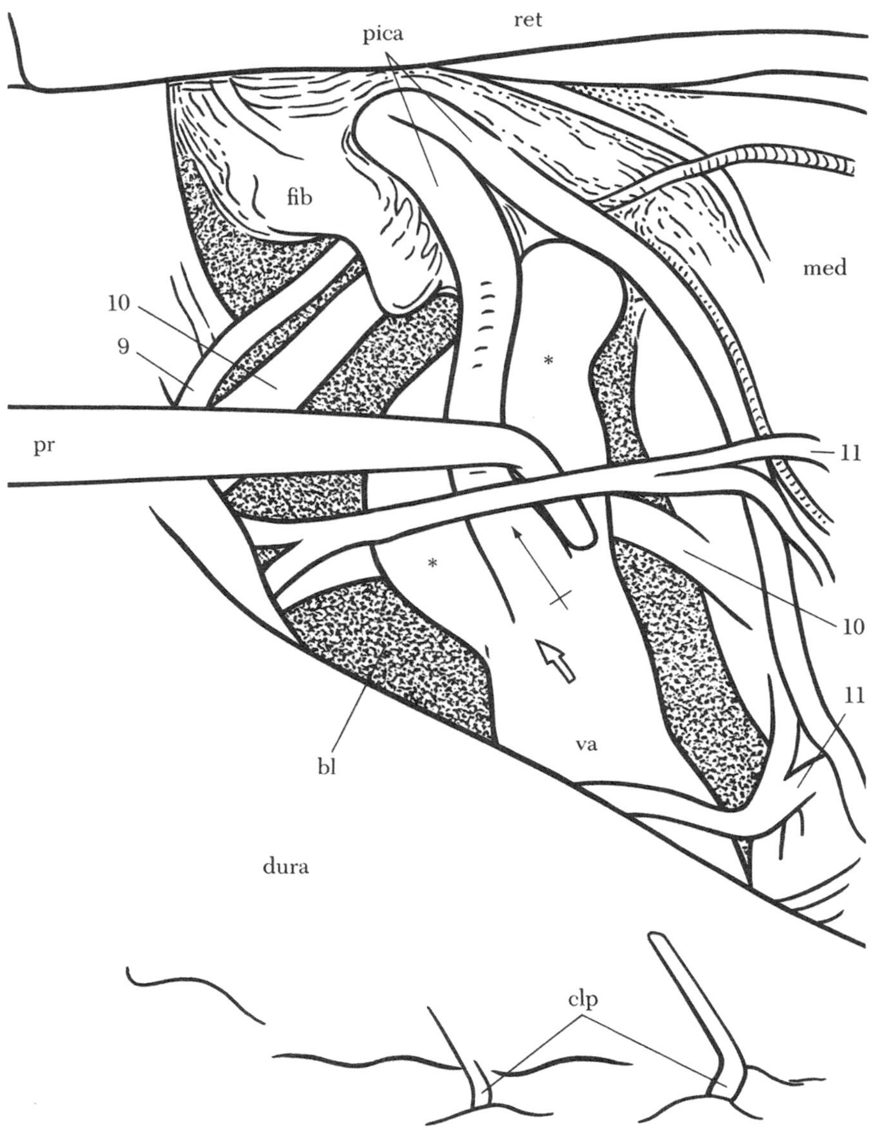

Fig. 39.5. Surgical photographs presented as if from the left side. Upon elevating the cerebellum with the retractor blade (*ret*), the aneurysm (*) is immediately seen overlying the vertebral artery (*va*) from which it arises. Its origin is at the take-off (*single-crossed arrow*) of the posterior inferior cerebellar artery (*pica*). A probe (*pr*) is crossing the jugular foramen and retracting the base of the aneurysm laterally. *9,* glossopharyngeal nerve; *10,* vagal rootlets; *med,* side of medulla oblongata; *dura,* dura at base of posterior fossa; *clp,* tantalum clips on dural edge; *bl,* blood from original hemorrhage; *fib,* fibrin clot enveloping CN-9, CN-10, and PICA. *Open arrow,* direction of blood flow. Same case as in Figs. 39.3, 39.4, and 39.6.

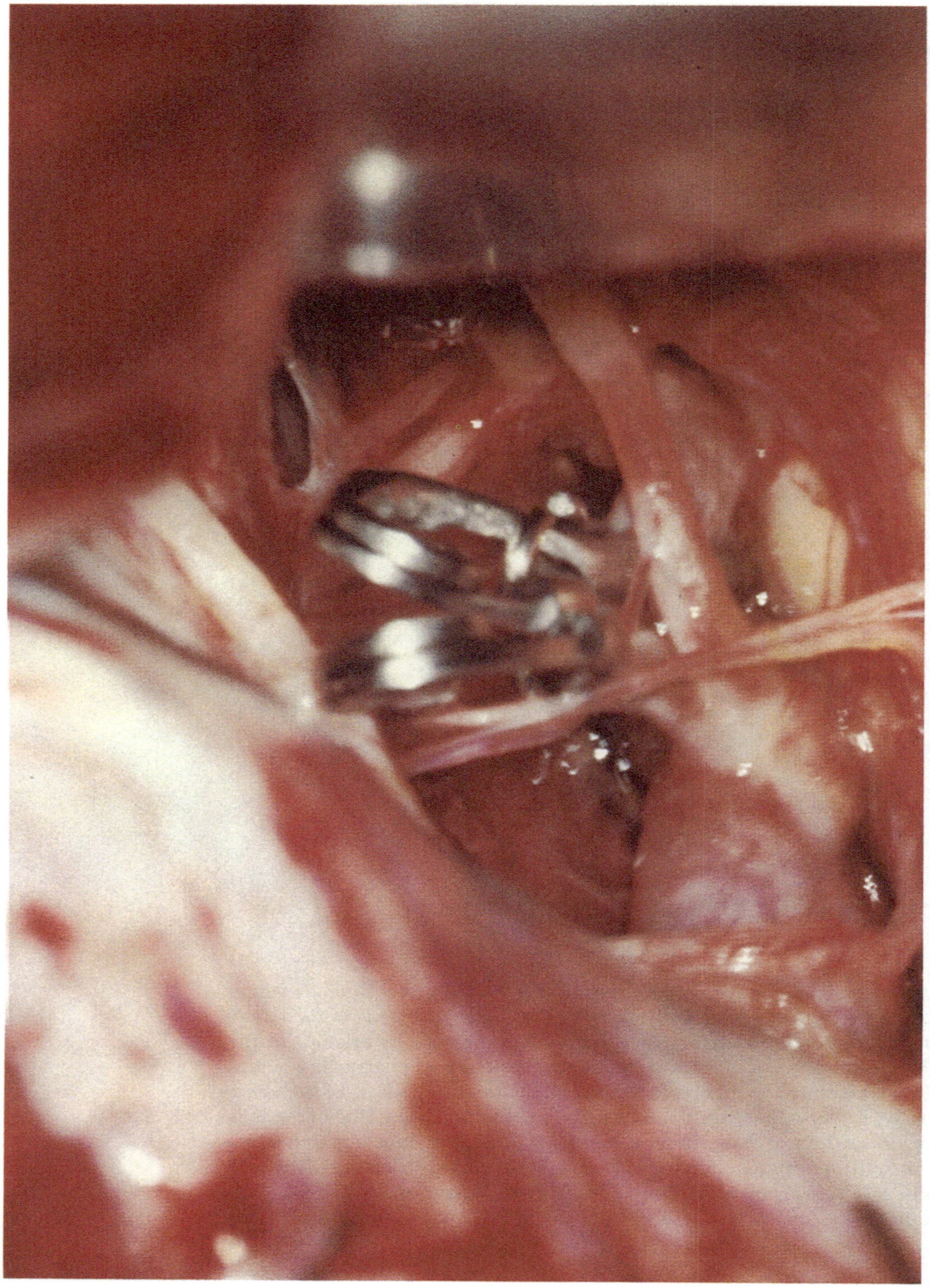

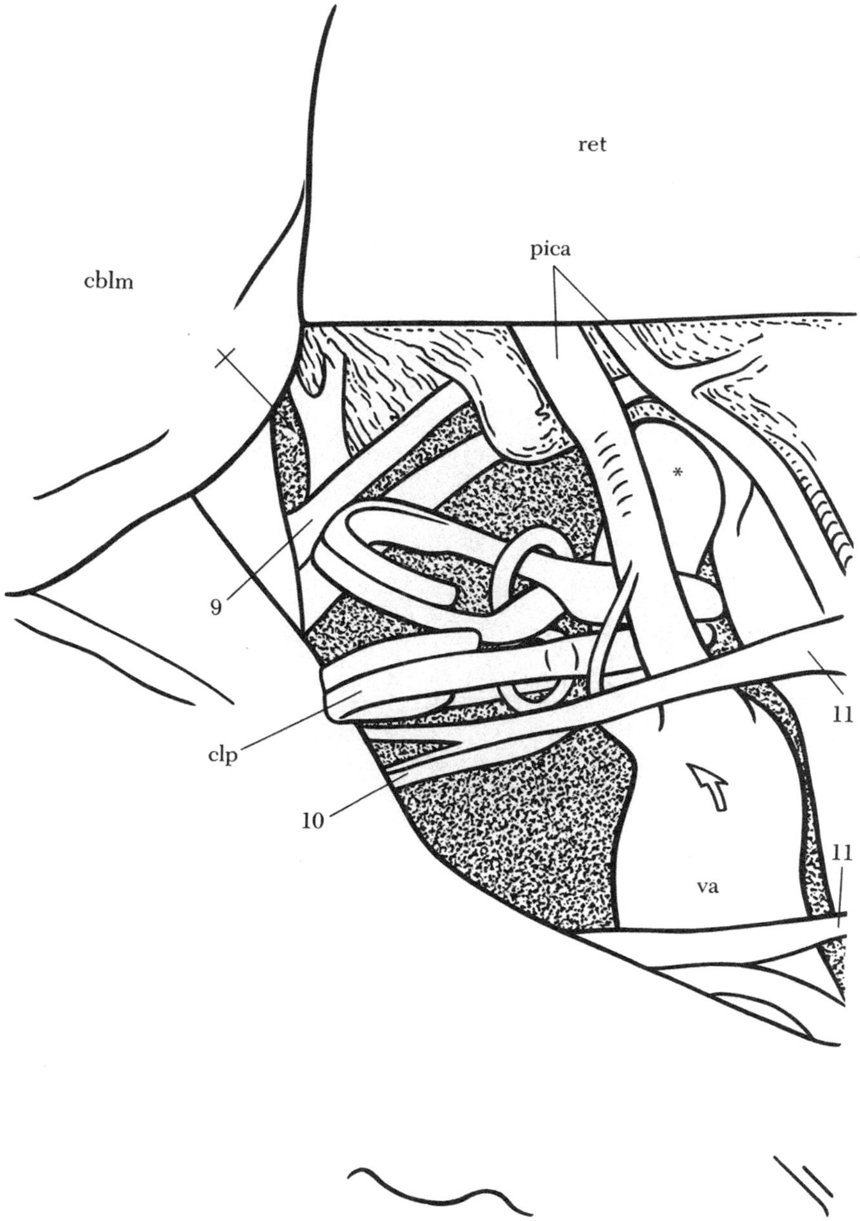

Fig. 39.6. Same case as in Figs. 39.3–39.5 after clipping of the aneurysm. *pica,* posterior inferior cerebellar artery; *, dome of clipped aneurysm; *ret,* retractor blade; *11,* spinal accessory rootlets; *va,* vertebral artery; *10,* vagal rootlet; *clp,* shanks of clips (Yaşargil spring clips) on neck of aneurysm; *9,* glossopharyngeal nerve; *cblm,* cerebellum retracted upward; *crossed arrow* points to opening in arachnoid membrane, on the other side of which is the cerebellopontine angle cistern. *Open arrow,* direction of blood flow.

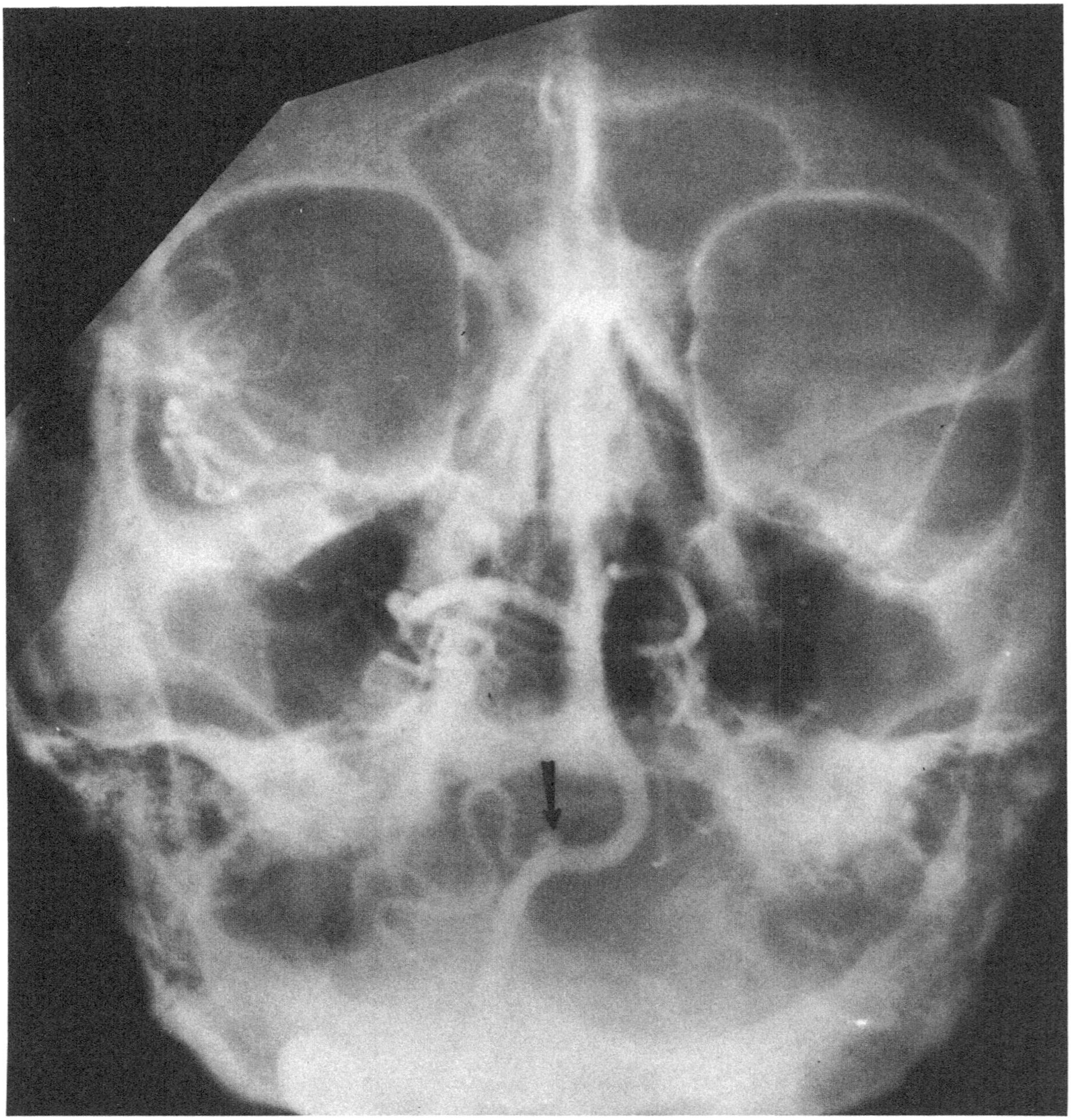

Fig. 39.7. Frontal view of small picaVAA which bled upon elevation of the cerebellum at surgery. Although the aneurysm was clipped successfully, the patient returned home with hoarseness and dysphagia due to CN-9 and CN-10 trauma.

BP should be maintained after clipping during surgery and for a few days afterward. This patient developed a transient, mild Wallenberg syndrome before discharge home. In such situations the surgeon must be confident that the contralateral VA is functioning well. Sugita et al. (6) recently developed a special clip for dealing with these localized fusiform aneurysms (Fig. 39.21).

Although the basic approach to the VAA is

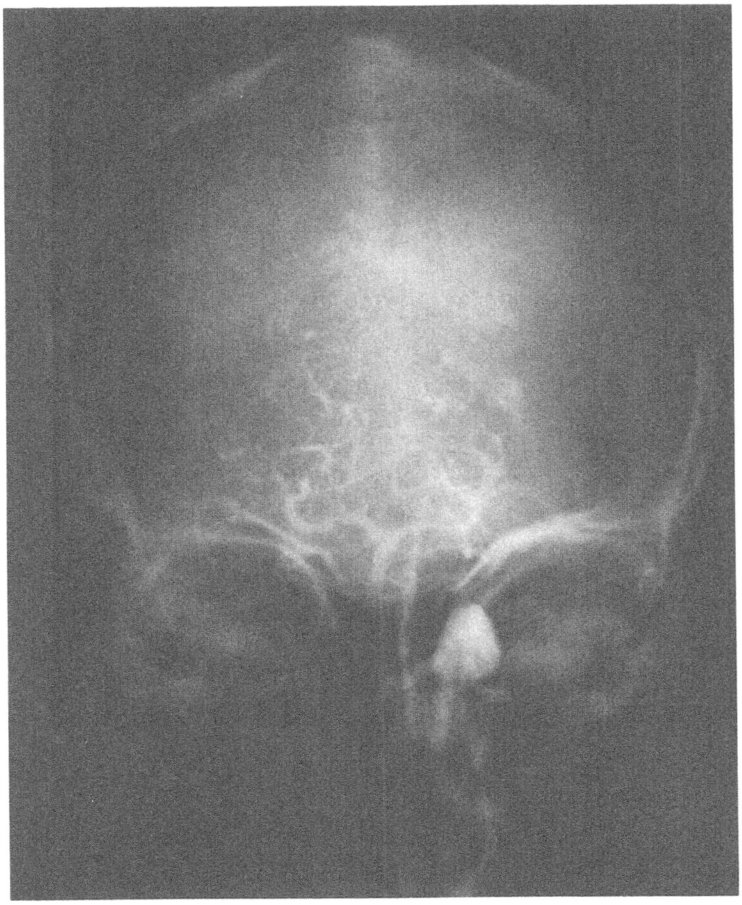

A

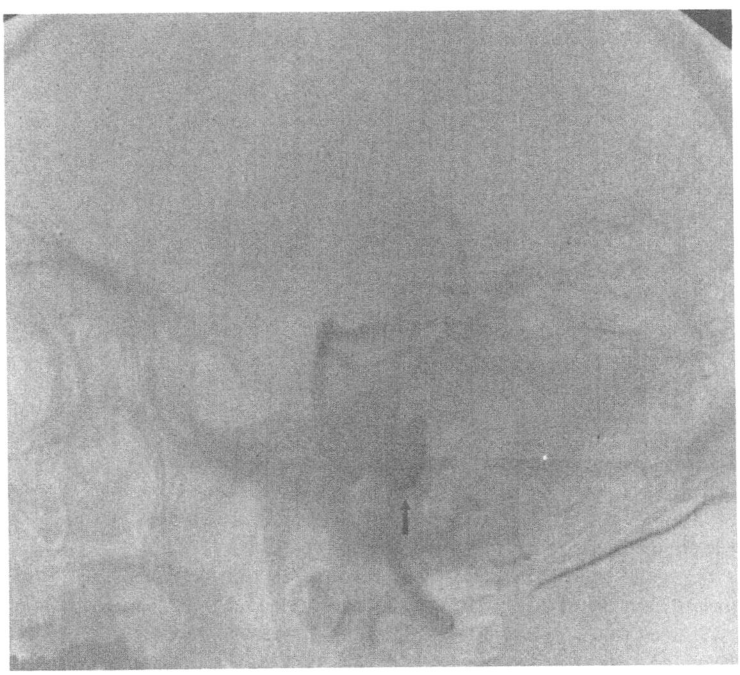

B

Fig. 39.8. **A** Frontal view of large picaVAA pointing laterally. **B** Lateral view of same with *arrow* pointing to origin of PICA. The aneurysm is fairly high up on the vertebral artery. Same case as in Figs. 39.9–39.12.

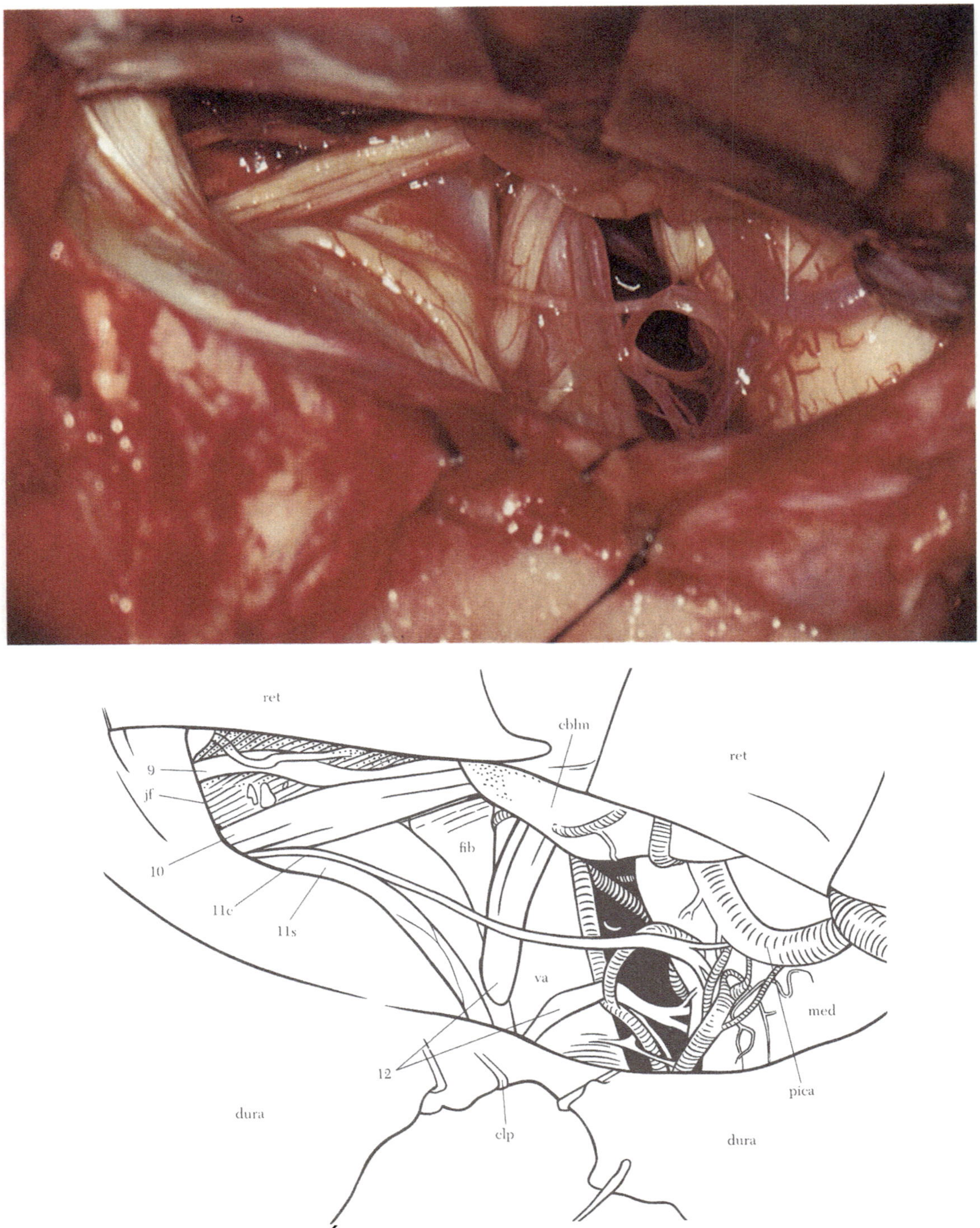

Fig. 39.9. Initial exposure of left cerebellomedullary angle. Same case as in Figs. 39.8 and 39.10–39.12. Photographed with Zeiss magnification dial set at No. 10. *fib,* fibrin clot hiding lateral side of origin of aneurysm; *cblm,* part of retracted cerebellum; *ret,* retractor blade; *pica,* descending loop of the posterior inferior cerebellar artery; *med,* medulla oblongata; *dura,* dural flap hanging down from cranial opening; *clp,* tantalum clip on dural edge; *va,* vertebral artery; *12,* rootlets of hypoglossal nerve; *11s,* rootlets of spinal portion of spinal accessory nerve; *11c,* rootlets of cranial portion of spinal accessory nerve; *10,* rootlets of vagus nerve; *jf,* jugular foramen; *9,* glossopharyngeal nerve.

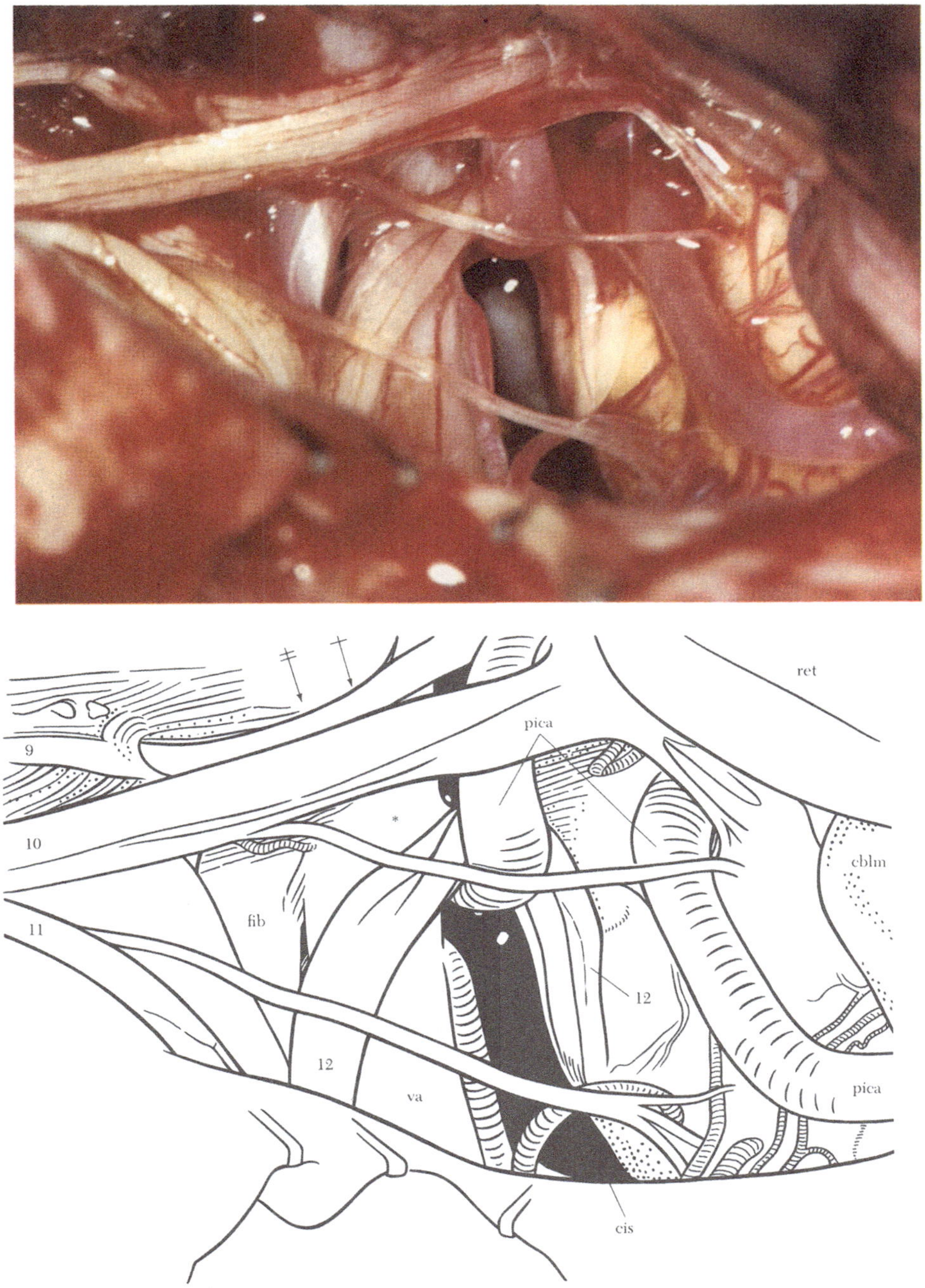

Fig. 39.10. Zeiss magnification dial set at the usual No. 16. Same case as in Figs. 39.8, 39.9, 39.11, and 39.12. Further cerebellar retraction reveals origin of the posterior inferior cerebellar artery. Note how the upper hypoglossal rootlets (*12*) gather together, loop around the origin of the posterior inferior cerebellar artery (*pica*), and then descend toward the anterior condyloid foramen (hypoglossal foramen). The dome of the aneurysm (*single-crossed arrow*) is hidden by blood (*double-crossed arrow*) and the rootlets of CN-9 and CN-10. *, junctional zone of the vertebral artery (*va*), the posterior inferior cerebellar artery (*pica*), and the neck of the aneurysm. *ret,* retractor blade; *cblm,* medial part of overhanging cerebellum; *cis* points to premedullary cistern; *11,* spinal accessory rootlets; *10,* vagal rootlets; *9,* glossopharyngeal nerve; *fib,* fibrin lateral to vertebral artery near origin of the aneurysm.

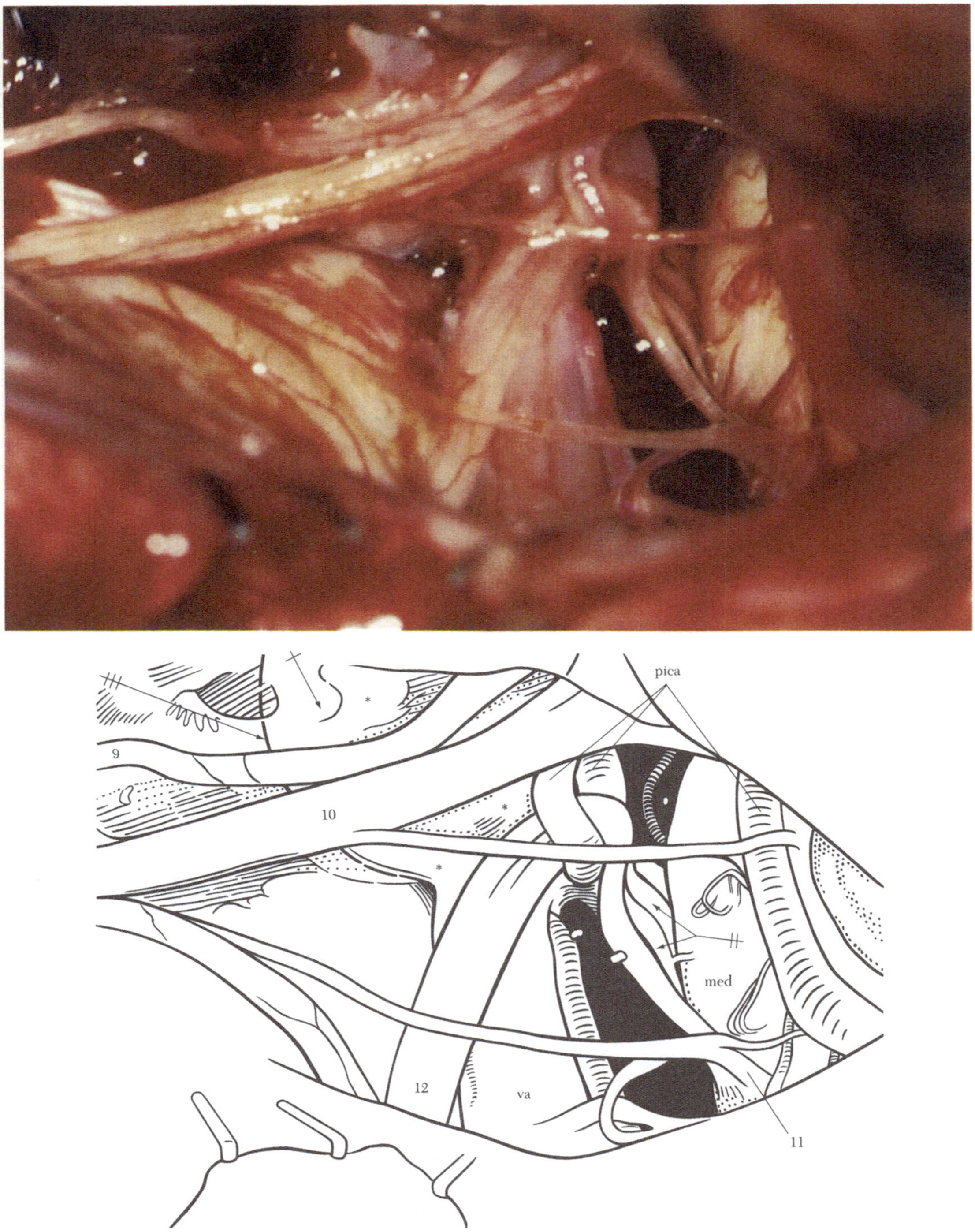

Fig. 39.11. After clearing away the fibrin, parts of the large neck and dome of the aneurysm (*) come into view. The glossopharyngeal (*9*) and vagus (*10*) nerves are adherent to the dome. Part of the dome is covered by blood laterally (*single-crossed arrow*). Note how four hypoglossal rootlets (*double-crossed arrows*) gather together from under the inferior olive of the medulla (*med*) and loop around the origin of the posterior inferior cerebellar artery (*pica*). *Triple-crossed arrow,* outline of lateral border of hidden aneurysm fundus; *11,* cranial origin of part of spinal accessory nerve; *12,* hypoglossal nerve; *va,* vertebral artery. Same case as in Figs. 39.8–39.10 and 39.12.

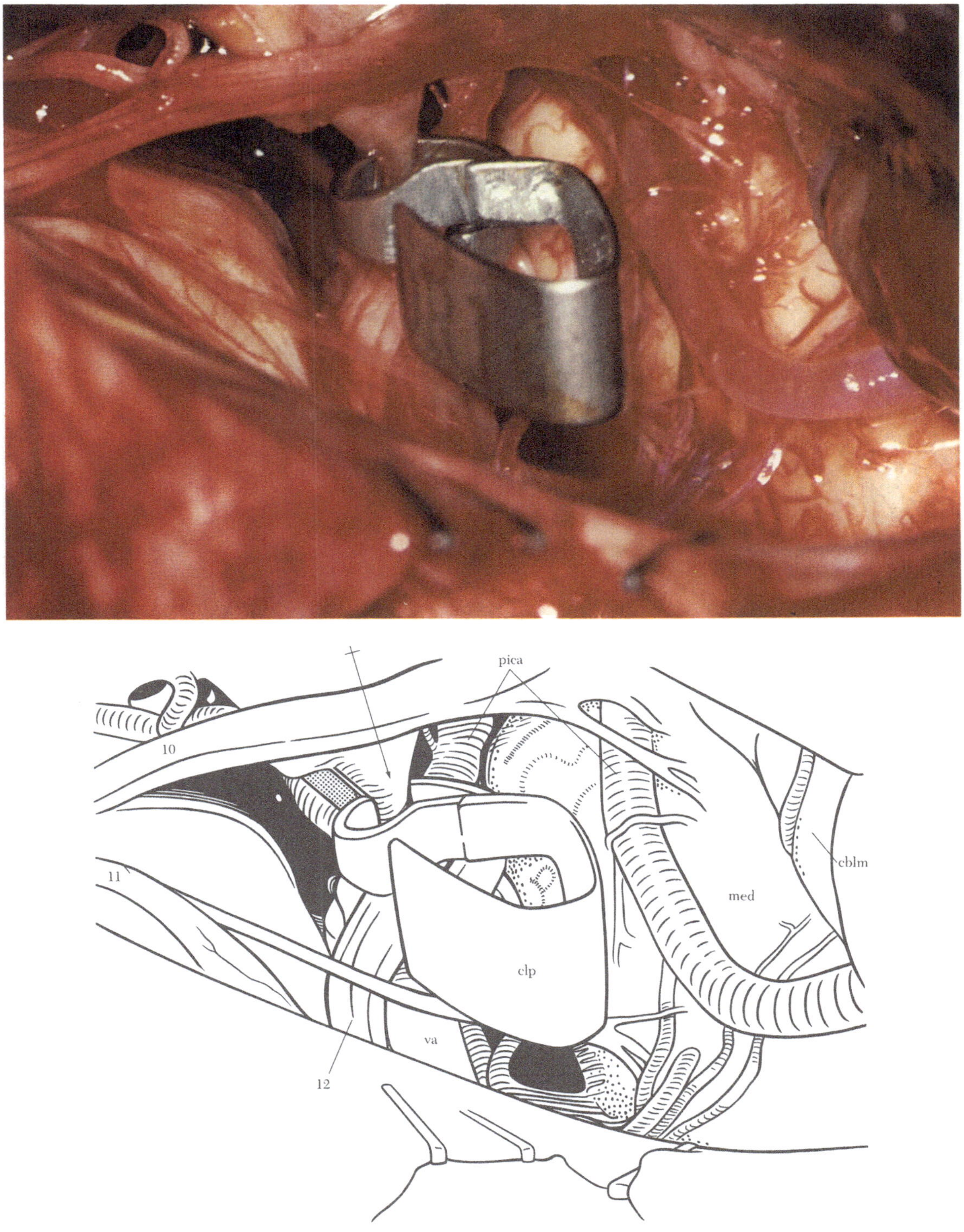

Fig. 39.12. Same case as in Figs. 39.8–39.11 after clipping. A long Drake clip (*clp*) finally secured broad base of aneurysm with successful clinical result. *Single-crossed arrow* extends from fundus to neck of aneurysm. *pica,* posterior inferior cerebellar artery; *cblm,* medial part of cerebellum hanging down; *med,* medulla oblongata; *va,* vertebral artery; *12,* hypoglossal nerve; *11,* spinal accessory nerve; *10,* vagus nerve.

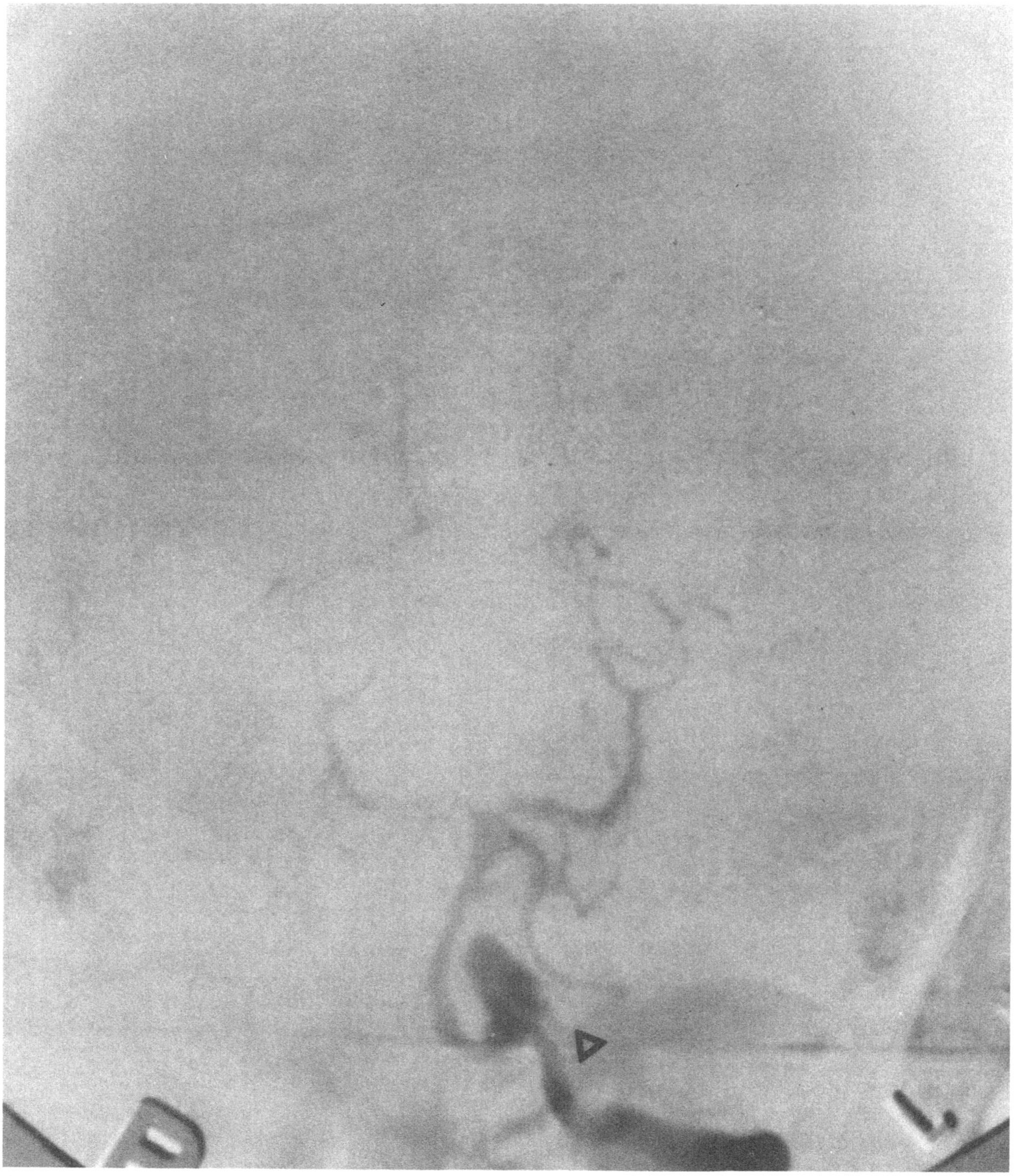

A

Fig. 39.13. **A** Frontal view of picaVAA. *Triangle,* PICA. **B** Oblique view of same. *Triangle,* PICA. Same case as in Figs. 39.14–39.18.

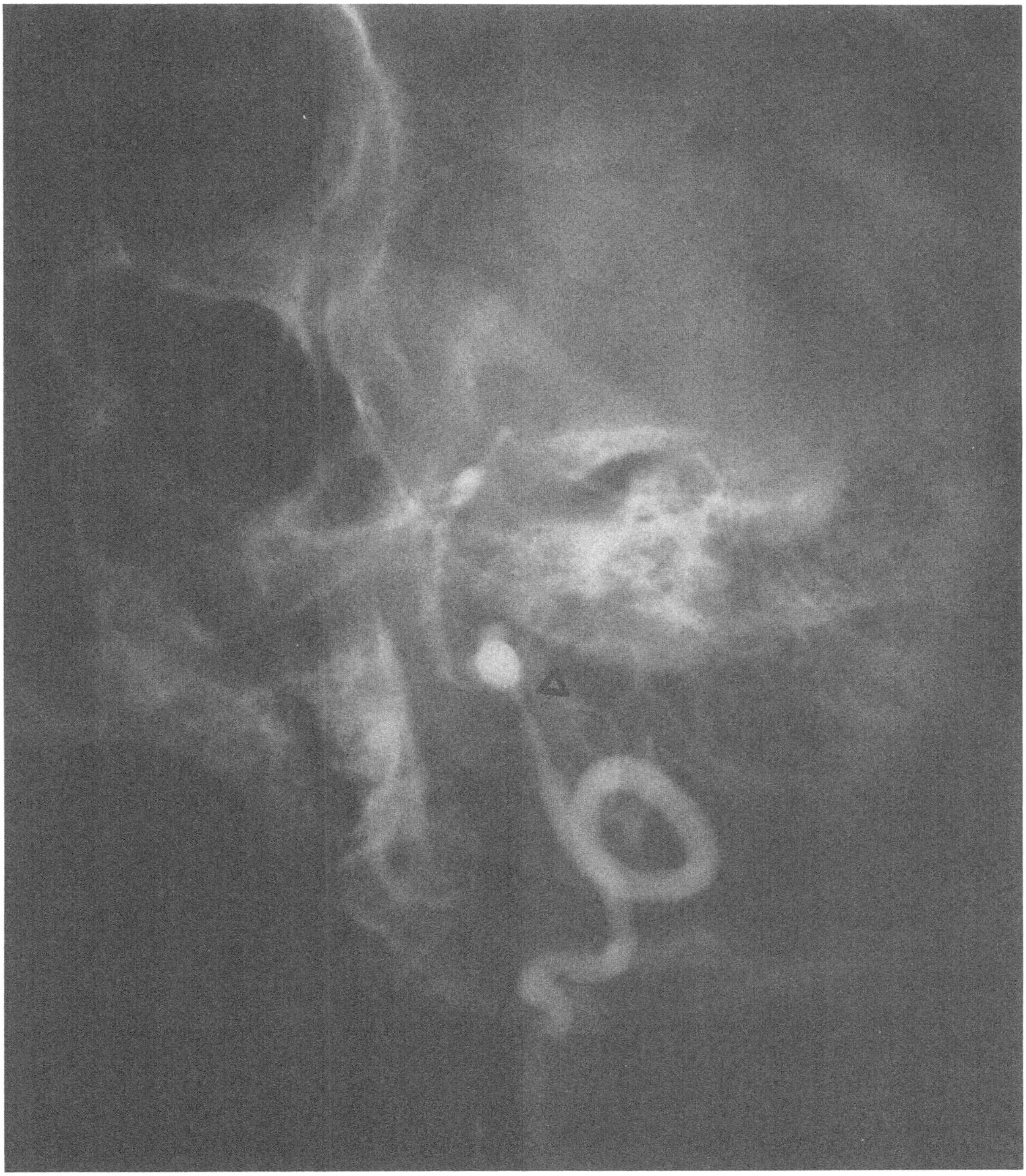

B

via a standard unilateral suboccipital craniotomy or craniectomy, there are some midline VAA and low-lying BAA which can be clipped after a transclival exposure (see Chapter 29). However, such an approach is time consuming, confining, and risky. With the advent of microtechnique even these difficult aneurysms often can be clipped satisfactorily by the suboccipital route or possibly a combined suboccipital-subtemporal route.

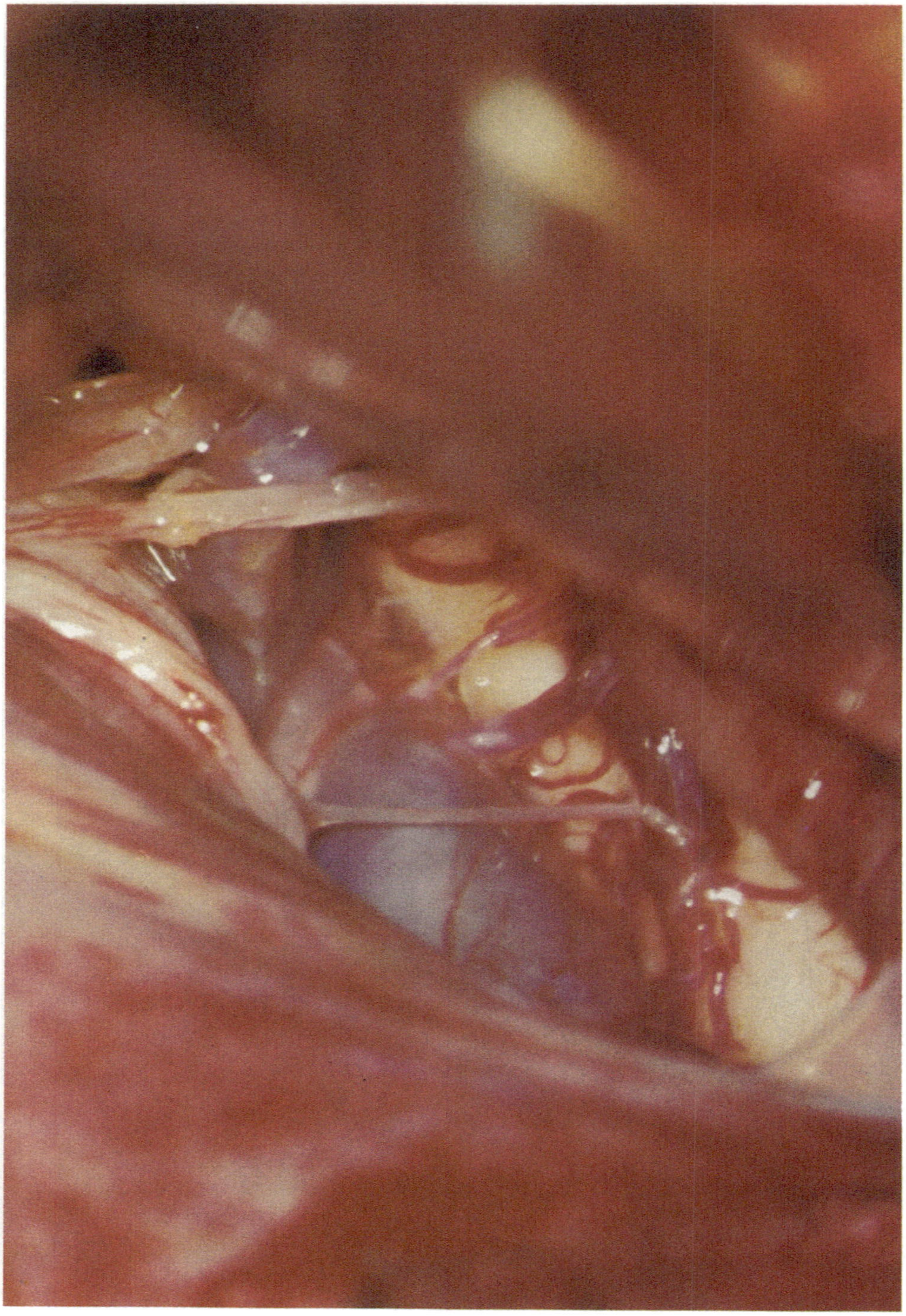

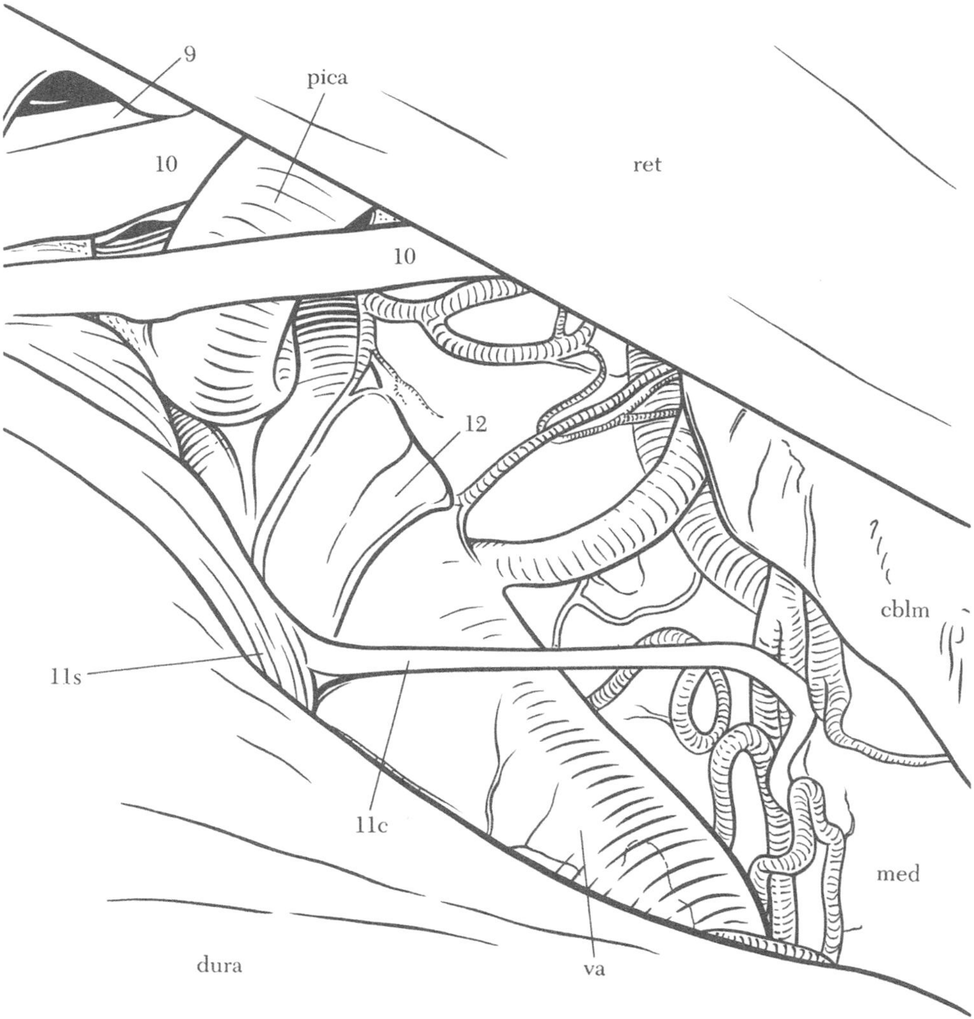

Fig. 39.14. Initial exposure of cerebellomedullary cistern on the left side. Same case as in Figs. 39.13 and 39.15–39.18. *9,* glossopharyngeal nerve; *10,* vagal rootlets; *pica,* loop of the posterior inferior cerebellar artery; *ret,* retractor; *cblm,* medial portion of elevated cerebellum; *12,* hypoglossal nerve coursing around the vertebral artery (*va*) toward the anterior condyloid foramen; *med,* medulla oblongata; *dura,* dura on floor of posterior fossa; *11c,* cranial portion of spinal accessory nerve; *11s,* spinal portion of spinal accessory nerve; *va,* vertebral artery. Note many lateral medullary branches of the vertebral artery.

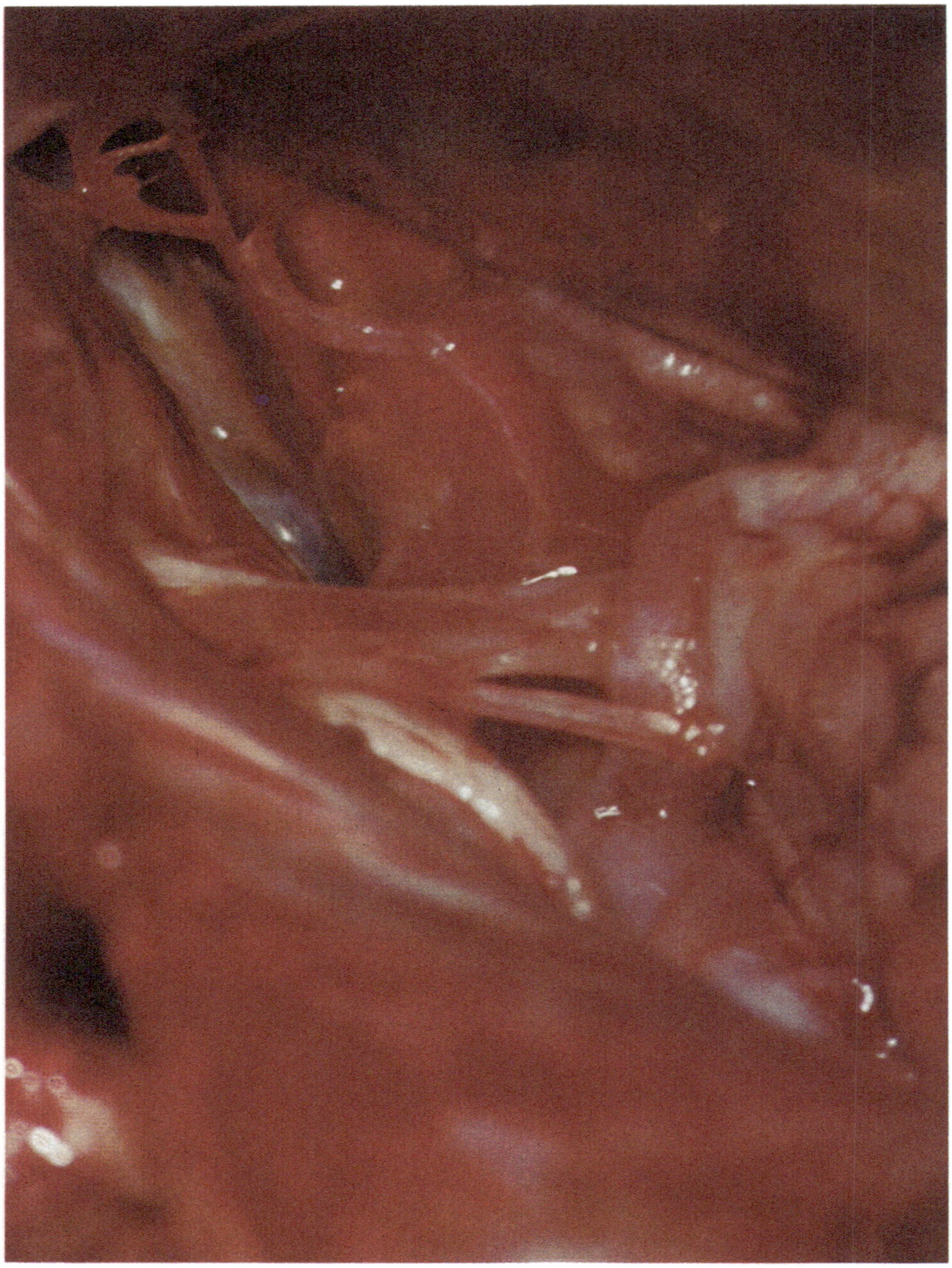

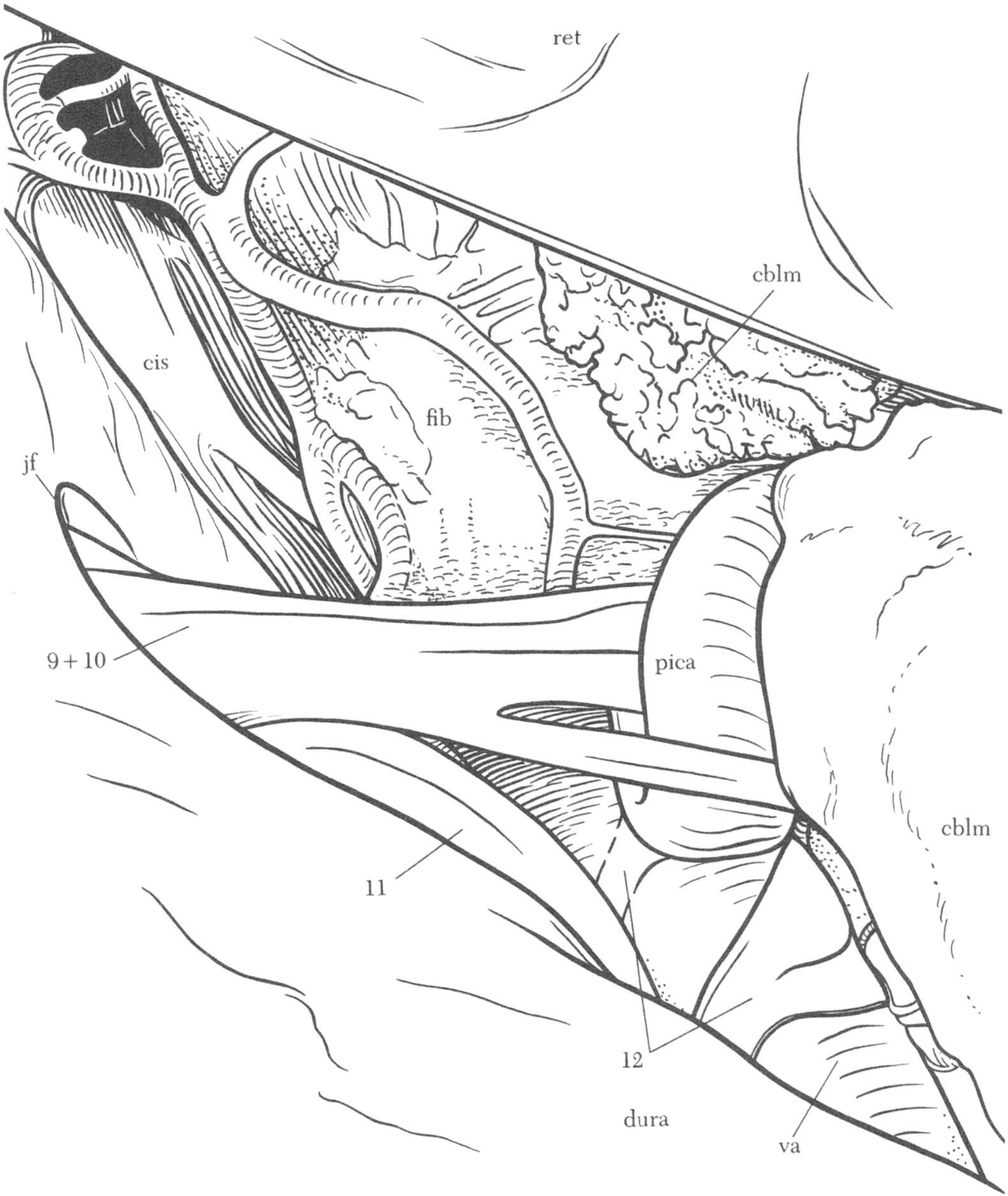

Fig. 39.15. Same case as in Figs. 39.13, 39.14, and 39.16–39.18. Further elevation of the cerebellum (*cblm*) by the retractor (*ret*) reveals fibrin (*fib*) from a recent bleed hiding the aneurysm. *pica,* posterior inferior cerebellar artery; *dura,* dura at base of skull; *va,* vertebral artery; *12,* hypoglossal nerve; *11,* spinal accessory nerve; *9 & 10,* glossopharyngeal and vagus nerves; *jf,* jugular foramen; *cis,* arachnoid membrane of cerebellopontine angle cistern (spinal fluid behind membrane gives bluish appearance).

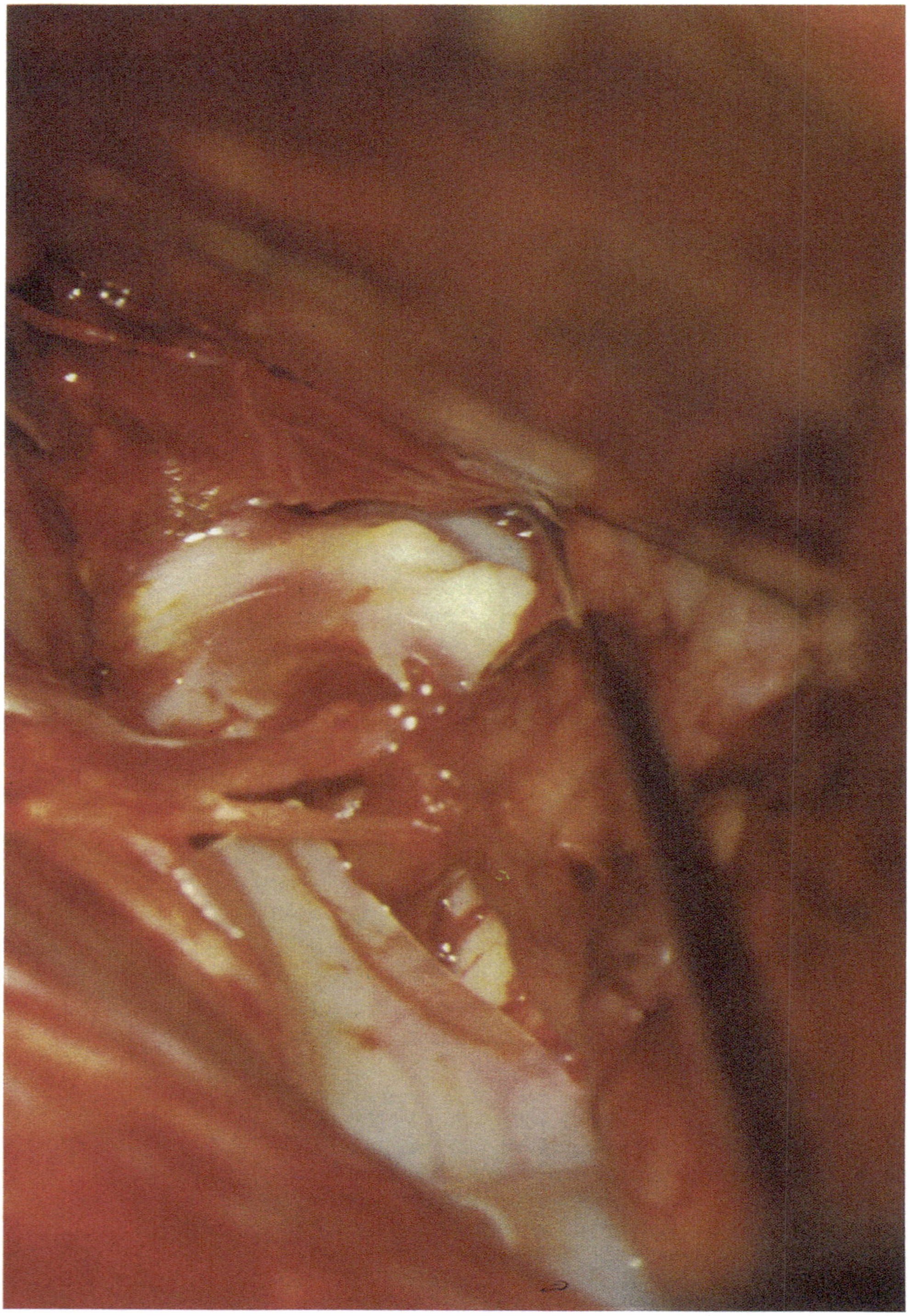

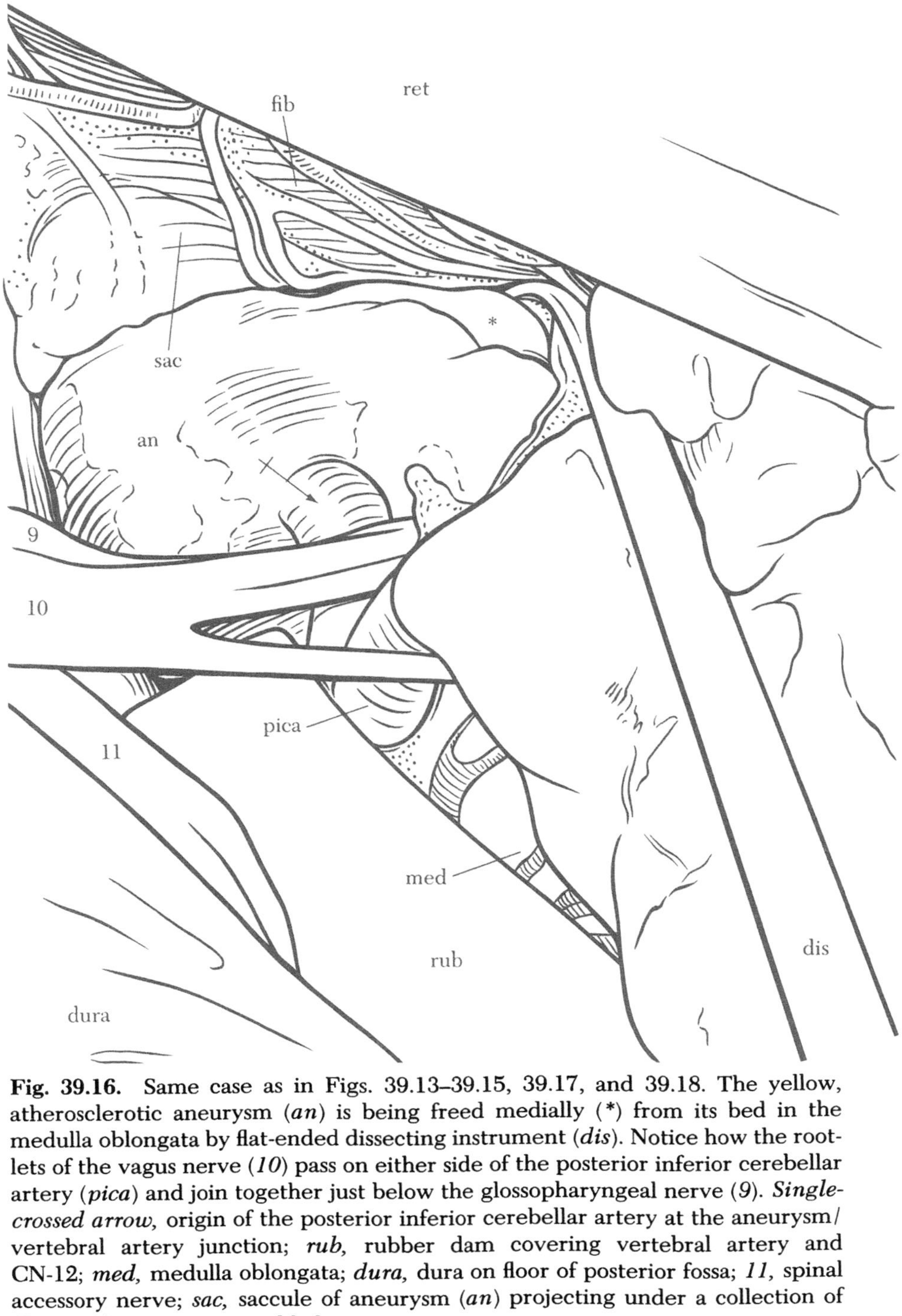

Fig. 39.16. Same case as in Figs. 39.13–39.15, 39.17, and 39.18. The yellow, atherosclerotic aneurysm (*an*) is being freed medially (*) from its bed in the medulla oblongata by flat-ended dissecting instrument (*dis*). Notice how the rootlets of the vagus nerve (*10*) pass on either side of the posterior inferior cerebellar artery (*pica*) and join together just below the glossopharyngeal nerve (*9*). *Single-crossed arrow,* origin of the posterior inferior cerebellar artery at the aneurysm/vertebral artery junction; *rub,* rubber dam covering vertebral artery and CN-12; *med,* medulla oblongata; *dura,* dura on floor of posterior fossa; *11,* spinal accessory nerve; *sac,* saccule of aneurysm (*an*) projecting under a collection of fibrin (*fib*); *ret,* retractor blade.

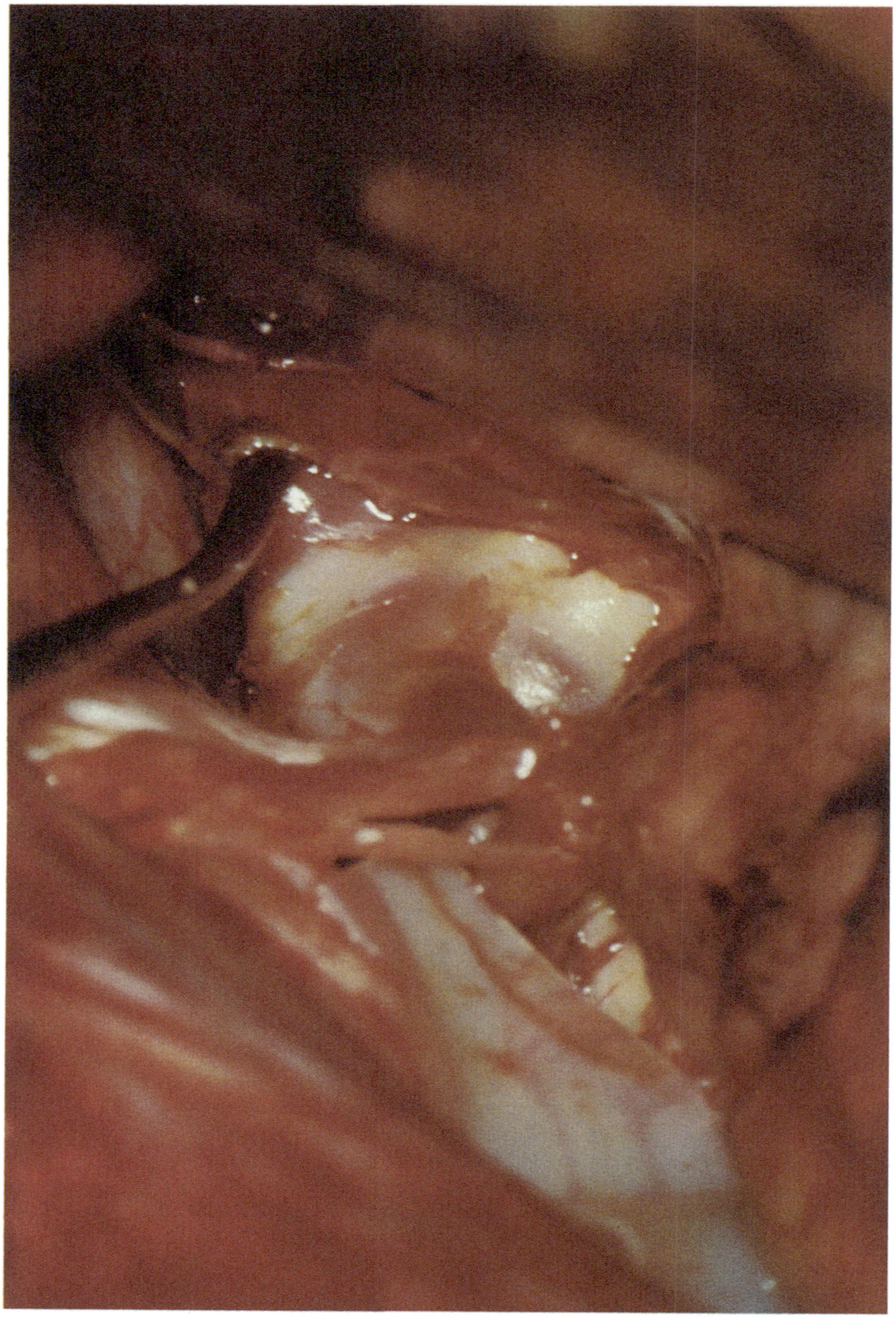

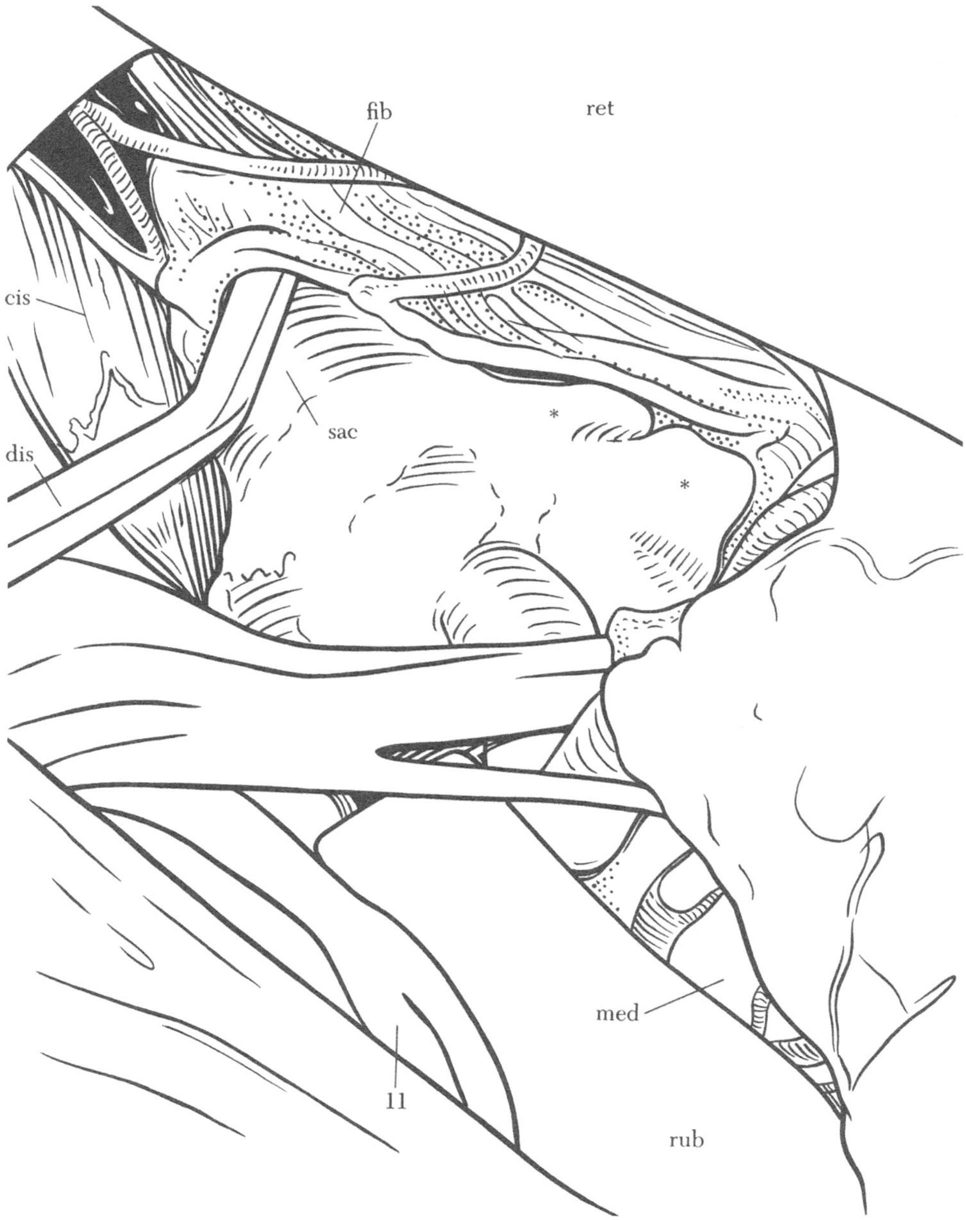

Fig. 39.17. Same case as in Figs. 39.13–39.16 and 39.18. The dissecting instrument (*dis*) is removing fibrin (*fib*) from the lateral saccule (*sac*) of the aneurysm. *, two atherosclerotic blisters on medial side of aneurysm; *med,* medulla oblongata; *rub,* rubber dam over the vertebral artery; *11,* spinal accessory nerve; *ret,* retractor blade; *cis,* arachnoid membrane of cerebellopontine angle cistern (no longer blue as in Fig. 39.15 because spinal fluid behind membrane was replaced with air).

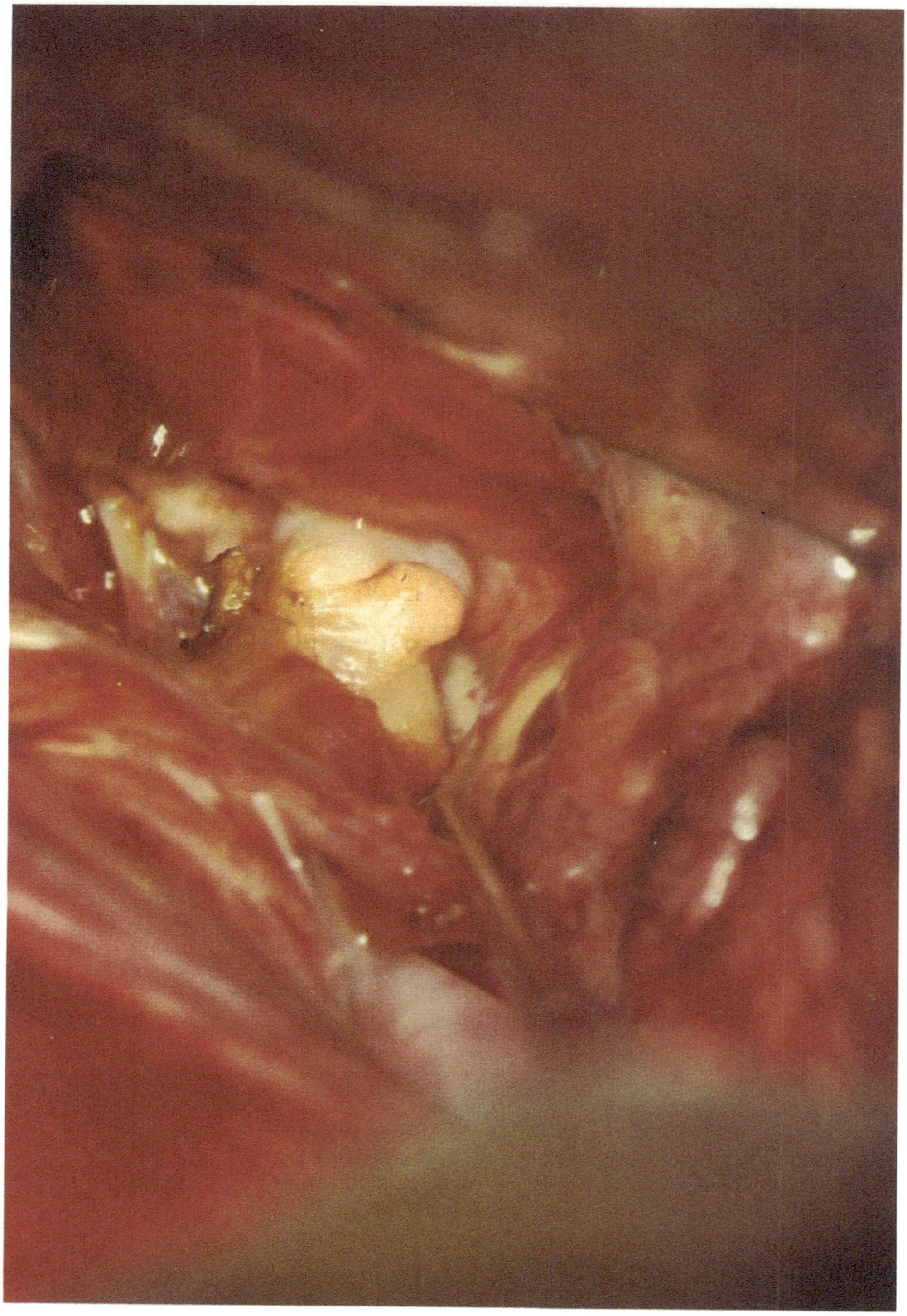

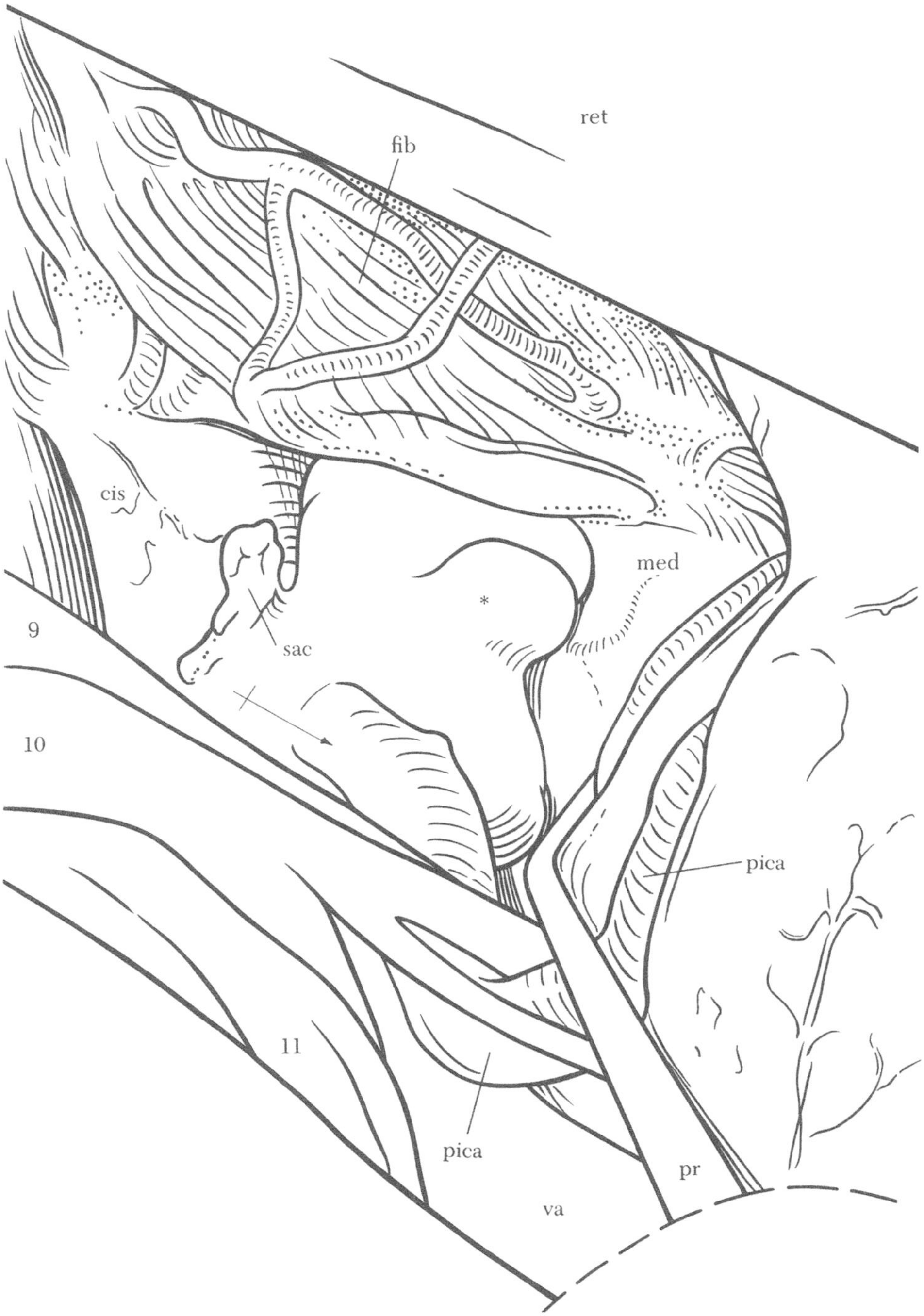

Fig. 39.18. Same case as in Figs. 39.13–39.17. The thin-walled saccule (*sac*) seen in Fig. 39.17 has been electrocoagulated and shrunken. Then the entire aneurysm was shrunken with bipolar electrocoagulation to allow successful clipping. *fib*, fibrin; *, atherosclerotic saccule; *med*, medulla oblongata where aneurysm had been compressing it. A probe (*pr*) is retracting portions of medial cerebellum, an arterial branch, and the posterior inferior cerebellar artery (*pica*). *va*, vertebral artery; *single-crossed arrow*, origin of the posterior inferior cerebellar artery (*pica*) from the vertebral artery and base of aneurysm. The cranial nerves (*9*, *10*, and *11*) are out of focus here. *cis*, arachnoid membrane of cerebellopontine angle cistern; the membrane is thickened in parts by adhesions.

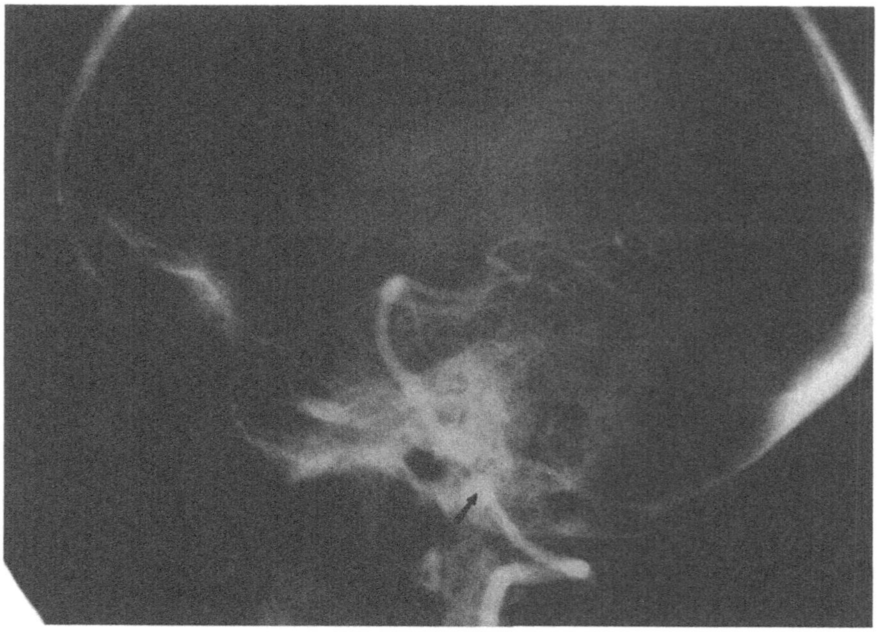

A

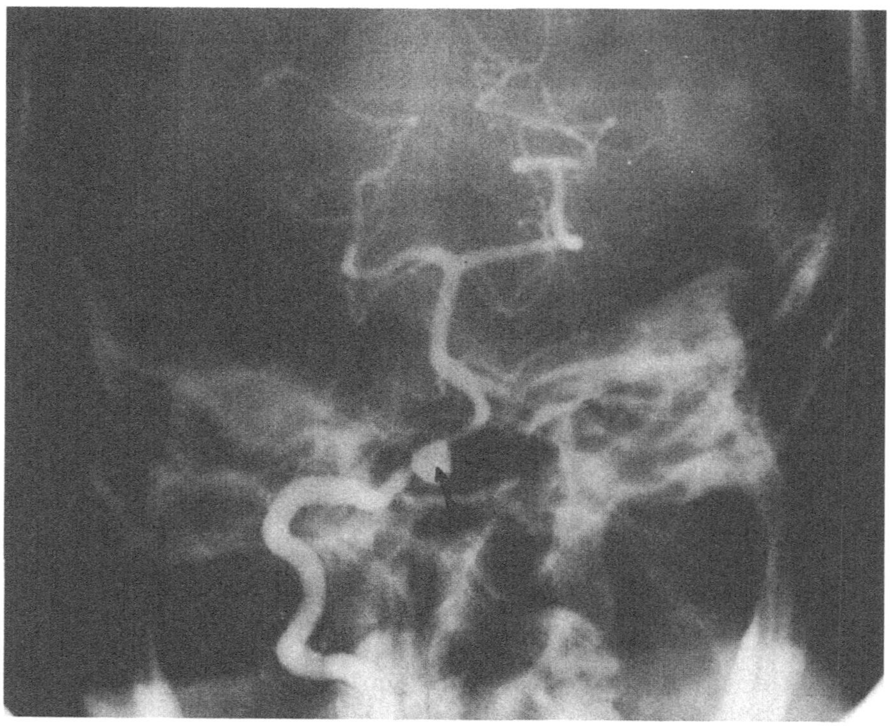

B

Fig. 39.19. A Lateral angiogram of picaVAA (*arrow*). There is adjacent spasm of the VA. B Frontal view of aneurysm (*arrow*). No neck is seen. Same case as in Fig. 39.20.

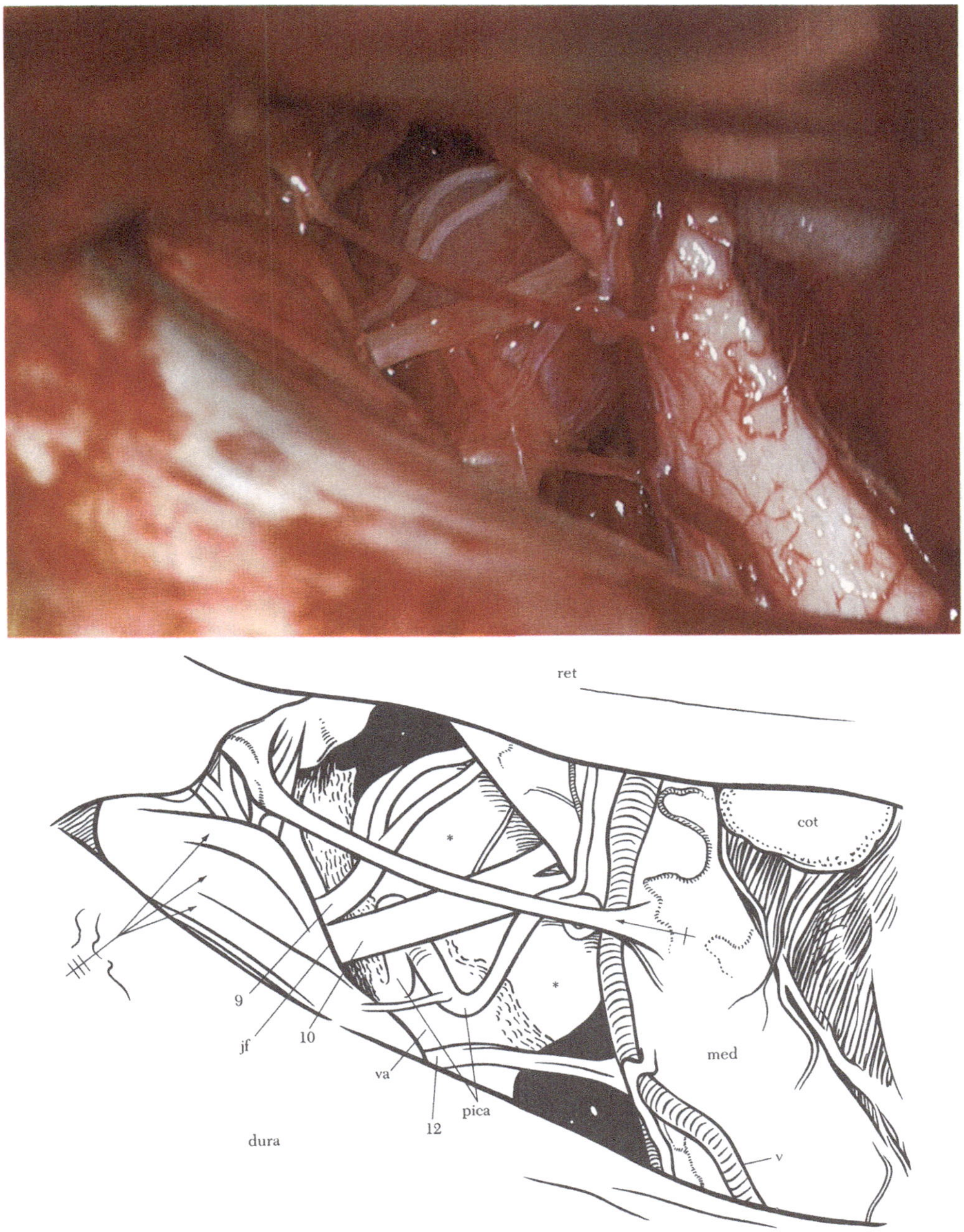

Fig. 39.20. Same case as in Fig. 39.19 (surgical photograph reversed to present as if on left side for consistency and anatomic orientation). This is a localized fusiform aneurysm (*) of the vertebral artery (*va*). Note rootlets of the glossopharyngeal nerve (*9*) and vagus nerve (*10*) coursing over aneurysm and entering the jugular foramen (*jf*). The *triple-crossed arrows* point to folds of dura on the lateral wall of the posterior fossa; these are not nerve roots. *ret,* retractor elevating the cerebellum; *cot,* edge of cottonoid strip; *single-crossed arrow,* unknown nerve rootlet (originates as would CN-11 but disappears superior to jugular foramen); *med,* medulla oblongata; *v,* vein; *pica,* small posterior inferior cerebellar artery arising at start of aneurysmal expansion; *va,* vertebral artery; *dura,* dura on lateral floor of posterior fossa. The patient was treated successfully by clipping the vertebral artery just proximal to the aneurysm.

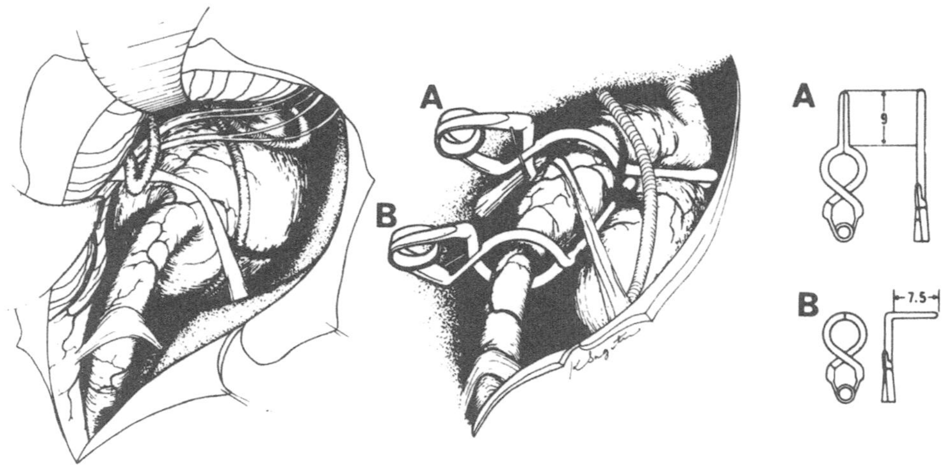

Fig. 39.21. Schematic drawings of operative views (right suboccipital craniotomy) illustrating fenestrated clips for fusiform vertebral artery aneurysms. This aneurysm was clipped using straight (**A**) and angled (**B**) fenestrated clips. From Sugita K, et al.: ref. 6.

Bibliography

1. Allcock JM: Aneurysms. In Newton TH, Pottes DG (eds.): Radiology of the Skull and Brain, Vol. 2, Book 4. St. Louis, Mosby, 1974, pp. 2435–2489
2. Drake CG: Management of aneurysms of posterior circulation. In Youmans JR (ed.): Neurological Surgery, Vol. 2, Philadelphia, Saunders, 1973, pp. 787–806
3. Drake CG: Surgical treatment of vertebrobasilar aneurysms. In Koos WT, Böck FW, Spetzler RF (eds.): Clinical Microneurosurgery. Stuttgart, Georg Thieme Verlag, 1976, pp. 213–219
4. Drake CG: The surgical treatment of vertebral-basilar aneurysms. Excerpta Med ICS No. 320:183–190, 1974
5. Karasawa J, Kikuchi H, Furuse S, et al.: Surgery of vertebral aneurysms of the origin of PICA Neurol Surg (Tokyo) 4:1157–1164, 1977
6. Sugita K, Kobayashi S, Inoue T, et al.: New angled fenestrated clips for fusiform vertebral artery aneurysms. J Neurosurg 54:346–350, 1981
7. Yaşargil MG, Fox JL: The microsurgical approach to acoustic neurinomas. Surg Neurol 2:393–398, 1974

Index

GPSR Compliance

The European Union's (EU) General Product Safety Regulation (GPSR) is a set of rules that requires consumer products to be safe and our obligations to ensure this.

If you have any concerns about our products, you can contact us on ProductSafety@springernature.com

In case Publisher is established outside the EU, the EU authorized representative is:

Springer Nature Customer Service Center GmbH
Europaplatz 3
69115 Heidelberg, Germany

Batch number: 10692513

Printed by Printforce, the Netherlands